CHEMICAL INDUCTION
OF CANCER

CHEMICAL INDUCTION OF CANCER

Modulation and Combination Effects

An Inventory of the Many Factors Which Influence Carcinogenesis

Joseph C. Arcos
Editor

Mary F. Argus
Yin-tak Woo
Associate Editors

Birkhäuser
Boston • Basel • Berlin

Joseph C. Arcos
U.S. Environmental Protection Agency
Washington, D.C. 20460, USA
Tulane University School of Medicine
New Orleans, LA 70112, USA

Mary F. Argus
U.S. Environmental Protection Agency
Washington, D.C. 20460, USA
Tulane University School of Medicine
New Orleans, LA 70112, USA

Yin-tak Woo
U.S. Environmental Protection Agency
Washington, D.C. 20460, USA

This volume was produced under the
editorial coordination of
Harriet D. Shields
Harriet Damon Shields & Associates
New York, NY 10010, USA

Library of Congress Cataloging-in-Publication Data

Chemical induction of cancer : modulation and combination effects : an
  inventory of the many factors which influence carcinogenesis /
  Joseph C. Arcos, editor ; Mary F. Argus, Yin-tak Woo, associate
  editors.
      p. cm.
    Includes bibliographical references and index.
    ISBN 0-8176-3766-4 (H : alk. paper). — ISBN 3-7643-3766-4 (alk.
paper)
    1. Chemical carcinogenesis. 2. Cancer—Etiology. I. Arcos,
Joseph C. II. Argus, Mary F. III. Woo, Yin-tak.
    [DNLM: 1. Neoplasms, Experimental—chemically induced.
2. Neoplasms—etiology. 3. Carcinogens. QZ 206 C516 1995]
RC268.6.C492 1995
616.88'4071—dc20
DNLM/DLC
for Library of Congress   94-29782
                                                           CIP

Printed on acid-free paper.

ISBN 0-8176-3766-4   Typeset by TechType, Inc., Upper Saddle River, NJ
ISBN 3-7643-3766-4   Printed and bound by Braun-Brumfield, Inc., Ann Arbor, MI

Printed in the United States of America.

9 8 7 6 5 4 3 2 1

This volume is dedicated

to

ERIC BOYLAND

ELIZABETH C. MILLER

and

JAMES A. MILLER

whose original and massive contributions
heralded the modern era
of chemical carcinogenesis research

and to

DIETRICH SCHMÄHL

pioneer on combination effects
in carcinogenesis

Contents

PREFATORY CHAPTER

**Multifactor Interaction Network of Carcinogenesis —
A "Tour Guide"**

Joseph C. Arcos and Mary F. Argus

PART 1

Cross-Reactions between Carcinogens. Modification of Chemical Carcinogenesis by Noncarcinogenic Agents

CHAPTER **4**

Inhibition of Chemical Carcinogenesis

Gary J. Kelloff, Charles W. Boone, Vernon E. Steele, Judith R. Fay, and Caroline C. Sigman

CHAPTER 5
Promotion and Cocarcinogenesis

INTRODUCTION **123**

Friedrich Marks, Michael Schwarz, and Gerhard Fürstenberger

SECTION I **Tumor Promotion in Skin**

Friedrich Marks and Gerhard Fürstenberger

SECTION II **Tumor Promotion in Liver**

Michael Schwarz

CHAPTER **6**

Computerized Data Management as a Tool to Study Combination Effects in Carcinogenesis

Yin-tak Woo, Gregg Polansky, Joseph C. Arcos, Jeff Stokes DuBose, and Mary F. Argus

CHAPTER **7**

Intercellular Communication: A Paradigm for the Interpretation of the Initiation/Promotion/Progression Model of Carcinogenesis

James E. Trosko, Chia-Cheng Chang, Burra V. Madhukar, and Emmanuel Dupont

APPENDIX TO PART 1

Chemical Cancerogenesis: Definitions of Frequently Used Terms

K. E. Appel, G. Fürstenberger, H. J. Hapke, E. Hecker, A. G. Hildebrandt,
W. Koransky, F. Marks, H. G. Neumann, F. K. Ohnesorge, and R. Schulte-Hermann

PART **2**

Exogenous Factors and Endogenous Biological Parameters That Modulate Chemical Carcinogenesis

CHAPTER **8**

Immunotoxicology of Chemical Carcinogens

Karen A. Sullivan and John E. Salvaggio

CHAPTER 9
The Effect of Diet on Tumor Induction

SECTION I. **Effect of Caloric (Energy) Restriction**
David Kritchevsky

SECTION II. **Modulation by Protein and Individual Amino Acids**
Erwin J. Hawrylewicz

SECTION III. **Modulation by Vitamins**

Edgar Petru, Yin-tak Woo, and Martin R. Berger

SECTION IV. **Modulation by Minerals**

Maryce M. Jacobs and Roman J. Pienta

CHAPTER **10**

The Effect of Animal Age on Tumor Induction

Yvonne Leutzinger and John P. Richie, Jr.

CHAPTER **12**

Effect of Genetic Susceptibility on Tumor Induction

Norman R. Drinkwater

CHAPTER **13**

Radiation Injury and Radiation Carcinogenesis with Special Reference to Combination Effects with Chemical Agents

Jeffrey L. Schwartz

CHAPTER **14**

Mechanisms of Viral Tumorigenesis and the Combination Effects of Viruses and Chemical Carcinogens

INTRODUCTION **509**
Joseph C. Arcos

SECTION I. **General Characteristics of Tumor Viruses. Viral and Cellular Oncogenes. Nonviral Oncogene Activators.**
Joseph C. Arcos, Lawrence R. Boone, and William C. Phelps

SECTION II. **Molecular Biology of Virally-Induced Cell Transformation and Tumorigenesis**

Lawrence R. Boone, K. Gregory Moore, William C. Phelps, and Yin-tak Woo

SECTION III. **Viral–Chemical Combination Effects in Tumorigenesis**
Yin-tak Woo

Contributors

Klaus E. Appel Max-von-Pettenkofer Institute, Federal Health Office, D-1000 Berlin 33, Germany (Append. to Part 1)

Joseph C. Arcos U.S. Environmental Protection Agency, Washington, DC 20460, USA, and Department of Medicine, Tulane University School of Medicine (Emeritus) (Chap. 1; Chap. 6; Chap. 14: Intro., Sect. I, and Closing Note; Editors' Notes to Chaps. 9, 11, and 15; Postscript.)

Mary F. Argus U.S. Environmental Protection Agency, Washington, DC 20460, USA, and Department of Medicine, Tulane University School of Medicine (Spec. Appt.) (Chap. 1; Chap. 6; Editors' Notes to Chaps. 9, 11, and 15)

Martin R. Berger Department of Carcinogenesis and Chemotherapy, German Cancer Research Center, D-6900 Heidelberg, Germany (Chap. 2; Chap. 9, Sect. III)

Charles W. Boone Chemoprevention Branch, DCPC, National Cancer Institute, Bethesda, MD 20892, USA (Chap. 4)

Lawrence R. Boone Division of Virology, Wellcome Research Laboratory, Burroughs Wellcome Co., Research Triangle Park, NC 27709, USA (Chap. 14: Sects. I and II)

Chia-Cheng Chang Department of Pediatrics & Human Development, Michigan State University College of Human Medicine, East Lansing, MI 48824, USA (Chap. 7)

Norman R. Drinkwater McArdle Laboratory for Cancer Research, University of Wisconsin Medical School, Madison, WI 53706, USA (Chap. 12)

Emmanuel Dupont Department of Pediatrics & Human Development, Michigan State University College of Human Medicine, East Lansing, MI 48824, USA (Chap. 7)

Emmanuel Farber Departments of Pathology and Biochemistry, Faculty of Medicine, University of Toronto, Toronto, Ontario M5S 1A8, Canada (Foreword)

Judith R. Fay CCS Associates, 1285 Hamilton Ave., Palo Alto, CA 94301, USA (Chap. 4)

Gerhard Fürstenberger Department of Biochemistry (Tissue-Specific Regulation), German Cancer Research Center, D-6900 Heidelberg, Germany (Chap. 5: Intro. and Sect. I; Append. to Part 1)

Hans-Jürgen Hapke Institute for Pharmacology & Toxicology, Veterinary University School, D-3000 Hanover, Germany (Append. to Part 1)

Erwin J. Hawrylewicz   Research Department, Mercy Hospital and Medical Center, Chicago, IL 60616, USA, and Department of Biological Chemistry, University of Illinois College of Medicine, Chicago, IL, USA (Chap. 9, Sect. II)

Erich Hecker   Department of Biochemistry, German Cancer Research Center, D-6900 Heidelberg, Germany (Append. to Part 1)

Alfred G. Hildebrandt   Institute for Medicinal Drugs, Federal Health Office, D-1000 Berlin 65, Germany (Append. to Part 1)

Maryce M. Jacobs   American Institute for Cancer Research, Washington, DC 20009; *corresp. to*: 1800 Old Meadow Rd./Unit 801, McLean, VA 22102, USA (Chap. 9, Sect. IV)

Gary J. Kelloff   Chemoprevention Branch, DCPC, National Cancer Institute, Bethesda, MD 20892, USA (Chap. 4)

Wolfgang Koransky   Institute for Toxicology and Pharmacology, University of Marburg, D-3550 Marburg, Germany (Append. to Part 1)

David Kritchevsky   Wistar Institute, Philadelphia, PA 19104, USA (Chap. 9: Sects. I and V)

Yvonne Leutzinger   American Health Foundation, Valhalla, NY 10595, USA (Chap. 10)

Jonathan J. Li   Hormonal Carcinogenesis Laboratory, Department of Pharmaceutical Sciences, College of Pharmacy, Washington State University, Pullman, WA 99165, USA; *Present address*: Div. Etiology & Prevention/Hormonal Cancer, Univ. Kansas Medical Ctr., Robinson 5008, 3901 Rainbow Blvd., Kansas City, KS 66160, USA (Chap. 11)

Sara A. Li   Hormonal Carcinogenesis Laboratory, Department of Pharmaceutical Sciences, College of Pharmacy, Washington State University, Pullman, WA 99165, USA; *Present address*: Veterans Administration Medical Ctr., Linwood Blvd., Kansas City, KS 64128, USA (Chap. 11)

Burra V. Madhukar   Department of Pediatrics & Human Development, Michigan State University College of Human Medicine, East Lansing, MI 48824, USA (Chap. 7)

Friedrich Marks   Department of Biochemistry (Tissue-Specific Regulation), German Cancer Research Center, D-6900 Heidelberg, Germany (Chap. 5: Intro. and Sects. I and IIIA & B; Append. to Part 1)

K. Gregory Moore   Department of Cell Biology, Upstate Biotechnology, Inc., 199 Saranac Avenue, Lake Placid, NY 12496, USA (Chap. 14, Sect. II)

Hans-Günter Neumann   Institute for Pharmacology, University of Würzburg, 8700 Würzburg, Germany (Append. to Part 1)

Friedrich K. Ohnesorge   Institute for Toxicology, University of Düsseldorf, D-4000 Düsseldorf, Germany (Append. to Part 1)

Edgar Petru   Department of Obstetrics and Gynecology, University of Graz, A-8036 Graz, Austria (Chap. 9, Sect. III)

William C. Phelps   Division of Virology, Wellcome Research Laboratory, Burroughs Wellcome Co., Research Triangle Park, NC 27709, USA (Chap. 14: Sects. I and II)

Roman J. Pienta   R. J. Pienta and Associates, 14113 Flint Rock Rd., Rockville MD 20853, USA (Chap. 9, Sect. IV)

Gregg Polansky   Science Applications International Corp., 1710 Goodridge Drive, McLean, VA 22102, USA (Chap. 6)

Arnold E. Reif   Department of Pathology, Boston University School of Medicine (Emeritus); *corresp. to*: 39 College Rd., Wellesley, MA 02181, USA (Chap. 3)

John P. Richie, Jr.,   American Health Foundation, Valhalla, NY 10595, USA (Chap. 10)

Jeffrey D. Saffer   Battelle–Pacific Northwest Laboratories, Richland, WA 99352, USA (Chap. 16)

John E. Salvaggio   Department of Medicine, Tulane University School of Medicine, New Orleans, LA 70112, USA (Chap. 8)

Rolf Schulte-Hermann   Institute for Tumorbiology/Cancer Research, University of Wien, A-1090 Wien, Austria (Append. to Part 1)

Jeffrey L. Schwartz   Biological and Medical Research Division, Argonne National Laboratory, Argonne, IL 60439, USA, and Department of Radiation Oncology, University of Chicago Medical School, Chicago, IL, USA (Chap. 13)

Michael Schwarz   Department of Experimental Pathology, German Cancer Research Center, D-6900 Heidelberg, Germany (Chap. 5: Intro. and Sect. II)

Caroline C. Sigman   CCS Associates, 1285 Hamilton Ave., Palo Alto, CA 94301, USA (Chap. 4)

Vernon E. Steele   Chemoprevention Branch, DCPC, National Cancer Institute, Bethesda, MD 20892, USA (Chap. 4)

Jeff Stokes DuBose   Viar & Co., Inc., 300 N. Lee St., Alexandria, VA 22314, USA (Chap. 6)

Karen A. Sullivan   Department of Medicine, Tulane University School of Medicine, New Orleans, LA 70112, USA (Chap. 8)

James E. Trosko   Department of Pediatrics & Human Development, Michigan State University College of Human Medicine, East Lansing, MI 48824, USA (Chap. 7)

Wolfgang H. Vogel   Department of Pharmacology, Jefferson Medical College, Philadelphia, PA 19107, USA (Chap. 15)

Bary W. Wilson   Battelle–Pacific Northwest Laboratories, Richland, WA 99352, USA (Chap. 16)

Yin-tak Woo   U.S. Environmental Protection Agency, Washington, DC 20460, USA (Chap. 6; Chap. 9, Sect. III; Chap. 14: Sects. II and III; Editors' Notes to Chaps. 9, 11, and 15)

Acknowledgments*

- *For substantive editorial assistance:*

Lorraine Hester   U.S. Environmental Protection Agency, Washington, DC, USA

To whom the Editors wish to express their special appreciation and indebtedness for her invaluable and indispensable help with editorial standardization, formatting, and upgrading of these chapters.

- *For editorial and production coordination, and more:*

Harriet D. Shields   Harriet Damon Shields & Associates, New York, NY, USA

Whom the Editors thank for the very high quality of editorial coordination and for her perseverant pursuit in overseeing the multitude of tasks in the production of this book. Beyond that, JCA and MFA wish to express their lasting indebtedness for her special caring in the birthing of this volume.

- *For critical, facilitating administrative actions:*

Edwin F. Beschler   Birkhäuser Publishers, Boston-Basel-Berlin

To whom the Editors wish to express their sincere thankfulness and indebtedness for his foresight and for repeatedly interceding in behalf of volumes of this series — previously as President of Academic Press and at present as Executive Vice President of Birkhäuser (Boston) — as well as for his truly compassionate support at a difficult, stressful stage in the production of this volume.

- *For scientific review, critique, and consultation:*

Donya Bagheri   CCS Associates, Palo Alto, CA, USA (Chap. 4)

L. Michelle Bennett   McArdle Laboratory, University of Wisconsin, Madison, WI, USA (Chap. 12)

Charles C. Brown   Biostatistics Branch, DCPC, National Cancer Institute, Washington, DC, USA (Chap. 3)

Ernest Clark   Division of Biostatistics, Tufts University School of Dental Medicine, Medford, MA, USA (Chap. 3)

Theodore Colton   Sect. Epidemiology and Biostatistics, Boston University School of Medicine, Boston, MA, USA (Chap. 3)

Mary K. Doeltz   CCS Associates, Palo Alto, CA, USA (Chap. 4)

Linda A. Doody   CCS Associates, Palo Alto, CA, USA (Chap. 4)

David J. Grdina   Argonne National Laboratory, Argonne, IL, USA (Chap. 13)

---

*Acknowledgments to grant or contract support, if any, are given in the respective chapters.

Melvin Griem   Argonne National Laboratory, Argonne, IL, USA (Chap. 13)

Debra Jaffe   Department of Radiation Oncology, University of Chicago, Chicago, IL, USA (Chap. 13)

Danuta Malejka-Giganti   Cancer Research Laboratory, Veteran Affairs Medical Center, Minneapolis, MN, USA (Prefatory Chap. & Chap. 11)

Stephen C. Nesnow   HERL, U.S. Environmental Protection Agency, Research Triangle Park, NC, USA (Prefatory Chap.)

Therese Poole   McArdle Laboratory, University of Wisconsin, Madison, WI, USA (Chap. 12)

James L. Repace   Division of Indoor Air, U.S. Environmental Protection Agency, Washington, DC, USA (Chap. 3)

Janet A. Springer   Division of Mathematics, U.S. Food and Drug Administration, Washington, DC, USA (Chap. 3)

Raymond W. Tennant   Laboratory of Environmental Carcinogenesis, NIEHS, Research Triangle Park, NC, USA (Chap. 14)

Michael D. Waters   HERL, U.S. Environmental Protection Agency, Research Triangle Park, NC, USA (Pref. Chap.)

John H. Weisburger   American Health Foundation, Valhalla, NY, USA (Chap. 10)

For editorial advice, technical/clerical assistance:

Lisa A. Costa   CCS Associates, Palo Alto, CA, USA (Chap. 4)

Zenaida C. Dingle   CCS Associates, Palo Alto, CA, USA (Chap. 4)

Barbara F. Doyle   U.S. Environmental Protection Agency, Washington, DC, USA (Prefatory Chap., Chap. 11, and Chap. 14)

Gloria Drayton-Miller   U.S. Environmental Protection Agency, Washington, DC, USA [Chaps. 2, 5, 8, 9(Sect.4), and 14]

Akiko Enami   Department of Pediatrics, Michigan State University College of Human Medicine, East Lansing, MI, USA (Chap. 7)

Bruce H. Gibson   AVI Multimedia, Inc., Alexandria, VA, USA (Pref. Chap.; cover art)

June Lear   Argonne Natl. Laboratory, Argonne, IL, USA (Chap. 13)

Beth Lockwood   Department of Pediatrics, Michigan State University College of Human Medicine, East Lansing, MI, USA (Chap. 7)

Jean McHugh   Department of Pediatrics, Michigan State University College of Human Medicine, East Lansing, MI, USA (Chap. 7)

David Nadziejka   Argonne Natl. Laboratory, Argonne, IL, USA (Chap. 13)

Elizabeth Nsubuga   Department of Pharmacology, Jefferson Medical College, Philadelphia, PA, USA (Chap. 15)

Christine Onaga   Univ. Wisconsin, Madison, WI, USA (Chap. 12)

William Paradee   Department of Pediatrics, Michigan State University College of Human Medicine, East Lansing, MI, USA (Chap. 7)

Heather Rupp   Department of Pediatrics, Michigan State University College of Human Medicine, East Lansing, MI, USA (Chap. 7)

Sandra J. Shafer   CCS Associates, Palo Alto, CA, USA (Chap. 4)

Lora R. Smith   CCS Associates, Palo Alto, CA, USA (Chap. 4)

Leona E. B. Tarrice   CCS Associates, Palo Alto, CA, USA (Chap. 4)

Ursula J. Vogel   Department of Pharmacology, Jefferson Medical College, Philadelphia, PA, USA (Chap. 15)

Nancy L. Wandler   CCS Associates, Palo Alto, CA, USA (Chap. 4)

A Quote from 1962

"In very large and richly cross-connected feedback systems, as the multiple control network of *normal* cell metabolism is now considered . . . there are various ways that *may* make regulation possible. . . . Sometimes control may follow unusual orientations in the network (alternative metabolic pathways). . . . But in all types of richly cross-connected feedback systems, whatever the ways of achieving regulation, a sufficient number of paths must remain functional if the system is to remain 'goal seeking'. . . . In the cell of a multicellular organism, this means the adjustment of its homeostasis to the tissue environment. Thus, in a controlled but self-maintaining system such as the cell, homeostasis may be adjusted despite the elimination of a *few* control channels, either by a more extensive use of alternative pathways or by possibly rebuilding altered nonfunctional channels. Cellular repair takes place, *in fact,* following radiation induced lesions of biochemical pathways supporting DNA synthesis . . . which seems to be subject to regulation, proceeding through reversible structural changes, by feedback mechanisms. . . . Numerous evidence, suggestive of cellular repair following lesions caused by chemical agents, is scattered in the literature.

"During the process of carcinogenesis, however, a limit may be reached in a number of cells where, because of the elimination of too many pathways, compensation or rebuilding may not be possible. Many altered cells will die because of structural alteration of a large number of metabolic pathways essential for synthetic reactions indispensable for the life of the cell. *In fact*, early stages of chemical carcinogenesis are known to coincide with notable cell death. . . . Those cells in which vital pathways have been only slightly damaged because of the random distribution of biochemical lesions in the cell population will, however, survive. This is consistent with the concept . . . supported recently . . . that the actually observable tumor incidence is a complex product of the cytotoxic and carcinogenic action of carcinogenic agents. That is, the cells that proliferate are those which, despite loss of native fine structural patterns of regulatory membranes (and perhaps of regulatory genes), survive the random selective action of cytotoxicity. These cells will then be unable to respond to the systemic or tissue chemical signals of the regulation of growth and division and will be, thus, tumor cells.

"Consistent with this thesis is the long period of time required for carcinogenesis by physical and simple chemical agents, because of the 'waste' (cell death) during random selection, due to the relative non-specificity of the cellular action. However, certain viruses may have sufficient structural complexity to be able to display a high degree of specificity toward cellular metabolic control sites. This is actually supported by the fact that oncogenic viruses produce tumors generally much more rapidly and specifically than physical or chemical carcinogens and without resorting to the prodution of 'waste' (cell death).

"From the phylogenetic standpoint, carcinogenesis represents a reverse process to evolutionary trend at the cell structural level. . . . *In fact,* the establishment of tissue homeostasis and its foundation in cell structure is a survival condition of whole organisms in evolutionary selection, resulting in cellular associations, differentiation and successively more and more complex morphological entities."

From Arcos, J.C., and Arcos, M.: "Molecular Geometry and Mechanisms of Action of Chemical Carcinogens". *In* Progr. Drug Res., E. Jucker, ed. Vol. 4, pp. 407–581, 1962, Birkhäuser (Basel).

Foreword

In the approach to the analysis of disease, including, of course, cancer, two major thrusts may be distinguished. These may be referred to, in shorthand, as *agents* and *processes*: the causative agents (chemical, microbial, physical, environmental, and psychosocial) and the organismic processes, initiated and furthered by the agents, culminating in observable pathology (at the macromolecular, cytological, histological, organ function, locomotor, and behavioral levels).

The past 25 years, since the appearance of the first volume of the predecessor series (1) authored by the Editors of this present volume, have seen an impressive number of studies on chemicals (and other agents) as etiologic factors in the induction of cancer. The major emphasis has been on the discovery of many chemical carcinogens of widely different structures, their metabolism by various tissues and cells, and, in turn, their molecular-biochemical effects on the cells. This rapidly expanded body of information, as effectively covered in the predecessor volumes, is an excellent entrée to the second half of the overall problem of chemical carcinogenesis, *the processes*. The active agents trigger a large array of molecular-biochemical alterations to which the target cells, target tissues, and target organisms respond in many select and common ways.

This second major aspect of the induction of cancer by chemicals (and by other agents) — the sequence of cellular and tissue changes clearly relevant to cancer — remains the challenge for the future. This will require studies of the meaningful and relevant interplay between the molecular-biochemical level of organization and the biological level. One key to this endeavour will be the development of rational hypotheses that offer a reasonable ground for understanding the functional physiological basis for each of the steps in the process leading to the emergence of cancer.

For example, what is (are) the nature of the new phenotype or phenotypes in the rare altered target cells after initiation and how is a differential effect created during promotion to induce clonal expansion of the different initiated cells? How many different patterns of phenotype might there be in the initiated cells in any single organ or tissue and how do these relate physiologically to the selections created during promotion by different promoting agents? At what step in the subsequent cellular evolution of the cells in the clonal expansions (such as papillomas, nodules, and polyps) does some degree of seemingly autonomous cell proliferation appear? Is this cell proliferation largely balanced by cell loss, such that the clonally expanded focal proliferations enlarge only very slowly? At what step does the discrepancy between cell proliferation and cell loss become exaggerated so as to favor the former? How do such possible changes in the precursor lesions to cancer relate mechanistically to the malignant behavior of a cancer?

The stage is now being set for the next major challenges and redirection of emphasis — from initiators to initiation, from promoters to promotion, etc. — from agent to processes — as well as for the analysis of the many factors that effectively modulate the process and often determine the emergence of clinically verifiable cancer. These challenges are major and will require novel approaches in research and new orientation in teaching.

The chapters in this volume introduce precisely this type of fundamental considerations that must be followed up and clarified if we are ever to understand the induction of cancer by chemicals and how the *process* might be interrupted so as to prevent cancer. The large amount of material covered in the volumes of the predecessor series selectively highlighted the major properties and metabolism of and tissue responses induced by chemical agents in a critical and meaningful way. Thus, it offers an excellent base and perspective for the future investigator interested in tackling, in detail, the *process-related sequence* or sequences leading to cancer. The development of rational, testable hypotheses that can explain each major step in chemical carcinogenesis will be awaited with great interest. This present unique volume adds an important dimension to the essential background for such future studies.

EMMANUEL FARBER
Departments of Pathology and of Biochemistry
Faculty of Medicine, University of Toronto
Toronto, Ontario, Canada

1. "Chemical Induction of Cancer": Vol. I, 1968, Chemical Background, General Characteristics of Tumors, Testing Procedures; Vol. IIA, 1974, Polynuclear Compounds; Vol. IIB, 1974, Aromatic Amines and Azo Compounds; Vol. IIIA, 1982, Aliphatic Carcinogens; Vol. IIIB, 1985, Aliphatic and Polyhalogenated Carcinogens; Vol. IIIC, 1988, Natural, Metal, Fiber and Macromolecular Carcinogens. Academic Press, New York/Orlando/San Diego.

Multifactor Interaction Network of Carcinogenesis – A "Tour Guide"

Joseph C. Arcos and Mary F. Argus

I. INTRODUCTION. THE INTERACTION NETWORK AS A GRAPH

Many exogenous and endogenous factors influence or in some instances can actually determine the outcome of the administration of a chemical carcinogen. The multiplicity of these factors outdates the classical concept that a given carcinogen is the sole etiological agent in the "causation of a cancer", except when under controlled laboratory conditions or resulting from well-defined occupational or lifestyle exposures. In the same framework the significance of the search for "threshold" of carcinogens acquires an illusory character unless nutritional, genetic, lifestyle, and stress factors, and exposure to radiations, viruses, and a host of environmentally occurring chemicals – such as immunotoxicants, modifiers of mixed-function oxidases (MFO) and of endocrine balance, and antagonists and/or synergists – are taken into account (*cf.* 1). In addition, the majority of the factors that can modulate carcinogenesis directly and indirectly (Table 1) influence the effect of each other, so that the totality forms a complex, interwoven interaction network.

The subsequent chapters discuss synergism, antagonism, inhibition, and promotion, as well as the host of exogenous and endogenous influencing factors – all parameters that can modify chemical carcinogenesis. Whenever possible the respective authors have endeavored to interpret the mechanisms of the effects in the backdrop of the known molecular events in the stages of carcinogenesis. The aim of this Prefatory Chapter is to highlight some of the major causal and physical *linkages* in the network of interactions between the modifying factors/parameters as depicted in Figure 1.

In the graph–theoretical sense this network is a typical directed graph, where the factors/entities represented are the "vertexes" and the arrows connecting them are the "directed edges" or "arcs". A directed graph is a structural model describing the relationships and the directions of the relationships between the vertexes (2-4). It is uniquely suited to represent a network of dynamic interactions – occurring often simultaneously between a large and complex set of elements – that either maintain a steady-state in some operational mode of behavior, or further the progress toward a particular endpoint or outcome (*e.g.*, 3, 5-7). As Figure 1 illustrates, there is substantial information on the directions of the causal effects operative in carcinogenesis; on the other hand, quantitative information about numerical weights appropriate for those relationships is virtually nil. However, because of natural delay of the causal effects in affecting the final outcome, as

TABLE 1. **Classes of Factors/Parameters That Can Modify Chemical Carcinogenesis**

- Interactions Between Carcinogenic Effects (in Multiple or Closely Sequential Exposure)
- Promoters/Cocarcinogens
- Inhibitors of Chemical Carcinogenesis
- Radiations (Ionizing and Nonionizing; Background, Occupational and Medical Exposure)
- Biological Age
- Endocrine Imbalance
- Diet (Composition, Calorie Level, Presence of Cooking-Generated and Naturally Occurring Mutagens)
- Oncogenic and "Helper" Viruses
- Immunotoxicants
- Mixed-Function Oxidase Modifiers (Inducers/Repressors)
- Physical Trauma/Irritation
- Electromagnetic Fields
- Stress
- Tissue Hypertrophy/Atrophy
- Physical Activity Level

in all complex systems, the *overall structure* of the graph is of primary importance for understanding the behavioral mode of the network (*cf.* 3, 5–7).

In spite of the high density of the linkages shown, it is emphasized that Figure 1 merely *illustrates* the enormous complexity of the process; this is because the linkages that could be shown are very far from being exhaustive. Moreover, the representation (as vertexes) of certain factors, for example, the autocrine- and paracrine-acting growth factors and other "tissue hormones"—which yet play critically important roles in cell transformation and tumorigenesis—were intentionally omitted; this is because the rich diversity of additional linkages of these hormone-like substances with the factors/entities already represented would have rendered the layout of the figure unmanageable.

II. REVIEW OF ELEMENTS OF THE NETWORK—AN ANALYSIS OF THEIR INTERRELATIONSHIPS

The *starred sequence* in Figure 1 symbolizes the (loosely defined) stages in cell transformation from normal to malignant at the gene and perigenetic level; by "perigenetic" is meant here segments of the cell machinery perceived to be directly linked to the maintenance of genomic stability, to gene expression, to signal transduction and intercellular communication, and to phenotypic cell behavior. According to current definitions (*e.g.*, Chapter 5, Section I): *initiation* represents the generation of genotypic alteration(s) inheritable at the level of the initiated cells; *conversion* represents induction of promotability; *promotion* consists of the stimulation and clonal expansion of initiated cells; and *progression* is the term covering the stimulation of benign/premalignant cells and (probably) further genotypic alterations leading to autonomous tumor cells. Although not included in the starred sequence, *hyperplastic foci* (showing histochemical alterations) that represent a preneoplastic state have been described extensively in rodent liver and in mammary gland as well.

Also not represented in the starred sequence is the ability to undergo *metastasis*, the ultimate stage beyond the attainment of malignancy by cytological and histopathological

FIGURE 1. [*See* pp. 4 and 5.] Multifactor interaction network in carcinogenesis based on some major identified relationships. An arrow pointing from one factor to another symbolizes that the effect of the latter is modified by the former. For example, "Diet Composition" affects "Membrane-lipids Composition", that alters "Receptor Mobility" which, in turn, modulates the functioning of "Membrane Receptors". Or an arrow may symbolize a segment of the actual sequence of a biological process involved directly or indirectly in the series of events leading to carcinogenesis. For example, "Genotoxic 'Complete' Chemical Carcinogens" are metabolized by the "Mixed-Function Oxidase (MFO) System"; this system represents molecular entities underlying "Activating Metabolism" and "Detoxifying Metabolism", the former yielding intermediates that are generally mutagenic ("Mutagens") leading to "Initiation/Mutagenesis" in DNA.

A dashed line-pair breaking an arrow symbolizes inhibition or blockage of the path by a factor which is at the origin of another arrow pointing *to the line-pair*. For example, increase of "Mitogenic Activity" by "Calorie Intake" is reduced/ blocked by "Physical Activity (Exercise)"; similarly, the effect of "Mitogenic Activity" in bringing about "Alterations of Signal Transduction Pathways & of Gene Expression" and its participation in "Initiation/Mutagenesis" may be blocked by certain "Inhibitors of Tumorigenesis".

The *starred sequence* from "Cells with Normal Genome" through "Malignant Cells" connected with *heavy arrows* represents changes at the gene and perigenetic levels during the phases of the carcinogenic process; for example, "Initiation/Mutagenesis" modifies DNA (or the entire genome) directly in what is the first stage toward malignancy. Converting agents (which bring about "Conversion") possibly affect DNA both directly and via "Alterations of Signal Transduction Pathways & of Gene Expression". "Promoters—Epigenetic Carcinogens" (and also "Genotoxic 'Complete' Chemical Carcinogens" *beyond* "Initiation") must act as converting, promoter, and progressor agents via "Alterations of Signal Transduction Pathways & of Gene Expression"; these changes culminate eventually in "Blockage of Intercellular Communication".

An arrow pointing *to another arrow* is unique to the starred sequence. It symbolizes the effect of a factor upon DNA (or the entire genome) in a particular phase of genetic/genomic changes. For example, "Chromosomal Translocation", "Insertion, Gene Amplification", and chromosomal changes brought about by "Electromagnetic Fields" do represent initial genomic changes toward malignancy even though not formally associated with the term "Initiation" of the conventional two-stage or multistage chemical carcinogenesis model. Activated "Nuclear Receptors" can act on DNA and influence all stages of the process *beyond* "Initiated Cells".

The progress toward malignancy through the stages of carcinogenesis, shown in the starred sequence, may be interrupted/blocked at all stages *beyond* "Initiated Cells" by a competent "Systemic Immune Network", which represents the total capability of the immune system ("immune surveillance") to detect and destroy emerging neoplastic cells (as well as microbial invaders). However, "Initiation/ Mutagenesis" cannot be blocked by the immune system because the covalent binding of locally present electrophiles to, or other direct effects (such as radiation target effects) upon, DNA are purely chemical/physico-chemical interactions which, if followed by cell division—triggered by "Mitogenic Activity" before DNA repair can take place—"lock in" as mutation. It is during the successive genomic alterations that may occur *after* "Initiation" that immunologically distinct epitopes begin to appear on the cell surface.

Branching of an arrow is indicated by a solid node at the point of branching; conversely, a single or multiple overpass where arrow lines cross indicates that the paths that cross represent different streams of effect/relationship and are unconnected. To exemplify the former, an arrow originating at "Diet Composition" branches off to "Mixed-Function Oxidase (MFO) System" and to "Induction/ Repression of MFOs"; the first branch represents the requirement of all nutrient categories for the functioning and sustained maintenance of the MFO system, the second branch represents the specific effects: MFO repression by carbohydrates, MFO induction by protein, and the induction/repression of MFO(s) by certain nonnutrient substances present in the diet.

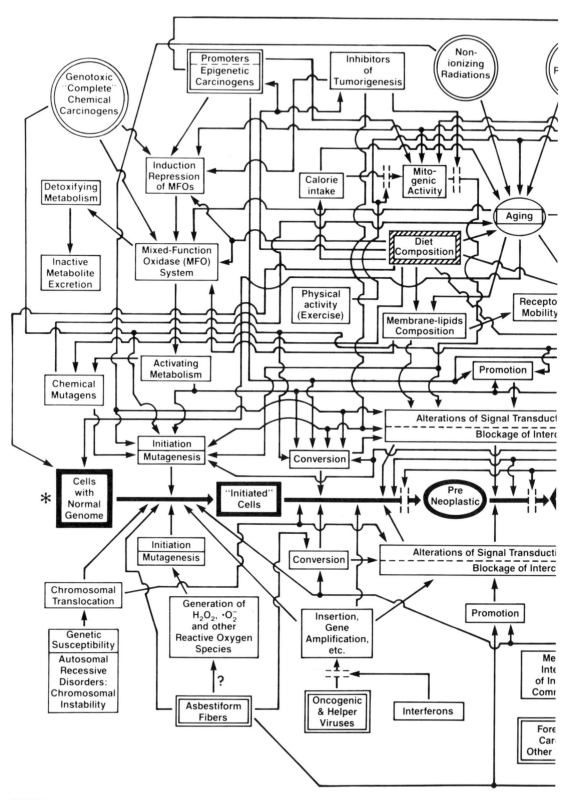

FIGURE 1.

4

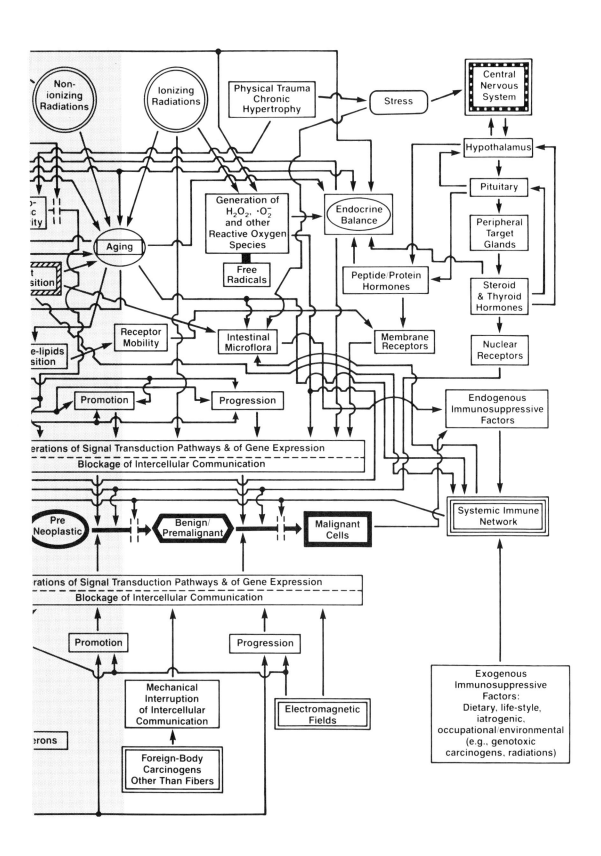

criteria. The ability to metastasize involves additional changes in DNA and probably the entire genome, that confer selective advantage; these changes allow increased expression of multiple gene products (8, 9) or bring about cooperative interaction between dominant and recessive genetic alterations (10). As with the genetic changes in the other stages of the carcinogenic process, the rate of alterations leading to invasiveness and to metastasis are also under the influence of a multiplicity of modulating factors; thus, it is abundantly documented that tumor foci (that have post-mortem been established to be malignant by histopathological criteria) can remain quasi-dormant for years or during a sizeable portion of the entire life span. The genetic nature of the establishment and augmentation of metastatic potential of tumor cells is further supported by the demonstration of the reversal of metastatic phenotype by gene transfer (11).

A. Varieties of Initiation Processes

"Initiation/Mutagenesis", the first stage in the *starred sequence*, represents target effect on critical DNA segment(s), such as the covalent binding of electrophiles (direct-acting carcinogens or metabolically generated reactive intermediates). The disruption of base-pairing due to binding of an electrophile will be "locked in" as a point mutation or frameshift mutation if—prompted by "Mitogenic Activity"—the cell replicates *before* DNA repair can take place.[1] Thus, the higher the rate of cell proliferation the greater the likelihood that a molecular lesion in DNA will be locked in as a mutation. The role of mitogenesis in mutagenesis and the importance of chronic mitogenesis in cancer have been discussed (12, 13).

The target of electrophile-produced "Initiation/Mutagenesis" may be a proto-oncogene (which thereby becomes activated to an oncogene) or a tumor-suppressor gene (which would become nonfunctional as a suppressor). The protein products of proto-oncogenes generally function as normal components of signal transduction pathways (STP). For example, Ras is a GTP/GDP actuated allosteric switch device (14); a diversity of G proteins are involved in the functioning of STP (15–17). Conversely, protein products of tumor-suppressor genes can act as phosphorylation/conformation–governed complexing agents to oncoproteins. For example, the p53 gene product, which is an antiproliferative device acting in the G_1-S boundary of the cell cycle (18a), represses the *hsp* 70 promoter gene by protein-protein interaction with the CCAAT binding factor (18b). Similarly, the K-*rev*-1 gene product (which contains a homologous sequence to the effector-binding region of the p21^{Ras} protein) blocks the action of the *ras* oncogene by binding to the Ras protein (19). Activation/mutation of proto-oncogenes can create abnormal bypasses in the STP and can eliminate or generate "cross-talk" between parallel pathways (20–22). At the same time, while the capacity for positive growth control at levels of proto-oncogenes is thus being abolished, the negative control of cell proliferation (23, 24) is also eliminated through mutation in the tumor-suppressor genes (21, 25, 26).

Another phenomenon participating in the maintenance of tissue size homeostasis is programmed cell death—apoptosis. Although there were preliminary data that promotion by the phorbol ester TPA involves the blockage of apoptosis (*rev.* 27), up to about 1992 little was known about the mechanism(s) how carcinogens/promoters/progressor agents affect, in general, the apoptotic process (28a).

Investigations summarized in 1993 (28b) provide powerful support that apoptosis— which together with cell proliferation are the competing phenomena governing tissue

---

[1]The terms "genotoxic" and "epigenetic" (or "nongenotoxic"), as generally used, denote categories of agents that are mutagenic and nonmutagenic, respectively, in different short-term tests. The limitations in attributing exact mechanistic meanings to these terms are discussed later in this chapter.

homeostasis—is under the control of oncogenes as well as tumor-suppressor genes. For example, the *bcl*-2 oncogene is potent in inhibiting apoptosis in B-cell lymphoma cells; there is, accordingly, a cooperative effect between *bcl*-2 and *myc*, in that transgenic mice that carry both oncogenes develop B-cell tumors much faster than animals that carry only *myc*. The *p53* tumor-suppressor gene, on the other hand, stimulates apoptosis, and activation of *p53* was observed to cause shrinkage of experimental colon tumors in animals. Mutation in *p53* abolishes its apoptosis-inducing ability.

"Initiation/Mutagenesis" may also result from other factors besides electrophilic organic chemicals/intermediates, for example, directly from the "Generation of H_2O_2, $\cdot O_2^-$ and Other Reactive Oxygen Species" including $HO\cdot$ radicals by "Ionizing Radiations", indirectly by *epigenetic* carcinogens that induce peroxisome proliferation[2] (32, 33), and possibly by "Asbestiform Fibers" (34–36). Induced peroxisomes appear to display an imbalance between fatty acid β-oxidation and catalase, and this results in increased release of H_2O_2 yielding reactive oxygen species which are mutagenic and clastogenic (32); these oxidants can also act as promoter and progressor agents (37, 38). In Salmonella tester strains, which contain no peroxisomes, peroxisome proliferators are nonmutagenic (32). Peroxisome proliferators act through activation of a nuclear receptor which is part of the "cross-talk" network of nuclear-receptor–using hormonal regulatory pathways (39, 40). Fatty acids bind and activate the same nuclear receptor and, indeed, high-fat diets (41) as well as vitamin E deficiency (42) have been shown to induce peroxisome proliferation.

Free radicals larger than $\cdot O_2^-$ or $HO\cdot$ are also generated by "Ionizing Radiations", and these can contribute to initiating mutagenesis. Ultraviolet radiation, a "Non-ionizing Radiation", induces a variety of photoproducts in DNA, *e.g.*, a thymidine-cytidine-6,4 dimer; if unrepaired or misrepaired these alterations are also expressed as mutations (43).

By a convention arising from the experimental design and extensive literature of "two-stage" and "multistage" carcinogenesis, the term "initiation" has come to be used to denote exclusively the cellular consequences of a point mutation or a frameshift mutation by a *genotoxic* carcinogen, yielding a convertible/promotable genotype. However, this limitation of the meaning of "initiation" to gene mutations appears to be too restrictive. Perhaps the term should be broadened to include large changes (such as chromosomal translocation, gene insertion, gene amplification, aneuploidy), which can yield promotable genotypes. Indeed, the significance of "chromosome mutations" for carcinogenesis has been discussed (*e.g.*, 44–47; *cf.* 48). Already in the earlier literature some so-called epigenetic carcinogens as well as asbestiform fibers were reported to induce chromosome mutations (*e.g.*, 46, 47, 49, 50), and different genotoxic carcinogens are known to also induce cytologically observable chromosomal aberrations beyond gene mutations. Moreover, in a recent extensive report the putative lack of mutagenicity of nongenotoxic carcinogens has been reexamined (51). The agents have been classified on the basis of the three genetic endpoints: gene mutation, chromosomal aberration, and aneuploidy. This massive reexamination of the data demonstrated that many of the putative nongenotoxic carcinogens that have been adequately tested in short-term bioassays are actually genotoxic by the above endpoint criteria (51). Perhaps the restrictiveness of the term "genotoxic", as used hitherto, provides a partial explanation for the number of putatively nongenotoxic carcinogens that were listed in a 1990 review (52).

Viral gene "Insertion, Gene Amplification" and virally-induced deletions and translocations are chromosome mutation-type large-scale genetic events and, thus, feed in at this first stage of the starred sequence. "Chromosomal Translocation" can also result from inherent chromosomal instability such as occurring in certain "Autosomal Recessive

---

[2]A similar mechanism may account for the carcinogenicity of another epigenetic carcinogen, metapyrilene, which has the unique property to induce the proliferation of mitochondria (22), sites of generation of hydrogen peroxide and its forerunner reactive oxygen species (29–31).

Disorders" (*e.g.*, 48). There are over 200 mutations which are predisposing factors to neoplastic diseases in humans (53). There is evidence (54) suggesting that the early cellular effects (chromosomal abnormalities, aberrations, and aneuploidy) of certain electromagnetic fields (microwaves; refs. 55, 56) may also feed in at this first stage of the sequence.

B. Beyond Initiation

Once cells have become "initiated", they can gradually advance toward malignancy.[3] The next stage, "Conversion", is the first that entails "Alterations of Signal Transduction Pathways". Possibly most if not all alterations in the STP along the way toward full cellular autonomy are eventually reflected in additional permanent changes in the genotype of the cells. Of course all genotypic changes, if reflected in germ cells—even though no somatic cells progress to autonomy/malignancy during the individual's life span—are inheritable. These predisposing genetic changes, which are cumulative, may be expressed, however, in the offspring (or in later generations) if appropriate and sufficient stimuli for conversion/promotion/progression are then present; this is the basis for the transgenerational transmission of cancer risk (*rev.* 59, 60).

Since all chemical and physical agents which are carcinogenic alone (genotoxic and epigenetic chemical carcinogens, radiations, and asbestiform fibers) must provide promoter/progressor stimulus toward the malignant transformation, they feed into the sequence—at and beyond "Conversion"—*also* via "Promotion" and "Progression"; some of these effects may reach the genome by way of the STP. Molecular input for tumor induction by certain steroids as well as by peroxisome proliferators would appear to bypass the STP, since the steroid receptors generally and receptors for peroxisome proliferators are located in the nucleus ("Nuclear Receptors"). Existing evidence (*rev.* 61) suggests that implanted platelets ("Foreign-Body Carcinogens") bring about malignancy via chronic "Mechanical Interruption of Intercellular Communication" between adjacent cell layers in subcutaneous tissue. Changes in the genome or in DNA proper (involving chromosome translocation, viral gene insertion, or virally-induced gene amplification)—through the interaction of the STP with an already altered genome—can and often do provide self-sustaining stimulus for progress toward full autonomy/malignancy without additional converting/promoter/progressor input. This is reminiscent of the synergistic nature of random genetic alterations, a phenomenon known for some years (58, *cf.* 62).

C. Repositories of Inheritable Epigenetic Information

It is possible that for some truly nongenotoxic "Epigenetic Carcinogens" the inheritable genomic imprinting lies exclusively in the structure and conformation of chromatin, rather than in DNA proper. As it has been restated, "more than DNA sequence information is transmitted from one cell generation to the next. What is transmitted is chromatin, a three-dimensional complex of DNA and proteins. Therefore, in addition to the instructions coded in the base sequence of DNA, genes can carry and transmit information embedded in the structure and conformation of chromatin. Such information is epigenetic information" (63). For example, one factor that appears to be epigenetically inherited in somatic cell lineages is the pattern of cytosine methylation (64, 65) and some changes in gene activity were correlated with changes in methylation

---

[3]Karyotypic instability that is observed in most (but not all) cancer cells is a contributing factor in the acceleration of evolution toward malignancy (48, 57) and it is likely that, in general, genetic instability gradually increases with the progressive accumulation of mutations (*cf.* 58).

patterns (66, 67). It is noteworthy in this connection that a high incidence of hepatic tumors are induced by maintaining rodents on a diet deficient in choline, the principal dietary source of methyl groups for transmethylation reactions (Chapter 9, Section III).

Another likely candidate as a carrier of inheritable cellular information is the mitochondria. Mitochondria are over 99% maternally inherited. In cell division, each of the two cells receives half of the original mitochondrial population. Any alteration of mitochondrial DNA (mtDNA) is, of course, a mutation in the literal sense of genetic terminology. However, by common parlance the term "genotoxic", as used in the field of carcinogenesis, has come to denote agents which are mutagenic specifically toward *nuclear* DNA (nDNA); in this sense, inheritable changes in mitochondria may be regarded as "epigenetic".

Although the maximum coding capacity of mtDNA is for only about 5000 amino acids (68), mtDNA genes share with nDNA genes the function of coding for the polypeptides making up the five enzyme complexes that carry out oxidative phosphorylation (OP) (69); OP is the main source of ATP needed for all energy-requiring cellular processes including DNA repair, an important component of genomic stability. Consistent with this, there is evidence that defects in OP are associated with a variety of degenerative processes (*rev.* 69). The inherent mutation rate of mtDNA is substantially higher than of most nDNA genes (69) and mtDNA is, precisely, the local target of oxidative damage by H_2O_2 and $\cdot O_2^-$ generated by the electron transport chain (29–31, *revs.* 70, 71); hence, the increasing defects of OP with age. Moreover, the preferential alkylation of mtDNA by a typical genotoxic carcinogen, *N*-methyl-*N*-nitrosourea, at a rate 3 to 7 times that of nDNA has been shown (72).

In addition to alterations of the OP enzyme complexes, defects in OP may also be due to alterations of the mitochondrial inner membrane which serves as a structural matrix for the OP complexes (73). A functional expression of the inner mitochondrial membrane (74) is electron transport $\leftrightarrow$ ATP hydrolysis linked "swelling" $\leftrightarrow$ "contraction" of mitochondria, which reflects ultrastructural transitions of the membrane (75, 76). These membrane transitions express a chemiosmotic regulatory modality of the rate of ATP synthesis through control of the degree of coupling (76, 77) of complex V (ATP synthase) to the electrochemical gradient in complexes I through IV (the electron transport chain) (78, 79). The degree of coupling is manifested in the Respiratory Control Index.

Defects in the OP enzyme complexes I through V and/or in the structure of the inner membrane can have a cascading effect on the progress of neoplastic change because: (a) decrease in the generation and availability of ATP will reduce the rate of DNA repair, (b) increasing "Generation of H_2O_2, $\cdot O_2^-$ and Other Reactive Oxygen Species" by a defective electron transport chain will act as mutagens toward mtDNA and as promoter and progressor agents toward nDNA also by virtue of their mutagenic effects (37, 38), and (c) mutations in both mtDNA and nDNA will, in turn, further increase the rate of defects generation in the OP enzyme complexes. Thus, the mitochondrial effects of genotoxic carcinogens (direct-acting or reactive metabolic intermediates) may represent an important (or for some agents the sole) *promoter component* of their mechanism of carcinogenic action. For certain epigenetic carcinogens (*e.g.*, the mitochondria proliferator, metapyrilene, and the uncoupler of oxidative phosphorylation, pentachlorophenol) mitochondria may represent the principal or exclusive effector sites.

The genotoxic potent hepatocarcinogen, 3'-methyl-4-dimethylaminoazobenzene (3'-Me-DAB) was probably the most extensively studied carcinogen for effects on the mitochondrial energy transduction system. During administration of 3'-Me-DAB, dramatic phase changes/restructuring occur in both the inner and outer mitochondrial membrane at the threshold of tumorigenesis (under the specific experimental conditions used). This restructuring was manifested by two marker phenomena: by very large changes in swelling $\leftrightarrow$ contraction response (80a–82) and by breaks in the Arrhenius plot of the outer-membrane–localized NADH–indophenol reductase (82). Throughout 3′-Me-DAB administration there is a progressive disappearance of the receptor sites for swelling-inducer agents, which are control sites for the rate of ATP synthesis, and these sites were virtually absent in mitochondria isolated from hepatoma nodules (81). Large changes in the respiratory control index, which closely paralleled the changes in the swelling ↔ contraction response, were observed, and tumor mitochondria were partially or totally uncoupled (83). There were extensive variations in the respiratory rate during restructuring, and tumor mitochondria showed a generally impaired respiration (83).

The electron transport chain appears to be normally a site of generation of H_2O_2 and reactive radical oxidant species (29–31, *revs.* 70, 71). Although there is no direct evidence for increase in the generation of oxidants in the mitochondria specifically during 3′-Me-DAB carcinogenesis, results by Vithayathil *et al.* (84a, *cf.* 76) suggest electron leak from the respiratory chain assembly resulting prom/from the effect of other carcinogens on mitochondria. It should be noted in this regard that the mitochondrial membrane(s) is a major site of covalent binding of 3′-Me-DAB in the target tissue (*cf.* 80a, 81, 84b), and the level of bound dye reaches a maximum closely before or at the tumorigenesis threshold (J.C. Arcos, unpublished).

D. Role and Control of Mixed-Function Oxidases

The majority of vertexes representing categories of carcinogens and exogenous and endogenous factors that modify carcinogenesis are shown above the starred sequence in Figure 1. The vertex "Genotoxic 'Complete' Chemical Carcinogens" covers the category of direct-acting carcinogens (including those activated by simple acid- or alkali-catalyzed hydrolysis) and of those requiring metabolic activation to ultimate reactive intermediates. Hence, this vertex feeds into the starred sequence (through "Initiation/Mutagenesis", "Conversion", "Promotion", and "Progression") directly, as well as via the vertex "Mixed-Function Oxidase (MFO) System" that leads to "Activating Metabolism". Metabolically activated carcinogenic intermediates are generally mutagenic, hence the bypass linkage "Chemical Mutagens"; this bypass also symbolizes the apparent fact that not all mutagens which are initiators are "complete" carcinogens. The second broad category of MFO function is "Detoxifying Metabolism" leading to "Inactive Metabolite Excretion".

The foremost control feature of the MFOs is their inducibility and repressibility (via modulation of gene expression and at post-transcriptional levels). Factors that influence the functioning of the MFO system can act: (a) in a general manner, such as biological "Aging" (85) or "Diet Composition", the latter representing requirement of *all* nutrient categories for the functioning and sustained maintenance of the MFOs (86–89) or (b) more specifically via "Induction/Repression of MFOs", such as: hormone effects summed under "Endocrine Balance" upon the MFOs; "Promoters" and "Inhibitors" that exert their effects via MFOs; those "Genotoxic 'Complete' Chemical Carcinogens" which are *also* inducers and/or repressors of MFOs (*e.g.*, certain polynuclear aromatic hydrocarbons); as well as the second branch of the arrow that originates at "Diet Composition", reflecting the presence in the diet of nonnutrient substances which can induce/repress MFOs (89) and the MFO induction by dietary protein and repression by carbohydrate (89, 90).

E. Promoters *versus* Epigenetic Carcinogens

Regarding the depiction of the vertex "Promoters—Epigenetic Carcinogens", it should be noted that the meaning of the terms "promoter" and "nongenotoxic (or epigenetic) carcinogen", and the understanding of their interrelationship, are at present in a state of considerable flux. Since the early realization that croton oil, a "pure promoter" extensively used in the 1950s, is, in fact, carcinogenic when applied alone (*e.g.*, 91, 93), a number of agents with promoter activity (*e.g.*, Tween 60 and 80, anthralin, phenol, 1,4-dioxane, apocholic acid, phenobarbital, *o*-phenylphenol, certain chlorinated pesticides, several naturally occurring complex compounds, 1,2,7,8-tetrachlorodibenzo-*p*-dioxin) were shown to induce tumors when administered/applied alone. Moreover, the phorbol ester, TPA, shows a clear dose–response relationship as a solitary carcinogen toward the mouse skin (94). A very substantial (if not total) overlap exists between the cellular and tissue effects and putative molecular mechanisms of action of "promoters" and "epigenetic carcinogens". There is possibly a paradigm-shift in the making (*e.g.*, 95–99) in that promotion and epigenetic carcinogenesis may come to be widely regarded as different operational features of the same broad category of agents.

F. Promoters, Inhibitors, Calorie Intake *versus* Rate of Cell Proliferation

Different "Promoters – Epigenetic Carcinogens" and "Inhibitors of Tumorigenesis" can each act through a variety of mechanisms. For example, some inhibitors exert their effect by blocking "Mitogenic Activity" which would further the "Alterations of Signal Transduction Pathways & of Gene Expression". Conversely, an important property of "Promoters" is "Mitogenic Activity", which is also increased by high "Calorie Intake" (a function of the "Diet Composition" and of its amount), by "Physical Trauma/Chronic Hypertrophy", as well as by the hormone levels ("Endocrine Balance") in the target tissue(s). Increase of "Mitogenic Activity" by "Calorie Intake" may, in turn, be blocked/reduced by "Physical Activity (Exercise)", using up calories; elevated calorie intake has, in fact, been termed "the most striking rodent carcinogen ever discovered" (13). The arrow coming from "Physical Activity (Exercise)" to the blockage break between "Calorie Intake" ⟶ "Mitogenic Activity" branches off and continues beyond the node to "Aging" and to "Endocrine Balance". However, some "Promoters – Epigenetic Carcinogens" may act, as we have seen earlier, through the "Generation of H_2O_2, $\cdot O_2^-$, and Other Reactive Oxygen Species," or through effect on the "Endocrine Balance".

G. The Neuroendocrine Interface. Factors Affecting Hormonal Regulatory Pathways

"Physical Trauma/Chronic Hypertrophy" also feeds into "Stress". In a broad sense stress ranges from psychosocial (*e.g.*, 100–104) through lifestyle/behavioral (*e.g.*, 105–108) to stress at tissue level (*e.g.*, 109–113). Sensory input perceived as "Stress" in the "Central Nervous System" (Chapter 15) is expressed via the autonomic nervous system, the hypothalamic–pituitary axis and its target glands, as well as via other arms of the endocrine system not represented in Figure 1. The levels of "Peptide/Protein Hormones" and of "Steroid Hormones" are maintained in a steady-state through the multiple feedback loops of the target glands to the pituitary and hypothalamus (Chapter 11, Section I). This steady-state – the "Endocrine Balance" – can rapidly shift because, for example, of "Stress"-induced neurological signals channeled via or originating from the "Central Nervous System", as well as because of increased/decreased hormone demand at the target tissues (change in demand, which itself may be generated by "Stress"). Chronic overstimulation of hormonal tissue targets by hormone administration or by persistent endocrine imbalance may lead to tumor induction (Chapter 11, Section II). Such endocrine perturbations can also modulate the action of nonhormone chemical carcinogens (Chapter 11, Section III).

The regulatory functions of hormones are carried out through actions on "Membrane Receptors" for "Peptide/Protein Hormones" and on "Nuclear Receptors" for "Steroid Hormones" as well as for thyroid hormones, retinoids, and 1,25-dihydroxycholecalciferol ("activated" vitamin D_3). "Cross-talk" between different hormonal regulatory pathways, mentioned in Section II.A. above, provides the diversity and specificity to regulate the myriad hormone responsive genes; there is evidence (39, 40) that in the nuclear receptor-using pathways "cross-talk" is carried out by heterodimer formation between receptors. Various isoforms of the 9-*cis*-retinoic acid receptor, RXR, appear to play key roles in this "cross-talk" between some essential nuclear receptors; RXR serves as common heterodimerization partner for peroxisome proliferator-activated receptor (PPAR), "activated" vitamin D_3 receptor (VDR), thyroid hormone receptor (TR) and all-*trans*-retinoic acid receptor (RAR) (39, 40). RXR and RAR are structurally and functionally distinct. In addition to the role of RXR in heterodimers, it also forms homodimers in response to activation by 9-*cis*-retinoic acid. The C-terminus of RXR and of other members of the nuclear receptor superfamily contains regions necessary for homo- and heterodimerization (39). Typically, members of the superfamily bind to the "hormone response element"-DNA sequence as dimers, to trigger gene expression. The structure of RXR has been investigated in some detail (114a).

Similar molecular mechanisms appear to account for "cross-talk" between STP involving cell membrane receptors. The protein products of the proto-oncogenes, *fos* and *jun*, that can regulate patterns of gene expression of many genes when induced by a great variety of extracellular stimuli, interact with the AP-1 binding site (found in the transcriptional control region of many genes) with much higher affinity when in the heterodimer form (114b).

Binding of carcinogens to nuclear receptors has been hypothesized to compete with the binding of their natural ligands and to result in aberrant regulation of transcription, preventing the differentiation-promoting effect of the natural ligands (*cf.* 115). The existence of a retinoic acid–inducible "cellular retinol-binding protein" (CRBP), a cytosolic nonenzymatic protein, the level of which is increased in squamous cell carcinomas, is consistent with the decreased terminal differentiation of these carcinoma cells (*rev.* 116); presumably CRBP competes with the nuclear receptor for the available retinol. It is noteworthy that CRBP is involved in the mechanism of toxicity by polyhalogenated hydrocarbons, creating a vitamin A deficient condition (117).

An interesting path traces the interlocking effects of "Diet Composition" on gene expression via STP. The effect of the nature of dietary lipids on the composition and functioning of the cell membrane and of endoplasmic membranes has been extensively documented (*e.g.*, 118–122). The "Membrane-lipids Composition" has a profound influence on membrane fluidity (118, 119, 123–125) which, in turn, modulates through "Receptor Mobility" the functions of "Membrane Receptors", the first components in the pathways of signal transduction. Another path in Figure 1, representing the effect of "Diet Composition" on normal gene expression, is via diet-mediated changes of chromatin structure which have a profound influence on the process of transcription (126).

H. Factors Affecting the Systemic Immune Network. The Neuroimmunoendocrine Interface

The "Systemic Immune Network" representing immune surveillance capability is affected by a multitude of factors, such as biological "Aging", "Diet Composition", and endogenous and exogenous "Immunosuppressive Factors". A variety of "Endogenous

Immunosuppressive Factors" (*e.g.*, α-globulin-like proteins, glycoproteins, tumor prostaglandins, 1-methyladenosine) are produced by "Malignant Cells" (127–137a).

There is a beginning of understanding of the complex mechanisms of tumor-induced impairment of the immune response. For example, unlike in normal mice, in tumor-bearing mice, the binding of ligand to T lymphocyte antigen receptor (TCR) triggered only a blunted release of intracellular Ca^{2+}, even though surface TCR density was normal and the cells had adequate intracellular Ca^{2+} stores (137b). This led to the discovery that protein tyrosine phosphorylation, the earliest demonstrable event in TCR-mediated signal transduction, shows an altered pattern in tumor-bearing mice, which was traced to the absence of certain protein components in the TCR. There was also reduced expression of p56^{lck} and p59^{fyn}, two *src* family protein tyrosine kinases, in T cells from tumor-bearing mice (137b). Such changes may account for some aspects of the immune defects in tumor-bearing hosts.

Immunosuppressive/mutagenic agents are also produced by the "Intestinal Microflora" (138–141); the absorption of these from the gut may be a function of biological aging, as there is an age-associated increase of intestinal absorption of macromolecules (142). The "Systemic Immune Network", in turn, determines the compatible microbial species composition of the intestinal microflora (139, 143), also modulated by "Stress" (144) and possibly by biological "Aging" (145). "Exogenous Immunosuppressive Factors" may be of dietary, lifestyle, iatrogenic, occupational, and environmental origin (*e.g.*, genotoxic carcinogens and ionizing radiations are immunosuppressive). There are, moreover, important signaling pathways between the neuroendocrine network and the immune network (*e.g.*, *revs.* 146–148), not represented in Figure 1. The immune system can be influenced by almost any type of endogenous and exogenous (xenobiotic) biological messenger molecule (148, 149).

A competent "Systemic Immune Network" may detect and destroy emerging neoplastic cells possibly at different stages of autonomy; this is symbolized in the graph by an arrow—originating at the Network and branching off at the three stages beyond "Initiation"—blocking the progress toward malignancy. However, the immune network may not prevent/block the stage of "Initiation" which is a chemically- or radiation-induced or genetically pre-programmed ("intrinsic mutagenesis", *e.g.*, 150, 151) structural change in DNA, not yet manifested at this first stage as immunologically distinct epitopes on the cell surface.

I. Central Role of the Effect of Aging

A vertex of central significance is biological "Aging", the rate of which is modulated by a variety of factors, including "Diet Composition", "Calorie Intake", "Physical Activity (Exercise)", and exposure to "Chemical Mutagens", "Non-ionizing Radiations" and "Ionizing Radiations". In turn, biological "Aging" influences many cellular processes, for example: (a) the "Endocrine Balance"; (b) the functions of the "Mixed-Function Oxidase (MFO) System" through different paths [*e.g.*, through "Endocrine Balance" via the "Induction/Repression of MFOs" linkage, through "Membrane-lipids Composition" (152) and through a direct path representing the aging-governed possible changes in membrane proteins (153)]; (c) the "Systemic Immune Network" (and, ancillarily linked to it, the microbial species distribution of the "Intestinal Microflora"); (d) the functions localized in the cell membrane (*e.g.*, receptor functions, membrane transport, and intercellular communication) and in the endoplasmic membranes (*e.g.*, the control of mitochondrial oxidative phosphorylation and of MFO functions, and membrane transport); (e) the stability and functioning of the genome through effect on nucleotide metabolism, on rate of methylation of bases, and on rate and fidelity of DNA repair.

J.   Generation of Reactive Radical Species and Damage to Membranes

A commonality of effect between aging, diet-induced changes in lipid composition, and/or membrane binding of reactive intermediates (mutagen/carcinogen) may be peroxidative damage to endoplasmic membranes (154, 155). This may lead to the creation or increase of electron leak from the electron transport chain (29–31, 76, 154, *rev.* 70) and other enzymatic processes and, in turn, to the generation or increased generation of H_2O_2, $\cdot O_2^-$, and higher free radicals (29–31, 84, 156, *rev.* 71); these can bring about cascading/synergistic alterations in the genome and the STP, and are immune modulators (*e.g.*, 35, 70, 157). The sum total of cellular aging is a generally impaired responsiveness to maintain homeostasis (158, 159) involving alterations in the actin cytoskeletal network (160), and leading at the systemic level to decreasing immune competence (127, 158, 161, 162).

K.   Aging, Cancer, and Loss of Homeostatic Functions

Both aging and neoplasia represent decrease in homeostatic regulatory functions. However, while in aging the gradual loss of cellular feedback competence spreads over all tissues and is (probably) genetically pre-programmed, neoplasia results from an *induced* "subversion of growth regulatory pathways" (20) generally assumed to occur initially in a few cells in a specific tissue target. "Induced" in this context signifies that neoplasia is brought about/enhanced by any means (including inheritable genetic/genomic predisposition to neoplasia) *other than* the genetic program of aging, which is the gradual, orderly, system-wide shut-down of homeostatic functions. However, because of partial overlap of the two processes (*e.g.*, in decrease of the fidelity of DNA replication and impairment of DNA repair, decrease of immune competence, structural alterations of the cell membrane and endoplasmic membranes), aging, the systemic phenomenon, will tend to amplify/ synergize any local tumorigenic factor(s) wherever it occurs; hence the general increase of "spontaneous" tumor incidence with age, in all species.

If a genetic program predetermining aging indeed exists, and represents a genetically determined rate of random mutations, the above argument is not invalidated, we believe, by the synergism between random genetic alterations (58, *cf.* 62). Such synergism simply points to the thermodynamic inescapability of the progressive effect of age on the cancer rate.

It remains that any tumorigenic potentiality present locally at a tissue site is generally the resultant of a number of factors in the system-wide network (Figure 1). These represent then a "spectrum of predisposing factors" *beyond* age—such as chemical and radiation exposures of environmental/occupational/lifestyle/medical origin, diet composition/calorie intake, genetic susceptibility (if any), endocrine balance, physical activity level, and stress, *acting interactively*. Could it be that the entire "spectrum of predisposing factors"—if maintained unchanged—is the basis underlying the view that "cancer is a systemic disease" (*e.g.*, 163), ensuring frequently the recurrence of a tumor locally or at a different site, a few years from the time of removal of the original tumor? In this light, the multifactor interaction network concept of carcinogenesis appears to open a new perspective on cancer prevention.

III. CLOSING NOTE

The total perspective summarized in this chapter prompts a reexamination of the prevailing notion of distinct "stages" in carcinogenesis and suggests the following hypothesis:

The genomes of species are endowed with a relatively high resilience to damage and degree of stability,[4] and this stability increases ascending the evolutionary ladder of complexity. This relative genomic stability, which provides a temporary permanence for inherited traits under stable environmental conditions, is the basis of the "punctuated equilibria" in neodarwinian evolutionary theory (*e.g.*, 166, 167).

Because of this relative stability, a stimulus of high energy (such as provided by genotoxic direct-acting agents or reactive metabolic intermediates, or by ionizing radiations) is required to bring about an initial perturbation (mutation) in the integrity of the genome. Once the genome has departed from the plateau of initial stability, there is increasing ease (karyotypic instability[5]) for the occurrence of progressive genomic structural changes through successive mutations by: covalent adduct formation through the *sustained* action of electrophilic agents (promotion component of the effect of "complete" carcinogens); radiations; potent hydrogen/hydrophobic bonding agents that can modify DNA conformation; gene translocations; gene amplification; insertion of mobile genetic elements of exogenous origin; etc. It is possible that agents that can modify DNA conformation without covalent interaction could also bring about *the initiating* mutation(s) *if* administered/applied at elevated levels and for a prolonged period of time (*e.g.*, dioxane, acetamide, nitrilotriacetic acid, phenobarbital, phenol). Consistent with this, a number of water-soluble carcinogens were found to be potent agents of protein denaturation (168–171), *i.e.*, have the capability to bring about random changes in the conformations of biological macromolecules. Thus, alternatively, the mode of action of such nongenotoxic agents (epigenetic carcinogens) may be via the induction of conformational changes in chromatin proteins and possibly in nuclear matrix proteins.

Some other nongenotoxic agents (nonmutagenic in Salmonella tester strains) may induce the initial mutations by indirect means (*e.g.*, through the generation of H_2O_2 and reactive oxygen species), such as peroxisome proliferators and metapyrilene, a mitochondria proliferator. Again, other agents that induce genomic alterations by indirect means may act via the heterodimerization "cross-talk" network of hormonal regulatory pathways (such as in carcinogenesis by steroid hormones). In addition to the successive alterations of the genome that can be brought about by specific chemical and physical agents, it is possible that the forward momentum of spontaneous genetic/genomic changes may become increasingly self-sustaining in accord with the synergistic nature of random genetic alterations (58, *cf.* 62) consistent with increasing karyotypic instability. Eventually, *in vivo*, an equilibrium *may* become established between the growth potential of the tumor and the "immune surveillance" capability of the systemic immune network, an unstable equilibrium modulated by the totality of factors in the interaction network.

The progressive accumulation of genomic alterations during the change from normal to malignant cells and then to metastasis is the underlying determinant of the histo-

---

[4]This notion was foreshadowed by Schrödinger (164), comparing the sequential, orderly structure of the genome to the periodicity of a crystal lattice (*cf.* 165).

[5]Followup of specific marker chromosomes (57) may not be an appropriate design to confirm karyotypic instability (or the lack of it) in carcinogenesis. This is because instability is likely to affect primarily regions of the genome containing induced alterations. Such regions may be selectively or randomly distributed through the genome and may vary, depending on the agent and the experimental conditions.

pathologically observable *continuum* of the transition. Thus the "stages" in carcinogenesis (initiation, conversion, promotion, progression) should be viewed as categories of conceptual and operational convenience—useful to provide a framework for systematic experimental approaches—rather than truly distinct biological/cytological categories.

U.S. GOVERNMENT COPYRIGHT LICENSE

The authors of this chapter are employees of the U.S. Government. Accordingly, the U.S. Government retains a nonexclusive, royalty-free license to reproduce the published form of the contribution, or allow others to do so, for U.S. Government purposes.

REFERENCES

1. Trosko, J. E., and Chang, C.-C.: Potential Role of Intercellular Communication in the Rate-Limiting Step in Carcinogenesis. *In* "Cancer and the Environment—Possible Mechanisms of Threshold for Carcinogens and Other Toxic Substances" (J. A. Cimino, H. B. Demopoulos, M. Kushner, H. Uehleke, B. L. Van Duuren, B. M. Wagner, and V. R. Young, eds.). Mary Ann Liebert, New York, 1983, p. 5.
2. Chartrand, G.: "Introductory Graph Theory". Dover, New York, 1977.
3. Laue, R.: "Elemente der Graphentheorie und ihre Anwendung in den biologischen Wissenschaften". Friedrich Vieweg, Braunschweig, Germany, 1971.
4. Harary, F.: "Graph Theory". Addison-Wesley, Reading, England, 1969.
5. Forrester, J. W.: "Principles of Systems". Wright-Allen Press, Cambridge, Massachusetts, 1968.
6. Forrester, J. W.: "World Dynamics". Wright-Allen Press, Cambridge, Massachusetts, 1971.
7. Meadows, D. H., Meadows, D. L., Randers, J., and Behrens, W. W., III: "The Limits to Growth". Signet/New American Library, New York, 1972.
8. Liotta, L. A.: Oncogene Induction of Metastases. *In* "Metastasis", Ciba Foundation Symp. No. 141. Wiley, New York, 1988, p. 94.
9. Tarin, D.: Molecular Genetics of Metastasis. *In* "Metastasis", Ciba Foundation Symp. No. 141. Wiley, New York, 1988, p. 149.
10. Egan, S. E., Wright, J. A., and Greenberg, A. H.: *Environ. Health Perspect.* **93**, 91 (1991).
11. Feldman, M., Gelber, C., Plaksin, D., Kushtai, G., and Eisenbach, L.: The Reversal of the Metastatic Phenotype by Gene Transfer. *In* "Metastasis", Ciba Foundation Symp. No. 141. Wiley, New York, 1988, p. 170.
12. Ames, B. N., and Swirsky-Gold, L.: *Mutat. Res.* **250**, 3 (1991).
13. Engelman, R. W., Day, N. K., and Good, R. A.: *Proc. Soc. Exp. Biol. Med.* **203**, 13 (1993).
14. Satoh, T., Nakafuku, M., and Kaziro, Y.: *J. Biol. Chem.* 1992 Minireview Compendium, p. 24149.
15. Iyengar, R., and Birnbaumer, L.: "G Proteins". Academic Press, San Diego, 1990.
16. Simon, M. I., Strathman, M. P., and Gautam, N.: *Science* **252**, 802 (1991).
17. Milligan, G., and Wakelam, M., eds.: "G Proteins—Signal Transduction and Disease". Academic Press, San Diego, 1992.
18a. Ullrich, S. J., Anderson, C. W., Mercer, W. E., and Appella, E., *J. Biol. Chem.* 1992 Minireview Compendium, p. 15259.
18b. Agoff, S. N., Hou, J., Linzer, D. I. H., and Wu, B.: *Science* **259**, 84 (1993).
19. Kitayama, H., Sugimoto, Y., Matsuzaki, T., Ikawa, Y., and Noda, M.: *Cell* **56**, 77 (1989).
20. Heldin, C.-H., Betsholtz, C., Claesson-Welsh, L. and Westermark, B.: *Biochim. Biophys. Acta* **907**, 219 (1987).
21. Stubblefield, E.: *Mol. Carcinogenesis* **4**, 257 (1991).
22. Schüller, H. M.: *Biochem. Pharmacol.* **42**, 1511 (1991).
23. Weinberg, R. A.: *Cancer Res.* **49**, 3713 (1989).
24. Boyd, J. A., and Barrett, J. C.: *Mol. Carcinogenesis* **3**, 325 (1990).
25. Bouck, N. P., and Benton, B. K.: *Chem. Res. Toxicol.* **2**, 1 (1989).
26. Weinberg, R. A.: *Mol. Carcinogenesis* **3**, 3 (1990).
27. Tomei, L. D.: Apoptosis—A Program for Death or Survival? *In* "Apoptosis—The Molecular Basis of Cell Death" (L. D. Tomei and F. O. Cope, eds.). Cold Spring Harbor Laboratory Press, New York, 1991, p. 279.

28a. Thompson, H. J., Strange, R., Schedin, P. J.: *Cancer Epidemiol., Biomarkers, Prevention* **1**, 597 (1992).
28b. Marx, J.: Research News *in Science* **259**, 760 (1993).
29. Boveris, A., Oshino, N., and Chance, B.: *Biochem. J.* **128**, 617 (1972).
30. Loschen, G. A., Azzi, A., Richter, C., and Flohe, L.: *FEBS Lett.* **41**, 68 (1974).
31. Konstantinov, A. A., Peskin, A. V., Popova, E. Y., Khomutor, G. B., and Runge, E. K.: *Biochim. Biophys. Acta* **894**, 1 (1987).
32. Reddy, J. K., Warren, J. R., Reddy, M. K., and Lalwain, N. D.: *Ann. N. Y. Acad. Sci.* **386**, 81 (1982).
33. Lazarow, P. B.: Catabolic Functions of Peroxisomes: Modification by Hypolipidemic Drugs. *In* "Cancer and the Environment – Possible Mechanisms of Threshold for Carcinogens and Other Toxic Substances" (J. A. Cimino, H. B. Demopoulos, M. Kushner et al., eds.). Mary Ann Liebert, New York, 1983, p. 101.
34. Archer, J.: *Med Hypotheses* **5**, 1257 (1979).
35. Mossman, B. T., and Landesman, J. M.: *Chest* **83**, Suppl. 50 (1983).
36. Mossman, B. T.: *Environ. Carcino. Rev.* **C6**, 151 (1988).
37. Cerutti, P., Larsson, R., and Krupitza, G.: Mechanisms of Oxidant Carcinogenesis. *In* "Genetic Mechanisms in Carcinogenesis and Tumor Progression" (C. C. Harris and L. A. Liotta, eds.). Wiley-Liss, New York, 1990, p. 69.
38. Cerutti, P.: Tumor Promotion by Oxidants. *In* "Theories of Carcinogenesis" (O. H. Iversen, ed.). Hemisphere, Washington, D.C. 1988, p. 221.
39. Kliever, S. A., Umesone, D. I., Mangelsdorf, R. M., and Evans, R. M.: *Nature* **355**, 446 (1992).
40. Kliever, S. A., Umesono, K., Noonan, D. J., Heyman, R. A., and Evans, R. M.: *Nature* **358**, 771 (1992).
41. Krahling, J. B., and Tolbert, N. E.: *Ann. N. Y. Acad. Sci.* **386**, 433 (1982).
42. Dabholkar, A. S.: *Ann. N.Y. Acad. Sci.* **386**, 475 (1982).
43. Kripke, M. L., Pitcher, H., and Longstreth, J. D.: *Environ. Carcino. Rev.* **C7**, 53 (1989).
44. Sasaki, M.: *Cytogenet. Cell Genet.* **33**, 160 (1982).
45. Sandberg, A. A.: *Cancer Genet. Cytogenet.* **8**, 277 (1983).
46. Barrett, J. C., Thomassen, D. G., and Hesterberg, J. W.: *Ann. N.Y. Acad. Sci.* **407**, 291 (1983).
47. Hesterberg, T. W., Oshimura, M., Brady, A. R., and Barrett, C. J.: Asbestos and Silica Induce Morphological Transformation of Mammalian Cells in Culture: A Possible Mechanism. *In* "Silica, Silicosis and Cancer" (D. F. Goldsmith, D. M. Winn, and C. M. Shy, eds.). Praeger, New York, 1986, p. 177.
48. Phillips, R. A.: The Genetic Basis of Cancer. *In* "The Basic Science of Oncology" (I. F. Tannock and R. P. Hill, eds.). Pergamon, New York, 1987, p. 24.
49. Oshimura, M., Hesterberg, T. W., Tsutsiu, T., and Barrett, J. C.: *Cancer Res.* **44**, 5017 (1984).
50. Barrett, J. C., Wong, A., and McLachlan, J. A.: *Science* **212**, 1402 (1981).
51. Jackson, M. A., Stack, H. F. and Waters, M. D.: *Mutat. Res.* **296**, 241 (1993).
52. Lijinsky, W.: *Environ. Carcino. Rev.* **C8**, 45 (1990).
53. Mulvihill, J. J.: Genetic Repertory of Human Neoplasia. *In* "Genetics of Human Cancer" (J. J. Mulvihill, R. W. Miller, and J. F. Fraumeni, Jr., eds.). Raven Press, New York, 1977, p. 137.
54. Balcer-Kubiczek, E. K., and Harrison, G. H.: *Carcinogenesis* **6**, 859 (1985).
55. Lin, J. C., and Peterson, W. D.: *J. Bioeng.* **1**, 471 (1977).
56. Alam, M. T., Barthaker, N., Lambert, N. G., and Kastiya, S. S.: *Can. J. Genet. Cytol.* **20**, 23 (1978).
57. Barrett, J. C., Tsutsui, T., Tlsty, T., and Oshimura, M.: Role of Genetic Instability in Carcinogenesis. *In* "Genetic Mechanisms in Carcinogenesis and Tumor Progression" (C. C. Harris and L. A. Liotta, eds.). Wiley-Liss, New York, 1990, p. 97.
58. Wright, S.: *Am. Naturalist* **90**, 5 (1956).
59. Tomatis, L., Narod, S., and Yamasaki, H.: *Carcinogenesis* **13**, 145 (1992).
60. Napalkov, N. P., Rice, J. M., Tomatis, L., and Yamasaki, H., eds.: "Perinatal and Multigeneration Carcinogenesis", IARC Sci. Publ. No. 96. Internat. Agency for Res. on Cancer, Lyon, 1989.
61. Woo, Y.-T., Lai, D. Y., Arcos, J. C., and Argus, M. F.: "Chemical Induction of Cancer – Structural Bases and Biological Mechanisms", Vol. IIIC: Natural, Metal, Fiber, and Macromolecular Carcinogens. Academic Press, San Diego, 1988, Chap. 5.5.3, p. 555.
62. Riley, P. A.: *Free Radical Res. Commun.* **11**, 59 (1990).
63. Jablonka, E., and Lamb, M. J.: *J. Theoret. Biol.* **139**, 69 (1989).
64. Holliday, R., and Pugh, J. E.: *Science* **187**, 226 (1975).
65. Riggs, A. D.: *Cytogenet. Cell Genet.* **14**, 9 (1975).
66. Razin, A., and Riggs, A. D.: *Science* **210**, 604 (1980).
67. Doerfler, W.: *Annu. Rev. Biochem.* **52**, 93 (1983).
68. Roodyn, D. B., and Wilkie, D.: "The Biogenesis of Mitochondria". Methuen, London, 1968, p. 12.
69. Wallace, D. C.: *Science* **256**, 628 (1992).
70. Simic, M. G.: *Environ. Carcino. Rev.* **C9**, 113 (1991).
71. Aust, S. D., Morehouse, L. A., and Thomas, C. E. J.: *Free Radical Biol. Med.* **1**, 3 (1985).

72. Wunderlich, V., Schütt, M., Böttger, M., and Graffi, A.: *Biochem. J.* **118**, 99 (1970).
73. Tzagoloff, A.: "Mitochondria". Plenum Press, New York, 1982.
74. Blondin, G. A., and Green, D. E.: *Proc. Natl. Acad. Sci. U.S.A.* **58**, 612 (1967).
75. Sordahl, L. A., Blailock, Z. R., Liebelt, A. G., Kraft, G. H., and Schwartz, A.: *Cancer Res.* **29**, 2002 (1969).
76. Arcos, J. C.: *J. Theoret. Biol.* **30**, 533 (1971).
77. Komai, H., Hunter, D. R., and Green, D. E.: *Ann. N. Y. Acad. Sci.* **227**, 175 (1974).
78. Capaldi, R. A., Halphen, D. G., Zhang, Y.-Z., and Yanamura, W.: *J. Bioenerg. Biomembr.* **30**, 291 (1988).
79. Senior, A. E.: *Physiol. Rev.* **68**, 177 (1988).
80a. Arcos, J. C., Griffith, G. W., and Cunningham, R. W.: *J. Biophys. Biochem. Cytol.* **7**, 49 (1960).
80b. Yamamoto, G., Utsumi, K., and Nishikaze, K.: *Acta Med. Okayama* **18**, 311 (1964).
81. Arcos, J. C., Mathison, J. B., Tison, M. J., and Mouledoux, A. M.: *Cancer Res.* **29**, 1288 (1969).
82. Bryant, G. M., Argus, M. F., and Arcos, J. C.: *Gann (Jpn. J. Cancer Res.)* **68**, 89 (1977).
83. Arcos, J. C., Tison, M. J., Gosch, H. H., and Fabian, J. A.: *Cancer Res.* **29**, 1298 (1969).
84a. Vithayathil, A. J., Ternberg, J. L., and Commoner, B.: *Nature* **207**, 1246 (1965).
84b. Yamada, T., Matsumoto, M., and Terayama, H.: *Exp. Cell Res.* **29**, 153 (1963).
85. Schmucker, D.: *Pharmacol. Rev.* **30**, 445 (1979).
86. Campbell, T. C., and Hayes, J. R.: *Pharmacol. Rev.* **26**, 171 (1974).
87. Mahaffey, K. R., and Vanderveen, J. E.: *Environ. Health Perspect.* **29**, 81 (1979).
88. Hayes, J. R., and Campbell, T. C.: Nutrition as a Modifier of Chemical Carcinogenesis. *In* "Carcinogenesis", Vol. 5: Modifiers of Chemical Carcinogenesis (T. J. Slaga, ed.). Raven Press, New York, 1980, p. 207.
89. Alvares, A. P., Kappas, A., Anderson, K. E., Pantuck, E. J., and Conney, A. H.: Nutritional Factors Regulating Drug Biotransformation in Man. *In* "Drug Action Modification — Comparative Pharmacology" (G. Olive, ed.), Vol. 8 *Adv. Pharmacol. Therap.* (Proc. 7th Int. Congr. Pharmacol., Paris, 1978). Pergamon, Oxford, 1979, p. 43.
90. Venkatesan, N., Arcos, J. C., and Argus, M. F.: *Cancer Res.* **30**, 2563 (1970).
91. Roe, F. J. C.: *Br. J. Cancer* **10**, 72 (1956).
92. Klein, M.: *Cancer Res.* **16**, 123 (1956).
93. Boutwell, R. K., Bosch, D., and Rusch, H. P.: *Cancer Res.* **17**, 71 (1957).
94. Iversen, O. H.: *Virchows Arch. (Cell Pathol.)* **49**, 129 (1985).
95. Sivak, A., Goyer, M. M., and Ricci, P. F.: Nongenotoxic Carcinogens: Prologue. *In* "Nongenotoxic Mechanisms in Carcinogenesis" (B. E. Butterworth and T. J. Slaga, eds.), Banbury Rept. #25. Cold Spring Harbor Laboratory publ. Cold Spring Harbor, New York, 1987, p. 1.
96. Chouroulinkov, I.: Initiation, Promotion: Working Concept, Biological and Toxicologicol. Interpretations of Carcinogenesis. *In* "Theories of Carcinogenesis" (O. H. Iversen, ed.). Hemisphere, Washington, D.C., 1988, p. 191.
97. Clayson, D. B.: *Mutation Res.* **221**, 53 (1989).
98. Roe, F. J. C.: *Mutagenesis* **4**, 407 (1989).
99. Grasso, P., Sharratt, M., and Cohen, A. J.: *Annu. Rev. Pharmacol. Toxicol.* **31**, 253 (1991).
100. Bahnson, C. B.: *Ann. N.Y. Acad. Sci.* **164**, 319 (1969).
101. Eaton, W. W., and Kessler, L. G.: *Am. J. Epidemiol.* **114**, 528 (1981).
102. de la Pena, A. M.: "The Psychobiology of Cancer — Automatization and Boredom in Health and Disease". Praeger, New York, 1983.
103. Dearfield, J. E., Shea, M., Kensett, M., Horlock, P., Wilson, R. A., and de Landsheere, C. M.: *Lancet* **2**, 1001 (1984).
104. Welgan, P., Meshkinpour, H., and Bealer, M.: *Gastroenterology* **94**, 1150 (1988).
105. Marshall, W. R., and Epstein, C. H.: *Addict. Behav.* **5**, 389 (1980).
106. Pocock, S. J., Shaper, A. C., Cook, D. G., Phillips, A. N., and Walker, M.: *Lancet* **2**, 197 (1987).
107. Schweiger, U., and Pirke, K. M.: "Cyclical Ovarian Function and Eating Behavior in Restrained and Unrestrained Eaters", 72nd Annu. Meet. Endocrine Soc., Atlanta, 1990, Abstract # 1158.
108. Hill, P.: *Nutrition* **7**, 385 (1991).
109. Hirohata, T.: *J. Natl. Cancer Inst.* **47**, 895 (1968).
110. Strickland, R. G., and McKay, I. R.: *Am. J. Dig. Dis.* **18**, 426 (1973).
111. Demopoulos, H. B., Pietronigro, D. D., and Seligman, M. L.: The Development of Secondary Pathology with Free Radical Reactions as a Threshold Mechanism. *In* "Cancer and the Environment — Possible Mechanisms of Threshold for Carcinogens and Other Toxic Substances" (J. A. Cimino, H. B. Demopoulos, M. Kushner, H. Uehleke, B. L. Van Duuren, B. M. Wagner, and V. R. Young, eds.). Mary Ann Liebert, New York, 1983, p. 173.
112. Linn, S.: DNA Damage and Stress Responses Caused by Oxygen Radicals. *In* "Biological Consequences

of Oxidative Stress—Implications for Cardiovascular Disease and Carcinogenesis" (L. Spatz and A. D. Bloom, eds.). Oxford Univ. Press, Oxford 1992, p. 107.

113. Colburn, N. H.: Gene Regulation by Oxygen Radicals and Other Stress Inducers: Role in Tumor Promotion and Progression. *In* "Biological Consequences of Oxidative Stress—Implications for Cardiovascular Disease and Carcinogenesis" (L. Spatz and A. D. Bloom, eds.). Oxford Univ. Press, Oxford 1992, p. 121.

114a. Lee, M. S., Kliever, S. A., Provencal, J., Wright, P. E., and Evans, R. M.: *Science* **260,** 1117 (1993).

114b. Abate, C., Rauscher F. J., III, Gentz, R., and Curran, T.: Fos and Jun Interact Through a Structural Motif Reminiscent of a Coil-Coil Structure. *In* "Genetic Mechanisms in Carcinogenesis and Tumor Progression" (C. C. Harris and L. A. Liotta, eds.). Wiley-Liss, New York, 1990, p. 1.

115. Vedeckis, W. V.: *Proc. Soc. Exp. Biol. Med.* **199,** 1 (1992).

116. Bowden, G. T., and Krieg, P.: *Environ. Health. Perspect.* **93,** 51 (1991).

117. Zile, M. H.: *Proc. Soc. Exp. Biol. Med.* **201,** 141 (1992).

118. Farias, R. N., Bloj, B., Morero, R. D., Sineris, F., and Trucco, R. E.: *Biochim. Biophys. Acta* **475,** 231 (1975).

119. Meir Shimitzky, ed.: "Physiology of Membrane Fluidity". CRC Press, Boca Raton, Florida, 1984.

120. Domke, I., and Weis, W.: *Ann. Nutr. Metab.* **28,** 261 (1984).

121. Gershwin, M. E., Beach, R. S., and Hurley, L. S.: "Nutrition and Immunity". Academic Press, Orlando, Florida, 1985.

122. Murphy, M. G.: *J. Nutr. Biochem.* **1,** 68 (1990).

123. Stier, A.: *Biochem. Pharmacol.* **25,** 109 (1976).

124. Cullis, P. R., and Hope, M. J.: Physical Properties and Functional Roles of Lipid Membranes. *In* "Biochemistry of Lipids in Membranes" (D. E. Vance and J. E. Vance, eds.). Benjamin/Cummings, Menlo Park, California, 1988, p. 25.

125. Eriksson, L. C., and Andersson, G. N.: *Crit. Rev. Biochem. Mol. Biol.* **27,** 1 (1992).

126. Castro, C. E., Armstrong-Major, J., and Ramirez, M. E.: *Federation Proc.* **45,** 2394 (1986).

127. Mullen, C. A., and Schreiber, H.: *Surv. Immunol. Res.* **4,** 264 (1985).

128. Chan, P. L., and Sinclair, N. R., St. C.: *J. Natl. Cancer Inst.* **48,** 162 (1972).

129. Grohman, J., and Nowotny, A.: *J. Immunol.* **104,** 1090 (1972).

130. Field, E. J., and Caspary, E. A., *Br. J. Cancer* **26,** 164 (1972).

131. Masaki, H., Takatsu, K., Hamaoka, T., and Kitagawa, M.: *Gann* **63,** 633 (1972).

132. Yamazaki, H., Nitta, K., and Umezawa, H.: *Gann* **64** 83 (1973).

133. Motoki, H., Kamo, I., Kikuchi, M., Ono, Y. and Ishida, N.: *Gann* **65,** 269 (1974).

134. Hrsak, I., and Mazotti, T.: *J. Natl. Cancer Inst.* **53,** 1113 (1974).

135. Peirce, G. E., and Devald, B. L.: *Cancer Res.* **35,** 2729 (1975).

136. Namba, M., Ogura, T., Hirao, F., and Yamamura, Y.: *Gann* **68,** 751 (1977).

137a. Ishida, N.: *Yakugaku Zasshi* **105,** 91 (1985).

137b. Mizoguchi, H., O'Shea, J. J., Longo, D. L., Loeffler, C. M., McVicar, D. W., and Ochoa, A. C.: *Science* **258,** 1795 (1992).

138. Abrams, G. D.: Impact of the Intestinal Microflora on Intestinal Structure and Function. *In:* "Human Intestinal Microflora in Health and Disease" (D. J. Hentges, ed.). Academic Press, New York, 1983, p. 292.

139. Berg, R. D.: Host Immune Response to Antigens of the Indigenous Intestinal Flora. *In* "Human Intestinal Microflora in Health and Disease" (D. J. Hentges, ed.). Academic Press, New York, 1983, p. 101.

140. Wilkins, T. D., and Van Fassell, R. L.: Production of Intestinal Mutagens. *In* "Human Intestinal Microflora in Health and Disease" (D. J. Hentges, ed.). Academic Press, New York, 1983, p. 265.

141. Galland, J.: The Effect of Intestinal Microbes on Systemic Immunity. *In* "Post-Viral Fatigue Syndrome (R. Jenkins and J. Mowbray, eds.). Wiley, New York, 1991, Chap. 28, p. 405.

142. Hollander, D., and Tarnawski, H.: *Gerontology* **31,** 133 (1985).

143. van der Waaij, D.: The Immunoregulation of the Intestinal Flora; Consequences of Decreased Thymus Activity and Broad-Spectrum Antibiotic Treatment. *In* "Chemotherapy and Immunity (G. Pulverer and J. Jeljaszewicz, eds.). Gustav Fischer Verlag, Stuttgart, 1985, p. 73.

144. Tannock, G. W.: Effect of Dietary and Environmental Stress on the Gastrointestinal Microflora. *In* "Human Intestinal Microflora in Health and Disease" (D. J. Hentges, ed.). Academic Press, New York, 1983, p. 517.

145. Gorbach, S. L., Nahas, L., Lerner, P. I., and Weinstein, L.: *Gastroenterology* **53,** 845 (1967).

146. Blalock, J. E., and Smith, E. M.: *Federation Proc.* **44,** 108 (1985).

147. Blalock, J. E., ed.: "Neuroimmunoendocrinology". Karger, Basel, 1988.

148. Sanders, V. M., Fuchs, B. A., Pruett, S. B., Kerkvliet, N. I., and Kaminski, N. E.: *Fundam. Appl. Toxicol.* **17,** 641 (1991).

149. Lynn, W. S., Wallwork, J. C., and Mathews, D.: *Clin. Biotechnol.* **3,** 39 (1991).

150. Rideout, W. M. III, Coetzer, G. A., Olumi, A. F., Spruck, C. H., and Jones, P. A.: 5-Methylcytosine as an Endogenous Mutagen in the p53 Tumor Suppressor Gene. *In* "Multistage Carcinogenesis" (C. C. Harris, S. Hirohashi, N. Ito, H. D. Pitot, T. Sugimura, M. Terada, and J. Yokota, eds.). CRC Press, Boca Raton, Florida, 1993.

151. Reid, T. M., Fry, M., and Loeb, L. A.: Endogenous Mutations and Cancer. *In* "Multistage Carcinogenesis" (C. C. Harris, S. Hirohashi, N. Ito, H. C. Pitot, T. Sugimura, M. Terada, and J. Yokota, eds.). CRC Press, Boca Raton, Florida, 1993.

152. Schmucker, D. L., Vessey, D. A., Wang, R. K., James, J. L., and Maloney, A.: *Mech. Aging Dev.* **27**, 207 (1984).

153. Cutler, R. G.: Longevity Is Determined by Specific Genes: Testing the Hypothesis. *In* "Testing the Theories of Aging" (R. C. Adelman and G. S. Roth, eds.). CRC Press, Boca Raton, Florida, 1982, p. 25.

154. Benzi, G., Curti, D., Pastoris, O., Marzatico, F., Villa, R. F., and Dagani, F.: *Neurochem. Res.* **16**, 1295 (1991).

155. Ursini, F., Maiorino, M., and Sevanian, A.: Membrane Hydroperoxides. *In* "Oxidative Stress – Oxidants and Antioxidants" (H. Siess, ed.). Academic Press, San Diego, 1991, p. 319.

156. McCord, J. M., and Fridovich, I.: *J. Biol. Chem.* **244**, 6049 (1969).

157. Sahu, S. C.: *Environ. Carcino. Rev.* **C9**, 83 (1991).

158. Hadley, E. C.: Genetic Alteration and the Pathology of Aging. *In* "Testing the Theories of Aging" (R. C. Adelman and G. S. Roth, eds.). CRC Press, Boca Raton, Florida, 1982, p. 115.

159. Derventzi, A., and Rattan, S. I. S.: *Mutat. Res.* **256**, 191 (1991).

160. Rao, K. M. K., and Cohen, H. J.: *Mutat. Res.* **256**, 139 (1991).

161. Am. Soc. Exp. Pathol. Symp.: "Immunopathology of Aging". *Federation Proc.* **33**, 2017 (1974).

162. Burnett, M. F.: "Immunology, Aging, and Cancer". Freeman, San Francisco, 1976.

163. Salomon, J.-C.: "Le Tissu Déchiré – Propos sur la Diversité des Cancers". Seuil, Paris, 1991, Chap. 19, p. 112.

164. Schrödinger, E.: "What Is Life? The Physical Aspect of the Living Cell". Cambridge Univ. Press, London, 1944.

165. Lima-de-Faria, A.: "Evolution Without Selection – Form and Function by Autoevolution". Elsevier, Amsterdam, 1988, p. 121.

166. Gould, S. J., and Eldredge, N.: *Paleobiology* **3**, 115 (1977).

167. Gould, S. J., and Eldredge, N.: *Syst. Zool.* **35**, 143 (1986).

168. Argus, M. F., Leutze, C. J., and Kane, J. F.: *Experientia* **17**, 357 (1961).

169. Argus, M. F., Arcos, J. C., Alam, A., and Mathison, J. H.: *J. Medicinal Chem.* **7**, 460 (1964).

170. Argus, M. F., Arcos, J. C., Mathison, J. H., Alam, A., and Bemis, J. A.: *Arzneimittel. Forsch (Drug Res.)* **16**, 740 (1966).

171. Bemis, J. A., Argus, M. F., and Arcos, J. C.: *Biochim. Biophys. Acta* **126**, 274 (1966).

Note added in Proof: 1. *Genetic Control of Metastatic Potential.* Besides the genes coding for metalloproteinase inhibitory proteins known to block metastasis [rev. L. A. Liotta: *Sci. Am.* **266**, 54 (1992)], the *nm23* gene coding for another metastasis-suppressor protein was subsequently identified in murine experimental systems [rev. P. S. Steeg *et al.*: *Cancer Cells* **3**, 257 (1991)]. Low *nm23* RNA levels correlate with histopathological criteria indicative of high metastatic potential in infiltrating human breast carcinomas [G. Bevilacqua *et al.*: *Cancer Res.* **49**, 5185 (1989)], and the level of *nm23* expression was proposed as prognostic marker for breast carcinoma patients [R. Barnes *et al.*: *Am. J. Pathol.* **139**, 245 (1991)]. It has been speculated [*cit.* J. Marx: *Science* **259**, 626 (1993)] that decreased *nm23* levels are associated with increased tumor cell motility. A malignant melanoma metastasis-regulatory/suppressor gene detected in human chromosome 6 may be identical with *nm23* or may represent another gene regulating it [D. R. Welch, pers. commun., May 1994; Welch *et al.*: *Oncogene* **9**, 255 (1994)].

2. *Significance of Nuclear Matrix Proteins (NMP).* The nuclear matrix is a network serving as molecular scaffolding, associated with DNA at different regions, and composed of nonchromatin proteins and RNAproteins. NMP are involved in the regulation of nuclear metabolism and are associated with actively transcribed genes [N. Ogden: *Biochem. J.* **267**, (1990); J. P. Bidwell *et al.*: *Proc. Nat. Acad. Sci. U.S.A. (PNAS)* **90**, 3162 (1993)]. NMP provide transport for, and represent sites of metabolism of, heterogenous nuclear RNA [S. Zeitlin *et al.*: *Mol. Cell Biol.* **7**, 111 (1987); *J. Cell Biol.* **108**, 765 (1989)]. Tissue specific NMP were identified in the rat, mouse, and human [E. G. Fey & S. Penman: *PNAS* **85**, 121 (1988); J. Stuurman *et al.*: *J. Biol. Chem.* **265**, 5460 (1990); R. H. Getzenberg & D. S. Coffey: *Mol. Endocrinol.* **4**, 1336 (1990)]. Specific NMP play a role in cell differentiation and transformation [J. P. Bidwell *et al.*, 1993, *loc. cit.*; C. Brancolini & C. Schneider: *PNAS* **88**, 6936 (1991); I. Greenfield *et al.*: *ibid.* p. 11217]. Tumor-specific NMP were detected in cancers of the human and rat prostate [A. W. Partin *et al.*: *Cancer Res.* **53**, 744 (1993); R. H. Getzenberg *et al.*: *ibid.* **51**, 6514 (1991)], human breast [P. S. Khanuja *et al.*: *Cancer Res.* **53**, 3394 (1993)] and human colon [S. K. Keesee *et al.*: *PNAS* **91**, 1913 (1994)]. Thus, NMP may also prove useful as a prognostic tool.

Cross-Reactions Between Carcinogens. Modification of Chemical Carcinogenesis by Noncarcinogenic Agents

CHAPTER **2**

Synergism and Antagonism Between Chemical Carcinogens[1]

Martin R. Berger

I. INTRODUCTION

Modern analytical methods have shown that the human environment is a source of ubiquitous exposure to low levels of naturally occurring and synthetic chemical carcinogens, which act either sequentially or simultaneously. This complex scenario has not adequately been modeled by routine testing for carcinogenicity in which relatively high doses of single agents have been used predominantly to establish the relative risk that chemical compounds may represent. This approach has been questioned for two reasons:

A. The multitude of chemical risk factors in carcinogenesis and their almost infinite number of possible interactive combinations have long been the major obstacle in handling this problem adequately and have led researchers rather to investigate monocausal relationships. However, the increment of cancer risk due to exposure to combinations of mixtures of even low levels of individual carcinogens may be much higher than expected. Consequently, the identification of consistent patterns of interactions between specific types of chemicals is of utmost importance for realistic hazard assessment, for regulation of chemicals, and for public health policy (1).

B. Recently it has been hypothesized that the "maximum tolerated dose" (or comparably high dose) generally used in bioassays may stimulate cell proliferation which, by itself, can lead to the development of cancer from previously initiated, but dormant cells; thus, this approach may result in the overestimation of potential cancer hazard (2).

This chapter is guided by certain definitions so as to avoid overlap with other chapters. The first is that only those chemicals have been considered which *alone* can induce tumors in experimental animals, *i.e.*, are "complete" carcinogens. Secondly, the joint action of two or more complete (solitary) carcinogens is termed syncarcinogenesis (*see* ref. 3 and "Appendix to Part 1"). Syncarcinogenesis can occur with similar or different organotropism and can involve genotoxic or epigenetic carcinogens. Syncarcinogenesis can occur either when two or more carcinogens are administered concurrently (simultaneously or in mixture) or when they are administered sequentially (one following the other); the time sequence of exposure is of no importance for syncarcinogenesis, as distinct from initiation–promotion in two-stage carcinogenesis. The effects of the

---

[1]Abbreviations used *see* p. 47.

individual components can be additive, overadditive, or subadditive. The latter two terms are synonyms for "synergistic" and "antagonistic", respectively.

The aim of this chapter is to provide an analysis of the general trend of interaction effects of complete chemical carcinogens which, if administered in combination, result in synergistic or antagonistic carcinogenic effects. A problem arises, however, from the different ways that the definitions of the terms "synergistic" and "antagonistic" have been used. Synergism resulted from combined exposure in a larger number of cases than could be anticipated from the separate effects of the component chemicals (4, 5). Conversely, this would mean that a lower number of cases of antagonism has been observed than would have been anticipated.

In the context of a recent comprehensive survey on binary combination effects of chemical carcinogens, the definitions of "synergism" and "antagonism" have been used in a broad sense (1). "Synergism" denotes the observation that a combination of carcinogens exerts an effect exceeding the arithmetic sum of the effects of the chemicals individually. However, the increased effect may be due to true synergistic action, but it may also result from the potentiation/promotion of the carcinogenic effect of one chemical by another chemical which by itself was not carcinogenic *under the specific conditions of the experiment*. As is to be expected, a clear distinction between "synergism" and "additivity" is not always possible because of the experimental design or inadequate statistical information in the original studies. "Antagonism" denotes the observation that the combination of carcinogens exerts an effect less than additive or even lower than the effect of one of the carcinogens singly.

II. SOURCES AND SELECTION OF DATA FOR ANALYSIS

Since data on combination effects of chemical carcinogens in laboratory animals are widely scattered in the literature, extensive use was made of a comprehensive survey, "Database on Binary Combination Effects of Chemical Carcinogens", which appeared in *Environmental Carcinogenesis Reviews* in 1988. The "Database" covers results available on combination experiments with two carcinogens reported until the end of 1987 (*see* ref. 1). The "Database" organizes the data—98% in rodent species—into ten structural classes according to "primary carcinogen" in binary combination. The term "primary carcinogen" does not imply any primacy in the combined mechanism of action, but is a semantic device for the classification of the data. The term "primary carcinogen" simply denotes the name of one of the two carcinogens which precedes the other in any *listed entry* of binary combination. Accordingly, in the "Database" (1) any given binary combination is listed under two classes, representing the class affiliations of the two chemicals in the combination. The ten structural classes of "primary carcinogens" are

    I. Polycyclic aromatic hydrocarbons
    II. Aromatic amines
   III. Azo dyes
   IV. Nitrosamines and nitrosamides
    V. Hydrazo and azoxy compounds
   VI. Carbamates
  VII. Halogenated compounds
VIII. Naturally occurring compounds
   IX. Inorganic carcinogens (metals, metalloids, and fibers)
    X. Miscellaneous compounds (including alkylating agents, aldehydes, peroxy compounds, phenolics, etc.)

For clarity of this overview, the selection of the data for analysis was carried out according to the following criteria:

a. All agents which are given in ref. (1) *in parentheses*, indicating suspected/but not proven carcinogenicity, were omitted from the overview.
b. Only the "primary carcinogens" that are "most common" in the tabulations of ref. (1) were included, *i.e.*, "primary carcinogens" with less than seven different combination effects are not discussed in this overview.
c. Only combination effects resulting in synergism or antagonism were included; they are organized and displayed in tables for each of the ten classes of carcinogens.
d. Only results of *in vivo* experiments were considered.

In addition to the data obtained from the survey of Arcos et al. (1), selected according to the above criteria, a literature search was performed to cover the time period from 1987 to 1992. Combination experiments reported during this time period, demonstrating synergism or antagonism for one of the agents listed as "primary carcinogen" in ref. (1) and selected for review in this chapter, were included in the tables together with their original literature references. Furthermore, several mechanistically informative combination experiments with three or more chemical carcinogens were included (Tables 16–18). The discussion of the tabulated data does not extend to all details of the experiments reviewed, but aims to give an analysis of the relationships between formal aspects and — as far as possible — to clarify discrepancies, *e.g.*, a secondary carcinogen being both synergistic and antagonistic with a given primary carcinogen, depending on the experimental conditions used.

III. OVERVIEW OF CARCINOGENIC EFFECTS OF SELECTED BINARY COMBINATIONS

Synergistic and antagonistic binary combination effects of polycyclic aromatic hydrocarbons (PAH) with other chemical carcinogens are exemplified in Tables 1 and 2. The most common organ showing synergistic or antagonistic interactions was the skin (owing to the most often used route of topical administration of PAH), followed by the mammary gland, the liver, and the respiratory tract. When the two modes of interaction are compared more antagonistic than synergistic combination effects are found, the ratio being 1.6 in favor of the former. The secondary carcinogens resulting in synergism were fairly scattered among all groups of carcinogens, whereas those resulting in antagonism clustered in Groups I and III, *i.e.*, PAH and azo dyes. This can be exemplified by the observation that only 3 (9%) of 34 secondary carcinogens causing synergism belong to the class of PAH (Table 1), but 16 (30%) of 54 chemicals causing antagonism (Table 2). This clustering supports the hypothesis that structurally similar compounds with varying carcinogenic potency may interact antagonistically in binary combinations because of competition for binding sites. One example of dose–dependently diverging results is the combination of 7,12-dimethylbenz[*a*]anthracene (DMBA) and *N*-methyl-*N*-nitrosourea (MNU), both of which induce tumors in the mammary gland when administered systemically (6). Low doses of MNU were found to cause synergism in the induction of mammary carcinomas (Table 1), whereas high doses of MNU were antagonistic (Table 2). The reason for this apparent discrepancy may be the cytotoxic action of MNU at high doses, which causes cell death, and thus overrides the consequences of its mutagenicity. A similar explanation obviously does not pertain to the synergism observed in the interaction of 3-methylcholanthrene (3-MC) with the three cytostatic agents cyclophosphamide, actinomycin D, and mitomycin C used at maximum tolerated doses (Table 1).

TABLE 1. **Synergistic Interactions of Selected Polycyclic Aromatic Hydrocarbons with a Second Carcinogen**

Primary carcinogen	Skin/local	Respiratory tract	Liver/ bile duct	Gastrointestinal tract	Urinary tract	Mammary gland
		Target organ with secondary carcinogen				
BaP	BeP[a] Cyclopenteno- [cd]pyrene CCl$_4$ Ni$_3$S$_2$	DEN[b] As$_2$O$_3$ Asbestos[c]	2-AAF[e]			
DMBA	7-Br-Me-BA 2-AAF DEHP Allylisothiocyanate As$_2$O$_3$ Urethan (52)	Asbestos[c] (61)				MNU[d] Reserpine DES
3-MC	DAS 4-NQO DMN Methylhydrazine Cyclophosphamide Actinomycin D Mitomycin C Chloramphenicol DDT TCDD	4-NQO[e] DMN[f]	DAB[e] 2-AAF[e]	2,7-FAA DMN	DMN	

Note: Unless individually referenced in parentheses, binary combination effects tabulated are taken from the database of Arcos *et al.* (1).

[a]BaP + TPA.
[b]BaP + Fe$_2$O$_3$.
[c]Chrysotile.
[d]Low doses.
[e]Based on two experiments.
[f]Based on three experiments.

Another formal discrepancy is displayed by 2,3,7,8-tetrachlorodibenzo-*p*-dioxin (TCDD), which can be both synergistic and antagonistic in carcinogenesis induced by 3-MC (compare Tables 1 and 2). This equivocal effect has its basis in the administration schedule of TCDD which, *when given together* with a high dose of 3-MC, causes more than additive tumor incidence in a 3-MC-resistant mouse strain (7), but suppresses tumorigenesis when given *prior to* a low dose of 3-MC (which is then followed by phorbol ester promotion) (8).

Synergistic and antagonistic binary combination effects of aromatic amines with other chemical carcinogens are presented in Tables 3 and 4. Due to the organ specificity of aromatic amines, the most common site of interactions is the liver, followed by the urinary tract, the mammary gland, and the gastrointestinal tract. The overall numbers of synergistic or antagonistic effects in these show no general predominance of either mode of interaction. Among the secondary carcinogens interacting synergistically with aromatic amines, a clustering of group IV agents, *i.e.*, of *N*-nitrosamines/*N*-nitrosamides, was discernible (6 of 27, *i.e.*, 22%; *see* Table 3). There appears to be no predominance of any chemical class among the secondary carcinogens in causing antagonism when in combination with aromatic amines (Table 4). The fact that the combination of 4-hydroxybutylbutylnitrosamine (4-HBBN) and 2-acetylaminofluorene (2-AAF) can show both synergism and antagonism in urinary bladder carcinogenesis is related to the periods

TABLE 2. Antagonistic Interactions of Selected Polycyclic Aromatic Hydrocarbons with a Second Carcinogen

Primary carcinogen	Target organ with second carcinogen						
	Skin/local	Liver	Mammary gland	Respiratory tract	Hematopoietic system	Zymbal's gland	Gastrointestinal tract
BaP	DB[a,c]A 3-OH-BaP[a,h] 4-NQO[b] Griseofulvin[c] TCDD[a,h]	3'-Me-DAB		Toxaphene			
DMBA	BaP BeP 3-MC[h] 6,8-DMBA DB[a,c]A DB[a,h]A DB[a,g]F Acridine orange Sulfur mustard[d] Chloroquine mustard Glycidaldehyde d,l-Diepoxybutane Actinomycin D[i] AFB$_1$ PCB TCDD[e]		BA 3-MC 6,8-DMBA 3,9-DMBA MDA Actinomycin D[h] Chloramphenicol Clofibrate Propylthiouracil DDT MNU[g]		DDT		
3-MC	DMBA[h] DB[a,g]F[h] Reserpine TCDD[f] As$_2$O$_3$	3'-Me-DAB[i] 4'-F-DAB 2',4'-di-F-DAB 2-AAF[h] 7-F-2-AAF Quinoline α-BHC	DMBA 2-AAF 7-F-2-AAF			2-AAF[h] 7-F-2-AAF	2-AAF 7-F-2-AAF

Note: Binary combination effects tabulated are taken from the database of Arcos et al. (1).
[a]BaP plus TPA, BaPdiol-epoxide plus TPA.
[b]BaP plus CO, 4-NQO plus CO.
[c]BaP plus CO.
[d]DMBA plus PMA.
[e]DMBA plus TPA.
[f]3-MC plus TPA.
[g]High doses.
[h]Based on two experiments.
[i]Based on four experiments.

27

TABLE 3. Synergistic Interactions of Selected Aromatic Amines with a Second Carcinogen

Primary carcinogen	Target organ with secondary carcinogen				
	Liver	Urinary tract	Thyroid	Gastrointestinal tract	Pancreas
2-AAF	BaP[a,e]	FANFT	Thiouracil		
	3'-Me-DAB[a,f]	4-HBBN[b,g]	Allylthiourea		
	trans-AAS	Lead subacetate			
	DES				
	DEN[g]				
	DBN				
	Di-*n*-amylnitrosamine				
	NNM				
	MNU[a]				
	1,2-DMH[a]				
	Methapyrilene				
	CCl$_4$[e]				
	DDT[e]				
	Azaserine				
	Tannic acid				
	Lead subacetate				
	EE (59)				
MDA	No data available				
FANFT		Cyclophosphamide		1,2-DMH	
QUINS				Snuff[d] (56)	Ethionine[c]
				Betel nut[d] (57)	Azaserine[c]

Note: Unless individually referenced in parentheses, binary combination effects tabulated are taken from the database of Arcos *et al.* (1).
[a]2-AAF plus CCl$_4$.
[b]4-HBBN plus 3,3'-DCB.
[c]4-Hydroxylaminoquinoline-*N*-oxide.
[d]4-Nitroquinoline-*N*-oxide.
[e]Based on two experiments.
[f]Based on three experiments.
[g]Based on four experiments.

of carcinogen administration. Only when both chemicals are given together does synergism become manifest (Table 3), whereas when 2-AAF is given *before or after* 4-HBBN administration there is a decrease in urinary bladder carcinoma incidence as compared to 4-HBBN alone (9). Another apparent discrepancy is the observation that the combination of 2-AAF with carbon tetrachloride (CCl$_4$) can result in both synergistically increased or antagonistically decreased hepatoma incidence. This differential in neoplastic expression has probably its basis in the regimens used, since a single peroral administration of a hepatonecrotic dose of CCl$_4$ was shown to result in increased incidence of liver cancer induced by 0.02% dietary 2-AAF (10), whereas prolonged subcutaneous application of lower CCl$_4$ doses to rats, as a pretreatment to a higher dose of 2-AAF (0.06% in the diet), was found to cause a lower incidence of liver cancer than 2-AAF alone (11).

Table 5 shows the synergistic and antagonistic combination effects of azo dyes with other chemical carcinogens. Consistent with the target organ specificity of azo dyes, virtually all combination effects observed were in the liver. The numbers of synergistic or antagonistic effects in Table 5 are comparably high, and thus show no general predominance of either mode of interaction. The secondary carcinogens leading to synergism, when combined with azo dyes, show no predominant distribution for any chemical class

TABLE 4.   Antagonistic Interactions of Selected Aromatic Amines with a Second Carcinogen

Primary carcinogen	Target organ with secondary carcinogen				
	Liver	Mammary gland	Urinary tract	Gastrointestinal tract	Zymbal's gland
2-AAF	3-MC	3-MC	4-HBBN	3-MC	3-MC
	4-AABP	DB[a,g]F	CCl_4		
	8-HQ[b]	PBB			
	Chloramphenicol				
	Nafenopin				
	CCl_4				
	α-BHC				
	PCB[b] (62)				
	Thiouracil[b]				
	DMN (63)				
MDA	EHEN	DMBA	EHEN		
	Quinoline		4-HBBN		
FANFT	No data available				
QUINS	3-MC[a]				
	MDA[a]				

Note: Unless individually referenced in parentheses, binary combination effects tabulated are taken from the database of Arcos *et al.* (1).

[a]Quinoline.

[b]Based on two experiments.

of agents. A minor clustering of PAH was, however, noticeable, leading to antagonistic combination effects. Regarding 4-dimethylaminoazobenzene (DAB) carcinogenesis antagonized by coadministration of 3-MC, this antagonism is due to the induction of azo dye *N*-demethylase and azo dye reductase by 3-MC (12), thereby increasing the rate of metabolic degradation of the dye to inactive metabolites. The same holds for the effect of 3-MC on 3'-methyl-4-dimethylaminoazobezene (3'-Me-DAB)-induced carcinogenesis (13).

Worthy of special mention are the two apparent discrepancies pertaining to ethionine and polychlorinated biphenyls (PCB), which can cause both synergistic and antagonistic interactions with azo dyes. For the combination of 3'-Me-DAB with PCB, *the sequence* of administration is of importance. Administration of PCB *following* 3'-Me-DAB results in synergistically increased liver cancer incidence, whereas administration of PCB *before or together with* 3'-Me-DAB produces an antagonistic effect (14). The antagonistic effect of PCB is so strong that even the synergistic effect of 3'-Me-DAB and diethylnitrosamine (DEN), displayed in Table 5, is antagonistically depressed when PCB are coadministered (15). Regarding the effect of the protein synthesis inhibitor, ethionine, on DAB carcinogenesis, a lower dose of ethionine (0.05% in diet) is associated with a synergistic combination effect (16), whereas the higher dose (0.1% in diet) is associated with an antagonistic effect.

Tables 6 and 7 present the synergistic and antagonistic combination effects of *N*-nitroso compounds with other chemical carcinogens. The multiple target organ specificity of this group is reflected by the elevated number of target sites in which combination effect is displayed, the most common being the liver, the urinary tract, and the respiratory tract. The overall number of synergistic interactions was considerably higher than that of antagonistic combination effects; the ratio is 3.6 in favor of the former. This predominance of synergism is also reflected by the frequency of combination effects of *N*-nitroso compounds with the other classes of carcinogens. Combinations with

TABLE 5. Synergistic and Antagonistic Interactions of Selected Azo Dyes with a Second Carcinogen

Primary carcinogen	Synergism		Antagonism	
	Target organ with secondary carcinogen			
	Liver	Zymbal's gland	Liver	Gonads
DAB	3'-Me-DAB		3-MC	Ethionine
	4'-Me-DAB[c]		3-Amino-1,2,4-triazole	
	DMN[c]		AF-2[c]	
	DEN		5-Nitro-2-furaldehyde semicarbazone	
	Ethionine		Trypan blue	
	CCl$_4$[c]		Ethionine[c]	
	Reserpine[d]		Thiouracil	
			Chloramphenicol[c]	
3'-Me-DAB	2-AAF[a,e]	3-ABT	3-MC[f]	
	4-Nitrostilbene		BaP	
	DAB		AF-2	
	2-Me-DAB		DES	
	DEN		Nitrogen mustard	
	Urethan		DEN + PCB	
	CCl$_4$[c]		γ-BHC	
	PCB		PCB	
	DDT		DDT	
			Chloramphenicol[c]	
			Yellow rice toxins[b]	
			NiCl$_2$	
			Ni(AcO)$_2$	

Note: Binary combination effects tabulated are taken from the database of Arcos *et al.* (1).
[a]2-AAF plus CCl$_4$ in one experiment.
[b]Yellow rice toxins include luteoskyrin, cyclochlorotine, islanditoxin, and rugulosin.
[c]Based on two experiments.
[d]Based on three experiments.
[e]Based on four experiments.
[f]Based on six experiments.

secondary carcinogens belonging to Groups VII (halogenated compounds) and VIII (naturally occurring compounds), for instance, generally resulted in synergistic, but only seldom in antagonistic combination effects. Generalizing from these observations — certainly limited by the relatively small number of experiments available in the literature — this would imply that *N*-nitroso compounds are a class of carcinogens which probably represent a greater hazard than others, because the majority of binary combinations tend to result in synergistic effects. Again, an apparent discrepancy should be mentioned. The effect of PCB, which were synergistic (Table 6) as well as antagonistic (Table 7) in DEN-induced liver carcinogenesis, paralleled the effect of PCB in azo dye-induced carcinogenesis. The modulation of carcinogenesis by PCB depended on the timing of exposure to the PCB, relative to the exposure to the other carcinogen, in a binary combination. Thus, a reduction in the number of DEN-induced hepatomas was seen in rats *preexposed* to or fed *together with* PCB (15, 17). In contrast, when PCB were fed *after* exposure of rats to DEN, enhancement of hepatocarcinogenesis was observed (18–20). Species specificity, however, complicates this scenario even further, since simultaneous exposure of trout to DEN and PCB resulted in a synergistic combination effect (21). The enzyme-inducing effect of PCB acting upon activating and/or detoxifying enzymes is possibly the basis for these differential effects.

Synergistic and antagonistic combination effects of selected hydrazo and azoxy

TABLE 6. Synergistic Interactions of Selected *N*-Nitroso Compounds with a Second Carcinogen

Primary carcinogen	Target organ with secondary carcinogen						
	Respiratory tract	Gastrointestinal tract	Liver	Urinary tract	Skin/local	Mammary gland	Hematopoietic system
Nitrosamines							
DMN	3-MC[c] PCB Benzene CdCl$_2$		AFB$_1$ CCl$_4$[c] Benzene CdCl$_2$[b] (54) 2-AAF (63)	Actinomycin D CCl$_4$[b] CdCl$_2$ (54)	3-MC	Estradiol valerate	
DEN	BaP+Fe$_2$O$_3$ Aniline DMN Formaldehyde AFB$_1$ CPFA	AFB$_1$	Aniline 2-AAF[d] CCl$_4$[c] DDT PCB[d] TCDD AFB$_1$ Wy-14,463 DEHP[b] Dipyrone	NaAsO$_2$			
EHEN			EE (59)	NTA CrCl$_3$ CdCl$_2$ NiCl$_2$ Basic lead acetate Unleaded gasoline (55) EE (59)			
4-HBBN				2-AAF o-Phenylphenol, Na Adriamycin Mitomycin C EE (59)			
Nitrosamides							
MNNG							
MNU				MMS	TCDD		
BNU			CCl$_4$ DES[b]			DMBA[a]	Haloperidol (51) CCl$_4$ Azathioprine

Note: Unless individually referenced in parentheses, binary combination effects tabulated are taken from the database of Arcos *et al.* (1).
[a]Low doses of MNU only.
[b]Based on three experiments.
[c]Based on two experiments.
[d]Based on four experiments.

TABLE 7. **Antagonistic Interactions of Selected *N*-Nitroso Compounds with a Second Carcinogen**

Primary carcinogen	Target organ with secondary carcinogen				
	Respiratory tract	Liver	Urinary tract	Mammary gland	Gastro-intestinal tract
Nitrosamines					
DMN	Estradiol valerate				
DEN	$CHCl_3$(49)	$CHCl_3$ (49) PCB[c] Reserpine $CdCl_2$[b] (54)			
EHEN		MDA	MDA		

4-HBBN			MDA
			DEN
			N-Nitroso-
			  piperidine
			N-Nitroso-
			  morpholine
			NTA (60)		

Nitrosamides					
MNNG					NTA (60)
MNU				DMBA[a]	
BNU	No data available				

Note: Unless individually referenced in parentheses, binary combination effects tabulated are taken from the database of Arcos *et al.* (1).
[a]High doses of MNU only.
[b]$CdCl_2$ pretreatment only.
[c]Based on two experiments.

TABLE 8. **Synergistic and Antagonistic Interactions of Selected Hydrazo and Azoxy Compounds with a Second Carcinogen**

Primary carcinogen	Synergism					Antagonism	
	Target organ with secondary carcinogen						
	Respiratory tract	Gastro-intestinal tract	Hemato-poietic system	Liver	Skin/local	Neurogenic tissue	Gastro-intestinal tract
1,2-DMH	3-MC	3-MC FANFT	3-MC	2-AAF	3-MC[a]		$CHCl_3$ (50)
MAMA		MMS CCl_4 1-HA (53)		MMS 1-HA (53)		ENU	

Note: Unless individually referenced in parentheses, binary combination effects tabulated are taken from the database of Arcos et al. (1).
[a]Methylhydrazine was the primary carcinogen.

compounds with other chemical carcinogens are given in Table 8. Consistent with the target organ specificity of this group of agents, the most common combination effects centered in the gastrointestinal tract and to a lesser extent in the liver. The majority of the 13 nonadditive interactions reported with this group of compounds are synergistic combination effects, as indicated by a ratio of 5.5 for synergisms over antagonisms.

TABLE 9. **Synergistic and Antagonistic Interactions of the Carbamate, Urethan, with a Second Carcinogen**

	Synergism			Antagonism	
	Target organ with secondary carcinogen				
Primary carcinogen	Hematopoietic/ lymphatic system	Skin/local	Respiratory tract	Skin/local	Mammary gland
Urethan	3-MC	Colchicine	3-MC	*n*-Butylcarbamate + CO	*n*-Butyl- carbamate
	DES	Cantharidin	CCl$_4$		
	Estradiol	Teflon	Chlordane		
	Zearalenone	DMBA (52)	Chlor- amphenicol		

Note: Unless individually referenced in parentheses, binary combination effects tabulated are taken from the database of Arcos *et al.* (1).

Again, as with *N*-nitroso compounds, this observation – if valid – may anticipate an elevated cancer hazard for this group of agents. However, the database is admittedly very small and therefore cannot be regarded as being representative.

Synergistic and antagonistic combination effects of selected carbamates with other chemical carcinogens are given in Table 9. The most common target organs of the combination effects were the skin, the hematopoietic/lymphatic system, and the respiratory tract. Since 8 of the 14 combination responses with other chemical carcinogens were synergistic, the ratio is 1.3 for the synergistic *over* antagonistic responses. The overall database is, however, very small and thus precludes definitive assumptions. *n*-Butylcarbamate, when coadministered with urethan (ethylcarbamate), was reported to antagonize skin tumorigenesis by urethan (22) and the two agents together induced a lower mammary tumor incidence than the sum of tumors by both individual agents alone (23). These observations, although contested (24), would parallel the observations on PAH, the carcinogenicity of which is antagonized by close structural homologs in binary combinations.

An important group of agents, in terms of potential human contact and exposure, are the halogenated compounds CCl$_4$, PCB, DDT, and TCDD. Tables 10 and 11 show the synergistic and antagonistic combination effects of these with some chemical carcinogens. According to the data available in these tables, 26 secondary carcinogens interacted synergistically and 14 interacted antagonistically, all target organs considered. The most common target organ was the liver, followed by the skin. Other target organs appeared to be of minor importance within the framework of the number of experiments reported. A predominance of synergistic interactions was discernible from the ratio of synergistic *over* antagonistic interactions, which was 1.7 for all sites and 3.8 specifically for liver. A significant proportion (37%) of secondary carcinogens interacting synergistically with halogenated compounds are *N*-nitroso compounds, thus indicating an elevated cancer risk for this type of combinations. Apart from this cluster, the distribution of secondary carcinogens, among all other chemical classes represented, was fairly scattered. Apparent discrepancies which need comment are 2-AAF (in combination with CCl$_4$), 3'-Me-DAB and DEN (both in combination with PCB) which combinations are synergistic (Table 10) as well as antagonistic (Table 11) in the liver, and 3-MC (in combination with TCDD) which displayed both interaction responses in the skin. In each of these experiments the sequence of administration was of importance. If the halogenated compound was given *prior to* the second carcinogen a decreased tumorigenesis resulted, whereas application

TABLE 10. Synergistic Interactions of Selected Halogenated Compounds with a Second Carcinogen

Primary carcinogen	Target organ with secondary carcinogen				
	Liver	Skin/ local	Urinary tract	Gastrointestinal tract	Respiratory tract
CCl$_4$	2-AAF[d]	BaP	DMN[d]	MAMA	
	2,7-FAA				
	DAB[d]				
	3'-Me-DAB[d]				
	DMN[a,f]				
	DEN[e]				
	MEN				
	BNU				
	AFB$_1$[d]				
	Petasitenine				
PCB[b]	3'-Me-DAB				DMN
	DEN[f]				
	α-BHC				
	β-BHC				
DDT	2-AAF[d]	3-MC			
	3'-Me-DAB				
	trans-AAS				
	DEN				
TCDD	DEN	MNNG			
		3-MC[c]			

Note: Binary combination effects tabulated are taken from the database of Arcos *et al.* (1).
[a]DMN precursors in one experiment.
[b]Arochlor 1254 or Kanechlor 300, 400, or 500.
[c]Strain differences observed.
[d]Based on two experiments.
[e]Based on three experiments.
[f]Based on four experiments.

simultaneously with or following the second carcinogen enhanced tumorigenesis (7, 8, 10, 11, 14, 15).

In Table 12 are summarized the available synergistic and antagonistic effects data on selected naturally occurring compounds (Group VIII) in combination with chemical carcinogens. Concluding from this admittedly very limited set of available data, an approximately equal number of secondary carcinogens lead to synergistic and to antagonistic effects. The most common target organ is the liver, followed by the skin and the mammary gland. There is a minor clustering of *N*-nitroso compounds (Group IV) and of naturally occurring compounds (Group VIII) as secondary carcinogens that lead preferentially to synergistic combinations.

Available data on synergistic and antagonistic effects of selected inorganic carcinogens in combination with other chemical carcinogens are summarized in Table 13. The majority of the number of combinations are synergistic; the ratio is 4.5 for the number of synergistic *over* antagonistic interactions, all target organs considered. The respiratory tract is the most common target organ. From this very limited set of data, among the secondary carcinogens involved in synergistic interactions PAH and *N*-nitroso compounds are predominant.

In the chemical class assignment for primary carcinogens (*see* I. Introduction), Class X "Miscellaneous Compounds" contains compounds that are represented in the "Database" (1) with only minor frequencies of entries. Synergistic and antagonistic interactions of these miscellaneous agents with other chemical carcinogens are listed in Tables 14 and

TABLE 11. Antagonistic Interactions of Selected Halogenated Compounds with a Second Carcinogen

Primary carcinogen	Target organ with secondary carcinogen					
	Liver	Urinary tract	Respiratory tract	Skin/local	Mammary gland	Hematopoietic tissue
CCl$_4$	2-AAF	2-AAF	Urethan			
PCB[a]	2-AAF[c] (62) 3'-Me-DAB DEN[c]			DMBA		
DDT	3'-Me-DAB			trans-AAS	DMBA[c]	DMBA[c]
TCDD				BaP + TPA[c] 3-MC + TPA[b] DMBA + TPA[d]		

Note: Unless individually referenced in parentheses, binary combination effects tabulated are taken from the database of Arcos et al. (1).
[a]Arochlor 1254 or Kanechlor 300, 400, or 500.
[b]TCDD prior to 3-MC; no effect otherwise.
[c]Based on two experiments.
[d]Based on three experiments.

TABLE 12. Synergistic and Antagonistic Interactions of Selected Naturally Occurring Compounds with a Second Carcinogen

Primary carcinogen	Synergism				Antagonism			
	Target organ with secondary carcinogen							
	Liver	Skin/local	Urinary tract	Mammary gland	Liver	Skin/local	Mammary gland	Respiratory tract
AFB$_1$	DEN[a] CCl$_4$[b] Dieldrin AFB$_2$ Ochratoxin CPFA[c] Ethionine				DES α-BHC	DMBA		
Actino-mycin D		3-MC	DMN			DMBA[d]	DMBA[b]	
Chloram-phenicol		3-MC			2-AAF[b] DAB[b] 3'-Me-DAB[b]		DMBA	Urethan
Reserpine	DAB			DMBA	2,7-FAA DEN	3-MC	MNU	

Note: Binary combination effects tabulated are taken from the database of Arcos *et al.* (1).
[a]DEN and AFB$_1$ combination also elicited synergistic response in the respiratory and gastrointestinal tracts.
[b]Based on two experiments.
[c]Based on three experiments.
[d]Based on four experiments.

15. The majority of the combinations show synergistic response, the ratio of synergistic *over* antagonistic interactions being 1.7. The most frequent target organ for both combination effects is the liver, followed by the skin and the urinary tract. Among the secondary carcinogens displaying antagonistic effects Group III agents (azo dyes) were most prevalent, whereas among those involved in synergisms Group IV agents (*N*-nitroso compounds) were most common.

TABLE 13. Synergistic and Antagonistic Interactions of Selected Inorganic Carcinogens with a Second Carcinogen

	Synergism			Antagonism	
	Target organ with a secondary carcinogen				
Primary carcinogen	Skin/ local	Respiratory tract	Urinary tract	Skin/ local	Liver
As$_2$O$_3$	DMBA	BaP	DEN[a]	3-MC	
Ni-compounds	BaP[b]		EHEN[c]		3'-Me-DAB[f,g]
Asbestos[d]		BaP[g] (61)	No data		
		DMBA	indicating		
		BHPN	antagonism		
		NHMI[e]			

Note: Unless individually referenced in parentheses, binary combination effects tabulated are taken from the database of Arcos *et al.* (1).
[a]Combination with NaAsO$_2$.
[b]Ni$_3$S$_2$ was used.
[c]NiCl$_2$ was used.
[d]Chrysotile.
[e]Asbestos plus CdCl$_2$.
[f]NiCl$_2$ and Ni(AcO)$_2$ were used.
[g]Based on two experiments.

IV. OVERVIEW OF CARCINOGENIC EFFECTS OF SELECTED MULTIPLE (NONBINARY) COMBINATIONS OF STRUCTURALLY-DEFINED CHEMICAL COMPOUNDS AND COMPLEX MIXTURES

Experimental studies involving the combination of more than two complete chemical carcinogens are by far less common than those on binary combinations. Because of the paucity of data, no attempt was made to organize the available experiments into chemical classes; rather, the available experiments were structured into categories according to the number of partners in the combination and the target organ specificities of the partners. Thus, experiments involving three carcinogens were described first, followed by those with more than three agents in combination. The tabulation of the results includes headings to indicate whether the combination effects occurred in the common target organs of the carcinogens or if additional new organ target(s) (for the mixture only) have appeared. Because of the low overall number of these experiments and because the experimental design did not always allow distinguishing between synergism or additivity or antagonism, the experiments which showed not entirely clearcut synergism or antagonism were not excluded from consideration.

Experiments on combination effects resulting from more than two chemical carcinogens with similar organotropy are given in Tables 16 and 17. As shown therein, the majority of interactions resulted in synergistic or additive effects, whereas antagonistic or mixed combination effects were rare. The most common target organs were the skin, the liver, and the urinary tract. Analysis of the types of combinations and the numbers of chemicals participating in them indicates that, when a large number of chemicals or even complex mixtures of certain carcinogens interact, unexpected combination effects can occur. The following is to highlight some of the challenges in the interpretation of the results.

As might be expected from their comparable metabolism and mechanism of action, simultaneous administration of three *N*-nitroso compounds with similar organotropy (liver), resulted in an additive combination effect toward this organ (25, 26). Since low to very low dosages were given in this experiment, a linear dose–response relationship was

TABLE 14. Synergistic Interactions of Miscellaneous Carcinogens with a Second Carcinogen

Primary carcinogen	Target organ with secondary carcinogen							
	Liver	Skin/local	Urinary tract	Gastrointestinal tract	Pancreas	Mammary gland	Hematopoietic/ lymphatic system	Prostate
Alkylating drugs	MAMA[a]	3-MC[b]	FANFT[b] MNU[a]	MAMA[a]				
Ethionine	DAB m-Toluylenediamine AFB$_1$				4-HAQO			
Estrogens	2-AAF[c] BNU[c,e] EHEN[d] (59) BHPN[d] (59) 2-AAF[d] (59) N-Pip[d] (59)			EHEN[d] (59)		DMBA[c] trans-AAS[c]	Urethan[c,d,e]	DMBA[d] (58)

Note: Unless individually referenced in parentheses, binary combination effects tabulated are taken from the database of Arcos *et al.* (1).
[a]Methyl methanesulfonate as primary carcinogen.
[b]Cyclophosphamide as primary carcinogen.
[c]Diethylstilbestrol as primary carcinogen.
[d]Estradiol as primary carcinogen.
[e]Based on two experiments.

TABLE 15. Antagonistic Interactions of Miscellaneous Carcinogens with a Second Carcinogen

Primary carcinogen	Target organ with secondary carcinogen				
	Skin/local	Liver	Gonads	Respiratory tract	Urinary tract
Alkylating drugs	DMBA + PMA[a] DMBA[c]	3'-Me-DAB[b]			
Ethionine		DAB[f] Trypan blue α-BHC	DAB		
Estrogens	trans-AAS[d]	3'-Me-DAB[d] AFB₁[d]		BHPN[e] (59)	4-HBBN[e] (59)

Note: Unless individually referenced in parentheses, binary combination effects tabulated are taken from the database of Arcos *et al.* (1).
[a]Sulfur mustard as primary carcinogen.
[b]Nitrogen mustard as primary carcinogen.
[c]Chloroquine mustard as primary carcinogen.
[d]Diethylstilbestrol as primary carcinogen.
[e]Ethinyl estradiol as primary carcinogen.
[f]Based on two experiments.

observed after fitting the data into an appropriate model (Figure 1.) However, simultaneous or sequential administration of three or four urinary bladder carcinogens, with *dissimilar* metabolism and mechanism of action, caused synergistic combination effects in their common target organ (Table 16; refs. 27, 28). In the framework of the multistage hypothesis of carcinogenesis, this difference appears to be consistent with the interpretation that carcinogens of similar potency acting at the same stage/site act additively, whereas carcinogens that act at different stages/sites will act multiplicatively (29).

This interpretation is not appropriate, however, to explain data from the experiments of Takayama et al. (30), who found a synergistic effect following administration of a combination of five heterocyclic amines, which yet belong to the same group of carcinogens and, therefore, act probably at the same stage of carcinogenesis. Although the validity of the observations of these authors appears to be limited, because the actual combination effect was compared to historical single agent studies and no dose–response relationships were determined, later studies corroborated the synergism concluded for liver tissue (Table 16; Refs. 31, 32). This instance of synergism, observed in the induction of liver cancer and preneoplastic foci of the liver, may be partially related to induction of the different enzymes involved in the metabolism of the carcinogens; indeed, the P-450 species involved in metabolic activation and their inducibility appear to be different for the individual heterocyclic amines (32, 33).

A multiple chemical combinations testing study by Fukushima et al. (34) (Table 17) was based on the assumption that if the individual role of a single carcinogen within a group of agents with similar organotropy is disregarded, then the influence of a short pretreatment with other carcinogens causing epithelial cell stimulation can be assessed. Pretreatment with such diverse carcinogens as DEN, MNU, and bis(2-hydroxypropyl)nitrosamine (BHPN), followed by five hepatocarcinogens which act at different stages of carcinogenesis, resulted only in an additive effect. It is possible that this result is simply the consequence of multiple binary interactions (some enhancing, some inhibiting) between agents of different organotropy in the set of chemicals administered, rather than attributable to the original assumption underlying the experiment.

Another mechanism potentially leading to unexpected results was addressed in an experiment by Springer et al. (35) (Table 17), who focused on the inhibition of

TABLE 16. Combination Effects Involving More Than Two Chemical Carcinogens with Similar Organotropy

Number of carcinogens	Carcinogens	Effect observed in target organs				Reference
		Liver	Urinary tract	Skin	Genital glands	
3	DEN +NDIEA +NPYR	Additive				(25, 26)
3	4-HBBN +2-AAF +3,3'-DCB		Synergistic			(27, 28)
3	4-HBBN → FANFT → 2-AAF		Synergistic			(28)
3	FANFT → 2-AAF → 3,3'-DCB		Synergistic			(28)
4	4-HBBN → FANFT → 2-AAF → 3,3'-DCB		Synergistic			(30)
5	Trp-P-1 +Trp-P-2 +Glu-P-2 +AαC+IQ	Synergistic		Synergistic[a]	Synergistic[b]	(30)
6	DEN[f] → (Trp-P-2 +Glu-P-1 +MeAαC +AαC+PhIP)	Synergistic[c,d]				(31)
6	DEN[f] → (Trp-P-1 + Glu-P-2+IQ +MeIQ+MIQx)	Synergistic[c,e]				(32)

Note: + = simultaneous administration; → = sequential administration.
[a]Male rats only.
[b]Female rats only.
[c]Foci only.
[d]High dose only.
[e]Low dose only.
[f]Plus partial hepatectomy.

PAH-induced carcinogenesis by a multiple combination of much weaker carcinogens or noncarcinogens of this same class. Single coadministration of benzo[*a*]pyrene (BaP) and coal-derived complex organic mixtures followed by phorbol ester (TPA) promotion for 24 weeks resulted in slightly to substantially decreased tumor-initiating activity as compared to administration of BaP alone. Since the degree of antagonism was related to the boiling point range used to segregate the complex mixtures (footnote b in Table 17), the mixture with the highest antagonistic potential (boiling point range: 750–800°F) was fractionated so as to obtain the chemical class fractions. Results from the testing of these fractions indicated that the aliphatic fraction and the hydroxylated PAH fraction ("aliphatics and olefins" and "HPAH" in Table 17) caused only modest decreases in initiating activity, whereas the other two chromatographic fractions, PAH and nitrogen-containing polynuclear aromatic compounds (NPAC), produced substantial decreases. In accordance with this, the combination effects of BaP with the first two fractions were considered additive, and the effects of the last two fractions antagonistic (Table 17). These results suggest that

TABLE 17. Combination Effects of Complex Mixtures and of More Than Two Structurally Defined Chemical Carcinogens with Similar Organotropy

Number of carcinogens	Carcinogens	Effect observed in target organs			Reference
		Liver	Skin	Respiratory tract	
8	(DEN + MNU + BHPN) → (2-AAF + DMN + 3'-Me-DAB + PB + TAA)	Additive			(34)
CM[a]	BaP[e] + coal-derived complex mixtures		Antagonistic/ additive		(35)
CM[a]	BaP[e] + coal-derived aliphatics and olefins		Additive		(35)
CM[a]	BaP[e] + coal-derived HPAH		Additive		(35)
CM[a]	BaP[e] + coal-derived PAH		Antagonistic		(35)
CM[a]	BaP[e] + coal-derived NPAC		Antagonistic		(35)
11	BaP + cigarette smoke condensate PAH		Additive		(36)
11	BaP + automobile exhaust condensate PAH		Additive		(36)
11	BaP + smokehouse soot and tar PAH		Additive		(36)
CM[a]	DPN + gasoline engine exhaust			Antagonistic/ synergistic[c]	(37)
CM[a]	DPN + diesel engine exhaust			Additive/ antagonistic[d]	(37)

Note: + = simultaneous administration; → = sequential administration.
[a]Complex mixture.
[b]Dependent on boiling point range during fractionation.
[c]Antagonism for lung tumors, synergism for nasal cavity tumors.
[d]Additivity for lung tumors (but synergism for squamous cell carcinoma of the lung), antagonism for nasal cavity tumors.
[e]BaP plus TPA.

the greatest antagonism is shown by classes of compounds with chemical structures most similar to that of BaP and that the fractions with the least structural similarity produce the least antagonistic effect.

A different result was observed in an experiment reported by Berger and Schmähl (36). In this study, administration of BaP was prolonged continuous and was given alone *or* together with mixtures of carcinogenic and/or noncarcinogenic polycyclic hydrocarbons, without promotion by TPA. As shown in Table 17 and Figures 2–4, additive syncarcinogenesis was observed when coadministering BaP and the mixtures of PAH, which mixtures were compounded so as to mimic cigarette smoke condensate, automobile exhaust condensate, and smokehouse soot plus tar. The main difference between this

FIGURE 1. Relationship between individual daily *N*-nitrosamine dose and time to death with liver tumors. The time that elapsed until 1% (square), 5% (bullet), or 10% (triangle) of the animals have died with liver tumor, due to the administration of diethylnitrosamine (DEN) (a), *N*-nitrosopyrrolidine (NPYR) (b), *N*-nitrosodiethanol-amine (NDIEA) (c), or their combination (d) is indicated by the broken, solid, and dashed straight line plots, respectively. All points are calculated from the proportional hazards model fitted to the single nitrosamines and their combination. [Adapted from M. R. Berger, D. Schmähl, and L. Edler, *Jpn. J. Cancer Res.* 81, 598 (1990).]

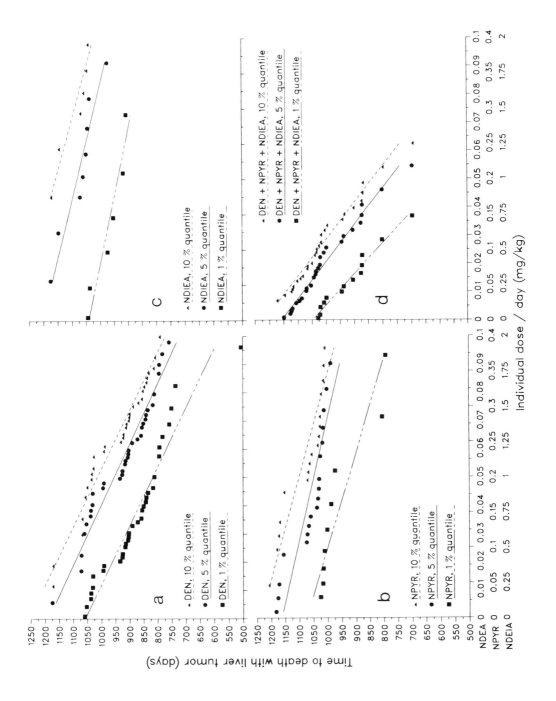

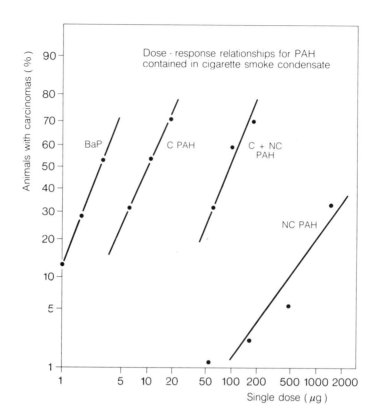

FIGURE 2. Incidence of malignant skin tumors following life-long painting of benzo[a]pyrene (BaP) and mixtures of carcinogenic polycyclic hydrocarbons (CPAH), noncarcinogenic PAH (NCPAH), and CPAH plus NCPAH, compounded to mimic cigarette smoke condensate, to the skin of NMRI mice. [Adapted from M. R. Berger and D. Schmähl: In "Combination Effects in Chemical Carcinogenesis" (D. Schmähl, ed.). VCH Publishers, Weinheim, Germany, 1988, p. 598.]

experiment, showing additivity, and the experiment by Springer et al. (35), showing antagonism, is clearly the administration period of BaP and of the PAH. Obviously, prolonged continuous application of the hydrocarbons leads to results different from a single administration followed by phorbol ester promotion. In the case of single administration of BaP, followed by TPA promotion, the profile of BAP-metabolite and DNA-adduct formation was altered by coadministration of complex coal-derived mixtures, and this probably was causally related to the observed antagonism. It is reasonable to draw the conclusion that prolonged continuous exposure to BaP and other PAH leads to a change in metabolic pattern which compensates for and overrides the (probable) competition between carcinogens underlying the antagonism observed by Springer et al. (35). Similarly challenging is the report by Heinrich et al. (37), who found antagonistic, additive, and synergistic effects in the respiratory tract after application of dipentylnitrosamine (DPN), which almost exclusively induced lung tumors after subcutaneous administration, and exposure to gasoline engine or diesel engine exhaust (Table 17). Remarkably, gasoline engine exhaust inhibited the development of tumors induced by DPN in the lung, but synergized tumor development in the nasal cavity, whereas diesel engine exhaust did not influence the overall lung tumor rate—with the exception of squamous cell carcinomas which were significantly increased relative to other histological lung tumor types—but decreased the tumor rate in the nasal cavity. This result may partly be explained by a different metabolism of DPN in the target cells of the lung and the nasal

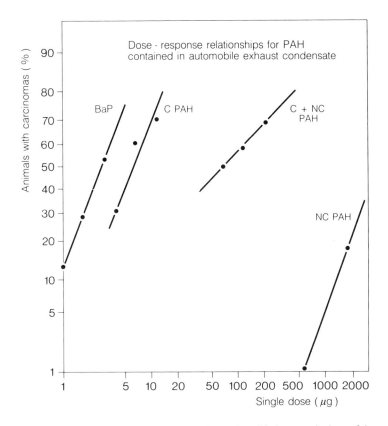

FIGURE 3. Incidence of malignant skin tumors following life-long painting of benzo[a]pyrene (BaP) and mixtures of carcinogenic polycyclic hydrocarbons (CPAH), noncarcinogenic PAH (NCPAH), and CPAH plus NCPAH, compounded to mimic automobile exhaust condensate, to the skin of NMRI mice. [Adapted from M. R. Berger and D. Schmähl: In "Combination Effects in Chemical Carcinogenesis" (D. Schmähl, ed.). VCH Publishers, Weinheim, Germany, 1988, p. 598.]

cavity, and partly by the differential retention of exhaust components in the upper and lower respiratory tracts of the rat.

Experiments illustrating the scant database on combination effects involving more than two chemical carcinogens with different organotropy are shown in Table 18. The most common target organs were the liver and the urinary tract. The overall number of these experiments is lower than those based on multiple combinations of carcinogens having a common target organ. This is possibly due to the assumption (when the experiments were designed) that, in general, syncarcinogenesis occurs only when the individual carcinogens have the same target organ (38). However, many carcinogens have a main target organ and, in addition, other target organs of minor importance. A typical combination, with some overlap in the target organ specificities, was used in a testing experiment (39) involving continuous exposure to low doses of DEN, 4-HBBN, and 4-dimethylaminostilbene (DAS). The principal targets of these carcinogens are the liver, the urinary tract, and the ear duct, respectively, and, in addition, the latter two agents also induce tumors in the liver to a minor extent. Remarkably, there were antagonistic interactions in all three target organs, and most prominent in the liver (39). A different result was obtained by Fukushima et al. (34), who observed a synergistic combination effect in the liver of rats after short pretreatment with DEN, MNU, and BHPN and subsequent exposure to the five *N*-nitroso compounds: 4-HBBN, dibutylnitrosamine

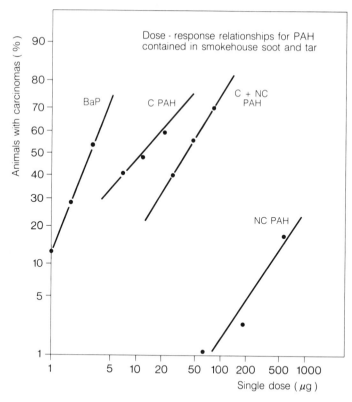

FIGURE 4.   Incidence of malignant skin tumors following life-long painting of benzo[a]pyrene BaP and mixtures of carcinogenic polycyclic hydrocarbons (CPAH), noncarcinogenic PAH (NCPAH), and CPAH plus NCPAH, compounded to mimic smokehouse soot plus tar, to the skin of NMRI mice. [Adapted from M. R. Berger and D. Schmähl: In "Combination Effects in Chemical Carcinogenesis" (D. Schmähl, ed.). VCH Publishers, Weinheim, Germany, 1988, p. 598.]

(DBN), N-ethyl-N-hydroxyethylnitrosamine (EHEN), N-methyl-N'-nitro-N-nitrosoguanidine (MNNG), and propylnitrosourea (PNU), which have various target organs. Interestingly, an additive combination effect was found in the urinary bladder of these rats, thus again demonstrating a mixed response. The same type of mixed response was seen when the aforementioned five N-nitroso compounds were given together with the five hepatocarcinogens 2-AAF, dimethylnitrosamine (DMN), phenobarbital (PB), 3'-Me-DAB, and thioacetamide (TAA). However, synergism in *both organs* (liver and urinary bladder) occurred when this treatment was supplemented by a short pretreatment with DEN, MNU, and BHPN (Table 18).

In an experiment of Takayama et al. (40), rats were administered simultaneously 40 carcinogens given at 1/50 of their respective TD_{50} (*i.e.*, the respective daily dose rates producing 50% tumor incidence after 2 years of treatment). The only two organs showing significantly elevated tumor incidences or incidences of neoplastic foci were the thyroid gland and the liver, respectively. Since 20 of the 40 carcinogens (50%) were known to target the liver and 5 (13%) the thyroid gland, it seemed rational to assume that a summation of individual effects led to this (probably) additive combination effect. Such an assumption is, however, inconsistent with the fact that the urinary tract is the usual target of 10 of the 40 carcinogens (25%) in the mixture and that the hematopoietic organs and the skin are the usual targets of 8 and 4 of the 40 carcinogens (20 and 10%), respectively. Thus, it is possible that antagonistic interactions may have suppressed the

TABLE 18. Combination Effects Involving More Than Two Chemical Carcinogens with Different Organotropy

| Number of carcinogens | Carcinogens | Effect observed in target organs | | | | |
		Liver	Urinary tract	Ear duct	Thyroid	Reference
3	DEN + HBBN + DAS	Antagonistic	Antagonistic	Antagonistic		(39)
8	(DEN + MNU + BHPN) → (HBBN + DBN + EHEN + MNNG + PNU)	Synergistic	Additive			(34)
10	HBBN + DBN + EHEN + MNNG + PNU + 2-AAF + DMN + PB + 3'-Me-DAB + TAA	Synergistic	Additive			(34)
13	(DEN + MNU + BHPN) → (HBBN + DBN + EHEN + MNNG + PNU + 2-AAF + DMN + PB + 3'-Me-DAB +TAA)	Synergistic	Synergistic			(34)
40	Simultaneous administration of various carcinogens	Additive			Additive	(40)

Note: + = simultaneous administration; → = sequential administration.

emergence of tumors in these organs. However, since the dosages used were far too low in comparison to those used in single-agent studies, the question whether or not such a mixed response actually occurred cannot be readily answered. This illustrates the difficulties in interpreting complex combination experiments with unexpected results.

V. CONSIDERATIONS ON THE MECHANISMS INVOLVED IN THE SYNERGISTIC AND ANTAGONISTIC INTERACTIONS OF CHEMICAL CARCINOGENS

A given chemical carcinogen can enhance or inhibit tumor induction by another chemical carcinogen through a variety of mechanisms at different stages within the process of carcinogenesis; these mechanisms include modification of carcinogen availability, biotransformation, adduct formation, reactive interactions, expression of cellular alteration, and neoplastic development (41). Another manner to categorize the various mechanisms leading to synergistic and antagonistic effects is to distinguish between: (i) chemical interactions which can change the composition as well as increase or decrease the toxicity of components of a mixture, (ii) toxicokinetic interactions which can alter the relationship of administered dose to target-site dose, and (iii) toxicodynamic interactions which can alter the relationship of target-site dose to magnitude of effect (42). It should be noted that the same agent (*e.g.*, a "secondary" carcinogen) can be *both* an enhancer and an inhibitor of the carcinogenic process, depending on the target organ and the experimental conditions of its interaction with the "primary" carcinogen, and can thus lead to so-called "mixed" responses in the same animal. A short overview of some known mechanisms of action leading to synergistic or antagonistic combination effects is given below by discussing three examples in greater detail.

A. The first example comes from the area of carcinogenesis by PAH. A reasonable number of studies have demonstrated that when a potent hydrocarbon is coadministered with a weak or inactive one, the latter will reduce the carcinogenicity of the combination compared to the potent hydrocarbon alone (Table 2). Early attempts to interpret this effect mechanistically focused on the notion of interaction at a receptor site, thereby assuming decreased availability of the more potent carcinogen at the target site. Since it is well established that PAH are procarcinogens which require metabolic activation to reactive species, antagonistic interaction is likely to be associated with the induction of activating enzymes (such as the mixed-function oxidases) and with the competition of structurally similar chemicals for active sites on metabolizing enzymes. For example, the weak carcinogen, benzo[e]pyrene (BeP) and the two noncarcinogenic PAH, pyrene and fluoranthene, all inhibit DMBA tumor initiation. Although these three PAH do inhibit initiation by DMBA, they produce a slight *increase* in the initiating activity of BaP. The weak carcinogen, BeP, strongly inhibits the covalent binding of DMBA to target-site DNA, but has no influence on BaP–DNA binding, although it brings about substantial changes in the metabolite and adduct profiles of BaP. These results seem to provide an explanation for the observed antagonism when combining BeP and DMBA and the synergism when combining BeP and BaP (35, 43). Similarly to the findings with binary mixtures, the initiating activity of BaP was antagonized when BaP was coadministered with certain coal-derived complex organic mixtures, which mixtures were shown to cause decreased DNA binding and adduct shifts of metabolites generated from BaP (Table 17 and ref. 35). The reduced binding of BaP to DNA probably resulted from altered rates and/or pathways of metabolism due to competition for active site(s) in the mixed-function oxidase system. It should be borne in mind, however, that such observations are generally restricted to experiments in which the influence of *repeated* carcinogen exposures and, hence, subsequent enzyme induction is removed by the use of an initiation–promotion protocol; in contrast, repeated coadministration of BaP with mixtures of 10 PAH leads to additive instead of antagonistic tumor expression (Table 17). It is noteworthy that the latter protocol mimics potential human exposure to PAH (*e.g.*, in tobacco products) more closely than the former protocol.

B. The second example concerns the influence of certain halogenated compounds (such as listed in Tables 10 and 11) on tumorigenesis induced by other chemical carcinogens. Exposure to halogenated compounds prior to a carcinogen results in an anticarcinogenic effect, whereas the inverse sequence of exposure causes increased expression of carcinogenesis. The postulated mechanism of action for the effect of administration of one of these halogenated compounds may be enzyme induction; for example, this leads to increased papilloma incidence when giving TCDD *together with* 3-MC (Table 1), and to decreased incidence of papillomas when giving it *prior to* 3-MC. TCDD is an extremely potent inducer of the mixed-function oxidase system which is capable of metabolizing lipophilic compounds to more polar products. One enzyme of this system, arylhydrocarbon hydroxylase, is well known to be involved in the activation of 3-MC to its ultimate carcinogen; alteration of the balance of metabolism by increased formation or increased metabolic inactivation of the ultimate carcinogen is probably the basis for the synergistic or antagonistic effects (44). Distinct from their effect as enzyme inducers, a number of polyhalogenated hydrocarbons (*e.g.*, PCB) are known to be nongenotoxic carcinogens. A synergistic effect observed when administering them following a genotoxic carcinogen suggests that modulation of the expression of DNA lesions ("indirect genotoxic effects") — which was postulated to be brought about by this type of agent — can enhance/multiply the DNA damage produced by genotoxic carcinogens (41, 45).

C. The third example highlights the importance of cell proliferation in combination effects. Carcinogenesis requires two or more genetic events such as point mutations, chromosomal rearrangements, insertions or deletions of genes, and gene amplification followed by cell proliferation for clonal expansion of initiated cells. Consequently, in a tissue which is the target of adduct formation, but which shows no proliferation, tumorigenesis is much less expressed than in a tissue with increased proliferation. Induction of proliferation leads, therefore, to a more than additive effect, whereas the opposite (*i.e.*, cytotoxicity) causes an antagonistic effect. Such results were observed when combining the rat mammary carcinogens DMBA with MNU, which is cytotoxic at high doses. Low noncytotoxic MNU doses led to increased proliferation and consequently to synergistic induction of carcinomas, whereas high cytotoxic MNU doses resulted in an antagonistic combination effect (6). Thus, the dose level, allowing *or* inhibiting cell proliferation, is a highly important variable.

The complexity of these mechanisms, as illustrated by the three examples, and the fact that the detailed mechanism(s) responsible for the induction of tumors is not yet known even for single chemicals (*e.g.*, 46), indicate that the prediction of the modes of interaction in multiple carcinogenic effects is unlikely to be possible in the near future. Computerized search systems for combination effects (*e.g.*, 47) will, however, provide useful tools for recognizing predominant types of interactions and, thus, facilitate structural analysis (48). Systematic synopsis of existing data periodically will, hence, be helpful in defining the most promising areas for future research.

Abbreviations Used: 2-AAF, 2-acetylaminofluorene; trans-AAS, *trans*-4-acetylaminostilbene; 4-AABP, 4-acetylaminobiphenyl; AαC, 2-amino-9*H*-pyrido[2,3-*b*]indole; AF-2, furylfuramide; AFB$_1$, aflatoxin B$_1$; AFB$_2$, aflatoxin B$_2$; As$_2$O$_3$, arsenic trioxide; BA, benz[*a*]anthracene; BaP, benzo[*a*]pyrene; BeP, benzo[*e*]pyrene; α-BHC, α-hexachlorocyclohexane*; β-BHC, β-hexachlorocyclohexane*; γBHC, γ-hexachlorocyclohexane*; BHPN, bis(2-hydroxypropyl)nitrosamine; BNU, *N-n*-butyl-*N*-nitrosourea; 7-Br-Me-BA, 7-bromomethylbenz[*a*]anthracene; CCl$_4$, carbon tetrachloride; CdCl$_2$, cadmium chloride; CO, croton oil; CPFA, cyclopropenoid fatty acids; DAB, 4-dimethylaminoazobenzene; DAS, 4-dimethylaminostilbene; DB[a,c]A, dibenz[*a,c*]anthracene; DB[a,h]A, dibenz[*a, h*]anthracene; DB[a,g]F, dibenz[*a,g*]fluorene; DBN, di-*n*-butylnitrosamine; 3,3'-DCB, 3,3'-dichlorobenzidine; DDT, 1,1,1-trichloro-2-bis-(*p*-chlorophenyl)ethane; DEN, diethylnitrosamine; DEHP, di(2-ethylhexyl)phthalate; DES, diethylstilbestrol; DMBA, 7, 12-dimethylbenz[*a*]anthracene; 3,9-DMBA, 3,9-dimethylbenz[*a*]anthracene; 6,8-DMBA, 6,8-dimethylbenz[*a*]anthracene; 1,2-DMH, 1,2-dimethylhydrazine; DMN, dimethylnitrosamine; DPN, dipentylnitrosamine; EE, ethinyl estradiol; EHEN, *N*-ethyl-*N*-hydroxyethylnitrosamine; ENU, *N*-ethyl-*N*-nitrosourea; 2,7-FAA, *N,N'*-2,7-fluorenylenebisacetamide; FANFT, *N*-[4-(5-nitro-2-furyl)-2-thioazolyl]formamide; 7-F-2-AAF, 7-fluoro-2-acetylaminofluorene; 4'-F-DAB, 4'-fluoro-4-dimethylaminoazobenzene; 2',4'-di-F-DAB, 2',4'-difluoro-4-dimethylaminoazobenzene; Glu-P-2, 2-amino-dipyrido[1,2-*a*:3',2'-*d*]imidazole; 1-HA, 1-hydroxyanthraquinone; 4-HAQO, 4-hydroxylaminoquinoline-1-oxide; 4-HBBN, 4-hydroxybutylbutylnitrosamine; HPAH, hydroxylated polycyclic aromatic hydrocarbons; 8-HQ, 8-hydroxyquinoline; IQ, 2-amino-3-methylimidazo[4,5-*f*]quinoline; MAMA, methylazoxymethanol acetate; 3-MC, 3-methylcholanthrene; MDA, methyl-

---

*The three isomers of hexachlorocyclohexane are generally known in the literature by their misnomer as benzenehexachloride. Hence, the abbreviation BHC.

enedianiline; MeAαC, 2-amino-3-methyl-9*H*-pyrido[2,3-*b*]indole; 2-Me-DAB, 2-methyl-4-dimethylaminoazobenzene; 3'-Me-DAB, 3'-methyl-4-dimethylaminoazobenzene; 4'-Me-DAB, 4'-methyl-4-dimethylaminoazobenzene; MEN, methylethylnitrosamine; MeIQ, 2-amino-3,4-dimethylimidazo[4,5-*f*]quinoline; MeIQx, 2-amino-3,8-dimethylimidazo-[4,5-*f*]quinoxaline; MMS, methyl methanesulfonate; MNNG, *N*-methyl-*N'*-nitro-*N*-nitrosoguanidine; MNU, *N*-methyl-*N*-nitrosourea; N-PIP, *N*-nitrosopiperidine; NDIEA, *N*-nitrosodiethanolamine; NHMI, *N*-nitrosoheptamethyleneimine; NNM, *N*-nitrosomorpholine; NPAC, nitrogen-containing polycyclic aromatic compounds; NPYR, *N*-nitrosopyridine; 4-NQO, 4-nitroquinoline-*N*-oxide; NTA, nitrilotriacetic acid; 3-OH-BaP, 3-hydroxybenzo[*a*]pyrene; PAH, polycyclic aromatic hydrocarbons; PBB, polybrominated biphenyls; PB, phenobarbital; PCB, polychlorinated biphenyls; PMA, phorbol myristate acetate; PhIP, 2-amino-1-methyl-6-phenylimidazo[4,5-*b*]pyridine; PNU, propylnitrosourea; QUINS, quinolines; TAA, thioacetamide; TCDD, 2,3,7,8-tetrachlorodibenzo-*p*-dioxin; TPA, 12-*O*-tetradecanoylphorbol-13-acetate; Trp-P-1, 3-amino-1,4-dimethyl-5*H*-pyrido[4,3-*b*]indole; Trp-P-2, 3-amino-1-methyl-5*H*-pyrido[4,3-*b*]-indole; Wy-14,643, [4-chloro-6-(2,3-xylidino)-2-pyrimidinylthio]acetic acid.

REFERENCES

1. Arcos, J. C., Woo, Y. T., and Lai, D. Y.: Database on binary combination effects of chemical carcinogens. *Environ. Carcino. Rev.* **C6**, No. 1 (1988), Special Issue. The data are organized under the following headings: record no.; carcinogen 1 (compound, route, dose level); carcinogen 2 (compound, route, dose level); species (sex); target tissue; effect; reference.
2. Ames, B. N.: *Environ. Mol. Mutagen.* **14**, Suppl. 16, 66 (1989).
3. Appel, K. E., Fürstenberger, G., Hapke, H. J., Hecker, E., Hildebrandt, A. G., Koransky, W., Marks, F., Neumann, H. G., Ohnesorge, F. K., and Schulte-Hermann, R.: *J. Cancer Res. Clin. Oncol.* **116**, 232 (1990).
4. Elashoff, R. M., Fears, T. R., and Schneiderman, M. A.: *J. Natl. Cancer Inst.* **79**, 509 (1987).
5. Reif, A. E.: *J. Natl. Cancer Inst.* **73**, 25 (1984).
6. Berger, M. R. and Künstler, K.: *Arch. Geschwülstforsch.* **53**, 423 (1983).
7. Kouri, R. E., Rude, T. H., Joglekar, R., Dansette, P. M., Jerina, D. M., Atlas, S. A., Owens, I. S., and Nebert, D. W.: *Cancer Res.* **38**, 2277 (1978).
8. DiGiovanni, J., Berry, D. L., Gleason, G. L., Kishore, G. S., and Slaga, T. J.: *Cancer Res.* **40**, 1580 (1980).
9. Ito, N., Matayoshi, K., Matsumura, K., Denda, A., Kani, T., Arai, M., and Makiura, S.: *Gann* **65**, 123 (1974).
10. Hasegawa, R., Tatematsu, M., Tsuda, H., Shirai, T., Hagiwara, A., and Ito, N.: *Gann* **73**, 264 (1982).
11. Oyasu, R.: *Gann* **54**, 339 (1963).
12. Miller, E. C., Miller, J. A., Brown, R. R., and MacDonald, J. C.: *Cancer Res.* **18**, 469 (1958).
13. Flaks, A., and Flaks, B.: *Carcinogenesis* **3**, 981 (1982).
14. Kimura, N. T., Kanematsu, T., and Baba, T.: *Z. Krebsforsch.* **87**, 257 (1976).
15. Makiura, S., Aoe, H., Sugihara, S., Hirao, K., Arai, M., and Ito, N.: *J. Natl. Cancer Inst.* **53**, 1253 (1974).
16. Takamiya, K. Chen, S. H., and Kitagawa, H.: *Gann* **64**, 363 (1973).
17. Nishizumi, M.: *Gann* **71**, 910 (1980).
18. Preston, B. D., Miller, J. P., Moore, R. W., and Allen, J. R.: *J. Natl. Cancer Inst.* **66**, 509 (1981).
19. Nishizumi, M.: *Cancer Lett.* **2**, 11 (1976).
20. Nishizumi, M.: *Gann* **70**, 835 (1979).
21. Shelton, D. W., Hendricks, J. D., and Baily, G. S.: *Toxicol. Lett.* **22**, 27 (1984).
22. Garcia, H.: *Biologica (Chile)* **36**, 11 (1963).
23. Garcia, H. and Guerrero, A.: *Proc. Soc. Exp. Biol. Med.* **132**, 422 (1969).
24. Pound, A. W.: *Br. J. Cancer* **26**, 216 (1972).
25. Berger, M. R., Schmähl, D., and Zerban, H.: *Carcinogenesis* **8**, 1635 (1987).
26. Berger, M. R., Schmähl, D., and Edler, L.: *Jpn. J. Cancer Res.* **81**, 598 (1990).
27. Tsuda, H., Miyata, Y., Murasaki, G., Kinoshita, H., Fukushima, S., and Ito, N.; *Gann* **68**, 183 (1977).
28. Tatematsu, M., Miyata, Y., Mizutani, M., Hamanouchi, M., Hirose, M., and Ito, N.: *Gann* **68**, 193 (1977).

29. Gart, J. J., Krewski, D., Lee, P. N., Tarone, R. E., and Wahrendorf, J.: "Statistical Methods in Cancer Research, Vol. II: The Design and Analysis of Long-Term Animal Experiments", IARC Sci. Publ. No. 79. IARC, Lyon, 1986, p. 155.
30. Takayama, S., Nakatsuru, Y., and Sato, S.: *Jpn. J. Cancer Res.* **78**, 1068 (1987).
31. Hasegawa, R., Shirai, T., Hakoi, K., Takaba, K., Iwasaki, S., Hoshiya, T., Ito, N., Nagao, M., and Sugimura, T.: *Jpn. J. Cancer Res.* **82**, 1378 (1991).
32. Ito, N., Hasegawa, R., Shirai, T., Fukushima, S., Hakoi, K., Takaba, K., Iwasaki, S., Wakabayashi, K., Nagao, M., and Sugimura, T.: *Carcinogenesis* **12**, 767 (1991).
33. Alexander, J., and Wallin, H.: *CRC Crit. Rev. Toxicol.* **20**, 143 (1990).
34. Fukushima, S., Shibata, M. A., Hirose, M., Kato, T., Tatematsu, M., and Ito, N.: *Jpn. J. Cancer Res.* **82**, 784 (1991).
35. Springer, D. L., Mann, D. B., Dankovic, D. A., Thomas, B. L., Wright, C. W., and Mahlum, D. D.: *Carcinogenesis* **10**, 131 (1989).
36. Berger, M. R. and Schmähl, D.: Combination effects of low doses of genotoxic carcinogens with similar organotropism. *In* "Combination Effects in Chemical Carcinogenesis" (D. Schmähl, ed.). VCH Publishers, Weinheim, 1988, p. 93.
37. Heinrich, U., Peters, L., Fuhst, R., and Mohr, U.: *Exp. Pathol.* **37**, 51 (1989).
38. Schmähl, D.: *Arch. Toxicol. Suppl.* **4**, 29 (1980).
39. Berger, M. R.: Untersuchungen zur Kombinationswirkung genotoxischer Karzinogene. *In* "Umwelt und Krebs" (Arbeitsgemeinschaft der Gross Forschung Einrichtung, ed.). Thenée Druck, Bonn, 1990, p. 42.
40. Takayama, S., Hasegawa, H., and Ohgaki, H.: *Jpn. J Cancer Res.* **80**, 732 (1989).
41. Williams, G. M.: *Fundam. Appl. Toxicol.* **4**, 325 (1984).
42. O'Flaherty, E. J.: *Toxicol. Ind. Health* **5**, 667 (1989).
43. Smolarek, T. A. and Baird, W. M.: *Cancer Res.* **46**, 1170 (1986).
44. World Health Organization: Environmental Health Criteria 88: Polychlorinated Dibenzo-para-dioxins and Dibenzofurans. WHO, Geneva, 1989.
45. Lutz, W. K. and Maier, P.: *Trends Pharmacol. Sci.* **9**, 322 (1988).
46. Swenberg, J. A., Fedtke, N., Fennell, T. R., and Walker, V. E.: Relationships between Carcinogen Exposure, DNA Adducts and Carcinogenesis. *In* "Progress in Predictive Toxicology" (D. B. Clayson, I. C. Munroe, P. Shubik, and J. A. Swenberg, eds.). Elsevier, Amsterdam, 1990, p. 161.
47. Polansky, G. and Woo, Y.-T.: *Environ. Carcino. Rev.* **C7**, 109 (1989).
48. Rao, V. R.: *J. Toxicol. Environ. Health* **33**, 237 (1991).
49. Klaunig, J. E:, Ruch, R. J., and Pereira, M. A.: *Environ. Health Perspect.* **69**, 89 (1986).
50. Daniel, F. B., Deangelo, A. B., Stober, J. A., Pereira, M. A., and Olson, F. R.: *Fundam. Appl. Toxicol.* **13**, 40 (1989).
51. Wunderlich, V., Fey, F., and Sydow, G.: *Neoplasma* **34**, 389 (1987).
52. Iversen, O. H.: *Carcinogenesis* **12**, 901 (1991).
53. Mori, Y., Yoshimi, N., Iwata, H., Tanaka, T., and Mori, H.: *Carcinogenesis* **12**, 335 (1991).
54. Wade, G. G., Mandel, R., and Ryser, H. J. P.: *Cancer Res.* **47**, 6606 (1987).
55. Short, B. G., Steinhagen, W. H. and Swenberg, J. A.: *Cancer Res.* **49**, 6369 (1989).
56. Johansson, S. L., Saidi, J., Oesterdahl, B. G., and Smith, R. A.: *Cancer Res.* **51**, 4388 (1991).
57. Tanaka, T., Kuniyasu, T., Shima, H., Sugie, S., Mori, H., Takahashi, M., and Hirono, I.: *J. Natl. Cancer Inst.* **77**, 777 (1986).
58. Shirai, T., Fukushima, S., Ikawa, E., Tagawa, Y., and Ito, N.: *Cancer Res.* **46**, 6423 (1986).
59. Shirai, T., Tsuda, H., Ogiso, T., Hirose, M., and Ito, N.: *Carcinogenesis* **8**, 115 (1987).
60. Fears, T. R., Elashoff, R. M., and Schneiderman, M. A.: *Toxicol. Ind. Health* **4**, 221 (1988).
61. Kimizuka, G., Ohwada, H., and Hayashi, Y.: *Acta Pathol. Jpn.* **37**, 465 (1987).
62. Hayes, M. H., Roberts, E., Safe, S. H., Farber, E., and Cameron, R. G.: *J. Natl. Cancer Inst.* **76**, 683 (1986).
63. Becker, F. F.: *Cancer Res.* **35**, 1734 (1975).

CHAPTER 3

Synergism in Carcinogenesis: Mathematical Approaches to Its Evaluation

Arnold E. Reif

Determination of the statistical validity of synergism between two carcinogens is conceptually complex. If the dose–response curves of two carcinogens are linear, then the two carcinogens would be in synergism if the tumor yield, when they are administered *together*, exceeded that obtained by the summation of the tumor yields from the separate testing of the two carcinogens at their respective single doses. For synergism to be established, the difference must be statistically significant.

The situation where the dose–response curves are linear represents, however, only a special case of the far more commonly encountered situation, in which the dose–response curve of one or both of the two interacting carcinogens is/are S-shaped, *i.e.*, nonlinear. The reason why distinguishing between linear and nonlinear dose–response curves is important is because doubling the dose of a carcinogen in the steep middle section of its S-shaped dose–response curve will *more than double* the tumor yield. Hence, two different carcinogens when administered together could falsely seem to be synergistic when, due to the nonlinearity of one or both of their dose–response curves, their combined effects appear to be enhanced *beyond* arithmetic additivity. This is the basis of the requirement to know the shape of the relevant portions of the *individual dose-response curves* of the two carcinogens. Thus, any general statement on synergism in carcinogenesis or equation for its quantification must include adequate consideration of the shapes of the curves. Moreover, for full validation of synergism, lifetime data are required to avoid a possible overturning of premature conclusions by late incidences.

This chapter updates the conceptual framework for statistical formalism on synergism in carcinogenesis published in 1984 (1). The various classes of synergism in carcinogenesis are illustrated using examples taken from animal model systems. These illustrative examples are used to deduce principles for experimental design for the substantiation of synergism in carcinogenesis. Finally, the mechanism of synergism in carcinogenesis, suggested by the statistical consideration of these examples, is discussed.

I. THEORETICAL BACKGROUND

As already stated above, synergism in carcinogenesis occurs when the combined action of two carcinogens results in a significantly larger effect than their expected additive effect, which depends critically on the shapes of their dose–response curves. Antagonism in carcinogenesis is defined identically, except that "larger" is replaced by "smaller"; therefore, it may be regarded as negative synergism.

A. Conditions for Substantiation of Synergism

There are three necessary conditions for rigorously defining synergism or antagonism in carcinogenesis:

1. Statistically significant validation of synergism defined according to the principle embodied in Equation 1 or its variants given below.
2. Adequate data on relevant portions of the dose–response curves of the two carcinogens administered singly. These data may stem from studies other than that under consideration.
3. Tumor incidence data extending to the end of the life span of all experimental or epidemiological subjects included in the study. [It should be pointed out that this condition is also in accordance with the recommendation (2) of the United Nations Scientific Committee on the Effects of Atomic Radiations.]

In practice, it is seldom possible to satisfy all three requirements. Therefore, to simplify the determination of synergism in carcinogenesis, five different categories or classes of synergism are considered, rather than the two classes proposed previously (1).

B. Classes of Synergism

The previous requirements for strict synergism (1,2,3) can seldom be attained in practice; thus, it is a too restrictive concept. Data covering the entire life span of all subjects are usually unavailable. However, a valid claim for strict synergism can be made by limiting it to the time interval for which data are available. In addition, classes of synergism of intermediate rigor, as "part-way stages", are far easier to attain, yet have scientific merit. These stages include the previously proposed concept of apparent synergism, but add an additional stage between apparent and strict synergism.

1. Suggestion of Synergism

Equation 1 or its variants give a positive result, but no statistical tests of synergism can be run, because of insufficient data. When results are left in this form, they constitute a claim without scientific validity. Yet, they may have scientific value in prompting that a more rigorous test for synergism be undertaken.

2. Apparent Synergism

Equation 1 or its variants give a positive result, and a valid test shows statistical significance. However, neither the study under consideration nor previous studies provide useful data on the shape of the relevant portions of the individual dose–response curves of the two carcinogens. Nor do the data extend to the end of the life span of all animals in all groups.

This is the situation with data available from most studies on synergism in carcinogenesis. While a statistically significant result does not constitute definitive proof of synergism, it does provide a scientifically valid conclusion within the context of the uncertainties caused by the lack of fulfillment of Conditions 2 and 3 above.

3. Probable Synergism

This new class is now added in recognition of the difficulty of gathering data to prove strict synergism and, thus, to accommodate studies which come close to strict synergism. The existence of probable synergism may be claimed if two additional conditions beyond those for apparent synergism are met: (a) synergism, as evaluated by Equation 1 or its variants, is not only statistically significant, but is also multiplicative or hypermultiplicative (as defined by Equation 2 below); and (b) there is evidence from the study under consideration (or from other studies) that each of the two carcinogens possess close to straight-line dose–response curves in the relevant response range. This range extends from the lowest response for the single administration of one carcinogen (at the same dose that was used for an apparently synergistic joint administration), to the highest response obtained for joint administration of the two carcinogens. In this case, fulfillment of Condition 3 is not required.

4. Strict Synergism

Strict synergism may be claimed if Conditions 1,2, and 3 above are all fulfilled. If data to the end of the life span of all subjects are unavailable, then the time interval for data collection, over which strict synergism has been proven, should be stated.

5. Absolute Synergism

This is particularly relevant to cases of viral tumorigenesis in which two separate oncogenes are required for tumor development. If there is no carcinogenic response unless both oncogenes are simultaneously present, then absolute synergism may be claimed.

The requirements for the classes of synergism discussed above are summarized in Table 1.

TABLE 1. Conventions for Substantiation of Synergism or Antagonism in Carcinogenesis

Column:	1	2	3	4
Class of Synergism or Antagonism	Statistical significance of Equation 1	High degree of synergism[a]	Adequate dose–response data	Lifetime data
1. Suggestion of synergism	No	—[b]	—	—
2. Apparent synergism	Yes[c]	—	—	—
3. Probable synergism	Yes	Yes	Probable[d]	—
4. Strict synergism	Yes	—	Yes	Yes
5. Absolute synergism	Yes	Yes	Yes	Yes

[a]The synergism is multiplicative or hypermultiplicative using Equation 2.

[b]A dash (—) means that either "Yes" or "No" is acceptable.

[c] "Yes" means data are available for the entire life span of all subjects. If such data are unavailable, then the time interval for data collection, over which strict synergism has been proven, should be stated.

[d] "Probable" means evidence exists that the relevant portions of the dose-response curves for separate application of each of the two carcinogens show close to linear relationships.

C. Significance of Linearity of Dose–Response Curves

In this subsection synergism is defined in mathematical terms. For simplicity, in-depth consideration of the statistical apparatus is deferred to Appendix I.

When the two carcinogens under study both have linear dose–response curves when applied singly, the definition of synergism is easily translated into an equation. Suppose that two carcinogens, A and B, act on four separate subgroups of a population, and cause a number of biological effects (incidence or death from cancer, or related effects) in each as follows: n_0 for the unexposed subgroup, n_A and n_B for the subgroups each exposed only to A or only to B, and n_{AB} for the subgroup exposed both to A and to B. Here, $n = x/m$, where x is the number of occurrences in a subgroup of m individuals. Then, by the above definition of synergism,

$$n_{AB} - n_0 > (n_A - n_0) + (n_B - n_0) \qquad \text{or} \qquad n_{AB} > n_A + n_B - n_0 \qquad (1)$$

Equation 1 states that for synergism, the effect in the group exposed to both carcinogens is larger than the addition of the effects in the two singly exposed groups; also, a correction for the spontaneous incidence in the unexposed group is applied to the effects observed in each group. If synergism is to be proven, then n_{AB} must be shown to be *significantly greater* than $n_A + n_B - n_0$. Furthermore, the two carcinogens are in antagonism when n_{AB} is *significantly smaller* than $n_A + n_B - n_0$.

This means, stated in a different way, that when the individual dose–response curves for each of the two carcinogens are linear, then doubling the dose of a carcinogen will double the biological response. If two such carcinogens are administered together then, *if* their biological effects are independent of each other, their effect will be expected to be the sum of their separate effects. In this case any increase in effect beyond additive will be due to synergism and any decrease to antagonism.

Another way to write Equation 1 is to divide both sides of the equation by its right-hand side, so that

$$\frac{n_{AB} - n_0}{n_A + n_B - 2n_0} > 1 \qquad (1a)$$

Thus, synergism exists if the left-hand side of this equation is significantly higher than 1, whereas antagonism exists if it is lower than 1, that is,

$$\frac{n_{AB} - n_0}{n_A + n_B - 2\,n_0} < 1 \qquad (1a')$$

When Equation 1 or 1a or 1a' (or 1b or 1b', *see below*) has been used, and the result obtained is statistically significant, the question of whether or not strict synergism or strict antagonism exists depends on whether or not all three conditions for the substantiation of synergism have been met.

D. Significance of Nonlinearity of Dose–Response Curves

In most situations in which two carcinogens are tested for synergism in experimental animals, the dose–response curves for one or both carcinogens are either nonlinear or unknown. In the latter case, the safe assumption is that they are nonlinear. If the dose–response curve of carcinogen A is S-shaped, then if it is applied alone at dose $2a$, which places its effect at a point on the early steep portion of the response curve, its effect will be considerably greater than twice its effect when applied at dose *a*. Suppose that a second carcinogen B exists, which at dose *b* produces the same type of tumor and with the same frequency as produced by carcinogen A at dose *a*. Then, if carcinogen A at dose *a* is applied jointly with carcinogen B at dose *b*, then — even if the two carcinogens do not interact when applied together — the situation will be the same as if carcinogen A were applied alone at a dose of 2*a*, that is, combined administration will produce an effect considerably greater than the sum of the effects of carcinogen A and B each administered alone at doses of *a* and *b*, respectively. Thus, to establish synergism or antagonism, it is essential to take into account the shape of the dose–response curves of the two carcinogens when tested individually.

One analytical method is the use of isobolic diagrams (1,2). However, the method is cumbersome and complex. In practice, it requires data for plotting complete dose–response curves for administration of carcinogens A, B, and AB, which are seldom available.

A far simpler method is substantiation of synergism over a specified response range. For each of two carcinogens considered singly, that range begins with the response to the lowest dose used in the joint administration with the other carcinogen. The range ends with the response to the highest dose used in the joint administration.

Noninteraction of two carcinogens A and B means that they are neither synergistic nor antagonistic when administered jointly. If carcinogens A and B are noninteractive, then they should have a purely additive effect when administered together. If their dose–response curves are nonlinear, this additive effect is obtained by moving up on the individual dose–response curves of each of the two carcinogens. This is carried out by reading off, from the individual dose–response curve of one of the carcinogens, say A, the effect expected from addition of a second carcinogen, B, which is noninteractive.

The equation used to substantiate synergism differs from Equation 1, in that it takes into account the nonlinearity of the dose–response curves of each of the two carcinogens. If n_0, n_A, n_B, and n_{AB} have the meanings defined above, then the response from a single dose *a* of carcinogen A will be $n_A - n_0$, and the corresponding response from a single dose *b* of carcinogen B will be $n_B - n_0$. The question that arises is what is the response to joint administration of A at dose *a* and B at dose *b* if A and B were noninteracting. In that case, addition of B at dose *b* would be equivalent to the addition of a quantity of A identical to that which would produce the response actually produced by single administration of B at dose *b*, namely, n_B. Therefore Equation 1 changes to

$$n_{AB} - n_0 > n_{A+B} - n_0 \quad \text{or} \quad n_{AB} > n_{A+B} \tag{1b}$$

To document antagonism, Equation 1b is rewritten as

$$n_{AB} < n_{A+B} \tag{1b'}$$

Equations 1b and 1b' represent the general forms of an equation to quantify synergism and antagonism in carcinogenesis. Equations 1a and 1a' are special cases, where $(n_{A+B} - n_0)$ is represented simply by $(n_A - n_0) + (n_B - n_0)$, since responses along straight-line dose–response curves are additive.

Synergism or antagonism can also be documented by a mathematical form obtained by dividing both sides of Equations 1b and 1b' by the right-hand side; for synergism:

$$\frac{n_{AB}}{n_{A+B}} > 1 \tag{1c}$$

and for antagonism:

$$\frac{n_{AB}}{n_{A+B}} < 1 \tag{1c'}$$

In Equations 1b through 1c', n_{A+B} represents the biological effect expected if A and B were acting jointly, in a purely additive manner (without displaying either synergism or antagonism). In that case, n_{A+B} can be read off on the dose–response curve for single administration of carcinogen A at the dose $(a + a_b)$, where a is the dose of carcinogen A used in joint application with B, and a_b is a dose of A producing the same biological effect as a single application of B at dose b (the dose at which B is used jointly with A). Thus, a_b "converts" the effect of carcinogen B into the corresponding effect of A, on the assumption that both A and B have identical biological effects. A correction for the spontaneous incidence n_0 is not required, because the effect at dose $(a + a_b)$ includes n_0 only once, as does the effect to the joint administration n_{AB}.

Equation 1c may also be written as

$$\frac{n_{AB}}{n_{B+A}} > 1 \tag{1d}$$

where n_{B+A} is analogous to n_{A+B}, however, read off on the dose–response curve of carcinogen B at the dose of $(b + b_a)$. Here, b_a is the dose of B read off on the dose–response curve of B, which produces the same effect as a single application of A at dose a.

Due to differences in the shapes of the dose–response curves for the two carcinogens, A and B, the value of n_{A+B} will not be identical to n_{B+A}. If the value of n_{AB} is significantly larger or smaller than either n_{A+B} *or* n_{B+A}, then statistical evidence for the existence of synergism or antagonism has been obtained.

In situations where the degree of synergism is expected to be very large, a significant result may be obtained if only a single value of n_{AB} is compared with n_{A+B} and n_{B+A}. Since this comparison has taken into account the nonlinear shapes of the distinct, individual dose–response curves of A and B, if this comparison gives a statistically significant result, then the conditions for substantiating strict synergism have been met. If the requirement of data collection to the end of the life span of all subjects has not been met, then the time period monitored should be stated.

Obviously, the chance for significance will be better in the situation where several values of n_{AB} have been tested. If n_{A+B} has been determined for three values of a and b, for instance, for $1(a + b)$, for $3(a + b)$, and for $9(a + b)$, then three sets of values of n_{AB}, of n_{A+B}, and of n_{B+A} will be obtained. In that case, units of $(a + b)$ can be plotted along the x-axis, and values of the biologic effects n along the y axis, to yield three curves, representing n_{AB}, n_{A+B}, and n_{B+A}. To substantiate synergism or antagonism, the method described above can be used with the separate three sets of data. Better, standard methods of regression analysis can be adapted to test whether or not the curve for n_{AB} differs significantly from that for either n_{A+B} or n_{B+A}. If the results are significant, then strict synergism has been substantiated.

E. Multiplicative Synergism

The concept that synergism in carcinogenesis may be multiplicative is simple in some situations. Two carcinogens display multiplicative synergism when the relative risk of the subgroup exposed to both agents is the product of the relative risks of the two subgroups, each having been exposed to only one of the two agents (4–6).

If the ratios of the biological effects that result from the single and joint administration of two carcinogens, A and B, are written as $R_A = n_A/n_0$, $R_B = n_B/n_0$, and $R_{AB} = n_{AB}/n_0$, then multiplicative synergism occurs when

$$R_{AB} = R_A \cdot R_B \qquad (2)$$

If the experimental value of R_{AB} is significantly higher than R_A. R_B, then the synergistic action may be called hypermultiplicative. An experimental value of R_{AB} that is significantly lower than R_A. R_B may still indicate synergism if

$$R_{AB} > R_A + R_B \qquad (3)$$

Equation 3 is equivalent to Equation 1 in implying the truth of Equation 1; however, the inverse is not true.

The values of n_0, n_A, n_B, and n_{AB} may be arranged in the form of a 2×2 table:

$$
\begin{array}{cc|c}
n_{AB} & n_B & \\
n_A & n_0 & R_A \\
\hline
& R_B & R_{AB}
\end{array}
$$

All four *n*-values represent experimental data and are independent of each other. In contrast to a conventional 2×2 table, the *R*-values represent the ratios defined above. The additional ratios n_{AB}/n_B and n_{AB}/n_A are not listed, since only three of the five possible ratios are independent of each other.

Equation 3 does not address issues involved in the substantiation of synergism, or (if ">" is replaced by "<" in Equation 3) of antagonism. Therefore, it is subject to the same qualifications as are other forms of Equation 1, *i.e.*, the need to involve consideration of the dose–response curves. These qualifications include the need to fulfill other necessary conditions discussed below.

As in the case of synergism deduced from Equation 1, statistically significant differences obtained from Equation 3 only suggest that the two carcinogens are acting in apparent synergism. If other data suggest that both carcinogens possess linear dose-response curves, then probable synergism has been demonstrated. If there is evidence that these curves really are linear, then strict synergism has been proven. If multiplicative or hypermultiplicative synergism can be proven to hold then, even in the absence of evidence for linearity of dose response of the two carcinogens singly, the chance that this could be due to reasons other than synergism seems small; hence, probable synergism may be claimed. Because existing epidemiological data often indicate multiplicative synergism (*see below*), this is a useful concept.

Examples for multiplicative synergism come from six different sets of epidemiological data (*in* Refs. 7–12) involving human exposure to two pulmonary carcinogens studied previously. In all six sets one of the carcinogens was cigarette smoke. This is consistent with the fact that cigarette smoking accounts for about 25% of all cancers in both sexes (13) and about 41% of all cancers in men (14); no other known carcinogen has as great an effect on the population. Another similarity among the six sets (7–12) is that all data on exposure to a single carcinogen cluster in the low dose-response range (1).

The record of statistical significance for these examples is, however, spotty. Only for the data in two studies (7,9) could clear statistical significance ($p < 0.01$) for synergism be demonstrated.

II. EXAMPLES OF SUBSTANTIATION OF CLASSES OF SYNERGISM

In this section, epidemiological data involving carcinogenesis in humans (7–12) as well as data from animal experimentation are used to illustrate the proving of classes of synergism.

A. Suggestion of Synergism (Class 1 Synergism)

Rothman and Keller (11) presented data on the relative risk of oral cancer, in population groups who did and who did not smoke and drink, in the four possible combinations of these lifestyle habits. The data document hypermultiplicative synergism as defined by use of Equation 2. However, the data cannot be used to evaluate statistical significance through use of Equations 4 and 5 (in Appendix I), since the numbers of subjects are missing. Therefore, the data merely suggest synergism, and a more complete study is needed before even Class 2 synergism can be substantiated by establishing statistical validity, as outlined below. Thus, studies that fit into this category have still substantial value in suggesting that a more incisive test be undertaken.

B. Apparent Synergism (Class 2 Synergism)

The report by Sharp and Crouse (15) of apparent synergism between radiation and 1,2-dimethylhydrazine in the induction of colon tumors in rats provides ideal data to illustrate substantiation of this finding. The data of the four groups studied in their first experiment (Table 2) give a strongly positive value for synergism using Equation 1. However, when these data are tested for significance by the use of Equations 4 and 5, the value of p is $\cong 0.10$, indicating a lack of or borderline statistical significance.

In a second experiment, rats of the same strain were exposed to three treatments with the same agents (Table 3.) The data obtained gave a stronger indication of synergism using Equation 1, and this finding was found to be highly significant ($p < 0.01$) when tested through Equations 4 and 5.

In addition, the authors presented data on tumor multiplicity in the animals with tumors. The group receiving both carcinogens had an average of 3.5 tumors per animal compared to 1.5 for the 1,2-dimethylhydrazine-treated group, whereas no tumors developed in the radiation-treated group (15). These additional results strongly support the finding of apparent synergism.

TABLE 2.   **Radiation plus 1, 2-Dimethylhydrazine (DMH)-Induced Colon Carcinogenesis in Fisher 344 Rats (Experiment I)[a]**

Group	Colon tumor incidence 8 months after treatment
Control	0/10
Single abdominal radiation exposure	1/14
Single DMH treatment	9/32
Radiation plus DMH treatment	20/35

Note: The radiation was 9 Gy of ^{60}Co, DMH was dosed at 150 mg/kg; in the coadministration group DMH was given 3.5 days after radiation.

[a]From the data of J. G. Sharp and D. A. Crouse [*Radiation Res.* **117**, 304 (1989)].

TABLE 3. Radiation plus 1, 2-Dimethylhydrazine (DMH)-Induced Colon Carcinogenesis in Fisher 344 Rats (Experiment II)[a]

Group	Colon tumor incidence 6 months after treatment
Control	—
Three abdominal radiation exposures	0/7
Three DMH treatments	2/38
Three radiation plus three DMH treatments	14/19

Note: Each radiation treatment was 9 Gy from a 4-MeV linear accelerator; each treatment with DMH was at the dose of 45 mg/rat. Radiation treatments were spaced 1 month apart, and in the coadministration group the DMH treatments were given 3.5 days after the radiation.

[a]From the data of J. G. Sharp and D. A. Crouse [*Radiation Res.* **117**, 304 (1989)].

C. Probable Synergism (Class 3 Synergism)

Probable synergism can be seen in the data of Hammond *et al.* (9) on synergism between exposure to asbestos and cigarette smoking in the development of lung cancer (Table 4.)

First, the data are strongly indicative of synergism when processed through Equation 1, and this synergism is highly significant ($p < 0.01$) when tested through the use of Equations 4 and 5. Second, the data fit multiplicative synergism defined by Equation 2. This evidence satisfies the requirements for probable synergism (*see* columns 1 and 2 in Table 1).

Regarding the shape of the dose–response curves of each of the two carcinogens tested separately, four different studies have shown a linear relationship between the number of cigarettes smoked daily and lung cancer incidence (16). While there is no direct data available regarding the shape of the dose–response curve for the inhalation of asbestos fibers, the following indirect evidence suggests that it may be a straight line in the narrow response range implicated (*see* Table 1, footnote d).

The only other type of carcinogenic agent (besides tobacco smoke) for which dose–response data on humans are available is radiation. Evidence that leukemia incidence following exposure to radiation is linear in the low-response range is highly persuasive (2). What scant evidence exists on dose response for other radiation-induced cancers in human populations also suggests that a linear relationship does exist in this range (2). Thus, for the few instances where a dose–response relationship for carcinogenesis in human populations is known, it is linear in the low-response range.

Secondly, a linear dose–response relationship would be expected in the low-response range, considering the wide range of susceptibilities to cancer induction in a population

TABLE 4. Synergism between Asbestos and Cigarette Smoke in the Production of Lung Cancer[a]

Group	Lung cancer
Control	28/37,000
Cigarette smoke	303/37,000
Asbestos exposure (workplace)	4/891
Both carcinogenic exposures	276/6,841

[a]From the data of E. C. Hammond, I. J. Selikoff, and H. Seidman [*Ann. N.Y. Acad. Sci.* **330**, 473 (1979)].

which is genetically highly diverse. A particular carcinogen may be considered as merely advancing the time of appearance of cancer induced through a combination of additional factors, such as genetic susceptibility and exposure to other environmental carcinogens (16). In a genetically heterogeneous population, susceptibility to lung cancer would be expected to follow a normal (Gaussian) distribution. Individuals most liable to develop a certain type of cancer would fall in the "tail" of highest susceptibility of the normal distribution curve of human susceptibility to that type of cancer (17). This "tail" would include (*see* Ref. 18) both the 0.3% of the population who carry the lung cancer–susceptibility gene reported by Sellers *et al.* (19,20) in homozygous form, as well as the 9.9% who carry it in heterozygous form. While the "tails" of a normal distribution curve are not flat, the rate of change in curvature is far smaller than the rate in the middle sections. Thus, the number of individuals who would develop cancer when exposed to increasing doses of a given carcinogen would be expected to increase in a roughly linear manner with carcinogen dose within a small segment of the low-response range. In the case of our data, this range is only 0.45–4.0%. Thus, there is either direct evidence (for tobacco) or indirect evidence (for asbestos) that the dose–response curves are close to linear in the relevant range. This satisfies the last requirement for probable synergism of column 3 in Table 1.

D. Strict Synergism (Class 4 Synergism)

Strict synergism exists if all three Conditions 1,2, and 3 for the substantiation of synergism are fulfilled. In contrast to the previous definition of strict synergism (1), there is, however, a way to circumvent the severe condition 3. If data to the end of the life span of all subjects are unavailable, then the time interval for data collection, over which strict synergism has been proven, must be stated.

Furthermore, instead of using the unwieldy method of isobolic diagrams (4) to establish strict synergism, the testing for synergism may be restricted to only a specified part of the dose–response range. In essence, the procedure involves application of Equation 1b to data read off on the nonlinear dose–response curves of the two carcinogens at appropriate points, as explained above under Section I.D. "Significance of Nonlinearity of Dose–Response Curves". The method requires a sufficient number of points for the individual dose responses of each of the two carcinogens alone so that the two dose–response curves can be drawn with adequate statistical precision in the relevant range. In Appendix I, a detailed example is given of the application of Equation 1b to such data and its test for statistical significance. The result of this testing should provide a statement on the probability that the strict synergism, if established, applies only over the specified dose ranges of the two carcinogens. If lifetime records cannot be obtained, then the time interval over which strict synergism exists should be stated. Some principles of experimental design are discussed below in Section III.D.

E. Absolute Synergism (Class 5 Synergism)

Corallini *et al.* (21) induced malignant sarcomas in 11 of 15 newborn Syrian hamsters by s.c. inoculation of a recombinant DNA that contained the early region gene of BK virus (BKV) plus the activated human c-Harvey-*ras* (c-Ha-*ras*) oncogene derived from the T24 bladder carcinoma. When, however, these two genes were inoculated separately into newborn hamsters, they were not oncogenic. Nor did the injection of a combination of the early region gene of BKV plus normal human c-Ha-*ras* proto-oncogene produce any tumors.

The data of Corallini *et al.* provide an example for the most potent form of synergism. Fitting these data into Equation 1a, one observes that the denominator becomes zero, since n_A, n_B, and n_0 all have a value of zero. Thus, the synergism evaluated by Equation 1a becomes infinitely large; hence, its designation as absolute synergism.

Cases may be encountered where the incidence of tumors elicited by chemical or physical carcinogens, administered alone, may be too low to give a valid dose–response curve. In such cases, statistical proof for absolute synergism is unattainable, but obtaining proof for probable synergism should be possible.

III. DISCUSSION

A. Definition and Statistical Considerations

Historically, approaches to the evaluation of synergism in carcinogenesis (*e.g.*, 1,3,22) were primarily concerned with finding a solution to the problem of testing for statistically valid synergism in situations where the dose–response curves of two carcinogens are nonlinear (S-shaped) rather than linear. Because the dose–response curves of many carcinogens are nonlinear, when two carcinogens are administered jointly and produce a response beyond the arithmetically additive there is a chance of attributing this excess response to synergism. However, such an increase could just as well be due to moving from the initial shallow region to the steep region of the dose–response curve of one of the two carcinogens, as the effective *total carcinogen dose* is increased by the presence of a second carcinogen.

Following the authoritative recommendations of the United Nations Scientific Committee (Annex L *in* Ref. 2), the evaluation of synergism should be based upon its definition according to Equation 1, or a close variant. If antagonism is understood as negative synergism, then any method that will substantiate synergism will also substantiate antagonism.

Definition of synergism by means of Equation 1 is empirical, and other rational definitions have been proposed. Reif and Colton (23) have used data of tumor latency, and of the time to death from tumor, to test for synergism. However, this method assumes a relationship between the time required for the appearance of a tumor (or the ability of the tumor to kill its bearer) and carcinogenic potency. While this assumption may be appropriate for a given set of conditions, it differs from the definition inherent in Equation 1. Therefore, this method should be avoided. Similarly, the use of other methods not directly based on the use of Equation 1 is not recommended. This includes nonidentical variants of Equation 1, as when curves are linearized (6), as well as the cumbersome method of isobolic diagrams (4). Instead, synergism should be tested over a specified portion of the dose–response range as indicated in Sections II.D above and III.C below.

The United Nations Scientific Committee's report (2) makes a strong case that any putative synergism in carcinogenesis should be tested by statistical methods. Even so, statistical significance should not be viewed as providing absolute certainty, but only as a probability estimate. The statistical significance of small numerical differences could still be due to chance. Similarly, a finding of negative statistical significance may have little practical value if the numerical difference being tested is large. Furthermore, the quantifiable variables tested comprise only a portion of the total. For these reasons, the actual risk ratios observed for particular study groups are as important as the significance test. The risk ratio data on human exposure to asbestos and cigarette smoke discussed in Section I.E bear this out.

For the examples on potentially synergistic carcinogenesis in humans, analyzed above in this chapter, the data are significant or suggestive that the risk for cancer in the group exposed to both carcinogens is multiplicative or hypermultiplicative, *i.e.*, is equal to or greater than the product of the risk ratios for the two groups exposed to the carcinogens singly (1). These results suggest, in turn, that all cases where two or more different types of carcinogens produce the same type of cancer should be investigated for the possibility of synergism.

The question arises then, that if such synergism is established, what action can be taken? It is this author's view that both current smokers as well as the 0.3% of people who test positive for the lung cancer–susceptibility gene (19) should be excluded from employment in uranium mining or asbestos working (24,25). The feasibility of such a policy could, of course, encounter strong societal backlash. Nonetheless, habitual smokers testing positive for the lung cancer–susceptibility gene should be warned and enjoined to stop smoking, irrespective of employment.

Synergism may exist between smoking and type of employment, posing an increased risk of cancer at sites other than those usually affected in smokers, that is, in the mouth, kidney, larynx, esophagus, bladder, and pancreas (26). Heavy consumption of alcohol should also be viewed as an unacceptable risk factor for employment in a type of work that carries an increased cancer risk due to synergism with alcohol intake (27).

B. On Interaction Between Initiation and Promotion in Epidemiological Data

By definition, complete carcinogens act both as initiators and as promoters (28). For this reason, effects ascribed to synergism actually may be the result of promotion. Cigarette smoke contains a complex mixture of complete carcinogens and promoters (29), and in both humans and animals the promotional effect appears to be predominant (30). Additive effects (31), apparent synergism, as well as inhibition (32) have all been observed in different studies on the interactive effects of inhalation of cigarette smoke and inhalation of radon and/or radon daughters. Yet all these results may represent valid observations of cancer incidence made *at different times* after exposure to radiation. In the study of Lundin *et al.* (7), observations made relatively early after radon exposure focus on the promotional effects of tobacco smoke on carcinogenesis initiated by radiation. The additive results found after a longer period (31) may indicate the gradual dying of cells initiated by radiation but not yet promoted by tobacco smoke. Finally, the lower cancer rate ("inhibition") observed after the longest follow-up time (32) is possibly indicative that the tumors induced by radiation had already been expressed in smokers, whereas those induced by radiation in nonsmokers were only now being expressed.

Whether or not this explanation is correct, the above data stress the importance of the time interval that elapses between the start of exposure to a carcinogen and the collection of data. Hence, the most complete picture is obtained when the data are collected at the end of the life span of all subjects. However, what happens earlier may also be of great interest. Finally, it should be pointed out that tobacco smoke is possibly not the only "complex carcinogen" that comprises so many different initiators and promoters and which has, consequently, a complicated time-dependent interaction with radiation.

C. Some Principles of Testing for Synergism in Animals

Tests of synergism in carcinogenesis are often performed in the high dose–response range, because this optimizes the chance that statistically significant differences between experimental groups will be obtained when relatively small numbers of animals are used.

Furthermore, the time required for tumor development is shorter. But even when the carcinogen doses are so elevated that all animals in every treated group develop tumors (*see in* Ref. 1, Table 10), data on the latent period or on the mean time to death *can* still be used for testing for synergism (23). However, such an approach involves questionable assumptions and is inconsistent with the definition of synergism in Equation 1.

Indeed, there are good reasons why high carcinogen dose levels should not be used in tests for synergism. For example, at high dose–response levels, radiations *inhibit* carcinogenesis, because the cytotoxic effects outweigh the carcinogenic effects. In addition, high doses of radiation shorten the life span and, as the result of both types of effects, tumor incidence is decreased (33). Similar considerations apply to the use of chemical carcinogens. To avoid such effects, which would invalidate the appropriateness of the experimental design and of the use of Equation 1, tumor incidence in any experimental group should not exceed approximately 80%. A further important consideration is that carcinogenesis in human populations generally occurs in the low dose–response range (2).

How can the conflicting requirements for experimental design of animal models be reconciled? As a compromise, for the combined administration of two carcinogens, the dose of each carcinogen should be that which produces a net tumor incidence of about 20%, when applied singly. The importance of the control group, for yielding the spontaneous incidence of the same type of tumor as elicited by the binary carcinogen combination, cannot be stressed enough. The dose–response curves for each of the two carcinogens must be established for the determination of strict synergism. If this is to be confined to a specified dose range, then this dose range should be limited to the range between the lower of the two tumor incidences for single exposure and the highest tumor incidence observed for joint action of the two carcinogens.

Brown (3) has suggested the use of Hewlett and Plackett's method (34) of plotting an envelope of additivity, for which Wahrendorf and Brown (35) have developed a statistical evaluation method. However, this requires documentation of the full range of the dose–response curves and sophistication in statistical analysis. In contrast, the here recommended methods fit more closely the practical needs of investigators in carcinogenesis. At any rate, a study can prove strict synergism only if it is extended to the end of the life span of all animals.

D. Comments on Experimental Design of Testing for Synergism

A preliminary experiment is necessary to investigate wide dose ranges for the three sets of administrations (carcinogens A and B given alone and together), and the magnitude of synergism as evaluated from Equation 1. If the synergism is large, then an intermediate scale experiment can be set up to provide data suitable for use in Equation 1b. The design could include a test of carcinogens A and B used separately at doses of $1a$, $3a$, and $9a$ and $1b$, $3b$, and $9b$, respectively, and together at $1(a + b)$ and $3(a + b)$. Here, $1a$ and $1b$ would be doses of carcinogens A and B, each chosen to produce a tumor incidence of 10–15% if both carcinogens are roughly equal in effectiveness. If B is far weaker than A, but effective in combined application, then that dose should be chosen as $1b$ (even though it would induce a far lower tumor incidence on separate application).

If preliminary tests suggest that the synergism is not very strong, then a more extensive definitive test is needed. Depending on the relative strengths of the two agents, the two carcinogens should be tested alone at doses arranged in a geometric series, for instance, at doses of $1a$, $3a$, $9a$, and $27a$ for A and of $1b$, $3b$, $9b$, and $27b$ for B. As above, $1a$ and $1b$ represent minimal doses of A and B that produce a significant tumor incidence, but if the two carcinogens are similar in strengths, then 1*a* and 1*b* should be chosen such that doses 3*a* and 3*b* produce roughly an equal incidence of tumors. In addition, the joint action of the two carcinogens should be tested at doses of 1*a* + 1*b*, 3*a* + 3*b*, and 9*a* + 9*b*. A test at doses of 27*a* + 27*b* is omitted, since for proper use of Equation 1b, the highest responses obtained for single administration of the two carcinogens should equal or exceed the highest response obtained for joint administration.

The advantage of this design of testing for synergism lies in its logical simplicity implicit in Equation 1b. If one of the carcinogens is so weak that an individual dose–response curve cannot be obtained, then the dose–response curve of the more potent carcinogen alone serves for comparison with combined administration.

E. Speculative Considerations on the Mechanism of Synergism

Carcinogenesis is a highly complex process that depends on the conditions of exposure to the active agents and on the reactions of the host to these agents. The conditions of exposure include factors such as the time sequence, dose, vehicle, route, and number/frequency of exposures to complete carcinogens, initiators, promoters, and inhibitors. The reactions of the host will be determined by its genetic susceptibility, its state of immune competence, age, diet, stress, and exposure to other carcinogens present in the environment (chemicals, radiations, and viruses). For chemical carcinogens, the host's reactions of metabolic disposition comprise transport, activation, conjugation, inactivation, and excretion of the agents (28,36,37). This network of interactive features and factors that determine the actual emergence of tumors (*see* Prefatory Chapter) provides many levels for potential interference with cellular homeostasis. Hence, the simultaneous (or closely sequential) administration of chemical carcinogens can result in additive, synergistic, or antagonistic effect, depending on their structures, relative doses, and route of administration.

Little is known about the mechanism(s) of synergism in carcinogenesis. However, since the malignant features of tumor cells are inheritable characteristics, and since the majority of (the genotoxic) carcinogens are known to interact with and bind to DNA, it is safe to conclude that DNA is central to the mechanism(s) of synergism. Specific regions in the genome, the oncogenes have been shown to play a key role in viral tumorigenesis and probably a similar central role in carcinogenesis by chemical agents (*see* Chapter 14). Cellular oncogenes are usually involved in mitogenic stimulation in normal cells, *i.e.*, they represent positive regulatory elements of cellular growth control (38). Chemical carcinogens and some of the carcinogenic viruses act through the activation of cellular oncogenes, resulting in altered and/or amplified expression (transcription/translation) of these genes. The various oncoproteins/growth factors that are generated interfere with the cellular signal transduction pathways of growth control and cell multiplication [*see* Chapters 5 (Section 1) and 14].

The tumor-suppressor genes (anti-oncogenes) discovered subsequently are a class of cellular genes whose normal function is to suppress signal transduction that leads to inappropriate cell proliferation, *i.e.*, they represent negative regulatory elements of cellular growth control (*e.g.*, 39). Existing data clearly indicate that the products of tumor-suppressor gene expression may interact with, modulate, or compete with onco-gene products at various points in the cascade of events leading to neoplastic transfor-mation; they presumably also function in the control of normal cell growth and differentiation, not only in cells with activated oncogenes (39). Hence, the functional loss of tumor-suppressor genes through mutation has been termed the "driving force in carcinogenesis" (40).

Many or most instances of malignant cell transformation entail the emergence of features of autocrine mitogenic stimulation, meaning that the cells will acquire the capability to synthesize growth factors as well as receptors to these factors, so that the cells become independent from the requirement for systemic and adjacent-cells–provided (*i.e.*, paracrine) growth factors. Since the altered/mutated oncogenes and tumor-suppressor genes — which underlie the emergence of these autocrine features — are inherent parts of the genome, the acquired malignant characteristics are inheritable.

The detailed mechanisms of promotion (Chapter 5) and of cell transformation (Chapter 14) provide an increasingly clear insight that cell transformation and carcinogenesis by chemical (but not always by viral) agents, is generally a multistep process. Several sequential genetic (and possibly epigenetic) alterations must occur for the fully malignant phenotype to emerge (*see also* Refs. 41–43). It has been documented (*e.g.*, 44) that differential gene expression — that is, shifts in expression pattern of genes — occurs during stages of carcinogenesis.

The results of Corallini *et al.* (21), which provide an illustration for the Class of Absolute Synergism (Section II.E), exemplify the cooperative action of two oncogenes. These authors found that combination of two different oncogenes injected into newborn Syrian hamsters produces a 73% incidence of malignant sarcomas, while injection at the same doses of either of the two oncogenes alone was not tumorigenic. This suggests that two activated oncogenes are necessary for the production of this type of tumor.

A multistep mechanism based on the activation of oncogenes may be applied to provide a rationale for the elevated lung cancer incidence of uranium miners (7) and asbestos workers (9) who smoke. In the first instance the carcinogens are radiation from radon and tobacco tar components from cigarette smoke, established to interact synergistically to induce lung cancer (*e.g.*, *rev.* 45). In the second instance the carcinogens are asbestos and the tar components from tobacco smoke. It should be noted that despite the apparent chemical inertness of asbestos fibers, there is evidence that asbestos fibers exhibit genotoxic properties and can induce chromosomal abnormalities, mutations, aneuploidy, and micronucleus induction; this is consistent with the relative ease of transport of the fibers through membranes, including the nuclear membrane (*rev.* Section 5.5 *in* ref. 46).

Suppose that lung carcinogenesis requires the action of three cellular genes: X, Y, and Z. Assume that the rate-limiting step in radiation (or asbestos) carcinogenesis is the activation of gene X, an oncogene, and for chemical carcinogenesis it is the activation of gene Y, a second oncogene. The third gene, Z, may also be an oncogene, however already in the activated state owing to a vertically transmitted oncogenic virus; another candidate for the role of Z is the lung cancer-susceptibility gene reported by Sellers *et al.* (19,20) or the gene discovered by Caporaso *et al.* (47), which strongly facilitates the activation of chemical carcinogens involved in lung carcinogenesis, present in the majority of the population.

Since the action of all three genes, X, Y, and Z, is required for lung carcinogenesis, only individuals who possess an oncogene Z in the activated form (or who possess an operationally equivalent gene) will be susceptible to the single or joint action of the two carcinogenic agents (acting on X and Y). In that case, each carcinogen would possess a higher capability to activate oncogenes that were not limiting in its own carcinogenic process. Thus, each carcinogen would provide the tumorigenic process generated by the other carcinogen with more than an additive contribution for completion of its rate-limiting step. Therefore, the combined action of the two carcinogens would be synergistic.

Alternatively, gene Y in this model may be a tumor-suppressor gene which normally down-regulates the expression of oncogene X. Thus, inactivation/mutation of this tumor-suppressor gene by the carcinogens, acting specifically on Y, will facilitate more than additively the completion of the rate-limiting step, *i.e.*, the expression of oncogene *X*.

These considerations suggest that synergism will occur in instances when the rate-limiting step in the production of a given type of tumor differs for two carcinogens. The rate-limiting steps for two carcinogens is likely to be different when the agents differ greatly in their chemical structure or physical nature (*e.g.*, radiation or asbestos fibers *vs* the complete carcinogens and promoters in cigarette smoke), because then their action is likely also to differ in the efficiency of activating oncogenes.

Oncogenes and tumor-suppressor genes represent, however, only one of the cellular operational levels providing mechanistic basis for synergism between carcinogens. Other possible levels include the induction and repression of the synthesis of mixed-function oxidases underlying the activation and detoxification of carcinogens, effects on the permeability of endocellular membranes, DNA repair, and effects on genes regulating immune response.

APPENDIX I: STATISTICAL SIGNIFICANCE

A. Significance of Linearity of Dose–Response Curves

The procedure (1,3,48,49) described here tests the statistical significance of data on the interaction of two carcinogens, both of which have linear dose–response curves, or are imputed to be linear. In this procedure, the critical ratio z is used to test whether ($n_{AB} - n_0$) significantly exceeds ($n_A - n_0$) + ($n_B - n_0$). Thus, the z-test examines the significance of a relationship that involves the interaction of the four groups AB, A, B, and 0, with fractional biological responses (such as tumor incidence) of, respectively, n_{AB}, n_A, n_B, and n_0, and groups sizes of m_{AB}, m_A, m_B, and m_0 individuals. The use of Student's t-test or Fisher's exact test as an alternative is questionable, because these were not designed to test the significance of interactions between groups.

For use in the z-test, we can define n of Equation 1 to mean $n = x/m$, where x is the number of occurrences among a subgroup of m individuals. Then,

$$z = \frac{(n_{AB} - n_A - n_B + n_0)}{[n_{AB}(1 - n_{AB})/m_{AB} + n_A(1 - n_A)/m_A + n_B(1 - n_B)/m_B + n_0(1 - n_0)/m_0]^{1/2}} \quad (4)$$

where

$$n_{AB} = x_{AB}/m_{AB} \qquad n_A = x_A/m_A \qquad n_B = x_B/m_B \qquad \text{and} \qquad n_0 = x_0/m_0 \quad (5)$$

The value of z is entered into a two-tailed normal table (a table of t) to obtain the probability p that the difference between the expected and observed effects could be fortuitous rather than due to synergism.

Statistical theory holds that the z-test is valid only if the variances of the various groups do not differ significantly when subjected to Bartlett's test. However, the data here deal with frequencies and ranges not involving variances. Therefore, Bartlett's test does not apply.

The results (summarized in Table 2) of the first experiment in the study by Sharp and Crouse (15) can be used to illustrate the simplicity of the above adaptation of the z-test. By Equation 5, $n_{AB} = 20/35$, $n_A = 1/14$, $n_B = 9/32$, and $n_0 = 0/10$. These fractions yield, respectively, 0.5714, 0.0714, 0.2812, and 0. Thus, the numerator of Equation 4 is (0.5714 − 0.0714 − 0.2812) or 0.2188, and the denominator is [0.5714(1 − 0.5714)/35

+ 0.0714(1 − 0.0714)/14 + 0.2812(1 − 0.2812)/32]$^{1/2}$ or 0.1343. Thus, $z =$ 0.2188/0.1343 or 1.629. Entering this value of z into a table of t at infinite degrees of freedom gives $p = 0.10$. Thus, the results of this first experiment lack statistical significance.

However, the data of Sharp and Crouse's second experiment (*in* Table 3) give $z = 4.5$ and $p < 0.01$ when tested by this method. This result establishes high statistical significance for synergism. Although no dose–response data were obtained in this study on the combined effect of radiation and the colon carcinogen, 1,2-dimethylhydrazine, the authors have provided statistical verification for Equation 1, thus indicating apparent synergism (Class 2 Synergism) (for which the requirements are summarized in Table 1). This is precisely their conclusion.

For the data of Hammond *et al.* (9) on the combined effect of asbestos exposure and cigarette smoking (Table 4), $z = 5.0$ and $p < 0.01$ (for discussion *see* Sections I.B.3 and II.C on "Probable Synergism").

B. Significance of Nonlinearity of Dose–Response Curves; Substantiation of Strict Synergism*

When the dose–response curves of the two carcinogens administered separately are nonlinear, use the method described for nonlinear dose–response curves and for Strict Synergism (Class 4 Synergism). To test for strict synergism, Colton's Equation 4 has been adapted to allow the testing of data inserted into Equation 1c or 1d. This adaptation corrects for the error introduced by use of the actual dose–response curve of one of the two carcinogens (namely, of carcinogen A) and consists of addition of the error term E_A:

$$z = \frac{(n_{AB} - n_{A+B})}{[n_{AB}(1 - n_{AB})/m_{AB} + n_A(1 - n_A)/m_A + n_B(1 - n_B)/m_B + n_0(1 - n_0)/m_0 + E_A]^{1/2}} \tag{6}$$

Even though the dose–response curves for the singly administered carcinogens are nonlinear, the same four results are tested (those for groups AB, A, B, and 0) as when both carcinogens possess straight-line response curves. The only difference is that the dose–response curve of A is utilized for readings at two different points.

The dose–response curve of carcinogen A (usually the more potent of the two carcinogens) should be plotted to yield a straight-line fit. Standard computer methods (*e.g.*, a Gompertz transformation performed using UCLA's BMPD program for curve fitting) can be used to fit a straight line to the data, which may be sigmoidal. The method used should be stated, but the error introduced by fitting data to a straight line is far smaller than the experimental error of each data point.

In order to tie the dose–response curve closely to the points P and Q at which readings are taken, the plotting should be restricted to points that run from the first one that lies below the lower read-off point P to the first one that lies above the higher read-off point Q (*see* Figure 1). Point P falls where the biological response produced by carcinogen B is plotted on the curve to read off the dose of A that produces the same (and thus equivalent) response as does B. Point Q represents the sum of this B-equivalent dose of A plus the actual applied dose of A. Then the biological response A + B, which is expected for joint action of the two carcinogens if they acted purely additively, is read off from the curve at Q.

The errors of these two readings P and Q are closely related to the errors of the experimental points on the curve, close to where these two readings are taken. If P or Q

---

*See "Note Added in Proof" in p. 71.

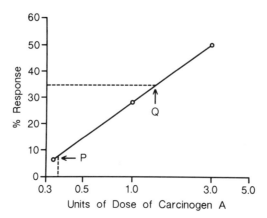

FIGURE 1. Use of the dose–response curve of carcinogen A for quantifying synergism in carcinogenesis by means of Equation 1b. If A and B acted additively, then the response of 7.1% produced by separate administration of carcinogen B, which plots at point P on the dose–response curve of A, is equivalent to 0.36 dose units of carcinogen A given alone. Then, for joint application of A and B, the expected additive response is that for 1.0 + 0.36 = 1.36 dose units of A; this is read off on the curve at point Q as 34.0%. This calculated response for additive action is then compared to the experimental response obtained for joint administration. The amount by which the experimental response exceeds the additive response quantifies synergism. This example is based on the data from Sharp and Crouse (15), complemented by addition of two hypothetical points at 0.33 and 3.0 units of A.

lies very close to one of those points, then the error reading for that point can be utilized. For instance, consider point 1, which is one of the points used to draw the dose–response curve A, and represents a fractional experimental response of n_{A1} for a group numbering m_{A1} individuals. For this point, the error term corresponding to those in Equation 6 is n_{A1} $(1 - n_{A1})/m_{A1}$. Equivalent error terms apply to other experimental points from which this curve was drawn. Then if point P falls very close to an experimental point such as point 1, its error term will be essentially identical to that for point 1, namely, $n_{A1} (1 - n_{A1})/m_{A1}$. On the other hand, if P lies intermediate between the two experimental points 1 and 2, then its error is obtained by prorating its fractional distance from those two points. For instance, if P lies one-fourth the distance beyond point 1 on the way to point 2, then its error term will be $0.75\, n_{A1} (1 - n_{A1})/m_{A1} + 0.25\, n_{A2} (1 - n_{A2})/m_{A2}$. In the case when point P lies a fractional distance f beyond p, and thus, lies between the experimental points p and q that were used to draw curve A, its error term will be

$$E_X = (1-f)n_{Ap}(1-n_{Ap})/m_{Ap}+f \cdot n_{Aq}(1-n_{Aq})/m_{Aq} \qquad (7)$$

Similarly, the error term for point Q can be estimated with Equation 7. Then the combined error term for the two readings P and Q is given by:

$$E_A = (E_X+E_Y)/1.414 \qquad (8)$$

Examples for the use of Equations 6, 7, and 8 follow. We shall use the data from the first experiment of Sharp and Crouse (Table 2) for single exposure to 1,2-dimethyl-hydrazine (carcinogen A) and single radiation exposure (carcinogen B). They evaluated the tumor incidence 8 months after application of the carcinogens to their four groups, which correspond to 0 (0/10), A (9/32), B (1/14), and AB (20/35). For the present example, assume that they had also used carcinogen A alone at doses of 1/3 and 3 times (*i.e.*, at

0.33 and 3.0 dose units, as contrasted with the dose of 1.0 unit that they actually used), and obtained tumor incidences of 2/32 and 5/10 at 8 months. In that case, a dose–response curve can be constructed for carcinogen A (1,2-dimethylhydrazine), based on these two supposed and on the one determined point. A straight line can be obtained by plotting, on semilogarithmic graph paper, the three doses (0.33,1.0, and 3.0 dose units of A) along the logarithmic x-axis and the three responses (6.25,28.1, and 50.0%) along the linear y-axis. Then the tumor incidence of 1/14 or 7.14% produced by carcinogen B (radiation) can be read off from the dose–response curve of A at point P, as being equivalent to that produced by 0.36 dose units of carcinogen A (*see* Figure 1). Then the effect of administering carcinogens A and B together should be 1.0 + 0.36 or 1.36 dose units, if they were acting purely additively. From the dose–response curve of A, 1.38 carcinogen units are read off at Q as giving a tumor incidence of 34.0%; thus $n_{A+B} = 0.340$.

The following values may now be substituted into Equation 6:

$$n_{AB} = 20/35 \quad \text{or} \quad 0.5714, \qquad n_{A+B} = 0.340, \qquad n_A = 1/14 \quad \text{or} \quad 0.0714,$$
$$n_B = 9/32 \quad \text{or} \quad 0.2812, \qquad \text{and} \qquad n_0 = 0.$$

Then,

$$z = (0.5714 - 0.340)/[0.5714(1 - 0.5714)/35 + 0.0714(1 - 0.0714)/14$$
$$+ 0.2812(1 - 0.2812)/32 + E_A]^{1/2}$$
$$= 0.2314/[0.0070 + 0.0047 + 0.0063 + E_A]^{1/2}$$
$$= 0.2314/[0.0180 + E_A]^{1/2}$$

In our example, subscript X is an indicator for a tumor incidence of 7.14%, which lies close to the assumed experimental result of 2 tumor-bearers out of 32 animals, or 6.25%. Then Equation 7 yields $E_X = (1.0)(0.0625)(1 - 0.0625)/32 = 0.0018$.

Point Q plots beyond point 2 on curve A, and lies at 0.21 of the total distance between points 2 and 3. In our example, experimental points 2 and 3 represent tumor incidences of, respectively, 9/32 (or 28.1%), and of 5/10 (or 50.0%). Then Equation 7 gives $E_Y = [(0.79)(0.281)(1 - 0.281)/32] + [(0.21)(0.500)(1 - 0.500)/10] = 0.0050 + 0.0053 = 0.0103$. Further, Equation 8 yields $E_A = (0.0018 + 0.0103)/1.414 = 0.0121/1.414 = 0.0086$. Substitution of this value of E_A into Equation 6 gives $z = 0.2314/[0.0180 + 0.0086]^{1/2} = 0.2314/[0.0266]^{1/2} = 1.42$. This value of z corresponds to $p < 0.20$, indicating that the synergism found is not statistically significant. With the assumption of straight-line dose–response curves for the two carcinogens, as for the data analyzed in the previous section, $p \cong 0.10$ was obtained. As expected, nonlinear dose–response curves make achievement of statistical significance more difficult. If this result had been statistically significant, it would have met the criteria for substantiating strict synergism.

C. If Tumor Incidence in the Control Group Is Unknown

In the situation where data for biological response are lacking for a control group, then the safest assumption that can be made is that this response (n_0) is zero. This assumption will not affect the validity of the statistical test of synergism, since $n_0 = 0$ makes it actually more difficult to obtain significance in this test than with any other value for n_0. The reason is that Equation 1 for the evaluation of synergism can be written in the form as it is found in the numerator of Equation 4, namely, as

$$(n_{AB} + n_0) - (n_A + n_B) > 0 \tag{1e}$$

Thus, the larger the value of n_0, the greater the value of $(n_{AB} + n_0) - (n_A + n_B)$, and thus the greater the synergism. An example (Table 5) will serve to verify this assumption.

TABLE 5.   **Data Demonstrating Optimal Significance of Synergism When Control Tumor Incidence n_0 is Zero**

Column:	1	2	3
	Tumor incidence	When $n_0 = 0/20$, $n - n_0$ is[a]	When $n_0 = 8/20$, $n - n_0$ is[a]
n_0	Unknown	—	—
n_A	9/20	9/20	1/20
n_B	9/18	9/20	1/20
n_{AB}	18/20	18/20	10/20
Numerator of Equation 4	—	0	0.4
z	—	0	1.96
p	—	—	0.05

[a]For the line beginning with n_A, $n - n_0$ means $n_A - n_0$, etc.

For the hypothetical data given in column 1, n_0 is unknown. If n_0 is 0/20 (column 2), then the numerator of Equation 5 is also zero and there is neither synergism nor antagonism. If n_0 is 8/20, then the numerator of Equation 4 indicates that there is synergism, and application of Colton's z-test shows that this is significant at the 5% level. If intermediate levels of n_0 rising from 0/20 to 8/20 are chosen, then intermediate values of z and of p are obtained. Thus, the value of n_0 that makes it most difficult to substantiate synergism statistically is when n_0 is zero.

In the above example (column 3 of table 5, where $n_0 = 8/20$), p is significant only when n_A and n_B are both 1/20, but not when either one has any higher value such as 2/10. In other words, the present statistical test is rather rigorous regarding the degree of synergism required for producing a significant result. In that case, one can be certain that strict synergism has really been substantiated. On the other hand, the power of this method to detect marginal levels of synergism is questionable.

An alternative test for the statistical validity of synergism based on probability theory is given in the review (2). However, there are conditions of experimental design under which the appropriateness of this test becomes questionable (1,3).

REFERENCES

1.   Reif, A. E.: *J. Natl. Cancer Inst.* **73**, 25 (1984).
2.   United Nations Scientific Committee on the Effects of Atomic Radiations: "Ionizing Radiation: Sources and Biological Effects". United Nations, New York, 1982, p. 727.
3.   Brown, C. C.: *J. Natl. Cancer Inst.* **74**, 730 (1985).
4.   Loewe, S: *Arzneim. Forsch.* **3**, 285 (1953).
5.   Valeriote, F., and Lin, H.: *Cancer Chem. Rep.* **59**, 895 (1975).
6.   Steel, G. C., and Peckham, M. J.: *Int. J. Radiat. Oncol. Biol. Phys.* **5**, 85 (1979).
7.   Lundin, F. E., Lloyd, J. W., Smith, E. M., Archer, V. E., and Holaday, D.A.: *Health Phys.* **16**, 571 (1969).
8.   Band, P., Feldstein, M., Saccomanno, G., Watson, L., and King, G.: *Cancer* **45**, 1273 (1980).
9.   Hammond, E. C., Selikoff, I. J., and Seidman, H.: *Ann. N.Y. Acad. Sci.* **330**, 473 (1979).
10.   Meurman, L. O., Kiviluoto, R., and Hakama, M.: *Ann. N.Y. Acad. Sci.* **330**, 491 (1979).
11.   Rothman, K. J., and Keller, A.: *J. Chronic. Dis.* **25**, 711 (1972).
12.   Kolonel, L. N.: *Cancer* **37**, 1782 (1976).
13.   American Cancer Society: "Cancer Facts and Figures 1983". American Cancer Society, New York, 1982, p. 14.
14.   Reif, A. E.: *Natl. Cancer Inst. Monogr.* **52**, 123 (1979).
15.   Sharp, J. G., and Crouse, D. A.: *Radiation Res.* **117**, 304 (1989),
16.   Reif, A. E.: *Oncology* **38**, 76 (1981).

17. Reif, A. E.: *Cancer* **57**, 2408 (1986).
18. Reif, A. E.: *J. Natl. Cancer Inst.* **83**, 64 (1991).
19. Sellers, T. A., Bailey-Wilson, J. E., Elston, R. C., Wilson, A. F., Elston, G. Z., Ooi, W. L., and Rothschild, H.: *J. Natl. Cancer Inst.* **82**, 1272 (1990).
20. Sellers, T. A., Bailey-Wilson, J. E., Elston, R. C., and Rothschild, H.: *J. Natl. Cancer Inst.* **83**, 65 (1991).
21. Corallini, A., Pagnani, M., Viadana, P., Camellin, P., Caputo, A., Reschiglian, P., Rossi, S., Altavilla, G., and Barbanti-Brodano, G.: *Cancer Res.* **47**, 6671 (1987)
22. Bois, F. Y., and Vasseur, P.: *J. Natl. Cancer Inst.* **74**, 729 (1985).
23. Reif, A. E., and Colton, T.: *Carcinogenesis* **5**, 837 (1984).
24. Knudson, A. G., Jr.: *New Engl. J. Med.* **301**, 606 (1979).
25. Fraumeni, J. F., Jr. (ed.): "Persons at High Risk of Cancer". Academic Press, New York, 1975.
26. U.S. Department of Health and Human Services: "The Health Consequences of Smoking. Cancer. A Report of the Surgeon General." Office on Smoking and Health, Rockville, Maryland, 1982.
27. McCoy, G. D., Hecht, S. S., and Wynder, E. L.: *Prev. Med.* **9**, 622 (1980).
28. Potter, V. R.: *Yale J. Biol. Med.* **53**, 367 (1980).
29. Wynder, E. L., and Hoffman, D.: *New Engl. J. Med.* **300**, 894 (1979).
30. Van Duuren, B. L., Sivak, A., Katz, C., and Melchionne, S.: *J. Natl. Cancer Inst.* **47**, 235 (1971).
31. Radford, E. P.: Radon Daughters in the Induction of Lung Cancer in Underground Miners. *In* "Banbury Report 9. Quantification of Occupational Cancer". (R. Peto and M. Schneiderman, eds.). Cold Spring Harbor Laboratory, Cold Spring Harbor, New York, 1981, p. 151.
32. Axelson, O., and Sundell, L.: *Scand. J. Environ. Health* **4**, 46 (1978).
33. Reif, A. E.: *Nature* **190**, 415, (1961).
34. Hewlett, P. S., and Plackett, R. L.: *Biometrics* **15**, 591 (1959).
35. Wahrendorf, J., and Brown, C. C.: *Biometrics* **36**, 653 (1980).
36. Farber, E.: *New Engl. J. Med.* **305**, 1379 (1981).
37. Pitot, H. C.: *Cancer* **49**, 1206 (1982).
38. Heldin, C. H., Betsholtz, C., Claesson-Welch, L., and Westermark, B.: *Biochim. Biophys. Acta* **907**, 219 (1987).
39. Boyd, J. A., and Barrett, J. C.: *Mol. Carcinogenesis* **3**, 325 (1990).
40. Bouck, N. P., and Benton, B. K.: *Chem. Res. Toxicol.* **2**, 1 (1989).
41. Land, H., Parada, L. F., and Weinberg, R. A.: *Nature* **304**, 596 (1983).
42. Whittemore, A. S.: *Adv. Cancer Res.* **27**, 55 (1978).
43. Holden, C.: *Science* **222** 602 (1983).
44. Bowden, G. T., and Krieg, P.: *Environ. Health Perspect.* **93**, 51 (1991).
45. Cothern, C. R.: *Environ. Carcino. Rev.* **C7**, 75 (1989).
46. Woo, Y. T., Lai, D. Y., Arcos, J. C., and Argus, M. F.: "Chemical Induction of Cancer, Vol. IIIC, Natural, Metal, Fiber, and Macromolecular Carcinogens". Academic Press, San Diego, 1988.
47. Caporaso, N. E., Tucker, M. A., Hoover, R. N., Hayes, R. B., Pickle, L. W., Issaq, H. J., Muschik, G. M., Green-Gallo, L., Buivys, D., Aisner, S., Resau, J. H., Trump, B. F., Tollerud, D., Weston, A., and Harris, C. C.: *J. Natl. Cancer Inst.* **82**, 1264 (1990).
48. Colton, T.: "Statistics in Medicine". Little, Brown, Boston, 1974, p. 163.
49. Hogan, M. D., Kupper, L. L., Most, B. M., and Haseman, J. K.: *Am. J. Epidemiol.* **108**, 60 (1978).

Note Added in Proof: The author has advised the Editors of a reinterpretation of the error term (or variance) in Equation 6 on p. 67. This variance should read E_A^2. Following up this reinterpretaion Equation 7 should read:

$$E_X^2 = (1-f)^2 n_{Ap}(1-n_{Ap})/m_{Ap} + f^2 \cdot n_{Aq}(1-n_{Aq})/m_{Aq}$$

and Equation 8 should read:

$$E_A^2 = (E_X^2 + E_Y^2)/2$$

where the denominator is the number of readings, 2 in this case.

Substitution of the same data from Sharp and Crouse into the modified Equation 6 yields $z = 1.58$, which corresponds to $p = 0.11$ rather than $p < 0.20$ on p. 69.

CHAPTER **4**

Inhibition of Chemical Carcinogenesis[1]

Gary J. Kelloff, Charles W. Boone, Vernon E. Steele, Judith R. Fay, and Caroline C. Sigman

I. INTRODUCTION

More than 1500 naturally occurring and synthetic chemicals have been tested for inhibition of chemically induced carcinogenesis in experimental models (1,2). Among the chemicals tested, representatives of numerous structural and biological activity classes have been found to be inhibitors. Examples of structural classes of inhibitors are arylalkyl isothiocyanates, cinnamyl compounds, flavonoids, glucarates, indoles, polyphenols, retinoids and carotenoids, and thiols and sulfides. Biological activity classes include antihormones, anti-inflammatory agents, antioxidants, arachidonic acid (AA) metabolism inhibitors, glutathione (GSH) inducers, ornithine decarboxylase (ODC) inhibitors, and protein kinase C (PKC) inhibitors. These chemicals and their likely mechanisms of activity are the subject of this chapter. Although the experimental systems used to evaluate inhibitory activity include various cell cultures and carcinogenesis-related endpoints (*e.g.*, mutagenicity, precancerous lesions, DNA binding, enzyme activities) other than the definitive appearance of tumors, much research on inhibition of chemical carcinogenesis is indeed carried out in animal models with tumors as the endpoints; this review concentrates on the results of these studies in animals.

Besides their utility in elucidating the process of carcinogenesis, there is a practical application of the inhibitors as cancer chemoprophylactic or chemopreventive agents. Sporn and Newton (3) coined the term chemoprevention to describe the administration of agents to prevent the induction or to inhibit or delay the progression of tumors. Wattenberg, who is to be credited for much of the research on inhibitors of carcinogenesis in animal models that is described in this chapter, also pioneered the study of inhibitors as chemopreventive agents (*e.g.*, 4–8). Since 1985, a great deal of progress has been made in development of chemopreventive agents for clinical use, and the Chemoprevention Branch of the National Cancer Institute has established a drug development program for chemopreventives. This program is summarized at the end of this chapter.

---

[1]For Abbreviations used, *see* p. 108.

II. EXPERIMENTAL SYSTEMS

Numerous animal models are used to study the inhibition of chemical carcinogenesis. Those that have been used frequently are listed in Table 1, along with the references. Most studies are carried out in rats, mice, or hamsters. Typically, a carcinogen is administered to the animal at a dose level high enough to induce a significant incidence of tumors in a specific target tissue. The carcinogen dose and treatment schedule are usually selected to ensure that the tumor incidence is not so high as to mask the potential of the inhibitor to reduce tumorigenicity. The inhibitor is administered before, simultaneously with, or after the administration of the carcinogen; or the administration of the inhibitors can be in any combination of these relative times, if administration is repeated. The relative timing of the administration of the carcinogen and the inhibitor can be useful in interpreting the

TABLE 1.   Animal Models for Studies of Carcinogenesis Inhibition

Organ Model	Species	Carcinogen	Endpoint: inhibition of	References
Buccal pouch	Hamster	DMBA	Squamous cell carcinoma, papilloma	135,136,147,314
Colon	Mouse	AOM, DMH, MAM	Adenocarcinoma, adenoma	41,86,105,133,148,153, 164,165,224,230,317,489, 491,497–499
	Rat	AOM, DMH, MAM, MNU	Adenocarcinoma, adenoma	19,101,149,232,318,319, 321,540,550
Esophagus	Rat	Nitrosamines	Squamous cell carcinoma, papilloma	87,107,157,322,523
Forestomach	Mouse	BaP	Squamous cell carcinoma, papilloma	45,82,88,91,97,156,166, 167,323,490,515,563,564
Liver	Rat	Various	Hepatocellular carcinoma, adenoma	106,157,324–326,456
Lung	Mouse	BaP, DMBA, NNK, urethan	Adenoma	44,45,49,60–62,88,91, 102,169,490,515,564
Mammary glands	Mouse	DMBA	Adenocarcinoma, adenoma	333–335,339,340,491,515
	Rat	DMBA	Adenocarcinoma, adenoma	5,62,77,79,97,153,155, 156,158–163,188,190,191, 233,234,252–254,258,295, 329–338,340–346,408,425, 430,431,490,491,515, 521,527,528,535
		MNU	Adenocarcinoma, adenoma	78,158,160,187,189,235, 236,252,255–258,408,501, 524,529
Pancreas	Hamster	BOP	Ductal adenocarcinoma, adenoma	327
Skin	Mouse	BaP, DMBA, 3-MC	Carcinoma, papilloma	37,38,52–54,63,64, 67–74,138–141,150,151, 184,199–207,209,226,237
		BaP/TPA, DMBA/TPA, DMBA/other promoters	Papilloma, carcinoma	238,241,251,439,450, 503,511,520,548,549
Urinary bladder	Mouse	OH-BBN	Transitional cell carcinoma	234,256,259,467,471,472
	Rat	MNU, OH-BBN	Transitional cell carcinoma	239,240,464–466,468–470, 517,518

Note: For additional examples, *see* Ref. 1 and Tables 3–9.

mechanism of inhibition. For example, a compound that inhibits when it is administered before the carcinogen, but not when it is given after the carcinogen treatment schedule is completed, most likely inhibits the initiation phase of carcinogenesis.

Typically the studies are carried out as long as needed for the carcinogen to induce a high tumor incidence. Because the activity of most of the carcinogens used is well known, these tests are usually shorter than chronic carcinogenicity studies. Most often, they are of 6 months to 1 year in duration. Inhibition is usually measured as the percentage by which the inhibitor lowers the incidence, multiplicity, or total number of tumors, or increases the latency of the induction of tumors. Sometimes such factors as tumor size and degree of invasiveness are considered. Results usually are determined by histopathological evaluation of the target tissues, although gross pathology may also be used. For example, rat mammary tumors are often detected by palpation, and mouse skin tumors are determined by visual observation.

Some general guidelines have been suggested for interpreting the results of testing a potential inhibitor of carcinogenesis (1). For a test to indicate an inhibitory effect, the chemical must cause a statistically significant ($p < 0.05$) decrease in tumor incidence, multiplicity, size, or invasiveness, or a statistically significant increase in tumor latency compared with the carcinogen controls. Tumor latency is measured as the time to appearance of the first tumor or the time to 50% tumor incidence. In the absence of statistics, at least a twofold decrease in incidence, multiplicity, size, or invasiveness, or a similar increase in latency, should be observed to confirm an inhibitory effect. A result is considered suggestive if no statistical analyses are performed, but the inhibition ranges from 35 to 50%. These criteria are for a *single* dose of a potentially inhibitory chemical. However, if at least three inhibitor doses are used and a dose response of inhibition is observed, the result may be considered positive even if the inhibition is not significant statistically and the twofold decrease (above) is not observed at any of the individual doses.

Regardless of the magnitude of the effect observed, other factors are considered in determining that a test is an adequate measure of inhibition. First, the numbers of animals in the treatment and control groups should be sufficient to demonstrate statistical significance. Animal survival in both test and control groups should be adequate to allow statistical evaluation, *i.e.*, the toxicities observed due to carcinogen or inhibitor treatment should not be so severe as to compromise the results of the study. Evidence of carcinogenicity should be established in concurrently run carcinogen-treated control animals. Examples of specific conditions that can call the adequacy of a test into question are: statistically significant lower body weights in animals treated with inhibitor compared with carcinogen controls; a relatively small number of animals used; and a lower than expected tumor incidence in the carcinogen control group. Body weight is a particularly meaningful and confounding factor in inhibition experiments, since decreased or delayed weight gain is a measure of slowed growth. Slowed growth alone can depress tumorigenicity without other specific effects of an inhibitor.

Table 1 exemplifies studies which were adequately conducted according to the criteria listed above. All discussions on inhibitors in this chapter refer to chemicals tested according to these criteria.

III. MECHANISMS OF INHIBITION

Figure 1 gives a schematic representation of the process of chemical carcinogenesis — the emergence and progression of a malignant tumor. The process starts with cells in normal tissue which are then initiated and gradually progress through the precancerous stage and finally into malignant (*i.e.*, invasive) cancer (9). Some of the mechanisms by which inhibitors of chemical carcinogenesis may act at various steps are indicated in Figure 1. These mechanisms have been the subject of several excellent reviews (particularly 6–8, 10–17) and are summarized below.

The activities represented in Figure 1 fall into general mechanistic groupings. Wattenberg (6–8) established first an organizational framework for the classification of inhibitors, based on the stage in carcinogenesis when they are effective. Inhibitors were divided into three categories: (a) compounds that prevent the formation of carcinogens from their precursors, and these may be termed "preventing agents", (b) compounds that inhibit carcinogenesis by preventing carcinogenic agents from reaching or reacting with critical targets in the tissues, *i.e.*, they perform a barrier function and hence have been termed "blocking agents"; and (c) inhibitors that act subsequent to exposure to carcinogenic agents and are termed "suppressing agents" because they act by suppressing the expression of neoplasia in cells that have been exposed to doses of carcinogens which would otherwise induce tumors. The classification used in the present chapter is a modification of Wattenberg's. Following the classification used here, *Blocking activities* are those which prevent a carcinogen from reaching or reacting with target sites. This includes such activities as prevention of carcinogen activation, enhancement of carcinogen detoxification, and inhibition of carcinogen–DNA adduct formation. *Antioxidant activities*, which may be either blocking or suppressing, include free radical and electrophile scavenging. In contrast to blocking activities, *Suppressing* or (as termed in this chapter) *Antiproliferative/antiprogression activities*, do not directly affect carcinogens. Rather, these activities inhibit cellular processes involved in the proliferation, or progression of genetic and other lesions, induced by carcinogens. Activities such as restoring normal cell growth and differentiation, and inhibition of the tissue destruction associated with carcinogenesis fall in this category. Table 2 lists the mechanisms of inhibition shown in Figure 1, grouped into these three general categories. The mechanisms of inhibition are not yet well understood; what is known of the action of carcinogenesis inhibitors is briefly reviewed below. It should be noted that a correlation with inhibition of carcinogenesis does not necessarily confirm that a given mechanism is the most important or the only mechanism by which carcinogenic activity is inhibited. As will become evident from the brief review below, many of the inhibitors have potential for acting by multiple mechanisms.

Where appropriate, data in Tables 3 to 9 are cited as supporting evidence for the discussion on mechanisms. These tables list inhibitors of chemical carcinogenesis classified by chemical structure (*e.g.*, retinoids/carotenoids, thiols/dithiolthiones/sulfides) and biological activity (*e.g.*, AA metabolism inhibitors, ODC inhibitors). The tables also summarize the inhibitory activities of the chemicals against carcinogenesis in animals (specifying the tissues, species, and carcinogens). Only results of studies considered to be adequate by the criteria described in Section II are cited in these tables. The inhibitors cited in the tables are discussed in more detail in Section IV.

A. Blocking Activities

1. Inhibition of Carcinogen Uptake

Inhibitors with this activity appear to react directly with putative carcinogens, either initiators or promoters. For example, calcium inhibits the promotion of colon

FIGURE 1. The various biological activities of tumorigenesis inhibitors modulate the carcinogenic process at different stages in the progress toward malignancy: a schematic representation.

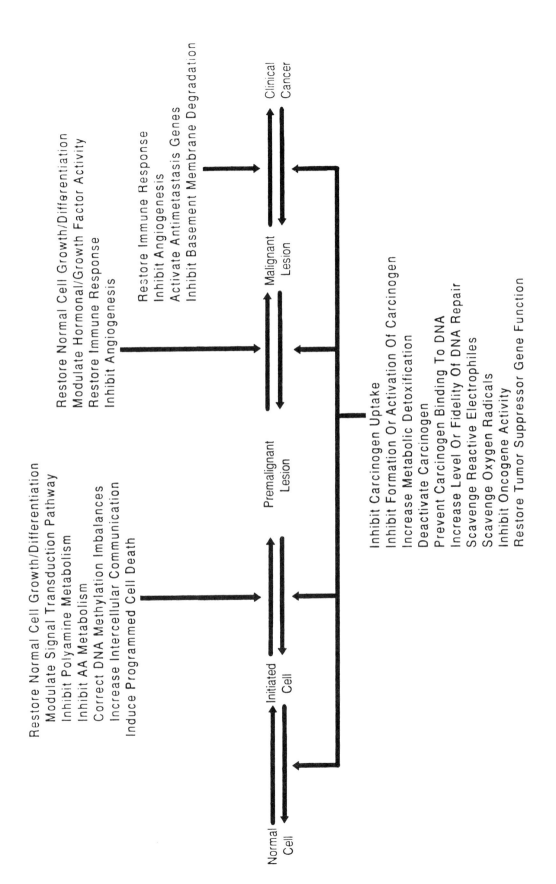

Restore Normal Cell Growth/Differentiation
Modulate Signal Transduction Pathway
Inhibit Polyamine Metabolism
Inhibit AA Metabolism
Correct DNA Methylation Imbalances
Increase Intercellular Communication
Induce Programmed Cell Death

Restore Normal Cell Growth/Differentiation
Modulate Hormonal/Growth Factor Activity
Restore Immune Response
Inhibit Angiogenesis

Restore Immune Response
Inhibit Angiogenesis
Activate Antimetastasis Genes
Inhibit Basement Membrane Degradation

Inhibit Carcinogen Uptake
Inhibit Formation Or Activation Of Carcinogen
Increase Metabolic Detoxification
Deactivate Carcinogen
Prevent Carcinogen Binding To DNA
Increase Level Or Fidelity Of DNA Repair
Scavenge Reactive Electrophiles
Scavenge Oxygen Radicals
Inhibit Oncogene Activity
Restore Tumor Suppressor Gene Function

Normal Cell

Initiated Cell

Premalignant Lesion

Malignant Lesion

Clinical Cancer

TABLE 2. **Possible Mechanisms of Inhibition of Chemical Carcinogenesis**

Blocking activities

Inhibit carcinogen uptake (*e.g.*, calcium)

Inhibit formation or activation of carcinogen (*e.g.*, allylic sulfides, arylalkyl isothiocyanates, aspirin, benzoflavones, disulfiram, indole-3-carbinol, polyphenols, vitamin C)

Deactivate carcinogen (*e.g.*, ellagic acid, GSH)

Increase metabolic detoxification by enzymatic reaction (*e.g.*, oltipraz, BHA)

Prevent carcinogen binding to DNA (*e.g.*, ellagic acid)

Increase level or fidelity of DNA repair (*e.g.*, coumarin, NAC, protease inhibitors)

Antioxidant activities

Scavenge reactive electrophiles (*e.g.*, GSH, 4-mercaptobenzenesulfonate, NAC, sodium thiosulfate)

Scavenge oxygen radicals (*e.g.*, BHA, BHT, β-carotene, CuDIPS, GSH, NAC, propyl gallate, vitamin E)

Inhibit arachidonic acid metabolism (*e.g.*, 4-bromophenacyl bromide, curcumin, flavonoids, glucocorticoids, NDGA, NSAIDs)

Antiproliferative/antiprogression activities

Modulate signal transduction (*e.g.*, 18β-glycyrrhetinic acid, NSAIDs, D,L-palmitoylcarnitine, tamoxifen)

Modulate hormonal/growth factor activity (*e.g.*, retinoic acid, tamoxifen)

Inhibit oncogene activity (*e.g.*, indomethacin, D-limonene, nerolidol)

Inhibit polyamine metabolism (*e.g.*, DFMO, 18β-glycyrrhetinic acid, GSH, NSAIDs, D,L-palmitoylcarnitine, tamoxifen)

Induce terminal differentiation (*e.g.*, calcium, DMSO, retinoids, vitamin D_3)

Restore immune response (*e.g.*, indomethacin, selenium, vitamin E)

Increase intercellular communication (*e.g.*, β-carotene, retinoic acid)

Restore tumor suppressor function

Induce programmed cell death (apoptosis) (*e.g.*, tamoxifen)

Correct DNA methylation imbalances (*e.g.*, folic acid, methionine)

Inhibit angiogenesis (*e.g.*, NSAIDs)

Inhibit basement membrane degradation (*e.g.*, protease inhibitors)

Activate antimetastasis genes

---

tumors induced in rats by azoxymethane (AOM) (18), by 1,2-dimethylhydrazine (DMH) (19), and by high dietary fat. It also inhibits colonic hyperproliferation induced in rats by *N*-methyl-*N'*-nitro-*N*-nitrosoguanidine (MNNG) (20), in mice by deoxycholic acid (21), fatty acids (22), or cholic acid (23), and in rats and mice by a Western "stress" diet, *i.e.*, a diet low in calcium and vitamin D and high in fat and phosphate (24). A partial explanation of these effects is that calcium binds to excess bile and free fatty acids that irritate the colon lumen and promote the formation of tumors (21,22,24,25).

2. Inhibition of the Formation or Activation of Carcinogens

Perhaps the best known inhibitor in this group is vitamin C. For example, in mice, vitamin C inhibits the induction of lung tumors by the combination of methylurea and nitrite, all compounds being administered orally (26). One of the activities of the vitamin is its reaction with nitrite at acidic pH (such as in the stomach after oral administration), thereby blocking the formation of potentially carcinogenic *N*-nitroso compounds (such as *N*-methyl-*N*-nitrosourea [MNU] formed from methylurea and nitrite) (13,27–32). Phenolic compounds such as gallic, ferulic, and caffeic acids (6,33) and vitamin E (6,34) prevent the formation of nitrosamines from their precursors by scavenging nitrite. Gallic acid inhibits the induction of lung tumors by morpholine and nitrite in strain A mice (26), demonstrating that such compounds inhibit the carcinogenicity of nitrosatable substrates in animals.

Another method of inhibiting formation of a carcinogen is prevention of metabolic activation of a procarcinogen. Many classes of inhibitors have this type of activity, including allylic sulfides, arylalkyl isothiocyanates, and flavonoids and other polyphenols. For example, the polyphenol, ellagic acid, is a well-known inhibitor of cytochrome P-450 enzymes that activate polycyclic aromatic hydrocarbon (PAH) carcinogens, such as benzo[a]pyrene (BaP) and 3-methylcholanthrene (3-MC). This inhibition is observed in the lungs of strain A mice (35,36) and in cultured mouse keratinocytes (37). In accord with this probable mechanism, ellagic acid inhibits PAH-induced skin tumors in mice by both topical (38) and oral administration (37).

Disulfiram and other carbamates inhibit the activation of DMH (39). Accordingly, these compounds inhibit the carcinogenicity of DMH in mouse colon (40,41). The arylalkyl isothiocyanates are also known to affect a number of activities associated with nitrosamine metabolism, including the crucial step of α-C-hydroxylation (42–44). These compounds are potent inhibitors of nitrosamine-induced tumors. Benzyl isothiocyanate inhibits the induction of forestomach tumors in mice by N,N-diethylnitrosamine (DEN) (45). Phenylethyl isothiocyanate (PEITC) inhibits the induction of lung tumors in mice and rats by N'-nitrosonornicotine (NNN) (44,46,47), and PEITC analogs with longer alkyl chains, such as phenylbutyl and, particularly, phenylhexyl isothiocyanate, are even more effective than their parent compound in inhibiting 4-(methylnitrosamino)-1-(3-pyridyl)-1-butanone (NNK)-induced lung tumors in mice (47–49).[2]

3. Deactivation of Carcinogens

Inhibitors can deactivate specific carcinogens by binding to them. This activity is a subset of the more general mechanism of electrophile scavenging described in Section III.B.1. Ellagic acid is a well-known example, which binds to BaP-diolepoxide, the activated form of BaP, thereby preventing BaP from binding to DNA (50). As already noted, ellagic acid protects against the carcinogenicity of BaP. GSH is a prototype of carcinogen scavengers. It reacts spontaneously or via catalysis by GSH S-transferases with numerous activated carcinogens, including MNNG, aflatoxin B$_1$ (AFB$_1$), and BaP-diolepoxide and other activated PAHs (10,51). Likewise, GSH protects against mouse skin tumors induced by 7,12-dimethylbenz[a]anthracene (DMBA)/12-O-tetradecanoylphorbol-13-acetate (TPA) (52–54), rat forestomach tumors induced by MNNG (55), and rat liver tumors induced by AFB$_1$ (56).

4. Increase of Detoxification by Enzymatic Reaction

Carcinogen detoxification is generally regarded as a very important mechanism of inhibition (6,8). Two metabolic pathways are critical. The first is the introduction or exposure of polar groups (*e.g.*, hydroxyl groups) on xenobiotic compounds via the Phase I metabolic enzymes, which are primarily the microsomal mixed-function oxidases. In many cases, the polar groups may become substrates for conjugation. The

---

[2]The acronym NNK for *Nicotine-derived Nitrosamino Ketone* — deeply embedded in the literature *before the exact structure of the compound was established* — is the term for one of the three products resulting from the nitrosation of nicotine, together with NNN (above) and NNA (*Nicotine-derived Nitrosamino Aldehyde*).

second pathway is via the Phase II metabolic enzymes, which are responsible for conjugation and the formation of glucuronides, GSH conjugates, and sulfates. Inhibitors of carcinogenesis that can act via this mechanism have been divided into two groups. Type A compounds are those that primarily enhance the activity of Phase II enzymes, particularly GSH S-transferases and also UDP-glucuronyltransferase (6,8,57,58). Type B inhibitors induce increases in microsomal mixed-function oxidase activities, while also increasing the activity of the major Phase II enzymes.

The best known examples of Type B inhibitors are the benzoflavones (6,8). 5,6-Benzoflavone inhibits the induction of tumors in rat liver by AFB_1 (59), mouse lung by BaP (60) and DMBA (61,62), rat mammary glands by DMBA (62), and mouse skin by BaP/croton oil (60) and by DMBA/TPA (63). 7,8-Benzoflavone inhibits the induction of mouse lung tumors by DMBA (61,64), hamster skin melanomas by DMBA or by DMBA/TPA (65), mouse skin tumors by various PAHs (66,67), particularly DMBA (64,68–70), and DMBA with promoters (63,67–69,71–74).

Another type of inhibition is modulation of the mixed-function oxidases involved in the metabolism of estrogens. Estrogenic activity is associated with the promotion of tumors, especially hormone-responsive mammary cancers, in animals (*e.g.*, 75–80) and humans (*e.g.*, 81). Indole-3-carbinol, a compound which occurs naturally in cruciferous vegetables, inhibits the induction of mammary tumors in rats (82,83), and it induces mixed-function oxidases (84). Particularly, it induces the activity of the enzymes responsible for 2-hydroxylation of estradiol, leading to increased excretion of estradiol metabolites (85).

Type A compounds are generally considered to be more desirable (of potential clinical usefulness) as inhibitors (6,8,58), since the enzymes in the microsomal mixed-function oxidase system induced by Type B agents are more likely to increase carcinogen activation. That is, the enzymes induced by Type B agents can catalyze aryl ring C-hydroxylation leading to the activation of PAHs, α-C-hydroxylation activating nitrosamines, and N-hydroxylation leading to activation of aromatic amines.

Among the Type A compounds, those that have received most attention as inhibitors of carcinogenesis are potent inducers of the GSH S-transferases. Prominent among these compounds are the allylic sulfides, natural products found in onion, garlic, and other members of the *Allium* genus. The best tested of these compounds, diallyl sulfide, inhibits the induction of tumors in mouse colon by DMH (86), rat esophagus by N-methylbenzylnitrosamine (MBN) (87), mouse forestomach by BaP (88), rat lung by various nitrosamines (89), and mouse lung by BaP (88) and NNK (90). Another GSH S-transferase inducer, oltipraz [5-(2-pyraziny)-4-methyl-1,2-dithiol-3-thione], is an antischistosomal agent related to dithiolthiones that occur naturally in cruciferous vegetables. Oltipraz has a wide spectrum of inhibitory activity. It inhibits the induction of mouse lung tumors by BaP, DEN, and uracil mustard (91). It also inhibits induction of rat liver tumors by AFB_1 (92) and rat colon tumors by AOM (93).

5. Prevention of Carcinogen Binding to DNA

The inhibition of nitroso compound carcinogenesis by ellagic acid has been attributed to blocking the methylation of guanine at the O^6 position (13,94,95). Presumably, this effect is due to ellagic acid binding to the duplex form of DNA (10,94).

6. Increase of the Level or Fidelity of DNA Repair

Three possible mechanisms that involve DNA repair have been suggested to explain carcinogenesis inhibition. First, an increase in the overall level of DNA repair is expected to minimize DNA damage caused by carcinogen binding. The antimutagenicity of coumarin has been attributed to this activity (10,96). Coumarin inhibits tumor induction in mouse forestomach by BaP and in rat mammary glands by DMBA (97). Second, the enzyme poly(ADP-ribosyl)transferase (ADPRT) is known to be involved in modulation of DNA damage (98,99), and the level of this enzyme is decreased in the presence of carcinogens (100). *N*-Acetyl-L-cysteine (NAC) prevents the decrease in ADPRT caused by the carcinogen 2-acetylaminofluorene (AAF) (100). NAC shows inhibitory activity in rat colon against DMH-induced tumors (101) and in mouse lung against urethan-induced tumors (102). The third mechanism is suppression of error-prone DNA repair. It is known that protease inhibitors depress error-prone repair in bacteria (103), and it has been suggested that they possibly prevent carcinogenesis by inhibiting an error-prone repair system activated by proteases that, in turn, are induced by tumor promoters (104). The protease inhibitor best studied as an inhibitor of carcinogenesis is the Bowman–Birk soybean trypsin inhibitor (BBI). It inhibits DMH-induced tumors in mouse colon (105) and liver (106), and MBN-induced tumors in rat esophagus (107).

B. Antioxidant Activities

1. Scavenging of Reactive Electrophiles

Potent nucleophiles that can react directly with carcinogens and other electrophiles may operate through this mechanism. The specific reaction of ellagic acid with BaP-diolepoxide is described in Section III.A.3. Other examples are GSH, 4-mercaptobenzenesulfonate, NAC, and sodium thiosulfate. 4-Mercaptobenzenesulfonate, administered intrarectally, inhibits colon and forestomach tumors induced by β-propiolactone (BPL) in mice (108). Sodium thiosulfate also inhibits BPL-induced forestomach tumors (108). The inhibitory activities of GSH and NAC are described in Sections III.A.3 and III.A.6, respectively.

2. Scavenging of Oxygen Radicals

There is abundant evidence that activated oxygen species (*i.e.*, singlet oxygen, peroxy radicals, superoxide anion, and hydroxyl radical) are involved in carcinogenesis (*e.g.*, 15,109,110). They are potentially involved both in initiation and in promotion and progression. For example, relevant to initiation, oxygen radicals can oxidize DNA bases (112), producing mutagenic lesions (*e.g.*, 113). Radicals also cause DNA strand breaks and chromosome deletions and rearrangements (114). Further, they participate in the activation of certain carcinogens (15,115). The best documented involvement in carcinogen activation is the role of peroxidation in activating BaP-7,8-diol to an intermediate that binds to DNA and is mutagenic in bacteria and mammalian cells (15). Kensler *et al.* (15) have listed carcinogens that form free radicals. Besides PAHs such as BaP, the list includes aromatic amines (*e.g.*, AAF, azo dyes), hydrazines (*e.g.*, DMH), nitrofurans (*e.g.*, *N*-[4-(5-nitro-2-furyl)-2-thiazolyl] formamide [FANFT]), and quinones.

Activated oxygen species most likely play an important role in tumor promotion and progression. Kensler *et al.* (15) have summarized the experimental evidence for this involvement: (a) Oxygen radical-generating systems (*e.g.*, superoxide anion generation via xanthine oxidase) show activities *in vitro* similar to those of known tumor promoters.

These activities include increasing transformation frequencies of fibroblasts and keratinocytes and increasing transcription of genes associated with early steps in cell proliferation, including c-*fos*, c-*myc*, c-*jun*, and ODC (116–118). (b) Inflammatory cells produce a wide range of reactive oxygen species, and there is evidence associating inflammation with cancers in various tissues including stomach, esophagus, colon/rectum, liver, pancreas, mouth, lung, skin, and bladder (119,120). (c) Conversely, tumor promoters stimulate the endogenous production of oxygen radicals in inflammatory cells and keratinocytes. (d) Tumor promoters inhibit endogenous activities that protect against oxidative damage, *e.g.*, GSH peroxidase (GSH-Px), catalase, and superoxide dismutase. (e) Free radical-generating agents such as benzoyl peroxide (121) and butylated hydroxytoluene (BHT) hydroperoxide (122) are tumor promoters in mouse skin.

There is direct evidence that scavenging of activated oxygen species is a mechanism for inhibiting carcinogenesis. That is, free radical scavengers do inhibit carcinogenesis induced by carcinogens known to induce activated oxygen species. For example, NAC and other thiols are known to react with hydroxyl radicals (13,123,124). The inhibitory activity of NAC is described in Section III.A.6. The reaction of β-carotene with singlet oxygen (*e.g.*, 125,126) and its participation in other free radical-trapping reactions (*e.g.*, 127–132) is well documented. β-Carotene inhibits DMH-induced colon tumorigenesis in mice (133) and DMBA-induced squamous cell carcinoma in rat salivary glands (134) and in hamster buccal pouch and forestomach (135). In mouse skin, it also inhibits DMBA-induced tumors (136) and DMBA-initiated tumors promoted by croton oil (137) or TPA (138,139).

Copper (II) 3,5-diisopropylsalicylic acid (CuDIPS), a superoxide dismutase mimetic, inhibits DMBA-induced (140) and DMBA/TPA-induced (141) tumors in mouse skin. Vitamin E (α-tocopherol) is known to scavenge peroxy radicals (*e.g.*, 13,110,142–145), singlet oxygen (*e.g.*, 146), and superoxide radicals (*e.g.*, 13). Vitamin E inhibits the induction of buccal pouch cancer in hamsters by DMBA (147) and the induction by DMH of colon tumors in mice (148) and of colon and small intestine tumors in rats (149). Like β-carotene, vitamin E inhibits tumors induced by DMBA/TPA (150) or DMBA/croton oil (151) in mouse skin.

Phenolic antioxidants (*see* Table 3) are known to scavenge peroxy radicals (13,15,152). Two phenolic antioxidants, BHT and butylated hydroxyanisole (BHA), have been studied extensively as inhibitors of chemical carcinogenesis. BHT inhibits DMH induction of colon tumors in mice (153), DMBA induction of ear duct tumors in rats (154,155), BaP and DMBA induction of forestomach tumors in mice (156), AAF induction of liver tumors in mice (157), DMBA induction of mammary gland tumors in rats (154,156,158–163), and DMBA induction with TPA promotion of skin tumors in mice (73). Likewise, BHA inhibits induction of colon tumors in mice by DMH (164,165), mouse forestomach tumors by BaP (156,166,167) and DMBA (156), and mammary gland tumors by DMBA (154–156,159). It also inhibits the induction of liver tumors in rats by ciprofibrate, a chemical known to increase cellular peroxy radicals (168), lung tumors in mice by DMBA, by dibenz[*a,h*]anthracene [DB(a,h)A], and by BaP (169). Another common phenolic antioxidant, propyl gallate, inhibits the induction of mammary gland tumors in rats by DMBA (161,163).

Nonphenolic antioxidants also scavenge oxygen free radicals. For example, GSH reacts with alkylperoxy radicals (15). The inhibitory activity of GSH against the promotion of DMBA-induced skin tumors by TPA is cited above.

Perhaps the most prominent oxygen free radical scavenging activity associated with inhibition of carcinogenesis is that of antioxidants which are potent inhibitors of AA metabolism. This activity is described below.

3. Inhibition of Arachidonic Acid (AA) Metabolism

Marnett (170) and Zenser and Davis (17) have recently reviewed the role of AA metabolism in carcinogenesis. Essentially, AA is metabolized to prostaglandins (PG), thromboxanes, leukotrienes, and hydroxyeicosatetraenoic acids (HETE) via oxidative enzymes. Activated oxygen species and alkylperoxy species are formed throughout this process; AA metabolism is increased during inflammation. There are two components of AA metabolism that have been associated strongly with carcinogenicity. Both can be inhibited by antioxidants and anti-inflammatory agents.

The first is the PG synthetic pathway and involves the enzyme PGH synthetase. This enzyme has two activities: cyclooxygenase, which catalyzes the formation of PGG_2 from arachidonic acid, and hydroperoxidase, which catalyzes the reduction of PGG_2 to PGH_2. To return to its native state, the hydroperoxidase requires a reducing cosubstrate, and carcinogens such as aromatic amines have been found to be appropriate substrates. According to the model proposed, during catalysis the carcinogens produce free radicals and electrophiles that can form adducts with DNA and, thus, initiate carcinogenesis. This process can be stopped at four steps: (a) at formation of PGG_2 via inhibition of cyclooxygenase, (b) by inhibition of peroxidase activity, (c) by prevention of formation of reactive intermediates, and (d) by scavenging reactive intermediates (*e.g.*, by GSH conjugation). Relevant to these potential mechanisms, cyclooxygenase inhibitors such as nonsteroidal anti-inflammatory drugs (NSAIDs such as aspirin, ibuprofen, indomethacin, piroxicam) and certain antioxidants, *e.g.*, nordihydroguaiaretic acid [NDGA], are effective inhibitors of carcinogenesis (*see* Table 4). Additionally, PGH_2 itself breaks down to form a direct-acting mutagen, malondialdehyde (170). Thus, inhibition of cyclooxygenase may directly prevent the formation of a potential carcinogen.

An interesting demonstration of this mechanism may be operative in the inhibition of nitrofuran carcinogenesis by aspirin. Aspirin inhibits the induction of bladder carcinoma in rats by FANFT (171,172). Aspirin inhibits PG synthesis in rat bladder, and PGH synthetase activities are known to catalyze the activation of FANFT to a carcinogen (173).

The second component of AA metabolism associated with carcinogenesis is the burst of PGH synthetase and lipoxygenase activities that are seen during inflammation and are stimulated by the tumor promoter TPA. The available evidence suggests that the immediate products of lipoxygenase activity, the HETE and their hydroperoxy precursors (HPETE), are more important to tumor promotion than are PGs. Compounds that inhibit lipoxygenase, such as vitamin E and esculetin, inhibit tumor promotion in mouse skin. Likewise, compounds that inhibit lipoxygenase, and that are stable one-electron donors which competitively inhibit the production of unstable free radicals and electrophiles by PGH synthetase (*e.g.*, curcumin, the flavonoids, and NDGA) also inhibit tumor promotion in mouse skin. Anti-inflammatory agents that predominantly inhibit cyclooxygenase (*e.g.*, aspirin) are not effective inhibitors of tumor promotion in mouse skin (17).

Another control point in the AA metabolic pathway is the release of AA from membrane phospholipids. This release is catalyzed by phospholipases. The predominant location of AA on phospholipids is position *sn*-2, and phospholipase A_2 catalyzes release of AA from this position. Phospholipase A_2 inhibitors such as glucocorticoids and 4-bromophenacyl bromide inhibit carcinogenesis (*see* Table 4). Note that these compounds also inhibit other enzymes in the AA pathway, and so their inhibition of carcinogenesis cannot be attributed directly to inhibition of phospholipase A_2. For instance, the glucocorticoids appear to inhibit the induction of PGH synthetase enzymes (170,174,175). Likewise, AA can be released from phospholipids by other mechanisms (*e.g.*, via phospholipase C and diacylglycerol lipase, and increases in intracellular calcium resulting in higher levels of phospholipase activity) (17).

AA metabolites, specifically PG, also are believed to be involved in signal transduction pathways (17,176,177). As discussed in Section III.C.1, changes in activities in these pathways appear to be integrally involved in the promotion and progression of tumors. Thus, inhibition of AA metabolism may play a role in controlling these aspects of carcinogenesis, as well as directly blocking carcinogens and tumor promoters. PGE$_2$ is known to suppress the immune response to certain tumor cells (170,178,179). Inhibitors of PGH synthetase may relieve this suppression (*see* Section III.C.6).

C. Antiproliferative/Antiprogression Activities

1. Modulation of Signal Transduction

Weinstein (11) characterized carcinogenesis as a progressive series of disorders in the function of signal transduction pathways; signal transduction is the cascade of molecular communication through which hormones and growth factors that regulate cell growth, proliferation, and differentiation communicate across cell membranes involving intermediary molecules known as second messengers (17). Whitfield (180) has provided a comprehensive review of signal transduction pathways (*see also* Chapters 5 [Section I], 11, and 14 of this volume). Most of the antiproliferative/antiprogression activities discussed in this chapter impact on some part of the signal transduction pathways. Second messengers include cyclic AMP, inositol 1,4,5-triphosphate, diacylglycerol, and, as mentioned above, PGs. One of the steps in signal transduction involves activation of the enzyme PKC by diacylglycerol. There is evidence that carcinogenesis may be suppressed by inhibiting this enzyme. Apparently, the tumor promoter TPA can replace diacylglycerol in activating PKC. Chemicals that inhibit PKC, such as D,L-palmitoylcarnitine, flavonoids, 18β-glycyrrhetinic acid, and *N*-(6-aminohexyl)-5-chloro-1-naphthalenesulfonamide (W-7), also inhibit TPA-induced tumor promotion in mouse skin.

Zenser and Davis (17) summarized the evidence that PGs are signal transduction intermediaries. This evidence includes increased PG synthesis observed during human keratinocyte proliferation (181), in the MDCK line of dog kidney cells treated with carcinogens and tumor promoters (182), in BALB/c 3T3 fibroblasts transformed by 3-MC (183), during tumor promotion in mouse skin (184), and in malignant tumors (17). Although this interpretation is speculative, it is possible that cyclooxygenase inhibitors such as the NSAIDs inhibit tumor promotion by inhibiting these proliferative activities associated with PGs.

2. Modulation of Hormonal/Growth Factor Activity

Chemicals may inhibit the cell growth and proliferation associated with carcinogenesis by directly regulating the induction and activity of specific hormones and growth factors that initiate steps in signal transduction. For example, antiestrogens such as tamoxifen and toremifene bind to estrogen receptors, preventing the binding and activity of estrogens (185,186). Both compounds inhibit carcinogen-induced, estrogen-sensitive tumors in rat mammary glands (187–192; *see* Section IV.A). Tamoxifen also inhibits the induction of kidney tumors in hamsters by estrogen (17β-estradiol) (80).

Transforming growth factor β (TGFβ) has antiproliferative activity in both normal and neoplastic cells *in vitro* (193) and in mammary glands (194,195) and liver (195,196) *in vivo.* Neoplastic cells, such as A549 human lung carcinoma cells, produce TGFβ, but usually in a latent form that cannot bind to its receptor; these cells are responsive to antiproliferative effects of activated TGFβ (193). There is evidence from studies in rat intestinal crypt epithelial cells that TGFβ may also promote differentiation (197). These observations suggest that chemicals that activate TGFβ could also control proliferation in carcinogenesis. Studies with human MCF-7 breast cancer cells and tamoxifen are interesting in this regard. These cells normally produce only small amounts of activated TGFβ, but production increases up to 20-fold by treatment with tamoxifen or its metabolite, 4-hydroxytamoxifen (193,198). Retinoic acid, which inhibits chemical carcinogenesis, particularly tumor promotion, in mouse skin (70,199–209) induces TGFβ-2 in mouse keratinocytes and in mouse skin *in vivo* after topical application (195,210). The increase in TGFβ-2 occurs post-transcriptionally. In vitamin A–deficient rats treated with retinoic acid, the level of expression of TGFβ correlates with tissue levels of retinoids in skin, intestines, and respiratory epithelia (195,211).

Insulin-like growth factor I (IGF-I) stimulates cell replication in various tumors (212,213). Particularly, human breast cancer cells have receptors for and excrete IGF-I (212,214). Tamoxifen lowers blood concentrations of IGF-I in breast cancer patients, suggesting that a component of its antitumor activity is inhibition of IGF-I (212,214).

3. Inhibition of Oncogene Activity

During the course of cell proliferation in carcinogenesis, numerous oncogenes are expressed, possibly as intermediates in the signal transduction pathways. The evidence for oncogene activity in signal transduction in carcinogenesis is based on the similarity of some of their products (protein kinases) to other intermediates (11). Some very interesting recent research demonstrates that compounds that inhibit oncogene activation also inhibit carcinogenesis. For example, *ras* oncogenes are expressed during mammary gland carcinogenesis induced by MNU (215) and, to a lesser extent, by DMBA (216). Gould and coworkers (217) showed that D-limonene inhibits the progression of mammary tumors induced in rats by MNU or DMBA; they also showed that D-limonene inhibits the farnesylation of small G proteins (21–26 kDa). These experimental data suggest that D-limonene inhibits this tumor progression by preventing oncogene activation through inhibiting post-translational farnesylation of the p21 *ras* protein (218).

Similarly, it has long been known that nerolidol inhibits conversion of farnesyl pyrophosphate to squalene (219), suggesting that this terpene may be a competitive inhibitor of other farnesylation reactions, such as that of *ras* products. Wattenberg (8,220) found that nerolidol effectively inhibits the proliferation and progression of colon carcinoma induced in rats by AOM.

Also, cyclooxygenase inhibitors may inhibit proliferation in carcinogenesis through inhibition of oncogene expression (17), although the evidence for this is less direct than for other effects of AA metabolism inhibitors. Expression of the oncogene c-*myc* occurs early in epidermal growth factor (EGF)-induced cell proliferation. PGs are required, but this requirement is not sufficient for c-*myc* expression and for the stimulation of DNA synthesis by EGF in BALB/c 3T3 cells (221). Indomethacin inhibits both DNA synthesis and oncogene expression in this system, and this inhibition is reversed by addition of PGG_2 (17,221,222).

In vitro studies indicate that inhibition of oncogene expression is a mechanism for the inhibitory activity of protease inhibitors (*see* Section IV.J.9 and Table 9) and retinoids (*see* Section IV.H and Table 7). For example, 6-aminocaproic acid, antipain, and leupeptin inhibit transformation of NIH-3T3 cells transfected with activated H-*ras* oncogene (223). 6-Aminocaproic acid inhibits DMH-induced colon tumors in rats (224); antipain inhibits urethan-induced tumors in mouse lung (225); and leupeptin inhibits DMBA/croton oil carcinogenesis in mouse skin (226). Antipain, leupeptin, and BBI suppress c-*myc* expression in normal proliferating mouse fibroblasts (223). The tumor inhibiting activity of BBI is summarized in Section III.A.6, as well as in Section IV.J.9 and Table 9). Retinoic acid also inhibits H-*ras*-induced transformation in NIH-3T3 cells (223), and it inhibits tumorigenicity in mouse skin (*see* Section IV.H and Table 7).

4. Inhibition of Polyamine Metabolism

Pegg (227) and subsequently Verma (16) have reviewed the evidence that polyamines play a significant role in cell proliferation, differentiation, and malignant transformation. The mode of action is not yet known, but it has been suggested that, as polycations, polyamines can stabilize DNA structures; indeed, they have been shown to affect DNA and protein synthesis (16,228). A critical step in polyamine biosynthesis is the synthesis of putrescine from ornithine, catalyzed by ODC. There is ample evidence that ODC participates in cell proliferation associated with carcinogenesis. For example, TPA and other tumor promoters increase ODC activity in skin, colon, bladder, and liver (16). In mouse skin, topically applied TPA causes an approximately 200-fold increase in ODC activity within 4.5 hours after treatment (16). The increase is dose dependent and correlates with the relative potency of the TPA doses to promote skin tumorigenesis. Also, increased ODC activity appears to be a specific marker of tumor promotion, since most hyperplastic agents that are not tumor promoters do not induce ODC (229).

Likewise, chemicals that inhibit the induction of or deactivate ODC also inhibit carcinogenesis (*see* Section IV.F and Table 6). Some of the most convincing results demonstrating that inhibition of ODC prevents carcinogenesis come from studies with 2-difluoromethylornithine (DFMO). DFMO is a specific, mechanism-based irreversible inhibitor of ODC; this means that DFMO is activated by ODC to a reactive form which, in turn, interacts with the enzyme and inactivates it (227). DFMO inhibits tumor induction by DMH in mouse colon (230), AOM in rat colon (231,232), DMBA (233,234) and MNU (189,235,236) in rat mammary glands, DMBA/TPA in mouse skin (204,237,238), N-butyl-N-(4-hydroxybutyl)nitrosamine (OH-BBN) in mouse urinary bladder (234), and MNU (239) and OH-BBN (240) in rat urinary bladder.

Verma and coworkers (207,241–244) found that ODC induction by TPA is regulated at the transcription level. PKC also appears to be involved (241,243), as are diverse intermediates induced by TPA, including PGs (245), other products of AA metabolism (246), and free radicals (247). Thus, chemicals that inhibit PKC and AA metabolism and those that scavenge free radicals may also inhibit the induction of ODC; hence, this mechanism may be involved in their inhibition of carcinogenesis. In this regard, several of the PKC inhibitors cited in Section III.C.1, including 18β-glycyrrhetinic acid and D,L-palmitoylcarnitine, inhibit ODC induction and tumor promotion in mouse skin. Inhibitors of AA metabolism, such as 4-bromophenacyl bromide, also inhibit both ODC induction and TPA-promoted mouse skin tumorigenesis, as do free radical scavengers such as GSH, the flavonoids, and CuDIPS (*see* Section III.B).

Vitamin A (retinol) and certain of its derivatives (*i.e.*, retinoids) inhibit carcinogenesis specifically during promotion (*see* Section IV.H and Table 7). There is evidence that the carcinogenesis inhibitory activity of these compounds may be mediated partially by regulation of ODC induction. In mouse skin, Verma *et al.* (201,248) found that the inhibition of ODC induction by retinoic acid and its analogs (such as 13-*cis*-retinoic acid, 13-*cis*-retinal, and 5,6-dihydroretinoic acid) correlates with their ability to inhibit TPA-induced tumor promotion. Analogs which do not inhibit ODC induction also do not inhibit tumor promotion. One of the most active retinoids is *all-trans-N*-(4-hydroxyphenyl)retinamide (4-HPR). This compound is a potent inhibitor of ODC induction (249) as well as of TPA promotion in mouse skin (250,251). It also inhibits mammary tumors in rats induced by DMBA (252–254) or MNU (252,255–258) and urinary bladder tumors in mice induced by MNU (256,259) when administered after carcinogen treatment is completed.

5. Induction of Terminal Differentiation

One of the steps in the proliferation of normal, regulated cells in epithelial tissues is terminal differentiation. In contrast, proliferating cancer cells have often totally lost the ability to differentiate (180). These cancer cells are either deficient in or incapable of responding to differentiation signals (180). Abundant evidence demonstrates that restoring the ability of abnormally proliferating cells to differentiate suppresses carcinogenesis. In fact, several classes of chemicals that inhibit carcinogenesis also induce differentiation. Retinoids are the best-studied example of such inhibitors (*see* Section IV.H and Table 7). For many years it has been known that vitamin A deficiency causes squamous metaplasia and keratinization, both of which are signs of uncontrolled proliferation (260). Studies in hamster trachea (261–263) and various cancer cells (264–272) show that the differentiated phenotype can be restored by treatment with retinoids. Evidence indicates that retinoids control differentiation via intracellular binding proteins (cellular retinol-binding protein and cellular retinoic acid–binding protein) and retinoid nuclear receptors (273–277).

Calcium and vitamin D_3 are well-known differentiation-inducing agents that also inhibit carcinogenesis (180; *see* Sections IV.J.2 and IV.J.11 and Table 9). Calcium induces differentiation in epithelial tissues (278), including rat esophagus (279), mouse skin (280), and human mammary gland (281,282) and colon (278). Vitamin D_3 induces differentiation in human colon (278,283), human and mouse myeloid leukemia cells (278,284–290), mouse skin cells (287), mouse melanoma cells (287), and other cells (287,291,292). It has been suggested that the effects of the two chemicals on differentiation may be mediated by the same signal transduction pathway, involving the vitamin D_3 nuclear receptor with calcium as the messenger (180,278).

Dimethylsulfoxide (DMSO) is another compound known to stimulate differentiation in many cells, including human leukemia and human colon, lung, and breast cancer cells (180,293,294). Calcium also appears to be involved in the differentiation-inducing activity of DMSO. It may act by raising cytosolic calcium levels, calcium-dependent endonuclease activity, and TGFβ-1 levels (180). DMSO inhibits DMBA-induced tumorigenesis in rat mammary glands (295) and TPA promotion of DMBA-induced mouse skin tumorigenesis (296).

6. Restoration of Immune Response

De Flora and Ramel (10) commented on the importance of the immune response in inhibiting carcinogenesis. For example, they described the results of Feramisco *et al.* (297), who found that antibodies to oncoproteins are important in the inhibition of cell transformation and of tumor growth.

PGE_2 is known to suppress immune response in certain tumor cells (170,178,179).

Cyclooxygenase inhibitors reduce immune suppression by tumor cells (298–308). Marnett (170) suggested that this effect on immune suppression may be part of the mechanism by which cyclooxygenase inhibitors reduce the rate of tumor growth, as seen in several animal tumor models, including colon and Lewis lung carcinoma (309).

Retinoids also are known to be immunostimulants (276,310). Retinoic acid increases cell-mediated and natural killer (NK) cell cytotoxicity; retinoids also cause some leukemia cells to differentiate to mature granulocytes comparable to mature neutrophils (265). Hill and Grubbs (276) suggested that these effects might be partially responsible for the activity of retinoids against established tumors.

Vitamin E added at pharmacological doses to normal, well-balanced animal diets causes increase in humoral antibody production, especially IgG; this effect has been observed repeatedly in chickens, mice, turkeys, guinea pigs, and rabbits (311). Vitamin E also stimulates cell-mediated immunity as evidenced by enhanced mitogenesis and mixed lymphocyte response in spleen cells from mice fed vitamin E (312). In particular, vitamin E prevents the carcinogen-induced decrease in the density of macrophage-equivalent cells (Langerhans cells) in the buccal pouch of DMBA-treated hamsters (313). Likewise, vitamin E inhibits the induction of tumors by DMBA in hamster buccal pouch (314,315). Moreover, locally injected vitamin E also causes the regression of DMBA-induced buccal pouch tumors, and the regression is associated with the induction of tumor necrosis factor-α in macrophages (316).

The role of selenium in mediating immune response suggests that the broad-spectrum activity of selenium in inhibiting chemical carcinogenesis may be due in part to stimulation of the immune system. Selenium compounds (*see* Section IV.J.10 and Table 9) prevent chemical carcinogenesis in mouse colon (317), rat colon and intestines (318–321), rat esophagus (322), mouse forestomach (323), mouse skin (151,150), rat liver (56,324–326), hamster pancreas (327), and rat stomach (328). The well-documented carcinogenesis-inhibiting activity of selenium is against the induction of DMBA-induced tumors in rat mammary glands (329–346) (*see also* Chapter 9 [Section 4] in this volume).

Kiremidjian-Schumacher and Stotzky (347) have reviewed the many effects selenium has on the immune system, including nonspecific, humoral, and cell-mediated immunity. In general, selenium deficiency causes immune suppression, while supplementation with low doses of selenium restores and increases immune response. Perhaps most important in inhibiting tumorigenesis is the effect of selenium on the cytotoxicity of immune system cells. Compared with normal cells, both T and NK lymphocytes from selenium-deficient mice have decreased ability to destroy tumor cells *in vitro*. Supplementation with 0.5 or 2 ppm selenium enhances the ability of rat NK cells to kill tumor cells. The role of immune stimulation in the inhibition of carcinogenesis by selenium has been studied only to a limited extent and has not been confirmed. However, the potent inhibitory activity of selenium compounds against the induction of tumors by DMBA in rat mammary glands is suggestive, since the immune suppressive effects of DMBA are well documented (348,349; *see also* Chapter 8).

7. Increasing Intercellular Communication

Gap junctions are the cell components that coordinate intercellular communication. They are composed of pores, or channels, in the cellular membranes that join channels of adjacent cells; these pores are regulated and, when open, allow passage of molecules up to about 1000 daltons in size (350,351). Bertram *et al.* (351), Loewenstein (352), and Mehta *et al.* (353,354) have proposed that gap junctions allow growth regulatory signals to move between cells. There is evidence from studies *in vitro* that inhibition of gap junctional intercellular communication occurs in the proliferative phase of carcinogenesis. Klaunig and Ruch (350) have reviewed this evidence. For example, they cited numerous reports that TPA, other phorbol ester tumor promoters, and mezerein inhibit gap junctional communication in Chinese hamster embryo V79 fibroblasts, mouse HEL-37 epidermal cells, human FL cells and fibroblasts, BALB/c 3T3 mouse fibroblasts, NIH-3T3 mouse fibroblasts, C3H10T1/2 mouse fibroblasts, rat liver epithelial cells, and primary hepatocytes. They noted that in several of the studies, the ability to inhibit intercellular communication correlates with tumor promoting activity *in vivo*. Also, TPA decreases the size and number of gap junctions in cells *in vitro* and in mouse skin. Furthermore, several nonphorbol tumor promoters and nongenotoxic carcinogens are inhibitors of gap junctional communication *in vitro*. The inhibitors of intercellular communication include such compounds as anthralin, benzoyl peroxide, bile acids, and phenobarbital.

Investigations by Bertram and coworkers using C3H10T1/2 cells support the concept that carcinogenesis may be inhibited by enhancing intercellular communication. They found that the carotenoids (355), such as β-carotene and canthaxanthine, and retinoids (356), such as vitamin A, enhance communication in C3H10T1/2 cells initiated by 3-MC. The enhancement of intercellular communication correlates with inhibition of malignant transformation of these cells. The carcinogenesis inhibitory activity of retinoids and carotenoids is summarized in Section IV.H and Table 7.

To date, there are only limited data suggesting the potential for inhibiting chemical carcinogenesis by the other antiproliferative/antiprogression mechanisms listed in Table 2, but the possibilities exist and warrant consideration.

8. Restoration of Tumor-Suppressor Function

Over the past few years, several "tumor-suppressor" genes have been identified. These genes are involved in controlling proliferation and differentiation in cells. In particular, their function is associated with control of abnormal growth in carcinogenesis. Mutated or otherwise dysfunctional forms of several of these genes have been implicated in pathogenesis by their presence in specific cancers. For example, dysfunctional forms of the tumor-suppressor gene, *rb*, are involved in retinoblastoma, osteosarcoma, and in tumors in the lung, bladder, prostate, and breast (357–361); of *p53* in adenocarcinomas in colon and breast, human T-cell leukemias, glioblastomas, sarcomas, and tumors in lung and liver (*e.g.*, 361–368); of *wt* in Wilm's tumor (369–371); and of *dcc* in colon tumors (372). Friedmann (367) has reviewed the studies demonstrating the potential for treating cancer patients with exogenous functional tumor-suppressor genes to inhibit tumor growth and spread. Possibly, it will be found that chemicals can modulate the expression and activity of tumor suppressors and inhibit carcinogenicity by this mechanism.

9. Induction of Programmed Cell Death (Apoptosis)

Apoptosis is a well-regulated function of the normal cell cycle; it requires gene transcription and translation (373,374). Tumor suppressors such as wild-type *p53* (375,376) and certain growth factors, particularly TGFβ-1 (374,377), have been implicated in the induction of apoptosis. Programmed cell death has become understood as the *complementation of mitosis* in the maintenance, growth, and involution of tissues: this is the process by which damaged and excessive cells are eliminated (374). Apoptosis is inhibited by tumor promoters such as TPA

(376,378,379) and phenobarbital (376,380) and other chemicals that stimulate cell proliferation, such as hormones (374,381–384). These data suggest, in turn, that induction of apoptosis may inhibit tumor formation. Moreover, chemicals that inhibit tumor promotion may act by inducing or preventing the inhibition of apoptosis. Although there is as yet no direct evidence that this mode of action is operative, pancreatic cancers were shown to regress in hamsters in which apoptosis is induced (374,385). Tamoxifen, as described in Section IV.A and Table 2, inhibits mammary gland tumors, and it also induces programmed cell death in human mammary cancer MCF-7 cells (374).

10. Correction of DNA Methylation Imbalance

Wainfan and Poirier (386) reviewed investigations indicating that changes in DNA methylation patterns are involved in carcinogenesis. Methyl-deficient diets cause fatty livers, increase cell turnover, and promote the development of carcinogen-induced liver tumors in rats and mice (386–390; *see also* Chapter 9 [Section III] in this volume). Conversely, methyl-rich diets (fortified with choline and methionine) prevent or reduce these effects (386,391–393). Changes in gene expression—increased expression of proto-oncogenes and decreased expression of growth factors and growth factor receptors in liver—appear in animals maintained on methyl-deficient diets (386,394–397). These effects are similar to those seen in rodents given tumor-promoting chemicals (386,398–400), and they are reversible upon providing methyl sources (386,401). Most importantly, increased proto-oncogene expression correlates with hypomethylation of the genes in animals fed methyl-deficient diets for 1 week or longer (386,395,401–403). Essentially, these observations support the hypothesis that hypomethylation of DNA results in alterations in the expression of genes involved in cell growth and regulation (386,390,392). This observation, in turn, supports the more general concept that changes in DNA methylation, including hypomethylation as well as mutation and steric blocking, can affect carcinogenesis (386,404–407). There is only very limited evidence associating chemicals that modulate DNA methylation with inhibition of carcinogenesis. Methionine, which is involved with choline, folic acid, and vitamin B_{12} in regulating intracellular methyl metabolism (386), inhibits DMBA- and MNU-induced mammary gland cancers in rats (408). Also, folic acid inhibits isoniazid-induced lung tumors in mice (409; *see also* Chapter 9 [Section II] in this volume).

11. Inhibition of Angiogenesis

Angiogenesis is the process leading to formation of new blood vessels. In normal tissue, it is a highly regulated process essential to reproduction, development, and wound repair (410). In carcinogenesis, it is required for tumor growth and is involved in metastasis (411). A study in transgenic mice (strain RIP1-Tag 2) indicates that angiogenesis may also occur before tumors are formed in hyperplasia (412). There is some indirect evidence that certain chemicals that inhibit carcinogenesis may inhibit angiogenesis. For example, PGE_1 and PGE_2 are angiogenic (413,414). Thus, compounds which inhibit PG synthesis (*see* Section III.B.3 and Table 4) may inhibit carcinogenesis through the inhibition of angiogenesis.

12. Inhibition of Basement Membrane Degradation

Tumor cells produce various enzymes that destroy the basement membrane which acts as a barrier against malignant cancer cells and prevents cancer spread. These enzymes include the proteases: collagenase, cathepsin B, and plasminogen activators (223,415). Protease inhibitors are known to act against the proteases thrombin and type IV collagenase, which are among the proteases hypothesized to participate in the destruction of basement membranes during invasion by cancer (223). Thus, the effect of protease inhibitors that inhibit carcinogenesis (*see* Sections III.A.6 and IV.J.9 and Table 9) may involve, at least in part, the inhibition of basement membrane degradation.

13. Activation of Antimetastasis Genes

In the past few years, evidence has accumulated that tumor invasion and metastasis are controlled by effector genes just as are the other phases of tumor cell proliferation (416). Several genes have been identified which are involved in the suppression of metastasis (416). One of these is *nm*23, which apparently produces nucleoside diphosphate kinase (417). Levels of *nm*23 correlate inversely with the prognosis and metastatic state of human breast cancer (418,419). Although there is no substantial evidence at present that chemicals which inhibit carcinogenesis do induce the antimetastasis genes, it is likely that agents which increase the expression of these genes or enhance the levels of their products (*e.g.*, nucleoside diphosphate kinase) inhibit tumor progression via these mechanisms.

IV. CHEMICAL AGENTS CLASSIFIED BY STRUCTURE OR BIOLOGICAL ACTIVITY THAT HAVE DISPLAYED INHIBITION OF CHEMICAL CARCINOGENESIS

Inhibitors of chemical carcinogenesis may be classified according to a tandem system: by chemical structural class and by biological activity(ies) initiated/amplified or reduced/suppressed by the agents; a summary listing of thus classified inhibitors of chemical carcinogenesis in animals are given in Tables 3 to 9. Within the classes, additional subdivisions by structure and biological activity are made. In all cases, the associations between the structures/activities and inhibition of chemical carcinogenesis have been inferred from experimental results. Many chemicals listed belong to more than one class and, hence, are referred to in more than one table. For chemicals belonging to multiple classes, the inhibition data are listed under the presently perceived predominant mode of action of the chemical. Wherever possible, structurally similar compounds are grouped together. Since the mechanisms of inhibition are at present not completely understood, the classifications by structure and activity should not be considered definitive. In some cases the inhibitory activities may be species- or tissue-specific, depending on factors such as pharmacokinetics, metabolic enzyme levels, and types of cellular receptors. It is useful to look at all the inhibition-correlated structural analogs and the respective activities for estimating the potential of a particular chemical to be an inhibitor of carcinogenesis.

Tables 3 to 9 should be considered representative rather than comprehensive of the chemicals and inhibitory activities, since only results of animal studies considered to be adequate by the criteria described in Section II are cited. For many of the chemicals discussed, as well as for other related chemicals, there are additional positive results that do not meet the criteria cited or that are not direct measures of inhibition of chemical carcinogenesis (but, for example, are measures of radiation-induced carcinogenesis or spontaneous tumors). For many of these chemicals, supporting data are available from tests of antimutagenicity, of inhibition of malignant transformation, of inhibition of cell proliferation, and other activities which are associated with inhibition of carcinogenesis, and some of these are discussed below in this section.

A. Antihormones

Hormones, particularly estrogens and glucocorticoids, play a cardinal role in the regulation of cell proliferation and of the various pathways involved in carcinogenesis (*see* Chapter 11 in this volume). For example, in both animals and humans estrogens promote carcinogenesis in the target tissues of this hormone, such as the mammary glands and the uterus. Androgens promote tumorigenesis by binding to androgen receptors, and testosterone is implicated in the promotion of prostate cancers. In animals, in addition to promoting prostate cancers, testosterone has also been implicated in the induction of tumors of the mammary gland and liver (420).

There are essentially two main types of antihormones: (a) hormonal antagonists (antiandrogens and antiestrogens) which act by interfering with binding of the hormone to its receptor, and (b) chemicals which affect the biosynthesis of hormones. Among the nonsteroidal antiestrogens, tamoxifen is by far the best studied. It is used clinically as adjuvant treatment in postmenopausal women (421,422). Initially, this clinical use was based on its efficacy of causing the regression of chemically induced mammary tumors as well as on its ability to inhibit DMBA-induced mammary tumors in rats and 17β-estradiol–induced renal tumors in hamsters (80,187–191,423–425). In mammary glands, it blocks estrogenic activity; on the other hand, in some tissues it appears to substitute for estrogen and has hormonal activity (186,426). The antiestrogenic activity of tamoxifen may also explain its other inhibitory effects on carcinogenesis-related activities, in particular its potent inhibition of PKC (11) and its induction of TGFβ (198). Other antiestrogens which inhibit DMBA-induced mammary tumors in rats include melatonin (1), toremifene (190), and "Antineoplaston A10" (191). The latter compound is also capable of inhibiting BaP- or urethan-induced lung carcinogenesis in mice (569,570).

At least three antiandrogens—3β-methylandrost-5-en-17-one, cyprosterone acetate, and flutamide—have demonstrated anticarcinogenic effects. The first two inhibit DMBA-induced skin carcinogenesis in mice with or without TPA as the promoter (1,496,502), whereas the latter inhibits DMBA-induced mammary carcinogenesis in rats (430).

A number of antihormones exert their activities via inhibiting the biosynthesis of hormones. One of the key enzymes involved in estrogen biosynthesis is aromatase, a cytochrome P-450–dependent enzyme that catalyzes the C-19 hydroxylation and subsequent oxidative cleavage of the androgens androstenedione and testosterone to estrone and estradiol, respectively (427,428). At least two specific inhibitors of aromatase have been tested and found to have inhibitory activity against carcinogenesis. 4-Hydroxy-androst-4-ene-3,17-dione, a suicide inhibitor of aromatase, inhibits DMBA-induced tumors in rat mammary gland (428). When administered after DMBA, it reduces tumor multiplicity and size and causes regression of existing tumors (430). CGS 18320b [butanedioic acid, complexed 1:2 with 4,4'-(1 *H*-imidazolylmethylene)-bis(benzonitrile)], a competitive inhibitor of aromatase, reduces tumor incidence in rat mammary glands, when administered at the same time as and after the carcinogen, DMBA (431). Aminoglutethimide, a nonspecific aromatase inhibitor which inhibits cytochrome P-450–dependent activities associated with the synthesis of cholesterol (429), also inhibits DMBA-induced mammary carcinogenesis (1). In addition, the tumorigenesis inhibitory activity of quercetin, curcumin (*see* Table 3), 7,8-benzoflavone (*see* Table 5), and indole-3-carbinol (*see* Table 9) may be due, at least in part, to their antihormonal activities.

B. Anti-inflammatory Agents

A variety of anti-inflammatory agents can inhibit chemical carcinogenesis. Like carcinogenesis, inflammation is associated with production of oxygen free radicals and cell proliferation. The mechanisms of inhibition of carcinogenesis by anti-inflammatory agents appear to involve inhibition of these activities. For example, the steroidal anti-inflammatory agents most likely work by binding to steroid receptors, thereby inducing proliferation control factors (*e.g.*, in activated T-cells) (432). They also interfere with leukotriene biosynthesis and thus in the generation of free radicals (17). The steroids and sterols that have been shown to inhibit PAH-induced skin carcinogenesis in mice include cortisone, hydrocortisone, prednisolone, dexamethasone, fluocinolone acetonide, 18β-glycyrrhetinic acid, oleanic acid, and ursolic acid (1,72,151,205,207,450). Among these, hydrocortisone also inhibits methylazoxymethanol (MAM)-induced colon carcinogenesis in rats (1). 18β-Glycyrrhetinic acid, a naturally occurring substance found in licorice root, has structural similarity to steroidal anti-inflammatory agents and may act by mechanisms similar to these compounds. Its relation to the steroids is supported by its mineralocorticoid activities (445) as well as those of its succinic acid ester, carbenoxolone (446,447). As an anti-inflammatory agent, 18β-glycyrrhetinic acid has been used at concentrations up to 2% in ointments for the treatment of various skin diseases (448). Both 18β-glycyrrhetinic acid and its saponin parent, glycyrrhizin, are tumorigenesis inhibitors in various animal models. Glycyrrhizin inhibits the development of liver tumors in mice and rats (*rev. in* 449), and 18β-glycyrrhetinic acid inhibits tumor promotion in mouse skin (449,450). The inhibitory activity in mouse skin is believed to be related to anti-inflammatory potential, as evidenced by inhibition of the inflammation associated with tumor promotion in this tissue (449). 18β-Glycyrrhetinic acid also inhibits other biological activities associated with tumor promotion, especially those mediated by signal transduction via PKC (449).

A number of antioxidants (curcumin, ethoxyquin, fumaric acid, quercetin) also possess anti-inflammatory activity and are inhibitors of chemical carcinogenesis (*see* Table 3). Among these, curcumin is of special interest. It is the major yellow pigment in turmeric and is obtained from the rhizome of the plant *Curcuma longa*. It is a potent antioxidant (433,434) and anti-inflammatory agent (435–438). It has tumor-inhibitory activity in the two-stage DMBA/TPA mouse skin model (439,440) and against the induction of skin tumors by BaP (438). Curcumin probably inhibits carcinogenesis by multiple mechanisms related to its antioxidant and anti-inflammatory properties. It inhibits AA metabolism in CD-1 mouse skin by blocking both the lipoxygenase and cyclooxygenase pathways (441,438). There is also evidence that it inhibits phospholipase A_2 (438). Its antioxidant activity is based on scavenging superoxide radicals (442). On topical application, curcumin inhibits TPA-induced DNA synthesis in mouse skin as measured by tritiated thymidine incorporation, demonstrating its effect against proliferation (439). It also inhibits the metabolic activation and DNA binding of PAH carcinogens (438,443,444).

C. Antioxidants

Some antioxidants which inhibit carcinogenesis are listed in Table 3. The mechanisms by which these compounds are expected to act are described in some detail in Section III.B and reviewed by Kensler *et al.* (15). Fumaric acid is a particularly interesting antioxidant

TABLE 3.   Antioxidants That Inhibit Chemical Carcinogenesis

Inhibitor	Target	Species	Carcinogen	References
Fatty acid/fatty alkyl compounds				
Ascorbyl palmitate, palmitic acid	Skin	Mouse	DMBA/TPA	1
Phenolic compounds: cinnamyl compounds				
Caffeic acid, ferulic acid	Forestomach	Mouse	BaP	563
	Skin	Mouse	DMBA/TPA	439
Chlorogenic acid	Intestines (NOS)	Hamster	MAM	1
	Lung	Mouse	BaP	1,571
	Skin	Mouse	DMBA/TPA	439
Curcumin	Skin	Mouse	DMBA/TPA	439
Phenolic compounds: flavonoids				
Morin	Skin	Mouse	BaP, DMBA/TPA	1
Myricetin	Lung	Mouse	BaP	1
	Skin	Mouse	BaP/TPA, DMBA/TPA, 3-MC, MNU/TPA	1
Quercetin	Lung	Mouse	BaP	1
	Skin	Mouse	BaP, BaP/TPA, DMBA/teleocidin, DMBA/TPA, 3-MC, MNU/TPA	1
Phenolic compounds: simple phenols				
BHT	Colon	Mouse	DMH	153
	Ear duct	Rat	AOM, DMBA	1,154,155
	Forestomach	Mouse	BaP, DEN, DMBA	1,156
	Liver	Rat	AAF	157
	Lung	Mouse	Isoniazid, urethan	1
	Mammary gland	Rat	DMBA	1,154,156, 158–163
	Skin	Mouse	DMBA/TPA	1,73
BHA	Colon	Mouse	DMH, MAM	1,164,165
	Forestomach	Mouse	BaP, DMBA	156,166,167
	Liver	Rat	Ciprofibrate, OH-EEN	1,168
	Lung	Mouse	Nitrosating compounds, PAH	1,169
	Mammary gland	Rat	DMBA	154–156,159
4-Methoxyphenol	Forestomach	Mouse	BaP, BPL	323,563,564
		Rat	MNNG	572
Phenolic compounds: polyphenols				
Ellagic acid	Lung	Mouse	BaP, DB(a,h)A-diolepoxide	1,571
	Skin	Mouse	BaP/TPA, 3-MC	1,37,38
Gallic acid	Lung	Mouse	Morpholine + sodium nitrite, nitrosopiperazine	26
NDGA	Colon	Rat	MAM	1
	Mammary gland	Rat	MNU	573
	Skin	Mouse	DMBA/TPA	1
Propyl gallate	Mammary gland	Rat	DMBA	161,163
Tannic acid	Skin	Mouse	BaP/TPA, DMBA/TPA, 3-MC, MNU/TPA	1

TABLE 3.   *(Continued)*

Inhibitor	Target	Species	Carcinogen	References
		Other		
CuDIPS	Skin	Mouse	DMBA, DMBA/TPA	140,141
DMSO	Mammary gland	Rat	DMBA	295
	Skin	Mouse	DMBA/TPA	296
Ethoxyquin	Ear duct	Rat	DMBA	154,155
	Forestomach	Mouse	BaP	156
	Liver	Rat	Ciprofibrate, DEN/AAF/PH, OH-EEN	1,168
	Mammary gland	Rat	DMBA	154–156
Fumaric acid	Forestomach, lung	Mouse	NFN	455
	Liver	Mouse	Thioacetamide	574
		Rat	Me-DAB, thioacetamide	456,457
Inositol hexaphosphate	Intestines (NOS)	Rat	AOM	1
Vitamin C	Colon	Mouse, rat	DMH	1,149
	Kidney	Hamster	DES, 17β-Estradiol	1
	Liver	Rat	AFB_1	56
	Lung	Mouse, rat	Secondary amines + sodium nitrite	1
	Mammary gland	Rat	DMBA	345
	Skin	Mouse	DMBA/TPA	575
	Stomach	Rat	MNNG	55
Vitamin E	Buccal pouch	Hamster	DMBA	314,315
	Colon	Mouse, rat	DMH	148,149
	Ear duct	Rat	DMBA	147,154,155
	Liver	Rat	AFB_1	56
	Skin	Mouse	DMBA/croton oil	150,151

Note: In addition to compounds listed in this table, fish oil, Ω-eicosapentaenoic acid (Table 4), some retinoids and carotenoids (Table 7), some thiols/dithiolthiones/sulfides and sodium selenite (Table 9) are also antioxidants.

in terms of its carcinogenesis-inhibitory activity. It is, of course, a metabolic intermediate in mammalian tissues (in the citric acid and urea cycles) and is a GRAS (generally recognized as safe) substance used commercially in foods and beverages as an antioxidant, acidulant, flavoring agent, and as a feed additive and cure accelerator (451). The tumor-inhibiting efficacy of fumaric acid was shown first by Kuroda and coworkers (452,453). They identified fumaric acid as the component of the herb *Capsella bursapastoris*, responsible for its antiproliferative and anti-inflammatory properties; this is the basis of the inhibition by this botanical of the growth of transplanted tumors in mice (452) and gastric ulcers in rats (453). *Capsella* also reduces the liver toxicity of the carcinogens mitomycin C and AFB_1 (454). In a series of studies, Kuroda *et al.* (455–457) showed that fumaric acid has chemopreventive activity in mouse forestomach (455), rat liver (456,457), and mouse lung (455); however, the mechanism of action of fumaric acid has not been elucidated. The studies cited above suggest that it probably interferes with later stages of carcinogenesis. In studies with the mouse forestomach, rat liver, and mouse lung, fumaric acid was active when given after carcinogen treatment.

D. Arachidonic Acid (AA) Metabolism Inhibitors

The potential role of inhibition of AA metabolism is discussed in detail in Sections III.B.3 and III.C. Inhibitors of cyclooxygenase and lipoxygenase inhibit AA metabolism,

TABLE 4.   Arachidonic Acid (AA) Metabolism Inhibitors That Inhibit Chemical Carcinogenesis

Inhibitor	Target	Species	Carcinogen	References
Fatty acid/fatty alkyl compounds				
Ω-Eicosapentaenoic acid	Colon	Rat	AOM	576
Fish oil	Mammary gland	Rat	DMBA	577
Nonsteroidal anti-inflammatory drugs (NSAID)				
Aspirin	Urinary bladder	Rat	FANFT/saccharin	172
Ibuprofen	Buccal pouch	Hamster	DMBA	1
	Colon	Rat	AOM	578
Indomethacin	Colon	Rat	DMH, MAM, MNU	1
	Esophagus	Mouse	DEN	1
	Mammary gland	Rat	DMBA	1
Piroxicam	Colon	Rat	AOM, MAM, MNU	1,578
Other cyclooxygenase inhibitor				
4-Bromophenacyl bromide	Skin	Mouse	DMBA/TPA	1

Note: The compounds listed in this table are inhibitors of cyclooxygenase, a key enzyme involved in AA metabolism. Inhibitors of lipoxygenase (e.g., esculetin [Table 5], β-carotene [Table 7] and of phospholipase A_1/A_2 (e.g., morin, vitamin E [Table 3] and some steroidal anti-inflammatories) are also AA metabolism inhibitors.

whereas inhibitors of phospholipase A_1/A_2 reduce the release of AA from membrane phospholipids. Some cyclooxygenase inhibitors which have been shown to prevent chemical carcinogenesis are listed in Table 4. In addition to these compounds, a variety of antioxidants (*e.g.*, BHT, curcumin, morin, myricetin, NDGA, quercetin; *see* Table 3), steroid/sterol anti-inflammatory agents (*e.g.*, fluocinolone acetonide, 18β-glycyrrhetinic acid, hydrocortisone; *see* Section IV.B), β-carotene (Table 7), and NAC (Table 8) are also inhibitors of cyclooxygenase. Lipoxygenase inhibitors include tamoxifen (*see* Section IV.A), esculetin (Table 5), β-carotene (Table 7), and a variety of antioxidants. 4-Bromophenacyl bromide and indomethacin are inhibitors of both cyclooxygenase and phospholipase A_1/A_2; other carcinogenesis inhibitors such as compound "W-7" (Table 7), morin, vitamin E (Table 3), fluocinolone acetonide, and dexamethasone (*see* Section IV.B) are also inhibitors of phospholipase A_1/A_2.

E. GSH Enhancers

The ability of compounds to inhibit by enhancing the detoxification and excretion of carcinogens is discussed in Section III.A.4. As noted therein, the induction of Phase II metabolizing enzymes that lead to conjugation and excretion of the carcinogens is likely to be more effective in inhibiting carcinogenesis than is induction of the Phase I enzymes. This is because the Phase I enzymes, of which the most important are the cytochrome P-450 enzymes involved in oxidation of aromatic compounds, also are involved in activation of proximate carcinogens. For example, two of the prominent Phase I enzymes are cytochrome P-450 IA1, which catalyzes the conversion of PAH to the electrophilic and carcinogenic diolepoxides, and cytochrome P-450 IA2, which is involved in *N*-hydroxylation of aromatic amines (58). In contrast, the Phase II enzymes are involved in: (a) raising the intracellular levels of GSH for scavenging electrophile carcinogens (*see* Section III.B.1), (b) the catalysis of the detoxification of carcinogens by conjugation with GSH (via GSH *S*-transferases) and glucuronic acid (via UDP glucuronyltransferase), and (c) inactivating carcinogens by hydrolysis (via epoxide hydrolases). Talalay (58) has also

TABLE 5.   GSH Enhancers That Inhibit Chemical Carcinogenesis

Inhibitor	Target	Species	Carcinogen	References
		Lactones		
α-Angelicalactone	Forestomach	Mouse	BaP	97
Coumarin	Forestomach	Mouse	BaP	97
	Mammary gland	Rat	DMBA	97
Esculetin	Skin	Mouse	BaP, DMBA/TPA	1
		Other		
5,6-Benzoflavone	Liver	Rat	AFB$_1$	59
	Lung	Mouse	BaP, DMBA	61,62
	Mammary gland	Rat	DMBA	62
	Skin	Mouse	BaP/croton oil	60
7,8-Benzoflavone	Lung	Mouse	DMBA, DMBA/TPA	61,64
	Skin	Hamster	DMBA, DMBA/TPA	65
		Mouse	DMBA, DMBA/TPA, DMBA/croton oil, other PAH	66–73
Kahweol palmitate	Mammary gland	Rat	DMBA	1

Note: In addition to the compounds listed in this table, some antioxidants (e.g., BHA, BHT, ethoxyquin, 4-methoxyphenol; see Table 3), disulfiram analogs, and thiol and selenium compounds (Tables 8 and 9) are also GSH enhancers.

noted the importance of NADPH:quinone reductase which catalyzes the reduction of quinones, thereby preventing their involvement in the induction of oxidative damage to cells. As is evident from Sections III.A.4 and III.B.1, the elevation of intracellular GSH and its participation in conjugation reactions via GSH *S*-transferase appear to be particularly important. Table 5 lists inhibitors of carcinogenesis that enhance the GSH level, induce GSH *S*-transferase, or both.

In addition to Table 5, several thiols and dithiolthiones (*see* Table 8), disulfiram analogs, and selenium compounds (*see* Table 9) are also GSH enhancers. The dithiolthione compound, oltipraz, in particular, is one of the best characterized in terms of linking its carcinogenesis inhibitory effect to the elevation of GSH level and induction of Phase II enzymes. Its activity in inhibiting carcinogenesis is summarized in Section III. Although the mechanism of this activity is not fully understood, the anticarcinogenic potential of oltipraz was first suggested by its chemoprotective, radioprotective, and antimutagenic properties. Ansher *et al.* (458) demonstrated that oltipraz protects against hepatotoxicity in mice induced by acetaminophen and carbon tetrachloride. The agent also inhibits AFB$_1$ hepatotoxicity and DNA adduct formation in rat liver (459). Orally administered oltipraz increases liver GSH levels and induces enzymes involved in electrophile detoxification, namely, GSH *S*-transferases, epoxide hydrolase, and NADPH:quinone reductase (458–461). It also reacts with hydrogen peroxide catalyzed by glutathione peroxidase (GSH-Px) and prevents the formation of other more reactive oxygen compounds (462). The chemopreventive and chemoprotective efficacy of oltipraz in liver has been attributed to these activities (92,458,463).

F.   Ornithine Decarboxylase (ODC) Inhibitors

ODC inhibitors that inhibit carcinogenesis are listed in Table 6. These include mechanism-based specific irreversible inhibitors (*e.g.*, DFMO) and nonspecific inhibitors of enzyme induction. The role of ODC inhibition in prevention of carcinogenesis and the mechanism of action of DFMO-type inhibitors are discussed in Section III.C.4.

TABLE 6. **Orinithine Decarboxylase (ODC) Inhibitors That Inhibit Chemical Carcinogenesis**

Inhibitor	Target	Species	Carcinogen	References
Mechanism-based irreversible inhibitors				
DFMO	Colon	Mouse	DMH	230
		Rat	AOM	231,232
	Mammary gland	Rat	DMBA, MNU	189,233–236
	Skin	Mouse	DMBA/TPA	204,237,238
	Urinary bladder	Mouse	OH-BBN	234
		Rat	MNU, OH-BBN	239,240
Other				
Nicotinamide/nicotinic acid	Esophagus	Rat	MBN	322
	Intestines (NOS)	Rat	Bracken fern	1
	Pancreas	Hamster	BOP	1
	Urinary bladder	Rat	Bracken fern	1

Note: A variety of inhibitors of enzyme induction (such as anti-inflammatory agents, antioxidants, AA metabolism inhibitors) are also ODC inhibitors (see text).

G. Protein Kinase C (PKC) Inhibitors

Inhibition of PKC as a measure of modulation of signal transduction to inhibit carcinogenesis is discussed in Section III.C.1. Several PKC inhibitors—chlorpromazine, D,L-palmitoylcarnitine, verapamil, compound "W-7", cromolyn sodium—have been shown to inhibit PAH-induced carcinogenesis in skin, buccal pouch, and injection site (1,241,580). Cromolyn sodium is also capable of inhibiting DMBA-induced mammary carcinogenesis (579). A number of antioxidants (*e.g.*, morin, myricetin, quercetin; *see* Table 3), tamoxifen (an antihormone; *see* Section IV.A), and 18β-glycyrrhetinic acid (an anti-inflammatory agent; *see* Section IV.B) are all known to inhibit PKC.

H. Retinoids/Carotenoids

Retinoids and carotenoids that inhibit carcinogenesis are listed in Table 7 (*see also* Chapter 9, Section III). Hill and Grubbs (276) recently reviewed the activity of retinoids which are among the most frequently studied inhibitors of chemical carcinogenesis. Most of the retinoids tested are retinoic acids and esters (*e.g.*, 13-*cis*-retinoic acid), retinamides (*e.g.*, 4-HPR), or retinyl ethers and hydrocarbons (*e.g.*, retinyl methyl ether). Retinoids are active against chemically-induced leukemias and lymphomas and cancers in various tissues including skin, buccal pouch, mammary gland, bladder, lung, colon, and pancreas. Most studies have been in mammary gland, skin, and bladder. Hill and Grubbs (276) described some potential tissue specificities of the retinoids based on their chemical structures. For example, they noted that retinoids active in skin have side-chains with free carboxylic acid groups or groups that are readily bioconverted to the acid. Retinamides and derivatives of retinol without carboxylic acid groups are most active in mammary tissue. Retinamides also are active in bladder. Furthermore, Hill and Grubbs noted that pharmacokinetics appears to be important in determining the tissue specificity of the inhibitory activity. 4-HPR (256) and 13-*cis*-retinoic acid (464–472) are active in bladder, and they have relatively long half-lives in this tissue. 13-*cis*-Retinoic acid is ineffective in lung, where its half-life is shorter. 4-HPR is active in mammary gland (252–258), where it accumulates.

Retinoids are active in the proliferation and progression stages of carcinogenesis (201,258,473). For example, in the two-stage mouse skin carcinogenesis model, they

TABLE 7.   Retinoids/Carotenoids That Inhibit Chemical Carcinogenesis

Inhibitor	Target	Species	Carcinogen	References
Retinoids				
N-Ethylretinamide	Urinary bladder	Mouse	OH-BBN	259,472
		Rat	OH-BBN	472
Etretinate	Colon	Mouse	DMH	1
	Skin	Mouse	DMBA/croton oil, DMBA/TPA	1
	Urinary bladder	Rat	OH-BBN	1
4-HPR	Mammary gland	Rat	DMBA, MNU	252–258
	Skin	Mouse	DMBA/TPA	250,251
	Urinary bladder	Mouse	OH-BBN	256
N-(2-Hydroxyethyl) retinamide	Liver, pancreas	Rat	L-Azaserine	581
	Urinary bladder	Mouse	OH-BBN	259
13-*cis*-Retinoic acid	Mammary gland	Rat	DMBA	253
	Skin	Mouse	BaP/TPA, DMBA/TPA	1,201,204,208
	Urinary bladder	Mouse	MNU, OH-BBN	464–472
all-*trans*-Retinoic acid	Skin	Mouse	DMBA/TPA, DMBA/ other promoters	70,199–209
Vitamin A	Forestomach	Hamster	BaP + hematite	1
	Mammary gland	Rat	DMBA, EE2, MNU	1,255,345
	Skin	Mouse	DMBA, DMBA/croton oil, DMBA/Phenol	1
	Urinary bladder	Rat	OH-BBN	1
Carotenoids				
Canthaxanthine	Buccal pouch	Hamster	DMBA	136
	Mammary gland	Rat	DMBA	582
	Skin	Mouse	BaP	137
	Urinary bladder	Mouse	BaP	583
β-Carotene	Buccal pouch	Hamster	DMBA	135,136
	Forestomach	Hamster	DMBA	135
	Liver	Rat	AFB$_1$	56
	Salivary gland	Rat	DMBA	134
	Skin	Mouse	DMBA, DMBA/croton oil, DMBA/TPA	137–139
Crocetin	Skin	Mouse	DMBA/croton oil	1,137

Note: See Chapter 9, Section III for discussion.

inhibit carcinogenesis only when they are administered together with a tumor promoter (70,474). Retinoids inhibit several activities involved in tumor promotion, including induction of ODC (201); they probably modulate signal transduction via their own cellular receptors (275). As discussed in Section III.C.5, they induce terminal differentiation in selected cells, and this activity is mediated via receptor binding (273–275). They also enhance intercellular communication and are immunostimulants (*see* Section III.C.6).

The most extensively studied carotenoid is β-carotene. Its activity in inhibiting carcinogenesis may be attributed in part to its bioconversion to vitamin A (475–478). Carotenoids possess the antiproliferative and antiprogression activities associated with retinoids. Moreover, β-carotene and other carotenoids are known to participate in electron transport during photosynthesis and to protect plants from oxidative damage (128,478,479). In general, the potent inhibitory activity of carotenoids against lipid oxidation in plants and animals has been well documented (130,355,478–481). Studies on the inhibition by carotenoids of malignant transformation of C3H10T1/2 cells suggest that, besides retinoid activity, the antioxidant activity of carotenoids is important in their anticarcinogenic effects (478). Carotenoids, but not retinoids, enhance aryl hydrocarbon hydroxylase activity in the large intestine (482), suggesting that the boosting of the detoxification of PAH carcinogens is a component factor of their anticarcinogenic activity. Another feature of the inhibitory action of carotenoids has been reported by Bertram and coworkers (355) who found that the potency of carotenoids in inhibiting malignant transformation of C3H10T1/2 cells parallels their potency in stimulating intercellular communication in these cells, but does not correlate with either antioxidant activity or ability to convert to retinoids. Instead they observed (483) that stimulation of intercellular communication correlates with the potency of the carotenoids to induce the synthesis of connexin 43, one of the protein components of gap junction structure.

I.   Thiols/Dithiolthiones/Sulfides

Numerous thiol-containing compounds and thiol derivatives such as dithiolthiones and disulfides inhibit chemical carcinogenesis in animal studies. These compounds are listed in Table 8.

Many of these compounds are presumed to be inhibitors because they enhance the formation of GSH (*see* Section IV.E). Some of these may act by increasing the intracellular pool of cysteine, a precursor of GSH. One such compound is NAC, which is

TABLE 8.   Thiols/Dithiolthiones/Sulfides That Inhibit Chemical Carcinogenesis

Inhibitor	Target	Species	Carcinogen	References
		Thiols		
S-Allyl-L-cysteine	Colon	Mouse	DMH	489
GSH	Liver	Rat	AFB$_1$	56
	Skin	Mouse	DMBA/TPA	52,54
	Stomach	Rat	MNNG	55
4-Mercaptobenzene-sulfonate	Colon, forestomach	Mouse	BPL	108
2-Mercaptoethane-sulfonate	Urinary bladder	Rat	Cyclophosphamide, OH-BBN	1
2-Mercaptoethyl-amine	Mammary gland	Rat	DMBA	1
	Stomach	Rat	MNNG	1
Methionine	Mammary gland	Rat	DMBA, MNU	408
NAC	Colon, intestines	Rat	DMH	101
	Lung	Mouse	Urethane	102
		Dithiolthiones		
Oltipraz	Colon, small intestine	Rat	AOM	93
	Forestomach	Mouse	BaP	91
	Liver	Rat	AFB$_1$	92
	Lung	Mouse	BaP, DEN, uracil mustard	91
		Sulfides		
Allyl methyl disulfide	Forestomach, lung	Mouse	BaP	88
Allyl methyl trisulfide	Forestomach	Mouse	BaP	1,88
Diallyl sulfide	Colon	Mouse	DMH	86
	Esophagus	Rat	MBN	87
	Forestomach	Mouse	BaP	88
	Lung	Mouse	BaP, NNK	88,90
	Lung, thyroid	Rat	DEN + MNU + DBN	89

readily deacetylated to form cysteine (484). The inhibition of carcinogenesis by NAC is summarized in Table 8 and in Section III.A.6. Besides preventing a decrease in ADPRT levels (as described in Section III), other activities also may contribute to the ability of NAC to inhibit carcinogenesis. It is an inhibitor of cyclooxygenase (485) and TPA-induced ODC activity (486). Its activity against ODC induction may be attributable to the increased level of GSH, that is, it may be the consequence of free-radical scavenging by GSH which, in turn, limits the cascade of activities associated with tumor promotion, including ODC induction.

The allylic sulfides (S-allyl-L-cysteine, allyl methyl disulfide, allyl methyl trisulfide, diallyl sulfide, diallyl trisulfide) may inhibit carcinogenesis at least in part through the inhibition of the activation of carcinogens (*see* Section III.A.2). Yang and coworkers found that diallyl sulfide inhibits cytochrome P-450 IIE1 (487), which is the enzyme likely to be responsible for activation of nitrosamine and hydrazine carcinogens (487,488). Correlating with this possible mechanism, diallyl sulfide inhibits the induction of tumors by nitrosamines in rat esophagus (87), mouse (90) and rat lung (89), and rat thyroid (89). Furthermore, diallyl sulfide inhibits carcinogenesis in the rat esophagus by MBN only during the initiation phase (488). The mechanism of action of allylic sulfides may also consist in enhancing the detoxification of carcinogens (*see* Section III.A.4). Like the thiols and dithiolthiones, these compounds are effective inducers of GSH S-transferases (488,489).

J. Other Chemical Classes Associated with Inhibition of Carcinogenesis

The chemicals in Table 9 represent other chemical structural types known to inhibit carcinogenesis. The classes summarized in Tables 3 to 9 generally are very broad, containing large numbers of chemicals of widely varying structures. In contrast, the classes grouped into Table 9 are far more specific; they consist of small numbers of chemicals, chemicals that are closely related structurally, or both (*e.g.*, dehydroepiandrosterone [DHEA] and DHEA analogs).

1. Arylalkyl Isothiocyanates

As shown in Table 9, several arylalkyl isothiocyanates inhibit mammary, fore-stomach, and lung tumors induced by PAH and nitrosamines in rats and mice (45,46,49,490,491). Several possible mechanisms have been suggested. For example (as noted in Section III.A.4), benzyl isothiocyanate is known to enhance GSH S-transferase activity (492), thus promoting the detoxification and excretion of carcinogens. These compounds also inhibit proliferation and progression, as indicated by the activity of benzyl isothiocyanate of preventing DMBA-induced mammary tumors when administered starting 1 week after the carcinogen (6). As described in Section III, a series of arylalkyl isothiocyanates with alkyl chains ranging from two carbons (PEITC) to six carbons (phenylhexyl isothiocyanate) inhibit the induction of lung tumors in mice by the tobacco-specific carcinogen NNK (46,49,492). Available evidence indicates that the primary mechanism of the inhibition of NNK carcinogenesis by arylalkyl isothiocyanates is the inhibition of NNK activation (47). In these studies, the structural similarity of the isothiocyanates to NNK and the length of the alkyl chain proved to be important determinants of the inhibitory potency. Inhibition increased as the alkyl chain was lengthened. Thus, phenylhexyl isothiocyanate, the most potent of the agents tested, is 50–100 times more potent than PEITC (49,492). Although the reasons for the effect of alkyl chain length have not been fully elucidated, increased lipophilicity and stability have been suggested to be the basis of the higher activity (47).

TABLE 9.   Other Chemical Structures/Activities Associated with Inhibition of Chemical Carcinogenesis

Inhibitor	Target	Species	Carcinogen	References
Arylalkyl isothiocyanates				
Benzyl isothiocyanate	Forestomach	Mouse	BaP, DEN, DMBA	45,490
	Lung	Mouse	BaP, DMBA	45,490
	Mammary gland	Rat	DMBA	490,491
PEITC	Forestomach	Mouse	DMBA,	490
	Lung	Mouse	DMBA, NNK	44,49,490
	Mammary gland	Rat	DMBA	490
Higher homologs[a]	Lung	Mouse	NNK	49
Calcium compounds				
Calcium acetate	Lung	Mouse	Lead subacetate, nickel acetate	584
Calcium carbonate	Colon	Rat	DMH	19
Calcium chloride	Intestines (NOS)	Rat	Bracken fern + thiamine hydrochloride	1
	Urinary bladder	Rat	Bracken fern + thiamine hydrochloride	1
Calcium lactate	Colon	Rat	AOM	18
DHEA/DHEA analogs				
DHEA	Colon, anus	Mouse	DMH	497–499
	Lung	Mouse	DMBA, urethan	495
	Mammary gland	Rat	MNU	501
	Skin	Mouse	DMBA, DMBA/TPA	496,502
	Thyroid	Rat	DHPN	500
Fluasterone (DHEA analog 8354)	Mammary gland	Rat	MNU	501
	Skin	Mouse	DMBA/TPA	511,585
Disulfiram/disulfiram analogs				
Carbon disulfide	Intestines (NOS)	Mouse	DMH	514
Bis(ethylxanthogen)	Colon	Mouse	DMH	41
Diethyldithiocarbamic acid	Colon	Mouse	DMH	41
	Skin	Mouse	DMBA/TPA, DMBA/TPA/mezerein	520
Disulfiram	Colon	Mouse	AOM	41
	Forestomach, lung	Mouse	BaP	1,515,516
	Intestines (NOS)	Mouse	DMH	1,40
		Rat	AOM	1
	Mammary gland	Rat	AAF, DMBA	515,519
	Skin	Mouse	DMBA/TPA	54
	Urinary bladder	Rat	BCPN, OH-BBN	517,518
Glucarates				
2,5-Di-O-acetyl-D-glucaro-1,4:6,3-dilactone	Mammary gland	Rat	DMBA	521
Glucaric acid, calcium salt	Colon	Rat	AOM	586
	Mammary gland	Rat	DMBA, MNU	1,254
Indoles				
3,3'-Diindolylmethane	Forestomach	Mouse	BaP	82
	Mammary gland	Rat	DMBA	82
Indole	Urinary bladder	Hamster	DBN	1
Indole-3-carbinol	Forestomach	Mouse	BaP	82
	Mammary gland	Rat	DMBA	82

TABLE 9.   *(Continued)*

Inhibitor	Target	Species	Carcinogen	References
	Molybdenum compounds			
Molybdate, ammonium	Esophagus	Rat	MBN	322
Molybdate, sodium	Esophagus, forestomach	Rat	NSEE	523
	Mammary gland	Rat	MNU	524
	Monocyclic terpenes/isoprenylation inhibitors			
D-Limonene	Lung	Mouse	Dibenzpyrene, NNK	1,526
	Mammary gland	Rat	DMBA, MNU	527–529,587
(−)-Menthol	Mammary gland	Rat	DMBA	587
Nerolidol	Colon	Rat	AOM	220
	Protease inhibitors			
Antipain	Lung	Mouse	Urethan	225
BBI	Colon	Mouse	DMH	105
	Esophagus	Rat	MBN	107
	Liver	Mouse	DMH	106
Leupeptin	Skin	Mouse	DMBA/croton oil	226
Soybean trypsin inhibitor	Pancreas	Hamster	BOP	588
TAME, TLCK, TPCK	Skin	Mouse	DMBA/croton oil	1
	Selenium compounds			
Benzyl selenocyanate	Colon	Rat	AOM	321
	Forestomach	Mouse	BaP	323
	Mammary gland	Rat	DMBA	535
Selenite, sodium	Colon	Mouse	DMH	317
		Rat	AOM, BOP, DMH	318–320,542
	Esophagus	Rat	MBN	322
	Liver	Rat	AAF, Me-DAB	324–326
	Mammary gland	Rat	AAF, DMBA, MNU	1,324,329–346
	Pancreas	Hamster	BOP	327
	Stomach	Rat	MNNG	328
D,L-Selenomethionine	Mammary gland	Rat	DMBA	340,341
p-Xylylselenocyanate	Colon	Rat	AOM	589
	Vitamin D_3 metabolites			
1,25-Dihydroxychole-calciferol	Skin	Mouse	DMBA/TPA	548,549
1-Hydroxychole-calciferol	Colon	Rat	MNU/lithocholic acid	550

[a]Includes phenylpropyl/butyl/pentyl/hexyl and 4-(3-pyridyl)butyl isothiocyanates.

2. Calcium Compounds

Several mechanisms have been suggested to explain the inhibition of carcinogenesis by calcium. The possibility that it acts via inhibiting dietary fat promotion of tumors, induced in rat colon by AOM and DMH, is discussed in Section III.A.1. According to the proposed mechanism, calcium binds to excess fat, forming a complex that is unavailable to the cells. Calcium is essential for maintaining cell structure and membrane function. Wargovich (493) suggested that calcium could prevent carcinogen-induced proliferation by restoring the integrity of carcinogen-produced cell damage. Most importantly, as a second messenger, calcium is involved in the regulation of cell functions; its role in cell proliferation and differentiation may be particularly important in the inhibition of carcinogenesis (19,180,278,493). Sitrin *et al.* (19) cited preliminary work indicating that calcium inhibits mutational activation of K-*ras* in

DMH-induced colon tumors. This suggests inhibition of oncogene activity as another potential mechanism of inhibition related to the cellular roles of calcium.

3. DHEA/DHEA Analogs

DHEA is an adrenocortical steroid. Although it has no known physiological function, it is a precursor for the synthesis of testosterone and estradiol and a potent inhibitor of glucose 6-phosphate dehydrogenase (G6PDH), the first enzyme in the pentose phosphate metabolic pathway, involved in the generation of extramitochondrial NADPH and ribose 5-phosphate (494). As seen in Table 9, DHEA inhibits the induction of tumors by a variety of carcinogens, including DMBA (495,496), DMH (497–499), and nitroso compounds (500,501). It is effective in colon (497–499), mammary gland (501), lung (495), skin (502,496), and thyroid (500). Its inhibitory activity may be attributed in part to interference with carcinogen activation and binding. Just as DHEA inhibits DMBA-induced tumors in skin, orally and topically administered DHEA inhibits binding of DMBA to DNA in mouse skin (502,503). Additionally, DHEA has antiproliferative/antiprogression activity, demonstrated by its inhibition of TPA-promoted DMBA induction of skin tumorigenesis in mice (502) and its inhibition of TPA-induced DNA synthesis in mouse skin (504).

Schwartz has elucidated the mechanism of the anticarcinogenic activity of DHEA. On the basis of his own research and that of others, he hypothesized that the interference with both carcinogen activation and tumor promotion caused by DHEA can be attributed to inhibition of G6PDH (494,505). First, blocking of carcinogen activation can result from lowering of the NADPH cellular pool consequent to the inhibition of G6PDH. The lowered NADPH pool, in turn, can decrease the activity of NADPH-dependent mixed-function oxidases which activate carcinogens. This mechanism is supported by the observation that cultured fibroblasts from individuals with the Mediterranean variant of G6PDH deficiency are less sensitive to the cytotoxic and transforming activities of BaP, and metabolize BaP less efficiently than cells from normal individuals. Furthermore, normal cells treated with DHEA lose their sensitivity to BaP, and neither DHEA nor G6PDH deficiency protects the cells from MNU, which does not require metabolic activation (506).

The decreased levels of NADPH and ribose-5-phosphate after inhibition of G6PDH can affect cell proliferation by limiting nucleotide biosynthesis (494). Several steps in nucleotide biosynthesis depend on NADPH, including the reduction of folic acid to its active form, tetrahydrofolic acid, and the formation of deoxyribonucleotide diphosphates from ribonucleotide diphosphates by ribonucleotide reductase. Supporting evidence for this mechanism includes the observations that nucleosides can overcome DHEA-induced inhibition of growth of cultured HeLa cells (507), of DNA synthesis and development of enzyme-altered foci in rat liver (508,509), and of differentiation of 3T3 preadipocytes (510). Also, in the DHEA-treated preadipocytes, 6-phosphonogluconate, the product of G6PDH activity, partially restores differentiation (510), and orally administered deoxynucleosides reverse the inhibition of TPA promotion in mouse skin by the DHEA analog, fluasterone (511).

4. Disulfiram/Disulfiram Analogs

These compounds appear to inhibit carcinogenesis primarily by inhibiting the metabolic activation of carcinogens by microsomal mixed-function oxidases (39,512).

The site of inhibitory activity of the disulfiram compounds, most important in terms of clinical potential, is the colon, where they inhibit the carcinogenicity of DMH, and to a lesser extent that of the oxidative metabolite of DMH, AOM (40,41,513). Disulfiram is known to inhibit the oxidation of both of these compounds *in vivo* (39; *see also* Section III.A.2). Studies on the mechanism of disulfiram activity have shown that the whole structure is not required for inhibitory activity. The disulfiram metabolite, carbon disulfide, inhibits DMH tumor induction in mouse colon (514). Disulfiram derivatives and analogs also inhibit other carcinogens requiring oxidative metabolic activation such as PAH (54,515,516), nitrosamines (517,518), and the aromatic amine, AAF (519). Interestingly, disulfiram derivatives and analogs also inhibit tumor progression and promotion; disulfiram inhibits the progression of DMBA/TPA-induced tumors (54) and diethyldithiocarbamic acid inhibits both TPA and mezerein promotion of DMBA-initiated tumors (520).

5. Glucarates

Glucarates inhibit the enzyme β-glucuronidase, which hydrolyzes glucuronide esters. This inhibition of β-glucuronidase increases the levels of glucuronide conjugates of certain carcinogens, thereby leading to excretion instead of activation of the carcinogens. The inhibitory activity of glucarates against DMBA-induced mammary tumors has been attributed to this mechanism (521,522). However, glucarates also inhibit carcinogens such as MNU and AOM that do not require activation; they are therefore not likely to be affected by detoxification reactions. Glucarates also inhibit the promotional phase of carcinogenesis. These effects are explained by another possible mechanism: inhibition of β-glucuronidase increases the excretion of steroid hormones and thereby decreases tumor-promoting activity in glucarate-treated animals (522).

6. Indoles

Indoles, including indole-3-carbinol and 3,3'-diindolyl-methane, occur in cruciferous vegetables such as Brussels sprouts, broccoli, and cauliflower (512). Wattenberg (512) noted that indoles enhance the activity of microsomal mixed-function oxidases and inhibit carcinogenesis, possibly by increasing the oxidative detoxification rate of carcinogens. For example, in the inhibition of DMBA-induced mammary tumorigenesis in rats, potency correlated with the induction of aryl hydrocarbon hydroxylase (82). The activity of indole-3-carbinol in altering the hydroxylation pattern of estrogen, so as to emphasize detoxification, is discussed in Section III.A.4.

7. Molybdenum Compounds

Thus far, carcinogenesis-inhibitory activity of molybdenum compounds has been observed only with nitroso carcinogens. The mechanism of the inhibitory activity of molybdenum compounds is not yet understood. One possibility is a role in the maintenance of cellular differentiation (523). Another, more specific potential mechanism may be operative in the inhibition of mammary gland tumorigenesis; Wei and coworkers (524) noted that molybdenum compounds can interfere with the activation of estrogen receptors.

8. Monocyclic Terpenes/Isoprenylation-Inhibiting Compounds

Monocyclic terpenes such as D-limonene have potentially several mechanisms of inhibition. When given before carcinogen treatment, D-limonene inhibits the activation of DEN (7). In tests limited to a small number of animals and by toxicity toward the treated animals (decreased body weight gain), D-limonene and D-carvone were found to inhibit DEN-induced carcinogenesis in the mouse forestomach and lung (7,525). In a subsequent study, D-limonene was found to inhibit NNK-induced carcinogenesis in mouse lung (7,526). D-Limonene also is known to induce GSH S-transferase activity (7). These carcinogen-blocking activities may provide a partial explanation for the activity of D-limonene against mammary gland tumorigenesis induced by DMBA (217,527,528) and by MNU (217,529). As discussed in Section III.C.3, inhibition of oncogene activity also has been implicated in the prevention of mammary gland tumorigenesis by D-limonene. Both the monocyclic terpene D-limonene (217,530) and other terpenes such as nerolidol (8) appear to inhibit post-translational isoprenylation of oncogene products. This activity could lead to suppression of tumor proliferation and progression.

9. Protease Inhibitors

Proteases act on specific amino acid residues—*e.g.*, chymotrypsin is specific for phenylalanine, tyrosine, and tryptophan, while trypsin is specific for lysine and arginine. Some are specific for certain proteins, *e.g.*, collagenase. Tumor cells contain more proteases than normal cells (415). Although they have been implicated in blocking carcinogenesis by inhibiting error-prone DNA repair (*see* Section III.A.6), protease inhibitors appear to affect primarily the progression phase of carcinogenesis. As discussed in Section III.C.12, tumor cells contain many proteolytic enzymes that are thought to be involved in invasion and metastasis. Protease inhibitors may protect against this activity. Protease inhibitors have also been implicated in the suppression of oncogene expression (*see* Section III.C.3). A preliminary study has provided some direct evidence that protease inhibition may inhibit carcinogenesis; in this study, BBI inhibited both DMBA-induced tumors and elevated serine protease activity in the buccal pouch of hamsters (531).

Two types of protease inhibitors are listed in Table 9. The first type comprises small peptides and other compounds that can react directly with specific protease receptors and compete with the protease substrates (415). Such inhibitors are leupeptin, N-α-tosyl-L-arginine methyl ester (TAME), N-α-tosyl-L-lysine chloromethyl ketone (TLCK), and N-α-tosyl-L-phenylalanine chloromethyl ketone (TPCK). Other types of inhibitors, such as BBI, probably act by deactivating proteases (415).

10. Selenium Compounds

Selenium compounds display blocking, antioxidant, and antiproliferative/antiprogression activities. Their blocking activities include effects on carcinogen metabolism and binding to DNA. For example, sodium selenite increases the rate of detoxification and decreases the rate of activation of AAF in rats (326,532,533). It also inhibits the carcinogenicity of AAF in the rat toward the mammary gland and the liver (324). Benzylselenocyanate, which inhibits the development of AOM-induced colon tumors in rats (321), increases the metabolic degradation of AOM and MAM to CO_2 (534). This increased metabolism, which reduces the level of carcinogen delivered to the colon via the bloodstream, accounts for the lowered tumor incidence. Sodium selenite inhibits binding of AFB_1 to calf thymus DNA and the binding of DMBA to rat mammary cells. Likewise, selenium inhibits AFB_1-induced liver tumorigenesis in rats (56). Selenium compounds inhibit DMBA-induced carcinogenesis in rat mammary glands (329–346,535) and sodium selenite inhibits the activation of BaP *in vitro* and the induction of injection site tumors by BaP in mice (536).

The antioxidant effects of selenium compounds appear to be related to selenium being a cofactor of the enzyme glutathione peroxidase (GSH-Px), which catalyzes the reduction of H_2O_2 and organic hydroperoxides (537–539). Several studies show, however, that the anticarcinogenic activity of selenium in mouse and rat mammary glands is not mediated by GSH-Px (320,540,541). On the other hand, in other tissues, such as colon (542), glandular stomach (328), and skin (538), GSH-Px is thought to play a role.

Several studies have shown antiproliferative effects of selenium as indicated by inhibition of cell growth (543,544). For example, selenium compounds inhibit DNA (544), RNA (545), and protein synthesis (546). Also, certain selenium compounds (selenium oxide, selenious acid, and selenic acid) inhibit PKC (544). The immunostimulating effects of selenium and their relationship to inhibition of carcinogenesis are discussed in Section III.C.6. Additional aspects of the carcinogenesis-modulating effects of selenium compounds are reviewed in Chapter 9, Section IV.

11. Vitamin D_3/Vitamin D_3 Analogs

Vitamin D_3 is involved in the regulation of cell growth and differentiation mediated via the control of calcium levels (*see* Chapter 11, Section I). Vitamin D_3 receptors have been identified in cells of several target organs, including the intestines, bone, kidney, and hematopoietic system (287,547). There is evidence demonstrating that the vitamin D_3 compounds can inhibit chemical carcinogenesis. As listed in Table 9, the vitamin D_3 metabolites, 1,25-dihydroxycholecalciferol (1,25-DHCC; the hormonally active form of vitamin D_3) and 1-hydroxycholecalciferol (1-HCC), are known to inhibit chemically-induced tumors in mouse skin (548,549) and rat colon (550), respectively. 1,25-DHCC and 1-HCC both inhibit tumor promoter–induced ODC activity *in vivo* in rat colon, liver, skin, and stomach (551) and mouse skin (287,552).

Several direct markers of the effect of activated vitamin D_3 on cellular proliferation and differentiation also suggest its potential cancer-preventing activity. 1,25-DHCC inhibits the rate of tumor growth (553–555) and increases survival time of mice inoculated with murine myeloid leukemia cells (556,557). It inhibits cell proliferation in numerous cell lines *in vitro* (554,555,558–561) and enhances differentiation of human promyelocytic (HL-60) cells (288,289), human myeloid leukemic blast cells (286), and P388D1-derived 3-MC-induced lymphoma cells (291).

V. CANCER CHEMOPREVENTION: THE APPLIED SCIENCE OF THE INHIBITION OF CARCINOGENESIS

As defined in the beginning of this chapter, chemoprevention is the use of natural or synthetic chemicals to prevent, delay the onset or slow the progress of, or reverse the neoplastic process. Chemoprevention is a logical use of inhibitors of chemical carcinogenesis, and it is the focus of most of the studies of inhibitors discussed in this chapter, spearheaded by Wattenberg's early and continuing research (*e.g.*, 4–8,45,88,490,

512,525,562–564). Chemopreventive agents are already producing promising clinical results. Hong and coworkers (565) showed that 13-*cis* retinoic acid prevents the appearance of second primary tumors in patients who had been treated for squamous cell cancers of the larynx, pharynx, or oral cavity. Several major clinical trials of cancer chemopreventive agents are presently in progress, including the highly publicized trial of tamoxifen against breast cancer in women at high risk (422,566).

The Chemoprevention Branch of the National Cancer Institute initiated in 1985 a systematic drug development program with clinical trials as the end stage. This program has been extensively described (*e.g.*, 567,568). The first step of the program is the survey and review of published literature and previous test results to identify candidates for development. The chemicals selected in this process are tested *in vitro* for activities related to inhibition of carcinogenesis (*e.g.*, ODC inhibition and enhancement of GSH level), *in vitro* for inhibition of malignant transformation and tumor phenotype expression, and in animal models to determine their potential efficacy. Those that are efficacious are reevaluated and submitted to preclinical toxicological testing and clinical trials, as appropriate. As of the time of this writing, more than 300 chemicals have entered the program: 198 are in *in vitro* tests, 129 are under testing in animal models, 22 are in toxicological tests, 10 are in Phase I clinical trials, and 17 are in Phase II and III clinical trials.

For this chapter, the progress in animal efficacy tests is of primary interest. In the program, most of the efficacy tests completed have been for inhibition of chemical carcinogenesis induced by the following carcinogens and in tissue targets: DEN in hamster lung, MNU in hamster trachea, MAM in mouse colon, AOM in rat colon, DMBA and MNU in rat mammary gland, OH-BBN in mouse urinary bladder, and DMBA/TPA in mouse skin. Among the 129 chemicals tested, several, including β-carotene, DFMO, 18β-glycyrrhetinic acid, 4-HPR, oltipraz, NAC, and piroxicam, are among those now in clinical trial.

At least two factors limit the potential usefulness of chemopreventives in clinical practice. One is that cancers are not reduced to zero by administration of these agents, another is toxicity. Several very promising agents are toxic at efficacious doses; however, the simultaneous or sequential administration of multiple inhibitors each at lower dose can increase the efficacy of chemoprevention and yet reduce overall toxicity. Such an approach uses differences in the mechanism of tumor inhibition among the agents to increase the inhibitory activity. Furthermore, the increased efficacy achieves desirable levels of cancer inhibition at lower and less toxic doses of the individual agents. For example, synergistic chemopreventive activity is seen with combinations of β-carotene and 4-HPR or vitamin A in hamster lung. DFMO is synergistic with 4-HPR in hamster lung and mouse bladder, with oltipraz in mouse bladder, and with piroxicam in rat colon. Also, 4-HPR is synergistic with oltipraz in hamster lung and mouse bladder, and with tamoxifen in rat mammary gland. The progress that has been made to date, due in large part to studies on the inhibition of chemical carcinogenesis in animals, clearly indicates that research on chemoprevention is on the threshold of beginning to yield practical clinical applications.

Abbreviations Used*: AA, arachidonic acid; AAF, 2-acetylaminofluorene; ADPRT, poly(ADP-ribosyl)transferase; AFB$_1$, aflatoxin B$_1$; AOM, azoxymethane; BaP, benzo[*a*]pyrene; BBI, Bowman–Birk soybean trypsin inhibitor; BCPN, 3-butyl-*N*-

---

*In two-stage carcinogenesis studies, the carcinogen and tumor promoter are represented as carcinogen/tumor promoter (*e.e.*, DMBA/TPA).

(3-carboxypropyl)nitrosamine; BHA, butylated hydroxyanisole; BHT, butylated hydroxytoluene; BOP, N-nitrosobis(2-oxopropyl)amine; BPL, β-propiolactone; CuDIPS, copper (II) 3,5-diisopropylsalicylic acid; DB(a,h)A, dibenz[a,h]anthracene; DBN, N, N-dibutylnitrosamine; DEN, N,N-diethylnitrosamine; DES, diethylstilbestrol; DFMO, 2-difluoromethylornithine; DHEA, dehydroepiandrosterone; DHPN, N, N-dihydroxy-dipropylnitrosamine; DMBA, 7,12-dimethylbenz[a]anthracene; DMH, 1,2-dimethyl-hydrazine; DMN, N,N-dimethylnitrosamine; DMSO, dimethylsulfoxide; EE2, 17α-ethinylestradiol; EGF, epidermal growth factor; FANFT, N-[4-(5-nitro-2-furyl)-2-thiazolyl]formamide; G6PDH, glucose-6-phosphate dehydrogenase; GSH, glutathione; GSH-Px, GSH peroxidase; HETE, hydroxyeicosatetraenoic acid; HPETE, hydroperoxy-eicosatetraenoic acid; 4-HPR, *all-trans-N*-(4-hydroxyphenyl)retinamide; IGF-1, insulin-like growth factor 1; MAM, methylazoxymethanol; MBN, N-methylbenzylnitrosamine; Me-DAB, 3'-methyl-N,N-dimethylaminoazobenzene; 3-MC, 3-methylcholanthrene; MNNG, N-methyl-N'-nitro-N-nitrosoguanidine; MNU, N-methyl-N-nitrosourea; NAC, N-acetyl-L-cysteine; NDGA, nordihydroguaiaretic acid; NFN, potassium 1-methyl-7-[2-(5-nitro-2-furyl)vinyl]-4-oxo-1,4-dihydro-1,8-naphthydridine-3-carboxylate; NK, natural killer; NNK, 4-(methylnitrosamino)-1-(3-pyridyl)-1-butanone; NOS, not otherwise specified; NSAID, nonsteroidal antiinflammatory drug; NSEE, N-nitrososarcosine ethyl ester; ODC, ornithine decarboxylase; OH-BBN, N-butyl-N-(4-hydroxybutyl)nitrosamine; OH-EEN, N-ethyl-N-hydroxyethyl-nitrosamine; PAH, polycyclic aromatic hydrocarbon; PEITC, phenethyl isothiocyanate; PG, prostaglandin; PH, partial hepatectomy; PKC, protein kinase C; TAME, N-α-tosyl-L-arginine methyl ester; TGF-β, transforming growth factor β; TLCK, N-α-tosyl-L-lysine chloromethyl ketone; TPCK, N-α-tosyl-L-phenyl-alanine chloromethyl ketone; TPA, 12-O-tetradecanoylphorbol-13-acetate; W-7, N-(6-aminohexyl)-5-chloro-1-naphthalenesulfonamide.

REFERENCES

1. Bagheri, D., Doeltz, M. K., Fay, J. R., Helmes, C. T., Monasmith, L. A., and Sigman, C. C.: *Environ. Carcino. Rev.* **C6**, No.3, Special Issue (1988–89).
2. CCS Associates: "Master List of Chemopreventive Agents," Prepared for Chemoprevention Branch, DCPC, NCI. NIH Contract No NO1-CN-25417. CCS Associates, Palo Alto, California December 1992.
3. Sporn, M. B., and Newton, D. L.: *Federation Proc.* **38**, 2528 (1979).
4. Wattenberg, L. W.: *Cancer Res.* **26**, 1520 (1966).
5. Wattenberg, L. W.: *Cancer Res.* **43**, 2448S (1983).
6. Wattenberg, L. W.: *Cancer Res.* **45**, 1 (1985).
7. Wattenberg, L. W.: *Cancer Res.* **52**, 2085S (1992).
8. Wattenberg, L. W.: Chemoprevention of Cancer by Naturally Occurring and Synthetic Compounds. *In* "Cancer Chemoprevention" (L. Wattenberg, M. Lipkin, C. W. Boone, and G. J. Kelloff, eds.). CRC Press, Boca Raton, Florida, 1992, p. 19.
9. Klingelhutz, A. J., Wu, S.-Q., Huang, J., and Reznikoff, C. A.: *Cancer Res.* **52**, 1631 (1992).
10. De Flora, S., and Ramel, C.: *Mutat. Res.* **202**, 285 (1988).
11. Weinstein, I. B.: *Mutat. Res.* **202**, 413 (1988).
12. Rotstein, J. B., and Slaga, T. J.: *Mutat. Res.* **202**, 421 (1988).
13. Hartman, P. E., and Shankel, D. M.: *Environ. Mol. Mutagen.* **15**, 145 (1990).
14. Weinstein, I. B.: *Cancer Res.* **51**, 5080 (1991).
15. Kensler, T. W., Trush, M. A., and Guyton, K. Z.: Free Radicals as Targets for Cancer Chemoprevention: Prospects and Problems. *In* "Cellular and Molecular Targets for Chemoprevention" (V. E. Steele, G. D. Stoner, C. W. Boone, and G. J. Kelloff, eds.) CRC Press, Boca Raton, Florida, 1992, p. 173.
16. Verma, A. K.: Ornithine Decarboxylase, a Possible Target for Human Cancer Prevention. *In* "Cellular and Molecular Targets for Chemoprevention" (V. E. Steele, G. D. Stoner, C. W. Boone, and G. J. Kelloff, eds.). CRC Press, Boca Raton, Florida, 1992, p. 207.

17. Zenser, T. V., and Davis, B. B.: Arachidonic Acid Metabolism. *In* "Cellular and Molecular Targets for Chemoprevention" (V. E. Steele, G. D. Stoner, C. W. Boone, and G. J. Kelloff, eds.). CRC Press, Boca Raton, Florida, 1992, p. 225.

18. Wargovich, M. J., Allnutt, D., Palmer, C., Anaya, P., and Stephens, L. C.: *Cancer Lett.* **53**, 17 (1990).

19. Sitrin, M. D., Halline, A. G., Abrahams, C., and Brasitus, T. A.: *Cancer Res.* **51**, 5608 (1991).

20. Reshef, R., Rozen, P., Fireman, Z., Fine, N., Barzilai, M., Shasha, S. M., and Shkolnik, T.: *Cancer Res.* **50**, 1764 (1990).

21. Wargovich, M. J., Eng, V. W. S., Newmark, H. L., and Bruce, W. R.: *Carcinogenesis* **4**, 1205 (1983).

22. Wargovich, M. J., Eng, V. W. S., and Newmark, H. L.: *Cancer Lett.* **23**, 253 (1984).

23. Bird, R. P., Schneider, R., Stamp, D., and Bruce, W. R.: *Carcinogenesis* **7**, 1657 (1986).

24. Newmark, H. L., and Lipkin, M.: *Cancer Res.* **52**, 2067S (1992).

25. Newmark, H. L., Wargovich, M. J., and Bruce, W. R.: *J. Natl. Cancer Inst.* **72**, 1323 (1984).

26. Mirvish, S. S., Cardesa, A., Wallcave, L., and Shubik, P.: *J. Natl. Cancer Inst.* **55**, 633 (1975).

27. Mirvish, S. S., Wallcave, L., Eagen, M., and Shubik, P.: *Science* **177**, 65 (1972).

28. Mirvish, S. S.: Ascorbic Acid Inhibition of *N*-Nitroso Compound Formation in Chemical, Food, and Biological Systems. *In* "Inhibition of Tumor Induction and Development" (M. S. Zedeck and M. Lipkin, eds.). Plenum Press, New York, 1981, p. 101.

29. Mirvish, S. S.: *Cancer* **58**, 1842 (1986).

30. Kyrtopoulos, S. A.: *Am. J. Clin. Nutr.* **45**, 1344 (1987).

31. Bartsch, H., Ohshima, H., and Pignatelli, B.: *Mutat. Res.* **202**, 307 (1988).

32. Mackerness, C. W., Leach, S. A., Thompson, M. H., and Hill, M. J.: *Carcinogenesis* **10**, 397 (1989).

33. Kuenzig, W., Chau, J., Norkus, E., Holowaschenko, H., Newmark, H., Mergens, W., and Conney, A. H.: *Carcinogenesis* **5**, 309 (1984).

34. Newmark, H. L., and Mergens, W.: α-Tocopherol (Vitamin E) and Its Relationship to Tumor Induction and Development. *In* "Inhibition of Tumor Induction and Development" (M. S. Zedeck and M. Lipkin, eds.). Plenum Press, New York, 1981, p. 127.

35. Dixit, R., Teel, R. W., Daniel, F. B., and Stoner, G. D.: *Cancer Res.* **45**, 2951 (1985).

36. Teel, R. W., Dixit, R., and Stoner, G. D.: *Carcinogenesis* **6**, 391 (1985).

37. Mukhtar, H., Das, M., and Bickers, D. R.: *Cancer Res.* **46**, 2262 (1986).

38. Mukhtar, H., Das, M., Del Tito, B. J., Jr., and Bickers, D. R.: *Biochem. Biophys. Res. Commun.* **119**, 751 (1984).

39. Fiala, E. S., Bobotas, G., Kulakis, C., Wattenberg, L. W., and Weisburger, J. H.: *Biochem. Pharmacol.* **26**, 1763 (1977).

40. Wattenberg, L. W.: *J. Natl. Cancer Inst.* **54**, 1005 (1975).

41. Wattenberg, L. W., Lam, L. K. T., Fladmoe, A. V., and Borchert, P.: *Cancer* **40**, 2432 (1977).

42. Chung, F.-L., Juchatz, A., Vitarius, J., and Hecht, S. S.: *Cancer Res.* **44**, 2924 (1984).

43. Chung, F.-L., Wang, M., and Hecht, S. S.: *Carcinogenesis* **6**, 539 (1985).

44. Morse, M. A., Amin, S. G., Hecht, S. S., and Chung, F.-L.: *Cancer Res.* **49**, 2894 (1989).

45. Wattenberg, L. W.: *Carcinogenesis* **8**, 1971 (1987).

46. Morse, M. A., Wang, C.-X., Stoner, G. D., Mandal, S., Conran, P. B., Amin, S. G., Hecht, S. S., and Chung, F.-L.: *Cancer Res.* **49**, 549 (1989).

47. Chung, F.-L.: Chemoprevention of Lung Carcinogenesis by Aromatic Isothiocyanates. *In* "Cancer Chemoprevention" (L. Wattenberg, M. Lipkin, C. W. Boone, and G. J. Kelloff, eds.). CRC Press, Boca Raton, Florida, 1992, p. 227.

48. Morse, M. A., Eklind, K. I., Amin, S. G., Hecht, S. S., and Chung, F-L.: *Carcinogenesis* **10**, 1757 (1989).

49. Morse, M. A., Eklind, K. I., Hecht, S. S., Jordan, K. G., Choi, C., Desai, D. H., Amin, S. G., and Chung, F.-L.: *Cancer Res.* **51**, 1846 (1991).

50. Sayer, J. M., Yagi, H., Wood, A. W., Conney, A. H., and Jerina, D. M.: *J. Am. Chem. Soc.* **104**, 5562 (1982).

51. Ketterer, B.: *Mutat. Res.* **202**, 343 (1988).

52. Perchellet, J.-P., Owen, M. D., Posey, T. D., Orten, D. K., and Schneider, B. A.: *Carcinogenesis* **6**, 567 (1985).

53. Perchellet, J.-P., Abney, N. L., Thomas, R. M., Guislain, Y. L., and Perchellet, E. M.: *Cancer Res.* **47**, 477 (1987).

54. Rotstein, J. B., and Slaga, T. J.: *Carcinogenesis* **9**, 1547 (1988).

55. Balansky, R. M., Blagoeva, P. M., Mircheva, Z. I., Stoitchev, I., and Chernozemski, I.: *J. Cancer Res. Clin. Oncol.* **112**, 272 (1986).

56. Nyandieka, H. S., Wakhis, J., and Kilonzo, M. M.: *Indian J. Med. Res.* **92**, 332 (1990).

57. Prochaska, H. J., and Talalay, P.: *Cancer Res.* **48**, 4776 (1988).

58. Talalay, P.: Chemical Protection Against Cancer by Induction of Electrophile Detoxication (Phase II)

Enzymes. *In* "Cellular and Molecular Targets for Chemoprevention" (V. E. Steele, G. D. Stoner, C. W. Boone, and G. J. Kelloff, eds.). CRC Press, Boca Raton, Florida, 1992, p. 193.

59. Gurtoo, H. L., Koser, P. L., Bansal, S. K., Fox, H. W., Sharma, S. D., Mulhern, A. I., and Pavelic, Z. P.: *Carcinogenesis* **6**, 675 (1985).
60. Wattenberg, L. W., and Leong, J. L.: *Cancer Res.* **30**, 1922 (1970).
61. Diamond, L., McFall, R., Miller, J., and Gelboin, H. V.: *Cancer Res.* **32**, 731 (1972).
62. Wattenberg, L. W., and Leong, J. L.: *Proc. Soc. Exp. Biol. Med.* **128**, 940 (1968).
63. Bowden, G. T., Slaga, T. J., Shapas, B. G., and Boutwell, R. K.: *Cancer Res.* **34**, 2634 (1974).
64. Goerttler, K., and Loehrke, H.: *Carcinogenesis* **7**, 1187 (1986).
65. Goerttler, K., Loehrke, H., Hesse, B., and Pyerin, W. G.: *Carcinogenesis* **3**, 791 (1982).
66. Coombs, M. M., Bhatt, T. S., and Young, S.: *Br. J. Cancer* **40**, 914 (1979).
67. DiGiovanni, J., Slaga, T. J., Viaje, A., Berry, D. L., Harvey, R. G., and Juchau, M. R.: *J. Natl. Cancer Inst.* **61**, 135 (1978).
68. Gelboin, H. V., Wiebel, F., and Diamond, L.: *Science* **170**, 169 (1970).
69. Kinoshita, N., and Gelboin, H. V.: *Cancer Res.* **32**, 1329 (1972).
70. Verma, A. K., Conrad, E. A., and Boutwell, R. K.: *Cancer Res.* **42**, 3519 (1982).
71. Kinoshita, N., and Gelboin, H. V.: *Proc. Natl. Acad. Sci. USA* **69**, 824 (1972).
72. Thompson, S., and Slaga, T. J.: *Eur. J. Cancer* **12**, 363 (1976).
73. Slaga, T. J., and Bracken, W. M.: *Cancer Res.* **37**, 1631 (1977).
74. Alworth, W. L., and Slaga, T. J.: *Carcinogenesis* **6**, 487 (1985).
75. Welsch, C. W., Adams, C., Lambrecht, L. K., Hassett, C. C., and Brooks, C. L.: *Br. J. Cancer* **35**, 322 (1977).
76. Welsch, C. W., Goodrich-Smith, M., Brown, C. K., and Wilson, M.: *Int. J. Cancer* **24**, 92 (1979).
77. Wolfrom, D. M., Rao, A. R., and Welsch, C. W.: *Breast Cancer Res. Treat.* **19**, 269 (1991).
78. Blask, D. E., Pelletier, D. B., Hill, S. M., Lemus-Wilson, A., Grosso, D. S., Wilson, S. T., and Wise, M. E.: *J. Cancer Res. Clin. Oncol.* **117**, 526 (1991).
79. Welsch, C. W., Goodrich-Smith, M., Brown, C. K., Greene, H. D., and Hamel, E. J.: *Carcinogenesis* **2**, 519 (1981).
80. Liehr, J. G., Sirbasku, D. A., Jurka, E., Randerath, K., and Randerath, E.: *Cancer Res.* **48**, 779 (1988).
81. Henderson, B. E., Ross, R. K., Shibata, A., Paganini-Hill, A., and Yu, M. C.: Environmental Carcinogens and Anticarcinogens. *In* "Cancer Chemoprevention" (L. Wattenberg, M. Lipkin, C. W. Boone, and G. J. Kelloff, eds.). CRC Press, Boca Raton, Florida, 1992, p. 3.
82. Wattenberg, L. W., and Loub, W. D.: *Cancer Res.* **38**, 1410 (1978).
83. Bradlow, H. L., Michnovicz, J. J., Telang, N. T., and Osborne, M. P.: *Carcinogenesis* **12**, 1571 (1991).
84. Bradfield, C. A., and Bjeldanes, L. F.: *Food Chem. Toxicol.* **22**, 977 (1984).
85. Michnovicz, J. J., and Bradlow, H. L.: *Nutr. Cancer* **16**, 59 (1991).
86. Wargovich, M. J.: *Carcinogenesis* **8**, 487 (1987).
87. Wargovich, M. J., Woods, C., Eng, V. W. S., Stephens, L. C., and Gray, K.: *Cancer Res.* **48**, 6872 (1988).
88. Sparnins, V. L., Barany, G., and Wattenberg, L. W.: *Carcinogenesis* **9**, 131 (1988).
89. Jang, J. J., Cho, K. J., Lee, Y. S., and Bae, J. H.: *Carcinogenesis* **12**, 691 (1991).
90. Hong, J.-Y., Wang, Z. Y., Smith, T. J., Zhou, S., Shi, S., Pan, J., and Yang, C. S.: *Carcinogenesis* **13**, 901 (1992).
91. Wattenberg, L. W., and Bueding, E.: *Carcinogenesis* **7**, 1379 (1986).
92. Roebuck, B. D., Liu, Y.-L., Rogers, A. E., Groopman, J. D., and Kensler, T. W.: *Cancer Res.* **51**, 5501 (1991).
93. Rao, C. V., Tokomo, K., Kelloff, G., and Reddy, B. S.: *Carcinogenesis* **12**, 1051 (1991).
94. Dixit, R., and Gold, B.: *IARC Sci. Publ.* **84**, 197 (1987).
95. Barch, D. H., and Fox, C. C.: *Cancer Res.* **48**, 7088 (1988).
96. Kada, T., Inoue, T., Ohta, T., and Shirasu, Y.: *Basic Life Sci.* **39**, 181 (1986).
97. Wattenberg, L. W., Lam, L. K. T., and Fladmoe, A. V.: *Cancer Res.* **39**, 1651 (1979).
98. Shall, S.: *Adv. Radiat. Biol.* **11**, 1 (1984).
99. Scovassi, A. I., Stefanini, M., Lagomarsini, P., Izzo, R., and Bertazzoni, U.: *Carcinogenesis* **8**, 1295 (1987).
100. Cesarone, C. F., Scovassi, A. I., Scarabelli, L., Izzo, R., Orunesu, M., and Bertazzoni, U.: *Cancer Res.* **48**, 3581 (1988).
101. Wilpart, M., Speder, A., and Roberfroid, M.: *Cancer Lett.* **31**, 319 (1986).
102. De Flora, S., Astengo, M., Serra, D., and Bennicelli, C.: *Cancer Lett.* **32**, 235 (1986).
103. Meyn, S. M., Rossman, T., and Troll, W.: *Proc. Natl. Acad. Sci. U.S.A.* **74**, 1152 (1977).
104. Baturay, N., and Kennedy, A. R.: *Cell Biol. Toxicol.* **2**, 21 (1986).

105. Weed, H. G., McGandy, R. B., and Kennedy, A. R.: *Carcinogenesis* **6**, 1239 (1985).
106. St. Clair, W. H., Billings, P. C., Carew, J. A., Keller-McGandy, C., Newberne, P., and Kennedy, A. R.: *Cancer Res.* **50**, 580 (1990).
107. von Hofe, E., Newberne, P. M., and Kennedy, A. R.: *Carcinogenesis* **12**, 2147 (1991).
108. Hochalter, J. B., Wattenberg, L. W., Coccia, J. B., and Galbraith, A. R.: *Cancer Res.* **48**, 2740 (1988).
109. Hochstein, P., and Atallah, A. S.: *Mutat. Res.* **202**, 363 (1988).
110. Simic, M. G.: *Mutat. Res.* **202**, 377 (1988).
111. Cerutti, P. A.: *Science* **227**, 375 (1985).
112. Imlay, J. A., and Linn, S.: *Science* **240**, 1302 (1988).
113. Basu, A. K., Loechler, E. L., Leadon, S. A., and Essigmann, J. M.: *Proc. Natl. Acad. Sci. U.S.A.* **86**, 7677 (1989).
114. O'Brien, P. J.: *Environ. Health Perspect.* **64**, 219 (1985).
115. Marnett, L. J.: *Carcinogenesis* **8**, 1365 (1987).
116. Zimmerman, R., and Cerutti, P.: *Proc. Natl. Acad. Sci. U.S.A.* **81**, 2085 (1984).
117. Nakamura, Y., Gindhart, T. D., Winterstein, D., Tomita, I., Seed, J. L., and Colburn, N. H.: *Carcinogenesis* **9**, 203 (1988).
118. Crawford, D., Zbinden, I., Amstad, P., and Cerutti, P.: *Oncogene* **3**, 27 (1988).
119. Demopoulos, H. B., Pietronigro, D. D., and Seligman, M. L.: *J. Am. Coll. Toxicol.* **2**, 173 (1983).
120. Weitzman, S. A., and Gordon, L. I.: *Blood* **76**, 655 (1990).
121. Slaga, T. J., Klein-Szanto, A. J. P., Triplett, L. L., Yotti, L. P., and Trosko, J. E.: *Science* **213**, 1023 (1981).
122. Taffe, B. G., Zweier, J. L., Pannell, L. K., and Kensler, T. W.: *Carcinogenesis* **10**, 1261 (1989).
123. Pryor, W. A.: *Free Rad. Biol. Med.* **4**, 219 (1988).
124. De Flora, S., Bennicelli, C., Zanacchi, P., D'Agostini, F., and Camoirano, A.: *Mutat. Res.* **214**, 153 (1989).
125. Foote, C. S., Chang, Y. C., and Denny, R. W.: *J. Am. Chem. Soc.* **92**, 5216 (1970).
126. Foote, C. S.: Quenching of Singlet Oxygen. *In* "Singlet Oxygen" (H. H. Wasserman, ed.). Academic Press, New York, 1979, p. 139.
127. Packer, J. E., Mahood, J. S., Mora-Arellano, V. O., Slater, T. F., Willson, R. L., and Wolfenden, B. S.: *Biochem. Biophys. Res. Commun.* **98**, 901 (1981).
128. Burton, G. W., and Ingold, K. U.: *Science* **224**, 569 (1984).
129. Cerutti, P. A., Nygaard, O. F., and Simic, M. G. (eds.): "Anticarcinogenesis and Radiation Protection". Plenum Press, New York, 1987, p. 41.
130. Krinsky, N. I.: *Free Radic. Biol. Med.* **7**, 617 (1989).
131. Burton, G. W.: *J. Nutr.* **19**, 109 (1989).
132. Rousseau, E. J., Davison, A. J., and Rosin, M. P.: *Environ. Mol. Mutagen.* **14**, 167, Abst. no. 485 (1989).
133. Temple, N. J., and Basu, T. K.: *J. Natl. Cancer Inst.* **78**, 1211 (1987).
134. Alam, B. S., and Alam, S. Q.: *Nutr. Cancer* **9**, 93 (1987).
135. Gijare, P. S., Rao, K. V. K., and Bhide, S. V.: *Nutr. Cancer* **14**, 253 (1990).
136. Schwartz, J. L., Sloane, D., and Shklar, G.: *Tumor Biol.* **10**, 297 (1989).
137. Mathews-Roth, M. M.: *Oncology* **39**, 33 (1982).
138. Steinel, H. H., and Baker, R. S. U.: *Cancer Lett.* **51**, 163 (1990).
139. Lambert, L. A., Koch, W. H., Wamer, W. G., and Kornhauser, A.: *Nutr. Cancer* **13**, 213 (1990).
140. Solanki, V., Yotti, L., Logani, M. K., and Slaga, T. J.: *Carcinogenesis* **5**, 129 (1984).
141. Kensler, T. W., Bush, D. M., and Kozumbo, W. J.: *Science* **221**, 75 (1983).
142. Burton, G. W., and Ingold, K. U.: *J. Am. Chem. Soc.* **103**, 6472 (1981).
143. McCay, P. B.: *Annu. Rev. Nutr.* **5**, 323 (1985).
144. Pryor, W. A.: *Basic Life Sci.* **39**, 45 (1986).
145. Cerutti, P. A., Nygaard, O. F., and Simic, M. G. (eds.): "Anticarcinogenesis and Radiation Protection". Plenum Press, New York, 1987, p. 47.
146. Gorman, A. A., and Rodgers, M. A. J.: *Chem. Soc. Rev.* **10**, 205 (1981).
147. Shklar, G., Schwartz, J., Trickler, D. P., and Niukian, K.: *J. Natl. Cancer Inst.* **78**, 987 (1987).
148. Cook, M. G., and McNamara, P.: *Cancer Res.* **40**, 1329 (1980).
149. Colacchio, T. A., Memoli, V. A., and Hildebrandt, L.: *Arch. Surg.* **124**, 217 (1989).
150. Shamberger, R. J.: *J. Natl. Cancer Inst.* **44**, 931 (1970).
151. Shamberger, R. J., and Rudolph G.: *Experientia* **22**, 116 (1966).
152. Twentyman, P. R., Fox, N. E., and White, D. J. G.: *Br. J. Cancer* **56**, 55 (1987).
153. Clapp, N. K., Bowles, N. D., Satterfield, L. C., and Klima, W. C.: *J. Natl. Cancer Inst.* **63**, 1081 (1979).
154. Hirose, M., Masuda, A., Inoue, T., Fukushima, S., and Ito, N.: *Carcinogenesis* **7**, 1155 (1986).
155. Ito, N., Hirose, M., Fukushima, S., Tsuda, H., Shirai, T., and Tatematsu, M.: *Food Chem. Toxicol.* **24**, 1071 (1986).

156. Wattenberg, L. W.: *J. Natl. Cancer Inst.* **48**, 1425 (1972).
157. Ulland, B. M., Weisburger, J. H., Yamamoto, R. S., and Weisburger, E. K.: *Food Cosmet. Toxicol.* **11**, 199 (1973).
158. King, M. M., McCay, P. B., and Kosanke, S. D.: *Cancer Lett.* **14**, 219 (1981).
159. McCormick, D. L., Major, N., and Moon, R. C.: *Cancer Res.* **44**, 2858 (1984).
160. King, M. M., and McCay, P. B.: *Cancer Res.* **43**, 2485s (1983).
161. King, M. M., Terao, J., Brueggemann, G., McCay, P. B., and Magarian, R. A.: *ACS Symp. Ser.* **277**, 131 (1985).
162. McCormick, D. L., May, C. M., Thomas, C. F., and Detrisac, C. J.: *Cancer Res.* **46**, 5264 (1986).
163. McCay, P. B., King, M. M., and Pitha, J. V.: *Cancer Res.* **41**, 3745 (1981).
164. Jones, F. E., Komorowski, R. A., and Condon, R. E.: *Surg. Forum* **32**, 435 (1981).
165. Jones, F. E., Komorowski, R. A., and Condon, R. E.: *J. Surg. Oncol.* **25**, 54 (1984).
166. Wattenberg, L. W., Jerina, D. M., Lam, L. K. T., and Yagi, H.: *J. Natl. Cancer Inst.* **62**, 1103 (1979).
167. Lam, L. K. T., and Hasegawa, S.: *Nutr. Cancer* **12**, 43 (1989).
168. Rao, M. S., Lalwani, N. D., Watanabe, T. K., and Reddy, J. K.: *Cancer Res.* **44**, 1072 (1984).
169. Wattenberg, L. W.: *J. Natl. Cancer Inst.* **50**, 1541 (1973).
170. Marnett, L. J.: *Cancer Res.* **52**, 5575 (1992).
171. Murasaki, G., Zenser, T. V., Davis, B. B., and Cohen, S. M.: *Carcinogenesis* **5**, 53 (1984).
172. Sakata, T., Hasegawa, R., Johansson, S. L., Zenser, T. V., and Cohen, S. M.: *Cancer Res.* **46**, 3903 (1986).
173. Cohen, S. M., Zenser, T. V., Murasaki, G., Fukushima, S., Mattammal, M. B., Rapp, N. S., and Davis, B. B.: *Cancer Res.* **41**, 3355 (1981).
174. Raz, A., Wyche, A., and Needleman, P.: *Proc. Natl. Acad. Sci. U.S.A.* **86**, 1657 (1989).
175. Bailey, J. M.: *Biofactors* **3**, 97 (1991).
176. Smith, W. L.: *Biochem. J.* **259**, 315 (1989).
177. Earnest, D. L., Hixson, L. J., Finley, P. R., Blackwell, G. G., Einspahr, J., Emerson, S. S., and Alberts, D. S.: Arachidonic Acid Cascade Inhibitors in Chemoprevention of Human Colon Cancer: Preliminary Studies. *In* "Cancer Chemoprevention" (L. Wattenberg, M. Lipkin, C. W. Boone, and G. J. Kelloff, eds.) CRC Press, Boca Raton, Florida, 1992, p. 165.
178. Goodwin, J. S., Bankhurst, A. D., and Messner, R. P.: *J. Exp. Med.* **146**, 1719 (1977).
179. Goodwin, J. S., Messner, R. P., and Peake, G. T.: *J. Clin. Invest.* **62**, 753 (1978).
180. Whitfield, J. F.: Calcium: Driver of Cell Cycles, Trigger of Differentiation, and Killer of Cells. *In* "Cellular and Molecular Targets for Chemoprevention" (V. E. Steele, G. D. Stoner, C. W. Boone, and G. J. Kelloff, eds.). CRC Press, Boca Raton, Florida, 1992, p. 257.
181. Pentland, A. P., and Needleman, P.: *J. Clin. Invest.* **77**, 246 (1986).
182. Levine, L., and Ohuchi, K.: *Cancer Res.* **38**, 4142 (1978).
183. Hong, S. L., Wheless, C. M., and Levine, L.: *Prostaglandins* **13**, 271 (1977).
184. Furstenberger, G., Gross, M., and Marks, F.: *Carcinogenesis* **10**, 91 (1989).
185. Gronemeyer, H., Benhamou, B., Berry, M., Bocquel, M. T., Gofflo, D., Garcia, T., Lerouge, T., Metzger, D., Meyer, M. E., Tora, L., Vergezac, A., and Chambon, P.: *J. Steroid Biochem. Mol. Biol.* **41**, 217 (1992).
186. Jordan, V. C.: *Cancer* **70**, 977 (1992).
187. Turcot-Lemay, L., and Kelly, P. A.: *Cancer Res.* **40**, 3232 (1980).
188. Sylvester, P. W., Aylsworth, C. F., Van Vugt, D. A., and Meites, J.: *Cancer Res.* **43**, 5342 (1983).
189. Thompson, H. J., and Ronan, A. M.: *Carcinogenesis* **7**, 2003 (1986).
190. Robinson, S. P., Mauel, D. A., and Jordan, V. C.: *Eur. J. Cancer Clin. Oncol.* **24**, 1817 (1988).
191. Hendry, L. B., and Muldoon, T. G.: *J. Steroid Biochem.* **30**, 325 (1988).
192. Moon, R. C., Kelloff, G. J., Detrisac, C. J., Steele, V. E., Thomas, C. F., and Sigman, C. C.: *Anticancer Res.* **12**, 1147 (1992).
193. Roberts, A. B., and Sporn, M. B.: *Adv. Cancer Res.* **51**, 107 (1988).
194. Silberstein, G. B., and Daniel, C. W.: *Science* **237**, 291 (1987).
195. Sporn, M. B., Roberts, A. B., Glick, A. B., Luckert, P. H., and Pollard, M.: Interactions of Retinoids and Transforming Growth Factor β in the Chemoprevention of Cancer. *In* "Control of Growth Factors and Prevention of Cancer" (M. B. Sporn, ed.). Springer-Verlag, New York, 1992, p. 37.
196. Russell, W. E., Coffey, R. J., Jr., Ouellette, A. J., and Moses, H. L.: *Proc. Natl. Acad. Sci. U.S.A.* **85**, 5126 (1988).
197. Kurokowa, M., Lynch, K., and Podolsky, D. K.: *Biochem. Biophys. Res. Commun.* **142**, 775 (1987).
198. Knabbe, C., Lippman, M. E., Wakefield, L. M., Flanders, K. C., Kasid, A., Derynck, R., and Dickson, R. B.: *Cell* **48**, 417 (1987).
199. Bollag, W.: *Experientia* **28**, 1219 (1972).
200. Verma, A. K., and Boutwell, R. K.: *Cancer Res.* **37**, 2196 (1977).

201. Verma, A. K., Shapas, B. G., Rice, H. M., and Boutwell, R. K.: *Cancer Res.* **39**, 419 (1979).
202. Slaga, T. J., Klein-Szanto, J. P., Fischer, S. M., Weeks, C. E., Nelson, K., and Major, S.: *Proc. Natl. Acad. Sci. U.S.A.* **77**, 2251 (1980).
203. Verma, A. K., Slaga, T. J., Wertz, P. W., Mueller, G. C., and Boutwell, R. K.: *Cancer Res.* **40**, 2367 (1980).
204. Verma, A. K., Duvick, L., and Ali, M.: *Carcinogenesis* **7**, 1019 (1986).
205. Tokuda, H., Ohigashi, H., Koshimizu, K., and Ito, Y.: *Cancer Lett.* **33**, 279 (1986).
206. Verma, A. K.: *Cancer Res.* **47**, 5097 (1987).
207. Verma, A. K.: *Cancer Res.* **48**, 2168 (1988).
208. Dawson, M. I., Chao, W. R., and Helmes, C. T.: *Cancer Res.* **47**, 6210 (1987).
209. Athar, M., Agarwal, R., Wang, Z. Y., Lloyd, J. R., Bickers, D. R., and Mukhtar, H.: *Carcinogenesis* **12**, 2325 (1991).
210. Glick, A. B., Flanders, K. C., Danielpour, D., Yuspa, S. H., and Sporn, M. B.: *Cell Regul.* **1**, 87 (1989).
211. Glick, A. B., McCune, B. K., Abdulkarem, N., Flanders, K. C., Lumadue, J. A., Smith, J. M., and Sporn, M. B.: *Development* **111**, 1081 (1991).
212. Pollak, M. N., Huynh, H. T., and Lefebvre, S. P.: *Breast Cancer Res. Treat.* **22**, 91 (1992).
213. Macaulay, V. M.: *Br. J. Cancer* **65**, 311 (1992).
214. Colletti, R. B., Roberts, J. D., Devlin, J. T., and Copeland, K. C.: *Cancer Res.* **49**, 1882 (1989).
215. Zarbl, H., Sukumar, S., Arthur, A. V., Martin-Zanca, D., and Barbacid, M.: *Nature* **315**, 382 (1985).
216. Vuorio, T, Warri, A, Sandberg, M, Alitalo, K and Vuorio, E: *Int. J. Cancer* **42**, 774 (1988).
217. Haag, J. D., Lindstrom, M. J., and Gould, M. N.: *Cancer Res.* **52**, 4021 (1992).
218. Crowell, P. L., Chang, R. R., Ren, Z., Elson, C. E., and Gould, M. N.: *J. Biol. Chem.* **266**, 17679 (1991).
219. Krishna, G., Whitlock, H. W., Jr., Feldbruegge, D. H., and Porter, J. W.: *Arch. Biochem. Biophys.* **114**, 200 (1966).
220. Wattenberg, L. W.: *Carcinogenesis* **12**, 151 (1991).
221. Nolan, R. D., Danilowicz, R. M., and Eling, T. E.: *Mol. Pharmacol.* **33**, 650 (1988).
222. Handler, J. A., Danilowicz, R. M., and Eling, T. E.: *J. Biol. Chem.* **265**, 3669 (1990).
223. Troll, W., and Kennedy, A. R.: *Cancer Res.* **49**, 499 (1989).
224. Corasanti, J. G., Hobika, G. H., and Markus, G.: *Science* **216**, 1020 (1982).
225. Nomura, T., Hata, S., Enomoto, T., Tanaka, H., and Shibata, K.: *Br. J. Cancer* **42**, 624 (1980).
226. Hozumi, M., Ogawa, M., Sugimura, T., Takeuchi, T., and Umezawa, H.: *Cancer Res.* **32**, 1725 (1972).
227. Pegg, A. E.: *Cancer Res.* **48**, 759 (1988).
228. Pegg, A. E., and McCann, P. P.: *Am. J. Physiol.* **243**, C212 (1982).
229. O'Brien, T. G.: *Cancer Res.* **36**, 2644 (1976).
230. Kingsnorth, A. N., King, W. W. K., Diekema, K. A., McCann, P. P., Ross, J. S., and Malt, R. A.: *Cancer Res.* **43**, 2545 (1983).
231. Rozhin, J., Wilson, P. S., Bull, A. W., and Nigro, N. D.: *Cancer Res.* **44**, 3226 (1984).
232. Nigro, N. D., Bull, A. W., and Boyd, M. E.: *Cancer Lett.* **35**, 153 (1987).
233. Fozard, J. R., and Prakash, N. J.: *Naunyn-Schmiedebergs Arch. Pharmacol.* **320**, 72 (1982).
234. Ratko, T. A., Detrisac, C. J., Rao, K. V. N., Thomas, C. F., Kelloff, G. J., and Moon, R. C.: *Anticancer Res.* **10**, 67 (1990).
235. Thompson, H. J., Meeker, L. D., Herbst, E. J., Ronan, A. M., and Minocha, R.: *Cancer Res.* **45**, 1170 (1985).
236. Thompson, H. J., Ronan, A. M., Ritacco, K. A., and Meeker, L. D.: *Carcinogenesis* **7**, 837 (1986).
237. Takigawa, M., Verma, A. K., Simsiman, R. C., and Boutwell, R. K.: *Biochem. Biophys. Res. Commun.* **105**, 969 (1982).
238. Takigawa, M., Verma, A. K., Simsiman, R. C., and Boutwell, R. K.: *Cancer Res.* **43**, 3732 (1983).
239. Homma, Y., Ozono, S., Numata, I., Seidenfeld, J., and Oyasu, R.: *Cancer Res.* **45**, 648 (1985).
240. Homma, Y., Kakizoe, T., Samma, S., and Oyasu, R.: *Cancer Res.* **47**, 6176 (1987).
241. Verma, A. K., Pong, R. C., and Erickson, D.: *Cancer Res.* **45**, 6149 (1986).
242. Gilmour, S. K., Verma, A. K., Madara, T., and O'Brien, T. G.: *Cancer Res.* **47**, 1221 (1987).
243. Hsieh, J. T., and Verma, A. K.: *Arch. Biochem. Biophys.* **262**, 326 (1988).
244. Hsieh, J. T., and Verma, A. K.: *Cancer Res.* **49**, 4251 (1989).
245. Verma, A. K., Ashendel, C. L., and Boutwell, R. K.: *Cancer Res.* **40**, 308 (1980).
246. Nakadate, T., Yamamoto, S., Ishii, M., and Kato, R.: *Cancer Res.* **42**, 2841 (1982).
247. Kozumbo, W. J., Seed, J. L., and Kensler, T. W.: *Cancer Res.* **43**, 2555 (1983).
248. Verma, A. K., Rice, H. M., Shapas, B. G., and Boutwell, R. K.: *Cancer Res.* **38**, 793 (1978).
249. Elegbede, J. A., Maltzman, T. H., Elson, C. E., Tanner, M. A., Verma, A. K., and Gould, M. N.: *Proc. Am. Assoc. Cancer Res.* **27**, 146, Abst. no. 576 (1986).
250. McCormick, D. L., and Moon, R. C.: *Cancer Lett.* **31**, 133 (1986).
251. McCormick, D. L., Bagg, B. J., and Hultin, T. A.: *Cancer Res.* **47**, 5989 (1987).

252. McCormick, D. L., Mehta, R. G., Thompson, C. A., Dinger, N., Caldwell, J. A., and Moon, R. C.: *Cancer Res.* **42**, 508 (1982).
253. Abou-Issa, H. and Duruibe, V. A.: *Biochem. Biophys. Res. Commun.* **135**, 116 (1986).
254. Abou-Issa, H. M., Duruibe, V. A., Minton, J. P., Larroya, S., Dwivedi, C., and Webb, T. E.: *Proc. Natl. Acad. Sci. U.S.A.* **85**, 4181 (1988).
255. Moon, R. C., Thompson, H. J., Becci, P. J., Grubbs, C. J., Gander, R. J., Newton, D. L., Smith, J. M., Phillips, S. L., Henderson, W. R., Mullen, L. T., Brown, C. C., and Sporn, M. B.: *Cancer Res.* **39**, 1339 (1979).
256. McCormick, D. L., Becci, P. J., and Moon, R. C.: *Carcinogenesis* **3**, 1473 (1982).
257. Silverman, J., Katayama, S., Radok, P., Levenstein, M. J., and Weisburger, J. H.: *Nutr. Cancer* **4**, 186 (1983).
258. Grubbs, C. J., Eto, I., Juliana, M. M., Hardin, J. M., and Whitaker, L. M.: *Anticancer Res.* **10**, 661 (1990).
259. Moon, R. C., McCormick, D. L., Becci, P. J., Shealy, Y. F., Frickel, F., Paust, J., and Sporn, M. B.: *Carcinogenesis* **3**, 1469 (1982).
260. De Luca, L. M.: *FASEB J.* **5**, 2924 (1991).
261. Newton, D. L., Henderson, W. R., and Sporn, M. B.: *Cancer Res.* **40**, 3413 (1980).
262. Huang, F. L., Roop, D. R., and De Luca, L. M.: *In Vitro Cell. Dev. Biol.* **22**, 223 (1986).
263. McDowell, E. M., Ben, T., Newkirk, C., Chang, S., and De Luca, L.: *Am. J. Pathol.* **129**, 511 (1987).
264. Huberman, E., and Callaham, M. F.: *Proc. Natl. Acad. Sci. U.S.A.* **76**, 1293 (1979).
265. Breitman, T. R., Selonick, S. E., and Collins, S. J.: *Proc. Natl. Acad. Sci. U.S.A.* **77**, 2936 (1980).
266. Honma, Y., Takenaga, K., Kasukabe, T., and Hozumi, M.: *Biochem. Biophys. Res. Commun.* **95**, 507 (1980).
267. Davies, P. J. A., Murtaugh, M. P., Moore, W. T., Jr., Johnson, G. S., and Lucas, D.: *J. Biol. Chem.* **260**, 5166 (1985).
268. Jetten, A. M., Anderson, K., Deas, M. A., Kagechika, H., Lotan, R., Rearick, J. I., and Shudo, K.: *Cancer Res.* **47**, 3523 (1987).
269. Jetten, A. M., and Shirley, J. E.: *Exp. Cell Res.* **156**, 221 (1985).
270. Hogan, B. L. M., Taylor, A., and Adamson, E.: *Nature* **291**, 235 (1981).
271. Carlin, B. E., Durkin, M. E., Benders, B., Jaffe, R., and Chung, A. E.: *J. Biol. Chem.* **258**, 7729 (1983).
272. Cooper, A. R., Taylor, A., and Hogan, B. L. M.: *Dev. Biol.* **99**, 510 (1983).
273. Bashor, M. M., Toft, D. O., and Chytil, F.: *Proc. Natl. Acad. Sci. USA* **70**, 3483 (1973).
274. Sani, B. P., and Hill, D. L.: *Cancer Res.* **36**, 409 (1976).
275. Sani, B. P., Singh, R. K., Reddy, L. G., and Gaub, M.-P.: *Arch. Biochem. Biophys.* **283**, 107 (1990).
276. Hill, D. L., and Grubbs, C. J.: *Annu. Rev. Nutr.* **12**, 161 (1992).
277. Sporn, M. B., and Roberts, A. B.: *Mol. Endocrinol.* **55**, 3 (1991).
278. Scalmati, A., Lipkin, M., and Newmark, H.: Relationships of Calcium and Vitamin D to Colon Cancer. *In* "Cancer Chemoprevention" (L. Wattenberg, M. Lipkin, C. W. Boone, and G. J. Kelloff, eds.). CRC Press, Boca Raton, Florida, 1992, p. 249.
279. Babcock, M. S., Marino, M. R., Gunning, W. T., III, and Stoner, G. D.: *In Vitro Cell Dev. Biol.* **19**, 403 (1983).
280. Hennings, H., Michael, D., Cheng, C., Steinert, P., Holbrook, K., and Yuspa, S. H.: *Cell* **19**, 245 (1980).
281. McGrath, C. M., and Soule, H. D.: *In Vitro Cell Dev. Biol.* **20**, 652 (1984).
282. Soule, H. D., and McGrath, C. M.: *In Vitro Cell Dev. Biol.* **22**, 6 (1986).
283. Cruse, J. P., Lewin, M. R., and Clark, C. G.: *Gut* **23**, 594 (1982).
284. Abe, E., Miyaura, C., Sakagami, H., Takeda, M., Konno, K., Yamazaki, T., Yoshiki, S., and Suda, T.: *Proc. Natl. Acad. Sci. U.S.A.* **78**, 4990 (1981).
285. Miyaura, C., Abe, E., Kuribayashi, T., Tanaka, H., Konno, K., Nishii, Y., and Suda, T.: *Biochem. Biophys. Res. Commun.* **102**, 937 (1981).
286. Koeffler, H. P., Hirji, K., Itri, L., and the Southern California Leukemia Group: *Cancer Treat. Rep.* **69**, 1399 (1985).
287. Kuroki, T., Chida, K., Hashiba, H., Hosoi, J., Hosomi, J., Sasaki, K., Abe, E., and Suda, T.: Regulation of Cell Differentiation and Tumor Promotion by 1α, 25-Dihydroxyvitamin D_3. *In* "Carcinogenesis—A Comprehensive Survey" (E. Huberman and S. H. Barr, eds.), Vol. 10. Raven Press, New York, 1985, p. 275.
288. Ostrem, V. K., and DeLuca, H. F.: *Steroids* **49**, 73 (1987).
289. Ostrem, V. K., Lau, W. F., Lee, S. H., Perlman, K., Prahl, J., Schnoes, H. K., DeLuca, H. F., and Ikegawa, N.: *J. Biol. Chem.* **262**, 14164 (1987).
290. Cruse, J. P., Lewin, M. R., and Clark, C. G.: *Clin. Oncol.* **10**, 213 (1984).
291. Goldman, R.: *Cancer Res.* **45**, 3118 (1985).
292. Friedman, E. A.: *Cancer Res.* **41**, 4588 (1981).

293. Carvalho, L., Foulkes, K., and Mickey, D. D.: *Prostate* **15**, 123 (1989).
294. Friedman, E. A.: A Primary Culture System of Human Colon Carcinoma Cells and Its Use in Evaluating Differentiation Therapy. *In* "Cell and Molecular Biology of Colon Cancer" (L. H. Augenlicht, ed.). CRC Press, Boca Raton, Florida, 1989, p. 69.
295. McCabe, D., O'Dwyer, P., Sickle-Santanello, B., Woltering, E., Abou-Issa, H., and James, A.: *Arch. Surg.* **121**, 1455 (1986).
296. Belman, S., and Troll, W.: *Cancer Res.* **34**, 3446 (1974).
297. Feramisco, J. R., Clark, R., Wong, G., Arnheim, N., Milley, R., and McCormick, F.: *Nature* **314**, 639 (1985).
298. Jaffe, B. M.: *Prostaglandins* **6**, 453 (1974).
299. Plescia, O. J., Smith, A. H., and Grinwich, K.: *Proc. Natl. Acad. Sci. U.S.A.* **72**, 1848 (1975).
300. Hial, V., Horakova, Z., Shaff, R. E., and Beaven, M. A.: *Eur. J. Pharmacol.* **37**, 367 (1976).
301. Grinwich, K. D., and Plescia, O. T.: *Prostaglandins* **14**, 1175 (1977).
302. Lynch, N. R., Castes, M., Astoin, M., and Salomon, J.-C.: *Br. J. Cancer* **38**, 503 (1978).
303. Bennett, A., Houghton, J., Leaper, D. J., and Stamford, I. F.: *Prostaglandins* **17**, 179 (1979).
304. Brunda, M. J., Herberman, R. B., and Holden, H. T.: *J. Immunol.* **124**, 2682 (1980).
305. Han, T., and Takita, H.: *Cancer* **46**, 2416 (1980).
306. Tilden, A. B., and Balch, C. M.: *Surgery* **90**, 77 (1981).
307. Balch, C. M., Dougherty, P. A., and Tilden, A. B.: *Ann. Surg.* **96**, 645 (1982).
308. Balch, C. M., Dougherty, P. A., Cloud, G. A., and Tilden, A. B.: *Surgery* **95**, 71 (1984).
309. Chiabrando, C., Broggini, M., Castagnoli, M. N., Donelli, M. G., Noseda, A., Visintainer, M., Garattini, S., and Fanelli, R.: *Cancer Res.* **45**, 3605 (1985).
310. Hill, D. L., and Grubbs, C. J.: *Anticancer Res.* **2**, 111 (1982).
311. Tengerdy, R. P.: Effect of Vitamin E on Immune Function. *In* "Vitamin E – A Comprehensive Treatise" (L. J. Machlin, ed.). Marcel Dekker, New York, 1980, p. 429.
312. Corwin, L. M., and Gordon, R. K.: *Ann. N.Y. Acad. Sci.* **393**, 437 (1982).
313. Schwartz, J., Odukoya, O., Stoufi, E., and Shklar, G.: *J. Dent. Res.* **64**, 117 (1985).
314. Shklar, G.: *J. Natl. Cancer Inst.* **68**, 791 (1982).
315. Trickler, D., and Shklar, G.: *J. Natl. Cancer Inst.* **78**, 165 (1987).
316. Shklar, G., and Schwartz, J.: *Eur. J. Cancer* **24**, 839 (1988).
317. Temple, N. J., and Basu, T. K.: *J. Natl. Cancer Inst.* **79**, 1131 (1987).
318. Jacobs, M. M.: *Cancer* **40**, 2557 (1977).
319. Jacobs, M. M., Jansson, B., and Griffin, A. C.: *Cancer Lett.* **2**, 133 (1977).
320. Birt, D. F., Lawson, T. A., Julius, A. D., Runice, C. E., and Salmasi, S.: *Cancer Res.* **42**, 4455 (1982).
321. Reddy, B. S., Sugie, S., Maruyama, H., El-Bayoumy, K., and Marra, P.: *Cancer Res.* **47**, 5901 (1987).
322. van Rensburg, S. J., Hall, J. M., and Gathercole, P. S.: *Nutr. Cancer* **8**, 163 (1986).
323. El-Bayoumy, K.: *Cancer Res.* **45**, 3631 (1985).
324. Harr, J. R., Exon, J. H., Whanger, P. D., and Weswig, P. H.: *Clin. Toxicol.* **5**, 187 (1972).
325. Griffin, A. C., and Jacobs, M. M.: *Cancer Lett.* **3**, 177 (1977).
326. Marshall, M. V., Arnott, M. S., Jacobs, M. M., and Griffin, A. C.: *Cancer Lett.* **7**, 331 (1979).
327. Birt, D. F., Julius, A. D., Runice, C. E., and Salmasi, S.: *J. Natl. Cancer Inst.* **77**, 1281 (1986).
328. Kobayashi, M., Kogata, M., Yamamura, M., Takada, H., Hioki, K., and Yamamoto, M.: *Cancer Res* **46**, 2266 (1986).
329. Ip, C., and Sinha, D.: *Carcinogenesis* **2**, 435 (1981).
330. Ip, C.: *Cancer Res.* **41**, 2683 (1981).
331. Ip, C.: *Cancer Res.* **41**, 4386 (1981).
332. Thompson, H. J., Meeker, L. D., Becci, P. J., and Kokoska, S.: *Cancer Res.* **42**, 4954 (1982).
333. Medina, D., and Lane, H. W.: *Biol. Trace Elem. Res.* **5**, 297 (1983).
334. Medina, D., Lane, H. W., and Shepherd, F.: *Carcinogenesis* **4**, 1159 (1983).
335. Medina, D., Lane, H. W., and Tracey, C. M.: *Cancer Res.* **43**, 2460S (1983).
336. Horvath, P. M., and Ip, C.: *Cancer Res.* **43**, 5335 (1983).
337. Ip, C.: *Cancer Lett.* **25**, 325 (1985).
338. Ip, C., and Daniel, F. B.: *Cancer Res.* **45**, 61 (1985).
339. Lane, H. W., and Medina, D.: *J. Natl. Cancer Inst.* **75**, 675 (1985).
340. Ip, C.: *J. Natl. Cancer Inst.* **77**, 299 (1986).
341. Ip, C., and White, G.: *Carcinogenesis* **8**, 1763 (1987).
342. Ip, C.: *Cancer Lett.* **39**, 239 (1988).
343. Ip, C and Ganther, H: *Carcinogenesis* **9**, 1481 (1988).
344. Ip, C.: *J. Natl. Cancer Inst.* **80**, 258 (1988).
345. Rao, A. R. N., Rao, A. R., Jannu, L. N., and Hussain, S. P.: *Jpn. J. Cancer Res.* **81**, 1239 (1990).
346. Ip, C., Hayes, C., Budnick, R. M., and Ganther, H. E.: *Cancer Res.* **51**, 595 (1991).

347. Kiremidjian-Schumacher, L., and Stotzky, G.: *Environ. Res.* **42**, 277 (1987).
348. Alfred, L. J., Wojdani, A., Nieto, M., Perez, R., and Yoshida, G.: *Immunology* **50**, 207 (1983).
349. Dean, J. H., Ward, E. C., Murray, M. J., Lauer, L. D., and House, R. V.: *Clin. Physiol. Biochem.* **3**, 98 (1985).
350. Klaunig, J. E., and Ruch, R. J.: *Lab. Invest.* **62**, 135 (1990).
351. Bertram, J. S., Hossain, M. Z., and Zhang, L. -X.: Use of Cell Culture Systems for Mechanistic Studies of Chemopreventive Agents. *In* "Cellular and Molecular Targets for Chemoprevention" (V. E. Steele, G. D. Stoner, C. W. Boone, and G. J. Kelloff, eds.), CRC Press, Boca Raton, Florida, 1992, p. 43.
352. Loewenstein, W. R.: *Biochim. Biophys. Acta* **560**, 1 (1979).
353. Mehta, P. P., Bertram, J. S., and Loewenstein, W. R.: *Cell* **44**, 187 (1986).
354. Mehta, P. P., Bertram, J. S., and Loewenstein, W. R.: *J. Cell Biol.* **108**, 1053 (1989).
355. Zhang, L. -X., Cooney, R. V., and Bertram, J. S.: *Carcinogenesis* **12**, 2109 (1991).
356. Hossain, M. Z., Wilkens, L. R., Mehta, P. P., Loewenstein, W., and Bertram, J. S.: *Carcinogenesis* **10**, 1743 (1989).
357. Knudson, A. G., Jr.: *Annu. Rev. Genet.* **20**, 231 (1986).
358. Lee, E. Y.-H. P., To, H., Shew, J.-Y., Bookstein, R., Scully, P., and Lee, W.-H.: *Science* **241**, 218 (1988).
359. Tang, A., Varley, J. M., Chakraborty, S., Murphree, A. L., and Fung, Y. -K. T.: *Science* **242**, 263 (1988).
360. Horowitz, J. M., Park, S.-H., Bogenmann, E., Cheng, J. -C., Yandell, D. W., Kaye, F. J., Minna, J. D., Dryja, T. P., and Weinberg, R. A.: *Proc. Natl. Acad. Sci. USA* **87**, 2775 (1990).
361. Marshall, C. J.: *Cell* **64**, 313 (1991).
362. Friedmann, T.: *Science* **244**, 1275 (1989).
363. Levine, A. J., and Momand, J.: *Biochim. Biophys. Acta* **1032**, 119 (1990).
364. Bressac, B., Galvin, K. M., Liang, T. J., Isselbacher, K. J., Wands, J. R., and Ozturk, M.: *Proc. Natl. Acad. Sci. U.S.A.* **87**, 1973 (1990).
365. Iggo, R., Gatter, K., Bartek, J., Lane, D., and Harris, A. L.: *Lancet* **335**, 675 (1990).
366. Mulligan, L. M., Matlashewski, G. J., Scrable, H. J., and Cavenee, W. K.: *Proc. Natl. Acad. Sci. U.S.A.* **87**, 5863 (1990).
367. Friedmann, T.: *Cancer* **70**, 1810 (1992).
368. Coles, C., Condie, A., Chetty, U., Steel, C. M., Evans, H. J., and Prosser, J.: *Cancer Res.* **52**, 5291 (1992).
369. Francke, U., Holmes, L. B., Atkins, L., and Riccardi, V. M.: *Cytogenet. Cell Genet.* **24**, 185 (1979).
370. Riccardi, V. M., Hittner, H. M., Francke, U., Yunis, J. J., Ledbetter, D., and Borges, W.: *Cancer Genet. Cytogenet.* **2**, 131 (1980).
371. Call, K. M., Glaser, T., Ito, C. Y., Buckler, A. J., Pelletier, J., Haber, D. A., Rose, E. A., Kral, A., Yeger, H., Lewis, W. H., Jones, C., and Housman, D. E.: *Cell* **60**, 509 (1990).
372. Fearon, E. R., and Vogelstein, B.: *Cell* **61**, 759 (1990).
373. Tornhamre, S., Gigou, A., Edenius, C., Lellouche, J. P., and Lindgren, J. A.: *FEBS Lett.* **307**, 78 (1992).
374. Bursch, W., Oberhammer, F., and Schulte-Hermann, R.: *Trends Pharmacol. Sci.* **13**, 245 (1992).
375. Yonish-Rouach, E., Resnitzky, D., Lotem, J., Sachs, L., Kimchi, A., and Oren, M.: *Nature* **352**, 345 (1991).
376. Oren, M.: *Cancer Metastasis Rev.* **11**, 141 (1992).
377. Oberhammer, F., Bursch, W., Parzefall, W., Breit, P., Erber, E., Stadler, M., and Schulte-Hermann, R.: *Cancer Res.* **51**, 2478 (1991).
378. McConkey, D. J., Hartzell, P., Jondal, M., and Orrenius, S.: *J. Biol. Chem.* **264**, 13399 (1989).
379. Lotem, J., Cragoe, E. J., Jr., and Sachs, L.: *Blood* **78**, 953 (1991).
380. Bursch, W., Paffe, S., Putz, B., Barthel, G., and Schulte-Hermann, R.: *Carcinogenesis* **11**, 847 (1990).
381. Wyllie, A. H., Kerr, J. F. R., and Currie, A. R.: *Int. Rev. Cytol.* **68**, 251 (1980).
382. Kyprianou, N., English, H. F., and Isaacs, J. T.: *Cancer Res.* **50**, 3748 (1990).
383. Bursch, W., Liehr, J. G., Sirbasku, D. A., Putz, B., Taper, H., and Schulte-Hermann, R.: *Carcinogenesis* **12**, 855 (1991).
384. Kyprianou, N., English, H. F., Davidson, N. E., and Isaacs, J. T.: *Cancer Res.* **51**, 162 (1991).
385. Szende, B., Zalatnai, A., and Schally, A. V.: *Proc. Natl. Acad. Sci. U.S.A.* **86**, 1643 (1989).
386. Wainfan, E., and Poirier, L. A.: *Cancer Res.* **52**, 2071S (1992).
387. Mikol, Y. B., Hoover, K. L., Creasia, D., and Poirier, L. A.: *Carcinogenesis* **4**, 1619 (1983).
388. Ghoshal, A. K., and Farber, E.: *Carcinogenesis* **5**, 1367 (1984).
389. Yokoyama, S., Sells, M. A., Reddy, T. V., and Lombardi, B.: *Cancer Res.* **45**, 2834 (1985).
390. Newberne, P. M., and Rogers, A. E.: *Annu. Rev. Nutr.* **6**, 407 (1986).
391. Brada, Z., Altman, N. H., Hill, M., and Bulba, S.: *Res. Commun. Chem. Pathol. Pharmacol.* **38**, 157 (1982).
392. Hoffman, R. M.: *Biochim. Biophys. Acta* **738**, 49 (1984).

393. Wainfan, E., and Dizik, M.: *Carcinogenesis* **8**, 615 (1987).
394. Hsieh, L. L., Wainfan, E., Hoshina, S., Dizik, M., and Weinstein, I. B.: *Cancer Res.* **49**, 3795 (1989).
395. Dizik, M., Christman, J. K., and Wainfan, E.: *Carcinogenesis* **12**, 1307 (1991).
396. Wainfan, E., Dizik, M., Sheikhnejad, G., and Christman, J. K.: *FASEB J.* **4**, A1043 (1990).
397. Cronin, G., Lyn-Cook, B., Zapisek, W., and Poirier, L.: *Proc. Am. Assoc. Cancer Res.* **32**, 147 Abst. 880 (1991).
398. Hsieh, L. L., Peraino, C., and Weinstein, I. B.: *Cancer Res.* **48**, 265 (1988).
399. Cote, G. J., Lastra, B. A., Cook, J. R., Huang, D.-P., and Chiu, J.-F.: *Cancer Lett.* **26**, 121 (1985).
400. Yaswen, P., Goyette, M., Shank, P. R., and Fausto, N.: *Mol. Cell. Biochem.* **5**, 780 (1985).
401. Dizik, M., Wainfan, E., Sheikhnejad, G., and Christman, J. K.: *Proc. Am. Assoc. Cancer Res.* **31**, 141, Abst. no. 837 (1990).
402. Wainfan, E., Dizik, M., Stender, M., and Christman, J. K.: *Cancer Res.* **49**, 4094 (1989).
403. Bhave, M. R., Wilson, M. J., and Poirier, L. A.: *Carcinogenesis* **9**, 343 (1988).
404. Holliday, R.: *Br. J. Cancer* **40**, 513 (1979).
405. Nyce, J., Weinhouse, S., and Magee, P. N.: *Br. J. Cancer* **48**, 463 (1983).
406. Weinstein, I. B., Gattoni-Celli, S., Kirschmeier, P., Hsiao, W., Horowitz, A., and Jeffrey, A.: *Federation Proc.* **43**, 2287 (1984).
407. Jones, P. A., and Buckley, J. D.: *Adv. Cancer Res.* **54**, 1 (1990).
408. Anisimov, V. N., Miretskii, G. I., Danetskaya, E. V., Troitskaya, M. N., and Ramzaev, P. V.: *Bull. Exp. Biol. Med.* **92**, 1424 (1981).
409. Maru, G. B., Sawai, M. M., and Bhide, S. V.: *J. Cancer Res. Clin. Oncol.* **97**, 145 (1980).
410. Folkman, J., and Shing, Y.: *J. Biol. Chem.* **267**, 10931 (1992).
411. Folkman, J.: *J. Natl. Cancer Inst.* **82**, 4 (1990).
412. Folkman, J., Watson, K., Ingber, D., and Hananhan, D.: *Nature* **339**, 58 (1989).
413. Form, D. M., and Auerbach, R.: *Proc. Soc. Exp. Biol. Med.* **172**, 214 (1983).
414. Graeber, J. E., Glaser, B. M., Setty, B. N. Y., Jerdan, J. A., Walenga, R. W., and Stuart, M. J.: *Prostaglandins* **39**, 665 (1990).
415. Hocman, G.: *Int. J. Biochem.* **24**, 1365 (1992).
416. Liotta, L. A., and Stetler-Stevenson, W. G.: *Cancer Res.* **51**, 5054s (1991).
417. Biggs, J., Hersperger, E., Steeg, P. S., Liotta, L. A., and Shearn, A.: *Cell* **63**, 933 (1990).
418. Hennessy, C., Henry, J. A., May, F. E. B., Westley, B. R., Angus, B., and Lennard, T. W. J.: *J. Natl. Cancer Inst.* **83**, 281 (1991).
419. Bevilacqua, G., Sobel, M. E., Liotta, L. A., and Steeg, P. S.: *Cancer Res.* **49**, 5185 (1989).
420. International Agency for Research on Cancer: *IARC Sci. Publ.* **21**, 33 (1979).
421. Rose, C., Thorpe, S. M., Andersen, K. W., Pedersen, B. V., Mouridsen, H. T., Blichert-Toft, M. and Rasmussen, B. B.: *Lancet* **01**, 16 (1985).
422. DeGregorio, M. W.: *J. NIH Res.* **4**, 84 (1992).
423. Jordan, V. C.: *Eur. J. Cancer* **12**, 419 (1976).
424. Welsch, C. W., Goodrich-Smith, M., Brown, C. K., Miglorie, N., and Clifton, K. H.: *Eur. J. Cancer* **17**, 1255 (1981).
425. Welsch, C. W., Goodrich-Smith, M., Brown, C. K., Mackie, D., and Johnson, D.: *Oncology* **39**, 88 (1982).
426. Jordan, V. C., and Murphy, C. S.: *Endocrin. Rev.* **11**, 578 (1990).
427. Kellis, J. T., Jr., Nesnow, S., and Vickery, L. E.: *Biochem. Pharmacol.* **35**, 2887 (1986).
428. Cole, P. A., and Robinson, C. H.: *J. Med. Chem.* **33**, 2933 (1990).
429. Brodie, A. M. H., Dowsett, M., and Coombes, R. C.: Aromatase Inhibitors as New Endocrine Therapy for Breast Cancer. *In* "Endocrine Therapies in Breast and Prostate Cancer" (C. K. Osborne, ed.). Kluwer Academic Publishers, Boston, 1988, p. 51.
430. Spinola, P. G., Marchetti, B., Merand, Y., Belanger, A., and Labrie, F.: *Breast Cancer Res. Treat.* **12**, 287 (1988).
431. Bhatnagar, A. S., Hausler, A., Schieweck, K., Browne, L. J., Bowman, R., and Steele, R. E.: *J. Steroid Biochem. Mol. Biol.* **37**, 363 (1990).
432. Haynes, R. C., Jr.: Adrenocorticotropic Hormone; Adrenocorticotropic Steroids and Their Synthetic Analogs; Inhibitors of the Synthesis and Actions of Adrenocortical Hormones. *In:* "The Pharmacological Basis of Therapeutics" (A. Goodman Gilman, T. W. Rall, A. S. Nies, and P. Taylor, eds.), 8th ed. McGraw-Hill, New York, 1990, p. 1431.
433. Sharma, O. P.: *Biochem. Pharmacol.* **25**, 1811 (1976).
434. Toda, S., Miyase, T., Arichi, H., Tanizawa, H., and Takino, Y.: *Chem. Pharm. Bull.* **33**, 1725 (1985).
435. Srimal, R. C., and Dhawan, B. N.: *J. Pharm. Pharmacol.* **25**, 447 (1973).
436. Rao, T. S., Basu, N., and Siddiqui, H. H.: *Indian J. Med. Res.* **75**, 574 (1982).
437. Mukhopadhyay, A., Basu, N., Ghatak, N., and Gujral, P. K.: *Agents Actions* **12**, 508 (1982).

438. Huang, M.-T., Lysz, T., Ferraro, T., and Conney, A. H.: Inhibitory Effects of Curcumin on Tumor Promotion in Mouse Epidermis. *In* "Cancer Chemoprevention" (L. Wattenberg, M. Lipkin, C. W. Boone, and G. J. Kelloff, eds.). CRC Press, Boca Raton, Florida, 1992, p. 375.
439. Huang, M.-T., Smart, R. C., Wong, C.-Q., and Conney, A. H.: *Cancer Res.* **48**, 5941 (1988).
440. Soudamini, K. K., and Kuttan, R.: *J. Ethnopharmacol.* **27**, 227 (1989).
441. Huang, M.-T., Lysz, T., Ferraro, T., Abidi, T. F., Laskin, J. D., and Conney, A. H.: *Cancer Res.* **51**, 813 (1991).
442. Srivastava, R.: *Agents Actions* **28**, 298 (1989).
443. Nagabhushan, M., and Bhide, S. V.: *Nutr. Cancer* **8**, 201 (1986).
444. Nagabhushan, M., Amonkar, A. J., and Bhide, S. V.: *Food Chem. Toxicol.* **25**, 545 (1987).
445. Reynolds, J. E. F., and Prasad, A. B. (eds.): "Martindale: The Extra Pharmacopoeia", 28th ed. The Pharmaceutical Press, London, 1982, p. 691.
446. Reynolds, J. E. F., and Prasad, A. B. (eds.): "Martindale: The Extra Pharmacopoeia", 28th ed. The Pharmaceutical Press, London, 1982, p. 77.
447. Brunton, L. L.: Drugs Affecting Gastrointestinal Function. *In*: "The Pharmacological Basis of Therapeutics" (A. Goodman Gilman, T. W. Rall, A. S. Nies, and P. Taylor, eds.), 8th ed. McGraw-Hill, New York, 1990, p. 897.
448. Reynolds, J. E. F., and Prasad, A. B. (eds.): "Martindale: The Extra Pharmacopoeia", 28th ed. The Pharmaceutical Press, London, 1982, p. 494.
449. Nishino, H.: Antitumor-Promoting Activity of Glycyrrhetinic Acid and Its Related Compounds. *In*: "Cancer Chemoprevention" (L. Wattenberg, M. Lipkin, C. W. Boone, and G. J. Kelloff, eds.), CRC Press, Boca Raton, Florida, 1992, p. 457.
450. Wang, Z. Y., Agarwal, R., Zhou, Z. C., Bickers, D. R., and Mukhtar, H.: *Carcinogenesis* **12**, 187 (1991).
451. Spencer, S. R., Wilczak, C. A., and Talalay, P.: *Cancer Res.* **50**, 7871 (1990).
452. Kuroda, K., Akao, M., Kanisawa, M., and Miyaki, K.: *Cancer Res.* **36**, 1900 (1976).
453. Kuroda, K., and Akao, M.: *Arch. Int. Pharmacodyn. Ther.* **226**, 324 (1977).
454. Kuroda, K., Akao, M., and Terao, K.: *Jpn. J. Cancer Res.* **77**, 750 (1986).
455. Kuroda, K., Kanisawa, M., and Akao, M.: *J. Natl. Cancer Inst.* **69**, 1317 (1982).
456. Kuroda, K., Terao, K., and Akao, M.: *J. Natl. Cancer Inst.* **71**, 855 (1983).
457. Kuroda, K., Terao, K., and Akao, M.: *J. Natl. Cancer Inst.* **79**, 1047 (1987).
458. Ansher, S. S., Dolan, P., and Bueding, E.: *Hepatology* **3**, 932 (1983).
459. Kensler, T. W., Egner, P. A., Trush, M. A., Bueding, E., and Groopman J. D.: *Carcinogenesis* **6**, 759 (1985).
460. Ansher, S. S., Dolan, P., and Bueding, E.: *Food Chem. Toxicol.* **25**, 45 (1986).
461. Kensler, T. W., Egner, P. A., Dolan, P. M., Groopman, J. D., and Roebuck, B. D.: *Cancer Res.* **47**, 4271 (1987).
462. Moldeus, P., Cotgreave, I. A., and Berggren, M.: *Respiration* **50**, 31 (1986).
463. Liu, Y. L., Roebuck, B. D., Yager, J. D., Groopman, J. D., and Kensler, T. W.: *Toxicol. Appl. Pharmacol.* **93**, 442 (1988).
464. Squire, R. A., Sporn, M. B., Brown, C. C., Smith, J. M., Wenk, M. L., and Springer, S.: *Cancer Res.* **37**, 2930 (1977).
465. Sporn, M. B., Squire, R. A., Brown, C. C., Smith, J. M., Wenk, M. L., and Springer, S.: *Science* **195**, 487 (1977).
466. Grubbs, C. J., Moon, R. C., Squire, R. A., Farrow, G. M., Stinson, S. F., Goodman, D. G., Brown, C. C., and Sporn, M. B.: *Science* **198**, 743 (1977).
467. Becci, P. J., Thompson, H. J., Grubbs, C. J., Squire, R. A., Brown, C. C., Sporn, M. B., and Moon, R. C.: *Cancer Res.* **38**, 4463 (1978).
468. Becci, P. J., Thompson, H. J., Grubbs, C. J., Brown, C. C., and Moon, R. C.: *Cancer Res.* **39**, 3141 (1979).
469. Tannenbaum, M., Tannenbaum, S., Richelo, B. N., and Trown, P. W.: *Scanning Electron Microsc.* **3**, 673 (1979).
470. Tannenbaum, M., Tannenbaum, S., Richelo, B. N., and Trown, P. W.: *Federation Proc.* **38**, 1073 (1979).
471. Becci, P. J., Thompson, H. J., Strum, J. M., Brown, C. C., Sporn, M. B., and Moon, R. C.: *Cancer Res.* **41**, 927 (1981).
472. Thompson, H. J., Becci, P. J., Grubbs, C. J., Shealy, Y. F., Stanek, E. J., Brown, C. C., Sporn, M. B., and Moon, R. C.: *Cancer Res.* **41**, 933 (1981).
473. Verma, A. K., Garcia, C. T., Ashendel, C. L., and Boutwell, R. K.: *Cancer Res.* **43**, 3045 (1983).
474. Schmähl, D., Krüger, C., and Preissler, P.: *Arzneimittel-Forsch.* **22**, 946 (1972).
475. Ullrey, D. E.: *J. Anim. Sci.* **35**, 648 (1972).
476. Bendich, A.: *Nutr. Cancer* **11**, 207 (1988).

477. Olson, J. A.: *J. Nutr.* **119**, 105 (1989).
478. Bertram, J. S., Pung, A., Churley, M., Kappock, T. J., Wilkins, L. R., and Cooney, R. V.: *Carcinogenesis* **12**, 671 (1991).
479. Goodwin, T. W. (ed.): "The Biochemistry of the Carotenoids", Vol. 1. Chapman & Hall, New York, 1980, p. 79.
480. Burton, G. W., Joyce, A., and Ingold, K. U.: *Arch. Biochem. Biophys.* **221**, 281 (1983).
481. Di Mascio, P., Kaiser, S., and Sies, H.: *Arch. Biochem. Biophys.* **274**, 532 (1989).
482. Edes, T. E., Thornton, W., and Shah, J.: *J. Nutr.* **119**, 796 (1989).
483. Zhang, L.-X., Cooney, R. V., and Bertram, J. S.: *Cancer Res.* **52**, 5707 (1992).
484. De Flora, S., Rossi, G. A., and De Flora, A.: *Respiration* **50**, 43 (1986).
485. Dorsch, W., Auch, E., and Powerlowicz, P.: *Int. Arch. Allergy Appl. Immunol.* **82**, 33 (1987).
486. Perchellet, E. M., Maatta, E. A., Abney, N. L., and Perchellet, J.-P.: *J. Cell. Physiol.* **131**, 64 (1987).
487. Brady, J. F., Li, D., Ishizaki, H., and Yang, C. S.: *Cancer Res.* **48**, 5937 (1988).
488. Wargovich, M. J.: Inhibition of Gastrointestinal Cancer by Organosulfur Compounds in Garlic. *In* "Cancer Chemoprevention" (L. Wattenberg, M. Lipkin, C. W. Boone, and G. J. Kelloff, eds.). CRC Press, Boca Raton, Florida 1992, p. 195.
489. Sumiyoshi, H., and Wargovich, M. J.: *Cancer Res.* **50**, 5084 (1990).
490. Wattenberg, L. W.: *J. Natl. Cancer Inst.* **58**, 395 (1977).
491. Wattenberg, L. W.: *Cancer Res.* **41**, 2991 (1981).
492. Chung, F.-L., Morse, M. A., and Eklind, K. I.: *Cancer Res.* **52**, 2719S (1992).
493. Wargovich, M. J.: *J. Am. Coll. Nutr.* **7**, 295 (1988).
494. Schwartz, A. G., Lewbart, M. L., and Pashko, L. L.: Inhibition of Tumorigenesis by Dehydroepiandrosterone and Structural Analogs. *In* "Cancer Chemoprevention" (L. Wattenberg, M. Lipkin, C. W. Boone, and G. J. Kelloff, eds.). CRC Press, Boca Raton, Florida, 1992, p. 443.
495. Schwartz, A. G., and Tannen, R. H.: *Carcinogenesis* **2**, 1335 (1981).
496. Pashko, L. L., Hard, G. C., Rovito, R. J., Williams, J. R., Sobel, E. L., and Schwartz, A. G.: *Cancer Res.* **45**, 164 (1985).
497. Nyce, J. W., Magee, P. N., and Schwartz, A. G.: *Ann. N. Y. Acad. Sci.* **397**, 317 (1982).
498. Schwartz, A. G., Nyce, J. W., and Tannen, R. H.: Inhibition of Tumorigenesis and Autoimmune Development in Mice by Dehydroepiandrosterone. *In* "Altered Endocrine Status During Aging" (V. J. Cristofalo, G. T. Baker, R. C. Adelman, and J. Roberts, eds.). Alan R. Liss, New York, 1984, p. 177.
499. Nyce, J. W., Magee, P. N., Hard, G. C., and Schwartz, A. G.: *Carcinogenesis* **5**, 57 (1984).
500. Moore, M. A., Thanavit, W., Tsuda, H., Sato, K., Ichihara, A., and Ito, N.: *Carcinogenesis* **7**, 311 (1986).
501. Ratko, T. A., Detrisac, C. J., Mehta, R. G., Kelloff, G. J., and Moon, R. C.: *Cancer Res.* **51**, 481 (1991).
502. Pashko, L. L., Rovito, R. J., Williams, J. R., Sobel, E. L., and Schwartz, A. G.: *Carcinogenesis* **5**, 463 (1984).
503. Paskho, L. L., and Schwartz, A. G.: *J. Gerontol.* **38**, 8 (1983).
504. Pashko, L. L., Schwartz, A. G., Abou-Gharbia, M., and Swern, D.: *Carcinogenesis* **2**, 717 (1981).
505. Schwartz, A. G., and Perantoni, A.: *Cancer Res.* **35**, 2482 (1975).
506. Feo, F., Pirisi, L., Pascale, R., Daino, L., Frassetto, S., Garcea, R., and Gaspa, L.: *Cancer Res.* **44**, 3419 (1984).
507. Dworkin, C. R., Gorman, S. D., Pashko, L. L., Cristofalo, V. J., and Schwartz, A. G.: *Life Sci.* **38**, 1451 (1986).
508. Garcea, R., Daino, L., Pascale, R., Frassetto, S., Cozzolino, P., Ruggiu, M. E., and Feo, F.: *Toxicol. Pathol.* **15**, 164 (1987).
509. Garcea, R., Daino, L., Frassetto, S., Cozzolino, P., Ruggiu, M. E., Vannini, M. G., Pascale, R., Lenzerini, L., Simile, M. M., Puddu, M., and Feo, F.: *Carcinogenesis* **9**, 931 (1988).
510. Gordon, G. B., Ahantz, L. M., and Talalay, P.: *Adv. Enzyme Regul.* **26**, 355 (1987).
511. Pashko, L. L., Lewbart, M. L., and Schwartz, A. G.: *Carcinogenesis* **12**, 2189 (1991).
512. Wattenberg, L. W.: Inhibitors of Chemical Carcinogens. *In* "Environmental Carcinogenesis. Occurrence, Risk Evaluation and Mechanisms" (P. Emmelot and E. Kriek, eds.). Elsevier, New York, 1979, p. 241.
513. Weinstein, I. B., Lee, L.-S., Fisher, P. B., Mufson, A., and Yamasaki, H.: The Mechanism of Action of Tumor Promoters and a Molecular Model of Two Stage Carcinogenesis. *In* "Environmental Carcinogenesis. Occurrence, Risk Evaluation and Mechanisms" (P. Emmelot and E. Kriek, eds.). Elsevier, New York, 1979, p. 265.
514. Suda, D., Schwartz, J., and Shklar, G.: *Carcinogenesis* **7**, 711 (1986).
515. Wattenberg, L. W.: *J. Natl. Cancer Inst.* **52**, 1583 (1974).
516. Borchert, P., and Wattenberg, L. W.: *J. Natl. Cancer Inst.* **57**, 173 (1976).
517. Irving, C. C., Tice, A. J., and Murphy, W. M.: *Cancer Res.* **39**, 3040 (1979).
518. Irving, C. C., Daniel, D. S., and Murphy, W. M.: *Carcinogenesis* **4**, 617 (1983).

519. Malejka-Giganti, D., McIver, R. C., and Rydell, R. E.: *J. Natl. Cancer Inst.* **64,** 1471 (1980).
520. Perchellet, J.-P., Abney, N. L., Thomas, R. M., Perchellet, E. M., and Maatta, E. A.: *Cancer Res.* **47,** 6302 (1987).
521. Walaszek, Z., Hanausek-Walaszek, M., and Webb, T. E.: *Carcinogenesis* **5,** 767 (1984).
522. Webb, T. E., Abou-Issa, H., Dwivedi, C., and Koolemans-Beynen, A.: Synergism Between Glucarate and Retinoids in the Rat Mammary System. *In* "Cancer Chemoprevention" (L. Wattenberg, M. Lipkin, C. W. Boone, and G. J. Kelloff, eds.). CRC Press, Boca Raton, Florida, 1992, p. 263.
523. Luo, X.-M., Wei, H.-J., and Yang, S. P.: *J. Natl. Cancer Inst.* **71,** 75 (1983).
524. Wei, H.-J., Luo, X.-M., and Yang, S. P.: *J. Natl. Cancer Inst.* **74,** 469 (1985).
525. Wattenberg, L. W., Sparnins, V. L., and Barany, G.: *Cancer Res.* **49,** 2689 (1989).
526. Wattenberg, L. W., and Coccia, J. B.: *Carcinogenesis* **12,** 115 (1991).
527. Elegbede, J. A., Elson, C. E., Qureshi, A., Tanner, M. A., and Gould, M. N.: *Carcinogenesis* **5,** 661 (1984).
528. Elson, C. E., Maltzman, T. H., Boston, J. L., Tanner, M. A., and Gould, M. N.: *Carcinogenesis* **9,** 331 (1988).
529. Maltzman, T. H., Hurt, L. M., Elson, C. E., Tanner, M. A., and Gould, M. N.: *Carcinogenesis* **10,** 781 (1989).
530. Gould, M. N.: *Proc. Am. Assoc. Cancer Res.* **32,** 474 (1991).
531. Messadi, D. V., Billings, P., Shklar, G., and Kennedy, A. R.: *J. Natl. Cancer Inst.* **76,** 447 (1986).
532. Daoud, A. H., and Griffin, A. C.: *Cancer Lett.* **5,** 231 (1978).
533. Besbris, H. J., Wortzman, M. S., and Cohen, A. M.: *J. Toxicol. Environ. Health* **9,** 63 (1982).
534. Joseph, C., Fiala, E. S., El-Bayoumy, K., and Sohn, O. S.: *Proc. Am. Assoc. Cancer Res.* **30,** 176, Abst. 697 (1989).
535. Nayini, J., El-Bayoumy, K., Sugie, S., Cohen, L. A., and Reddy, B. S.: *Carcinogenesis* **10,** 509 (1989).
536. Witting, C., Witting, U., and Krieg, V.: *J. Cancer Res. Clin. Oncol.* **104,** 109 (1982).
537. Wendel, A.: Glutathione Peroxidase. *In* "Enzymatic Basis of Detoxication" (W. B. Jakoby, ed.), Vol. 1. Academic Press, New York, 1980, p. 333.
538. Perchellet, J.-P., Perchellet, E. M., Orten, D. K., and Schneider, B. A.: *Cancer Lett.* **26,** 283 (1985).
539. Machlin, L. J., and Bendich, A.: *FASEB J.* **1,** 441 (1987).
540. Jacobs, M. M., Forst, C. F., and Beams, F. A.: *Cancer Res.* **41,** 4458 (1981).
541. Medina, D.: *Adv. Exp. Med. Biol.* **206,** 465 (1986).
542. Reddy, B. S., Sugie, S., Maruyama, H., and Marra, P.: *Cancer Res.* **48,** 1777 (1988).
543. Milner, J. A.: *Adv. Exp. Med. Biol.* **206,** 449 (1986).
544. Medina, D., and Morrison, D. G.: *Pathol. Immunopathol. Res.* **7,** 187 (1988).
545. Fico, M. E., Poirier, L. A., Watrach, A. M., Watrach, M. A., and Milner, J. A.: *Cancer Res.* **46,** 3384 (1986).
546. LeBoeuf, R. A., and Hoekstra, W. G.: *Federation Proc.* **44,** 2563 (1985).
547. Sandgren, M. E., Bronnegard, M., and DeLuca, H. F.: *Biochem. Biophys. Res. Commun.* **181,** 611 (1991).
548. Wood, A. W., Chang, R. L., Huang, M.-T., Uskokovic, M., and Conney, A. H.: *Biochem. Biophys. Res. Commun.* **116,** 605 (1983).
549. Chida, K., Hashiba, H., Fukushima, M., Suda, T., and Kuroki, T.: *Cancer Res.* **45,** 5426 (1985).
550. Kawaura, A., Tanida, N., Sawada, K., Oda, M., and Shimoyama, T.: *Carcinogenesis* **10,** 647 (1989).
551. Hashiba, H., Fukushima, M., Chida, K., and Kuroki, T.: *Cancer Res.* **47,** 5031 (1987).
552. Chida, K., Hashiba, H., Suda, T., and Kuroki, T.: *Cancer Res.* **44,** 1387 (1984).
553. Cohen, S. M., Saulenas, A. M., Sullivan, C. R., and Albert, D. M.: *Arch. Ophthalmol.* **106,** 541 (1988).
554. Colston, K. W., Berger, U., and Coombes, R. C.: *Lancet* **1,** 188 (1989).
555. Kizaki, M., and Koeffler, H. P.: 1, 25-Dihydroxyvitamin D_3 and Hematopoietic Cells: Applications to Cancer Therapy. *In* "Vitamins and Cancer Prevention" (S. A. Laidlaw and M. E. Swendseid, eds.). Wiley-Liss, New York, 1991, p. 91.
556. Honma, Y., Hozumi, M., Abe, E., Konno, K., Fukushima, M., Hata, S., Nishi, Y., DeLuca, H. F., and Suda, T.: *Proc. Natl. Acad. Sci. U.S.A.* **80,** 201 (1983).
557. Pols, H. A. P., Birkenhager, J. C., Foekens, J. A., and van Leeuwen, J. P. T. M.: *J. Steroid Biochem.* **37,** 873 (1990).
558. Koeffler, H. P., Amatruda, T., Ikekawa, N., Kobayashi, Y., and DeLuca, H. F.: *Cancer Res.* **44,** 5624 (1984).
559. Gross, M., Kost, S. B., Ennis, B., Stumpf, W., and Kumar, R.: *J. Bone Mineral Res.* **1,** 457 (1986).
560. Abe, J., Morikawa, M., Miyamoto, K., Kaiho, S., Fukushima, M., Miyaura, C., Abe, E., Suda, T., and Nishii, Y.: *FEBS Lett.* **226,** 58 (1987).
561. Tanaka, Y., Higgins, P. J., and Jubiz, W.: *Biochem. Pharmacol.* **38,** 449 (1989).
562. Wattenberg, L. W., and Fiala, E. S.: *J. Natl. Cancer Inst.* **60,** 1515 (1978).

563. Wattenberg, L. W., Coccia, J. B., and Lam, L. K. T.: *Cancer Res.* **40**, 2820 (1980).
564. Wattenberg, L. W., Borchert, P., Destafney, C. M., and Coccia, J. B.: *Cancer Res.* **43**, 4747 (1983).
565. Hong, W. K., Lippman, S. M., Itri, L. M., Karp, D. D., Lee, J. S., Byers, R. M., Schantz, S. P., Kramer, A. M., Lotan, R., Peters, L. J., Dimery, I. W., Brown, B. W., and Goepfert, H.: *New Engl. J. Med.* **323**, 795 (1990).
566. Fisher, B.: *Proc. Am. Assoc. Cancer Res.* **33**, 567 (1992).
567. Kelloff, G. J., Malone, W. F., Boone, C. W., Sigman, C. C., and Fay, J. R.: *Semin. Surg. Oncol.* **17**, 438 (1990).
568. Kelloff, G. J., Boone, C. W., Malone, W. F., and Steele, V.: Recent Results in Preclinical and Clinical Drug Development of Chemopreventive Agents at the National Cancer Institute. *In* "Cancer Chemoprevention" (L. Wattenberg, M. Lipkin, C. W. Boone, and G. J. Kelloff, eds.). CRC Press, Boca Raton, Florida, 1992, p. 41.
569. Kampalath, B. N., Liau, M. C., Burzynski, B., and Burzynski, S. R.: *Drugs Exp. Clin. Res.* **13**, 51 (1987).
570. Eriguchi, N., Hara, H., Yoshida, H., Nishida, H., Nakayama, T., Ohishi, K., Tsuda, H., Inoue, S., and Ikeda, I.: *Nippon Gan Chiryo Gakki Shi (J. Jpn. Soc. Cancer Ther.)* **23**, 1560 (1988).
571. Lesca, P.: *Carcinogenesis* **4**, 1651 (1983).
572. Hirose, M., Fukushima, S., Kurata, Y., Tsuda, H., Tatematsu, M., and Ito, N.: *Cancer Res.* **48**, 5310 (1988).
573. McCormick, D. L., and Spicer, A. M.: *Cancer Lett.* **37**, 139 (1987).
574. Akao, M., and Kuroda, K.: *Chem. Pharm. Bull. Tokyo.* **38**, 2012 (1990).
575. Smart, R. C., and Crawford, C. L.: *Am. J. Clin. Nutr.* **54**, 1266s (1991).
576. Minoura, T., Takata, T., Sakeguchi, M., Takada, H., Yamamura, M., Hioki, K., and Yamamoto, M.: *Cancer Res.* **48**, 4790 (1988).
577. Karmali, R. A., Donner, A., Gobel, S., and Shimamura, T.: *Anticancer Res.* **9**, 1161 (1989).
578. Reddy, B. S., Tokumo, K., Kulkarni, N., Aligia, C., and Kelloff, G.: *Carcinogenesis* **13**, 1019 (1992).
579. Ionov, I. D.: *Int. J. Cancer* **41**, 777 (1988).
580. Satyamoorthy, K., and Perchellet, J.-P.: *Cancer Res.* **49**, 5364 (1989).
581. Curphey, T. J., Kuhlmann, E. T., Roebuck, B. D., and Longnecker, D. S.: *Pancreas* **3**, 36 (1988).
582. Grubbs, C. J., Eto, I., Juliana, M. M., and Whitaker, L. M.: *Oncology* **48**, 239 (1991).
583. Pamukcu, A. M., Yalciner, S., and Bryan, G. T.: *Cancer* **40**, 2450 (1977).
584. Poirier, L. A., Theiss, J. C., Arnold, L. J., and Shimkin, M. B.: *Cancer Res.* **44**, 1520 (1984).
585. Schwartz, A. G., Fairman, D. K., Polansky, M., Lewbart, M. L., and Pashko, L. L.: *Carcinogenesis* **10**, 1809 (1989).
586. Dwivedi, C., Oredipe, O. A., Barth, R. F., Downie, A. A., and Webb, T. E.: *Carcinogenesis* **10**, 1539 (1989).
587. Russin, W. A., Hoesly, J. D., Elson, C. E., Tanner, M. A., and Gould, M. N.: *Carcinogenesis* **10**, 2161 (1989).
588. Furukawa, F., Imaida, K., Okamiya, H., Shinoda, K., Sato, M., Imazawa, T., Hayashi, Y., and Takahashi, M.: *Carcinogenesis* **12**, 2123 (1991).
589. Reddy, B. S., Rivenson, A., Kulkarni, N., Upadhyaya, P., and El-Bayoumy, K.: *Cancer Res.* **52**, 5635 (1992).

CHAPTER **5**

Promotion and Cocarcinogenesis

Contents: **Introduction.**   **Section I:** Tumor Promotion in Skin.   **Section II:** Tumor Promotion in Liver. **Section IIIA:** Note on Multistage Carcinogenesis in Other Organs and *in Vitro*. **Section IIIB:** Note on Tumor Promoters, Cocarcinogens, and Nongenotoxic Carcinogens.

Introduction

Friedrich Marks, Michael Schwarz, and Gerhard Fürstenberger

In experimental animals, tumors can be induced according to different protocols. Solitary carcinogenesis involves the application/administration of only one carcinogenic agent, given either once in a single high dose or repeatedly in several small doses. Solitary carcinogens, either as such or after metabolic transformation, can induce tumors by themselves, without the cooperative action of any other chemical agent. Generally, solitary carcinogens bind covalently to DNA and tend to induce DNA repair—they are genotoxic. A protocol of multistage carcinogenesis, in contrast, is based on the *cooperative action* of two or more different agents, each of which is unable by itself to induce the development of tumors when the experimental conditions are carefully controlled. Multistage models of carcinogenesis which have been developed for various animal species and tissues (1,2) provide methodological tools for mechanistic investigations, since tumor development is a complex process that can be subdivided into stages so as to yield to analysis on the cellular and molecular level. The operational concepts, initiation and promotion, are based historically on observations made in the framework of the two-stage mouse skin carcinogenesis protocol.

During the last decades, a large variety of agents of differing chemical structures have been found to exhibit promoting activity in carcinogen-initiated mouse skin; the investigations of the structure–activity relationships of their effects have greatly increased our knowledge about some of the mechanisms of their action. However, because humans are not usually exposed to most of these agents, the toxicological relevance of the majority of these compounds appears to be limited. In the case of tumor promotion in liver, on the other hand, the question of toxicological significance is of utmost importance. This is because many drugs and environmentally occurring chemicals to which humans are exposed were found to promote hepatocarcinogenesis in rodents (and may even induce tumors when administered alone at sufficiently high dose levels, without any prior exposure of the animals to an initiating carcinogen). Thus, animal models play an important role as *in vivo* test systems for the identification of environmentally occurring and also endogenously generated agents that contribute to different stages of carcinogenesis. Since human carcinogenesis, as carcinogenesis in animal models, also proceeds in stages (3,4) detailed investigations of the molecular and cellular mechanisms involved, as well as the identification of the relevant environmental and endogenous factors, are needed.

REFERENCES

1. Slaga, T. J.: "Mechanisms of Tumor Promotion", Vols. I–IV. CRC Press, Boca Raton, Florida, 1983–84.
2. Yamagiwa, K., and Ichikawa, K.: *Gann* **8**, 11 (1914).
3. Kennedy, A. R.: Relevance of Tumor Promotion to Carcinogenesis in Human Populations. *In* "Carcinogenesis", Vol. 8: Cancer of the Respiratory Tract (N. J. Mass, D. G. Kaufman, J. M. Siegfried, V. E. Steele, and S. Nesnow, eds.). Raven Press, New York, 1985, p. 431.
4. Day, N. E.: Epidemiological Evidence of Promoting Effect. The Example of Breast Cancer. *In* "Carcinogenesis," Vol. 7: Cocarcinogenesis and Biological Effects of Tumor Promoters (E. Hecker, N. E. Fusenig, W. Kunz, F. Marks, and H. W. Thielmann, eds.). Raven Press, New York, 1982, p. 183.

Tumor Promotion in Skin[1]

Friedrich Marks and Gerhard Fürstenberger

I. MULTISTAGE CARCINOGENESIS IN SKIN: HISTORICAL BACKGROUND AND BASIC CONCEPTUAL DEVELOPMENTS

The skin of rodents (especially of mice) is the oldest and until recently the most often used system for mechanistic studies on chemical carcinogenesis and for the bioassay of chemicals for carcinogenic activity. This is because this system provides special advantages such as the high sensitivity of the mouse skin to carcinogenic agents, the ease of manipulation, and the availability of different inbred mouse strains with graded susceptibilities. It is only relatively recently that the increasing use of other models such as the liver, the bladder, and a variety of cell and tissue culture systems has begun.

A. From Coal Tar Painting to the Initiation-Promotion Experiment

Studies on skin carcinogenesis have provided several important landmarks in cancer research. In 1914 Yamagiwa and Ichikawa's approach (1) to the induction of skin cancer in rabbits by prolonged application of coal tar opened the era of animal experimentation aimed at the exploration of the carcinogenic effects of chemicals. It was observed that coal tar-induced skin carcinomas developed in a stepwise manner, starting with an early inflammatory reaction and epidermal hyperplasia. Repeated application of the carcinogenic agent for many weeks resulted in the emergence of benign tumors (papillomas), a few of which eventually progressed to carcinomas. Following Virchow's famous postulate (2), these early investigators regarded the inflammatory response as providing an important condition for tumorigenesis, especially since irritating procedures such as application of unsaturated fatty acids, turpentine, chloroform, or wounding could accelerate the emergence of tumors in coal tar-painted skin (3,4). Later on the conclusion was reached that irritation *alone* was insufficient to induce neoplastic growth.

In the early 1940s, Rous and coworkers (5,6) proposed to distinguish two stages in experimental skin tumorigenesis, which they have termed initiation and promotion. They noted that initiation required only a limited duration of treatment of the animal skin with coal tar or benzo[a]pyrene (BaP). The papillomas thus elicited generally disappeared when the treatment was stopped. Their regrowth could be "promoted", however, at the

---

[1]For abbreviations used *see* p. 173.

same sites by a subsequent treatment with a skin irritant or by wounding. Without prior initiation the promoting treatment did not exhibit a significant tumorigenic effect. This result could only be explained by the assumption that—despite a complete regression of the visible papillomas—a few initiated cells irreversibly remained in the epidermis, which, when promoted, gave rise to new tumors.

At about the same time, croton oil, the highly irritating seed oil of the Euphorbiacea *Croton tiglium*, was found to contain extremely potent skin tumor promoters (7) which were later identified as phorbol esters, with 12-*O*-tetradecanoylphorbol-13-acetate (TPA; also called phorbol myristate acetate, PMA) being the prototype of these esters (8,9). In the meantime, many other types of skin tumor promoters have been identified in different natural products (*e.g.*, 10). Based on the work of Rous and coworkers, Mottram (11) and Berenblum and Shubik (12) introduced the standardized methodology of two-stage carcinogenesis in mouse skin which is still in use today. This consists of a single application of an initiator, usually a polycyclic aromatic hydrocarbon, such as 7,12-dimethylbenz[*a*]anthracene (DMBA), followed by repeated chronic treatment with a promoting agent (in earlier days croton oil, today mostly a phorbol ester) twice a week.

B. Initiation–Promotion in Mouse Skin: An Experimental Model

For a long time, initiation and promotion were operationally defined terms; their definition was based on a distinct experimental approach designed so that both processes could be clearly distinguished and experimentally characterized. Outside of these experimental conditions, the situation becomes less clear, since nature does not provide "pure" initiators and "pure" promoters (13,14).

Practically all initiating agents are solitary ("complete") carcinogens, which produce tumors in the absence of promotion, provided they are applied in a sufficient dose over a long enough period of time. Whether or not a promoting component is inherent in this carcinogenic activity and, if so, whether or not it follows the same mechanistic pathways as in the initiation–promotion process, is a matter of continuous debate.

On the other hand, the important fact must be borne in mind that every promoting agent induces a few tumors if applied long enough. Therefore, promoters have to be classified, in the strict sense of the word, as solitary carcinogens, albeit weak ones (13). This has created a long-lasting but rather fruitless debate about the reality and significance of tumor promotion, in general. Since none of the specific gene mutations and interactions with DNA—thought to be involved in initiation by solitary carcinogens—have been observed with promoters, their carcinogenic action is generally assumed to follow an epigenetic mechanism, whatever this means. The idea that in such cases "spontaneously" initiated cells are promoted is as easy to propose as it is impossible to prove. Presently, we observe something like a renaissance of Virchow's postulate in that an intense debate about the carcinogenic effects of cellular hyperproliferation is taking place. There is increasing evidence that a chronic dysregulation of cell cycle control—brought about either by a mutation of the relevant control genes or by permanent mitogenic stimulation—provides an important condition for carcinogenesis (15). It is one of the main characteristics of skin tumor promoters that they, in fact, induce permanent epidermal hyperproliferation and sustained hyperplasia when chronically applied.

When certain conditions such as use of an animal strain with a low rate of "spontaneous" skin tumor development, a low dose of the initiating carcinogen (said to be "subthreshold"), and a well-controlled regimen of the promoter application are observed, initiator and promoter act in an almost perfect cooperative manner, *i.e.*, the carcinogenic effect of each agent alone is so low that it does not significantly contribute to the final result and may thus be neglected. This provides an analytical model which allows the stepwise induction of tumors proceeding *via* the stages: (a) initiation, (b) promotion, and (c) malignant progression. Whether or not the observations thus made are relevant for an understanding of neoplastic processes in other tissues, and in humans, is another question which will be discussed below.

The fundamental observations (16a,16b,17) made by applying the Berenblum–Mottram scheme of initiation–promotion in mice may be summarized as follows. Under the described conditions initiation leads to histopathologically undetectable alterations in epidermal cells. These alterations are, however, virtually irreversible, since between initiation and promotion the experiment can be interrupted for any period of time without a substantial decrease in tumor incidence. Such irreversibility is consistent with the idea that initiation is due to gene mutations, probably occurring in an epidermal stem cell compartment (*see below*). This concept has now gained considerable support by the demonstration of a point-mutated, *i.e.*, activated H-*ras* proto-oncogene in skin tumors, generated through the two-stage protocol (18). In contrast to initiation, promotion has been found to be a reversible process. That is, when the time interval between two subsequent promoter applications is increased from 3 days up to more than 1 week, tumor incidence is drastically reduced. Moreover, contrary to the effect of an initiator, the effect of repeated promoter treatments is not additive. When the overall total dose of a promoter is split into several smaller doses, given in shorter time intervals, tumor incidence drops considerably. Tumors are found to develop only when the initiating carcinogen is applied *prior* to the promoter, but not vice versa — *i.e.*, a promoter does not act additively with the initiator but completes a process started with initiation — thus indicating that the mechanism of promotion must be different from that of initiation (19).

The above conclusion has been supported not only by mechanistic studies but also by a detailed analysis of the dose–response relationships showing a distinct no-effect level only for promoters, but not for initiators (20). Later, the Berenblum–Mottram scheme was refined by subdividing the stage of promotion into two different steps (21,22), by introducing a new stage called "conversion" (23), and by manipulating the progression from the benign to the malignant state (24). The entire process of carcinoma development in skin can now be studied through at least four separate but sequential stages (Figure 1).

It has been argued that the skin model is only of rather limited value since it describes first of all the development of benign rather than malignant tumors. Indeed, the dose of the promoter and the duration of promoter treatment have no effect on the rate of malignant progression (24). On the other hand, carcinoma development is practically nil in initiated skin *without* promotion. This indicates that promotion is a prerequisite for malignant progression, probably because the carcinomas develop from papillomas, the development of which, in turn, depends on promotion (*see below*). If malignant progression is the result of additional genotoxic effects as generally assumed, the probability of those effects to occur will be much higher in rapidly proliferating cell clones such as papillomas (being the result of a clonal expansion of initiated cells) than in single initiated cells.

Most interestingly, the whole process of skin tumorigenesis can be interrupted in its early stages, *i.e.*, before malignant carcinomas appear. In other words, the prevention or inhibition of promotion brings the development of cancer to a halt. If these observations can be extended to the human situation and to other organs, they may turn out to be of extreme practical relevance in that the identification of environmental tumor promoters and the investigation of their mechanism of action may provide a possibility of cancer prevention, in particular in an environment which cannot be entirely "cleansed" from carcinogenic hazards.

From the experimental point of view, the mouse skin model provides an additional

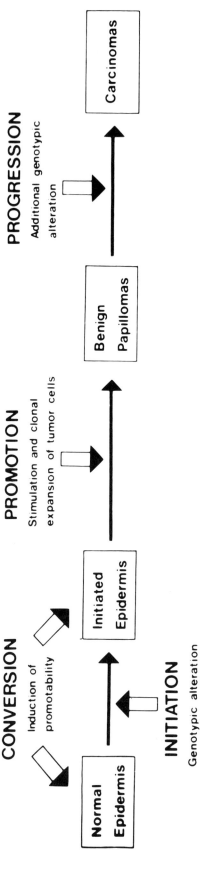

FIGURE 1. The stages of experimental skin carcinogenesis. Current concepts on the mechanisms of initiation, promotion, and progression are represented; the conversion stage is only operationally defined, due mainly to a lack of knowledge about the mechanisms involved. For details *see* text. [Adapted from F. Marks and G. Fürstenberger: *In* "Concepts and Theories in Carcinogenesis" (A. P. Maskens, P. Ebbesen, and A. Burny, eds.). Elsevier, Amsterdam, 1987, p. 169.]

advantage. Today it is generally accepted that cancer results from an accumulation of genetic defects. Recently, there has been much excitement over the so-called "Vogelstein model", which suggests that fully malignant colorectal cancer of man is due to both mutation of proto-oncogenes and inactivation of tumor suppressor genes (26). At first glance it appears as if this model has now outdated the classical animal model of skin carcinogenesis. It must not be overlooked, however, that the Vogelstein model — like any model of human carcinogenesis — is more or less a *descriptive* model dealing with *already existing* pathological states, whereas the skin model makes possible all kinds of experimental interventions and gradual procedures, thus permitting a much deeper analysis of the basic *mechanisms* of tumor induction and tumor development. Moreover, the animal skin model offers the rather unique possibility of being able to alternate between *in vivo* and *in vitro* conditions. The *in vitro* cultivation of skin cells has reached a high standard by now and allows a detailed analysis of those biochemical and cellular alterations, which are either the result of the critical gene mutations occurring during the process of carcinogenesis, or which facilitate the manifestation and expression of those genetic alterations.

C. Conversion and Promotion ("Two-Stage Tumor Promotion")

As already mentioned, the great majority of papillomas produced in mouse skin under the standard conditions of an initiation–promotion experiment do not show growth autonomy, but disappear after promoter treatment has been stopped, especially in the early phase of the experiment (27).

At first glance, this observation seems to provide a rather trivial explanation of promotion as a continuous stimulation of cellular proliferation in epidermis, which is required to make the nonautonomous papillomas visible at all. Such an interpretation is in accordance with the fact that all skin tumor promoters are strong irritant mitogens and that the generation of sustained epidermal hyperplasia is a prerequisite for promotion (*see below*).

However, the finding that not every agent which induced epidermal hyperplasia is a good promoter raised serious doubts about this simplistic concept. It was found, moreover, that such apparently nonpromoting skin mitogens could nevertheless "complete" the tumorigenic effect of a limited, insufficient promoter treatment (17). To explain this situation, Boutwell (17) postulated that promotion consists of two different events which he called "conversion" (the promoting effect proper) and "propagation" (the chronic mitogenic component). Later this concept was adopted by Slaga et al. (21) using Sencar mice with TPA as a converting agent and mezerein as a propagating agent, as well as by Fürstenberger *et al.* (22) using NMRI mice with the two phorbol esters, TPA and 12-*O*-retinoylphorbol-13-acetate (RPA), as converting and propagating agents, respectively. A distinction between "complete" and "incomplete" tumor promoters was made concomitantly with the introduction of the concept of "two-stage promotion". Besides a clastogenic effect to be discussed below, no clear-cut qualitative differences seem to exist between both types of agents in inducing skin inflammation and epidermal hyperplasia, including associated biochemical events such as ornithine decarboxylase (ODC) and protein kinase C (PKC) activation, eicosanoid release, and others (22,28–37). In addition, both propagation and conversion are equally sensitive to several inhibitors (antipromoters) such as retinoic acid (38), steroidal (39) and nonsteroidal antiphlogistic drugs (40), cyclosporins (41), hydroxyurea (42), antioxidants (43), inhibitors of arachidonic acid metabolism (44), and protease inhibitors (45).

In contrast to the initiated state, the converted state is reversible, exhibiting a half-life of 10–12 weeks in NMRI mice (23) and 2–4 weeks in Sencar mice (46). This is much longer than the time required for regression of the hyperproliferative state induced by a single phorbol ester application, thus supporting Boutwell's hypothesis (17) that conversion and propagation are based on different mechanisms.

The sequence of initiating and converting treatments is inversible (23,47), whereas the noninversibility of the initiation–promotion sequence is considered to be one of the fundamental characteristics of the classical two-stage experiment (12,17,19), that is, only preexisting initiated cells can be promoted. Consequently, conversion is not the first phase of promotion, but has to be regarded as a distinct, separate stage of the carcinogenic response. We have suggested, therefore, that the concept of "two-stage tumor promotion" be abandoned and the term promotion be reserved for what has been hitherto called propagation (23). Accordingly, one may distinguish two types of promoters: convertogenic ("complete") promoters and nonconvertogenic ("incomplete") promoters. It has been argued that the term "conversion" is ambiguous, since it can be confounded with the "conversion of the benign into the malignant" state. To avoid such semantic confusion, the latter process should be termed "malignant progression" as suggested by Foulds (48).

The cautionary note, that special experimental conditions must be observed to obtain a clear-cut separation of the stages initiation and promotion, is also relevant for conversion and promotion, since "pure" convertogenic and "pure" promoting agents do not exist; thus, TPA—as mentioned above—seems to be equipotent as both a convertogenic and a promoting agent. In addition, RPA (49) and some other agents such as 4-O-methyl-TPA and the ionophor A23187 (45) have been shown to be convertogenic agents in the Sencar mouse strain, but not in the NMRI strain (22).

The approach of experimental three-stage carcinogenesis in mouse skin is schematically summarized in Figure 2.

II. SKIN TUMOR PROMOTERS

Investigations into the mechanism of tumor promotion and conversion in mouse skin have been carried out mostly using phorbol esters, such as TPA. Recently, several other compounds have been identified as skin tumor promoters. Progress in the mechanistic understanding of promoter action now allows classifying these agents according to their molecular mechanism of action into those which interact directly with intracellular signalling pathways and those which seem to induce more unspecific tissue damage and evoke a wounding tissue response.

A. Tumor Promotion by Specific Interactions with Intracellular Signaling

Several skin tumor promoters have been shown to interact rather specifically with pathways of intracellular signal transduction (Table 1). The most prominent representatives of this group are the so-called diacylglycerol (DAG) agonists, also called TPA-type promoters. These agents bind to and activate the enzymes of the PKC family by mimicking the effect of the intracellular second messenger DAG. TPA-type promoters comprise a series of natural products derived from various organisms. They include also

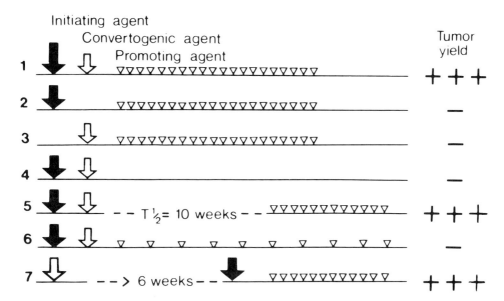

FIGURE 2. Multistage tumorigenesis in mouse skin. Each symbol represents a single local treatment of dorsal mouse skin. Tumor development occurs upon sequential treatment with an initiating, a converting (convertogenic), and a promoting agent — for example, 7,12-dimethylbenz[a]anthracene, phorbol ester TPA, and phorbol ester RPA (lines 1–4). While the initiated state is irreversible, and the converted state exhibits a half-life of several weeks (line 5), the effect of a single promoter treatment is quickly reversible (line 6). Line 7 schematizes the approach of "inverted sequence", i.e., where conversion is brought about prior to initiation. Instead of by chemical agents, conversion and promotion can also be brought about by skin wounding (see in Ref. 50).

staurosporine and related compounds, which are known as PKC inhibitors (61); actually, these compounds behave as mixed DAG agonists–antagonists in that they exhibit some ambivalent effects: on one hand they display some tumor-promoting capability of their own, while on the other hand, they inhibit tumor promotion by phorbol ester or teleocidin (62,63).

Within the class of the TPA-type tumor promoters a correlation between the affinity for PKC and the tumor-promotion efficacy has been found (64), whereas convertogenic potency is apparently not directly related to PKC activation (28). It should be pointed out, in this connection, that even compounds which do not interact directly with PKC have been identified as being converting agents, including 4-O-methyl-TPA and the ionophore A23187 in Sencar mouse skin (46), as well as transforming growth factor β (TGFβ) (65) and methyl methanesulfonate (66) in NMRI mouse skin. Moreover, nonpromoting phorbol esters carrying short acyl residues, such as phorbol-12,13-diacetate, inhibit TPA-induced conversion and promotion in doses which are far below those required for competitive PKC binding (67).

Another group of promoters interacting with intracellular signaling is represented by the phosphoprotein phosphatase inhibitors (59,68), with okadaic acid being a prototype. These agents bind to and inhibit specifically the phosphoprotein phosphatases 1 and 2A, but not the enzymes 2B and 2C (69). They do not interact with PKC. Thus, both inducers of protein phosphorylation and inhibitors of protein dephosphorylation are found among the most potent skin tumor promoters. The skin tumor promoter palytoxin (60) also interacts with intracellular signaling, perhaps by stimulating the Na^+ influx (70).

TABLE 1.   Selected Skin Tumor Promoters Known to Interact with Cellular Signaling

Agent	Chemical structure	Biological effect	Promoting efficacy	References
Phorbol ester (TPA)	Diterpene ester	DAG[a] agonist	Strong	51–53
Teleocidin	Indole alkaloid	DAG agonist	Strong	54
Aplysiatoxin	Polyacetate	DAG agonist	Strong	55,56
sn-1,2-Didecanoyl glycerol[b]	Diacylglycerol	DAG agonist	Moderate	57
Staurosporine	Alkaloid	PKC[c] inhibitor	Moderate	58
Okadaic acid	Polyether	Proteinphosphatase inhibitor	Strong	59
Palytoxin	Polyalcohol	Activation of Na^+ channel	Weak	60

[a]Diacylglycerol.
[b]sn, stereospecific numbering,
[c]Protein kinase C.

B. Tumor Promotion *via* Nonspecific Tissue Damage

Nonspecific tissue damage is also an efficient skin tumor promoter. Nonspecific tissue damage can be brought about by chemical irritation as well as by other means, such as ultraviolet (UV) radiation and mechanical wounding (Table 2).

UV light, in particular UV-B, is a well-established skin carcinogen and initiator. Recently, UV-A exposure has been associated with skin tumor promotion (90). If this finding is confirmed, it may well lead to a reevaluation of the risks of outdoor habits and artificial tanning devices, let alone the problem of ozone layer destruction.

As early as in the era of experimental coal tar carcinogenesis it was observed that

TABLE 2.   Selected Skin Tumor Promoters Hypothesized to Act by Inducing Tissue Damage and Wound Response

Agent	Promoting efficacy	References
Benzoyl peroxide	Moderate	71
t-Butylhydroperoxide	Moderate	72
Anthralin	Moderate	73
Chrysarobin	Moderate	73
Thapsigargin	Moderate	74
A23187	(Conversion)	46
Acyl esters	Weak	75
n-Dodecane	Weak	76,77
Phenols	Weak	78
Na laurylsulfate	Weak	79
Iodoacetic acid	Weak	80
1-Fluoro-2,4-dinitrobenzene	Moderate	81
Benzo[*a*]pyrene	Moderate	82
7-Bromomethylbenz[*a*]anthracene	Strong	83
Methyl methanesulfonate	Moderate	66
Citrus oil	Weak	84
Tobacco extract	Weak	85
Tobacco smoke condensate	Moderate	86
Mechanical wounding	Strong	87–89
UV radiation	Moderate	90

wounding accelerated the development of skin tumors. Later it was shown that both repeated incisions and abrasions of initiated mouse skin exhibited a strong tumor-promoting (87–89), but no initiating, effect (91). Superficial skin damage, however, as caused by tape-stripping of the horny layer, did not promote papilloma development (88), although it evoked a pronounced hyperplastic response of skin. A single wounding by incision of initiated mouse skin also induces conversion, as shown by papilloma development upon subsequent treatment with an "incomplete" promoter such as RPA (29,65).

The convertogenic and promoting effectiveness of wounding is expected to provide the key for an in-depth understanding of skin tumorigenesis (31); accordingly, tumorigenesis may proceed along inherently "normal" endogenous pathways involved in tissue repair and regeneration. Such regeneration processes are controlled by a complex interaction between various tissues and cell types, which communicate with each other by cytokines and lipid mediators (as discussed in greater detail below). Such factors may fulfill the role of endogenous tumor promoters, at least after tissue damage. Two putative wound factors, *i.e.*, TGFα and TGFβ, have indeed been shown to induce conversion in initiated mouse skin in a synergistic manner, when injected together intracutaneously (65).

Nonspecific "chemical wounding" may also explain the tumor-promoting effect of several skin irritants. The most prominent candidates for such a mechanism of action are provided by those skin tumor promoters which either generate the endogeneous production of free radicals or decompose themselves so as to yield free radicals, such as peroxides, hydroperoxides, or anthrone derivatives (Table 2). Free radical generation has indeed been postulated to provide a critical event in tumor promotion (92–97). Regarding conversion, evidence is growing for the role of hydroperoxides and free radicals, generated along the arachidonic acid cascade, as clastogenic agents (66,98). As already mentioned, chromosomal damage appears to correlate with conversion.

"Ca^{2+} effectors" such as A23187 (99) and thapsigargin (74,100) are strong inducers of epidermal hyperplasia and skin inflammation *in vivo*. While A23187 facilitates the Ca^{2+} transport across the plasma membrane (101), thapsigargin, a plant poison (74), inhibits the intracellular Ca^{2+} sequestration, resulting in an increase of the cytoplasmic Ca^{2+} level (102). Thapsigargin is a weak convertogenic skin tumor promoter (74), whereas A23187 has been shown to exhibit convertogenic activity in Sencar mouse skin (46). Both agents do not interact directly with PKC (74,103), which does not exclude, however, the possibility of an indirect PKC activation; this is because an elevation of the cytoplasmic Ca^{2+} level in keratinocytes has been shown to lead to an activation of phospholipase C, resulting in a release of DAG and inositol-1,4,5-triphosphate (IP_3) (104). At least for thapsigargin, evidence has been provided, however, that the tumor-promoting effect of this agent may be due to nonspecific tissue damage (100).

Without claiming completeness, several other skin tumor promoters are summarized in Table 2. These include the weakly promoting long-chain fatty acids (as acyl esters), alkanes, detergents, and the SH-reagent iodoacetic acid. In the rather high dosages required for tumor promotion these agents induce both skin inflammation and epidermal hyperplasia (75–80). Although no data on the mechanism of action of these promoters are available, it may be hypothesized that their effects are also due to cytotoxicity evoking a wound response. This assumption may also apply to the promoting action of 1-fluoro-2,4-dinitrobenzene (81) and of those polycyclic hydrocarbons which, while being inactive as initiators, exhibit distinct promoting effectiveness (82,83). The alkylating agent, methyl methanesulfonate, has been found to be a convertogenic skin tumor promoter under conditions in which it does not exhibit any initiating potential (66). This and the often-postulated tumor-promoting effect of many other potent carcinogens may also result from chronic cytotoxicity evoking a regenerative reaction in skin.

C. Skin Tumor Promoters Involved in the Etiology of Human Cancer

Most skin tumor–promoter chemical compounds used for experimental purposes are rather exotic chemicals of remote origin with which man is not usually expected to come in contact. There are, however, a few exceptions and in rare instances even epidemiological evidence indicating that skin tumor promoters play a role in the etiology of some human cancers. Among these are plant-derived tumor promoters of the diterpene ester type, closely related to the phorbol esters (105). The exposure of humans to these agents results from the utilization of Euphorbiaceae and Thymelaeaceae as ornamental plants, from their mass cultivation for the production of industrial oleochemicals (106), from the use of plant extracts in folk and officinal medicine, and from the occasional contamination of honey and milk with diterpene-type tumor promoters derived from food plants (105). The epidemiologically well-documented high incidence of esophageal cancer among blacks and creoles in Curaçao has been proposed to be partially due to the irritating and promoting activity identified in tea made from the leaves of the Euphorbiaceae *Croton flavens* (107). This tea is a common everyday beverage of this Caribbean population. Pickled vegetables consumed in Linxian County, China—again an area with a high incidence of esophageal cancer—contain Roussin red methyl ester[$Fe_2(SCH_3)_2(NO)_3$; RRME], a definite mouse skin tumor promoter (108). The elevated intake of pickled vegetables and high incidences of esophageal cancer coincide also in several other Chinese counties (108), suggesting that a promoting effect of chronic irritation is involved. Whether or not the well-documented association between esophageal cancer and the habitual drinking of strong alcoholic beverages in combination with smoking may be explained in an analogous way remains to be shown. In particular, tobacco extracts (85) and tobacco smoke condensate (86) have been shown to exhibit skin tumor–promoting capability in animals; this may well represent a component of their carcinogenic potential in humans. Other agents which promote tumorigenesis in animal skin are in dermatologic or cosmetic use. These include citrus oil (84), benzoyl peroxide (71), and anthralin (73). Whether or not these promoters represent significant health risk is at present unclear, because exposure to these compounds has not yet been submitted to detailed epidemiological evaluation.

III. THE RESPONSE OF THE SKIN TO TUMOR PROMOTERS

The most characteristic response of skin to exposure to a tumor promoter is the emergence of tumors, provided that initiation has occurred before. This long-term process is, however, preceded by a series of typical alterations at the tissue, cellular, and subcellular levels. These short-term responses seem to be unspecific, since they are also observed after some physical or chemical irritation which has no promoting capability. Nevertheless, they include several effects which clearly correlate with both promoting and convertogenic activity and may provide a clue to the cellular and molecular mechanisms involved.

A. Tumor Development

1. Papillomas and Carcinomas

Papillomas provide the majority of neoplastic lesions generated in the mouse skin through the initiation–promotion protocol. Papillomas are by no means undifferentiated clumps of epidermal tumor cells, but highly organized cauliflower-like structures consisting of several epithelial and dermal projections which are connected with the underlying skin by a "stalk" (Figure 3). Each of the projections contains a layer of connective tissue covered by hyperplastic epithelium. This morphology indicates that the development of papillomas depends on a delicate interplay between the transformed epithelium and the corresponding mesenchyme, which cannot be elucidated by focusing the investigative efforts exclusively on the epidermis.

Similar to normal epidermis, the epithelium of papillomas is clearly stratified in a stratum basale exhibiting a high number of mitotic cells, a stratum spinosum, and a stratum corneum together with a thick orthokeratotic horny layer. Upon initiation with DMBA this papilloma type becomes visible in the skin of promotion-sensitive mouse strains such as NMRI (53), CD-1 (110), Ha/ICR (111), and Sencar (112) after 6–8 weeks of treatment with a potent skin tumor promoter such as the phorbol ester TPA. Maximal papilloma incidence (5–15 per animal, depending on the dose of the initiator) is reached after 12–20 weeks of treatment, consisting of one to three weekly applications of the promoter (Figure 4).

The papillomas generated by DMBA/TPA treatment of mouse skin show two distinct growth variants: (a) nonautonomous or conditional papillomas which regress after completion of treatment with the promoter, and (b) autonomous or persisting papillomas, which grow independently of further promoter application. In CD-1 mice 60–70% (113,114) and in Ha/ICR mice even 80–90% (ref. 111, *see also* Figure 4) of the papillomas were reported to be nonautonomous. Persisting papillomas seem to develop stepwise from nonautonomous papillomas (115). A certain population may also derive directly from initiated cells without passing through the nonautonomous stage (114,116). Starting from the assumption of a clonal origin of the tumors (117), the heterogeneity of papillomas may be due either to an initiation of different target cells (*i.e.*, keratinocytes in different stages of differentiation) or to differences in the molecular lesions induced by

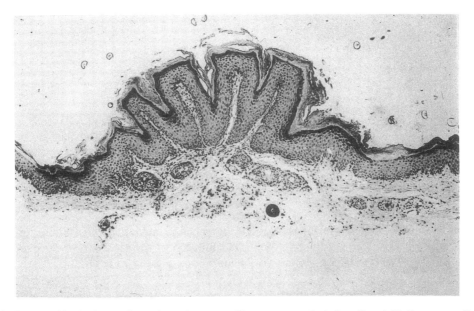

FIGURE 3. Vertical section through a papilloma generated by the initiation–promotion protocol (DMBA/TPA treatment) in NMRI mouse skin. [Adapted from F. Marks and G. Fürstenberger: *Carcinogenesis* **11**, 2085 (1990).]

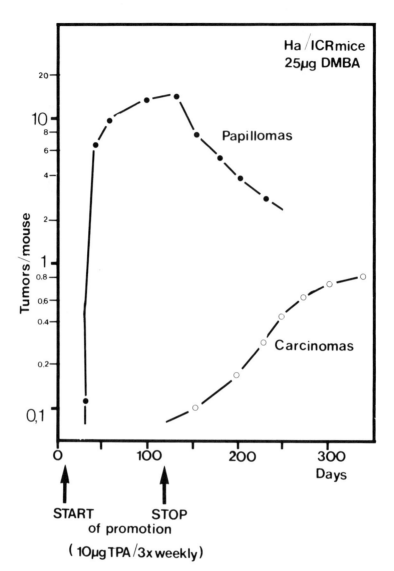

FIGURE 4.   Multistage carcinogenesis in Ha/ICR mouse skin. DMBA (25 μg/animal) was topically applied for initiation at day 0 followed by TPA treatment (10 μg/animal, three times per week) for promotion. The diagram shows the characteristic time course for rapid papilloma development (becoming visible after 6 weeks) and the delayed appearance of carcinomas. Furthermore, it illustrates the regression of papillomas and the promoter independence of carcinoma development, seen upon termination of promoter treatment. [Data from F. J. Burns, M. Vanderlaan, A. Sivak, and R. E. Albert: *Cancer Res.* **36**, 1422 (1976).]

the initiating carcinogen (24,118–121). The latter may include genetic alterations in addition to the most frequently observed point mutation of the H-*ras* proto-oncogene in codon 61, which is found already in the nonautonomous papillomas (18,122,123).

In promotion-sensitive mouse strains such as CD-1 (114), NMRI (53), Sencar (124), or Ha/ICR (ref. 111, Figure 4), the first carcinomas appear after promotion for 20–25 weeks and seem to derive mainly from autonomous papillomas (111,114). For instance, for Sencar mice the progression rate was highest for the early papillomas, becoming visible after promotion for 5 weeks and belonging mainly to the autonomous type (refs. 114 and 116; *see also* Table 3). Also, histopathological studies indicate papillomas to be

TABLE 3. **Responsiveness of Different Mouse Strains to Skin Carcinogenesis According to the Standardized Initiation-Promotion Protocol**

Strain	Tumor-bearing animals (%)	Papillomas/ animal[a]	References
Sencar	100	220	140
NMRI	100	8.6	
CD-1	75	4.8	140
C57BL/6	3.3	0.03	141

Note. Initiation was accomplished by a single topical application of DMBA (10 nmoles for Sencar, CD-1, NMRI; 400 nmoles for C57BL/6); for promotion the animals were topically treated with 8.5–10 nmoles TPA twice weekly for 15 weeks.

[a]Total number of papillomas divided by number of animals in group.

premalignant lesions being in continuous progression to the malignant state. Thus, in Sencar mice progressive dysplastic alterations leading up to carcinomas *in situ* were observed during promotion (125). After TPA treatment for 40 weeks, morphological symptoms of focal development of intrapapillomatous carcinomas were found in 25% of the benign tumors (125). According to such results, estimates for the progression rate as derived from animal experiments (126) seem to be too low, mainly because carcinomas have to grow to a substantial size in order to yield an unequivocal histopathological diagnosis, and most of the animals die from the most rapidly developing carcinomas.

The histopathological alterations progressing toward the malignant state are accompanied by an increase of the number of chromosomal abnormalities. Thus, early papillomas are mostly diploid, whereas the cells of late papillomas and carcinomas exhibit an increasing tendency to become aneuploid (127). Moreover, more specific chromosomal alterations, such as trisomies and loss of heterozygosity, have been observed in papillomas generated through the initiation–promotion protocol (128,129). The reason for this chromosomal instability—that is, whether it is an inherent property of papilloma cells or evoked by chronic promoter treatment—is not known. The clastogenic effect of TPA was demonstrated in mouse keratinocytes *in vivo* and *in vitro*, and was found to correlate with conversion (66,98). It must not be overlooked, however, that conversion represents an early stage of carcinogenesis, whereas the chromosomal abnormalities mentioned above become apparent only at a later stage (109).

The concept of the premalignant nature of papillomas is also supported by biochemical studies. The enzyme γ-glutamyl transferase (GGT) has been found to be consistently expressed in epidermal carcinomas generated by DMBA/TPA treatment, but not in normal or short-term TPA-treated interfollicular Sencar mouse epidermis. Enzyme expression occurred sporadically in papillomas, and the number of GGT-positive papillomas increased in the course of promotion (115,130). A similar result was obtained for the aberrant expression of keratin 13, which is expressed in papillomas and carcinomas, but not in normal or short-term TPA-treated NMRI mouse skin (131).

Taken together, these studies indicate that the majority of papillomas generated in mouse skin according to the initiation–promotion protocol provide a heterogeneous population of premalignant lesions. Papillomas generated in solitary carcinogenesis may also progress to malignancy. However, most of the carcinomas arising under such conditions obviously have not passed through the benign state (132).

2. Species and Strain Differences

Mouse skin has proved to be highly sensitive to the effects of carcinogens applied according to the protocols of both solitary carcinogenesis and initiation–promotion (133–135). As far as the combined DMBA/TPA treatment is concerned, mice appear to be considerably more responsive than rats (134,136), hamsters (134,137), and rabbits (133,138), whereas guinea pigs appear to be practically insensitive (133,138). Moreover, in the different species, different tumor types are induced (121,134): for instance, papillomas and squamous cell carcinomas in mice, rats, and the European hamster, but melanotic melanomas in the Syrian hamster (139). It is still not known whether these species differ in their responsiveness to the promoter or the initiating carcinogen.

Despite the high sensitivity of mice in general, the successful generation of skin tumors according to the initiation–promotion protocol critically depends on the mouse strain. Sencar mice (which, *in fact*, were bred for this purpose) exhibit the highest responsiveness to DMBA/TPA treatment, followed by the sensitive strains CD-1, NMRI, and DBA/2, whereas BALB/c, C3H, and C57BL/6 have proved to be rather resistant (Table 3 and Refs. 124,140–143). A distinct difference in promotability between Sencar and C57BL/6 mice was also found for the promoter, benzoyl peroxide, whereas responsiveness toward chrysarobin is almost identical in both mouse strains (141,143).

Comparable strain differences were not found in response to solitary carcinogenesis (143), including the potential of keratinocytes to metabolically activate DMBA (143,144), to produce and repair DMBA–DNA adducts (143), to generate mutagenic DMBA metabolites (144), and to respond to the directly acting initiator *N*-methyl-*N'*-nitro-*N*-nitrosoguanidine (MNNG) (143,145). These results clearly indicate that the above-mentioned mouse strains differ in their sensitivity to phorbol ester-induced tumor promotion, rather than in their responsiveness to initiator-induced gene mutation. Such strain and species differences in promotability are not due to the different abilities of keratinocytes to inactivate the tumor promoter (143,146), but may be most often related to the course of the hyperplastic response evoked by promoter treatment (*see below*).

Cross-breeding experiments between phorbol ester-sensitive DBA/2 and resistant C57BL/6 mice indicate that promotability is determined by multiple dominant genetic loci (145). A special case of genetic determination of promotability is provided by the tumor-promoting effect of 2,3,7,8-tetrachlorodibenzo-*p*-dioxin (TCDD) that has been observed only in the skin of hairless HRS/J mice, which is homozygous for the *hr* locus (*hr/hr*, Ref. 147), but not in other mouse strains.

Strain differences have also been found for the process of conversion. Thus the diterpene ester, mezerein, is a nonconvertogenic promoter in Sencar mouse skin (21), but inactive in NMRI mouse skin (22), whereas the phorbol ester RPA is a convertogenic promoter for Sencar (49), but a nonconvertogenic promoter for NMRI mouse skin (22).

3. Tissue Specificity

The major target tissues for phorbol ester-type promoters are keratinizing stratified epithelia, such as found in skin, esophagus, forestomach, and vagina; in contrast, glandular epithelia such as found in stomach or mammary gland are not responsive (134).

Other target cells for skin tumor promoters are dermal melanocytes, since the Syrian hamster (139) as well as BDF1 and C57BL/6 mice (148,149) respond to DMBA/TPA treatment by melanoma development, as mentioned above. Benzoyl peroxide also promotes melanoma growth in the skin of Syrian hamsters (150).

Okadaic acid type compounds have been found to exhibit tumor-promoting efficacy in both squamous and glandular epithelia of mice (151). Phorbol, the parent diterpene alcohol of phorbol esters, is inactive in mouse skin but is a promoter toward the mouse lung and liver (152) as well as toward the rat mammary gland (153). Whether or not this is due to a local esterification of phorbol is not known. Skin tumor promoters which are active also in the liver include TCDD (147,154) and di(2-ethylhexyl)phthalate, a peroxisome proliferator (155,156). In contrast, butylated hydroxytoluene (BHT) a promoter in lung and liver (157–159), inhibits phorbol ester–induced tumor promotion in the skin (160), whereas sodium o-phenylphenate, a nongenotoxic bladder carcinogen, has been proven to be a potent skin tumor promoter (161). Characteristic promoters of rat liver carcinogenesis (such as phenobarbital) and of rat colon carcinogenesis (such as lithocholic acid) have been shown to be inactive in mouse skin (162,163).

In general, tissue specificity seems to be more pronounced for tumor promoters compared to genotoxic carcinogens, probably due to the different mechanisms of promoter action in the different tissues. Investigation of the nature of tissue specificity of skin tumor promoters is hampered by the high toxicity of most of these agents, which frequently excludes chronic systemic application.

B. Morphological and Cytological Responses

Acute inflammation and epidermal hyperplasia (hyperplastic transformation, *see* Ref. 30) are the general short-term responses of the skin to mechanical and chemical irritation and provide, at the same time, essential but not sufficient conditions for tumor promotion (29). Actually, all skin tumor promoters are strong irritants (63,164–170), with the only exception being TCDD, which in its specific target strain, HRS/J, does not evoke an acute inflammatory response (147). Promoter-induced skin inflammation involves erythema and edema formation, as well as infiltration of the skin by leukocytes (164,165). At least for the phorbol esters, the ability to evoke this response seems to correlate with tumor-promoting efficacy in mouse strains of differing sensitivities toward promoters (164,166,167). Upon repeated TPA applications, a decrease of the dermal granulocytes concomitant with an infiltration of the skin by lymphocytes and macrophages has been observed, indicating a transition from acute to chronic inflammation (168).

Other morphological alterations induced by phorbol esters in skin include a hypertrophic enlargement of epidermal cells that becomes significant within 12 hours, epidermal hyperplasia (*i.e.*, increase of the cell number and of the number of nucleated cell layers) after 48–96 hours (30,164,165,170), and the appearance of cells with cytoplasmic and nuclear vacuoles and pyknotic nuclei which may indicate sublethal or perhaps even lethal cell damage. Indeed, 10–30% of the basal keratinocytes obtained from TPA-treated mouse skin were found to be stainable by trypan blue (169).

Most of these responses are rather unspecific and are evoked also by nonpromoting irritants (30,170,171), as well as by nonpromoting mechanical irritation such as removal of the horny layer (30). However, while mouse skin seems to become refractory to these substances and manipulations after a few treatments, tumor-promoting irritants and mechanical injury—such as deep-skin wounding (29,87,88) or abrasion (172)—are able to produce a lasting hyperplasia which does not disappear even during long-term treatment. Actually, the development of a sustained hyperplastic state due to repeated treatments at proper time intervals seems to be a critical condition for tumor promotion (77,167,173,175,178,179). If the time interval is too short, a subsequent treatment may coincide with a phase of refractoriness in the tissue (174–177); if the time interval is too long, the skin gets the opportunity to recover from the first "hyperplasiogenic" stimulus before the second treatment occurs. In both cases sustained hyperplasia cannot be maintained. Thus, in the skin of promoter-sensitive mice, synthetic diacylglycerols exhibit promoting potential only when they are applied at short time intervals, which allows a sustained epidermal hyperplasia to be maintained (57,180). An analogous observation has been made with "promoter-resistant" C57BL/6 mice, in which TPA exhibits considerable promoting efficacy when it is applied *daily* instead of at 3- to 7-day intervals, which is sufficient for "promoter-sensitive" mouse strains (181). Thus, the differences in both the promoting potentials of the chemical agents used and the susceptibility to promotion of the different species/strains employed is a very important consideration in experimental design. This has to be borne in mind when using animal models for the identification of environmentally occurring skin tumor promoters.

Hyperplastic transformation may thus be considered as a reliable indicator of promoting efficacy *only* if one can be certain that the skin does not become refractory to the stimulus upon repeated treatments.[2] This rule is not valid for the conversion stage, since this stage of skin tumorigenesis does not require chronic treatment, but can be induced by a single or only a few applications of the proper agent (21,22,109). Another response which shows quite a good correlation with tumor promotion is the *de novo* formation of hair follicles, observed after promoter treatment of both the mouse tail (183,184) and the mouse back skin (168). This response indicates metaplastic processes resembling those arising upon wounding, to be involved in tumor promotion.

Impairment of intercellular communication via gap junctions (*i.e.*, metabolic cooperation, electrical coupling, and capability of dye transfer between cells) represents another cellular parameter of tumor promotion observed with different types of tumor promoters *in vitro* (185–189) and *in vivo* (190). Since this effect is also observed upon skin wounding, it is probably closely related to regenerative processes. This conclusion may also apply to the induction of so-called dark cells [*i.e.*, keratinocytes with a compact chromatin structure and a high density of free ribosomes (191)], which was repeatedly shown to correlate with the tumor-promoting efficacy of phorbol esters (191), acyl peroxides, anthrone derivatives (167), and mechanical abrasion (192).

While hyperplastic transformation, the inhibition of intercellular communication, and the appearance of dark cells do not provide reliable parameters of conversion, chromosomal damage has been reported to be induced in keratinocytes *in vitro* (98), in mouse epidermis *in vivo* (66), and in HeLa cells (193) only by convertogenic promoters, such as TPA and methylmethane sulfonate, but not by the nonconvertogenic promoters RPA and "Ti8". (The latter nonconvertogenic promoter, "Ti8", is a TPA-derivative isolated from certain Euphorbia species.) Phorbol esters such as TPA have been found to cause chromosomal aberrations also in yeast (194) and human leukocytes (195), and related genetic changes such as sister chromatid exchange (196) and DNA single-strand breaks in leukocytes (197) and keratinocytes (198–201), as well as to cause the replication of endogenous and integrated viral genomes (202–205).

C. Biochemical Responses

Tumor-promoting agents of different chemical structures evoke a series of biochemical responses in mouse skin which are first of all related to their mitogenic effects. These include the activation of cell cycle–related genes such as c-*fos*, c-*myc*, and c-*jun*, the phosphorylation and *de novo* synthesis of histones, induction of DNA synthesis, etc. In the following, some molecular events which have been found to correlate with promoting and convertogenic potential will be discussed in more detail.

---

[2]An exception to this rule seems to be the guinea pig skin in which TPA induces sustained epidermal hyperplasia, but does not promote the emergence of tumors (182). It is not known whether this is due to the resistance of the tissue to the promoter or to the initiator.

1. Activation of Protein Kinase C

Some of the most potent skin tumor promoters are at the same time agonists of the second messenger, DAG, and as such are strong and specific activators of the enzymes of the PKC family (Table 1).

Since PKCs play a key role in the transduction of numerous extracellular signals (hormones, neurotransmitters, cytokines, etc.) into the interior of the cell (206), these TPA-type tumor promoters — by making a shortcut in such cascades of intracellular signaling — are expected to induce dramatic and unpredictable responses resulting in serious consequences for the social behavior of the cell.

As far as the TPA-type tumor promoters are concerned, the hypothesis that PKC activation is critically involved in cellular responses such as gene activation (207), ODC induction (208), eicosanoid release (209), etc., is as easily at hand as it is difficult to prove. A series of genes has been found to be regulated by a "TPA responsive element" (TRE; *see* Ref. 207), which is identical with the binding site for the transcription factor AP-1 (shown to be a dimer of the c-*fos* and c-*jun* proteins). The c-*jun* protein becomes dephosphorylated upon TPA treatment of cells (210), indicating that AP-1 is, if at all, an indirect rather than a direct substrate of PKC. The facts that PKC is a ubiquitous enzyme and that the AP-1 binding site is a rather abundant gene regulatory element provide the basis for the wide spectrum of phorbol ester effects on all kinds of cells and tissues. However, which of those effects provide insight that furthers the understanding of skin tumor promotion remains, in most cases, an open question. It is nevertheless of importance that, when topically applied, DAG derivatives exhibit both a hyperprolifera-tive and a tumor-promoting effect in mouse epidermis *in vivo* (57,180,211). Moreover, a role of PKC in skin tumor promotion is underlined by the fact that PKC inhibitors such as palmitoyl carnitine (212,213), glycyrrhetinic acid (214,215), quercetin (28,216), and staurosporine (62) exhibit antipromoting capability *in vivo*.

The obvious idea that strain and species differences in promotability could be due to differences in epidermal PKC expression could not be verified experimentally (217,218), although it should be pointed out that the differences in the PKC isoenzyme pattern (219–222) have not been investigated in detail. In particular, the roles of the Ca^{2+}-independent PKC-isoforms delta and eta, which are predominantly expressed in epidermis (223,224), are not known. Moreover, differences in intracellular PKC translocation and down-regulation could play a role (225–227). The complexity of the situation may be illustrated by the fact that bryostatin, a macrocyclic lactone derived from marine organisms, interacts with PKC as strongly as TPA without exhibiting, however, any skin tumor–promoting capability. Actually, bryostatin *inhibits* promotion by TPA of skin tumorigenesis (228–231).

Such observations have raised some doubts as to whether or not PKC-catalyzed protein phosphorylation is involved in tumor promotion. As an alternative explanation, PKC effects independent from protein phosphorylation have been taken into consideration. Such an effect is the phorbol ester–induced down-regulation of PKC (232–234), which results in an almost complete, but transient disappearance of the enzyme from epidermis within a few hours (223,226). This down-regulation has been proposed to provide the driving force for hyperplastic development and tumor promotion, in particular since PKC has been found to exert negative feedback effects on mitogenesis-related components of intracellular signal transduction (such as growth factor receptors and phospholipase C) (227). On the other hand, a severe and chronic hyperplastic state as observed in psoriatic skin is accompanied only by partial down-regulation of PKC (235). Moreover, the observation that the nonpromoting PKC activator bryostatin induces PKC down-regulation just as phorbol esters (229,230,236), and the nature of the kinetics of PKC down- and compensatory up-regulation in TPA-treated mouse skin, are consistent with the conclusion that PKC activation rather than permanent down-regulation is involved in each of the successive treatments required for promotion (unpublished). Finally, the potent tumor promoter okadaic acid does not induce PKC down-regulation (unpublished), but enhances intracellular protein phosphorylation by inhibiting phospho-protein phosphatases.

Whether or not cellular target proteins — other than PKC — for TPA-type promoters are involved in skin tumor promotion remains to be shown. A high-affinity binding protein for TPA has been recently found in Hl60 lymphocytes and HeLa cells (237). This protein does not exhibit kinase activity, but translocates, upon phorbol ester binding, from the cytoplasm into the nucleus. Another non–PKC-binding protein for TPA, called N-chimaerin, has been found in neuronal cells (238). A distinct structural element ("zinc finger") has been proposed to be involved in the interaction between phorbol esters and PKC (222). Thus, any protein containing such a structure may be expected to be a potential target for TPA-type tumor promoters.

PKC activation provides only one branch of the phosphatidylinositol–bisphosphate cascade of intracellular signal transduction (239). The other branch, *i.e.*, IP_3-mediated Ca^{2+} release, is apparently not influenced by TPA-type tumor promoters. Ca^{2+}-dependent reactions, such as the activation of phospholipase A2 (240), ODC induction (241), and the activation of protein kinase III (242), nevertheless play an important role in hyperplastic growth and tumor promotion in skin. Protein kinase III is a calmodulin-regulated enzyme with pronounced specificity for the ribosomal elongation factor EF2 (243). Rapid phosphorylation–dephosphorylation of EF2 has been found to be a critical initial event in mitogenic stimulation (244) and is also seen in TPA-treated mouse epidermis (245). The antihyperplastic and antipromoting effects of the immunosuppressing drugs such as cyclosporine (242), didemnin (246), and FK506 (247) are probably due to an inhibition of this and other calmodulin-dependent processes by these agents.

2. Effect on the Biosynthesis of Eicosanoids

Induction of arachidonic acid metabolism has been suggested to represent a charac-teristic biochemical marker indicative of tumor-promoting capability (64). Indeed, phorbol esters (248) and other skin tumor promoters (64,249) induce the release of arachidonic acid from cellular phospholipids in a wide variety of cell types, including keratinocytes *in vitro* (250) and mouse epidermis *in vivo* (251). Arachidonic acid is subsequently metab-olized to prostaglandins (PGs) and hydroperoxy- and hydroxyeicosatetraenoic acids (HPETE and HETE; *see* reviews *in* Refs. 252–254).

Prostaglandin E_2 (PGE_2) has been identified as a mediator of several phorbol ester effects *in vivo*, such as induction of ODC activity (255) and DNA synthesis and mitosis (250,254) in the mouse epidermis. No pronounced differences were found between "promotable" and "nonpromotable" mouse strains as far as the TPA-induced release of eicosanoids from epidermal cells is concerned (251). Inhibitors of PG synthase, such as indomethacin, turned out to be potent antihyperplastic and antipromoting agents in TPA-treated CD-1 and NMRI mouse skin (253,256). Interestingly, in NMRI mice only PGE_2 was able to overcome the inhibition of epidermal cell proliferation that was induced by a single promoter treatment, whereas the antipromoting effect of indomethacin was specifically abolished by $PGF_{2\alpha}$ (256). This result indicates that the release of PGE_2 is required for bringing normal skin into the hyperplastic state, whereas the maintenance of epidermal hyperplasia as brought about by repeated stimulation is under the control of $PGF_{2\alpha}$. Contrary to its inhibitory effects in CD-1 and NMRI mice, indomethacin has been shown to augment the TPA effect on tumor development in Sencar mice (253,181). Thus, strain differences seem to include also more subtle biochemical parameters.

Among the arachidonic acid metabolites generated along the lipoxygenase pathways, 12-HPETE/12-HETE predominates in untreated mouse epidermis, whereas in TPA-treated epidermis the additional formation of 5-HPETE and in particular of 8-HPETE/8-HETE has been described (35,257). Actually, the 8-lipoxygenase pathway, opened by a transient *de novo* synthesis of the enzyme, seems to be the major route of arachidonic acid metabolism in TPA-treated NMRI mouse skin, but it plays only a minor role in normal epidermis (253). The distinct differences in 8-HETE formation *in vivo* between "promotable" SSJN and Sencar mice and "nonpromotable" C57BL/6J mice (258), as well as the strong overproduction of 8-HETE in papillomas of NMRI mice (259), possibly indicate a relationship between 8-lipoxygenase induction and tumor promotion. Moreover, the lipoxygenase inhibitor nordihydroguaiaretic acid (258,260), as well as the inhibitor eicosa-5,8,11,14-tetraynoic acid (ETYA), applied in a dose which inhibits rather selectively lipoxygenase-catalyzed reactions (98,181,256), proved to be potent inhibitors of tumor promotion in CD-1, Sencar, and NMRI mouse skin.

In NMRI mice, ETYA also inhibits conversion and the corresponding clastogenic effect of TPA (66). HPETE and HETE have indeed been found to induce chromosomal damage in C3H10T1/2 fibroblasts (261) and primary mouse keratinocytes (240), indicating a possible mediator function of these eicosanoids for the clastogenic and convertogenic action of TPA. It has been postulated (109) that unsaturated structural elements found in nonconvertogenic promoters scavenge clastogenic mediators, such as free radicals and active oxygen species, which are generated in the course of eicosanoid formation. The introduction of the nonconvertogenic TPA derivative, RPA, into experimental usage was, indeed, based on a study showing that the insertion of conjugated double bonds into the long-chain fatty acyl moiety of a tumor-promoting phorbol ester results in strongly weakening the convertogenic component, without impairing the hyperplasiogenic component of its activity (67). The TPA-derivative promoter from certain Euphorbia species, "Ti8", carries four conjugated double bonds in the acyl side-chain (262); this compound exhibits an "incomplete" (nonconvertogenic) tumor-promoting efficacy when tested on initiated NMRI mouse skin (263,264). The almost complete lack of a convertogenic effect of the semisynthetic RPA in NMRI mouse skin is also the consequence of the double bond system of the retinoyl residue, rather than of an intrinsic antipromoting retinoic acid activity (which could not be demonstrated for either RPA or for Ti8).

Since eicosanoids are derived from fatty acids, experiments were undertaken to investigate the possible modulation of multistage skin carcinogenesis by dietary fat. While in Sencar mice the tumor incidence was found to increase in parallel with overall fat consumption, no reduction of papilloma incidence was observed in animals fed ω3-polyunsaturated fatty acids (265). On the other hand, the ω3-polyunsaturated fatty acids were found to protect rats from mammary carcinogenesis, probably because these fatty acids are poor substrates for eicosanoid-forming enzymes, and the corresponding ω3-prostanoids are biologically rather inactive (266). However, a diet rich in the congeneric ω6-polyunsaturated fatty acids (*i.e.*, linoleic acid) does inhibit skin tumor emergence (267); this is perhaps due to the antiproliferative effect of 13-hydroxy octadecadienoic acid, which is generated in considerable amounts in the epidermis of mice fed an ω6-rich diet (268).

3. Effect on the Generation of Reactive Oxygen Species

Reactive oxygen species are typical byproducts of eicosanoid metabolism which are generated in the course of peroxide reduction (269,270). They include superoxide anion radicals, hydrogen peroxide, hydroxyl radicals, and singlet oxygen, and may cause the formation of lipid, peroxylipid, and alkoxylipid radicals in cells. It has been proposed that such radicals play an essential role in the process of carcinogenesis, in particular in tumor promotion (*see* reviews *in* Refs. 92–97).

A chemiluminescence response observed immediately after TPA treatment of keratinocytes has been attributed to oxidants generated in the course of eicosanoid metabolism (271), and this effect was more pronounced with keratinocytes from promotion-sensitive Sencar mice than with keratinocytes from "nonpromotable" C57BL/6J mice (272). When tumor promoters such as phorbol esters (273), DAG, anthrone derivatives, or mezerein (274) were applied onto mouse skin *in vivo*, a distinct increase of the hydrogen peroxide level in epidermis could be measured, which correlated with the promotability of different mouse strains (274). Moreover, a subpopulation of hydrogen peroxide–producing keratinocytes was found in TPA-treated mouse epidermis (275). Reactive oxygen, in this case superoxide anion radicals as source for the much more agressive hydroxyl radicals, is also produced *via* the xanthin oxidase reaction, which is activated in keratinocytes by phorbol esters in connection with their hyperplasiogenic action (276,277). Reactive oxygen species are also released from the cells of the inflammatory skin infiltrate. Again, some relationship with promotability seems to exist, since macrophages from Sencar mice were found to secrete four times more H_2O_2 as compared with macrophages from C57BL/6J mice (278). An analogous gradation of leukocyte activation was observed with phorbol esters that have different promoting efficacies, but has not been observed with promoters which directly give rise to radicals, such as anthrone derivatives and acylperoxides (97,167,278). Both oxygen radical generation by inflammatory cells and skin tumor promotion are efficiently inhibited by protease inhibitors, indicating an interrelationship which is not yet fully understood (93,279,280).

Additional evidence for a critical role of free radicals in skin tumor promotion is provided by the potent antipromoting effects of antioxidant and radical-scavenging agents such as phenolic compounds (72,281–283), ascorbate (284), retinoids (38), and agents which increase the intracellular level of reduced glutathione (285), as well as by the tumor-promoting efficacy of free radical–generating compounds such as organic peroxides (72,97,286). Such peroxides also stimulate the malignant progression of papillomas (287) without displaying, however, a significant activity as initiators or solitary carcinogens (288).

There is some evidence that free radicals influence the cascades of intracellular signal transduction. Thus, acylhydroperoxides have been shown to activate PKC (289). Since they are found as esters in membrane phospholipids and as DAG, they are likely to modify the lipid-binding regulatory domain of PKC. The occurrence of a modified – *i.e.*, Ca^{2+}-independent and phospholipid-independent – form of PKC was indeed found in oxidant-treated C6 glioma and B16 melanoma cells (290). Prolonged treatment with oxidant resulted in complete inactivation of PKC (290), *i.e.*, in a situation analogous to the phorbol ester–induced down-regulation of the enzyme.

Tumor promoters have been shown to interact with the prooxidant state of cells, which is regulated by enzymes such as superoxide dismutase (SOD), catalase, and peroxidases as well as by the availability of radical scavengers and reducing agents such as glutathione, α-tocopherol, ascorbic acid, and retinoids. In TPA-treated mouse skin *in vivo*, a decrease of the epidermal SOD and catalase (291) and glutathione peroxidase (292) activities was observed and the intracellular level of oxidized glutathione was noted to rise fourfold (293).

4. Induction of Ornithine Decarboxylase

Ornithine decarboxylase (ODC), which catalyzes the formation of putrescine from ornithine, is the rate-limiting enzyme of polyamine biosynthesis. Since the induction of this enzyme is commonly observed upon application of tumor promoters such as phorbol esters (294,295), anthrone derivatives (73), and organic peroxides (296) onto the mouse skin, it has been proposed that it provides a critical event in skin tumor promotion. Moreover, inhibitors of induction and activation of ODC, such as ornithine analogs (297) and retinoids (177), are found among the most potent antipromoting agents. ODC induction involves the *de novo* synthesis of both mRNA and protein (298). In epidermal tumors an ODC-isoform, somewhat differing from phorbol ester–induced ODC in normal skin, is constitutively overexpressed (299). ODC activity is induced in mouse epidermis by both convertogenic and nonconvertogenic tumor promoters (21,29,33) as well as by superficial skin wounding (29,88), but not by nonhyperplasiogenic mitogens such as 4-*O*-methyl-TPA; this indicates that the response is related to the hyperplastic transformation of skin. On the other hand, several tumor-promoting (and hyperplasiogenic) agents such as thapsigargin, staurosporin, and palytoxin apparently lack ODC-inducing capability (63). Moreover, TPA has been shown to induce ODC in promotion- and hyperplasia-"resistant" C57BL/6 mice to the same degree as in sensitive SSJN (300) and DBA/2 mice (301). Finally, retinoids inhibit the induction of ODC but not the hyperplastic transformation of skin by TPA (302), whereas glucocorticoids exhibit an antihyperplastic effect without impairing ODC induction (303). Both agents are strong antipromoters in mouse skin. Thus, induction of ODC seems to be involved only in the response of skin to a limited class of promoting and hyperplasiogenic agents, rather than being inseparably linked to the mechanism of hyperplastic transformation; thus, induction of ODC does not provide a general biochemical marker of tumor promotion. It is, nevertheless, remarkable that alterations in ODC regulation, as observed in phorbol ester–treated mouse skin, are also found in human epithelial tumors (304).

IV. THE BIOLOGICAL NATURE OF SKIN TUMOR PROMOTION AND CONVERSION

It is the authors' view that the wound response provides the clue for an understanding of skin tumor promotion and conversion (30,31,109,305–307). Wounding is a potent tumor-promoting stimulus in the skin, and the morphological and biochemical responses of the skin to treatment with tumor promoters very closely resemble the wound response. Moreover, in skin, the induction of a wound response can overcome not only the latency of neoplasia but also the latency of other genetically determined diseases such as eczema, psoriasis (Köbner's phenomenon), and common warts. *Vice versa*, tumor promotion by wounding has also been reported for many other tissues, including crown gall tumorigenesis in plants. Thus, the induction of a wound response either by mechanical injury, UV irradiation, or chemical irritation may provide a general mechanism by which genetically determined but latent hyperproliferative states can be expressed.

While healthy tissue returns to normality after some time (*i.e.*, a wound heals), in these diseases the hyperproliferative state, once induced, continues endlessly in a self-perpetuating manner. Thus, it is the mechanism of termination rather than that of induction where the defect due to genetic changes lies. It has been said that a tumor resembles a wound that does not heal (308) or, *vice versa*, that a wound resembles a tumor that heals itself (309). Such ideas are by no means new but can be traced back to Rudolf Virchow's concept (2), which was most insightfully formulated by Orth (310) in postulating cancer to be the result of permanently repeated and disturbed tissue regeneration ("Krebs ist das Ergebniss immer wiederholter und gestörter Regeneration", *quoted from* Ref. 310).

A. Skin Tumor Promotion as the Consequence of a Chronic Regenerative Reaction

A characteristic event involved in the wound response is the hyperplastic transformation of the skin, that is, simultaneous acute inflammatory reaction and epithelial hyperplasia (30). As already mentioned, this response is induced by all skin tumor promoters.

Hyperplastic transformation has been proposed (306) to result from a complex stimulatory process called keratinocyte activation (311). In contrast to the earlier concept of a passive role seen for the keratinocytes in protecting the body from injury and water loss, the role of keratinocytes is now understood as a signaling interface between the surrounding environment and the body (312)—to translate a wide variety of harmful environmental stimuli into endogenous signals which then activate internal defense mechanisms. These include attraction and activation of leukocytes and lymphocytes; activation of the immune system; effects on blood flow, on coagulation, and on the complement system; and epidermal hyperproliferation—all triggered by wounding or by other kinds of injury involving the likelihood of tissue damage and microbial invasion. Since these responses are controlled by a complex mix of mediators and cytokines, a "pseudo wound reaction" may also be evoked by a direct interaction of an irritant with the pathways of intracellular signaling and signal transduction.

The ability to produce and release such wound factors (as well as to express the corresponding receptors) together with cell adhesion molecules (such as ICAM-1) upon exogeneous stimulation, are the main characteristics of an activated keratinocyte (313). Some of the cytokines, such as TGFα, TGFβ, interleukin-1 (Il-1), and others, are subject to autoinduction, thus providing a strong amplification mechanism and allowing autocrine stimulation of keratinocytes (312,314). In addition, cytokines may induce each other, for example Il-1 and TGFα (315), or stimulate the production of other mediators such as Il-1, TGFα, bradykinin, eicosanoids, and others (*see* Refs. 253,316).

The effects of the cytokines and mediators released from the activated keratinocyte are manifold, including autocrine mitogenic activation [as has been shown for TGFα, fibroblast growth factor b (bFGF), Il-1, Il-3, and others] or inhibition of keratinocytes [as by TGFβ, tumor necrosis factor (TNFα), γ-interferon, catecholamines, and "chalones"; *see* Refs. 307,317], the recruitment of the cells of the inflammatory infiltrate and of T-lymphocytes [as carried out by TGFβ, Il-1, Il-6, Il-8, PDGF, 12-HETE, and leukotriene B_4 (LTB$_4$); *see* Refs. 311,315,316,318], and effects on blood vessels and connective tissue such as fibrosis, angiogenesis, and remodelling of the extracellular matrix [as induced by TGFβ, platelet-derived growth factor (PDGF), bFGF, TGFα, epidermal growth factor (EGF); *see* Ref. 319]. The cells of the inflammatory infiltrate, as well as various nonepidermal cells residing in skin, are additional producers of cytokines and other mediators, many of which may act back on the keratinocytes. Thus, upon external stimulation a complex "cytokine network" develops rapidly between the different compartments of the injured tissue. This network integrates the function of the various cell types which are involved in defense and tissue repair. Both induction of an inflammatory infiltrate and the effects on dermis and blood vessels give rise to the formation of granulation tissue or — in the case of carcinogenesis — to the so-called stroma reaction, which is a most critical condition of tumor growth (109,320).

While for most of the epidermal cytokines induction of *de novo* synthesis seems to be necessary upon injury and irritation, bFGF, TGFβ, Il-1α, and the eicosanoids are already found in or around unstimulated keratinocytes, but probably in an inactive form, either as biosynthetic precursors or trapped by the extracellular matrix. There is evidence that activation and release take place immediately upon wounding or irritation (311,321,322) and that these factors may trigger the subsequent reactions; Il-1α probably acts as an inducer of epidermal hyperplasia (322) and TGFβ as an inducer of epidermal cell migration and of the stroma reaction (323–325), as well as a mediator of conversion in skin carcinogenesis (*see below*).

Both cytokines share these actions with the eicosanoids. As already mentioned, PG formation in mouse epidermis is critical for epidermal hyperplasia and tumor promotion *in vivo*, whereas the accompanying inflammatory reaction is rather controlled by lipoxygenase-generated arachidonic acid metabolites such as the leukotactic agents, 12-HETE and LTB$_4$. Moreover, lipoxygenase-derived eicosanoids seems to mediate both phorbol ester–induced clastogenesis and conversion.

The induction of the eicosanoid cascade in skin is a general and immediate response to all kinds of irritants, to UV irradiation, and to mechanical wounding. Eicosanoid formation in keratinocytes has also been shown to be induced by wound factors such as EGF, TGFα, Il-1, bradykinin, histamine, thrombin, bFGF, and probably many others. Actually, phospholipase A$_2$, the key enzyme of eicosanoid production in keratinocytes, has been found to be activated along multiple pathways of intracellular signal transduction (306,326). These observations indicate a role of eicosanoids as mediators of cytokine actions, which remains to be proven, however. Conversely, eicosanoids may be involved in cytokine release and production.

The bewildering multiplicity of interactions within the cutaneous cytokine network indicates that there are various pathways rather than one principal route for keratinocyte activation. Thus, the destruction of epidermal cells may result in the release of preformed mediators (such as Il-1) which then trigger the response, whereas primary wound factors [such as thrombin, platelet-activating factor (PAF), adenosine nucleotides, kinins, complement factors] may be released from nonepidermal sources and trigger cytokine and mediator release from keratinocytes along the physiological pathways of intracellular signal transduction. Finally, a direct interaction of exogenous stimuli with the cellular elements of signal transduction (for instance, PKC in the case of the TPA-type tumor promoters) should also be considered. All these interactions may lead to keratinocyte activation and — as a secondary consequence — even to the destruction of keratinocytes, for instance, through the release of clastogenic arachidonic acid metabolites and highly reactive oxygen radicals from keratinocytes and invading leukocytes.

Thus, if tumor promotion is understood as a permanent hyperproliferative process proceeding along the endogeneous pathways of tissue regeneration and wound healing (31,139), it becomes readily understandable why certain nonspecific irritants, UV radiations, and mechanical trauma, as well as agents which specifically interact with intracellular signal transduction, can all exhibit tumor promotion on the skin. In terms of the end result, it is irrelevant at which point of the cytokine network the triggering event has occurred.

The common denominator seems to be that keratinocyte activation results in hyperplastic transformation and that the promoting treatment is carried out in such a manner that the response leads to sustained hyperplasia.

B. Conversion and Wound Response

As was discussed above, in initiated mouse skin a chronic stimulation of epidermal cell proliferation is not sufficient for inducing the onset of the emergence of papillomas, which process actually requires an additional stimulus called conversion (109). Conversion depends on the induction of epidermal DNA synthesis (42); it can be brought about by mechanical wounding (29) or by the injection of wound factors such as TGFα plus TGFβ (65); and it correlates with chromosomal damage (66,98), *i.e.*, it is probably closely connected with the mechanism of regeneration (109).

Induction of promotability is the operational definition of conversion, since without convertogenic treatment chronic hyperplasiogenic stimulation does not result in the appearance of visible tumors. Conversion must override the "nonpromotability" of initiated cells which may be due to local growth restraints or to some kind of latency (this means the inability of the initiated cell to spontaneously express its neoplastic phenotype or to respond to the mitogenic stimulus of the promoter).

The significance of "growth restraint" and "latency" for the dynamics of an initiated cell is that its proliferative and functional behavior would be indistinguishable from that of a normal keratinocyte; thus, the cell would not gain any advantage over its healthy neighbors, *unless* it became "converted". The mechanism of this may reside, for instance, in the activation of genes coding for proteins which are involved in the transduction of mitogenic signals and in the control of tissue homeostasis, that is, in the regulation of the state between proliferation and terminal differentiation. Instead of transient activation by a convertogenic stimulus such genes may also undergo permanent activation by mutation. Promotable and nonpromotable cell mutants have indeed been generated *in vitro* (327). Whether or not such observations are truly relevant to conversion *in vivo* remains to be elucidated.

The selective advantage that both the activation of initiated cells and the removal of local growth restraints would provide is to favor the clonal expansion of initiated cells. This is actually supported by the finding that phorbol ester tumor promoters, such as TPA, induce terminal differentiation in normal keratinocytes *in vitro* (328–332), with the exception of a small subpopulation (333), whereas transformed keratinocytes are more resistant to this effect (334,335). To explain this result as well as the persistence of the initiated state, initiation is generally assumed to occur in a population of epidermal stem cells that are protected from terminal differentiation in order to fulfill their biological role in tissue regeneration. This putative identity of "initiated cells" as mutated stem cells could, of course, also explain their possible insensitivity to the mitogenic stimulus of a nonconvertogenic promoter. So-called "label-retaining cells" (336,337) and dark cells (338) – thought to represent epidermal stem cells – differ, indeed, in their response to convertogenic and nonconvertogenic tumor promoters in that only convertogenic promoters seem to stimulate their proliferation *in vivo* (339); *also*, in keratinocyte cultures the putative stem cells can be triggered into terminal differentiation by RPA but not by TPA (328,340). Moreover, a resistance to hyperplastic transformation and conversion has been observed in newborn mouse epidermis, indicating that both responses are subject to ontogenic development (341).

Clonal selection could also explain the convertogenic effect of the TGFs, provided that a difference in TGF sensitivity between normal and initiated keratinocytes exists (so that the initiated cells would be less sensitive to the growth-inhibitory effect of TGFβ and perhaps more sensitive to the growth-stimulatory effect of TGF α, as compared to normal cells) (342). However, growth factors might also activate initiated cells to express their neoplastic phenotype and mitogen responsiveness.

A difficulty in logic to be overcome by the concepts of activation and selection of initiated cells is the problem of the inversion of the initation–conversion sequence (23,109). How can an as yet nonexisting cell type be selected or how can a phenotype be expressed when the corresponding genotype does not yet exist but is induced only several weeks later? The only and admittedly highly speculative explanation would be that conversion creates a situation in the tissue that allows a spontaneous phenotype expression of the neoplastic genotype as soon as the latter has been created by the mutagenic event of initiation.

The inversion of the initiation–conversion sequence has been taken as an indication for a mutagenic event to be involved not only in initiation but also in conversion. In particular the clastogenic effect, which seems to correlate with conversion, has been speculated to include more specific genetic changes, such as loss or inactivation of tumor suppressor genes which would hinder the expression of the neoplastic phenotype in initiated cells (343). However, at present this hypothesis lacks any experimental support. Moreover, the chromosomal damage observed appears to be too severe to be compatible with survival of the cells. It may thus be considered to provide a symptom of tissue damage and cell death rather than of specific mutagenic events. Such an explanation would also be more consistent with the strong convertogenic effect of skin wounding and of the wound factors TGFα and TGFβ.

It is hoped that an elucidation of the physiological function of the TGFs in skin will provide the key for an in-depth understanding of conversion. While TGFα most probably provides the mitogenic stimulus on which conversion is *dependent* (42,65), the action of TGFβ may be directly related to the convertogenic effect proper. While the role of TGFβ in normal skin physiology could not yet be identified, its role as a wound hormone is established by a steadily increasing body of evidence. Its major function seems to be the control of dermal–epidermal interaction. Thus, TGFβ stimulates the formation of granulation tissue by inducing cytotactic and angiogenetic processes, the remodeling of the extracellular matrix, as well as the process of re-epithelization (344–346). While granulation tissue provides a substratum for the re-epithelization of a wound, TGFβ has been shown to stimulate epidermal cell migration also directly, probably by inducing the formation of both a fibronectin matrix (347–349) and the expression of fibronectin receptors in keratinocytes (350). Also, TGFβ transiently inhibits proliferation and terminal differentiation of migrating cells. Later, this inhibition is followed by a compensatory hyperproliferation at the wound edges (351). This direct effect of TGFβ on keratinocytes may well include stem cell activation or even temporal dedifferentiation, which are cellular events regarded to be critical in tumorigenesis (336–340,352).

Both the morphology of papillomas (*see* Figure 3) and the convertogenic and tumor-promoting effect of skin wounding indicate, indeed, an important role of dermal–epidermal interactions in skin tumorigenesis. Among these interactions the formation of stroma resembling the formation of granulation tissues is probably a most critical one, since it provides the energy supply and the waste disposal for the developing tumor. For this reason, in the absence of stroma, solid tumors are unable to grow beyond a size of 1–2 mm (308). The "nonpromotability" of initiated cells, which has to be overridden by conversion, could well be due to the restricted ability of those cells to release stroma-inducing signals, such as TGFβ. Actually, a convertogenic promoter, such as TPA, has been found to induce TGFβ formation in mouse epidermis much stronger than the nonconvertogenic promoter, RPA (342). In the case of multistage skin tumorigenesis this would mean that a permanent proliferative stimulation of initiated cells, such as by

RPA treatment, would not be sufficient to bring about the emergence of visible papillomas, but only of invisible minitumors, unless sufficient stroma formation is induced either by injection of TGFβ or by additional treatment with convertogenic agents. The stroma-inducing effect of convertogenic agents may be due to a more nonspecific tissue injury, the symptoms of which are chromosal damage followed by an endogenous release of wound factors, including TGFβ and stem cell activation. Thus, a convertogenic promoter may induce a complete wound response, for instance by way of its clastogenic capability, whereas a nonconvertogenic promoter mainly activates the hyperproliferative and inflammatory components of the wound response possibly by specifically interacting with the mechanisms of cellular signaling and signal transduction. Such a concept could readily explain both the reversibility of the converted state as well as the inverted conversion–initiation sequence: for tumorigenesis *the persistence* of the stroma reaction is critical, but the sequence appears not to be significant—the stroma bed may be formed before or after initiation.

The formation of minitumors postulated to occur in the absence of a convertogenic stimulus may also explain the phenomenon of "spontaneous conversion". It has been observed that when the time between initiation and the beginning of promotion is prolonged up to several weeks, a convertogenic treatment becomes more and more dispensable (23,353), indicating that conversion proceeds *spontaneously*, although at a slow rate in initiated skin. These observations were used by some investigators to deny the existence of a discrete conversion stage (*e.g.*, 353). On the other hand, under such conditions of delayed promotion the latency period of tumor development was shown to be decreased (17,353,354), and this is consistent with minitumor formation. Minitumors may become increasingly promotable without additional convertogenic treatment, provided that they develop sufficient potential to overcome local growth restraints. This potential may be based on the generation of stroma-inducing cytokines and autocrine growth factors, such as TGFβ and TGFα produced in the course of keratinocyte activation by the promoter.

V. CONCLUDING REMARKS

The mouse skin model of multistage carcinogenesis is not a model of normal life scenarios nor does it reflect carcinogenesis in humans. Instead it provides an artificial system which allows the experimental dissection of the complex process of carcinogenesis into defined stages, thus aiming at a detailed analysis of the cellular and molecular mechanisms involved. The mouse skin model may also be used for the detection of environmental and endogenous tumor promoters. Considering the tissue specificity of promoters, such a practical application may have, however, rather strict limitation, *i.e.*, limitation to those agents which promote tumorigenesis in skin and closely related epithelia. Pronounced species and strain differences in promotability, which are still not fully understood, indicate another type of serious limitation; however, this can be overcome, at least partially, by proper adjustment of the experimental conditions. Altogether, these restrictions indicate considerable problems as far as the extrapolation of results to humans is concerned.

Confining the discussion to the mouse skin model, convincing evidence is now available that tumor promotion depends on repeated hyperplastic transformation of skin resulting in sustained epidermal hyperplasia. Agents which evoke such a response have to be considered as potential skin tumor promoters. This conclusion cannot be extrapolated, however, to convertogenic efficacy, which may be related to clastogenesis and endogenous TGFβ release—although additional experimental support for this is required.

A key to the understanding of skin tumor promotion and conversion is provided by the wound response. Wounding is a strong promoting and convertogenic stimulus, and this effect can be, at least partially, simulated by intracutaneous injection of putative "wound hormones", such as TGFα and TGFβ. Hyperplastic transformation of skin is a characteristic component of the wound response, and the tumor-promoting effect of numerous agents may be due to their ability to evoke this response chronically because of nonspecific cytotoxicity ("chemical wounding"). This may also apply to UV irradiation, the UV-A component of which has been recently suggested to be a tumor-promoting stimulus. Other promoters such as the DAG agonists and the protein phosphatase inhibitors may evoke a *quasi*-wound response, by interacting with and thereby disturbing the complex network of inter- and intracellular signaling on which the wound response depends.

While skin tumor promotion proper may be understood as the result of prolonged regenerative hyperproliferation, the process of conversion cannot yet be fully explained. The apparent correlation of chromosomal damage with conversion may be interpreted as being a symptom of more severe cytotoxicity, resulting in cell death and a more pronounced wound response. The convertogenic efficacy of wounding and of TGFβ injection may be taken as an indication that the induction of stroma reaction is critically involved in conversion. In addition, a disequilibrium between stimulatory (TGFα) and inhibitory (TGFβ) signals may provide a selective advantage for initiated keratinocytes, provided that their responsiveness to such signals differs, even though only slightly, from that of normal cells.

The multistage approach to experimental skin carcinogenesis has provided convincing evidence that tumor development in epithelia is due to a series of genetic disorders (355), the induction and expression of which is strongly promoted by permanently repeated and disturbed regenerative processes (2,15,310).

REFERENCES

1. Yamagiwa, K., and Ichikawa, K.: *Gann* **8**, 11 (1914).
2. Virchow, R.: "Die Krankhaften Geschwülste". Hirschfeld, Berlin, 1863.
3. Twort, C. C., and Ing, H. R.: *Z. Krebsforsch.* **27**, 309 (1928).
4. Deelman, H. T.: *Z. Krebsforsch.* **21**, 220 (1924).
5. Rous, P., and Kidd, J. G.: *J. Exp. Med.* **73**, 365 (1941).
6. Friedwald, W. F., and Rous, P.: *J. Exp. Med.* **80**, 102 (1944).
7. Berenblum, I.: *Cancer Res.* **1**, 44 (1941).
8. Van Duuren, B. L.: *Progr. Exp. Tumor Res.* **11**, 31 (1969).
9. Hecker, E., and Schmidt, R.: *Progr. Chem. Org. Natur. Prod.* **31**, 378 (1974).
10. Fujiki, H., Suganuma, M., Tahira, T., Yoshioka, A., Nakayasu, M., Endo, Y., Shudo, K., Takayama, S., Moore, R. E., and Sugimura, T.: New Classes of Tumor Promoters: Teleocidin, Aplysiatoxin, and Palytoxin. *In* "Cellular Interactions by Environmental Tumor Promoters" (H. Fujiki, E. Hecker, R. E. Moore, T. Sugimura, and I. B. Weinstein, eds.). Japan. Sci. Soc. Press, Tokyo/VNU Science Press, Utrecht, 1984, p. 37.
11. Mottram, J. C.: *J. Pathol. Bacteriol.* **56**, 181 (1944).
12. Berenblum, I., and Shubik, P.: *Br. J. Cancer* **1**, 383 (1947).
13. Iversen, O. H., and Astrup, E. G.: *Cancer Invest.* **2**, 51 (1984).
14. Marks, F., and Fürstenberger, G.: Multistage Carcinogenesis in Animal Skin. *In* "Theories of Carcinogenesis" (O. H. Iversen, ed.). Hemisphere, Washington, D. C., 1988, p. 179.
15. Preston-Martin, S., Pike, M. C., Ross, R. K., Jones, P. A., and Henderson, B. E.: *Cancer Res.* **50**, 7415 (1990).
16a. Berenblum, I.: *Adv. Cancer Res.* **2**, 129 (1954).
16b. Berenblum, I.: Sequential Aspects of Chemical Carcinogenesis: Skin. *In* "Cancer: A Comprehensive Treatise" (F. F. Becker, ed.), Vol. 1. Plenum Press, New York, 1975, p. 323.

17. Boutwell, R. K.: *Progr. Exp. Tumor Res.* **4**, 207 (1964).
18. Balmain, A., and Brown, L.: *Adv. Cancer Res.* **51**, 147 (1988).
19. Berenblum, I., and Haran, N.: *Br. J. Cancer* **9**, 268 (1955).
20. Hecker, E., and Rippmann, F.: *Naunyn-Schmiedebergs Arch. Pharmacol.* **338**, (Suppl.), R11 (1988).
21. Slaga, T. J., Fischer, S. M., Nelson, K., and Gleason, G. L.: *Proc. Natl. Acad. Sci. U.S.A.* **77**, 3659 (1980).
22. Fürstenberger, G., Berry, D. L., Sorg, B., and Marks, F.: *Proc. Natl. Acad. Sci. U. S. A.* **78**, 7722 (1981).
23. Fürstenberger, G., Kinzel, V., Schwarz, M., and Marks, F.: *Science* **230**, 76 (1985).
24. Hennings, H., Shores, R., Wenk, M. L., Spangler, E. F., Tarone, R., and Yuspa, S. H.: *Nature* **304**, 67 (1983).
25. Marks, F., and Fürstenberger, G.: From the Normal Cell to Cancer, the Multistep Process of Experimental Skin Carcinogenesis. *In* "Concepts and Theories in Carcinogenesis" (A. P. Maskens, P. Ebbesen, and A. Burny, eds.). Elsevier, Amsterdam, 1987, p. 169.
26. Fearon, E. R., and Vogelstein, B.: *Cell* **61**, 759 (1990).
27. Burns, F. J., Albert, R. E., and Altshuler, B.: Cancer Progression in Mouse Skin. *In* "Mechanisms of Tumor Promotion" (T. J. Slaga, ed.), Vol. II. CRC Press, Boca Raton, Florida, 1984, p. 18.
28. Gschwendt, M., Horn, F., Kittstein, W., Fürstenberger, G., Besemfelder, E., and Marks, F.: *Biochem. Biophys. Res. Commun.* **124**, 63 (1984).
29. Fürstenberger, G., and Marks, F.: *J. Invest. Dermatol.* **81**, 157s (1983).
30. Marks, F.: Hyperplastic Transformation, the Response of the Skin to Irritation and Injury. *In* "Skin Pharmacology and Toxicology" (C. L. Galli, D. M. Marinovich, and C. N. Hensby, eds.), NATO Adv. Study Inst. Life Sci. Ser. A., Vol. 181. Plenum Press, New York, 1990, p. 121.
31. Marks, F., Fürstenberger, G., Gschwendt, M., Rogers, M., Schurich, B., Kaina, B., and Bauer, G.: The Wound Response as a Key Element for an Understanding of Multistage Carcinogenesis in Skin. *In* "Chemical Carcinogenesis" (F. Feo, P. Pani, A. Columbano, and R. Garcea, eds.). Plenum Press, New York, 1988, p. 217.
32. Gschwendt, M., Horn, F., Kittstein, W., Fürstenberger, G., Besemfelder, E., and Marks, F.: *Biochem. Biophys. Res. Commun.* **124**, 63 (1984).
33. Rose-John, S., Fürstenberger, G., Krieg, P., Besemfelder, E., Rincke, G., and Marks, F.: *Carcinogenesis* **9**, 831 (1988).
34. Schwarz, M., Peres, O., Kunz, W., Fürstenberger, G., Kittstein, W., and Marks, F.: *Carcinogenesis* **5**, 1663 (1984).
35. Gschwendt, M., Fürstenberger, G., Kittstein, W., Besemfelder, E., Hull, W. E., Hagedorn, H., Opferkuch, H. J., and Marks, F.: *Carcinogenesis* **7**, 449 (1986).
36. Gschwendt, M., Kittstein, W., and Marks, F.: *Cancer Lett.* **22**, 219 (1984).
37. Gschwendt, M., Kittstein, W., and Marks, F.: *Cancer Lett.* **25**, 177 (1984).
38. Verma, A. K.: *Cancer Res.* **47**, 5097 (1987).
39. Schwarz, J. A., Viaje, A., and Slaga, T. J.: *Chem.-Biol. Interact.* **17**, 331 (1977).
40. Fürstenberger, G., Gross, M., and Marks, F.: *Carcinogenesis* **10**, 91 (1989).
41. Gschwendt, M., Kittstein, W., and Marks, F.: *Carcinogenesis* **8**, 203 (1987).
42. Kinzel, V., Loehrke, H., Goerttler, K., Fürstenberger, G., and Marks, F.: *Proc. Natl. Acad. Sci. U. S. A.* **81**, 5858 (1984).
43. Perchellet, J. P., and Perchellet, E. M.: *Free Radicals Biol. Med.* **7**, 377 (1989).
44. Fischer, S. M., Mills, G. D., and Slaga, T. J.: *Carcinogenesis* **3**, 1243 (1982).
45. Slaga, T. J., Fischer, S. M., Weeks, C. E., and Klein-Szanto, A. J. P.: Cellular and Biochemical Mechanisms of Mouse Skin Tumor Promoters. *In* "Reviews in Biochemical Toxicology" (E. Hodgson, J. Bend, and R. M. Philpot, eds.), Vol. 3. Elsevier/North-Holland, New York, 1981, p. 231.
46. Slaga, T. J., Fischer, S. M., Weeks, C. E., Klein-Szanto, A. J. P., and Reiners, J.: *J. Cell. Biochem.* **18**, 99 (1982).
47. Ordman, A. B. Cleaveland, J. S., and Boutwell, R. K.: *Cancer Lett.* **29**, 79 (1985).
48. Foulds, L.: *Cancer Res.* **14**, 327 (1954).
49. Fischer, S. M., Hardin, L., Klein-Szanto, A. J. P., and Slaga, T. J.: *Cancer Lett.* **27**, 323 (1985).
50. Marks, F.: Skin Cancer (excluding melanomas). *In* "Pharmacology of the Skin II" (M. E. Greaves and S. Schuster, eds.), Handbook of Experimental Pharmacology, Vol. 87/II. Springer-Verlag, Berlin, 1989, p. 165.
51. Castagna, M., Takai, Y., Kaibuchi, K., Sano, K., Kikkawa, V., and Nishizuka, Y.: *J. Biol. Chem.* **257**, 7847 (1963).
52. Ashendel, C. L.: *Biochim. Biophys. Acta* **822**, 219 (1985).
53. Hecker, E., Adolf, W., Hergenhahn, M., Schmidt, R., and Sorg, B.: Irritant Diterpene Ester Promoters of Mouse Skin: Contributions to Etiologies of Environmental Cancer and to Biochemical Mechanisms of Carcinogenesis. *In* "Cellular Interactions by Environmental Tumor Promoters" (H. Fujiki, E. Hecker, R.

E. Moore, T. Sugimura, and I. B. Weinstein, eds.). Japan. Sci. Soc. Press, Tokyo/VNU Science Press, Utrecht, 1984, p. 3.

54. Fujiki, H., Mori, M., Nakayasu, M., Terade, M., Sugimura, T., and Moore, R. E.: *Proc. Natl. Acad. Sci. U.S.A.* **78**, 3872 (1981).
55. Fujiki, H., and Sugimura, T.: *Adv. Cancer Res.* **49**, 223 (1987).
56. Fujiki, H., Iyegami, K., Hakii, H., Suganuma, M., Yamaizumi, Z., Yamamoto, K., Moore, R. E., and Sugimura, T.: *Jpn. J. Cancer Res. (Gann)* **76**, 257 (1985).
57. Smart, R. C., Mills, K. J., Hansen, L. A., and Conney, A. H.: *Cancer Res.* **49**, 4455 (1989).
58. Yoshizawa, S., Fujiki, H., Suguri, H., Suganuma, M., Nakayasu, M., Matsushima, R., and Sugimura, T.: *J. Cancer Res. Clin. Oncol.* **50**, 4974 (1990).
59. Suganuma, M., Fujiki, H., Suguri, H., Yoshizawa, S., Hirota, M., Nakayasu, M., Ojika, M., Wakamatsu, K., Yamada, K., and Sugimura, T.: *Proc. Natl. Acad. Sci. U.S.A.* **85**, 1768 (1988).
60. Fujiki, H., Suganuma, M., Nakayasu, M., Hakii, H., Horituchi, T., Takayama, S., and Sugimura, T.: *Carcinogenesis* **7**, 707 (1986).
61. Tamaoki, T., Nomoto, H., Takahashi, I., Kato, Y., Morimoto, M., and Tonnita, F.: *Biochem. Biophys. Res. Commun.* **135**, 397 (1986).
62. Yamada, S., Hirota, K., Chida, K., and Kuroki, T.: *Biochem. Biophys. Res. Commun.* **157**, 9 (1988).
63. Fujiki, H., Suganuma, M., Suguri, H., Yoshizawa, S., Hirota, M., Takagi, K., and Sugimura, T.: Diversity in the Chemical Nature and Mechanism of Tumor Promoters. *In* "Skin Carcinogenesis, Mechanisms and Human Relevance" (T. J. Slaga, A. J. P. Klein-Szanto, R. K. Boutwell, D. F. Stevenson, H. L. Spitzer, and B. D'Motto, eds.). Alan R. Liss, New York, 1989, p. 281.
64. Fujiki, H., Suganuma, M., and Sugimura, T.: *Environ. Carcino. Rev.* **C7**, 1 (1989).
65. Fürstenberger, G., Rogers, M., Schnapke, R., Bauer, G., Höfler, P., and Marks, F.: *Int. J. Cancer* **43**, 915 (1989).
66. Fürstenberger, G., Schurich, B., Kaina, B., Petrusevska, R. T., Fusenig, N. E., and Marks, F.: *Carcinogenesis* **10**, 749 (1989).
67. Marks, F., and Fürstenberger, G.: Multistage Tumor Promotion in Skin. *In* "Cellular Interactions by Environmental Tumor Promoters" (H. Fujiki, E. Hecker, R. E. Moore, T. Sugimura, and I. B. Weinstein, eds.). Japan. Sci. Soc. Press, Tokyo/VNU Science Press, Utrecht, 1984, p. 273.
68. Fujiki, H., Suganuma, M., Suguri, H., Yoshizawa, S., Tagaki, K., Uda, N., Wakamatsu, K., Amada, K., Murata, M., Yasumoto, T., and Sugimura, T.: *Jpn. J. Cancer Res. (Gann)* **79**, 1089 (1988).
69. Haystead, T. A. J., Sim, A. T. R., Carling, D., Honnor, R. C., Tsukitani, Y., Cohen, P., and Hardie, D. G.: *Nature* **337**, 78 (1989).
70. Muramatsu, I., Nishio, J., Kigoshi, S., and Uemura, D.: *Br. J. Pharmacol.* **93**, 811 (1988).
71. Klein-Szanto, A. J. P., and Slaga, T. J.: *J. Invest. Dermatol.* **79**, 30 (1982).
72. Slaga, T. J., Solanki, V., and Logani, M.: Studies on the Mechanism of Action of Antitumor Promoting Agents: Suggestive Evidence for the Involvement of Free Radicals in Promotion. *In* "Radioprotectors and Anticarcinogens" (O. F. Nygaard and M. C. Simic, eds.). Academic Press, New York, 1983, p. 471.
73. DiGiovanni, J., Kruszewski, F. H., Coombs, M. M., Blatt, T. S., and Pezeslik, A.: *Carcinogenesis* **9**, 1437 (1988).
74. Hakii, H., Fujiki, H., Suganuma, M., Nakayasu, N., Tahira, T., Sugimura, T., Scheuer, P. J., and Christensen, S. B.: *J. Cancer Res. Clin. Oncol.* **111**, 177 (1986).
75. Arffman, E., and Glavind, J.: *Experientia* **27**, 1465 (1971).
76. Sice, J.: *Toxicol. Appl. Pharmacol.* **9**, 70 (1966).
77. Miller, M. L., Andringa, A., and Baxter, C. S.: *Carcinogenesis* **9**, 1959 (1988).
78. Boutwell, R. K., and Bosch, D. K.: *Cancer Res.* **19**, 413 (1959).
79. Setälä, K., Setälä, H., and Holsti, P.: *Science* **120**, 1075 (1954).
80. Gwynn, P. H., and Salaman, N. H.: *Br. J. Cancer* **7**, 482 (1953).
81. Bock, F. G., Fjelde, A., Fox, H. W., and Klein, E.: *Cancer Res.* **29**, 179 (1969).
82. Slaga, T. J., Jecker, L., Bracken, W. M., and Weeks, C. E.: *Cancer Lett.* **7**, 51 (1979).
83. Scribner, N. K., and Scribner, J. D.: *Carcinogenesis* **1**, 97 (1980).
84. Roe, F. J. C., and Pierce, W. E. H.: *J. Natl. Cancer Inst.* **24**, 1389 (1960).
85. Bock, F. G., Moors, G. E., Crouch, S. K.: *Science* **145**, 231 (1964).
86. Van Duuren, B. C., and Goldschmidt, B. M.: *J. Natl. Cancer Inst.* **56**, 1237 (1976).
87. Hennings, H., and Boutwell, R. K.: *Cancer Res.* **30**, 312 (1970).
88. Clark-Lewis, I., and Murray, A. W.: *Cancer Res.* **38**, 494 (1978).
89. Argyris, T. S.: *CRC Crit. Rev. Toxicol.* **14**, 211 (1986).
90. Matsui, M. S., and Deleo, V. A.: *Cancer Cells* **3**, 8 (1991).
91. Hasegawa, R., St. John, M., Tibbels, T. S., and Cohen, S. M.: *J. Invest. Dermatol.* **88**, 653 (1987).
92. Copeland, E. S.: *Cancer Res.* **43**, 5631 (1983).
93. Troll, W., and Wiesner, R.: *Annu. Rev. Pharmacol. Toxicol.* **25**, 509 (1985).

94. Cerutti, P.: *Science* **227**, 375 (1985).
95. Kensler, T. W., and Taffe, B. G.: *Adv. Free Radical Biol. Med.* **2**, 347 (1986).
96. Perchellet, J. P., and Perchellet, E. M.: *Free Radical Biol. Med.* **7**, 377 (1989).
97. Kensler, T. W., Egner, P. A., Taffe, B. G., and Trush, M. A.: Role of Free Radicals in Tumor Promotion and Progression. *In* "Skin Carcinogenesis: Mechanisms and Human Relevance" (T. J. Slaga, A. J. P. Klein-Szanto, R. K. Boutwell, D. E. Stevenson, H. L. Spitzer, and B. D'Motto, eds.). Alan R. Liss, New York, 1989, p. 223.
98. Petrusevska, R. T., Fürstenberger, G., Marks, F., and Fusenig, N. E.: *Carcinogenesis* **9**, 1207 (1988).
99. Marks, F., Fürstenberger, G., and Kownatzki, E.: *Cancer Res.* **41**, 696 (1981).
100. Marks, F., Hanke, B., Thastrup, O., and Fürstenberger, G.: *Carcinogenesis* **12**, 1491 (1991).
101. Pressman, B. C.: *Annu. Rev. Biochem.* **45**, 501 (1976).
102. Thastrup, O., Cullen, P. J., Drobak, B., Hanley, M. R., and Dawson, A. P.: *Proc. Natl. Acad. Sci. U.S.A.* **87**, 2466 (1990).
103. Gschwendt, M., Kittstein, W., Horn, F., Leibersperger, H., and Marks, F.: *J. Subcell. Biochem.* **40**, 295 (1989).
104. Jaken, S., and Yuspa, S. H.: *Carcinogenesis* **9**, 1033 (1988).
105. Hecker, E.: *J. Cancer Res. Clin. Oncol.* **99**, 102 (1981).
106. Hecker, E., and Sosath, S.: *Interdisc. Sci. Rev.* **14**, 241 (1989).
107. Hecker, E., Lutz, D., Weber, J., Goerttler, K., and Morton, J. F.: Multistage tumor development in the human esophagus—the first identification of cocarcinogens of the tumor promoter type as principal carcinogenic risk factors in a local life style cancer. *In* Proc. 13th Int. Cancer Congr., Part B, "Biology of Cancer". Alan R. Liss, New York, 1983, p. 219.
108. Liv, J. G., and Li, M.: *Carcinogenesis* **10**, 617 (1989).
109. Marks, F., and Fürstenberger, G.: *Carcinogenesis* **11**, 2085 (1990).
110. Slaga, T. J., Scribner, J. D., Thompson, S., and Viaje, A.: *J. Natl. Cancer Inst.* **57**, 1145 (1976).
111. Burns, F. J., Vanderlaan, M., Sivak, A., and Albert, R. E.: *Cancer Res.* **36**, 1422 (1976).
112. Slaga, T. J., and Nesnow, S.: Sencar Mouse Skin Carcinogenesis. *In* "Handbook of Carcinogen Testing" (H. A. Milan and E. K. Weisburger, eds.). Noyes Publications, Park Ridge, New Jersey, 1985, p. 231.
113. Verma, A. K., and Boutwell, R. K.: *Carcinogenesis* **1**, 271 (1980).
114. Hennings, H., Shores, R., Mitchell, P., Spangler, E. F., and Yuspa, S. H.: *Carcinogenesis* **6**, 1607 (1985).
115. Aldaz, C. M., Conti, C. J., Carder, F., Trono, D., Roop, D. R., Chesner, J., Whitehead, T., and Slaga, T. J.: *Cancer Res.* **48**, 3253 (1988).
116. Hennings, H.: Malignant Conversion: The First Stage in Progression from Benign to Malignant Tumors. *In* "Skin Carcinogenesis, Mechanisms and Human Relevance" (T. J. Slaga, A. J. P. Klein-Szanto, R. K. Boutwell, D. E. Stevenson, H. L. Spitzer, and B. D'Motto, eds.). Alan R. Liss, New York, 1989, p. 95.
117. Deamant, F. D., and Janacone, P. M.: *J. Cell Sci.* **88**, 305 (1987).
118. Scribner, J. D., Scribner, N. K., McKnight, B., and Mottet, N. K.: *Cancer Res.* **43**, 2034 (1983).
119. Burns, F., Allert, R., Altshuler, B., and Morris, F.: *Environ. Health Perspect.* **50**, 309 (1983).
120. Argyris, T. S.: *NCI Monogr.* **10**, 33 (1963).
121. Klein-Szanto, A. J. P.: Pathology of Human and Experimental Skin Tumors. *In* "Skin Tumors: Experimental and Clinical Aspects" (C. J. Conti, T. J. Slaga, and A. J. P. Klein-Szanto, eds.). Raven Press, New York, 1989, p. 19.
122. Balmain, A., and Pragnell, J. B.: *Nature* **303**, 72 (1983).
123. Brown, K., Buchmann, A., and Balmain, A.: *Proc. Natl. Acad. Sci. U.S.A.* **87**, 538 (1990).
124. Hennings, H., Devor, D., Wenk, M. L., Slaga, T. J., Former, B., Colburn, N. H., Bowden, G. T., Elgjo, K., and Yuspa, S. H.: *Cancer Res.* **41**, 773 (1981).
125. Aldaz, C. M., Conti, C. J., Klein-Szanto, A. J. P., and Slaga, T. J.: *Proc. Natl. Acad. Sci. U.S.A.* **84**, 2029 (1987).
126. Aldaz, C. M., and Conti, C. J.: The Premalignant Nature of Mouse Skin Papillomas: Histopathology, Cytogenetic and Biochemical Evidence. *In* "Skin Tumors: Experimental and Clinical Aspects" (C. J. Conti, T. J. Slaga, and A. J. P. Klein-Szanto, eds.). Raven Press, New York, 1989, p. 227.
127. Conti, C. J., Aldaz, C. M., O'Connell, J. F., Klein-Szanto, A. J. P., and Slaga, T. J.: *Carcinogenesis* **7**, 1845 (1986).
128. Aldaz, C. M., Trono, D., Larcher, F., Slaga, T. J., and Conti, C. J.: *Mol. Carcinogenesis* **2**, 22 (1989).
129. Bremner, R., and Balmain, A.: *Cell* **61**, 407 (1990).
130. DeYoung, L. M., Richards, W. L., Bonzels, W., Tsai, L. L., and Boutwell, R. K.: *Cancer Res.* **38**, 3697 (1978).
131. Nischt, R., Roop, D. R., Mehrel, T., Yuspa, S. H., Rentrop, M., Winter, H., and Schweizer, J.: *Mol. Carcinogenesis* **1**, 96 (1988).
132. Chiba, M., Maley, M. A., and Klein-Szanto, A. J. P.: *Cancer Res.* **46**, 259 (1986).

133. Shubik, P.: *Cancer Res.* **10**, 13 (1950).
134. Goerttler, K., Loehrke, H., Schweizer, J., and Hesse, B.: Diterpene Ester-Mediated Two-Stage Carcinogenesis. *In* "Cocarcinogenesis and Biological Effects of Tumor Promoters" (E. Hecker, N. E. Fusenig, W. Kunz, F. Marks, and H. W. Thielmann, eds.), Carcinogenesis, Vol. 7. Raven Press, New York, 1982, p. 75.
135. Slaga, T. J., and Fischer, S. M.: *Progr. Exp. Tumor Res.* **26**, 85 (1983).
136. Goerttler, K., Loehrke, H., Schweizer, J., and Hesse, B.: *Virchows Arch. (Pathol. Anat.)* **385**, 181 (1980).
137. Goerttler, K., Loehrke, H., Schweizer, J., and Hesse, B.: *Carcinogenesis* **5**, 521 (1984).
138. Berenblum, I.: *J. Natl. Cancer Inst.* **10**, 167 (1949).
139. Goerttler, K., Loehrke, H., Schweizer, J., and Hesse, B.: *Cancer Res.* **40**, 155 (1980).
140. DiGiovanni, J., Prichett, W. P., Decina, P. C., and Diamond, L.: *Carcinogenesis* **5**, 1493 (1984).
141. Reiners, J. J., Nesnow, S., and Slaga, T. J.: *Carcinogenesis* **5**, 301 (1984).
142. DiGiovanni, J., Slaga, T. J., and Boutwell, R. K.: *Carcinogenesis* **1**, 381 (1980).
143. Naito, M., and DiGiovanni, J.: Genetic Background and Development of Skin Tumors. *In* "Skin Tumors: Experimental and Clinical Aspects" (C. J. Conti, T. J. Slaga, and A. J. P. Klein-Szanto, eds.). Raven Press, New York, 1989, p. 187.
144. Phillips, D. H., Grover, P. I., and Sims, P.: *Int. J. Cancer* **22**, 487 (1978).
145. DiGiovanni, J., Naito, M., and Chenicek, K. J.: Genetic Factors Controlling Susceptibility to Skin Tumor Promotion in Mice. *In* "Tumor Promoters: Biological Approaches for Mechanistic Studies and Assay Systems" (C. J. Barrett, E. Langenbach, and E. Gilmore, eds.). Raven Press, New York, 1988, p. 51.
146. Barrett, J. C., Brown, M. T., and Sisskin, E. E.: *Cancer Res.* **42**, 3098 (1982).
147. Poland, A., Palen, D., and Glover, E.: *Nature* **300**, 271 (1982).
148. Kanno, J., Matsubara, O., and Kasuga, T.: *Acta Pathol. Jpn.* **36**, 1 (1986).
149. Berkelhammer, J., and Oxenhandler, R. W.: *Cancer Res.* **47**, 1251 (1987).
150. Schweizer, J., Loehrke, H., Lutz, E., and Goerttler, K.: *Carcinogenesis* **8**, 479 (1987).
151. Fujiki, H.: *Mol. Carcinogenesis* **5**, 16 (1992).
152. Armuth, V., and Berenblum, J.: *Cancer Res.* **32**, 2259 (1972).
153. Armuth, V., and Berenblum, J.: *Cancer Res.* **34**, 2704 (1974).
154. Pitot, H. C., Goldsworthy, T., Campbell, H. A., and Poland, A.: *Cancer Res.* **40**, 3616 (1980).
155. Diwan, B. A., Ward, J. M., Rice, J. M., Colburn, N. H., and Spangler, E. F.: *Carcinogenesis* **6**, 343 (1985).
156. Ward, J. M., Rice, J. M., Creasia, D., Lynch, P., and Rigap, C.: *Carcinogenesis* **4**, 1021 (1983).
157. Witschi, H. P.: Enhancement of Tumor Formation in Mouse Lung. *In* "Mechanisms of Tumor Promotion," Vol. 1, Tumor Promotion in Internal Organs" (T. J. Slaga, ed.). CRC Press, Boca Raton, Florida, 1983, p. 71.
158. Peraino, C., Fry, R. J. M., Staffeldt, E., and Christopher, J. P.: *Food Cosmet. Toxicol.* **15**, 93 (1977).
159. Pitot, H. C., and Campbell, H. A.: Quantitative Studies on Multistage Hepatocarcinogenesis in the Rat. *In* "Tumor Promoters: Biological Approaches for Mechanistic Studies and Assay Systems" (R. Langenbach, E. Elmore, and J. C. Barrett, eds.). Raven Press, New York, 1988, p. 79.
160. Slaga, T. J., and Butler, A. P.: Cellular and Biochemical Changes During Multistage Skin Tumor Promotion. *In* "Cellular Interactions by Environmental Tumor Promoters" (H. Fujiki, E. Hecker, R. E. Moore, T. Sugimura, and I. B. Weinstein, eds.). Japan. Sci. Soc. Press, Tokyo/VNU Science Press, Utrecht, 1984, p. 291.
161. Takahashi, M., Sato, H., Toyoda, K., Furukawa, F., Imaida, K., Hasegawa, R., and Hayoshi, Y.: *Carcinogenesis* **10**, 1163 (1989).
162. Graube, B. D., Peraino, C., and Fry, R. J. M.: *J. Invest. Dermatol.* **64**, 258 (1975).
163. Glauert, H. P., and Bernik, M. R.: *Chem. Pathol. Pharmacol.* **22**, 609 (1978).
164. Klein-Szanto, A. J. P.: Morphological Evaluation of Tumor Promoter Effects on Mammalian Skin. *In* "Mechanisms of Tumor Promotion", Vol. II, Tumor Promotion and Skin Carcinogenesis (T. J. Slaga, ed.). CRC Press, Boca Raton, Florida, 1984, p. 41.
165. Bach, H., and Goerttler, K.: *Virchows Arch. B. Cell. Pathol.* **8**, 196 (1971).
166. Lewis, J. G., and Adams, D. O.: *Proc. Am. Assoc. Cancer Res.* **27**, 146 (1986).
167. Naito, M., Naito, Y., and DiGiovanni, J.: *Carcinogenesis* **8**, 1807 (1987).
168. Aldaz, C. M., Conti, C. J., Gimenez, J. B., Slaga, T. J., and Klein-Szanto, A. J. P.: *Cancer Res.* **45**, 2753 (1985).
169. Klein-Szanto, A. J. P., Chiba, M., Lee, S. U., Conti, C. J., and Thetford, D.: *Carcinogenesis* **5**, 1459 (1984).
170. Argyris, T. S.: *CRC Crit. Rev. Toxicol.* **14**, 211 (1985).

171. Argyris, T. S.: Epidermal Tumor Promotion by Damage in the Skin of Mice. *In* "Skin Carcinogenesis: Mechanisms and Human Relevance" (T. J. Slaga, A. J. P. Klein-Szanto, R. K. Boutwell, D. E. Stevenson, H. L. Spitzer, and B. D'Motto, eds.). Alan R. Liss, New York, 1989, p. 63.

172. Argyris, T. S., and Slaga, T. J.: *Cancer Res.* **41**, 5193 (1981).

173. Sisskin, E. E., Gray, T., and Barrett, J. C.: *Carcinogenesis* **3**, 403 (1982).

174. Takigawa, M., Simsiman, R. C., and Boutwell, R. K.: *Cancer Res.* **46**, 106 (1986).

175. Fisher, S. M., Jasheway, D. W., Klann, R. C., Butler, A. P., Patrick, K. F., Baldwin, J. K., and Cameron, G. S.: *Cancer Res.* **49**, 6693 (1989).

176. Sisskin, E. E., and Barrett, J. C.: *Cancer Res.* **41**, 346 (1981).

177. Verma, A. K., Shapas, B. G., Rice, H. M., and Boutwell, R. K.: *Cancer Res.* **39**, 419 (1979).

178. Naito, M., Chenicek, K. J., Naito, Y., and DiGiovanni, J.: *Carcinogenesis* **9**, 639 (1988).

179. Hasper, F., Müller, G., and Schweizer, J.: *Cancer Res.* **42**, 2034 (1982).

180. Smart, R. C., Huang, T. M., Monteiro-Riviere, N. A., Wong, C. Q., Mills, K. J., and Conney, A. H.: *Carcinogenesis* **9**, 2221 (1988).

181. Fischer, S. M., Cameron, G. S., Baldwin, J. K., Jasheway, D. W., Patrick, K. E., and Belway, M. A.: The Arachidonic Acid Cascade and Multistage Carcinogenesis in Mouse Skin. *In* "Skin Carcinogenesis: Mechanisms and Human Relevance" (T. J. Slaga, A. J. P. Klein-Szanto, R. K. Boutwell, D. E. Stevenson, H. L. Spitzer, and B. D'Motto, eds.). Alan R. Liss, New York, 1989, p. 249.

182. Bourin, M. C., Delescluse, C., Fürstenberger, G., Marks, F., Schweizer, J., Klein-Szanto, A. J. P., and Prunieras, M.: *Carcinogenesis* **3**, 671 (1982).

183. Schweizer, J., and Marks, F.: *Cancer Res.* **37**, 4195 (1977).

184. Schweizer, J.: *Experientia* **35**, 1651 (1979).

185. Yotti, L. P., Chang, C. C., and Trosko, J. E.: *Science* **206**, 1089 (1979).

186. Trosko, J. E., Chang, C. C., and Medcalf, A.: *Cancer Invest.* **1**, 511 (1983).

187. Yamasaki, H.: Short-Term Assays to Detect Tumor-Promoting Activity in Environmental Chemicals. *In* "Skin Carcinogenesis: Mechanisms and Human Relevance" (T. J. Slaga, A. J. P. Klein-Szanto, R. K. Boutwell, D. E. Stevenson, H. L. Spitzer, and B. D'Motto, eds.). Alan R. Liss, New York, 1989, p. 265.

188. Fitzgerald, B. J., Knowles, S. E., Ballard, F. J., and Murray, A. W.: *Cancer Res.* **43**, 3614 (1983).

189. Trosko, J. E., and Chana, C. C.: Role of Intercellular Communication in Tumor Promotion. *In* "Mechanisms of Tumor Promotion," Vol.IV, Tumor Promotion and Skin Carcinogenesis (T. J. Slaga, ed.), CRC Press, Boca Raton, Florida, 1984, p. 119.

190. Kalimi, C. H., and Sirsat, S. M.: *Cancer Lett.* **22**, 343 (1984).

191. Klein-Szanto, A. J. P., Major, S. K., and Slaga, T. J.: *Carcinogenesis* **1**, 399 (1980).

192. Klein-Szanto, A. J. P.: Morphological Evaluation of the Effects of Carcinogens and Promoters. *In* "Skin Carcinogenesis: Mechanisms and Human Relevance" ((T. J. Slaga, A. J. P. Klein-Szanto, R. K. Boutwell, D. E. Stevenson, H. L. Spitzer, and B. D'Motto, eds.). Alan R. Liss, New York, 1989, p. 45.

193. Färber, B., Petrusevska, R. T., Fusenig, N. E., and Kinzel, V.: *Carcinogenesis* **10**, 2345 (1989).

194. Parry, J. M., Parry, E. M., and Barrett, J. C.: *Nature* **294**, 144 (1981).

195. Emerit, J., and Cerutti, P. A.: *Nature* **293**, 144 (1981).

196. Kinsella, A. R., and Radman, M.: *Proc. Natl. Acad. Sci. U.S.A.* **75**, 6149 (1978).

197. Birnboim, H. C.: *Science* **211**, 1247 (1982).

198. Dutton, R. D., and Bowden, G. T.: *Carcinogenesis* **6**, 1279 (1985).

199. Hartley, J. A., Gibson, N. W., Zwelling, L. A., and Yuspa, S. H.: *Cancer Res.* **45**, 4864 (1985).

200. Dzarlieva, R. T., and Fusenig, N. E.: *Cancer Lett.* **16**, 7 (1982).

201. Dzarlieva-Petrusevska, R. T., and Fusenig, N. E.: *Carcinogenesis* **6**, 1447 (1985).

202. Imbra, R. J., and Karin, M.: *Nature* **323**, 555 (1986).

203. Fisher, P. B., Weinstein, I. B., Eisenberg, D., and Grinsberg, H. S.: *Proc. Natl. Acad. Sci. U.S.A.* **75**, 2311 (1978).

204. zur Hausen, H., O'Neill, F. J., and Freese, U. K.: *Nature* **272**, 373 (1978).

205. zur Hausen, H., Bornkamm, G. W., Schmidt, R., and Hecker, E.: *Proc. Natl. Acad. Sci. U.S.A.* **76**, 782 (1979).

206. Woodgett, J. R., Hunter, T., and Gould, K. L.: Protein Kinase C and Its Role in Cell Growth. *In* " Cell Membranes. Methods and Reviews" (E. Elson, W. Frazier, and L. Glaser, eds.). Plenum Press, New York, 1988, p. 215.

207. Rahmsdorf, H. J., and Herrlich, P.: *Pharmacol. Therap.* **48**, 157 (1990).

208. Verma, A. K., Pong, R. C., and Erickson, D.: *Cancer Res.* **46**, 6149 (1986).

209. Emilsson, A., Wijhander, J., and Sundler, R.: *Biochem. J.* **239**, 685 (1986).

210. Boyle, W. J., Smeal, T., Defize, L. H. K., Angel, P., Woodgett, J. R., Karin, M., and Hunter, T., *Cell* **64**, 573 (1991).

211. Smart, R. C., Huang, M. T., and Conney, A. H.: *Carcinogenesis* **7**, 1865 (1986).

212. Nakadate, T., Yamamoto, S., Aizu, F., and Kato, R.: *Cancer Res.* **46**, 1589 (1986).

213. Nakadate, T., and Blumberg, P.: *Cancer Res.* **47**, 6537 (1984).
214. Nishino, H., Kitagawa, K., and Iwashima, A.: *Carcinogenesis* **5**, 1529 (1984).
215. Kitagawa, K., Nishino, H., and Iwashino, A.: *Oncology* **43**, 127 (1986).
216. Kato, R., Nakadate, T., Yamamoto, S., and Sugimura, T.: *Carcinogenesis* **4**, 1301 (1983).
217. Blumberg, P. M., Delclos, K. B., and Jaken, S.: Tissue and Species Specificity for Phorbol Ester Receptors. *In* "Organ and Species Specificity in Chemical Carcinogenesis" (R. Langenbach, S. Nesnow, and J. Rice, eds.). Plenum Press, New York, 1983, p. 201.
218. Wheldrake, J. F., Marshall, J., Pauli, J., and Murray, A. W.: *Carcinogenesis* **3**, 805 (1982).
219. Coussens, L., Parker, P. J., Rhee, L, Yang-feng, T. L., Chen, E., Waterfield, M. D., Franke, U., and Ullrich, A.: *Science* **233**, 859 (1986).
220. Nishizuka, Y.: *Nature* **334**, 662 (1988).
221. Kikkawa, U., Ogita, K., Shearman, M. S., Ase, K., Segikuchi, K., Naor, Z., Kishimoto, A., Nishizuka, Y., Saito, N., Tanaka, C., Ono, Y., Fujiki, T., and Igarashi, K.: *Cold Spring Harbor Symp. Quant. Biol.* **13**, 97 (1988).
222. Gschwendt, M., Kittstein, W., and Marks, F.: *Trends Biochem. Sci.* **16**, 167 (1991).
223. Leibersperger, H., Gschwendt, M., Gernold, M., and Marks, F.: *J. Biol. Chem.* **266**, 14778 (1991).
224. Osada, S., Mizuno, K., Saido, T. C., Akita, Y., Suzuki, K., Kuroki, T., and Ohno, S.: *J. Biol. Chem.* **265**, 22434 (1990).
225. Homma, Y., Henning-Chubb, C. B., and Huberman, E.: *Proc. Natl. Acad. Sci. U.S.A.* **83**, 7316 (1986).
226. Fournice, A., and Murray, A. W.: *Nature* **330**, 767 (1987).
227. Droms, K. A., and Malkinson, A. M.: *Mol. Carcinogenesis* **4**, 1 (1991).
228. Kraft, A. S., Smith, J. B., and Berko, R. L.: *Proc. Natl. Acad. Sci. U.S.A.* **83**, 1334 (1986).
229. Hennings, H., Blumberg, P. M., Pettit, G. R., Herald, C. L., Shores, R., and Yuspa, S. H.: *Carcinogenesis* **8**, 1343 (1987).
230. Gschwendt, M., Fürstenberger, G., Rose-John, S., Rogers, M., Kittstein, W., Pettit, G. R., Herald, C. L., and Marks, F.: *Carcinogenesis* **9**, 555 (1988).
231. Blumberg, P. M., Pettit, G. R., Warren, B. S., Szallasi, A., Schumann, L. D., Sharkey, N. A., Nakakuma, H., Dell'Aquita, M. L., and deVries, D. J.: The Protein Kinase C Pathway in Tumor Promotion. *In* "Skin Carcinogenesis: Mechanisms and Human Relevance" (T. J. Slaga, A. J. P. Klein-Szanto, R. K. Boutwell, D. E. Stevenson, H. L. Spitzer, and B. D'Motto, eds.). Alan R. Liss, New York, 1989, p. 201.
232. Pear, C., and Parker, P. J.: *FEBS Lett.* **284**, 120 (1991).
233. Freisewinkel, I., Riethmacher, D., and Stabel, S.: *FEBS Lett.* **280**, 262 (1991).
234. Lindner, D., Gschwendt, M., and Marks, F.: *Biochem. Biophys. Res. Commun.* **176**, 1227 (1991).
235. Horn, F., Marks, F., Fisher, G. J., Marcelo, C. L., and Voorhees, J. J., *J. Invest. Dermatol.* **88**, 220 (1987).
236. Kraft, A. S., Baker, V. V., and May, W. S.: *Oncogene* **1**, 111 (1987).
237. Hashimoto, Y., and Shudo, K.: *Jpn. J. Cancer Res.* **82**, 665 (1991).
238. Ahmed, S., Kozuma, R., Monfries, C., Hall, C., Lim, H. H., Smith, P., and Lim, L.: *Biochem. J.* **272**, 767 (1990).
239. Berridge, M. J.: *Biochim. Biophys. Acta* **907**, 33 (1987).
240. Ganss, M., Seemann, D., Fürstenberger, G., and Marks, F.: *FEBS Lett.* **143**, 54 (1982).
241. Verma, A. K. and Boutwell, R. K.: *Biochem. Biophys. Res. Commun.* **101**, 375 (1982).
242. Gschwendt, M., Kittstein, W., and Marks, F.: *Skin Pharmacol.* **1**, 84 (1988).
243. Nairn, A. C. and Palfrey, H. C.: *J. Biol. Chem.* **262**, 17299 (1987).
244. Palfrey, C., Nairn, A. C., Muldoon, L. L., and Villereal, M. L.: *J. Biol. Chem.* **262**, 9785 (1987).
245. Gschwendt, M., Kittstein, W., and Marks, F.: *Biochem. Biophys. Res. Commun.* **153**, 1129 (1988).
246. Gschwendt, M., Kittstein, W., and Marks, F.: *Cancer Lett.* **34**, 187 (1987).
247. Gschwendt, M., Kittstein, W., and Marks, F.: *J. Immunol.* **179**, 1 (1989).
248. Levine, L.: *Adv. Cancer Res.* **35**, 49 (1981).
249. Levine, L. and Fujiki, H.: *Carcinogenesis* **6**, 1631 (1985).
250. Fürstenberger, G., Richter, H., Fusenig, N. E., and Marks F.: *Cancer Lett.* **11**, 191 (1981).
251. Fürstenberger, G. and Marks, F.: *Biochem. Biophys. Res. Commun.* **92**, 749 (1980).
252. Fürstenberger, G. and Marks, F.: Prostaglandins, Epidermal Hyperplasia and Skin Tumor Promotion. *In* "Arachidonic Acid Metabolism and Tumor Promotion" (S. M. Fischer and T. J. Slaga, eds.). Martinus Nijhoff, Boston, 1985, p. 49.
253. Fischer, S. M.: Arachidonic Acid Metabolism and Tumor Promotion. *In* "Arachidonic Acid Metabolism and Tumor Promotion" (S. M. Fischer and T. J. Slaga, eds.). Martinus Nijhoff, Boston, 1985, p. 21.
254. Fürstenberger, G.: Role of Eicosanoids in Mammalian Skin Epidermis. *In* "Cell Biology Reviews". Springer Int., Univ. of the Basque Country, Bilbao, Spain, 1990.
255. Verma, A. K., Ashendel, C. L., and Boutwell, R. K: *Cancer Res.* **40**, 708 (1980).

256. Fürstenberger, G., Gross, M., and Marks, F.: *Carcinogenesis* **10**, 91 (1989).
257. Fürstenberger, G., Gschwendt, M., Hagedorn H., and Marks, F.: Modulation of the Conversion Stage of Multistage Carcinogenesis in Mouse Skin by Eicosanoids. *In* "Prostaglandins and Cancer Research" (E. Garaci, R. Paoletti and M. G. Santoro eds.). Springer-Verlag, Berlin, 1987, p. 48.
258. Fischer, S. M., Baldwin, J. K., Jasheway, D. W., Patrick, K. E., and Cameron, G. S.: *Cancer Res.* **48**, 658 (1988).
259. Lehmann, W. D., Stephan, M., and Fürstenberger, G.: *Anal. Biochem.* **204**, 158 (1992).
260. Kato, R., Nakadate, T., and Yamamoto, S.: Involvement of Lipoxygenase Products of Arachidonic Acid in Tumor-Promoting Activity of TPA. *In* "Eicosanoids and Cancer" (H. Thaler-Dao, A. Crastes de Paulet, and R. Paoletti, eds.). Raven Press, New York, 1984, p. 101.
261. Ochi, E., and Cerutti, P. A.: *Proc. Natl. Acad. Sci. U.S.A* **84**, 990 (1987).
262. Fürstenberger, G. and Hecker, E.: *J. Nat. Prod. (Lloydia)* **49**, 386 (1986).
263. Marks, F., Bertsch, S., and Fürstenberger, G.: *Cancer Res.* **39**, 4183 (1979).
264. Hecker, E.: *Toxicol. Pathol.* **15**, 245 (1987).
265. Locniskar, M., Belury, M., Cumberland, A. G., Patrick, K. E., and Fischer, S. M.: *Carcinogenesis* **11**, 1641 (1990).
266. Abou-El-Ela, S. H., Prasse, K. W., Farrel, R. L., Carroll, K. K., Wade, A. E., and Bunce, O. R.: *Cancer Res.* **49**, 1434 (1989).
267. Leyton, L., Lee, M. L., Locniskar, M., Belury, M. A., Slaga, T. J., Bechtel, D., and Fischer, S. M.: *Cancer Res.* **51**, 907 (1991).
268. Nolan, R. D., Danilowicz, R. M., and Eling, T. E.: *Mol. Pharmacol.* **33**, 650 (1988).
269. Siess, H., Wefers, H., and Cadenas, E.: Photoemission in Lipid Peroxidation and PG_2-Reduction and During Quinone Redox Cycling: Involvement of Singlet Oxygen. *In* "Eicosanoids and Cancer" (H. Thaler-Dao, A. Crastes de Paulet, and R. Paoletti eds.). Raven Press, New York, 1984, p. 11.
270. Marnett, L.: *Carcinogenesis* **8**, 1365 (1987).
271. Fischer, S. M., and Adams, L. M.: *Cancer Res.* **45**, 3110 (1985).
272. Fischer, S. M., Baldwin, J. K., and Adams, L. M.: *Carcinogenesis* **7**, 915 (1986).
273. Perchellet, E. M., Abney, L. N., and Perchellet, J. P.: *Cancer Lett.* **42**, 169 (1988).
274. Perchellet, E. M., and Perchellet, J. P: *Cancer Res.* **49**, 6193 (1989).
275. Robertson, F. M., Bearis, A. J., Oberyszyn, T. M., O'Connell, S. M., Dokidos, A., Laskin, D. L., Laskin, J. D., and Reiners, J. J.: *Cancer Res.* **50**, 6062 (1990).
276. Reiners, J. J., Pence, P. C., Barcus, M. C. S., and Cartu, A. R.: *Cancer Res.* **47**, 1775 (1987).
277. Pence, B. C., and Reiners, J. J.: *Cancer Res.* **47**, 6388 (1987).
278. Lewis, J. G., and Adams, D. O.: *Cancer Res.* **46**, 5696 (1986).
279. Goldskin, B. D., Witz, G., Ammeroso, M., and Troll, W.: *Biochem. Biophys. Res. Commun.* **88**, 804 (1979).
280. Troll, W., Klassen, A., and Janoff, A.: *Science* **169**, 1211 (1970).
281. Kozumbo, W. J., and Cerutti, P. A.: Antioxidants as Antipromoters. *In* "Antimutagenesis and Anticarcinogenesis Mechanisms" (D. M. Shankel, P. E. Hartman, T. Kada, and A. Hollander, eds.). Plenum Press, New York, 1986, p. 491.
282. Nakadate, T., Yamamoto, S., Aizu, E., and Kato, R.: *Gann* **75**, 214 (1984).
283. Huang, M. T., Smart, R. C., Wong, Ch. Q., and Conney, A. H.: *Cancer Res.* **48**, 5941 (1988).
284. Smart, R. C., Huang, M. T., Han, Z. T., Kaplan, M. C., Focella, A., and Conney, A. H.: *Cancer Res.* **47**, 6633 (1987).
285. Perchellet, J. P., Owen, M. D., Posey, T. D., Orten, D. K., and Schneider, B. A.: *Carcinogenesis* **6**, 567 (1985).
286. Taffe, B. G., Takahashi, N., Kensler, T. W., and Mason, R. P.: *J. Biol. Chem.* **62**, 12143 (1987).
287. O'Connell, J. F., Klein-Szanto, A. P. J., DiGiovanni, D. M., Fries, J. W., and Slaga, T. J.: *Cancer Res.* **46**, 2863 (1986).
288. Watts, P.: *Food Chem. Toxicol.* **23**, 957 (1985).
289. O'Brian, C. A., Ward, N. E., Weinstein, I. B., Bull, A. W., and Marnett, L.: *Biochem Biophys. Res. Commun.* **155**, 1374 (1988).
290. Gopalakrishna, R., and Anderson, W.: *Proc. Natl. Acad. Sci. U.S.A.* **86**, 6758 (1989).
291. Solanki, V., Rana, R. S., and Slaga, T. J.: *Carcinogenesis* **2**, 1141 (1981).
292. Perchellet, J. P., Perchellet, E. M., Orten, D. K., and Schneider, B. A.: *Cancer Lett.* **26**, 283 (1985).
293. Perchellet, J. P., Perchellet, E. M., Orten, D. K., and Schneider, B. A.: *Carcinogenesis* **7**, 503 (1986).
294. O'Brien, T. G.: *Cancer Res.* **36**, 2644 (1976).
295. Boutwell, R. K.: *Adv. Polyamine Res.* **4**, 127 (1983).
296. Athar, M., Raza, H., Bickers, D. R., and, Mukhtar, H.: *J. Invest. Dermatol.* **94**, 162 (1990).
297. Weeks, C. E., Herrmann, A. L., Nelson, F. R., and Slaga, T. J.: *Proc. Natl. Acad. Sci. U.S.A.* **79**, 6028 (1982).

298. Gilmour, S. K., Verma, A. K., Madara, T., and O'Brien, T. G.: *Cancer Res.* **47,** 1221 (1987).
299. O'Brien, T. G., Madara, T., and Holmes, M.: *Proc. Natl. Acad. Sci. U.S.A.* **84,** 9448 (1986).
300. Fischer, S. M., Jasheway, D. W., Klaun, R. C., Butler, A. P., Patrick, K. E., Baldwin, J. K., and Cameron, G. S.: *Cancer Res.* **49,** 6693 (1989).
301. Mills, K. J., and Smart, R. C.: *Carcinogenesis* **10,** 833 (1989).
302. Takigawa, M., Boutwell, R. K., and Verma, A. K.: Evidence That an Elevated Level of Ornithine Decarboxylase May Be Essential to Tumor Promotion by Phorbol Esters. *In* "Polyamines: Basic and Clinical Aspects" (K. Imahori, F. Suzuki, O. Suzuki, and U. Bachrach, eds.). Japan Sci. Soc. Press, Tokyo/VNU Science Press, Utrecht, 1985, p. 1.
303. Slaga, T. J., Fischer, S. M., Weeks, C. E., and Klein-Szanto A. J. P.: Cellular and Biochemical Mechanisms of Mouse Skin Tumor Promoters. *In* "Reviews in Biochemical Toxicology" (E. Hodgson, J. Bend, and R. M. Philpot eds.). Elsevier North-Holland, New York, 1981, p. 231.
304. O'Brien, T. G., Dzaubow, L., Dlugosz, A. A., Gilmour, S. K., O'Donnell, K., and Hietal, O.: Regulation of Ornithine Decarboxylase in Normal and Neoplastic Mouse and Human Epidermis. *In* "Skin Carcinogenesis: Mechanisms and Human Relevance" (T. J. Slaga, A. J. P. Klein-Szanto, R. K. Boutwell, D. E. Stevenson, H. L. Spitzer, and B. D'Motto eds.). Alan R. Liss, New York, 1984, p. 213.
305. Marks, F., Fürstenberger, G., Gschwendt, M.: Skin Tumour Promotion and the Wound Response: Two Sides of a Coin. *In* "The Environmental Threat to the Skin" (R. Marks and G. Plewig, eds.). Dunitz, London, 1992, p. 297.
306. Marks, F., and Fürstenberger, G.: *Environ. Health Perspect.* **101** (Suppl. 5), 95 (1993).
307. Marks, F.: Neoplasia and the Wound Response: the Lesson Learned from the Multistage Approach of Skin Carcinogenesis. *In* "Growth Regulation and Carcinogenesis" (W. Paukovits, ed.). CRC Press, Boca Raton, Florida, 1991, p. 54.
308. Dvorak, H. F.: *N. Engl. J. Med.* **315,** 1650 (1986).
309. Haddow, A.: *Adv. Cancer Res.* **16,** 181 (1972).
310. Orth J.: *Z. Krebsforsch.* **10,** 42 (1911).
311. Kupper, T. S.: *J. Invest. Dermatol.* **94,** 146s (1990).
312. Milestone, L. M. and Edelson, R. L. (eds.): "Endocrine, Metabolic and Immunologic Functions of Keratinocytes." *Ann. N. Y. Acad. Sci.* **548** (1988).
313. Nickoloff, G. J., Griffiths, C. E. M., and Barker, J. N. W. N.: *J. Invest. Dermatol.* **99,** 151s (1990).
314. Luger, T. A. and Schwartz, T.: *J. Invest. Dermatol.* **95,** 100s (1990).
315. Lee, S. W., Morhenn, V. B., Ilnicka, M., Eugui, E. M., and Allison, A. C.: *J. Invest. Dermatol.* **97,** 106 (1991).
316. Fürstenberger, G. and Marks, F.: The Role of Eicosanoids in Normal, Hyperplastic and Neoplastic Growth. *In* "Eicosanoids and the Skin" (T. Ruzicka, ed.). CRC Press, Boca Raton, Florida, 1990, p. 107.
317. McKay, I. A. and Leigh, I. M.: *Br. J. Dermatol.* **124,** 513 (1991).
318. Barker, J. N. W. N., Mitra, R. S., Griffiths, C. E. M., Dixit, V. M., and Nickoloff, B. J.: *Lancet* **337,** 211 (1991).
319. Folkman, J. and Klagsbrun, M.: *Science* **235,** 442 (1987).
320. Folkman, J.: *Adv. Cancer Res.* **43,** 175 (1985).
321. Kane, C. J. M., Hebda, P. A., Mansbridge, J. N., and Hanawalt, P. C.: *J. Cell Physiol.* **148,** 157 (1991).
322. Robertson, F. M., Oberyszyn, A. S., Bijur, G. N., and Oberyszyn, T. M.: *Proc. Am. Assoc. Cancer Res.* **33,** 180 (1992).
323. Glick, A. B., Sporn, M. B., and Yuspa, S. H.: *Carcinogenesis* **4,** 210 (1991).
324. Coffey, R. J., Sipes, N. J., Bascom, C. C., Graves-Deal, R., Pennington, C. Y., Weissmann, B. E., and Moses, H. J.: *Cancer Res.* **48,** 1596 (1988).
325. Barnard, J. A., Lyons, R. M., and Moses, H. L.: *Biochim. Biophys. Acta* **1032,** 79 (1990).
326. Kast, R., Fürstenberger, G., and Marks, F.: *Eur. J. Biochem.* **202,** 941 (1991).
327. Colburn, N., Talmadye, C. B., and Gindhart, T. J.: *Mol. Cell. Biol.* **3,** 1182 (1983).
328. Yuspa, S. H., Hennings, H., and Lichti, U.: *J. Supramol. Struct.* **17,** 245 (1981).
329. Parkinson, E. K.: *Br. J. Cancer* **52,** 479 (1985).
330. Yuspa, S. H., Ben, T., and Hennings, H.: *Carcinogenesis* **4,** 1413 (1983).
331. Parkinson, E. K. and Emmerson, A.: *Carcinogenesis* **3,** 525 (1982).
332. Reiners, J. J. and Slaga, T. J.: *Cell* **32,** 247 (1983).
333. Yuspa, S. H., Ben, T., Hennings, H., and Lichti, U.: *Cancer Res.* **42,** 2344 (1982).
334. Parkinson, E. K., Grabham, P., and Emmerson, A.: *Carcinogenesis* **4,** 857 (1983).
335. Yuspa, S., H., Kulesz-Martin, M., Ben, T., and Hennings, H.: *J. Invest. Dermatol.* **81,** 162s (1983).
336. MacKenzie, I. C. and Bickenbach, J. R.: Patterns of epidermal cell proliferation. *In* "Carcinogenesis. Vol. 7: Cocarcinogenesis and Biological Effects of Tumor Promoters" (E. Hecker, N. E. Fusenig, W. Kunz, F. Marks, and H. W. Thielmann, eds.). Raven Press, New York, 1982, p. 311.
337. Morris, R. J.: *J. Invest. Dermatol.* **84,** 277 (1985).

338. Klein-Szanto, A. J. P., and Slaga, T. J.: *Cancer Res.* **41**, 4437 (1981).
339. McCutcheon, J. A., Bickenbach, J. R. and MacKenzie, J. C.: *J. Dermatol. Res.* **64**, 298 (1985).
340. Parkinson, E. K., Pera, M. F., Emmerson, A., and Gorman, P. A.: *Carcinogenesis* **5**, 1071 (1984).
341. Fürstenberger, G., Schweizer, J., and Marks F.: *Carcinogenesis* **6**, 289 (1985).
342. Krieg, P., Schnapke, R., Fürstenberger, G., Vogt, I., and Marks, F.: *Mol. Carcinogenesis* **4**, 129 (1991).
343. Kaina, B.: *Teratogenesis, Carcinogenesis, Mutagenesis* **9**, 331 (1989).
344. Roberts, A. E., Sporn, M. B., Assoian, R. K., Smith, J. M., Roche, N. S., Wakefield, L. M., Heine, U. I., Liotta, L. A., Falanger, V., Kelert, J. H., and Fanci, A. S.: *Proc. Natl. Acad. Sci. U.S.A.* **83**, 4167 (1986).
345. Winter, G.: Epidermal Regeneration Studied in the Domestic Pig. *In* "Epidermal Wound Healing" (H. J. Maibach and D. T. Rovee, eds.). Year Book Medical Publishers, Chicago, 1982.
346. Hebda, P. A.: *J. Invest. Dermatol.* **91**, 440 (1988).
347. Clark, R. A. F., Lanigan, J. M., DellaPelle, P., Mansean, E., Dvorak, H. F., and Colvin, R. B.: *J. Invest. Dermatol.* **79**, 264 (1982).
348. Takashima, A. and Grinnell, F.: *J. Invest. Dermatol.* **85**, 304 (1985).
349. Wikner, N. E., Persichitte, K. A., Baskin, J. B., Nielsen, L. D., and Clark, R. A. F.: *J. Invest. Dermatol.* **91**, 207 (1988).
350. Ignotz, R. A. and Massagué, J.: *Cell* **51**, 189 (1987).
351. Bascom, C. C., Sipes, N. J., Coffey, R. J., and Moses, H. L.: *J. Cell. Biochem.* **39**, 25 (1989).
352. Marks, F., Bertsch, S., and Schweizer, J.: *Bull Cancer* **65**, 207 (1978).
353. Hennings, H. and Yuspa, S. H.: *J. Natl. Cancer Inst.* **74**, 735 (1985).
354. Loehrke, H., Schweizer, J., Dederer, E., Hesse, B., Rosenkranz, G., and Goerttler, K.: *Carcinogenesis* **4**, 771 (1983).
355. Boyd, J. A., and Barrett, J. C.: *Pharmacol Ther.* **46**, 469 (1990).

Tumor Promotion in Liver[1]

Michael Schwarz

I. STAGES IN HEPATOCARCINOGENESIS

The concepts of initiation and promotion in liver must be viewed in the backdrop of some basic observations on stages in hepatocarcinogenesis. As originally described independently by two groups (1,2), small foci of cells, hereafter called altered hepatic foci (AHF), appear in the liver shortly after exposure of experimental animals to a hepato-carcinogen. AHF are characterized by increases or decreases in the activity and/or level of a large variety of different enzymes and cellular substrates which can be used as markers for their identification. Among many others, these include the enzymes γ-glutamyl transferase (GGT) (3–5), adenosine triphosphatase (6–10), glucose-6-phosphatase (2), various cytochrome P-450 species (11,12), epoxide hydrolase (12), glucuronyl transferase (13), the placental form of glutathione transferase (14,15), and cellular glycogen content (16,17). The enzyme, glutathione transferase P, may even be used to detect single enzyme-altered liver cells (18). For recent summaries on enzyme changes in AHF reported in the literature, *see* references (19,20). AHF have been shown to be monoclonal in origin (21–23) and display, in comparison to their surrounding normal hepatocytes, increased cell proliferation (24–29). Accumulating evidence suggests that at least some of the AHF represent precursor lesions which are causally related to the carcinogenic process in liver. This is substantiated by the sequential appearance of AHF and tumors, by the similarity of many marker enzyme changes in both lesions (31), by the observation of "foci within foci" (31–33), and by the observation of quantitative relationships between the development of AHF and the later manifestations of hepatic tumors (10,34–36). Thus, chemically-induced hepatocarcinogenesis in rodents has turned out to be an extremely useful tool for the investigation of qualitative and quantitative changes that are of relevance during carcinogenesis (5,10,20,33,35,37–42).

II. LIVER TUMOR PROMOTERS

Research on tumor promotion in liver has been pioneered by Peraino and coworkers (43), who demonstrated that continuous treatment of rats with phenobarbital (a drug used as an anticonvulsant in the treatment of epilepsy) subsequent to a brief exposure of the

---

[1]For Abbreviations used *see* p. 173.

animals to 2-acetylaminofluorene (2-AAF) strongly increases the incidence of liver tumors when compared with rats given the initiating carcinogen alone (43). In subsequent studies carried out in many laboratories around the world, a large number of chemicals have been identified which have promoting activity in rodent liver. A list of representative examples is shown in Table 1.

Additional agents or treatments found to enhance hepatocarcinogenesis in an overadditive way, when administered subsequent to an initiating carcinogen (*i.e.*, which possess some kind of promoting activity), include: certain bile acids (54,61,62); plant products such as indole-3-carbinol (63); carbon tetrachloride (64–66) or chloroform (67); certain carcinogens such as 2-AAF (62,69,70), 4-dimethylaminoazobenzene (71), or 3′-methyl-4-dimethylaminoazobenzene (62); diets containing high levels of orotic acid (72), sucrose (73) or fructose (74); diets deficient in choline (68,75); and surgical manipulations such as partial hepatectomy (66,67) or portacaval anastomosis (78).

III. SPECIFICITY OF LIVER TUMOR PROMOTERS

Liver tumor promoters generally exhibit a high organ specificity. For example, phenobarbital, which is effective as a promoter in the liver of mice and rats, does not promote tumor development in bladder, lung, or skin of rats (79). It does, however, promote rat thyroid tumorigenesis (80,81). Inversely, saccharin, a bladder tumor promoter in rats, does not promote liver tumors in this species (79). Polyhalogenated biphenyls increase the frequency of liver adenomas and carcinomas in rats given *N*-ethyl-*N*-hydroxyethylnitrosamine as initiator, but have no effect on renal carcinogenesis initiated by this carcinogen (82). While the predominant target for the promoting activity of dibenzo-*p*-dioxins, dibenzofurans, polychlorinated biphenyls (PCB), and polybrominated biphenyls in rodents appears to be the liver (51,83), promotion of skin papilloma development has also been observed in certain strains of mice (84). The mechanisms of organ specificity are not entirely understood. It is remarkable, however, that promoting activity is generally associated with an increase in DNA synthesis and the induction of a pleiotropic cellular response in the respective target organs (85).

The vast majority of studies on tumor promotion in liver have been conducted in rodents. Most chemicals listed in Table 1 that were tested for promoting activity in rats and mice were effective as promoters in both species. Additional animal species have also been investigated, although not systematically. PCB, for example, promote hepatocarcinogenesis in rodents as well as in the rainbow trout (83). Indole-3-carbinol, a metabolite

TABLE 1. Some Compounds with Hepatic Tumor-Promoting Activity

Group	Prototype compound	References
Barbiturates	Phenobarbital	5,9,34,41,43–46
Different structurally unrelated chlorinated pesticides	2,2-Bis (*p*-chlorophenyl)-1,1,1-trichloroethane (DDT),	44
	α-hexachlorocyclohexane (α-BHC)[a]	47
Polyhalogenated biphenyls	3,3′,4,4′-Tetrachlorobiphenyl	48–50
Dibenzo-*p*-dioxins	2,3,7,8-Tetrachlorodibenzo-*p*-dioxin (TCDD)	51
Sex hormones	Ethinyl estradiol	52–56
Peroxisome proliferators	Clofibrate, di(2-ethylhexyl) phthalate (DEHP), Wy-14,643	57–60

[a]The acronym for α-benzenehexachloride, the *misnomer* term under which α-hexachlorocyclohexane ("Lindane") is widely known.

from cruciferous vegetables, promotes aflatoxin B_1-initiated hepatocarcinogenesis in both rats and trout (63). Phenobarbital enhances the formation of diethylnitrosamine (DEN)-induced liver tumors in patas monkeys (86,87). Similar to what is seen with 12-*O*-tetradecanoylphorbol-13-acetate (TPA) and other skin tumor promoters in different animal species, however, particular species appear not to be susceptible to promotion by certain liver-specific tumor promoters. This is best illustrated by the apparent lack of promoting activity of phenobarbital and DDT in the Syrian golden hamster (66,87,88).

Besides species differences, strong variations of promotability are frequently observed between different strains of animals and, within one and the same strain, between the two genders. Phenobarbital promotes the formation of AHF and/or liver tumors in DEN- or ethylnitrosourea-pretreated male BALB/c, Swiss, C3H, and DBA mice, while no enhancing effects were seen in male C57BL mice even after prolonged treatment with the tumor promoter for up to 45 weeks (89–91). Upon closer inspection, the effects of phenobarbital on hepatocarcinogenesis in mice become even more complex. While promotion of liver tumorigenesis was observed in male B6C3F1 mice pretreated with DEN at 4 weeks of age (90), the barbiturate inhibited the carcinogenic response in liver of mice that were given the initiator on day 15 after birth (90,92). Thus, whether phenobarbital functions as a promoter or an inhibitor of hepatocarcinogenesis may depend not only on the strain, but also on the age of mice at the time of initiation with the carcinogen (92).

Pronounced sex differences in the response of rats and mice to liver tumor promoters have been demonstrated. Promotion of AHF by Clophen A 50, a commercial PCB mixture, is much more pronounced in female rats when compared with males (93). This result correlates well with the frequently noted sex dependence of the tumorigenicity of PCB, indicating that females are more sensitive than males (83). Similarly, 2,3,7,8-tetrachlorodibenzo-*p*-dioxin (TCDD) has been found to be hepatocarcinogenic in female but not in male rats (94). This effect seems to be mediated by ovarian hormones, since surgical removal of the ovaries decreases the promoting effect of TCDD on the evolution of AHF in rats that were given DEN as initiator (95). While female rats appear to be more sensitive to promotion by dibenzo-*p*-dioxins and PCB, quite the opposite is the case with the peroxisome proliferator nafenopin (60). Strong sex dependence of promotion of hepatocarcinogenesis in the mouse by phenobarbital has also been observed. While continuous administration of the drug *inhibits* hepatocarcinogenesis in DEN-pretreated (day 15) B6C3F1 male mice, the drug *enhances* liver tumor formation in female mice of this strain under the identical treatment protocol (96). Partial hepatectomy promotes tumorigenesis in livers of male, but not of female, C57BL mice (77,97). The susceptibility to hepatocarcinogenesis is generally higher in male when compared with female mice. This has been attributed to indirect promotional activity of testosterone; male mutants lacking a functional androgen receptor develop much fewer liver tumors upon single carcinogen injection than the corresponding wild-type mice (98).

IV. EFFECTIVENESS OF PROMOTER AS CARCINOGEN WITHOUT INITIATOR; EFFECT OF REVERSION OF THE INITIATION–PROMOTION SEQUENCE

In the multistage model of carcinogenesis, promoters are considered to represent cancer risk factors that are capable of triggering the preferential multiplication of initiated cells without having the potential to initiate alone the process of carcinogenesis (41). Thus, promoters should be inactive at increasing the risk of cancer when given alone. However, administration of high doses of many of the agents in Table 1 has been repeatedly demonstrated to increase the incidence of liver tumors in long-term exposed animals *not* given any carcinogen as initiator (99–103). This has led to the suggestion that these compounds may be regarded as weakly carcinogenic agents (42). This latter supposition cannot be readily ruled out. Although most promoters such as phenobarbital or dieldrin do not seem to react with DNA and lack direct genotoxic activity in *in vitro* and *in vivo* mutagenicity assays (104–106), indirect DNA-damaging activity may occur in some instances. Clastogenic effects have been observed in livers of rats treated with phenobarbital and PCB (107); TCDD and orotic acid have been reported to induce DNA single strand breaks in rat liver (108,109) and long-term exposure of rats to peroxisome proliferators resulted in the formation of 8-hydroxydeoxyguanosine and 5-hydroxyde-oxyuridine in liver DNA (110,111), effects that may be mediated by the formation of reactive oxygen species. Thus, "pure" promoters devoid of any tumor-initiating activity may actually not exist. In fact, discussion about the existence or nonexistence of "pure" promoting agents may be rather academic and outside the reach of scientific investigation. However, as pointed out by Schulte-Hermann (85), the uncertainty about the existence of "pure" promoters should not becloud the fact that there is overwhelming evidence for the existence of the process of promotion, mechanistically different from that of initiation.

Within the framework of multistage models of carcinogenesis, an alternative explanation for the increases in tumor incidence in the livers of animals treated solely with tumor promoters is that these agents may promote tumor precursor populations that arise *spontaneously* as a function of age. In fact, the presence of spontaneously occurring AHF in the livers of rats has been repeatedly reported (112–114) and has been related to the tumorigenic activity of promoters in this target organ (41,85). Since the total number of enzyme-altered precursor cells expands with animal age as a result of increases in AHF number and concomitant growth of these lesions, tumor promoters, when present as single risk factors, should be more effective in aged when compared with young animals. This has in fact been shown to be the case with a variety of different agents including phenobarbital (112,115,116) and the peroxisome proliferators nafenopin (114), Wy-14,643 (117) and di(2-ethylhexyl)phthalate (DEHP) (116).

Differences in the frequency of spontaneously emerging preneoplastic liver lesions between certain strains of mice may also be related to the well-known differences in their susceptibility to liver tumorigenesis mediated by tumor promoters. The tumorigenic activity of dietary phenobarbital in liver of C3H/He mice has been first described by Peraino and coworkers (99). Its tumorigenic activity has been causally linked to the promoter activity of this barbiturate toward spontaneously initiated cells present in this particular strain of mice, characterized by a comparatively high background incidence of spontaneous liver tumors (97). In a more recent experiment reported by Becker (103), the cumulative background liver tumor incidence of about 40% seen in untreated B6C3F1 mice was increased to 80% by dietary phenobarbital treatment, whereas no liver tumors were observed in both untreated *and* phenobarbital-treated C57BL/6N mice, a comparatively "insensitive" strain of mice (97). An enhancement of spontaneous liver tumor incidence mediated by DDT (101) and dieldrin (100) has also been observed in the highly susceptible CF1 mice. Quantitative analyses demonstrated that approximately 60% of untreated control animals developed liver tumors at the end of their lives; treatment with dieldrin led to dose-related increase (above this baseline) in the cumulative incidence of liver tumors, combined with a shortening of the median tumor induction times (118). Interestingly, mutational activation of the c-Ha-*ras* proto-oncogene is a frequent genetic alteration in liver tumors of "sensitive" mouse strains, but is infrequent in "insensitive" strains, suggesting some correlation between mutational activation of the *ras* gene and susceptibility to hepatocarcinogenesis (119).

In summary, these data support the concept that the tumorigenic activity of nondirectly genotoxic liver tumor promoters, which is observed after prolonged treatment with high doses in aged animals and in animals characterized by a high background liver tumor rate, is due to promotion of spontaneously occurring preneoplastic cell populations.

Another observation appears to contradict, however — at least at the first glance — the existence of mechanistic differences between the actions of tumor initiators and promoters in liver. In fact, quantitative analyses of the number and size of AHF produced in rodent liver in sequential carcinogen/promoter treatment protocols indicate promoter-mediated increases not only in the growth kinetics of foci — which is to be expected — but also in the number of foci per liver (5,34,120). In principle, this could be a reflection of the potency of the promoters to initiate the formation of (additional) liver foci. A variety of considerations have to be taken into account, however: a.) A source of error, unfortunately not generally recognized, is that omission of stereological procedures for evaluating the (three-dimensional) number of foci per unit liver from the number and size of their transections can generate false-positive results with regard to foci number (121). Thus, any promoter-mediated increase in the mean size of AHF — which is a hallmark of promoting activity — will, for simple statistical reasons, proportionally increase the frequency of countable focal transections, often referred to as "foci/cm^2"; b.) Even when using appropriate stereology, increases in the number of AHF may only be apparent since — again — due to the growth-stimulatory activity of promoters, small, otherwise undetectable foci may pass over the limits of detection and thus become countable; c.) Finally, various liver tumor promoters have been demonstrated to directly affect the activity of certain marker enzymes used for AHF identification. This is particularly true for the marker enzyme GGT, which is strongly increased in activity by phenobarbital and other tumor promoters in normal liver cells *in vitro* (122) and *in vivo* (123) and in cells located within AHF (6,124). Weak phenotypic expression of marker enzymes in liver foci in animals not treated with promoters and in animals withdrawn from treatment with the promoting agent may thus lead to underestimation of the actual number of lesions (26).

While tumor promoters enhance carcinogenicity toward the liver when given subsequent to a hepatocarcinogen, they frequently reduce carcinogenicity when administered shortly before or simultaneously with a liver carcinogen (9,43,125–128). It is generally assumed that these effects are due to interference with the metabolic activation of the carcinogens (9,129) although other plausible explanations may also exist (130). In addition, experiments have been described in which the initiation–promotion sequence was reversed and a longer time interval between both treatments was chosen to eliminate any direct interference. In these studies neither enhancement nor inhibition of carcinogenesis was noted (131,132).

V. MECHANISMS OF TUMOR PROMOTION IN LIVER

A. Role of Liver Growth, Cell Proliferation, and Cell Death

In analogy to the activity of phorbol esters in mouse skin, liver tumor promoters increase the frequency of liver tumors and shorten, in a dose-dependent manner, the median induction times (133). Both effects can be explained on the basis of multi/two-stage models of carcinogenesis which include as important factors the rates of proliferation and death of tumor precursor populations (10,20,35,134,135). In these models, tumor promoters function by clonal expansion of initiated cells — liver cells in AHF — by increasing their proliferation and/or decreasing their death rates (134,135), both of which increase the probability of additional (genetic) changes leading to malignant cell populations. The important impact of cell proliferation during the promotional phase of carcinogenesis has been stressed by many authors (26,35,37–41,68,85,134–143).

In principle, there exist two basic mechanisms by which promoters could increase the pool of initiated cells: they could either act directly by stimulating their proliferation or decreasing their death rate or both. These effects will be discussed below in more detail. Alternatively, in the "resistant hepatocyte model" developed by Farber and associates (4,37–40), initiated liver cells are generated by brief exposure of animals to a carcinogen such as DEN; they are subsequently selected for rapid proliferation so as to form hyperplastic nodules by exposure to dietary 2-AAF and to a stimulus for hepatocyte proliferation, such as partial hepatectomy or CCl_4 administration (28,68). The selective toxicity of 2-AAF toward normal hepatocytes observed in this system may be explained by both a decreased uptake of this compound by initiated hepatocytes (144) and by a decrease of the generation in the initiated cells of carcinogen metabolites of elevated toxicity (145). Thus, resistance appears to provide the initiated cells with a selective growth advantage in a toxic environment. In fact, preneoplastic cell populations in liver are generally characterized by decreased levels in monooxygenase activity, combined with increased levels of detoxifying Phase II enzymes (11–15,146–149). Differential toxicity, resulting in the selective outgrowth of initiated hepatocytes, may be mediated by many different hepatotoxins such as CCl_4, nitrosamines, and aromatic amines (35,70,71,150) and may represent a general phenomenon (at higher doses) with most hepatotoxins that require metabolic activation. Other mechanisms of differential toxicity are of relevance for agents such as phalloidin (151), orotic acid (72), or diets deficient in choline (68,75). However, most of these effects may well be restricted to those dose levels of the selective agents where cytotoxic effects resulting in regenerative liver growth come into play (137,150,152). Although agents like 2-AAF can strongly enhance the carcinogenic activity of another agent in liver (when administered, for example, in an experimental setting so as to "promote" hepatocarcinogenesis initiated by DEN – as discussed above), the term "promoter" should, in general, be avoided since – by definition – "promoters" should lack initiating capability and direct genotoxic potential. It should be remembered that 2-AAF, which was used in a variety of initiation–promotion studies including the pioneering studies of Peraino and coworkers (43) *as an initiator*, certainly does not fulfill this requirement.

Most of the agents listed in Table 1 belong to a second group of chemicals which enhance hepatocarcinogenesis when given during the promotional phase of the carcinogenic process without showing overt hepatotoxicity. A common denominator of these agents is their ability to induce liver growth (9,25,26,34,45,47,50,56,69,85,130,153,154). This effect is assumed to represent an adaptive response of the organ to meet increased functional demands and is fully reversible upon withdrawal of the inducing agent (153,154). The increase in liver growth may be mediated both by hyperplasia (*i.e.,* increase in cell number) and hypertrophy (*i.e.,* increase in cell size), the latter often coupled with polyploidization of the liver cells (154–156). Although all tumor promoters listed in Table 1 induce an increase in DNA synthesis in liver cells (both normal and initiated) when administered at sufficiently high dose levels, this effect is generally not lasting, but persists only during the first days of treatment until the liver mass has reached a new elevated plateau. The percentage of hepatocytes that enter a phase of increased DNA synthesis decreases to control levels both in normal liver tissue and in AHF upon continuous treatment with agents such as phenobarbital, α-BHC[2], some steroid hormones, and the peroxisome proliferators nafenopin, clofibric acid, and DEHP (25,56,136,157,158). Some other tumor promoters, including the peroxisome proliferator

---

[2]α-Benzenehexachloride, widely used misnomer term for α-hexachlorocyclohexane.

Wy-14,643 (158,159), ethinyl estradiol (160), and TCDD (95), appear to induce persistent increase in DNA synthesis, which probably reflects regenerative cell turnover associated with hepatotoxicity.

The mechanisms of promoter-mediated stimulation of proliferation are only partially understood. In principle, liver-enlarging tumor promoters could directly stimulate hepatocyte proliferation similar to the physiological peptide growth factors such as epidermal growth factor (EGF), transforming growth factor α, hepatocyte growth factor, acidic fibroblast growth factor, hepatopoietin B, and hepatocyte stimulatory substance (161). Alternatively, tumor promoters could act indirectly by inducing endogenous hepatocyte growth factors or modulating their receptor activity, by exhibiting co-mitogenic activity with such growth factors, or by inhibiting negative growth control functions (161).

A decrease in EGF receptor binding associated with autophosphorylation and internalization of the receptor has been observed in liver plasma membranes following exposure of rats and mice to TCDD (162,163). Similarly, 3,3′,4,4′-tetrachlorobiphenyl and phenobarbital decreased EGF receptor binding in cultured hepatocytes (164,165). A diminution in binding capacity of hepatic estrogen and glucocorticoid receptors has also been reported to occur in TCDD–treated mice (166). Decreases in EGF receptor binding have been observed in regenerating liver and in persistent liver nodules (167,168) and are reminiscent of responses characteristic of excess EGF (169). Decreases in receptor binding may render preneoplastic and neoplastic liver cells less responsive to environmental signals (168). The significance of the observed EGF receptor changes, however, remains unclear since a variety of liver tumor promoters, including 3,3′,4,4′-tetrachlorobiphenyl and phenobarbital, neither affected the number of hepatic EGF receptors when administered *in vivo* (162) nor increased the receptor levels (170).

A variety of studies have shown cooperative effects between liver tumor promoters and peptide growth factors in the induction of hepatocyte proliferation in primary culture (141,164,170,171). Co-mitogenic effects of estrogens may also explain the ineffectiveness of TCDD to increase the labeling index of hepatocytes and to promote hepatocarcinogenesis in ovariectomized rats when compared with intact rats (95).

Finally, tumor promoters may inhibit negative control pathways of hepatocyte proliferation. The activity of transforming growth factor β (TGFβ) in this respect has been known for some time (161,172,173) and the inhibition by estradiol of TGF β–mediated negative growth control was reported (141). TGFβ induces cell death in cultured rat hepatocytes (174), which most probably represents apoptosis (programmed cell death) (175). Liver tumor promoters decrease the rate of apoptosis of cells in AHF (26,176,177). Stoppage of promoter treatment results in a rapid wave of death in both normal and initiated cells (26,176–178).

In summary, liver tumor promoters affect the rates of proliferation and of death of normal and initiated hepatocytes. Both, increases in proliferation and decreases in death rates of the initiated cells contribute to the observed changes in the growth behavior of AHF during promoter treatment, which may ultimately result in an earlier appearance of more malignant cell populations (143,179).

B. Changes in Gap-junction–Mediated Intercellular Communication

Hepatocyte proliferation is not only controlled by the growth factors and hormones described above, but also by direct cell-to-cell coupling via gap junctions which allows the transfer of ions and low–molecular weight molecules (*see* recent reviews 180–182).

Gap-junction–mediated intercellular communication can be measured by a variety of different methods, such as the test for metabolic cooperation, electric coupling, and dye transfer between cells (183). Tumor cells generally show decreased levels of intercellular communication and may thus be liberated from growth constraints delivered by their surrounding normal counterparts (180–184). In addition, a selective interruption of gap-junction–mediated cell-to-cell communication between tumor and normal cells has been observed (185). *See also* Chapter 7 in this volume.

Tumor promoters are capable of inhibiting gap-junction–mediated intercellular communication. This has been first described independently by Yotti et al. (186) and Murray and Fitzgerald (187) in 1979 for phorbol ester–type tumor promoters. In subsequent studies, a large number of promoting agents, including many liver-specific tumor promoters, have been investigated for their ability to inhibit intercellular communication. These include phenobarbital (188,189), pesticides such as DDT (188–190), aldrin (191) and lindane (189), various polyhalogenated biphenyls (192) and peroxisome proliferators such as DEHP (193), nafenopin, and clofibric acid (194). There are some remarkable exceptions: TCDD does not interfere with metabolic cooperation in V79 cells (195). It has been pointed out, however, that V79 cells may not be the appropriate test cells in this respect, because they are not the target cells for promotion by dibenzodioxins (181). In fact, some target cell specificity has been observed for phenobarbital, which inhibits gap-junction–mediated intercellular communication in rat hepatocytes, but not in 3T3 cells, when both cell types are cocultured (181).

Lack of interference with intercellular communication, which is seen with some, but not other, polyhalogenated biphenyls, has been suggested to be related to differences in the mechanism of tumor promotion by these chemicals (180). Thus, 3,3′,4,4′-tetrachloro-biphenyl and 3,3′,4,4′,5,5′ hexabromobiphenyl, both 3-methylcholanthrene (3-MC)-type inducers of cytochrome P-450 and potent promoters of hepatocarcinogenesis in rats (50,196), did not inhibit gap-junction–mediated intercellular communication (181,192). In contrast, phenobarbital-type inducers of cytochrome P-450 such as 2,2′,4,4′,5,5′-hexachlorobiphenyl, 2,3,4,4′,5-pentachlorobiphenyl, and 2,2′,4,4′,5,5′-hexabromo-biphenyl, all effective liver tumor promoters in rats (49,50,196), were also effective in interrupting cell-to-cell communication via gap junctions (181,192). While promotion by 3-MC inducer-type polyhalogenated biphenyls has been suggested to occur by an indirect mechanism only at those dose levels associated with overt hepatotoxicity, polyhalogenated biphenyls of the phenobarbital inducer-type may act by directly stimulating the proliferation of initiated hepatocytes (196). Inhibition of intercellular communication by 3-MC inducer-type polyhalogenated biphenyls may thus only occur at doses associated with cell killing. In this respect, it is interesting to note that a reduction in gap-junction proteins has been observed during regenerative liver cell growth following partial hepatectomy (197).

Decrease in the expression of gap-junction proteins may be a general cause for inhibition of intercellular communication between adjacent cells. Such decrease has been observed in rat liver tumors (198,199) as well as in subpopulations of AHF (199). Phenobarbital and DDT treatment of rats induced structural changes in hepatocyte gap junctions, which may be associated with inhibitory effects of these agents on intercellular communication (188). Similarly, phenobarbital caused a reduction of gap junction proteins in AHF of mouse liver (200). While only very few foci expressed decreased levels of gap junction proteins in the absence of phenobarbital, most foci displayed decreased levels—as shown by immunohistochemical staining—after a 28-day treatment with the tumor promoter. In AHF this effect was mostly reversible upon phenobarbital withdrawal, but not in hepatomas (200).

C. Role of Reactive Oxygen Species

Evidence in favor of the hypothesis that reactive oxygen species may be involved in the process of tumor promotion originated from studies on the action of phorbol ester–type tumor promoters in mouse skin, as has been discussed in detail in Section I of this chapter. There are at least two lines of evidence to suggest that oxygen radicals may also play some role during tumor promotion in liver. First, antioxidants generally decrease the preneoplastic or neoplastic response in liver when given during the promotional phase of hepatocarcinogenesis. For example, 11 out of 22 compounds found to inhibit hepatocarcinogenesis, when given subsequent to an initiating dose of DEN, were antioxidants (62). Second, a large number of tumor promoters have been demonstrated to increase the formation of hydrogen peroxide and superoxide anion radicals, and induce lipid peroxidation in livers of exposed rodents. Measurements were performed in liver subcellular fractions or by determining ethane exhalation *in vivo*. Such promoters include PCB (50,201), TCDD (108,202), barbiturates (203) and peroxisome proliferators (204–206). Often, however, the effects were very weak and were only seen at extraordinarily high doses. This is especially true for certain PCB (201) and TCDD, where negative results have also been reported (207). Most pronounced effects are seen with peroxisome proliferators, which are assumed to enhance the production of H_2O_2 in rodent liver by increasing peroxisomal enzyme systems involved in the β-oxidation of lipids (205,206). Generation of reactive oxygen species may also be mediated by cytochrome P-450–dependent liver monooxygenases (203). Many liver tumor promoters are inducers of liver monooxygenases. Positive correlations between induction of cytochrome P-450 and promoting activity have been observed within series of structural analogs of polyhalogenated biphenyls (50) and barbiturates (81,87,208). Moreover, the dose-response curves for the induction of cytochrome P-450 by 2,4,8,-trichlorodibenzofuran in rat liver and promotion of AHF in this organ were very similar (209). Finally, phenobarbital does not induce cytochrome P-450 in hamsters, a species also not susceptible to promotion by this compound (87). However, since certain other liver tumor promoters, such as the synthetic estrogens, do not significantly induce cytochrome P-450, the induction of liver monooxygenases does not appear to be necessary for tumor promotion in this organ (56,210).

Although reactive oxygen species may be involved in tumor promotion in liver, their exact mechanism of action remains unclear. As has been discussed above, in principle they could act either directly on initiated cells by modifying the expression of genes controlling their proliferation and/or differentiation, or indirectly by decreasing the growth rate of surrounding normal cells *via* selective toxicity. The observation of decreased levels of lipid peroxidation in AHF when compared with the surrounding tissue is in favor of the latter assumption (211). Similarly, in livers of peroxisome proliferator–treated rats, lipofuscin deposits, which are indicative of lipid peroxidation, were much more frequent in normal hepatocytes than in cells of AHF (212). Differences in the intracellular glutathione (GSH) levels between normal and tumor precursor cells could account for selective toxicity during oxidative stress. Increase in the activity of the enzyme GGT in AHF may—by enhancing their intracellular GSH level—provide the focal cells a selective advantage in a toxic environment, while at the same time GSH may be depleted in the surrounding GGT-negative cells (213). In fact, increased GSH levels have been observed in cells of AHF (214), and GGT-positive hepatocytes appear to be less susceptible to oxidative stress than GGT-negative ones (215). Although selective toxicity appears to be a plausible explanation for reactive oxygen-mediated promoting effects, there are other findings which contradict this idea. During rat hepatocarcinogenesis, the levels of chemiluminescence, indicative of reactive oxygen species, were always higher in tissue homogenates from liver nodules when compared with homogenates from the normal surrounding tissue, and the highest chemiluminescence levels were seen in the nodular tissue during phenobarbital treatment (216). This relative increase in reactive oxygen generation was already present in small AHF and correlated well with induction of cytochrome P-450 in these lesions (216). Reactive oxygen may lead to the formation of 8-hydroxydeoxyguanosine and 5-hydroxydeoxyuridine in DNA, as was observed in rat liver following treatment with peroxisome proliferators (110,111,206) and may cause misreading during DNA replication (217). Whether or not mutational changes in DNA are of any relevance during the promotional phase of hepatocarcinogenesis, however, remains unclear (218).

VI. QUANTITATIVE ASPECTS OF TUMOR PROMOTION IN LIVER

The stereological analysis of AHF offers a valuable tool to study the initiating and promoting potencies of liver cancer risk factors (5,20,34,35,41,51,71,120,121,142, 143,150,179,219). Since AHF are monoclonal in origin (21–23), the number of foci gives a rough estimate of the initiating potency of a test agent (35,71,150,219). By contrast, promoter-mediated clonal expansion of cells within AHF leads to changes in the *size distribution* of these lesions in liver (35,71,150,219). Under those circumstances, where evidence has accumulated from previous experiments that an agent under investigation does not significantly increase the number of AHF when administered without prior initiation, *i.e.*, does not or only very weakly initiate AHF formation, changes in the volume fraction (%) of AHF in liver produced by promoters in initiation–promotion experiments may serve as a rough measure of their promoting activity. Accordingly, a promotion index has been recently defined by Pitot and coworkers (219) as:

$$\text{Promotion index} = V_f/V_c \times \text{mmol}^{-1} \times \text{weeks}^{-1}$$

where V_f is the total volume fraction of AHF in livers of animals that were given an initiator followed by the test agent, V_c the total volume fraction in animals treated with the initiator alone, and the dose used and the duration of treatment are expressed in mmoles and weeks. The promotion indices for a number of xenobiotics are listed in Table 2.

This simple equation displays some shortcomings which have been pointed out by the authors themselves (219): for example, both dose and time response of promotion may not be linear, and the strain and sex of test animals as well as differences in the initiation–promotion protocols used in different laboratories may affect the experimental outcome. This explains the wide variations in the magnitude of the promotion index as determined for a given compound in different experiments (*see* Table 2). Despite these obvious shortcomings, the promotion index provides a semiquantitative measure of the relative promoting potencies of different agents. The search continues for a more accurate definition of the promoting potency using more complex mathematical treatment, such as described recently by Luebeck *et al.* (143) and Moolgavkar and coworkers (179,220).

The dose–response characteristics of various liver tumor promoters have been repeatedly investigated (34,51,120,133,209,219,221). In most of these initiation–promotion studies, saturation of promoter effectiveness was observed at high doses, which may be interpreted as a reflection of the limited number of initiated cells accessible for promotion (34,120,133,219). Nonlinearity of promoting efficacy has also been observed within low promoter dose range (34,120,133,221). From this, it has been concluded that promoters may possess no-effect or threshold levels of activity (34,120,133,221–224).

TABLE 2. Promotion Index of Some Selected Liver Tumor Promoters

Promoter[a]	Promotion Index[b]	Rat strain	Sex	References
TCDD	1.0×10^6	Fisher	f	219
	2.8×10^7	S.D.	f	51
3,3',4,4'-TCBP	182	Wistar	f	50
3,3',4,4'-TBBP	5,400	Wistar	f	50
Phenobarbital	6	Fisher	f	219
	75	S.D.	f	219
	13	Wistar	f	51
	30[c]	Fisher	m	54
	10[c]	Fisher	m	62
Barbital	0.8[c]	Fisher	m	62
Ethinyl estradiol	2,300[c]	Fisher	m	54
	1,100[c]	Fisher	m	62
	19,000	S.D.	f	157
Wy-14,643	63	Fisher	m	59,219
Nafenopin	48	Wistar	f	60
α-BHC	6[c]	Fisher	m	62
Dieldrin	57[c]	Fisher	m	62

[a]*Abbreviations used*: TCDD for 2,3,7,8-tetrachlorodibenzo-*p*-dioxin; TCBP for tetrachlorobiphenyl; TBBP for tetrabromobiphenyl; BHC for benzenehexachloride, the misnomer term generally used to designate hexachlorocyclohexane ("Lindane").

[b]The promotion index has been defined by Pitot and coworkers (219) as: $V_f/V_c \times$ mmole^{-1} $\times$ weeks^{-1}, where V_f is the volume fraction of altered hepatic foci in livers of animals that received the initiator followed by the test agent, while V_c is the volume fraction of controls given the initiator only.

[c]Rats underwent partial hepatectomy during promoter treatment.

However, nonlinearity can not be taken as proof for threshold, since all cancer risk factors, independent of their mode of action, may exhibit this kind of dose–response characteristic at very low doses when administered during the promotional phase subsequent to an initiator.

In analogy to the phorbol esters in mouse skin, a variety of liver-specific tumor promoters act at very low, hormone like concentrations. In fact, specific high-affinity receptors have been described for dibenzo-*p*-dioxins, dibenzofurans, certain PCB (225), estrogens (226), and peroxisome proliferators (227) and it is likely that the promoting effects are (indirectly) mediated *via* receptor binding. Whether or not threshold concentrations exist for receptor-mediated processes is a matter of debate (137,228).

The influence of the duration of promoter treatment on hepatocarcinogenesis has been investigated in several studies (34,51,63,120,229,231). Mostly, although not always, prolongation of the treatment period led to increases in the number of AHF and their volumetric fraction in liver, as well as to increases in the incidence and multiplicity of adenomas and carcinomas. The fact that the *number* of AHF increases only during the first months of continuous treatment, reaching a plateau from there on (34,120), is one of the strong arguments in favor of the existence of mechanistic differences in the action of initiators and promoters. Very short periods of promoter exposure appear to be ineffective in enhancing hepatocarcinogenesis (229,230).

In contrast to initiation, tumor promotion may include some reversible component. This assumption originated from studies in mouse skin which showed a.) a strong decrease in promoter effectiveness upon partitioning into intermittent exposures a total dose that is active in continuous treatment, and b.) a pronounced decrease in the number of benign papillomas after stoppage of promoter treatment (232,233). Similarly, a decrease in the number of detectable AHF and liver nodules after withdrawal of the promoting stimulus has also been observed in liver (26,34,37–40,234–237). This effect of "reversibility" is most dramatically seen in experimental protocols employing differential toxicity as a means to generate a selective pressure (4,37–40,237,238) and may include phenomena that have been variously named "remodeling", "redifferentiation", and "phenotypic maturation" (40,234,237,238). Increase in the rate of apoptosis after the cessation of promoter treatment (26,85,176,177) may lead to the extinction of a certain proportion of AHF. A decrease in AHF number, however, has not been consistently detected (120) and stop experiments with phenobarbital indicated that the *volume fraction* of AHF, which reflects the total number of initiated cells in liver, may still increase after promoter withdrawal (34,50,239) and even more dramatically after its readministration (239). This may be interpreted that although some AHF phenotypically "normalize" during promoter-free treatment periods, they retain a potential to reexpress the altered phenotype. This would also explain why there was no dramatic decrease, or none at all, in experiments with intermittent promoter exposure (34,63,240). A concept that may be useful to consider at this point is the following. Within the framework of mathematical carcinogenicity models (134,135,137) any promoter-mediated expansion of the pool of initiated cells, even if temporally limited to the period of direct exposure, would seem to be inevitably associated with an increase in the overall risk of cancer, thus pointing towards an irreversible component of promotion.

VII. RELEVANCE OF LIVER TUMOR PROMOTERS TO HUMANS

The question as to whether or not agents that promote hepatocarcinogenesis in rodents increase the risk of cancer in humans has been addressed in a large number of epidemiological studies. Exposure of individuals to TCDD, the most powerful tumor promoter in rodent liver, may be associated with only a very slight increase in overall cancer mortality (241,242). Liver tumors, however, were not among the cancers that were found to be possibly elevated (241,242). Similarly, as recently reviewed by Silberhorn and coworkers (83), there is no convincing evidence that polyhalogenated biphenyls increase the risk of hepatocellular cancer in humans. Treatment of patients, hospitalized for epilepsy, with phenobarbital, phenytoin, and other anticonvulsants does not appear to be associated with increased liver cancer incidence (243–246). The carcinogenic and/or promoting activity of peroxisome proliferators in rodent liver is most likely linked to their ability to stimulate the proliferation of peroxisomes. The presence of this latter activity is questionable in humans (248). An exception may be represented by synthetic estrogens in oral contraceptives which, when taken for prolonged periods of time, may lead in a small percentage of women to benign hepatic adenomas (248,249) and possibly also to carcinomas (250). The fact that some of the adenomas regress upon cessation of oral contraceptive treatment (251) supports a promoter-like action of the synthetic steroids.

Primary hepatocellular carcinoma (HCC) is among the ten most important human cancers worldwide (252). Its frequency distribution, however, varies considerably between different geographical areas in the world. While the incidence of HCC is comparatively low in most industrialized countries, there are certain areas of high risk in southern Africa and southern China, where both hepatitis B virus and aflatoxins are suspect etiological risk factors (253). While aflatoxins may act by generating mutations in relevant cell regulatory genes, such as p53 (254–256), the role of hepatitis B virus is less clear. Recent studies with transgenic mice, that overproduce the hepatitis B virus large envelope polypeptide and accumulate large quantities of hepatitis B surface antigen in the hepatocytes, demonstrate a strong correlation between the induction of prolonged hepatocellular injury and HCC development (257). Thus, induction of chronic liver cell necrosis and regeneration caused by viral infection or other stimuli such as alcohol abuse (258), glycogen storage disease (259), primary biliary cirrhosis (260) or, in the case of the LEC rat, by inheritance of a genetic disorder (261) may—in analogy to the effect of wounding in mouse skin (*see* preceding Section)—provide a "promoting" stimulus that may well favor the outgrowth of preneoplastic cell populations and the acquisition of secondary genetic events associated with cell transformation (137,152,257).

Abbreviations Used in Sections I and II: 2-AAF, 2-acetylaminoflourene; AHF, altered hepatic foci; BaP, benzo[*a*]pyrene; bFGF, fibroblast growth factor b; BHA, butylhydroxyanisol; BHC, benzenehexachloride (misnomer term used for hexachlorocyclohexane); BHT, butylated hydroxytoluene; DAG, diacylglycerol; DEN, diethylnitrosamine; DEHP, di(2-ethylhexyl)phthalate; DMBA, 7,12-dimethylbenz[*a*]anthracene; EGF, epidermal growth factor; ETYA, eicosa-5,8,11,14-tetraynoic acid; GGT, γ-glutamyl transferase; GSH, glutathione; HCC, hepatocellular carcinoma; HETE, hydroxyeicosatetraenoic acids; HPETE, hydroperoxyeicosatetraenoic acids; Il-1, interleukin-1; IP_3, inositol-1,4,5-triphosphate; LTB_4, leukotriene B_4; 3-MC, 3-methylcholanthrene; MNNG, *N*-methyl-*N'*-nitro-*N*-nitrosoguanidine; ODC, ornithine decarboxylase; PAF, platelet-activating factor; PCB, polychlorinated biphenyls; PDGF, platelet-derived growth factor; PG, prostaglandin; PKC, protein kinase C; PMA, phorbol myristate acetate; RPA, 12-*O*-retinoylphorbol-13-acetate; RRME, Roussin red methyl ester; SOD, superoxide dismutase; TCDD, 2,3,7,8-tetrachlorodibenzo-*p*-dioxin; TGFα or β, transforming growth factor α or β; TPA, 12-*O*-tetradecanoylphorbol-13-acetate; TNF, tumor necrosis factor; TRE, TPA-responsive element; UV, ultraviolet.

REFERENCES

1. Bannasch, P., and Müller, H. A.: *Arzneim.-Forsch.* **14**, 805 (1964).
2. Gössner, W., and Friedrich-Freksa, H.: *Z. Naturforsch.* **B19**, 862 (1964).
3. Kalengayi, M. M., Ronchi, G., and Desmet, V. J.: *J. Natl. Cancer Inst.* **55**, 579 (1975).
4. Solt, D., and Farber, E.: *Nature* **263**, 701 (1976).
5. Pitot, H. C., Barsness, L., Goldsworthy, T., and Kitagawa, T.: *Nature* **271**, 456 (1978).
6. Schauer, A., and Kunze, E.: *Z. Krebsforsch.* **70**, 252 (1968).
7. Börner, P., and Gössner, W.: *Z. Naturforsch. B* **23**, 1085 (1968).
8. Kitagawa, T.: *Gann* **62**, 207 (1971).
9. Kunz, W., Appel, K. E., Rickart, R., Schwarz, M., and Stöckle, G. Enhancement and Inhibition of Carcinogenic Effectiveness of Nitrosamines. *In* "Primary Liver Tumors" (H. Remmer, H. M. Bolt, P. Bannasch, and H. Popper, eds.). MTP Press, Int. Medical Publishers, Lancaster, U.K., 1978, p. 261.
10. Emmelot, P., and Scherer, E.: *Biochim. Biophys. Acta* **605**, 247 (1980).
11. Aström, A., de Pierre, J. W., and Eriksson, L.: *Carcinogenesis* **4**, 577 (1983).
12. Buchmann, A., Kuhlmann, W., Schwarz, M., Kunz, W., Wolf, C. R., Moll, E., Friedberg, T., and Oesch, F.: *Carcinogenesis* **6**, 513 (1985).
13. Bock, K. W., Lilienblum, W., Pfeil, H., and Erickson, L.C.: *Cancer Res.* **42**, 3747 (1982).
14. Sato, K., Kitahara, A., Satoh, K., Ishikawa, T., Tatematsu, M., and Ito, N.: *Gann* **75**, 199 (1984).
15. Tatematsu, M., Tsuda, H., Shirai, T. Masui, T., and Ito, N.: *Toxicol. Pathol.* **15**, 60 (1987).
16. Bannasch, P.: *Recent Resu. Cancer Res.* **19**, 1 (1968).
17. Bannasch, P., Mayer, D., and Hacker, H. J.: *Biochim. Biophys. Acta* **605**, 217 (1980).
18. Moore, M. A., Nakagawa, K., Satoh, K., Ishikawa, T., and Sato, K.: *Carcinogenesis* **8**, 483 (1987).
19. Peraino, C., Richards, W. L., and Stevens, F. J.: Multistage Carcinogenesis. *In* "Mechanisms of Tumor Promotion" (T. J. Slaga, ed.). CRC Press, Boca Raton, Florida, 1983, p. 1.
20. Pitot, H. C.: *Annu. Rev. Pharmacol. Toxicol.* **30**, 465 (1990).
21. Scherer, E., and Hoffmann, M.: *Eur. J. Cancer* **7**, 369 (1971).
22. Rabes, H. M., Bücher, T., Hartmann, A., Linke, I., and Dünnwald, M.: *Cancer Res.* **42**, 3220 (1982).
23. Weinberg, W. C., Berkwits, L., and Innaccone, P. M.: *Carcinogenesis* **8**, 565 (1987).

24. Scherer, E., and Emmelot, P.: *Eur. J. Cancer* **11**, 689 (1975).
25. Schulte-Hermann, R., Ohde, G., Schuppler, J., and Timmermann-Trosiener. I.: *Cancer Res.* **41**, 2556 (1981).
26. Schulte-Hermann, R., Timmermann-Troisiener, I., Barthel, G., and Bursch, W.: *Cancer Res.* **50**, 5127 (1990).
27. Rabes, H. M., Scholze, P., and Jantsch, B.: *Cancer Res.* **32**, 2577 (1972).
28. Rotstein, J., Sarma, D. S. R., and Farber, E.: *Cancer Res.* **46**, 2377 (1986).
29. Bannasch, P.: *J. Gastroenterol. Hepatol.* **5**, 149 (1990).
30. Goldfarb, S., and Pugh, T. D.: *Cancer Res.* **41**, 2092 (1981).
31. Potter, V. R.: *Carcinogenesis* **3**, 1375 (1981).
32. Potter, V. R.: *Cancer Res.* **44**, 2733 (1984).
33. Scherer, E.: *Arch. Toxicol. Suppl.* **10**, 81 (1987).
34. Kunz, H. W., Tennekes, H. A., Port, R. E., Schwarz, M., Lorke, D, and Schaude, G.: *Environ. Health Perspect.* **50**, 113 (1983).
35. Schwarz, M., Pearson, D., Buchmann, A., and Kunz, W.: The Use of Enzyme-Altered Foci for Risk Assessment of Hepatocarcinogens. *In* "Biologically Based Methods for Cancer Risk Assessment" (C. Travis, ed.), NATO ASI Series. Plenum, New York, 1989, p. 31.
36. Vesselinovitch, S. D., and Mihailovitch, N.: *Cancer Res.* **43**, 4253 (1983).
37. Farber, E., *Cancer Res.* **33**, 2537 (1973).
38. Farber, E.: *Biochim. Biophys. Acta* **605**, 149 (1980).
39. Farber, E., and Cameron, R.: *Adv. Cancer Res.* **31**, 125 (1980).
40. Farber, E.: *Cancer Res.* **44**, 4217 (1984).
41. Pitot, H.C., and Sirica, A. E.: *Biochim. Biophys. Acta* **605**, 191 (1980).
42. Bannasch, P.: *Carcinogenesis* **7**, 689 (1986).)
43. Peraino, C., Fry, R. J. M., and Staffeldt, E.: *Cancer Res.* **31**, 1506 (1971).
44. Peraino C., Fry, R. J. M., Staffeldt, E., and Christopher, E.: *Cancer Res.* **35**, 2884 (1975).
45. Kunz, H. W., Schwarz, M, Tennekes, H., Port, R., and Appel, K. E.: Mechanism and Dose-Time Response Characteristics of Carcinogenic and Tumor Promoting Xenobiotics in Liver. *In* "Tumorpromotoren: Erkennung, Wirkungsmechanismen und Bedeutung" (K. E. Appel and A. G. Hildebrandt, eds.), BGA-Schriften 6, MMV Medizin. Verl., Munich, 1985, p. 76.
46. Kitagawa, T., and Sugano, H.: *Gann* **69**, 679 (1978).
47. Schulte-Hermann, R., and Parzefall, W.: *Cancer Res.* **41**, 4140 (1981).
48. Deml, E., and Oesterle, D.: *Carcinogenesis* **3**, 1449 (1982).
49. Jensen, R. K., Sleight, S. D., Goodman, J. I., Aust, S. D., and Trosko, J. E.: *Carcinogenesis* **3**, 1183 (1982).
50. Buchmann, A., Ziegler, S., Wolf, A., Robertson, L. W., Durham, S. K., Schwarz, M.: *Toxicol. Appl. Pharmacol.* **111**, 454 (1991).
51. Pitot, H. C., Goldsworthy, T., Campbell, H. A., and Poland, A.: *Cancer Res.* **40**, 3616 (1980).
52. Taper, H. S.: *Cancer* **42**, 462 (1978).
53. Yager, J. D., and Yager, R.: *Cancer Res.* **40**, 3680 (1980).
54. Cameron, R. G., Imaida, K., Tsuda, H., and Ito, N.: *Cancer Res.* **42**, 2426 (1982).
55. Yager, J. D., Campbell, H. A., Longnecker, D. S., Roebuck, B. D., and Benoit, M. C.: *Cancer Res.* **44**, 3862 (1984).
56. Ochs, H., Düsterberg, B., Günzel, P., and Schulte-Hermann, R.: *Cancer Res.* **46**, 1224 (1986).
57. Mochizuki, Y., Furukawa, K., and Sawada, N.: *Carcinogenesis* **3**, 1027 (1982).
58. Ward, J. M., Rice, J. M., Creasia, D., Lynch, P., and Riggs, D.: *Carcinogenesis* **4**, 1021 (1983).
59. Glauert, H. P., Beer, D., Rao, M. S., Schwarz, M., Xu, Y.-D., and Goldsworthy, T. L.: *Cancer Res.* **46**, 4601 (1986).
60. Kraupp-Grasl, B., Huber, W., Putz, B., Gerbracht, U., and Schulte-Hermann, R.: *Cancer Res.* **50**, 3701 (1990).
61. Tsuda, H., Masui, T., Imaida, K., Fukushima, S., and Ito, N.: *Gann* **75**, 871 (1984).
62. Ito, N., Tsuda, H., Tatematsu, M., Inoue, T., Tagawa, Y., Aoki, T., Uwagawa, S., Kagawa, M., Osigo, T., Masui, T., Imaida, K., Fukushima, S., and Asamoto, M.: *Carcinogenesis* **9**, 387 (1988).
63. Dashwood, R. H., Fong, A. T., Williams, D. E., Hendricks, J. D., and Bailey, G. S.: *Cancer Res.* **51**, 2362 (1991).
64. Dragani, T. A., Manenti, G., and Porta, G. D.: *Cancer Lett.* **31**, 171 (1986).
65. Columbano, A., Ledda-Columbano, G. M., Ennas, M. G., Curto, M., Chelo, A., and Pani, P.: *Carcinogenesis* **11**, 771 (1990).
66. Tanaka, T., Mori, H., and Williams, G. M.: *Carcinogenesis* **8**, 1171 (1987).
67. Deml, E., and Oesterle, D.: *Cancer Lett.* **29**, 59 (1985).
68. Columbano, A., Rajalakshmi, S., and Sarma, D. S. R.: *Cancer Res.* **41**, 2079 (1981).

69. Schwarze, P. E., Petterson, E. O., Shoaib, M. C., and Seglen, P. O.: *Carcinogenesis* **5**, 1267 (1984).
70. Kuchlbauer, J., Romen, W., and Neumann, H.-G.: *Carcinogenesis* **9**, 1337 (1985).
71. Schwarz, M, Pearson, D., Port, R., and Kunz, W.: *Carcinogenesis* **5**, 725 (1984).
72. Rao, P. M., Nagamine, K., Ho, R.-K., Roomi, M. W., Laurier, C., Rajalakshmi, S., and Sarma, D. S. R.: *Carcinogenesis* **4**, 1541 (1983).
73. Hei, T. K., and Sudilovsky, O.: *Cancer Res.* **45**, 2700 (1985).
74. Enzmann, H., Ohlhauser, D., Dettler, T., and Bannasch, P.: *Carcinogenesis* **10**, 1247 (1989).
75. Yokoyama, S., Sells, M. A., Reddy, T. V., and Lombardi, B.: *Cancer Res.* **45**, 2834 (1985).
76. Pound, A. W., and McGuire, L. J.: *Br. J. Cancer* **37**, 595 (1978).
77. Hanigan, M. H., Winkler, M. L., and Drinkwater, N. R.: *Carcinogenesis* **11**, 589 (1990).
78. Preat, V. P., Pector, J. C., Taper, H., Lans, M., de Gelache, L., and Roberfroid, M.: *Carcinogenesis* **5**, 1151 (1984).
79. Nakanishi, K., Fukushima, S., Hagiwara, A., Tamano, S., and Ito, N.: *J. Natl. Cancer. Inst.* **68**, 497 (1982).
80. Hiasa, Y., Kitahori, Y, Konishi, N., Enoki, N., and Fujita, T.: *Carcinogenesis* **4**, 935 (1982)
81. Diwan, B. A., Rice, J. M., Nims, R. W., Lubet, R. A., Hu, H., and Ward, J. M.: *Cancer Res.* **48**, 2492 (1988).
82. Hirose, M., Shirai, T., Tsuda, H., Fukushima, S., Ogiso, T. and Ito, N.: *Carcinogenesis* **2**, 1299 (1981).
83. Silberhorn, E. M., Glauert, H. P., and Robertson, L. W.: *CRC Crit. Rev. Toxicol.* **20**, 439 (1990).
84. Poland, A., Palen, D., and Glover, E.: *Nature* **300**, 271 (1982).
85. Schulte-Hermann, R.: *Arch. Toxicol.* **57**, 147 (1985).
86. Palmer, A. E., Rice, J. M., Ward, J. M., Oshima, M., Cicmanek, J. L., Dove, L. F., and Lynch, P. H.: *Proc. Am. Assoc. Cancer Res.* **25**, 560 (1984).
87. Lubet, R. A., Nims, R. W., Ward, J. M., Rice, J. M., and Diwan, B. A.: *J. Am. Coll. Toxicol.* **8**, 259 (1989).
88. Stenbäck, F., Mori, H., Furuya, K., and Williams, G. M.: *J. Natl. Cancer Inst.* **76**, 327 (1986).
89. Pereira, M. A., Knutsen, G. L., and Herren-Freud, S. L.: *Carcinogenesis* **6**, 203 (1984).
90. Pereira, M. A., Klaunig, J. E., Herren-Freud, S. L., and Ruch, R. J.: *J. Natl. Cancer Inst.* **77**, 449 (1986).
91. Diwan, B. A., Rice, J. M., Oshima, M., and Ward, J. M.: *Carcinogenesis* **7**, 215 (1986).
92. Klaunig, J. E., Weghorst, C. M., and Pereira, M. A.: *Toxicol. Appl. Pharmacol.* **90**, 79 (1987).
93. Deml, E., and Oesterle, D.: *Carcinogenesis* **3**, 1449 (1982).
94. Kociba, R. J., Keyes, D. G., Beyer, J. E., Carreon, R. M., Wade, C. E., Dittenber, D. A., Kalnins, R. P., Frauson, L. E., Park, C. N., Barnard, S. D., Hummel, R. A., and Humiston, C. G.: *Toxicol. Appl. Pharmacol.* **46**, 279 (1978).
95. Lucier, G. W., Tritscher, A., Goldsworthy, T., Foley, J., Clark, G., Goldstein, J., and Maronpot, R.: *Cancer Res.* **51**, 1391 (1991).
96. Weghorst, C. M., and Klaunig, J. E.: *Carcinogenesis* **10**, 609 (1989).
97. Drinkwater, N. R., Hanigan, M. H., and Kemp, C. J.: Genetic and Epigenetic Promotion of Murine Hepatocarcinogenesis. *In* "Mouse Liver Carcinogenesis: Mechanisms and Species Comparisons" (D. E. Stevenson, J. A. Popp, J. M. Ward, R. M. McClain, T. J. Slaga, and H. C. Pitot, eds.). Alan R. Liss, New York, 1990, p. 163.
98. Kemp, C. J., Leary, C. N., and Drinkwater, N. R.: *Proc. Natl. Acad. Sci. U.S.A* **86**, 7505 (1989).
99. Peraino, C., Fry, R. J. M., and Staffeldt, E.: *J. Natl. Cancer Inst.* **51**, 1349 (1973).
100. Walker, A. I. T., Thorpe, E., and Stevenson, D. E.: *Food Cosmet. Toxicol.* **11**, 415 (1973).
101. Tomatis, L., Turosov, V., Day, N., and Charles, R. T.: *Int. J. Cancer* **10**, 489 (1972).
102. Rossi, L., Ravera, M., Repetti, G. and Santi, L.: *Int. J. Cancer* **19**, 179 (1977).
103. Becker, F. F.: *Cancer Res.* **45**, 768 (1985).
104. Ashby, J.: *Mutagenesis* **1**, 3 (1986).
105. Fox, T. R., Schumann, A. M., Watanabe, P. G., Yano, B. L., Maher, V. M. and McCormick, J. J.: *Cancer Res.* **50**, 4014 (1990).
106. Bauer-Hofmann, R., Buchmann, A., Mahr, J., Kress, S., and Schwarz, M.: *Carcinogenesis* **13**, 477 (1992).
107. Sargent, L. M., Sattler, G. L., Roloff, B., Xu, Y., Sattler, C. A., Meisner, L., and Pitot, H. C.: *Cancer Res.* **52**, 955 (1992).
108. Wahba, Z. Z., Lawson, T. W., Murray, W. J., and Stohs, S. J.: *Toxicology* **58**, 57 (1989).
109. Rao, P. M., Rajalakshmi, S., Alam, A., Sarma, D. S. R., Pala, M. and Parodi, S.: *Carcinogenesis* **6**, 765 (1985).
110. Kasai, H., Okada, Y., Nishimura, S., Rao, M. S., and Reddy, J. K.: *Cancer Res.* **49**, 2603 (1989).
111. Srinivasan, S., and Glauert, H. P.: *Carcinogenesis* **11**, 2021 (1990).
112. Schulte-Hermann, R., Timmermann-Trosiener, I., and Schuppler, J.: *Cancer Res.* **43**, 839 (1983).
113. Popp, J. A., Scortichini, B. H., and Garvey, L. K.: *Fund. Appl. Toxicol.* **5**, 314 (1985).

114. Kraupp-Grasl, B., Huber, W., Taper, H., and Schulte-Hermann, R.: *Cancer Res.* **51**, 666 (1991).
115. Ward, J. M.: *J. Natl. Cancer Inst.* **71**, 815 (1983).
116. Ward, J. M., Diwan, B. A., Lubet, R. A., Hennemann, J. R., and Devor, D.: Liver Tumor Promoters and Other Mouse Carcinogens. *In* "Mouse Liver Carcinogenesis: Mechanisms and Species Comparisons" (D. E. Stevenson, J. A. Popp, J. M. Ward, R. M. McClain, T. J. Slaga, and H. C. Pitot, eds.). Alan R. Liss, New York, 1990, p 85.
117. Cattley, R. C., Marsman, D. S., and Popp, J. A.: *Carcinogenesis* **12**, 469 (1991).
118. Tennekes, H. A., van Ravenzwaay, B., and Kunz, H. W.: *Carcinogenesis* **6**, 1457 (1985).
119. Buchmann, A., Bauer-Hofmann, R., Mahr, J., Drinkwater, N. R., Luz, A., and Schwarz, M.: *Proc. Natl. Acad. Sci. U.S.A.* **88**, 911 (1991).
120. Goldsworthy, T., Campbell, H. A., and Pitot, H. C.: *Carcinogenesis* **5**, 67 (1984).
121. Campbell, H. A., Pitot, H. C., Potter, V. R., and Laishes, B. A.: *Cancer Res.* **42**, 465 (1982).
122. Edwards, A. M., and Lucas, C. M.: *Carcinogenesis* **6**, 733 (1985).
123. Roomi, M. W., and Goldberg, D. M.: *Biochem. Pharmacol.* **30**, 1563 (1981).
124. Sirica, A. E., Jicinsky, J. K., and Heyer, E. K.: *Carcinogenesis* **5**, 1737 (1984).
125. Kunz, W., Schaude, G., and Thomas, C.: *Z. Krebsforsch.* **72**, 291 (1969).
126. Hoch-Ligeti, C., Argus, M. F., and Arcos, J. C.: *J. Natl. Cancer. Inst.* **40**, 535 (1968).
127. McLean, A. E. M., and Marshall, A.: *Br. J. Pathol.* **52**, 322 (1971).
128. Argus, M. F., Hoch-Ligeti, C., Arcos, J. C., and Conney, A. H.: *J. Natl. Cancer Inst.* **61**, 441 (1978).
129. Lai, D. Y., Myers, S. C., Woo, Y.-T., Green, E. J., Friedman, M. A., Argus, M. F., and Arcos, J. C.: *Chem.-Biol. Interact.* **28**, 107 (1979).
130. Schwarz, M., Buchmann, A., Klormann, H., Schrenk, D., and Kunz, W.: *Cancer Res.* **45**, 2020 (1985).
131. Schwarz, M., Bannasch, P., and Kunz, W.: *Cancer Lett.* **21**, 17 (1983).
132. Williams, G. M., and Furuya, K.: *Carcinogenesis* **5**, 171 (1984).
133. Peraino, C., Staffeldt, E., Heugen, D. A., Lombard, L. S., Stevens, F. J., and Fry, R. J. M.: *Cancer Res.* **40**, 3268 (1980).
134. Moolgavkar, S. H., and Knudson A. G., Jr.: *J. Natl. Cancer Inst.* **66**, 1037 (1981).
135. Moolgavkar, S. H.: *Environ. Health Perspect.* **50**, 285 (1983).
136. Schulte-Hermann, R., Timmermann-Trosiener, I., and Schuppler, J.: *Carcinogenesis* **7**, 1651 (1986).
137. Cohen, S. M., and Ellwein, L. B.: *Science* **249**, 1007 (1990).
138. Büsser, M.-T., and Lutz, W. K.: *Carcinogenesis* **8**, 1433 (1987).
139. Loury, D. J., Goldsworthy, T. L., and Butterworth, B. E.: The Value of Measuring Cell Replication as a Predictive Index of Tissue-Specific Tumorigenic Potential. *In* "Banbury Report 25: Nongenotoxic Mechanisms in Carcinogenesis" (B. E. Butterworth and T. J. Slaga, eds.). Cold Spring Harbor Laboratory, Cold Spring Harbor, New York, 1987, p. 119.
140. Butterworth, B. E., and Goldsworthy, T. L.: *Proc. Soc. Exp. Biol. Med.* **198**, 683 (1991).
141. Yager, J. D., Zurlo, J., and Ni, N.: *Proc. Soc. Exp. Biol. Med.* **198**, 667 (1991).
142. Pitot, H. C., Neveu, M. J., Hully, J. R., Rizvi, T. A., and Campbell, H.: Multistage Hepatocarcinogenesis in the Rat as a Basis for Models of Risk Assessment of Carcinogenesis. *In* "Scientific Issues in Quantitative Cancer Risk Assessment" (S. H. Moolgavkar, ed.). Birkhäuser, Boston, 1990, p. 69.
143. Luebeck, E. G., Moolgavkar, S. H., Buchmann, A., and Schwarz, M.: *Toxicol. Appl. Pharmacol.* **111**, 469 (1991)
144. Farber, E., Parker, S., and Gruenstein, M.: *Cancer Res.* **36**, 3879 (1976).
145. Farber, E.: *Cancer Res.* **28**, 1859 (1968).
146. Roomi, M. W., Ho, R. K., Sarma, D. S. R., and Farber, E.: *Cancer Res.* **45**, 564 (1985).
147. Buchmann, A., Schwarz, M., Schmitt, R., Wolf, C. R., Oesch, F., and Kunz, W.: *Cancer Res.* **47**, 2911 (1987).
148. Kunz, H. W., Buchmann, A., Schwarz, M., Schmitt, R., Kuhlmann, W. D., Wolf, C. R., and Oesch, F.: *Arch. Toxicol.* **60**, 198 (1987).
149. Tsuda, H., Moore, M. A., Asomoto, M., Inoue, T., Fukushima, S., Ito, N., Satoh, K., Amelizad, Z., and Oesch, F.: *Carcinogenesis* **8**, 711 (1987).
150. Schwarz, M., Buchmann, A., Robertson, L., and Kunz, W.: Cell proliferation and hepatocarcinogenesis. *In* "Scientific Issues in Quantitative Cancer Risk Assessment" (S. H. Moolgavkar, ed.) Birkhäuser, Boston, 1990, p. 96.
151. Tsukuda, H., Sawada, N., Mitaka, T., and Gotoh, M.: *Carcinogenesis* **7**, 335 (1986).
152. Ames, B. N., and Gold, L. S.: *Proc. Natl. Acad. Sci. U.S.A.* **87**, 7772 (1990).
153. Kunz, W., Schaude, G., Schimmassek, H., Schmid, W., and Siess, M.: Proc. Eur. Soc. Study Drug Tox. VII (*Exerpta Med. Int. Congr. Ser.*) **115**, 138 (1966).
154. Schulte-Hermann, R.: *CRC Crit. Rev. Toxicol.* **3**, 97 (1974).
155. Van Ravenszwaay, B., Tennekes, H., Stöhr, M., and Kunz, W.: *Carcinogenesis* **8**, 265 (1987).
156. Van Ravenszwaay, B., and Kunz, W.: *Br. J. Cancer* **58**, 52 (1988).

157. Yager, J. D., Roebuck, B. D., Paluszcyk, L., and Memoli, V. A.: *Carcinogenesis* **7**, 2007 (1986).
158. Marsman, D. S., Cattley, R. C., Conway, J. G., and Popp, J. A.: *Cancer Res.* **48**, 6739 (1988).
159. Eacho, P. I., Lanier, T., and Brodhecker, C. A.: *Carcinogenesis* **12**, 1557 (1991)
160. Mayol, X., Perez-Tomas, R., Cullere, X., Romero, A., Estadella, M. D., and Domingo, J.: *Carcinogenesis* **12**, 1133 (1991).
161. Michalopoulos, G.: *FASEB J.* **4**, 176 (1990).
162. Madhukar, B. V., Brewster, D. W., and Matsumura, F.: *Proc. Natl. Acad. Sci. U.S.A.* **81**, 7407 (1984).
163. Lin, F. H., Clark, G., Birnbaum, L. S., Lucier, G. W., and Goldstein, J. A.: *Mol. Pharmacol.* **39**, 307 (1991).
164. Wölfe, D., Münzel, P., Fischer, G., and Bock, K. W.: *Carcinogenesis* **9**, 919 (1988).
165. Eckl, P. M., Meyer, S. A., Whitcombe, W. R., and Jirtle, R. L.: *Carcinogenesis* **9**, 479 (1988).
166. Lin, F. H., Stohs, S. J., Birnbaum, L. S., Clark, G., Lucier, G. W., and Goldstein, J. A.: *Toxicol. Appl. Pharmacol.* **108**, 129 (1991).
167. Rubin, R. A., O'Keefe, E. J., and Earp, H. S.: *Proc. Natl. Acad. Sci U.S.A.* **79**, 776 (1982)
168. Harris, L., Preat, V., and Farber, E.: *Cancer Res.* **47**, 3954 (1987).
169. Lee, L. S., and Weinstein, B.: *Proc. Natl. Acad. Sci. U.S.A.* **76**, 5168 (1979).
170. Shi, Y. E., and Yager, J. D.: *Cancer Res.* **49**, 3574 (1989).
171. Yosof, Y. A. M., and Edwards, A. M.: *Carcinogenesis* **11**, 761 (1990).
172. Russell, W. E., Coffey, R. J., Ouellette, A. J. and Moses, H. L.: *Proc. Natl. Acad. Sci. U.S.A.* **85**, 5126 (1988).
173. Carr, B. I., Hayashi, I., Branum, E. L., and Moses, H. L.: *Cancer Res.* **46**, 2330 (1986).
174. Oberhammer, F., Bursch, W., Parzefall, W., Breit, P., Stadler, M., and Schulte-Hermann, R.: *Cancer Res.* **51**, 2478 (1991).
175. Oberhammer, F. A., Pavelka, M., Sharma, S., Tiefenbacher, R., Purchio, A. F., Bursch, W., and Schulte-Hermann, R.: *Proc. Natl. Acad. Sci. U.S.A.,* **88**, 5408 (1992).
176. Bursch, W., Lauer, B., Timmermann-Trosiener, I., Barthel, G., Schuppler, J., and Schulte-Hermann, R.: *Carcinogenesis* **5**, 453 (1984).
177. Bursch, W., Paffe, S., Putz, B., Barthel, G., and Schulte-Hermann, R.: *Carcinogenesis* **11**, 847 (1990).
178. Columbano, A., Ledda-Columbano, G. M., Coni, P. P., Faa, G., Liguori, C., Santa Cruz, G., and Pani, P.: *Lab. Invest.* **52**, 670 (1985).
179. Moolgavkar, S. H., Luebeck, G., and de Gunst, M.: Two Mutation Models for Carcinogenesis: Relative Roles of Somatic Mutations and Cell Proliferation in Determining Risk. *In* "Scientific Issues in Quantitative Cancer Risk Assessment" (S. H. Moolgavkar, ed.), Birkhäuser, Boston, 1990, p. 136.
180. Trosko, J. E., and Chang, C.-C.: Nongenotoxic Mechanisms in Carcinogenesis: Role of Inhibited Intercellular Communication. *In* "Banbury Report 31: Carcinogen Risk Assessment: New Directions in the Qualitative and Quantitative Aspects" (R. W. Hart and F. D. Hoerger, eds.). Cold Spring Harbor Laboratory, Cold Spring Harbor, New York, 1988, p. 139.
181. Fitzgerald, D. J., and Yamasaki, H.: *Terato. Carcino. Mutagen.* **10**, 89 (1990).
182. Klaunig, J. E., and Ruch, R. J.: *Lab. Invest.* **62**, 135 (1990).
183. Yamasaki, H.: Role of GAP Junctional Intercellular Communication in Malignant Cell Transformation. *In* "Modern Cell Biology: GAP Junctions" (E. L. Hertzberg and R. G. Johnson, eds.). Alan R. Liss, New York, 1988 p. 449.
184. Loewenstein W. R.: *Biochim. Biophys. Acta* **560**, 1 (1979).
185. Enomoto, T., and Yamasaki, H.: *Cancer Res.* **44**, 5200 (1984).
186. Yotti, L. P., Chang, C. C., and Trosko, J. E.: *Science* **206**, 1089 (1979).
187. Murray, A. W., and Fitzgerald, D. J.: *Biochem Biophys. Res. Commun.* **91**, 395 (1979).
188. Sugie, S., Mori, H., and Takahashi, M.: *Carcinogenesis* **8**, 45 (1987).
189. Klaunig, J. E., Ruch, R. J., and Weghorst, C. M.: *Toxicol. Appl. Pharmacol.* **102**, 553 (1990).
190. Flodström, S., Hemming, H., Wärngard, L., and Ahlborg, U. G.: *Carcinogenesis* **11**, 1413 (1990).
191. Jone, C., Trosko, J. E., and Chang, C. C.: *In vitro Cell Develop. Biol.* **23**, 214 (1987).
192. Tsushimoto, G., Trosko, J. E., Chang, C. C., and Aust, S. D.: *Carcinogenesis* **3**, 181 (1982).
193. Klaunig, J. E., Ruch, R. J., Deangelo, A. B., and Kaylor, W. H.: *Cancer Lett.* **43**, 65 (1988).
194. Schulz, N. E., Gray, T. J. B., and Klaunig, J. E.: *Toxicologist* **10**, 122 (1989).
195. Lincoln D. W., II, Kampcik, S. J., and Gierthy, J. F.: *Carcinogenesis* **8**, 1817 (1987).
196. Jensen, R. K., and Sleight, S. D.: *Carcinogenesis* **7**, 1771 (1986).
197. Traub, O., Drüge, P. M., and Willecke, K.: *Proc. Natl. Acad. Sci.* USA **80**, 755 (1983).
198. Mesnil, M., Fitzgerald, D. J., and Yamasaki, H.: *Mol. Carcinogenesis* **1**, 79 (1988).
199. Beer, D. G., Neveu, M. J., Paul, D. L., Rapp, U. R., and Pitot, H. C.: *Cancer Res.* **48**, 1610 (1988).
200. Klaunig, J. E.: *Proc. Soc. Exp. Biol. Med.* **198**, 688 (1991).
201. Droga, S., Filser, J. G., Cojocel, C., Greim, H., Regel, U., Oesch, F., and Robertson, L. W.: *Arch. Toxicol.* **62**, 369 (1988).

202. Stohs, S. J., Hassan, M. Q., and Murray, W. J.: *Biochem. Biophys. Res. Commun.* **111**, 854 (1983).
203. Hildebrandt, A. G., Speck, M., and Roots, I.: *Biochem. Biophys. Res. Commun.* **54**, 968 (1973).
204. Goel, S. K., Lalwani, N. D., and Reddy, J. K.: *Cancer Res.* **46**, 1324 (1986).
205. Reddy, J. K., and Lalwani; N. D.: *CRC Crit. Rev. Toxicol.* **12**, 1 (1983).
206. Reddy, J. K., and Rao, M. S.: *Mutation Res.* **214**, 63 (1989).
207. Robertson, L. W., Regel, U., Filser, J. G., and Oesch, F.: *Arch. Toxicol.* **57**, 13 (1985).
208. Nims, R. W., Devor, D. E., Hennemann, J. R., and Lubet, R. A.: *Carcinogenesis* **8**, 67 (1987).
209. Deml, E., Wiebel, F. J., and Oesterle, D.: *Toxicology* **59**, 229 (1989).
210. Schulte-Hermann, R., Ochs, H., Bursch, W., and Parzefall, W.: *Cancer Res.* **48**, 2462 (1988).
211. Benedetti, A., Malvalsi, G., Fulceri, R., and Comporti, M.: *Cancer Res.* **44**, 5712 (1984).
212. Rao, M. S., Lalwani, N. D., Scarpelli, D. G., and Reddy, J. K.: *Carcinogenesis* **3**, 1231 (1982).
213. Hanigan, M. H., and Pitot, H. C.: *Carcinogenesis* **6**, 165 (1985).
214. Deml, E., and Oesterle, D.: *Cancer Res.* **40**, 490 (1980).
215. Stenius, U., Rubin, K., Gullberg, D., and Högberg, J.: *Carcinogenesis* **11**, 69 (1990).
216. Scholz, W., Schütze, K., Kunz, W., and Schwarz, M.: *Cancer Res.* **50**, 7015 (1990).
217. Kuchino, Y., Mori, F., Kasai, H., Inoue, H., Iwai, S., Miura, K., Ohtsuka, E., and Nishimura, S.: *Nature* **327**, 77 (1987).
218. Pitot, H. C.: *Proc. Soc. Exp. Biol. Med.* **198**, 661 (1991).
219. Pitot, H. C., Goldsworthy, T. L., Moran, S., Kennan, W.; Glauert, H. P., Maronpot, R. R., and Campbell, H. A.: *Carcinogenesis* **8**, 1491 (1987).
220. Moolgavkar, S. H., Luebeck, E. G., DeGunst, M., Port, R. E., and Schwarz, M.: *Carcinogenesis* **11**, 1271 (1990).
221. Oesterle, D., and Deml, E.: *Carcinogenesis* **5**, 351 (1984).
222. Takano, T., Tatematsu, M., Hasegawa, R., Imaida, K., and Ito, N.: *Gann* **71**, 580 (1980).
223. Mochizuki, Y., Furukawa, K., Sawada, N., and Gotoh, M.: *Gann* **72**, 170 (1981).
224. Maekawa, A., Onodera, H., Ogasawara, H., Matsushima, Y., Mitsumori, K., and Hayashi, Y.: *Carcinogenesis* **13**, 501 (1992).
225. Poland, A., Glover, E., and Kende, A. S.: *J. Biol. Chem.* **251**, 4936 (1976).
226. Toft, D., Shyamala, G., and Gorski, J.: *Proc. Natl. Acad. Sci. U.S.A.* **57**, 1740 (1967).
227. Issemann, I., and Green, S.: *Nature* **347**, 645 (1990).
228. Lutz, W. K.: *Carcinogenesis* **11**, 1243 (1990).
229. Peraino, C., Fry, R. I. M., and Staffeldt, E.: *Cancer Res.* **37**, 3623 (1977).
230. Preat, V., Lans, M., de Gerlache, J., Taper, H., and Roberfroid, M.: *Carcinogenesis* **8**, 333 (1987).
231. Jensen, R. K., Sleight, S. D., and Aust, S. D.: *Carcinogenesis* **5**, 63 (1984).
232. Boutwell, R. K.: *Progr. Exp. Tumor Res.* **4**, 207 (1964).
233. Boutwell, R. K.: *CRC Crit. Rev. Toxicol.* **2**, 419 (1974).
234. Tatematsu, M., Nagamine, Y., and Farber, E.: *Cancer Res.* **43**, 5049 (1983).
235. Moore, M., Hacker, H.-J., and Bannasch, P.: *Carcinogenesis* **4**, 595 (1983).
236. Glauert, H. P., Schwarz, M., and Pitot, H. C.: *Carcinogenesis* **7**, 117 (1986).
237. Kitagawa, T.: *Gann* **62**, 207 (1971).
238. Enomoto, K., and Farber, E.: *Cancer Res.* **42**, 2330 (1982).
239. Hendrich, S., Glauert, H. P., and Pitot, H. C.: *Carcinogenesis* **7**, 2041 (1986).
240. Xu, Y.-D., Dragan, Y. P., Young, T., and Pitot, H. C.: *Carcinogenesis* **12**, 1009 (1991).
241. Fingerhut, M. A., Halperin, W. E., Marlow, D. A., Piacitelli, L. A., Honchar, P. A., Sweeney, M. H., Greife, A. L., Dill, P. A., Steenland, K., and Suruda, A. J.: *New Engl. J. Med.* **324**, 212 (1991).
242. Johnson, E. S.: *Toxicology* **21**, 451 (1992).
243. Clemmensen, J., Fuglsang, V., and Plum, C. M.: *Lancet* **1**, 705 (1977).
244. Ohlsen, J. H., Boice, J. D., Jr., Jensen, J. P. A., and Fraumeni, J. F., Jr.: *J. Natl. Cancer Inst.* **81**, 803 (1989).
246. McLean, E. M., Driver, H., and McDanell, R.: *Bull. Cancer* **77**, 505 (1990).
247. Stott, W. T.: *Reg. Toxicol. Pharmacol.* **8**, 125 (1988).
248. Baum, J., Holtz, F., Bookstein, J. J., and Klein, E. W.: *Lancet* **2**, 926 (1973).
249. Edmondson, H. A., Henderson, B., and Benton, B.: *New Engl. J. Med.* **249**, 470 (1976).
250. Palmer, J. R., Rosenberg, L., Kaufmann, D. W., Warshauer, M. E., Stolley, P., and Sharpiro, S.: *Am. J. Epidemiol.* **130**, 878 (1989).
251. Edmondson, H. A., Reynolds, T. B., Henderson, B., and Benton, B.: *Ann. Int. Med.* **86**, 180 (1977).
252. Parkin, D. M., Läära, E., and Muir, C. S.: *Int. J. Cancer* **41**, 184 (1988).
253. Bosch, F. X., and Munoz, N.: Epidemiology of Hepatocellular Carcinoma. *In* "Liver Cell Carcinoma" (P. Bannasch, D. Keppler, and G. Weber, eds.). Kluwer Academic Publishers, Dordrecht, 1988, p. 3.
254. Bressac, B., Key, M., Wands, J., and Oztürk, M.: *Nature* **350**, 429 (1991).

255. Hsu, I. C., Metcalf, R. A., Sun, T., Welsh, J. A., Wang, N. J., and Harris, C. C.: *Nature* **350**, 427 (1991).
256. Oztürk, M.: *Lancet* **338**, 1356 (1991).
257. Chisari, F. V., Klopchin, K., Moriyama, T., Pasquinelli, C., Dunsford, H. A., Sell, S., Pinkert, C. A., Brinster, R. L., and Palmiter, R. D.: *Cell* **59**, 1145 (1989).
258. Lieber, C. S., Garro, A., Leo, M. A., Mak, K. M., and Worner, T.: *Hepatology* **6**, 1005 (1986).
259. Niederau, C., Fisher, R., Sonneberg, A., Stremmel, W., Trampisch, H. J., and Strohmeyer, G.: *N. Engl. J. Med*. **313**, 1256 (1985).
260. Melia, W. M., Johnson, P. J., and Neuberger, J.: *Gastroenterology* **87**, 660 (1984).
261. Masuda, R., Yoshida, M. C., Sakai, M., Dempo, K., and Mori, M.: High Susceptibility to Spontaneous Development of Hepatocellular Carcinoma in LEC rats. *In* "The LEC Rat" (M. Mori, M. C. Yoshida, N. Takeichi, and N. Taniguchi, eds.). Springer Verlag, Tokyo, 1991, p. 54.

Note on Multistage Carcinogenesis in Other Organs and *in Vitro*

Friedrich Marks

As the previous two sections in this chapter indicated, the mouse skin and the rat liver were the most widely used systems for studies on tumor promotion. Other organs in which the initiation–promotion stages of carcinogenesis have been studied are the colon, the pancreas, the mammary glands, the kidneys, the respiratory tract, the thyroid, and the urinary bladder. Although, of course, the tumorigenic agents employed in these studies are different from those used in skin and liver, the conclusions drawn are, in general, the same. These conclusions include strong mutual enhancement of the effects ("synergism") between initiators and promoters, requirement of prolonged promoter treatment, and relationship between promotion and cellular hyperproliferation as induced, *e.g.*, by chronic mechanical or chemical injury. For these reasons tumor promotion in other organs will be dealt with only very briefly. Readers seeking more information on tumor promotion in different organs are referred to Refs. 1–8.

Many of the studies on the identification of tumor promoters in tissues other than skin and liver have furnished suggestive (but mostly circumstantial) evidence for the tumor-promoting effect of a great variety of environmental factors. For example, in rodents, diets high in fat and low in fiber have been repeatedly found to have an enhancing effect on colorectal carcinogenesis, which may be interpreted as promotion (9–12); this is discussed in greater detail in Chapter 9, sections I, II and V. More clearly delineated experimental evidence exists for the tumor-promoting effect of bile acids in the colon (9,13). By "clearly delineated" is meant that some bile acids have also been found to enhance the chemical transformation of C3H 10T1/2 fibroblasts *in vitro* (14) and to stimulate protein kinase C (15), that is, to display the behavior of phorbol ester–type promoters. Besides bile acids, some fatty acid metabolites, such as acylhydroperoxides, have been suspected of promoting activity in the gastrointestinal tract of rats (16). Since the secretion of bile acids is a function of the level of fat intake, these observations are consistent with human epidemiological evidence of a correlation between high-fat diet and colon cancer incidence. Another probable promoting factor, both in experimental and human colorectal carcinogenesis, appears to be ethanol (17). These findings are evidently of utmost importance for an understanding of the etiology of human colorectal cancer.

Dietary factors have been also suspected to act as tumor promoters in pancreatic carcinogenesis (18,19) and mammary carcinogenesis (*rev. in* ref. 8). However, definitive evidence based on standardized initiation-promotion protocols is not yet available. The rodent mammary gland provides a model for investigations on the putative tumor-promoting action of steroid sex hormones and prolactin.

Several studies on respiratory tract carcinogenesis indicate the promoting effect of asbestos and tobacco smoke in tracheal and bronchial mucosa (20,21). It is difficult, however, to distinguish a clearcut promoter action from a syncarcinogenic effect of such agents. Experiments using heterotypic transplants and organ cultures of tracheal mucosa showed that this tissue is sensitive to the tumor promoting effect of phorbol esters (20-22). Interestingly, also phorbol (the parent alcohol of the phorbol esters) promotes dimethyl-nitrosamine-induced lung carcinogenesis in mice when administered systemically (23). Since in the skin phorbol is inactive, the mechanism of its effect in the lung remains obscure. Environmental agents such as ozone, SO_2 and NO_2 as well as other lung-damaging chemicals have been suspected to promote tumor development in lung parenchyma, and a rather good correlation between hyperproliferation/hyperplasia and tumor development has been found in this tissue (24,25). The antioxidant, butylated hydroxytoluene (BHT), is one of the very few agents which have been tested in mice for lung tumor-promoting capability under the experimental conditions of the initiation-promotion protocol (26). Interestingly, BHT, in contrast to its effect in lung, exhibits an antipromoting effect in the mouse skin and has been reported to be anticarcinogenic in many other tissues (27).

Induction of kidney tumors using the initiation–promotion protocol has been repeatedly reported (28). The promoters used include sodium barbital (29,30) and metabolites thereof (31), as well as trisodium nitrilotriacetate (30), a constituent of detergents. Barbital and phenobarbital (inactive in the kidney) have been shown to promote tumorigenesis in the thyroid gland (32–34).

The use of the urinary bladder in experimental multistage carcinogenesis studies has become well known following the discovery of the tumor promoting effect of artificial sweeteners such as saccharin and cyclamate, as well as of tryptophan, and of the close relationship of this promoting effect to epithelial hyperproliferation (35–39). Chronic hyperproliferation also represents the common denominator of promotion resulting from vitamin A deficiency and from irritation by urinary calculi.

More recently, the possible role of promoting factors in virus-induced carcinogenesis has attracted increasing attention, since in most cases the development of virus-induced tumors has been found actually to be a multifactorial process. Illustrative examples are the role of certain papilloma virus types in the etiology of genital cancer (40,41) and the Burkitt lymphoma, which is caused by the combined action of Epstein-Barr virus and malaria parasites. Thus, it remains an open question which of the two cooperating agents represents the tumor-promoting factor (42). The interaction of viruses and chemical agents in tumor induction is discussed in some detail in Chapter 14.

For most of the organ systems mentioned above (and including skin) *in vivo* studies on initiation-promotion have been complemented and extended by appropriate *in vitro* systems, *i.e.*, cell and tissue cultures. The *in vitro* markers generally employed to ascertain tumor promotion in a two-stage experiment are the appearance of the typical symptoms of neoplastic transformation in culture, such as anchorage-independent growth, immortality, and tumorigenicity ("tumor take") upon transplantation into thymus-deficient "nude" mice. Although a clearcut extrapolation of *in vitro* observations to the *in vivo* process remains, in principle, problematic, the *in vitro* approach of multistage carcinogenesis has significantly contributed to a better understanding of the molecular mechanisms of initiation and promotion. For a detailed discussion of the voluminous literature of two-stage carcinogenesis *in vitro*, the reader is referred to a selection of reviews and books (*see* Refs. 2–8 and 43–52).

REFERENCES

1. Slaga, T. J. (ed.): "Mechanisms of Tumor Promotion, Vol. I: Tumor Promotion in Internal Organs". CRC Press, Boca Raton Florida, 1983.
2. Hecker, E., Fusenig, N. E., Kunz, W., Marks, F., and Thielmann, H. W. (eds.): "Cocarcinogenesis and Biological Effects of Tumor Promoters," Carcinogenesis – a Comprehensive Survey, Vol. 7. Raven Press, New York, 1982.
3. Fujiki, H., Hecker, E., Moore, R. E., Sugimura, T., and Weinstein, I.B. (eds.): "Cellular Interactions by Environmental Tumor Promoters". Japan. Sci. Soc. Press, Tokyo/VNU Science Press, Utrecht, 1989.
4. Börzsönyi, M., Day, N. E., Lapis, K., and Yamasaki, H. (eds.): "Models, Mechanisms and Etiology of Tumor Promotion". IARC, Lyon, 1984.
5. Slaga, T. J., Sivak, A., and Boutwell, R. K. (eds.): "Mechanisms of Tumor Promotion and Cocarcinogenesis", Carcinogenesis – a Comprehensive Survey, Vol. 2. Raven Press, New York 1978.
6. Ito, N., and Sugano, H. (eds.): "Modification of Tumor Development in Rodents", *Progr. Exp. Tumor Res.* **33**. Karger, Basel, 1991.
7. Langenbach, R., Elmore, E., and Barrett, J. C. (eds.): "Tumor Promoters: Biological Approaches for Mechanistic Studies and Assay Systems", *Progr. Cancer Res. Therap.* **34**. Raven Press, New York, 1988.
8. Peraino, C., and Jones, C. A.: The Multistage Concept of Carcinogenesis. *In*: "The Pathobiology of Neoplasia" (A. E. Sirica, ed.). Plenum Press, New York, 1988, p. 131.
9. Reddy, B. S.: Tumor Promotion in Colon Carcinogenesis. *In*: "Mechanisms of Tumor Promotion" (T. J. Slaga, ed.), Vol. 1. CRC Press, Boca Raton, Florida, 1983, p. 107.
10. Reddy, B. S., and Maeura, Y: *J. Natl. Cancer Inst.* **72**, 745 (1984).
11. Reddy, B. S., Tanaka, T., and Simi, B.: *J. Natl. Cancer Inst.* **75**, 791 (1985).
12. Abraham, S. (ed.): "Carcinogenesis and Dietary Fat", Kluwer, Dodrecht, The Netherlands, 1989.
13. Cohen, B. I., and Mosbach, E. H.: Effect of Bile Acids and Sterols in Animal Models of Colorectal Cancer. *In* "Calcium, Vitamin D, and Prevention of Colon Cancer" (M. Lipkin, H. L. Newmark, and G. Kelloff, eds.). CRC Press, Boca Raton, Florida, 1991, p. 209.
14. Kaibara, N., Yurugi, E., and Koga, S.: *Cancer Res.* **44**, 5482 (1984).
15. Fitzer, C. J., O'Brien, C. A., Guillem, J. G., and Weinstein, I. B.: *Carcinogenesis* **8**, 217 (1987).
16. Bull, A. W., Nigro, N. D., Golembieski, W. A., Crissman, J. D., and Marnett, L. J.: *Cancer Res.* **44**, 4924 (1984).
17. Garro, A. J., and Lieber, C. S.: *Annu. Rev. Pharmacol. Toxicol.* **30**, 219 (1990).
18. Roebuck, B. D., Longnecker, D. S., and Yager, J. D.: Initiation and Promotion in Pancreatic Carcinogenesis. *In* "Mechanisms of Tumor Promotion" (T. J. Slaga, ed.), Vol. I. CRC Press, Boca Raton, Florida, 1983, p. 151.
19. Pour, P.M.: Modification of Tumor Development in the Pancreas. *In* "Modification of Tumor Development in Rodents" (N. Ito and H. Sugano, eds.), *Progr. Exp. Tumor Res.* **33**, Karger, Basel, 1991, p. 108.
20. Steele, V. E., and Nettesheim, P.: Tumor Promotion in Respiratory Tract Carcinogenesis. *In* "Mechanisms of Tumor Promotion" (T. J. Slaga, ed.), Vol. I. CRC Press, Boca Raton, Florida, 1983, p. 91.
21. Mass, M. J., Kaufman, D. G., Siegfried, J. M., Steele, V. E., and Nesnow, S. (eds.): "Cancer and the Respiratory Tract: Predisposing Factors." Carcinogenesis – a Comprehensive Survey", Vol. 8. Raven Press, New York, 1985.
22. Nettesheim, P., Walker, C. L., Ferriola, P., and Steigerwalt, R.: *In vivo* and *in vitro* studies of multistage transformation of airway epithelium. *In* "Cell Transformation and Radiation-Induced Cancer" (K. H. Chadwick, C. Seymour, and B. Barnhart, eds.), Hilger, Bristol, 1989, p. 147.
23. Armuth, V., and Berenblum, I.: *Cancer Res.* **32**, 2259 (1972).
24. Witschi, H. P.: Enhancement of Tumor Formation in Mouse Lung. *In* "Mechanisms of Tumor Promotion" (T. J. Slaga, ed.), Vol. I. CRC Press, Boca Raton, Florida, 1983, p. 71.
25. Witschi, H. P.: Models of Lung Tumor Development in Rats, Hamsters and Mice. *In* "Modification of Tumor Development in Rodents" (N. Ito and H. Sugano, eds.), *Progr. Exp. Tumor Res.* **33**, Karger, Basel, 1991, p. 132.
26. Witschi, H. P., Williamson, D., and Loek, S.: *Pharmacol. Therap.* **42**, 89 (1989).
27. Ito, N., and Hirose, M.: *Adv. Cancer Res.* **53**, 247 (1989).
28. Hiasa, Y., and Ito, N.: *CRC Crit. Rev. Toxicol.* **17**, 279 (1987).
29. Diwan, B. A., Oshima, M., and Rice, J. M.: *Carcinogenesis* **10**, 183 (1989).
30. Hagiwara, A., Diwan, B. A., and Ward, J. M.: *Fundam. Appl. Toxicol.* **13**, 332 (1989).
31. Diwan, B. A., Nims, R. W., Ward, J. M., Hu, H., Lubet, R. A., and Rice, J. M.: *Carcinogenesis* **10**, 189 (1989).
32. Hiasa, Y., Kitahori, Y., Oshima, M., Fujita, T., Yuasa, T., Konishi, N., and Miyashiro, A.: *Carcinogenesis* **3**, 1187 (1982).

33. Tsuda, H., Fukushima, S., Imaida, K., Kurata, Y., and Ito, N.: *Cancer Res.* **43**, 3292 (1983).
34. Diwan, B. A., Palmer, A. E., Oshima, M., and Rice, J. M.: *J. Natl. Cancer Inst.* **75**, 1099 (1985).
35. Hicks, R. M.: Promotion in Bladder Cancer. *In:* "Cocarcinogenesis and Biological Effects of Tumor Promoters" (E. Hecker, N. E. Fusenig, W. Kunz, F. Marks, and H. W. Thielmann, eds.), Carcinogenesis—a Comprehensive Survey, Vol. 7. Raven Press, New York, 1982, p. 139.
36. Cohen, S. M., Murasaki, G., Ellwein, L. B., and Greenfield, R. E.: Tumor Promotion in Bladder Carcinogenesis. *In:* "Mechanisms of Tumor Promotion" (T. J. Slaga, ed.), Vol. 1. CRC Press, Boca Raton, Florida, 1983, p. 131.
37. Cohen, S. M.: *Food Chem. Toxicol.* **23** 521 (1985).
38. Ellwein, L. B., and Cohen, S. M.: *CRC Crit. Rev. Toxicol.* **20**, 311 (1989).
39. Fukushima, S.: Modification of Tumor Development in the Urinary Bladder. *In* "Modification of Tumor Development in Rodents" (N. Ito and H. Sugano, eds.), *Progr. Exp. Tumor Res.* **33**, Karger, Basel, 1991, p. 154.
40. zur Hausen, H.: Similarities of Papilloma Virus Infections with Tumor Promoters. *In:* "Cellular Interactions by Environmental Tumor Promoters" (H. Fujiki, E. Hecker, R. E. Moore, T. Sugimura, and I. B. Weinstein, eds.), Japan. Sci. Soc. Press, Tokyo/VNU Science Press, Utrecht, 1984, p. 147.
41. zur Hausen, H.: *Mol.* Carc. **1**, 147 (1988).
42. Facer, C. A., and Playfair, J. H. L.: *Adv. Cancer Res.* **53**, 33 (1989).
43. Bohrman, J. S.: *CRC Crit. Rev. Toxicol.* **11**, 121 (1982).
44. Slaga, T. J. (ed.): "Mechanisms of Tumor Promotion, Vol. III: Tumor Promotion and Carcinogenesis in Vitro". CRC Press, Boca Raton, Florida, 1984.
45. Diamond, L.: *Pharmacol. Therap.* **26**, 89 (1984).
46. Barrett, J. C., and Tennant, R. W. (eds.): "Mammalian Cell Transformation", Carcinogenesis—A Comprehensive Survey, Vol. 9. Raven Press, New York, 1985.
47. Huberman, E., and Barr, S. H. (eds.): "The Role of Chemicals and Radiation in the Etiology of Cancer", Carcinogenesis—a Comprehensive Survey, Vol. 10. Raven Press, New York, 1985.
48. Barrett, J. C., and Fletcher, W. F.: Cellular and Molecular Mechanisms of Multistep Carcinogenesis in Cell Culture Models. *In* "Mechanisms of Environmental Carcinogenesis" (J. C. Barrett, ed.). CRC Press, Boca Raton, Florida, 1987, p. 73.
49. Colburn, N. H.: The Genetics of Tumor Promotion. *In* "Mechanisms of Environmental Carcinogenesis" (J. C. Barrett, ed.). CRC Press, Boca Raton, Florida, 1987, p. 81.
50. Colburn, N. H. (ed.): "Genes and Signal Transduction in Multistage Carcinogenesis". Dekker, New York, 1989.
51. Conti, C. J., Slaga, T. J., and Klein-Szanto, A. J. P. (eds.): "Skin Tumors: Experimental and Clinical Aspects", Carcinogenesis—a Comprehensive Survey, Vol. 11. Raven Press, New York, 1989.
52. Knowles, M. A.: Transformation of Cells in Culture. *In* "Chemical Carcinogenesis and Mutagenesis I" (G. S. Cooper and P. L. Grover, eds.). Springer-Verl., Berlin, 1990, p. 211.

SECTION **IIIB**

Note on Tumor Promoters, Cocarcinogens, and Nongenotoxic Carcinogens

Friedrich Marks

In the early literature the terms promotion and cocarcinogenesis were frequently used as synonyms. Promotion was regarded by a number of authors as a special case of cocarcinogenesis. Today, most authors prefer to make a strict distinction between the two terms (1). *Promotion* is defined both operationally on the basis of the initiation–promotion protocol (as characterized by a defined regimen and sequence of manipulations) and mechanistically on the basis of a distinct conception of the underlying mechanisms (*i.e.*, clonal expansion of tumor cells as a condition for a further progression to the malignant state). In contrast, the term cocarcinogenesis is less precisely defined. *Cocarcinogenesis* comprises any process which augments initiation and which may take place generally before or simultaneously with initiation. It comprises effects which, for example, entail the facilitation of penetration and metabolic activation of the initiating carcinogen or an impairment of protective mechanisms such as immune surveillance, excretion, or cell death. In addition, cocarcinogenic factors may produce changes in the target cells—such as increased DNA synthesis or diminished DNA repair—which help the genetic changes involved in initiation to become manifest.

As discussed in Section I of this chapter, long-term cellular hyperproliferation resulting in sustained hyperplasia and resembling a regenerative process appears to represent the general histopathological symptom or even the precondition of tumor promotion in most tissues. Such a reaction may be induced either by nonspecific irritation or by more specific molecular interactions of the promoter with the cellular pathways of mitogenesis and growth control.

In this regard a remarkable similarity exists between tumor promoters and the so-called nongenotoxic carcinogens (2–4). The latter comprise a wide variety of agents which have been found to cause cancer in different organs (especially in rodents), although they do not exhibit any mutagenic activity, thought to be characteristic for initiating carcinogens. It has been proposed that nongenotoxic carcinogens render cells "more vulnerable either to the action of endogenous or environmental mutagens or to defects in cell reproduction" (3) by keeping them in an abnormally high proliferative state, thus providing the condition for a stepwise progression to malignancy (4). The same definition may be applied to both tumor promotion and certain types of cocarcinogenesis. Actually, prototypes of tumor promoters such as the phorbol esters, phenobarbital, butylhydroxyanisol (BHA), asbestos, saccharin, and many others have been also classified as nongenotoxic carcinogens (3).

Many nongenotoxic carcinogens share with agents designated by consensus as "tumor promoters" not only the ability to induce regenerative hyperproliferation, but also the requirement of long-term application, the phenomenon of lower threshold in their dose–response curves, and strong synergistic action with mutagenic carcinogens (3). Thus, at a closer focus, the distinction between "tumor promoters" and many "nongenotoxic carcinogens" may appear to be purely semantic rather than conceptual.

REFERENCES

1. Appel, K. E., Fürstenberger, G., Hapke, H. J., Hecker, E., Hildebrandt, A. G., Koransky, W., Marks, F., Neumann, H. G., Ohnesorge, F. K., and Schulte-Hermann, R.: *J. Cancer Res. Clin. Oncol.* **116**, 232 (1990).
2. Clayson, D. B.: *Mutat. Res.* **221**, 53 (1989).
3. Grasso, P., Sharratt, M., and Cohen, A. J.: *Annu. Rev. Pharmacol. Toxicol.* **31**, 253 (1991).
4. Roe, F. J. C., *Mutagenesis* **4**, 407 (1989).

CHAPTER **6**

Computerized Data Management as a Tool to Study Combination Effects in Carcinogenesis

*Yin-tak Woo, Gregg Polansky, Joseph C. Arcos,
Jeff Stokes DuBose, and Mary F. Argus*

I. INTRODUCTION

Humans and animals are exposed, either sequentially or simultaneously, to combinations of a variety of chemical agents which include low doses of naturally occurring and synthetic chemical carcinogens as well as carcinogenesis-modifying agents such as inhibitors and promoters. Assessment of the potential cancer hazard of exposure to environmentally occurring complex chemical mixtures/combinations is a difficult and challenging toxicological problem and a subject of major current concern to both the scientific and regulatory communities (*e.g.*, 1–3). Besides the usual problems associated with risk assessment of individual chemicals, there are three major obstacles associated with mixtures: (a) the impossibility of testing myriads of possible combinations of chemicals, (b) the lack of a universally accepted index for quantitative measurement of cancer risk of chemical carcinogens, and (c) the uncertainty of the possible outcomes of interactions among the various constituents of the mixture.

Despite this uncertainty, there is clear realization that the toxicologic evaluation of complex chemical mixtures is becoming an increasingly important requirement for the hazard assessment of environmental sites (*e.g.*, 4). The epitome of this troublesome uncertainty is the problem of assessing the relative hazard that hazardous wastes disposal sites represent (*e.g.*, 5) and, hence, the priority to be assigned for clean up and decontamination. Beyond this very acute example, the problem also surfaces in connection with the hazard represented by industrial effluents, pollutants in water and air, industrial products consisting of mixtures of chemicals, as well as complex human and veterinary medicinal preparations.

Other than testing a specific chemical mixture, there are currently no systematic methods available to assess the cancer risk of complex chemical mixtures or to study/express combination effects. The basic additivity model has hitherto been virtually the only method used for risk assessment of chemical mixtures (*e.g.*, 6). This method is based on the assumptions that: (a) the concentrations of various chemical carcinogens

185

present in environmental mixtures are usually relatively low with respect to the dose–response curve and (b) the effects of constituents of a chemical mixture do not interact with each other. Under these conditions, the individual effects of various constituents present in the mixture can be combined in an arithmetically additive manner to provide an estimate of the overall effect. The major scientific shortcoming of this method is that it does not account for interaction effects—among various constituents of the mixtures—which can cause significant deviation from the hazard/risk calculated using an additivity model.

During the past 8 years, the U.S. Environmental Protection Agency (EPA) and the National Cancer Institute (NCI) have been involved in systematically compiling databases on combined effects of binary mixtures of carcinogens (7), carcinogens and inhibitors (8), and carcinogens and promoters (9); these databases provide crucial information needed for mixture assessment. In this chapter, we describe a pragmatic approach of managing and integrating the information extracted from these databases, coupled with mathematical, statistical, and toxicological considerations, to develop a computerized system, the Integral Search System (ISS), capable of predicting/ranking the potential cancer hazard of complex chemical mixtures.

II. COMBINATION EFFECTS CATEGORIES: DEFINITIONS

One of the most difficult problems of the assessment of risk of complex mixtures is the presence of a variety of interaction effects. Considering a mixture which contains carcinogens as well as carcinogenesis inhibitors and promoters, there can be four types of interaction effects in the set of binary pairings of all chemicals present in a complex mixture:

A. When both chemicals are *established carcinogens*, the combined effect (*see* Reference 7 for database; *see also* Chapter 2 of this monograph) may be

(i) **additivity,** when the combined effect represents the arithmetic sum of the effects determined with each chemical agent individually (*i.e.*, the two chemical agents act independently of each other and there is no interaction between the individual effects)

(ii) **synergism,** when the combined effect is significantly greater than the arithmetic sum of the effects when exposure is to each chemical individually; or

(iii) **antagonism,** when the combined effect is less than additive or may even be below the effect of the least potent agent.

B. **Inhibition,** when exposure is to an established carcinogen at an effective dose, together with or preceded or followed by exposure to a noncarcinogenic chemical agent that is an inhibitor of the carcinogenic response (*see* Reference 8 for database; *see* also Chapter 4 of this monograph).

C. **Promotion/cocarcinogenesis,** when exposure is to an established carcinogen at subcarcinogenic ("subthreshold") dose(s) or to a very weak carcinogen, and this exposure is followed by (in the case of promoter) or simultaneous with (in the case of cocarcinogen) exposure to a noncarcinogenic chemical agent that significantly enhances the carcinogenic response (*see* Reference 9 for database; *see also* Chapter 5 of this monograph).

Among the four types of interactions, "synergism" and "promotion/cocarcinogenesis" exert hazard-enhancing effects beyond the expected level using the additivity model, whereas "antagonism" and "inhibition" have the opposite effects (*i.e.*, are hazard reducing). Each of these four effects represents a Standard Response Category (SRC).

III. CONCEPTUAL PRINCIPLES INVOLVED IN THE DEVELOPMENT OF ISS

The scientific principles underlying and assumptions used in the development of ISS are: (a) the cancer hazard/risk of any complex chemical mixture can be estimated by calculating the sum of the cancer risks of individual carcinogenic constituents present in the mixture followed by correction for the interaction effects which may cause deviation from additivity, (b) the overall interaction effect of a mixture can be approximated by integrating the individual interaction effects of each of all binary pairs of constituents present in the mixture, and (c) in the absence of actual interaction data, the interaction effect of a binary pair of chemicals may be inferred from the predominant interaction effect between the binary pair of chemical classes to which the chemicals belong.

Essentially, ISS consists of two major components: (a) a component to calculate the "Inherent (Cancer) Hazard" of the mixture based on the additivity model and (b) a "Hazard Modification" component to modify the "Inherent Hazard" by a "Weighting Ratio" calculated by analyzing and integrating the possible interaction effects of all the binary pairs of individual constituents of the mixture.

A. The "Inherent Cancer Hazard" Component

This component provides the mechanism for calculating the "Inherent Hazard" of the mixture by using the additivity model. It is based on the assumption that the individual effects of various constituents present in the mixture can be combined in an arithmetically additive manner to provide an estimate of the overall effect. Ideally, the additive effect should be calculated by taking the concentration of each chemical constituent into consideration (*i.e.*, total effect $= \Sigma$ concentration$_i$ $\times$ potency$_i$). However, realistically, for the overwhelming majority of environmental mixtures, information on the concentrations of constituents is either incomplete or nonexistent. Thus, in ISS, at its present stage of development, the overall effect is calculated by summing the potencies of individual constituents (*i.e.*, total effect $= \Sigma$ potency$_i$).

There is no consensus on a universally accepted index for the potency of carcinogens. In ISS, for carcinogens with sound dose–response data, the "Slope Factor" (q_1^*) has been used as an index of relative potency. The Slope Factor (q_1^*) is the slope of the straight line from the upper bound risk at zero dose to the dose producing an upper bound risk of 1%. It expresses the cancer risk (proportion of population affected) per unit of dose (in mg/kg/day or mmole/kg/day) (*e.g.*, 10, 11). The q_1^* values can be calculated using commercially available software (*e.g.*, "Global 86"). The q_1^* values of a number of carcinogens are available in an on-line database such as the U.S. EPA's Integrated Risk Information System (12).

For carcinogens with no q_1^* values and for chemicals strongly suspected to be carcinogenic, structure–activity relationship (SAR) analysis may be used to provide a rough estimate of their relative potencies. SAR analysis (*e.g.*, 13) has been successfully used at the U.S. EPA (*e.g.*, 14–16) to screen for potential cancer hazard of new/untested chemicals.[1] Typically, a narrative term, known as "Concern Level", ranging from Low to High, is assigned to a chemical to rank its potential cancer hazard, based on SAR analysis and available data, by a panel of experts at the U.S. EPA (the "Structure Activity Team", or SAT). Six Concern Level terms have been used; Table 1 shows some representative

---

[1]A knowledge–rule-based artificial intelligence expert system ("OncoLogic"), which embodies the SAR evaluation process of the Structure Activity Team, is currently being developed in cooperation between the U.S. EPA and Logichem, Inc. (Boyertown, PA 19512). This system can generate Concern Level ratings for chemicals to serve as input for the ISS system.

TABLE 1.   Concern Levels Established for Some Representative Carcinogens, Using Structure Activity Relationship (SAR) Analysis, by EPA's Structure Activity Team

Representative carcinogens	Concern Levels
Benzo[*a*]pyrene; 7,12-dimethylbenz[*a*]anthracene; benzidine; 1,2-dimethylhydrazine; diethylnitrosamine; 2,3,7,8-tetrachlorodibenzo-*p*-dioxin	High
Dibenz[*a,h*]anthracene; vinyl chloride; *N*-nitrosopiperidine; methylethylnitrosamine	High moderate
Dibenz[*a,j*]anthracene; chloroethane; *N*-nitrosopyrrolidine	Moderate
Vinylidene chloride; trimethyl phosphate; benz[*a*]anthracene; urethan	Low moderate
Benzo[*e*]pyrene; vinylidene fluoride; butylated hydroxytoluene; 12-*O*-tetradecanoylphorbol-13-acetate; phenol	Marginal
Di-*n*-octylnitrosamine; perylene; pyrene	Low

carcinogens in each of these Concern Level categories. The use of SAR analysis allows us to bring virtually any type of compound into this hazard assessment framework.

To allow conversion between the q_1^* values and the Concern Level scale, a Correspondence Table[2] (*see* Table 2) has been developed using 134 carcinogens, for which q_1^* values have been determined, as a training set, to reach a reasonably even distribution of the q_1^* values among the Concern Level terms. This conversion table renders it possible to calculate the arithmetic sum of the potencies of all carcinogenic constituents of a mixture, from either the q_1^* values or from the Concern Level terms, to give the "Inherent Hazard". Since interaction often modifies hazard by orders of magnitude, the "Inherent Hazard" must be converted to a linearized scale (Exponent Index) before the operation of the "Weighting Ratio" upon the "Inherent Hazard".

B. The "Hazard Modification" Component

One of the unique and powerful features of ISS is its capability to provide an estimate of the overall interaction effect of a mixture based on available interaction data and chemical class assignments. As discussed in Section II, there are four SRCs for interactions among chemicals that may cause deviation from the basic additivity model: synergism (syn), promotion (pro), antagonism (ant), and inhibition (inh). The former two represent "hazard-amplifying" interactions, while the latter two represent "hazard-reducing" interactions. Depending on the relative balance of the totality of hazard-amplifying and hazard-reducing interaction effects, the "Inherent Hazard" level may be accordingly modified upward or downward. Two important and reasonable assumptions have been made: (a) the overall interaction effect can be calculated by integrating the individual interaction effects of all the binary pairs of various constituents of the mixture and (b) in the absence of interaction data on any given binary pair of chemicals, the interaction of the binary pair can be approximated by the predominant interaction effect associated with the binary pair of chemical classes (see Appendix A for a list of the chemical classes in the ISS) to which each chemical belongs.

The "Hazard Modification" component consists of five segments/modules: (i) a computer program to generate all possible binary pairings of chemical constituents of a mixture, (ii) a Master Database which represents the integration of the three U.S. EPA and NCI databases (7–9) on binary interaction of carcinogen with carcinogen/promoter/inhibitor; (iii) search capabilities to locate interaction "hits" (H_A) for each binary pair of chemicals; (iv) mathematical formalism to calculate the adjusted "inferred"

---

[2]Besides q_1^* values and SAR Concern Levels, other alternative indexes/scales (*e.g.*, TD$_{50}$, reference dose) may also be used when sufficient data are available.

TABLE 2. Correspondence Between the Scales of Slope Factors, Exponent Indexes, and Concern Level Terms

Slope Factor[a]	Exponent index[b]	Concern Level[c]
0 to $< 5 \times 10^{-5}$	0 to < 1	Low
5×10^{-5} to $< 5 \times 10^{-1}$	1 to < 4	Marginal
5×10^{-1} to $< 5 \times 10^{0}$	4 to < 6	Low moderate
5×10^{0} to $< 5 \times 10^{1}$	6 to < 8	Moderate
5×10^{1} to $< 5 \times 10^{2}$	8 to < 10	High moderate
5×10^{2} to $\approx 5 \times 10^{7}$	10 to ≈ 14	High

[a]Slope Factor (q_1^*) expressed as cancer risk (proportion of population affected) per mmole/kg/day.

[b]A linear scale of hazard indicators which parallels the ranking sequence of the exponents of the Slope Factors.

[c]A narrative representation of hazard concern levels of chemicals based on SAR analysis.

values (H_B) for each pair of chemicals for which (iii) above can not locate interaction(s) in (ii), but for which interaction can be inferred from class membership in a pair of structural or functional classes (*i.e.*, to which the chemicals belong); and (v) mathematical formalism to calculate the "Weighting Ratio". These modules and their relationships are discussed below in some detail:

a. The number (N) of combinations (binary, ternary, etc.) that can occur between n individual chemicals present in a mixture is given by the factorial formula:

$$N = \frac{(n - 0)(n - 1)(n - 2) \cdots [n - (k - 1)]_k}{k!} \quad (1)$$

where k is the multiplicity of the combination. For binary mixtures ($k = 2$), it can be shown that the number of binary pairings increases rapidly with the number of chemicals (*e.g.*, $N = 45$ for 10 chemicals; $N = 4950$ for 100 chemicals). Owing to the speed of computers, it is feasible to establish binary pairing between any number n of identified compounds in a mixture. ISS contains a program [module (i)] that generates such a set of binary pairs, which is then used by module (iii) to search for interaction "hits" in module (ii).

b. The ISS Master Database [module (ii)] integrates standardized data from the three U.S. EPA and NCI databases (7–9) on binary interactions of carcinogen with either another carcinogen, a promoter, or an inhibitor; the Database contains carcinogenesis binary combination effects data on over 2000 chemicals distributed over 60 structural/functional classes. The Database is structured to allow searching by specifying binary pairs of individual chemical names, as well as binary pairs of chemical class terms. It should be noted that during the process of integrating the three databases into the Master Database, a distinction is made between record counts and analytical counts (or frequency of occurrence counts). A record count represents the total number of *all entries* in a given SRC, including multiple entries, for any pair of compounds. Since the multiple entries merely represent redundancy (*i.e.*, are only confirmatory of the same interaction for any pair of compounds in a given SRC), the record count is reduced to an analytical count of 1 to prevent undue overrepresentation. For the tallying of H_A and calculation of H_B described below, only the analytical counts are used.

c. The ISS search program [module (iii)] is designed to search for matching pairs between the set of binary pairs generated in (i) and those present in the Master Database [module (ii)] to locate interaction "hits" of the four SRCs (*i.e.*, syn, pro, ant, inh) that may cause deviation from the basic additivity model. For each binary pair of individual chemicals, a "name pair" hit is registered if interaction data on this specific pair are located in the Master Database. The number of "name pair" hits of the mixture is then tallied to give the total number (H_A) of "name pair" hits for each of the four SRCs.

d. For each binary pair with no "name pair" hit, ISS continues to search for interaction hits associated with the binary pair of structural/functional classes ("class pair" hits) to which the chemicals belong. Since "class pair" hits only represent possible interaction based on class membership, they are given less weight than "name pair" hits. For each SRC, the raw score of the total number of "class pair" hits is tallied and then statistically adjusted in module (iv) to give the "class pair" inferred value (H_B). The statistical adjustment of raw score of "class pair" hits involves consideration of the number of documented interactions between each class pair in the ISS Database, the distribution of the type of SRC effect within a class–class interaction, and the representativeness of classes in the ISS Database (see Appendix B of this chapter). The equation derived for these adjustments is

$$H_{B \text{ effect } x,y} = \left[\frac{(O_{\text{effect}})^2}{E_{\text{effect}} (n_x + n_y)} \right]_{\text{Lim} \longrightarrow 1} \tag{2}$$

where $H_{B \text{ effect } x,y}$ = the inferred value of a class pair interaction effect (synergism, promotion, antagonism, or inhibition) for a class x–class y interaction.

O_{effect} = an observed (counted) number of interactions for the effect between class x and class y.

E_{effect} = an estimated number of interactions for the effect between class x and class y.

n_x = the number of compounds in class x.

n_y = the number of compounds in class y.

The maximum limiting value of 1 has been placed on each $H_{B \text{ effect } x, y}$ because the contribution of a class pair interaction calculated inferred value should not exceed that of a name pair "hit".

For each SRC, the total interaction effect of the mixture with respect to that particular SRC is the sum of H_A and H_B; *e.g.*:

$$H_{\text{syn}} = H_{A \text{ syn}} + H_{B \text{ syn}} \tag{3}$$

e. Module (v) carries out the calculation of the Weighting Ratio (*WR*), which embodies the hazard modification trend due to interactions between mixture constituents. The extent of hazard modification is dependent on relative balance between hazard-amplifying and hazard-reducing interactions. This is represented in its general form as:

$$WR = \frac{\text{hazard-amplifying interaction effects}}{\text{hazard-reducing interaction effects}} \tag{4}$$

The algebraic form of *WR* is given by the equation:

$$WR = \frac{1 + (pH_{\text{syn}} + qH_{\text{pro}})}{1 + (rH_{\text{ant}} + sH_{\text{inh}})} \tag{5}$$

where the p, q, r, and s are "hazard-modification effectiveness coefficients", which reflect the effectiveness of the four types of combination effects to modify the "Inherent Hazard" level of chemicals. These coefficients are empirical and reflect the perspective of the entire combination effects literature (as well as the user's conceptual biases). It is the authors' present view that $p = 0.3$, $q = 0.7$, $r = 0.3$, and $s = 0.6$ are reasonable values. However, it is only through extended testing of this system and additional experimental data, becoming available in the future, that an increasingly accurate set of values for these coefficients will be reached.

The presence of the unit number in both the numerator and the denominator of the *WR* provides an algebraic formalism that will yield a working and realistic *WR* value even in limit circumstances when the hazard amplifying/reducing ratio would become a 0/x or x/0 type of expression, either as a result of actual data or because of partial absence of data. Furthermore, this formalism yields $WR = 1$ (and will leave therefore the "Inherent Hazard" invariant) either when the hazard amplifying/reducing ratio would be 1 because of complete balance of hazard amplifying/reducing effects or when it would be 0 because of total absence of data on combination effects.

Substituting for H_{effect} terms, the explicit form for WR is

$$WR = \frac{1 + p(H_{\text{A syn}} + H_{\text{B syn}}) + q(H_{\text{A pro}} + H_{\text{B pro}})}{1 + r(H_{\text{A ant}} + H_{\text{B ant}}) + s(H_{\text{A inh}} + H_{\text{B inh}})} \tag{6}$$

where $H_{\text{A syn}}$ = the count of name pair hits for synergism
   $H_{\text{A pro}}$ = the count of name pair hits for promotion
   $H_{\text{A ant}}$ = the count of name pair hits for antagonism
   $H_{\text{A inh}}$ = the count of name pair hits for inhibition
   $H_{\text{B syn}}$ = the class pair inferred values for synergism
   $H_{\text{B pro}}$ = the class pair inferred values for promotion
   $H_{\text{B ant}}$ = the class pair inferred values for antagonism
   $H_{\text{B inh}}$ = the class pair inferred values for inhibition
   p, q, r, s = hazard modification effectiveness coefficients for the four SRCs syn, pro, ant, and inh, respectively

Combining the outputs from the "Inherent Hazard" component and the "Hazard Modification" component, the Relative Hazard Ranking value of any complex mixture with known constituents can now be computed by multiplying the "Inherent Hazard" (expressed in Exponent Index Unit) of the mixture by the "Weighting Ratio". The numerical value thus obtained can be directly used for cancer hazard ranking, or converted back to a Concern Level term using the conversion table (Table 2).

IV. SYSTEM OVERVIEW AND APPLICATION TO SAMPLE MIXTURES

ISS is a menu-driven, user-friendly software system that can be used effectively with only minimal computer training. It is designed to be used on any IBM PC compatible (preferably AT) computer with at least 512 KB memory and a hard disk with 10 MB of free disk space. The software was written in Clipper (Nantucket Software) using dBase III plus database files. Over 14,000 lines of source codes were used to write this program.

Figure 1 presents the system logic flowchart which entails: (a) steps for the evaluation of the "Inherent Hazard" of the mixture, (b) steps for binary pairing by chemical names and chemical Class Term Assignments (CTA), and (c) steps for search for "hits" in the ISS Master Database and for computation of a "Weighting Ratio" for adjusting the "Inherent Hazard".

Once the list of chemical names of the compounds in a mixture is established and the Slope Factors or Concern Level terms are introduced, the program computes the "Inherent Hazard". The compounds are then paired into all of the possible binary combinations of names. The ISS uses these name pairs to search for matching pairs present in the Database. If a specific name pair is found in the Database, that specific interaction (or interactions) is counted as a name "hit" and the search for that name pair is terminated.

Since evidently not all possible chemical name pairs can be found in the ISS Database, it is most probable that in any run of the program no interaction "hit" will be registered for many name pairs. Each of these chemical name pairs is then "translated" into its chemical class pair, so that a class interaction search can be carried out. If any interaction

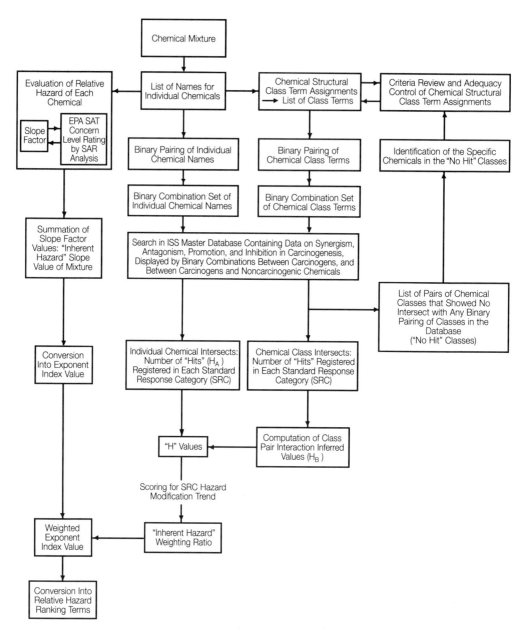

FIGURE 1. ISS System Logic Flowchart. [The Standard Response Categories (SRCs) are synergism (syn), antagonism (ant), inhibition (inh), and promotion/cocarcinogenesis (pro). EPA SAT = U.S. Environmental Protection Agency Structure–Activity Team; SAR = structure–activity relationship.]

exists between the two classes representing a pair, the extent of interaction is calculated and that inferred value is regarded as a class pair "hit"; the search for that class pair is then terminated.

As a safeguard against the possibility that some chemicals may have been missed (in a search by chemical class search criterion), because of improper or incomplete CTA, the system provides a listing of those pairs of chemical classes that did not intersect with any binary pair of classes in the Master Database ("no hit" classes). The chemicals in the "no hit" classes are identified and rerouted for "Criteria Review and Adequacy Control of Chemical Structural Class Assignment" (*see* Fig. 1) so as to allow verification of the correctness of the CTA, and the search may be repeated using the new CTA (if any). To avoid overrepresentation of any given binary pair of chemicals, the chemical class assignment is limited to no more than two.

The use of and hazard ranking values yielded by the ISS program are illustrated here by the *WR* values computed by the system for 6 sample mixtures. Table 3 summarizes the results of the ISS-generated hazard modification *WR* for these mixtures. Mixture #1, a polynuclear aromatic hydrocarbon (PAH) mixture containing two potent carcinogens (benzo[*a*]pyrene and 7,12-dimethylbenz[*a*]anthracene) and three weak or inactive compounds, has a *WR* of 0.63, indicating that the combined effect is expected to be less than that calculated by using the additivity model. This is consistent with data review that the predominant interaction among PAHs is antagonism (17; *see also* Chapter 2 of this monograph) and the experimental findings (*e.g.*, 18) that PAH mixtures tend to have lower carcinogenic potential than that expected by summing the carcinogenic potencies of individual PAHs. Not all PAH mixtures are expected to interact identically. This can in fact be shown with the ISS system. A slight change in the chemical composition of mixture #1 (replace 3,9-dimethylbenz[*a*]anthracene with cyclopenta[*c,d*]pyrene) yields a mixture (#2) with a higher *WR* of 0.81, reflecting a partial offsetting of the predominant antagonism among PAHs by the known synergistic interaction (19) between the specific binary pair of benzo[*a*]pyrene and cyclopenta[*c,d*]pyrene.

In addition to PAH mixtures, a mixture (mixture #3) which contains two potent PAH carcinogens (7,12-dimethylbenz[*a*]anthracene and 3-methylcholanthrene) and three active aromatic amine or azo dye carcinogens (2-acetylaminofluorene, 3'-methyl-4-dimethyl-aminoazobenzene, methylenedianiline) also yields a *WR* less than 1, indicating that the hazard-reducing interactions outweigh hazard-amplifying interactions. This is consistent with the finding that antagonism prevails in the class pair of PAH and aromatic amine/azo dye carcinogens (17).

In contrast to the dominance of hazard-reducing interactions in mixtures #1 to 3, the *WR* of mixtures #4 to 6 exceeds 1.0, indicating that the combined effect is expected to be greater than that calculated by using the additivity model. The ISS-generated screen which shows the interaction profile that yields a *WR* of 1.5 for mixture #4 is Figure 2. There are

TABLE 3. ISS-Generated Hazard Modification Weighting Ratios of Selected Sample Mixtures

Mixture	Constituent chemicals in mixture	Weighting Ratio
#1	Benz[*a*]anthracene; benzo[*a*]pyrene; 7,12-dimethylbenz[*a*]anthracene; 3,9-dimethylbenz[*a*]anthracene; pyrene	0.63
#2	Benz[*a*]anthracene; benzo[*a*]pyrene; 7,12-dimethylbenz[*a*]anthracene; cyclopenta[*c,d*]pyrene; pyrene	0.81
#3	7,12-dimethylbenz[*a*]anthracene; 3-methylcholanthrene; methylenedianiline; 2-acetylaminofluorene; 3'-methyl-4-dimethylaminoazobenzene	0.83
#4	Benz[*a*]anthracene; benzo[*a*]pyrene; butylated hydroxytoluene; 2,3,7,8-tetrachlorodibenzodioxin; diethylnitrosamine	1.50
#5	Benz[*a*]anthracene; benzo[*a*]pyrene; 2,3,7,8-tetrachlorodibenzodioxin; diethylnitrosamine	1.91
#6	Benz[*a*]anthracene; croton oil; phenol; pyrene; urethan	2.52

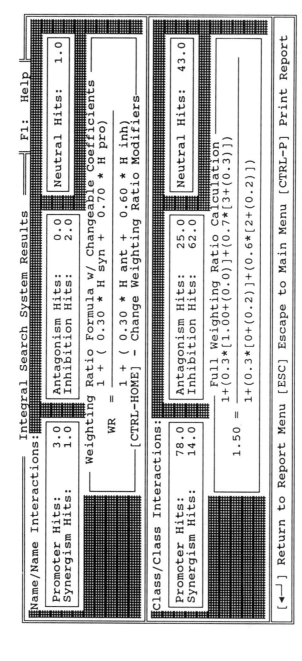

FIGURE 2. Printout of the ISS screen showing the profile of Name Pair and Class Pair interaction "hits" and calculation of the Weighting Ratio (*WR*) for mixture #4. (See Table 3 for composition of mixture #4.)

194

seven "name pair" hits[3] – four hazard-enhancing (three promotion and one synergism), two hazard-reducing (two inhibition) and one neutral (*i.e.*, additive) – and a variety of "class pair" hits. The totality of these hits yields an overall WR of 1.5. Most of the hazard-reducing interactions are attributable to the presence of butylated hydroxytoluene (BHT). Indeed, deletion of BHT from mixture # 4 yields a mixture (mixture #5) with a substantially higher WR of 1.91.

The ISS-generated WR for mixture #6 is 2.52, mainly because of multiple promotion hits with few or no hazard-reducing hits. The impact of applying this WR to the assessment of potential cancer hazard is depicted in Figure 3. There are no q_1^* values available on any of the compounds in mixture # 6. SAR considerations assign (*see* Table 1) a Concern Level of Low to pyrene and of Low Moderate to both benz[*a*]anthracene and urethan. Phenol and croton oil (even though the latter is a powerful promoter) have Concern Level ratings of marginal as *complete* carcinogens. With the use of the Correspondence Table (Table 2), these Concern Levels are converted to estimated q_1^* values (1×10^0 for Low Moderate and 1×10^{-2} for Marginal) for calculation of the "Inherent Hazard". The additivity model yields an "Inherent Hazard" q_1^* of 2.02×10^0, which is still in the Low Moderate range. However, after operating the WR of 2.52 upon the respective exponent index (5.21), the final adjusted estimated overall cancer hazard becomes 4.06×10^6 in q_1^* units, which is in the High concern range. This example illustrates the importance of taking interaction effects into account in assessing the potential cancer hazard of mixtures.

V. CLOSING NOTE

ISS is a unique computerized system capable of giving approximate, but realistic assessments of the potential cancer hazard of chemical mixtures. The information is useful for hazard ranking and for identifying research gaps.

Since the conceptual assumptions made in developing ISS have important implications for the hazard assessment of complex mixtures, it is the authors' hope that this conceptual framework will stimulate research to test these assumptions. The ISS represents the first scientific attempt where the totality of known interactions in chemical carcinogenesis was made to bear on the cancer hazard assessment of complex chemical mixtures. It is, however, most certainly not the last word in this assessment, as these conceptual insights will continue to develop.

It should also be borne in mind that no conceptual sophistication of any hazard ranking procedure can remedy the considerable uncertainties that often surround the experimental data on which the ranking is based. Great approximations, tenuous extrapolations, imperfect/incomplete study designs, and enormous data gaps are sometimes encountered in the literature on the carcinogenic effects of chemical combinations. Moreover, among the masses of data that have been analyzed for constructing the ISS Master Database, studies involving dose–response relationship of the interacting partners of chemicals are so scarce as to be virtually nonexistent; yet, this can be of critical importance in some instances where, depending on experimental conditions and levels of the interacting compounds, the same combination may be hazard-amplifying or hazard-reducing (*cf*. 21). Furthermore, there is no standard or accepted method of evaluation/ expression for the intensity of the different combination responses. All these uncertainties and limitations must be kept in mind in the area of carcinogenic effects of chemical combinations.

---

[3]The actual records of interaction data can be retrieved using the databases (7-9) or search software (17,20).

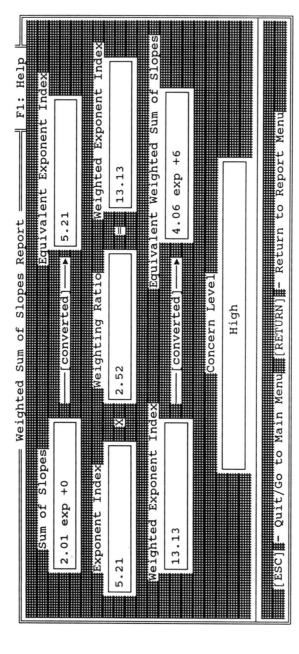

FIGURE 3. Printout of the ISS screen showing application of the Weighting Ratio to modify the sum of Slope Factors (q_1^*) calculated by using the additivity model to arrive at the final Concern Level for mixture #6. (See Table 2 for the Concern Level/q_1^*/Exponent Index correspondence table and Table 3 for composition of mixture #6).

APPENDIX A: LIST OF STRUCTURAL AND FUNCTIONAL CLASSES OF CHEMICALS IN ISS

1   Aldehydes
2   Aliphatic amines and amides
3   Aliphatic di-/tri-carboxylic acids and derivatives
4   Aliphatic and cycloaliphatic hydrocarbons
5   Alkenylbenzenes, cinnamyl and related compounds
6   Alkyl sulfides, sulfoxides, and sulfones
7   Amino acids and related compounds
8   Antioxidants and free radical scavengers (not including retinoids)
9   Aromatic amines (including nitroarenes)
10 Arylcarboxylic/arylalkylcarboxylic acids and derivatives
11 Azo dyes
12 Barbiturate derivatives and analogs
13 Benzene, naphthalene, and alkyl derivatives
14 Benzodiazepine derivatives
15 Benzothiazine/phenothiazine derivatives and analogs
16 Benzoxazin/phenoxazin derivatives and analogs
17 Branched (omega $-$ 1) carboxylic acids and derivatives
18 Carbamates, ureas, and thioanalogs
19 Choline and derivatives, phospholipids
20 Croton oil, phorbol esters, and related compounds
21 Cyanates and thiocyanates
22 Direct-acting alkylating, arylating, and acylating agents
23 Estrogenic and androgenic compounds
24 Fibrous materials
25 Flavonoids and other benzopyran derivatives
26 Haloalkanes and haloalkenes
27 Halogenated aromatics and analogs
28 Hydrazo and azoxy compounds and derivatives
29 Indoles and compounds containing indole substructure
30 Inorganic salts of alkali and alkaline earth metals
31 Lactones, lactams, anhydrides, cyclic imides, and coumarins
32 Macrocyclic ethers and esters
33 Metals/metalloids complexes, chelates, organic salts, and organometallics
34 Metals/metalloids, inorganic
35 Methylxanthines and other purine/pyrimidine/pyrazine compounds
36 Mycotoxins
37 Nitrosamines and nitrosamides
38 Ornithine decarboxylase inhibitors
39 Peroxides and peroxy compounds, other oxidizing agents
40 Peroxisome proliferators
41 Phenolic compounds
42 Polycyclic aromatic hydrocarbons (homo- and hetero-)
43 Polyhalogenated cycloaliphatics
44 Polymeric substances (natural and synthetic), nonfibrous
45 Protease inhibitors
46 Pyrazole/imidazole derivatives
47 Pyridine/quinoline derivatives
48 Pyrrolizidine alkaloids

49   Quinones
50   Retinoids and carotenoids
51   Selenium compounds
52   Simple alcohols, dihydroxy compounds, and glycerols
53   Steroids (excluding sex hormones), cholesterol, bile acids, and related
54   Straight chain aliphatic fatty acids, esters, and derivatives
55   Sulfhydryl reactors, mercapto, and related compounds
56   Sulfonamides
57   Surfactants
58   Terpenes and terpenoid compounds
59   Unidentified class
60   Chelating agents
61   Polyhydroxy compounds and polyacetates

APPENDIX B: DERIVATION OF CLASS HIT VALUES (H_B) AS INFERENCES FROM CLASS INTERACTIONS[4]

1.   General Principles

The inferred value (H_B) of an interaction between any two compounds is a function of the intersection of the two classes in which the compounds have class membership and which classes have documented interactions between them:

$$H_{B \text{ effect } x,y} = f (\text{class x} \cap \text{class y}) \tag{B1}$$

where $H_{B \text{ effect } x,y}$ = the class pair interaction value for compounds x and y, where "effect" is in any of the SRCs
    class x   = the class in which compound "x" is a member
    class y   = the class in which compound "y" is a member

The maximum value of $H_{B \text{ effect } x,y}$ should not exceed 1. Since a class pair is the representation of a single name pair, a class pair should only be counted as some number from 0 to 1, but not more than 1 (for any given effect). This simulates the effect that one name pair should have on the Weighting Ratio Formula, but limits the relative impact of a class pair which should carry less weight in the calculation than a name pair.

H_B should be dependent on the number of documented interactions between two classes of compounds in the ISS Database. In any interaction category a class pair with 20 entries, for example, is better documented than a similar class pair with 5 entries.

H_B is also dependent on the distribution of effects within a class intersection. If a class intersection exhibits a greater number of instances of promotion than of synergism, a greater inferred value of promotion than of synergism should reflect this distribution.

The direct and indirect variables extracted from the class–class interactions are (a) the counts of synergism, promotion, antagonism, and inhibition interactions found in each

---

[4]From User's Manual for "The Integral Search System for Cancer Hazard Ranking of Complex Chemical Mixtures", EPA/SAIC, Washington, D.C./Falls Church, Virginia, 1994.

class intersection; (b) the number of chemical names found in each class; (c) the sum of the numbers of all interactions found in each class intersection; (d) the numbers of interactions in the database summed following interaction categories; and (e) the sum total of *all* interactions documented in the database.

These variables are used to calculate the inferred H_B values for undocumented name pair interactions. Using these variables, the joint frequency distribution statistical inference method allows the evaluation of the current distribution of interactions for class intersections. This simple method relies on column and row margin sums from a matrix to evaluate the distribution as illustrated by the example below.

2. The Class Pair Interaction Matrix

A matrix is generated by the ISS software using the variables summarized above. One axis of the matrix lists the intersecting classes of the database. The other axis lists the types of effects within each of the intersections. The matrix can provide margin values (sums of categories) by class and effect for each of the categories.

Table B1 is an example of an observed class–class interaction matrix generated within the ISS. The matrix is generated by scanning the entire interaction database within the ISS and counting the interaction types by class. This observed class–class interaction matrix is not used directly to determine H_B.

This example illustrates that in the first row (Class 1:Class 2 intersection) there are three records in the ISS Database where a class 1 compound interacted with synergism to a class 2 compound; nine records where a class 1 compound interacted with promotion to a class 2 compound; four records on antagonism; and two records on inhibition. The total number of documented interactions between all of the class 1 compounds and all of the class 2 compounds is 18. The last column is the sum of the numbers of chemical compounds listed in class 1 and class 2.

The margin values (boldfaced numbers) in Table B1 are the sums of each of the categories. The row margin values are the sums of the numbers of all known interactions between one class and another. The column margin values are the sums of the numbers of all known interaction effects within each interaction category throughout the entire database.

TABLE B1. Example of the Observed Values from the ISS Database

Classes involved in each interaction (class pairs)	Number of synergism interactions	Number of promotion interactions	Number of antagonism interactions	Number of inhibition interactions	Sum of numbers of interactions	Sum of number of compounds in classes by class pair
Class 1:Class 2	3	9	4	2	**18**	22
Class 1:Class 3	5	3	6	0	**14**	27
Class 1:Class 4	0	3	4	8	**15**	32
Class 2:Class 3	2	6	0	3	**11**	33
Class 2:Class 4	7	2	5	0	**14**	26
... (all others)	...	...	...	...	...	...
Sum of number of interactions by category	**124**	**85**	**77**	**56**	**342**	

Note: The boldfaced numbers indicate sums of the categories and are not part of the matrix itself.

3. Absolute Cell Frequencies and Expected Cell Values

Expected values, assuming equality of frequency distributions of all interactions, can be calculated for each cell (interaction count) of Table B1. This expected value, known as the absolute cell frequency, E, is given by the formula:

$$E = \frac{RC}{T} \tag{B2}$$

where E = the expected value
R = the sum of the row in which the cell resides (row margin value)
C = the sum of the column in which the cell resides (column margin value)
T = the sum total of all interactions in the database (sum of row or column values)

Example:

For Class 1:Class 2 synergism, the expected value equals the row margin value, times the column margin value, divided by the sum of all of the interactions in the database. Application of Equation B2 to the Class 1:Class 2 synergism cell in Table B1 yields:

$$6.53 = \left(\frac{18 \times 124)}{342} \right)$$

Table B2 shows the expected values of each of the interactions for each of the classes.
Comparison of Table B1 with Table B2 indicates how much the observed values deviate from the expected values. This deviation is given by the formula:

$$\text{Cell Deviation} = \frac{O_{\text{cell}}}{E_{\text{cell}}} \tag{B3}$$

where O_{cell} = the observed value of the cell (Table B1)
E_{cell} = the expected value of the cell (Table B2)

TABLE B2. Expected Values of Interactions

Classes involved in each interaction (class pairs)	Number of synergism interactions	Number of promotion interactions	Number of antagonism interactions	Number of inhibition interactions	Sum of number of interactions	Sum of number of compounds in classes by class pair
Class 1:Class 2	6.53	4.47	4.05	2.95	**18**	22
Class 1:Class 3	5.07	3.47	3.15	2.29	**14**	27
Class 1:Class 4	5.43	3.72	3.38	2.45	**15**	32
Class 2:Class 3	3.98	2.73	2.48	1.80	**11**	33
Class 2:Class 4	5.07	3.47	3.15	2.29	**14**	26
... (all others)	...	...	...	...	...	...
Sum of number of interactions by category	**124**	**85**	**77**	**56**	**342**	

Note: The boldfaced numbers indicate sums of the categories and are not part of the matrix itself.

If the observed data always followed an equal frequency distribution, this ratio in Equation B3 would always equal 1. When the observed data are less than the expected, Equation B3 will yield <1, indicating that the distribution is skewed away from the probability that an interaction could be found if two more compounds were investigated. When the observed value is higher than the expected, Equation B3 will yield >1 and indicate that the distribution is skewed toward the probability that an interaction could be found if two more compounds were investigated. Thus, the values yielded by Equation B3 represent a good inference for interaction and it is therefore used to modify the class intersection data.

4. Representativeness of Classes in the Database

All of the possible interactions between compounds have not been investigated. If those inquiries had been made, there would be no reason for the ISS. This statement may seem obvious, but it points out that the representativeness of the current database must be evaluated when determining whether or not the data are sufficient to infer an accurate value of an interaction. A complete statistical evaluation of the probability of an undocumented interaction falling within one effect or another would be highly desirable, but may not be any more accurate than a simple function which estimates the real value for H_B.

The representativeness of a class intersection can be estimated as the ratio of the number of observed interactions of each effect to the sum of the number of chemical compounds (chemical names) in the pair of classes in which the effect occurred:

$$R = \frac{O_{\text{effect}}}{n_x + n_y} \qquad \text{(B4)}$$

where R = the representativeness of a cell with respect to the possible interaction categories
    O_{effect} = the observed count of the interactions for an effect
    n_x = the number of compounds in class x
    n_y = the number of compounds in class y

5. Calculation of H_B Values

The function for determining the H_B value for a cell may be derived from the ratio for frequency distribution deviation (Equation B3) and the ratio of representativeness of the database (Equation B4). Combination of these terms yields the equation:

$$H_{\text{B effect x,y}} = \left[\frac{O_{\text{effect}}}{E_{\text{effect}}} \right] \left[\frac{O_{\text{effect}}}{(n_x + n_y)} \right] \qquad \text{(B5)}$$

where $H_{\text{B effect x,y}}$ is the inferred value of a class pair interaction effect (synergism, promotion, antagonism, or inhibition) for a class x–class y interaction
    O_{effect} is an observed (counted) number of interactions for the effect between class x and class y
    E_{effect} is an estimated number of interactions for the effect between class x and class y
    n_x is the number of compounds in class x
    n_y is the number of compounds in class y

Since — as mentioned above in "General Principles" — the contribution of a class pair interaction calculated inferred value should not exceed that of a name pair "hit", the maximum value allowed for $H_{B \text{ effect } x,y}$ should have the limit of 1. Incorporation of this requirement into Equation B5 and combining terms yield the equation:

$$H_{B \text{ effect } x,y} = \left[\frac{(O_{\text{effect}})^2}{E_{\text{effect}} (n_x + n_y)} \right]_{\text{Lim} \rightarrow 1} \tag{B6}$$

6. Preparing an Inferred H_B Values Class Matrix; the Use of These Values in the Weighting Ratio

Using Equation B6 for calculating the class interaction inference values, a class matrix for inference values is prepared. The expected values class matrix in Table B2 yields the inference values matrix in Table B3.

H_B values can thus be determined for each interaction type. The function has the form:

$$H_{B \text{ effect}} = H_{B \text{ effect } 1,2} + H_{B \text{ effect } 1,3} + \ldots + H_{B \text{ effect } x,y} \tag{B7}$$

where "effect" represents interactions in any of the SRCs.

For example, from the class matrix in Table B3, the H_B values for each SRC can be calculated as the sum of the inferred values of class pairs in each interaction type: $H_{B \text{ syn}} = 0.31$; $H_{B \text{ pro}} = 1.40$; $H_{B \text{ ant}} = 0.78$; $H_{B \text{ inh}} = 1.02$. These values are the sums of the inferred values of class pair interactions for five pairs of classes (derived from five chemical name pairs), each contributing a value below 1. These H_B values are substituted along with H_A values (actual name pair hits) into the Weighting Ratio (*WR*) equation,

$$WR = \frac{1 + p(H_{A \text{ syn}} + H_{B \text{ syn}}) + q(H_{A \text{ pro}} + H_{B \text{ pro}})}{1 + r(H_{A \text{ ant}} + H_{B \text{ ant}}) + s(H_{A \text{ inh}} + H_{B \text{ inh}})} \tag{B8}$$

to provide the output from the "Hazard Modification" component for combining with the output from the "Inherent Hazard" component to generate the final concern level.

TABLE B3. Inferred H_B Values for the Example ISS Class Matrix

Classes involved in each interaction	Synergism interactions	Promotion interactions	Antagonism interactions	Inhibition interactions
Class 1:Class 2	0.06	0.82	0.18	0.06
Class 1:Class 3	0.18	0.10	0.42	0.00
Class 1:Class 4	0.00	0.08	0.15	0.81
Class 2:Class 3	0.03	0.40	0.00	0.15
Class 2:Class 4	0.04	0.00	0.03	0.00
Sum of inferred interaction values by category	0.31	1.40	0.78	1.02

Note: All values have been rounded to two decimal places.

Disclaimer. The scientific views expressed in this article are solely those of the authors and do not necessarily reflect the views or policies of the U.S. EPA or of Science Applications International Corporation (SAIC).

REFERENCES

1. National Academy of Sciences: "Complex Mixtures". National Academy Press, Washington, D.C., 1988.
2. Schmähl, D.: "Combination Effects in Chemical Carcinogenesis". VCH Publishers, Weinheim, Germany, 1988.
3. Calabrese, E. J.: "Multiple Chemical Interactions". Lewis Publishers, Chelsea, Michigan, 1991.
4. Silkworth, J. B., Cutler, D. S., and Sack, G.: *Fundam. Appl. Toxicol.* **12**, 303 (1989).
5. Rodericks, J. V.: *Hazardous Waste* **1**, 333 (1984).
6. U.S. Environmental Protection Agency: Proposed Guidelines for the Health Risk Assessment of Chemical Mixtures. *Fed. Register* **50** (6), 1170 (1985).
7. Arcos, J. C., Woo, Y.-T., and Lai, D. Y.: Database on Binary Combination Effects of Chemical Carcinogens. *Environ. Carcino. Rev.* **C6**, No. 1, Special Issue, 1988.
8. Bagheri, D., Doeltz, M. K., Fay, J. R., Helmes, C. T., Monasmith, L. A., and Sigman, C. C.: Database of Inhibitors of Carcinogenesis. *Environ. Carcino. Rev.* **C6**, No. 3, Special Issue, 1988/89.
9. Rao, V. R., Woo, Y.-T., Lai, D. Y., and Arcos, J. C.: Database on Promoters of Chemical Carcinogenesis. *Environ. Carcino. Rev.* **C7**, No. 2, Special Issue, 1989.
10. Crump, K. S.: *J. Environ. Pathol. Toxicol.* **5**, 675 (1981).
11. Crump, K. S., and Allen, B. C.: *Am. Stat.* **19**, 442 (1985).
12. U.S. Environmental Protection Agency: *Fed. Register* **53** (106), 20162 (1988).
13. Woo, Y.-t., Lai, D. Y., Arcos, J. C., and Argus, M. F: General Principles for the Prediction of Potential Carcinogenic Activity of Chemical Compounds. *In* "Chemical Induction of Cancer – Structural Bases and Biological Mechanisms", Vol. IIIC. Academic Press, San Diego, 1988, Appendix V, p. 741.
14. Arcos, J. C.: *J. Am. Coll. Toxicol.* **2**, 131 (1983).
15. Di Carlo, F. J., Bickart, P., and Auer, C. M.: *Drug Metab. Rev.* **17**, 171 (1986).
16. Auer, C. M., and Gould, D. H.: *Environ. Carcino. Rev.* **C5**, 29 (1987).
17. Polansky, G., and Woo, Y.-t.: *Environ. Carcino. Rev.* **C7**, 109 (1989).
18. Springer, D. L., Mann, D. B., Dankovic, D. A., Thomas, B. L., Wright, C. W., and Mahlum, D. D.: *Carcinogenesis* **10**, 131 (1989).
19. Cavalieri, E., Munhall, A., Rogan, E., Salmasi, S., and Patil, K.: *Carcinogenesis* **4**, 393 (1983).
20. Polansky, G., Woo, Y.-t., Arcos, J. C., and Argus, M. F.: Development of a Promoter Carcinogen Interaction Database Software System and Its Use in Data Analysis. *In* "Proceedings of 4th International Conference on the Combined Effects of Environmental Factors" (L. D. Fechter, ed.). Johns Hopkins Univ. Sch. Hyg. & Public Health publisher, Baltimore, 1991, p. 9.
21. Farber, E. *Tumor Biol.* **9**, 165 (1988).

CHAPTER **7**

Intercellular Communication: A Paradigm for the Interpretation of the Initiation/Promotion/Progression Model of Carcinogenesis

James E. Trosko, Chia-Cheng Chang,
Burra V. Madhukar, and Emmanuel Dupont

> *. . . during the critical periods, the cancer cells*
> *are susceptible to the influence of the host and are*
> *restrained by the normal cells. The basis for this is*
> *the fact that the normal sequel to an injury is*
> *growth which reaches a certain level and then*
> *stops when the injury has been repaired. . . . This*
> *growth must stop by some self-regulatory process*
> *which is possessed by normal cells but is not*
> *possessed by tumor cells.*
>
> V. R. Potter (1)

I. INTRODUCTION: CANCER AS A PROBLEM OF HOMEOSTATIC DYSFUNCTION

The insight provided by this quotation of Potter seems to have been lost or overshadowed by recent spectacular advances in the molecular biology of cancer. This is illustrated by the statement, "Understanding the cellular basis of cancer means being able to describe the biochemistry of the regulated pathways between cell surface and nucleus that control cell growth" (2). In spite of the success in elaborating the identity and structure of many oncogenes and their cellular products, as well as elucidating the details of several transmembrane signaling mechanisms, Varmus (3) has recently stated: "The hopes . . . must be balanced against pessimism borne of two long-standing frustrations in oncogenetics: (a) the failure to identify the relevant targets for the neoplastic action of oncogenes, even when the oncoproteins have provocative biochemical properties, such as protein kinase or guanine nucleotide binding activity . . . " .

Fundamentally, one might ask "why, with so much success on the molecular level, do we not have an understanding of how oncogenes function?" The answer seems to be because the bulk of the cancer research effort has been guided by a reductionist rather than an interactive or holistic approach. Cancer seemed to be a problem *within* a cell, rather than a "problem of cell interaction, not only within tissues, but with distant cells in other tissues" (4).

In reaction to the current pressure to approach the solution to the understanding of the "mechanism" of carcinogenesis only by means of molecular biology, Levitt (5) stated, "As a matter of fact, a number of areas crucial to our understanding of cellular homeostasis—the key to unraveling the biology of cancer—are not ready to make the transition to the molecular phase of investigation".

To begin to view the cancer problem from another perspective, one must recognize that multicellular organisms, including rats and humans, are the result of a hierarchical organization of levels (*e.g.*, cells, tissues, organs, systems) held together by various homeostatic or cybernetic mechanisms. Claude Bernard and W. B. Cannon were the first to introduce the cybernetic or homeostatic control concept of living organisms on the physiological level (6,7).

The objective of this Chapter is to examine several paradigms associated with the understanding of the cancer problem at some level and to integrate these paradigms into one which reflects cancer as a problem of homeostatic dysfunction. Toward this aim the initiation/promotion/progression theory of carcinogenesis (8), the oncogene concept (9), the paradigm of "carcinogenesis as mutagenesis" (10), "cancer as a disease of differentiation" (11) or "oncogeny as partially blocked or blocked ontogeny" (12), cancer as a stem cell disease (13), and the concept of intercellular communication (14) will be examined.

II. THE NATURAL HISTORY OF CARCINOGENESIS

The objective of the scientific method is to explain observations in order to make useful and testable predictions. In order to formulate a theory of carcinogenesis, a tremendous number of observations must be examined in order to generate a meaningful theory.

From experimental studies in animals, epidemiological examination of human cancers, and recent oncogene research, it has been concluded that the conversion of a normal cell to a metastasizing, invasive cancer cell is not the result of a single step (15). The multistep carcinogenic process seems to involve the evolution of phenotypes, including the inability to terminally differentiate (11,16), the loss of growth control (17) or contact inhibition (18), the inability to perform normal gap–junctional intercellular communication (19), and to migrate to distal tissues and to invade these tissues (20).

The tumor, once formed, appears to be clonally derived from the single errant stem cell (21). However, the clonal expansion during the multistep carcinogenic process involves acquisition of many phenotypes within the tumor, possibly due to additional genetic and/or epigenetic changes (22).

The operational concepts of initiation, promotion, and progression were derived from observations on experimental animals (23) (Figure 1). The multistage nature of carcinogenesis in studies on mouse skin carcinogenesis and, more recently, in liver and bladder (24) indicated very discrete and distinctive characteristics associated with the different phases of carcinogenesis. Although the operational concepts of initiation/promotion/progression do not imply any particular mechanism of action, it is clear that the mechanisms underlying these three stages are different (25).

Assuming the initiation event takes place in a single stem or progenitor cell, the experimental observations suggest strongly that the event is ostensibly *irreversible*. True

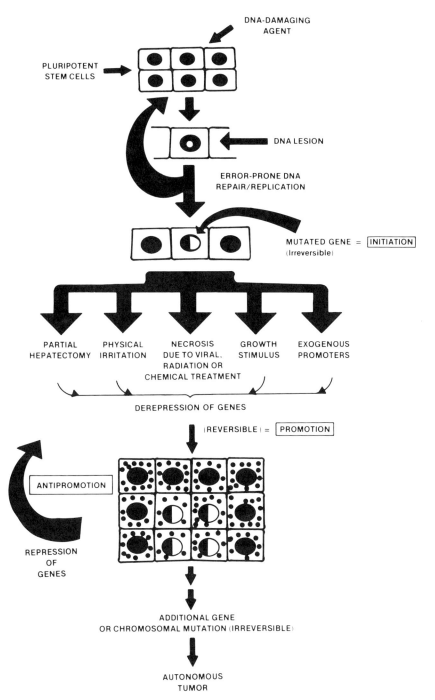

FIGURE 1.   Multiple modes by which initiated cells can be promoted. Promotion is conceptualized as a process allowing cells with a specific carcinogen-induced mutation to multiply, enabling them to reach either a "critical mass" in order to become resistant to the antiproliferative influences of normal cells or to increase the chance that one of these mutated cells would accumulate a second mutation. [From J. E. Trosko and C. C. Chang: *Med. Hypoth.* **6**, 455 (1980), with permission.]

mutagens (as opposed to false positive mutagens) are good initiators (26) and "complete carcinogens", when given at high enough concentrations or doses (27). This is consistent with the idea that *mutagenesis* is the underlying mechanism of initiation (25,28).

Tumor promotion is a potentially interruptible or reversible process which increases the frequency and speeds up the earlier appearance of tumors in a carcinogen-initiated animal (29). It is generally assumed that during the promotion process the single initiated stem cell, which is unable to terminally differentiate, but which can self-renew, is clonally amplified. Consequently, papillomas in the skin, enzyme-altered foci in the liver, and polyps in the colon may each be viewed as the tissue manifestation of a single stem cell which—when stimulated to proliferate during the tumor promotion process—accumulates in the tissue. Therefore, promotion must involve, among some other distinctive events, a *mitogenic* stimulus (30). It is interesting to note recent attempts to use "mitogenesis" as a biomarker for the mechanisms of action of some so-called "nongenotoxic" carcinogens (31–33). Unfortunately, no attempt has been made to distinguish the capabilities of a chemical to differentially stimulate initiated cells *versus* normal cells to enter mitosis, since there are reports of some chemicals which can stimulate the general proliferation of a tissue, but do not promote tumors of that tissue (34).

Progression has been viewed as that process which converts a promoter-dependent, premalignant, initiated cell to a malignant and tumor promoter independent cell. Since promoters, which act operationally as mitogens, rather than as mutagens (30), do not appear to be good agents to convert premalignant to malignant cells as are mutagens (35), one could speculate that at least another additional genetic mutation is necessary.

Predictions based on this model have been made in the case of the genetically predisposed human syndrome, retinoblastoma (36), and for the experimentally induced skin and liver cancers (35–40). Results seem to indicate that *at least* two genetic mutations are needed. From many recent studies, the "second" mutation seems to involve a deletion of a normal "suppressor" type gene (41,42). However, it would be premature to conclude that all second event mutations involve deletion mutations or, in fact, that two genetic events are sufficient for all types of tumors (43).

Of those genes which appear to be involved in carcinogenesis, oncogenes have recently been targeted. By definition, oncogenes are DNA sequences with a proven cancer association, which appear to function primarily in the regulation of cellular proliferation and differentiation (44). Attempts have been made to integrate the oncogene theory into the initiation/promotion/progression model (45,46). However, because of the lack of understanding of not only how various oncogenes function, but also of the *biological* consequences that might occur during the initiation/promotion/progression phases, no specific assignment of the various oncogenes in this model is possible at present.

Although altered oncogene expression, amplification of certain oncogenes/products, and mutations of certain oncogenes have been associated with some animal and human cancers, no universal pattern has yet emerged (9,44,47).

Mutations and, therefore, mutagens have been implicated in carcinogenesis, particularly in the initiation and possibly the progression phases, with the demonstration of the human genetic predisposition syndromes (*e.g.*, xeroderma pigmentosum) (48) and with experimental carcinogenesis studies using physical and chemical mutagens (49). The association of the mutated *ras* genes also lend support to the idea that mutations contribute to carcinogenesis (50). However, carcinogenesis is more than mutagenesis, which, in part, explains the lack of concordance between the National Toxicology Program's bioassay results and short-term tests to detect potential carcinogens by their presumptive mutagenicity in these tests (32,51). Many nonmutagenic chemicals, *e.g.*, 2,3,7,8-tetrachlorodibenzo-*p*-dioxin, saccharin, polybrominated biphenyls, and reserpine, are "carcinogenic" in animals. In addition, many so-called "mutagens" are not carcinogenic in bioassay tests. These observations do pose a challenge to the paradigm of "carcinogens as mutagens" (52). However, due to limitations of both the bioassay protocol and all the short-term tests for mutagenicity, plus the omission of non-genotoxic mechanisms in the theory of carcinogenesis, confusion reins in the understanding of the cancer problem (53,54). This point is the critical thesis of the remainder of this chapter, in that the mechanism underlying tumor promotion appears to be a nonmutagenic process.

The idea that cancer is a stem cell disease or a disease of differentiation needs to be considered in view of the preceding ideas. Initiation is speculated to prevent a stem cell from terminally differentiating (14,26,28,55–58) (Figure 2). Evidence has been generated using mouse skin cells, exposed to initiators, that noninitiated keratinocytes can differentiate under certain conditions *in vitro*, whereas initiation induces differentiation-resistant cells. These cells do, however, have self-renewal capabilities. Therefore, one of the earliest steps (*i.e.*, initiation) in the multistage carcinogenesis process is to prevent a stem cell from differentiation, possibly by mutating those oncogenes that regulate terminal differentiation, but not those that affect proliferation. This view runs counter to the notion that one of the important, if not the earliest, step in carcinogenesis is the immortalization of a normal cell (59,60). Our view is that a *normal* stem cell is *immortal* (*i.e.*, has the ability of continuous self-renewal) and one of the earliest steps (*i.e.*, initiation) is to block or partially block the ability of the cell to terminally differentiate (61).

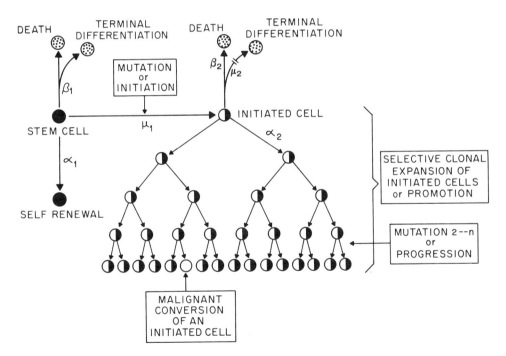

FIGURE 2. The initiation/promotion/progression model of carcinogenesis. β_1 = rate of terminal differentiation and death of stem cell; β_2 = rate of death, but not of terminal differentiation of the initiated cell (*see* break in arrow); α_1 = rate of cell division of stem cells; α_2 = rate of cell division of initiated cells; μ_1 = rate of the molecular event leading to initiation (*i.e.*, possibly mutation); μ_2 = rate at which second event occurs within an initiated cell. [From J. E. Trosko *et al.*: Modulation of gap junction intercellular communication by tumor promoting chemicals, oncogenes and growth factors during carcinogenesis. *In* "Gap Junctions" (E. Hertzberg and R. Johnson, eds.). Alan R. Liss, New York, 1988, with permission.]

The stem cell concept of cancer has been based on a variety of observations. These include (a) the similarity between stem cells and tumor cells, such as tissue origin, extensive proliferative potential, and tissue-specific differentiation potential; (b) the implication of small target size for tumor control with radiotherapy; (c) the demonstration that clonogenic potential, self-renewal capacity, and cell differentiation are restricted to subpopulations of cells in tumors; (d) the ability to induce terminal differentiation of some neoplastic cells *in vitro* by natural differentiation-inducing factors or by exogenous chemical compounds (12,61,62). The demonstration, that a small subpopulation of less differentiated and contact insensitive cells is more susceptible to neoplastic transformation than populations of cells depleted of these "presumptive" stem-like cells (63) again is consistent with the stem-cell origin of cancer.

The preceding suggest that all of these theories of carcinogenesis have an element of correctness about them. The question that remains is: Can they be integrated into a meaningful theory which not only explains the observations but also leads to important predictions and practical implications for prevention and management of cancer? At least one concept, that of intercellular communication, seems to relate to each of these theories of carcinogenesis.

III. INTERCELLULAR COMMUNICATION: A PROCESS TO ENSURE HOMEOSTASIS

The orchestration of diverse functions of multitypes of cells within multicellular organisms occurs via the process of intercellular communication. Intercellular communication is mediated by molecular information transfer between and within tissues. The control of cell proliferation and of cell differentiation, and the regulation of the functions of differentiated cells are carried out by the transfer of growth factors, hormones, neurotransmitters, etc. from one type of cell to another cell type over space and distance ("systemic communication") (12) or by the channeling of ions and other small–molecular–weight substances through a membrane–bound protein structure, the gap junction ("local communication") (64,65) (Figure 3).

Clearly, some of these molecular signals act as growth factors to those cells able to receive and respond to the signals (*i.e.*, via receptors); other signals exist that suppress the proliferation of the stem or progenitor cells, *e.g.*, chalones or growth suppressors (66). Intercellular communication, either systemic or via gap junctions, can control cell differentiation as seen, for example, in the control of germ cell maturation in the ovary (67). Also, the regulation of higher order functions in differentiated cells appears to be under the control of intercellular communication, as has been noted in the pancreas (68).

The balance of positive and negative signals to regulate stem, progenitor, and differentiated cells appears to be very different for the different organ systems (*i.e.*, closed *versus* open systems). Organs, such as the kidney or liver, must have strict regulation of cell proliferation to maintain a steady-state size (Figure 4). On the other hand, the constant loss of cells from the epithelial layers of skin or the gastrointestinal tract must promote a signal for the stem cells to self-renew and to differentiate. However, if a more differentiated cell type lineage produces a negative growth factor or suppressor signal which acts on the stem cell of the series, then the loss of differentiated cells by normal attrition, the lack of production of suppressor signal by the differentiated progeny, or the inability of certain stem cells to receive or respond to suppressor signals would lead to the proliferation of stem cells into other stem cells (renewal) and into daughter cells destined to differentiate. Once the critical mass of differentiated cells is reached, the suppressor

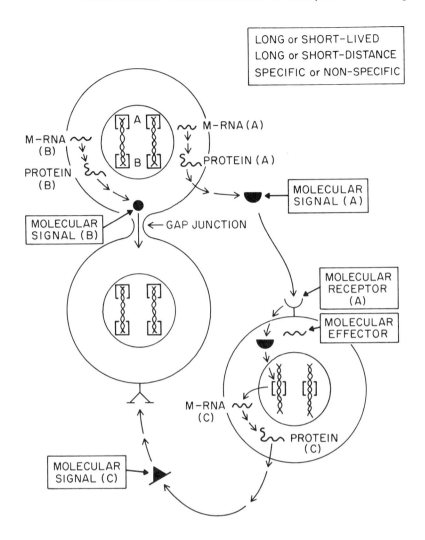

CELL—CELL COMMUNICATION

FIGURE 3.   This diagram illustrates two general forms of intercellular communication. One involves the production and transmission of "signal" molecules via permeable intercellular junctions between coupled cells. [From J. E. Trosko and C. C. Chang: *In* "SCOPE 26, Methods for Estimating Risk of Chemical Injury: Human and Non-Human Biota Ecosystems" (V. B. Vouk, G. C. Butler, D. G. Hoel, and D. B. Peakall, eds.). John Wiley, Chichester, England, 1985, p. 181, with permission.]

concentration will come to inhibit stem cell proliferation. Control of normal embryonic growth and wound healing could be explained by this concept.

In general, gap–junctional communication has been correlated with growth control and differentiation (by ionic and chemical metabolic coupling) in nonexcitable cells that may proliferate, with the control of organ function such as the synchronizing of heart and uterine muscle fibers, with the ionic and nutrient dependence of nonproliferating, excitable brain cells (69), and with embryonic development (70) and the wound healing or regenerative process (71).

In addition, it now appears clear that systemic cell-to-cell communication regulates local or gap–junctional communication as is evidenced by hormone (72), neurotransmitter (73), and growth factor (74,75) modulation of gap junctions.

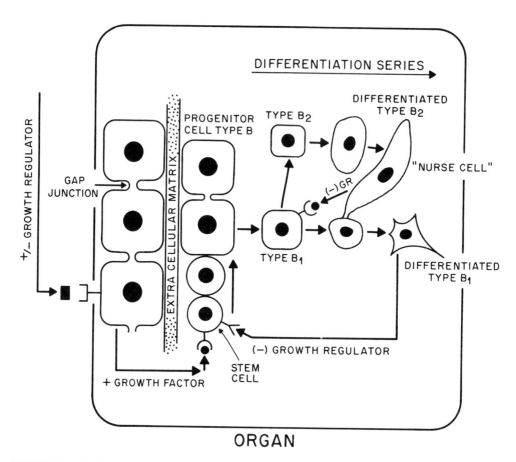

ORGAN

FIGURE 4. A diagram to illustrate the interrelationship of intercellular communication by positive and negative growth regulators on stem cell growth and differentiation and intercellular communication via gap junctions in a closed organ system. [From J. E. Trosko and C. C. Chang: *In* "Biologically Based Methods for Cancer Risk Assessment" (C. C. Travis, ed.). Plenum Press, New York, 1989, p. 165, with permission.]

In the early embryo, where cell proliferation is the primary function of the fertilized cell, few if any gap junctions are seen (76). The fertilized egg is a pluripotent stem cell. Only at the point of a "division of labor" in the blastula are gap junctions seen and differentiation of tissues can take place. Since the adult animal must maintain a pool of stem cells and regulate their proliferation, one might speculate that it is carried out by negative growth regulators rather than via gap junctions. In several reported examples (63,77), human breast epithelial and fetal kidney epithelial, presumptive stem cells were shown not to have gap–junctional intercellular communication. Differentiated normal human kidney epithelial cells do, however, have functional gap junctions (63,77).

IV. DYSFUNCTIONAL GAP–JUNCTIONAL COMMUNICATION DURING CARCINOGENESIS

Growth control in normal cells of solid tissues is associated with the phenomenon of contact inhibition (78). One of the universal phenotypes of malignant cells is the loss of contact inhibition (18).

If one assumes that gap–junctional communication is the mediating process for contact inhibition, then the observations that most cancer cells have some defect in intercellular communication, either because of their inability to adhere (*i.e.*, loss of cell adhesion molecules) or of some defect in the gap junction structure or its regulation, tend to support the assumption.

Moreover, since tumor cells are characterized by their loss of growth control and of their inability to terminally differentiate, the role of gap junctions is further implicated because gap junctions have been linked with the normal differentiation process of developing cells (70).

More direct evidence *in vivo* has shown that many tumor tissues have cells with decreased frequencies of gap junctions (79–87), although there have been several reports from both *in vitro* and *in vivo* studies which indicate that some cells from tumors have both normal appearing and functional gap junctions (19,88). The hypothesis that the lack of gap–junctional communication is important in carcinogenesis might seem to be challenged by these observations. However, the observation of the phenomenon of "selective" lack of cell communication between transformed and normal cells (89) might resolve the apparent contradiction. It has previously been noted that selective communication exist between various kinds of normal cells from different tissues or species (88,90). The most relevant observation is, however, that carcinogen-induced cell transformation *in vitro*, leads to cells in the transformed foci which are able to perform gap junctional communication with each other, but not with their *normal* neighbors (89).

We have demonstrated in our laboratory that several human tumor cells (human teratocarcinoma, human osteosarcoma, and Wilm's tumor cells) also possess the ability to communicate with each other, but not with their normal neighbors (unpublished results). The possible explanation for this phenomenon of selective communication may be that (a) cell adhesion molecules differ between cell types, (b) cells expressing different gap junction genes cannot couple, or (c) some structural alteration is made in the transformed cell which allows homologous but not heterologous coupling. Kanno *et al.* (91) have shown that antibodies directed to a cell adhesion molecule could prevent gap–junctional communication in one cell type. There are tumor cells which do not communicate homologously as well as heterologously; this feature tends to be associated with the ability of tumors to metastasize (92–94).

V. CHEMICAL INHIBITION DURING TUMOR PROMOTION

After the conceptualization that the carcinogenic process is distinguished by initiation, promotion, and progression phases (8), another series of events implicated the importance of cell-to-cell communication in carcinogenesis. Yotti *et al.* (95) and Murray and Fitzgerald (96) showed that the mouse skin tumor promoter, 12-tetradecanoyl-phorbol-13-acetate, inhibits gap–junctional communication *in vitro*. The demonstration that the inhibition is reversible and has thresholds (an important observation, since tumor promotion *in vivo* has been shown to be reversible and to have threshold levels) was validated using several different techniques to measure gap junction function, for example, metabolic cooperation (95–98), electrocoupling (99), dye injection (99), scrape loading/dye transfer (100), and fluorescence recovery after photobleaching (101). As a result of these studies, a wide spectrum of chemicals, such as natural plant and animal toxins, drugs, environmental pollutants, dietary constituents, solvents, heavy metals, growth factors, hormones, and neurotransmitters, known to be physiological modulators, tumor promoters, and/or a wide variety of toxicants (*e.g.*, teratogens, immune modulators, neuro-reproductive toxicants), have been shown to inhibit gap–junctional intercellular communication (102).

It has also been shown that the tumor promoting phorbol ester reduces the frequency of gap junctions *in vitro* in Chinese hamster cells (103) and in mouse skin *in vivo* (104). A reduction in gap junction frequency has been noted, using monoclonal antibodies to gap junction proteins (86) and freeze fracture analysis (87), in hepatocarcinomas of initiated/promoted rats. Decreased gap junction mRNA has been observed in primary tumors of initiated/promoted rat livers (105).

Partial hepatectomy, a tumor promoting stimulus, has been associated with a decreased amount of gap junctions during the regenerative growth phase (71). It has to be stressed that any means by which cells are removed (*i.e.*, surgery), killed (*i.e.*, burns, freezing, exposure to cytotoxicants), or by which physical barriers are placed between cells (*i.e.*, plastic sheets or solid metal), cell communication via gap junctions is, by definition, disrupted. Cell removal or cell death is the signal to induce compensatory or regenerative hyperplasia in the surviving stem or progenitor cells by allowing cells to escape the "contact inhibiting" or antimitotic effect of the surrounding and communicating normal cells. In the case of the liver, different types of injury could influence the source of the cells which repopulate the tissue. Partial hepatectomy, which does not injure the surviving cells, serves to stimulate the proliferation of preexisting hepatocytes. On the other hand, cell killing by agents, such as carbon tetrachloride (a cytotoxic, nongenotoxic chemical) and chemical carcinogens do injure the hepatocytes. In these cases, the oval cell of the liver, which might not metabolize these chemicals, would be forced to proliferate and differentiate. This, of course, is based on the assumption that the oval cell is a stem or progenitor cell of the hepatocytes (106–108). Therefore, if the stem cell theory of cancer is correct, hepatocarcinogenesis studies will have to focus on the oval cell rather than on the differentiated hepatocytes. This hypothesis has major risk assessment implications. For example, the number of oval cells in the liver would affect the probability of a given dose of carcinogen to produce a cancer. If the stem cell was previously initiated, regardless of how hepatocytes were removed or killed, promotion would occur.

Chemical tumor promoters and any tissue regenerative–inducing conditions are, by definition, "mitogens", in that they would allow the selective growth and accumulation of the initiated stem cell.

VI. ONCOGENES/ANTIONCOGENES OR TUMOR SUPPRESSOR GENES AND INTERCELLULAR COMMUNICATION

Cellular oncogenes seem to be those genes related to growth factors, growth factor receptors, signal transduction elements, and transcription and replication elements (9). These oncogenes seem to be related to the regulation of cell growth (50) and development and differentiation (109,110). This observation is reminiscent of the cellular consequences after exposure to chemical tumor promoters which can induce cell proliferation in one cell type, yet induce differentiation in other cell types (111).

We have speculated that if chemical tumor promoters act as growth and differentiation regulators, in part by their ability to inhibit intercellular communication, then possibly oncogenes might exert similar effects in the same manner. This prediction has been tested and the results appear to be consistent with the hypothesis. The *src, ras, raf,* and *mos* oncogenes (112–118), as well as the polyomavirus middle T gene (119), have been shown in several *in vitro* cell systems to be acting like the phorbol esters, in that gap–junctional intercellular communication is dysfunctional in all these systems.

The stable loss of gap–junctional communication has been correlated with tumor metastasis (20,53,93), and reversible inhibition of cell communication has been linked to the tumor promotion phase (102). Since transformed cells, *in vitro*, seem to be suppressed by surrounding and communicating normal cells and show selective communication at the morphologically transformed stage (89), one may speculate that the initiation phase is related to those oncogenes which prevent terminal differentiation, rather than to those that affect gap–junctional communication. Attempts to date to assign which oncogene, when altered, affects which stage of the multistage nature of carcinogenesis have not yet resolved the issue (*see* Reference 46).

It is this area of cancer research which has caused a "crisis in paradigms". The paradigm of "carcinogen as mutagen" has forced many cancer researchers to think that just because a chemical "causes" cancers in rodents, it must therefore be a genotoxic agent (54). To illustrate the problem, furan and furfural can induce liver tumors in mice (120). DNA from these tumors, as well as from spontaneous tumors in these mice, were shown by transfection to transform NIH 3T3 cells. Activated H-*ras* was found in the transforming DNA of both the spontaneous and furan/furfural–induced tumors. After analysis of the mutation spectrum in the H-*ras* DNA of the spontaneous and induced tumors, the researchers inferred that furan and furfural were mutagenic, in spite of the fact that there is no evidence that these chemicals are mutagenic in short-term tests for genotoxicity. Recently, Wilson *et al.* (121) have shown that these chemicals acted more as "mitogens" than as "mutagens". They interpreted their results as indicating that furan, by forcing cell proliferation, spontaneous mutations in the H-*ras* oncogene occurred. Conceivably, there is the possibility that spontaneous mutations occurred and that, in a microenvironment of furan/furfural, only cells with a certain class of H-*ras* mutations had a selective proliferative advantage.

A more radical challenge to the "carcinogen as mutagen" paradigm has been produced by Brookes (122) and others (123,124), who have noted that several "classic carcinogens" (*e.g.*, 7,12-dimethylbenz[*a*]anthracene, 3-methylcholanthrene), while able to transform cells so as to display mutated *ras* oncogenes, may not have been responsible for the induction of those mutations. Although several possible traditional explanations — based on the belief that these carcinogens must be acting as genotoxic agents — exist, there is also the possibility that many classic "complete carcinogens" are really promoters of pre-existing spontaneously mutated or initiated cells, and that these chemicals are promoters or mitogens rather than mutagens. One could argue, however, that there exist all kinds of evidence showing that (a) these chemicals induce DNA damage; (b) DNA lesions can be identified; (c) DNA repair can be induced; and (d) using known metabolites of these chemicals, mutations can be induced *in vitro*. One must bear in mind that if the evidence is derived from *in vivo* liver, then hepatocytes were the source of the DNA not the stem cells. Furthermore, if metabolites or artificial metabolizing systems were used *in vitro*, then the reactions may have no relevance to the *in vivo* target cells, which are probably nonmetabolizing stem cells.

There have been various attempts to assign specific oncogenes to a particular phase of carcinogenesis. In that context the study of Kumar *et al.* (125) provides some basis for postulating the role of various oncogenes and cell–cell communication. In their studies, they noted that activated H-*ras* and K-*ras* oncogenes could be found in normal mammary glands 2 weeks after carcinogen treatment and before the onset of neoplasia. Only after exposure to estrogen did these latent activated *ras* oncogenes lead to neoplasia. Our own studies have shown that while the expression of both the H-*ras* and *raf* oncogenes are associated with reduced gap junction function in a normal rat liver epithelial cell line and that the cells are tumorigenic (126,127), the presence of both expressed *myc* and *ras* or *raf* led to almost complete reduction of cell–cell communication and greatly enhanced tumorigenicity.

These observations lead to the speculation that the expression of an activated oncogene, in and of itself, is insufficient for either blockage of gap junction function or for tumorigenicity (128,129) and that interactions with other gene products (read antioncogene or tumor suppressor gene products) can modulate or neutralize their effect. As an example, lovastatin, by preventing the functioning of the H-*ras* oncogene product (binding to plasma membrane), could prevent the inhibition of gap junction by the H-*ras* oncogene (130). Conceivably, there are endogenous products, which are natural metabolites of certain genes, that can mimic the action of lovastatin.

To further support this concept, earlier studies had shown that phorbol esters, which are powerful inhibitors of gap junction function, synergistically interact with H-*ras* transfected but not transformed cells to bring about transformation (131). In this case, the phorbol ester, an exogenous tumor promoter, acted as a surrogate *myc*-type of oncogene.

Together these observations suggest that it is the combination of interactions of either or both multiple oncogene products with a cell or agents external to the cell (hormones, growth factors, or tumor promoting chemicals) that is needed to cause the cell to proliferate and to block terminal differentiation. Therefore, a unifying process linking these diverse factors together is the capability of down-regulation of gap junctions. Clearly, without the ability to down-regulate these structures, cells would be contact inhibited and be able to terminally differentiate.

VII. MODULATION OF GAP–JUNCTIONAL INTERCELLULAR COMMUNICATION BY GROWTH FACTORS

By definition, growth regulators are those extracellular substances which can (a) induce contact-inhibited, quiescent cells to enter the mitogenic phase of the cell cycle; (b) prevent potentially dividing cells from dividing; (c) induce undifferentiated cells to differentiate; and (d) stimulate differentiated cells to perform their cellular functions. If gap junctions are, in part, necessary for maintaining contact inhibition, one would predict that growth factors would modulate gap junction function. In addition, hormones, known to promote cell proliferation or induce differentiation or induce differentiated cells to function, would also be predicted to up- or down-regulate gap junction function. Neurotransmitters, by inducing differentiated functions, may also be predicted to be modulators of gap junction function.

Hormones were the first growth regulators to modulate gap junction function (72). More recently, several growth regulators, *e.g.*, epidermal growth factor (EGF), transforming growth factor β bovine pituitary extract, fetal calf serum factors, and neurotransmitters (73–75), were shown to down-regulate gap junctions.

Growth factors and hormones have been shown to act as tumor promoters *in vivo* (132–138) and *in vitro* (139,140).

VIII. ALTERED GAP JUNCTION FUNCTION AND "PARTIALLY BLOCKED ONTOGENY" DURING CARCINOGENESIS

Gap junctions have been implicated in the three primary functions of cells of multicellular organisms, from fertilization of the egg to the adaptive functions of a mature organism: (a) the control of proliferation of the single zygotic cell, (b) demarcation of areas of differentiation; and (c) the adaptive control of functions in differentiated cells. Consider now that chemical tumor promoters, which act to affect proliferation and differentiation, inhibit intercellular communication; that several growth factors, which also affect proliferation and differentiation, can act as tumor promoters and inhibit gap junction function; and that several oncogenes, which are linked to growth control and differentiation, seem to affect gap junction function as a part of their oncogenic function. These considerations suggest a common mechanism which could integrate all these factors influencing carcinogenesis (45).

Inhibition of gap–junctional communication, by chemical tumor promoters, by endogenous growth factors and hormones, or by expressed oncogenes, would facilitate the expansion of initiated cells, allowing these cells — unable to terminally differentiate because of the initiation event ["oncogeny as partially blocked ontogeny" (12)] — to escape the suppressing effect of surrounding and communicating normal cells. Gap–junctional communication would resume after cessation of exposure to exogenous chemical tumor promoters and endogenous growth factors. This presumably would interrupt the tumor promotion process (141). It is only after additional genetic events ("hits"; mutations), which would stabilize the inhibition of gap junctions, that the cells would become independent of exogenous tumor promoting (*i.e.*, gap junction–down-regulating) stimulus. However, in the case of altered oncogene expression or function, the inhibition of intercellular communication would be rather stable (as long as there is no expressed tumor-suppressor gene) and not dependent on regular exogenous exposure. In the case where the oncogene and tumor-suppressor gene might negate each other, exogenous tumor promoters might override the effect of the tumor-suppressor gene (131).

Finally, a common assumption regarding cancer cells must now be examined in order to perceive cancer as a disease of differentiation, namely that carcinogenesis involves the induction of immortalization of normal cells. With the demonstration that transfection or normal cells with the *myc* oncogene allowed "immortalization" but not transformation of normal mortal cells (59,60), came the observation that these cells could then be made tumorigenic after transfection with the *ras* oncogene.

An alternative view has been proposed, based on the observation that presumptive normal human kidney and breast epithelial stem cells do not have functional gap junction communication (63,77). This has led to the hypothesis that stem cells, which, of course, are undifferentiated, are epigenetically unable to have gap–junctional communication with their differentiated daughter cells. Since terminal differentiation can be viewed as a "mortalization" process, the stem cell can be viewed as immortal. In the normal nongrowing state of tissues, an equilibrium is maintained between the stem cells and their terminally differentiated daughter cells by the production of negative growth regulators which suppresses the stem cells. If there is a loss of differentiated cells (*i. e.*, a loss of negative growth regulators) or a gain of positive growth factors external to the tissue, then the stem cells divide to self-renew and to form progenitor cells for differentiation. The equilibrium is reestablished once enough differentiated cells are produced.

If immortal stem cells are initiated then, upon stimulation to proliferate/differentiate, the cells can self-renew but will be unable to differentiate (or become "mortalized") because of the genetic block ["oncogeny as partially blocked oncogeny" (12)]. We can infer from these experimental studies that the initiated cells can self-renew, but do not differentiate, and can be suppressed by surrounding normal and communicating cells; therefore, since cells in transformed foci can perform gap–junctional intercellular communication with each other, the initiated state probably does not involve total inhibition of the gap–junction–mediated communication function. It could, however, involve selective transfer of message or how that message is interpreted by the receiving cells.

Defects in cell adhesion molecules or possibly the nonfunctionality of different gap junction proteins might be an intermediate consequence of the carcinogenic process indicated by the "selective" communication properties of many transformed cells. When gap–junctional communication is sufficiently disrupted, the ability of the cells to maintain contact inhibition for controlling growth and for providing stimulus for differentiation is lost.

IX. THE INTEGRATION OF EXTRACELLULAR–INTRACELLULAR–INTERCELLULAR COMMUNICATION MECHANISMS FOR MAINTAINING HOMEOSTASIS

Since developmental (*i.e.*, genetic) factors, hormones, neurotransmitters, activated oncogenes, and growth factors, as well as a wide range of exogenous chemicals, can modulate gap junction function, a major question that now needs to be answered is: what is (are) the mechanism(s) by which these gap junction modulators work? Clearly, the answer must await experimental elucidation. However, one view is already available, namely, there are multiple mechanisms (Figure 5).

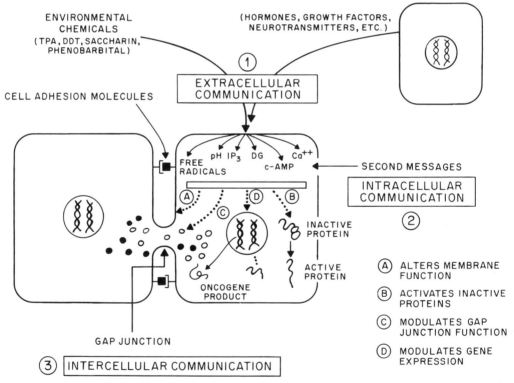

FIGURE 5. A heuristic scheme characterizing the postulated link between extracellular communication and intercellular communication via various intracellular trans-membrane signalling mechanisms. It provides an integrating view of how the neuroendocrine-immune system ("mind or brain/body connection") and other multisystem coordinations could occur. While not shown here, activation or altered expression of various oncogenes (and "antioncogenes") could also contribute to the regulation of gap junction function. [From J. E. Trosko, C. C. Chang, B. V. Madhukar, and S. Y. Oh: *In Vitro Toxicol.* **3**, 9 (1990), with permission.]

Changes in intracellular pH, Ca^{++}, as well as asymmetric voltages between cells have been associated with altered gap–junctional coupling (142). The phorbol esters, which exert their pleiotropic biological effects by activating the Ca^{++}-dependent, phospholipid-sensitive protein kinase C (PKC) (143), also have been implicated in the modulation of gap junction function, possibly through phosphorylation of the gap junction protein or one of the regulatory proteins (144). It has been demonstrated that PKC can phosphorylate a gap junction protein in a cell free system (145).

An increase in gap–junctional coupling has been observed when the activation of a cAMP-dependent protein kinase occurred in uncoupled rat liver and lens cells (146,147). Several reports have shown that when cells were exposed to agents which raised the intracellular cAMP levels, an increase in gap junctions or gap–junctional communication occurred (148–152).

These observations underscore a major concept that when *extracellular* signals trigger *intracellular* messages, *intercellular* communication can occur. In addition, they suggest a sophisticated regulation of gap junctions by a coupled phosphorylation/dephosphorylation system. The molecular structures of the different gap junction proteins, as well as the different physiological status of different cells (*e.g.*, liver oval cells *versus* hepatocytes), might explain differential responses to chemical modulators of gap junctions.

Clearly, there are other mechanisms by which gap junctions can be regulated. It has been shown that carbon tetrachloride inhibits gap–junctional communication, not by an increase in intracellular free Ca^{++} or acidity or by changing the phosphorylated state of the main gap junction protein, but apparently by free radical oxidation of sulfhydryl groups needed for gap junction coupling (153). As evidence that PKC phosphorylation is not the only mechanism to modulate gap junction coupling, it has been shown that cells that were made refractory to phorbol esters (*i. e.*, no PKC was available in the cells), did have their gap–junctional communication down-regulated by non-PKC stimulators, such as 1,1'-(2,2,2-trichloroethylidene) bis (4-chlorobenzene) [DDT] (154,155).

While the induction of free radical generation by phorbol ester (156) suggests that the effect on gap junction function might be mediated by an oxidative mechanism, this seems improbable since the high amount of free radicals required to block gap junction function makes it unlikely that noncytotoxic levels of phorbol ester would work via this mechanism (157).

In those cases where a non-PKC inducing chemical inhibits gap junction function by either increasing intracellular acidity or free Ca^{++}, a fine line must exist between the adaptive/reversible responses these changes would elicit in the physiological state of the cell and the nonadaptive/irreversible effect it would have on the ability of the cell to survive (25). The transfer of toxic substances to nondamaged cells would be prevented when a free radical–generating chemical uncouples the changed cell (153).

The effect of chemicals, such as heptanol, which rapidly and reversibly inhibit gap–junctional communication in pancreatic cancer cells, suggests yet another possible mechanism of regulating gap junctions, since heptanol does not seem to work via alteration of cytosolic pH, free Ca^{++}, or cAMP content.

Several expressed oncogenes [*e.g.*, *src*, *ras*, *raf*, *mos* (112–118)] and certain growth factors [*e.g.*, EGF and transforming growth factor β (74,75)] have been associated with the decrease of gap junction function. The receptor for EGF and the *src* gene product, pp60, are tyrosine kinases. Again, these observations suggest that phosphorylation of gap junction proteins at the tyrosine residues might regulate the function of gap junctions. Alternatively, these factors might interfere with gap junction function by increasing the production of inositol triphosphate and diacylglycerol, the breakdown products of phosphoinositide metabolism. The subsequent release of free calcium from its pools, in turn, may block cell–cell communication.

Because of the fact that gap junctions can be modulated by so many diverse chemicals which have important adaptive and non-adaptive effects, and because gap junctions play a critical role in the regulation of cell proliferation and differentiation, one may speculate that during the course of evolution, gap junctions had to be sensitive to many intracellular changes in order to allow the cell to survive and function. As a means to provide differential regulation and sensitivity to both endogenous and exogenous chemicals, a family of gap junction proteins, sharing a high degree of sequence homology, has evolved (158). The tissue specificity of chemical tumor promoters and selective communication in premalignant foci could be explained by the differential responses of gap–junctional regulation in cells having different expressed gap junction genes. In the former case, specific chemicals could regulate a particular gap junction protein in one cell type by triggering a second message system, but not another. In the latter case, the presence of the 43 kDa gap junction protein in the cells of a preneoplastic lesion might prevent the coupling with hepatocytes containing connexin 32.

All of these observations, showing that many second messengers could modulate gap junction function, could provide an integrating mechanistic link in the neuroendocrine-immune system or in any multisystem network (159–162). *Extracellular* communication, as mediated by peptide hormones, neurotransmitters, growth factors and growth regulators, affects *intracellular* communication of distal cells by triggering transmembrane signaling mechanisms (*i.e.*, alterations in intracellular free Ca^{++}, pH, activation of protein kinases), which, in turn, modulates gap junction *intercellular* communication. The maintenance of homeostasis in an organism can then be explained when cells of one organ or tissue can, by communicating via positive or negative molecular messages, increase or decrease intercellular communication in another organ or tissue. The coupling or uncoupling of cells in excitable or nonexcitable cells would have different kinds of physiological consequences, depending on the circumstances. The end result, at least for adaptive responses, would be the stimulation of cell growth, induction of differentiation, or modulation of a differentiated function in excitable or nonexcitable cells. By inhibiting gap–junctional intercellular communication via extracellular communicating signals, the intracellular regulatory signals can be increased. Therefore, in order to affect changes in quiescent cells, the extracellular signals must (a) affect membrane function to let in ions and substrate molecules needed for mitogenesis or differentiation to occur; (b) prevent loss of transmembrane regulatory molecules by blocking gap–junctional transfer; (c) activate inactive enzymes; and (d) modulate gene expression. Persistent disruption of this interconnected homeostatic network at any level (extracellular, intracellular, intercellular) could prevent growth control, and the ability of cells to differentiate and to perform synchronized differentiated functions. Cancer, as a disease of homeostasis, can thus be explained by this hypothesis.

X. MODULATION OF GAP–JUNCTIONAL COMMUNICATION AND ITS IMPLICATIONS FOR THE PREVENTION AND TREATMENT OF CANCER

Given the multistage nature of carcinogenesis and the assumption that mutations might be involved in the initiation and progression stages, while inhibition of intercellular communication plays a role in the tumor promotion phase, one would predict that the minimal exposure to environmental mutagens would go a long way to reduce the risk to cancer. Yet we know we can never reduce mutations in any gene to a zero level, since every gene has a finite chance of spontaneously mutating every time a cell divides.

Since promotion must involve the clonal expansion of an initiated cell, any endogenous or exogenous mitogenic stimulus, if persisting for a long period of time, could act as a potential promoter. Consequently, in growing organisms (such as in a young child) or in continuously proliferating tissues, the induction of an initiated stem cell would be exposed to its own endogenous promoting stimulus. On the other hand, in tissues of slow cell turnover (as in older adults) initiated stem cells would be exposed to chronic and sufficient levels of external agents which could promote by inhibiting intercellular communication. After genetic changes have occurred in the initiated/promoted cell population which changes lead to permanently decreased gap–junctional communication, the need for external promoters has ceased. One could envisage that such genetic changes yield alteration(s) of oncogene expression for increased growth factor receptors, for decreased growth suppressor receptors, or for the production of growth factors; these would enhance autonomous cell growth by the continuous inhibition of intercellular communication.

Because gap–junctional intercellular communication is fundamental to the normal functioning of all tissues, chronic inhibition of this critical function would lead to dramatic physiological consequences. For example, transgenic mice, which carries and expresses a fusion gene of the transcription I regulatory sequence of the atrial natriuretic factor and the SV40 T antigen (an oncoprotein), display both, tumors in the atrium *and* cardiac arrhythmias (163). Clearly, normal gap junction function would be expected for both growth control and atrial conduction, and its inhibition would be predicted to contribute to both of these diverse disease states. Azarnia and Loewenstein (119) have shown that the T antigen (both large and small) could alter junctional permeability. Thus, it seems logical to speculate that these two very different chronic diseases share a common etiology: the inhibition of gap junction function.

Since many cancer cells do not have normal gap–junctional communication, either because of some loss of cell adhesion molecules or because of dysfunctional gap junctions, a rational approach to cancer chemotherapy may be to search for drugs which would restore gap communication in these aberrant stem cells (164,165). By allowing these tumor cells to communicate with normal cells, these stem-like cells may be induced to terminally differentiate.

Lastly, with the introduction of the concept of antioncogenes or tumor-suppressor genes (166–168), it seems logical that, since certain oncogenes have the ability to down-regulate gap–junctional communication, these tumor-suppressor genes must code for proteins that either prevent the down-regulation of gap junction function or up-regulate gap junctions (127).

ACKNOWLEDGMENTS

This chapter was written during a period of research support through grants from the National Cancer Institute (CA21104), the U.S. Air Force Office of Scientific Research (AFOSR-89-0325), and the National Institute of Environmental Health Sciences (1P42ESO4911).

REFERENCES

1. Potter, V. R.: *Science* **101**, 105 (1945).
2. Hunter, T.: *Nature* **322**, 14 (1986).
3. Varmus, H. E.: *Science* **238**, 1337 (1987).
4. Potter, V. R.: Biochemistry of Cancer. *In* "Cancer Medicine" (J. Holl and E. Frei, eds.). Lea and Febiger, Philadelphia, Pennsylvania, 1973, p. 178.
5. Levitt, M. L.: *Cell Growth Differ.* **1**, 311 (1990).

6. Iverson, O. H.: The Chalones. *In* "Handbook of Experiments of Pharmacology" (R. Baserga, ed.). Springer-Verlag, Berlin, 1981, p. 491.

7. Iverson, O. H.: Cybernetic Aspects of the Cancer Problem. *In* "Progress in Biocybernetics" (N. Wiener and J. P. Schade, eds.). Elsevier, Amsterdam, 1965, p. 76.

8. Pitot, H. C., Goldsworthy, T., and Moran, S.: *J. Supramol. Struct. Cellul. Biochem.* **17**, 133 (1981).

9. Bishop, J. M.: *Cell* **42**, 23 (1985).

10. Ames, B. N., Durston, W. E., Yamasaki, E., and Lee, F. D.: *Proc. Natl. Acad. Sci. U.S.A.* **70**, 2281 (1973).

11. Markert, C.: *Cancer Res.* **28**, 1908 (1968).

12. Potter, V. R.: *Br. J. Cancer* **38**, 1 (1978).

13. Till, J. E.: *J. Cell. Physiol.* **1**, 3 (1982).

14. Potter, V. R.: *Prog. Nucleic Acid Res. Mol. Biol.* **29**, 161 (1983).

15. Cairns, J.: *Nature* **225**, 197 (1975).

16. Potter, V. R.: *Cancer Res.* **44**, 2733 (1984).

17. Loewenstein, W. R.: *Biochim. Biophys. Acta* **560**, 1 (1979).

18. Borek, C., and Sachs, L.: *Proc. Natl. Acad. Sci. U.S.A.* **56**, 1705 (1966).

19. Kanno, Y.: *Jpn. J. Physiol.* **35**, 693 (1985).

20. Nicolsin, G. L.: *Cancer Res.* **47**, 1473 (1987).

21. Fialkow, P. J.: *Am. Rev. Med.* **30**, 135 (1979).

22. Kerbel, R. S., Frost, P., Liteplo, R., Carlow, D. A., and Elliott, B. E.: *J. Cell. Physiol.* **3**, 87 (1984).

23. Slaga, T. J., Fischer, S. M., Weeks, C. E., Klein-Szanto, A., and Reiners, J.: *J. Cell. Biochem.* **18**, 99 (1982).

24. Slaga, T. J. (ed.): "Mechanisms of Tumor Promotion" Vol. 1. CRC Press, Boca Raton, Florida, 1983.

25. Trosko, J. E., and Chang, C. C.: Implications for Risk Assessment of Genotoxic and Non-genotoxic Mechanisms in Carcinogenesis. *In* "SCOPE 26, Methods for Estimating Risk of Chemical Injury: Human and Non-Human Biota Ecosystems" (V. B. Vouk, G. C. Butler, D. G. Hoel and D. B. Peakall, eds.). Wiley, Chichester, England, 1985, p. 181.

26. Trosko, J. E., and Chang, C. C.: *Med. Hypoth.* **6**, 455 (1980).

27. Trosko, J. E., Jone, C., and Chang, C. C.: *Ann. N.Y.. Acad. Sci.* **407**, 316 (1983).

28. Potter, V. R.: *Carcinogenesis* **2**, 3175 (1981).

29. Pitot, H. C., and Sirica, A. E.: *Biochim. Biophys. Acta* **605**, 191 (1980).

30. Trosko, J. E., Chang, C. C., and Medcalf, A.: *Cancer Invest.* **1**, 511 (1983).

31. Loury, D. J., Goldsworthy, T. L., and Butterworth, B. E.: The Value of Measuring Cell Replication as a Predictive Index of Tissue-Specific Tumorigenic Potential. *In* "Nongenotoxic Mechanisms in Carcinogenesis" (B. E. Butterworth and T. J. Slaga, eds.), Banbury Report 25. Cold Spring Harbor Laboratory, Cold Spring Harbor, New York, 1987, p. 119.

32. Ames, B. N., and Gold, L. S.: *Proc. Natl. Acad. Sci. U.S.A.* **87**, 7772 (1990).

33. Cohen, S. M., and Ellwein, L. B.: *Science* **249**, 1007 (1990).

34. Wada, S., Hirose, M., Takahashi, S., Okazaki, S., and Ito, N.: *Carcinogenesis* **71**, 1891 (1990).

35. Hennings, H., Shores, R., Wenk, M. L., Spangler, E. F., Tarone, R., and Yuspa, S. H.: *Nature* **304**, 67 (1983).

36. Moolgavkar, S. H., and Knudson, A. G.: *J. Natl. Cancer Inst.* **66**, 1037 (1981).

37. Reddy, A. L., and Fialkow, P. J.: *Carcinogenesis* **8**, 1455 (1987).

38. Quintanilla, M., Brown, K., Ramsden, M., and Balmain, A.: *Nature* **322**, 78 (1986).

39. Fry, R. J. M., Rey, R. D., Grube, D., and Staffeldt, E.: Studies on the Multistage Nature of Radiation Carcinogenesis. *In* "Carcinogenesis" (H. Hecker, N. E. Fusenig, W. Kunz, F. Marks, and H. N. Thielmann, eds.). Raven Press, New York, 1982, p. 155.

40. Scherer, E., Feringa, A. W., and Emmelot, P.: Initiation-Promotion-Progression. Induction of Neoplastic Foci Within Islands of Precancerous Liver Cells in the Rat. *In* "Models, Mechanisms and Etiology of Tumor Promotion" (M. Börzsönyi, N. E. Day, K. Lapis, and H. Yamasaki, eds.). IARC, Lyon, France, 1984, p. 57.

41. Orkin, S. H., Goldman, D. S., and Sallan, S. E.: *Nature* **309**, 172 (1984).

42. Koufos, A., Hansen, M. F., Copeland, N. G., Jenkins, N. A., Lampkin, B. C., and Cavenee, W. K.: *Nature* **316**, 330 (1985).

43. Marx, J.: *Science* **244**, 1386 (1989).

44. Goyns, M. H.: *Cancer J.* **1**, 183 (1986).

45. Trosko, J. E., Jone, C., and Chang, C. C.: Oncogenes, Inhibited Intercellular Communication and Tumor Promotion. *In* "Cellular Interactions by Environmental Tumor Promoters" (H. Fujiki, E. Hecker, R. E. Moore, T. Sugimura, and I. B. Weinstein, eds.). Japan Sci. Soc. Press, Tokyo, Japan, 1984, p. 101.

46. Trosko, J. E., Chang, C. C., and Madhukar, B. V.: Chemical and Oncogene Modulation of Intercellular Communication in Tumor Promotion. *In* "Biochemical Mechanisms and Regulation of Intercellular

Communication" (H. A. Milman and E. Elmore, eds.). Princeton Scientific Publishers, Princeton, New Jersey, 1987, p. 209.

47. Nishimura, S., and Sekiya, T.: *Biochem. J.* **243**, 313 (1987).
48. Trosko, J. E., Riccardi, V. M., Chang, C. C., Warren, S., and Wade, M.: Genetic Predisposition to Initiation or Promotion Phases in Human Carcinogenesis. *In* "Biomarkers, Genetics and Cancer" (H. Anton-Guirgis and H. T. Lynch, eds.). Van Nostrand-Reinhold, New York, 1985, p. 13.
49. Yuspa, S. H., and Morgan, D. L.: *Nature* **293**, 72 (1981).
50. Bishop, J. M.: *Science* **235**, 305 (1987).
51. Tennant, R. W., Margolin, B. H., Shelby, M. D., Zeiger, E., Haseman, J. K., Spalding, J., Caspary, W., Resnick, M., Stasiewicz, S., Anderson, B., and Minor, R.: *Science* **236**, 933 (1987).
52. Trosko, J. E., and Chang, C. C.: Non-genotoxic Mechanisms in Carcinogenesis: Role of Inhibited Intercellular Communication. *In* "New Directions in the Qualitative and Quantitative Aspects of Carcinogen Risk Assessment" (R. Battey, ed.), Banbury Report 31. Cold Spring Harbor Laboratory, Cold Spring Harbor, New York, 1989, p. 139.
53. Trosko, J. E.: *Environ. Mutagen.* **6**, 767 (1984).
54. Trosko, J. E.: *J. Am. Coll. Toxicol.* **8**, 1121 (1989).
55. Miller, D. R., Viaje, A., Aldaz, C. M., Conti, C. V., and Slaga, T. J.: *Cancer Res.* **47**, 1935 (1987).
56. Kawamura, H., Strickland, J. E., and Yuspa, S. H.: *Cancer Res.* **45**, 2748 (1985).
57. Scott, R. E., and Maercklein, P. B.: *Proc. Natl. Acad. Sci. U.S.A.* **82**, 2995 (1985).
58. Yuspa, S. H., Kilkenny, A. E., Stanley, J., and Lichti, U.: *Nature* **314**, 459 (1985).
59. Newbold, D. F., and Overell, R. W.: *Nature* **304**, 648 (1983).
60. Land, H., Parada, L. F., and Weinberg, R. A.: *Nature* **304**, 596 (1983).
61. Trosko, J. E., and Chang, C. C.: *Toxicol. Lett.* **49**, 283 (1989).
62. Buick, R. N., and Pollak, M. N.: *Cancer Res.* **44**, 4909 (1984).
63. Chang, C. C., Trosko, J. E., El-Fouly, M. H., Gibson-D'Ambrosio, R. E., and D'Ambrosio, S. M.: *Cancer Res.* **47**, 1634 (1987).
64. MacDonald, C.: *Essays Biochem.* **21**, 80 (1985).
65. Pitts, J. D., and Finbow, M. E.: *J. Cell Sci.* **4**, 239 (1986).
66. Potter, V. R.: *Oncodev. Biol. Med.* **2**, 243 (1981).
67. Schultz, R. M.: *Biol. Reprod.* **32**, 27 (1985).
68. Meda, P., Kohen, E., Kohen, C., Rabinovitch, A., and Orci, L.: *J. Cell Biol.* **92**, 221 (1982).
69. Peracchia, C., and Girsch, S. J.: *Am. J. Physiol.* **248**, 765 (1985).
70. Lo, C. W.: Communication Compartmentation and Pattern Formation in Development. *In* "Gap Junctions" (M. V. L. Bennett and D. C. Spray, eds.). Cold Spring Harbor Laboratory, Cold Spring Harbor, New York, 1985, p. 251.
71. Dermietzel, R., Yancey, S. B., Traub, O., Willecke, K., and Revel, J. P.: *J. Cell Biol.* **105**, 1925 (1987).
72. Larsen, W. J., and Risinger, M. A.: *Mod. Cell Biol.* **4**, 151 (1985).
73. Neyton, J., and Trautman, A.: *J. Physiol.* (*London*) **377**, 283 (1986).
74. Madhukar, B. V., Oh, S. Y., Chang, C. C., Wade, M. H. and Trosko, J. E.: *Carcinogenesis* **10**, 13 (1989).
75. Maldonado, P. E., Rose, B., and Loewenstein, W. R.: *J. Membr. Biol.* **106**, 203 (1988).
76. Lo, C. W., and Gilula, N. B.: *Cell* **18**, 411 (1974).
77. Chang, C. C., Nakatsuka, S., Kalimi, G., Trosko, J. E., and Welsch, C. W.: *J. Cell. Biochem.*, *Suppl.* **14B**, 331 (1990).
78. Levine, E. M., Becker, Y., Boone, C. W., and Eagle, H.: *Proc. Natl. Acad. Sci. U.S.A.* **53**, 350 (1965).
79. Alroy, J.: *Vet. Pathol.* **16**, 693 (1979).
80. Pauli, B. U., and Weinstein, R. S.: *Experientia* **37**, 248 (1981).
81. Schindler, A. M., Amaudruz, M. A., Kocker, O., Riotton, G., and Gabbiani, G.: *Acta Cytol.* **26**, 466 (1982).
82. Larsen, W. J.: *Tissue Cell* **15**, 645 (1983).
83. Swift, J. G., Mukherjee, T. M., and Rowland, R.: *J. Submicrosc. Cytol.* **15**, 799 (1983).
84. Horak, E., Lelkes, G., and Sugar, J.: *Br. J. Cancer* **49**, 637 (1984).
85. Weinstein, R. S., Merk, F. B., and Alroy, J.: *Adv. Cancer Res.* **23**, 23 (1976).
86. Janssen-Timmen, U., Traub, O., Dermietzel, R., Rabes, H. M., and Willecke, K.: *Carcinogenesis* **7**, 1475 (1986).
87. Sugie, S., Mori, H., and Takahashi, M.: *Carcinogenesis* **8**, 45 (1987).
88. Fentman, I. S., Hurst, J., Ceriani, R. L., and Taylor-Papadimitriou, J.: *Cancer Res.* **39**, 4739 (1979).
89. Yamasaki, H., Hollstein, M., Mesnil, M., Martel, N., and Aguelon, A. M.: *Cancer Res.* **47**, 5658 (1987).
90. Pitts, J. D., and Kour, E.: *Exp. Cell Res.* **156**, 439 (1985).
91. Kanno, Y., Sasaki, Y., Shiba, Y., Yoshida-Noro, C., and Takeichi, M.: *Exp. Cell Res.* **152**, 270 (1984).
92. Nicolson, G. L., Dulski, K. M., and Trosko, J. E.: *Proc. Natl. Acad. Sci. U.S.A.* **85**, 473 (1988).

93. Iijima, N., Yamamoto, T., Inoue, K., Soo, S., Matsuzawa, A., Kanno, Y., and Matsui, Y.: *Jpn. J. Exp. Med.* **39**, 205 (1969).
94. Hamada, J., Takeichi, M., and Kobayashi, H.: *Cancer Res.* **48**, 5129 (1988).
95. Yotti, L. P., Chang, C. C., and Trosko, J. E.: *Science* **206**, 1089 (1979).
96. Murray, A. W., and Fitzgerald, D. J.: *Biochem. Biophys. Res. Commun.* **91**, 395 (1979).
97. Jone, C., Trosko, J. E., and Chang, C. C.: *In Vitro Cell. Dev. Biol.* **23**, 214 (1987).
98. Kavanagh, T. J., Chang, C. C., and Trosko, J. E.: *Cancer Res.* **46**, 1359 (1986).
99. Enomoto, T., Sasaki, Y., Shiba, Y., Kanno, Y., and Yamasaki, H.: *Proc. Natl. Acad. Sci. U.S.A.* **78**, 5628 (1981).
100. El-Fouly, M. H., Trosko, J. E., and Chang, C. C.: *Exp. Cell Res.* **168**, 422 (1987).
101. Wade, M. H., Trosko, J. E., and Schindler, M.: *Science* **232**, 525 (1986).
102. Trosko, J. E., and Chang, C. C.: Nongenotoxic Mechanisms in Carcinogenesis: Role of Inhibited Intercellular Communication. *In* "Carcinogen Risk Assessment: New Directions in the Qualitative and Quantitative Aspects" (R. W. Hart and F. G. Hoerger, eds.), Banbury Report 31. Cold Spring Harbor Laboratory, Cold Spring Harbor, New York, 1988, p. 139.
103. Yancey, S. B., Edens, J. E., Trosko, J. E., Chang, C. C., and Revel, J. P.: *Exp. Cell Res.* **139**, 329 (1982).
104. Kalimi, G. H., and Sirsat, S. M.: *Carcinogenesis* **5**, 1671 (1984).
105. Beer, D. G., Neveu, M. J., Paul, D. L., Rapp, U. R., and Pitot, H. C.: *Cancer Res.* **48**, 1610 (1988).
106. Fausto, N.: Oval Cells and Liver Carcinogenesis: An Analysis of Cell Lineages in Hepatic Tumors Using Oncogene Transfection Techniques. *In* "Mouse Liver Carcinogenesis: Mechanisms and Species Comparisons" (D. E. Stevenson, J. A. Popp, J. M. Ward, R. M. McClain, T. J. Slaga, and H. C. Pitot, eds.). Alan R. Liss, Inc., New York, 1990, p. 325.
107. Sirica, A. E., Mathis, G. A., Sano, N., and Elmore, L. W.: *Pathobiology* **58**, 44 (1990).
108. Sell, S.: *Cancer Res.* **50**, 3811 (1990).
109. Adamson, E. D.: *Development* **99**, 449 (1987).
110. Ohlsson, R. I., and Pfeifer-Ohlsson, S. B.: *Exp. Cell Res.* **173**, 1 (1987).
111. Yamasaki, H.: Modulation of Cell Differentiation by Tumor Promoters. *In* "Mechanisms of Tumor Promotion" (T. J. Slaga, ed.), Vol. IV. CRC Press, Boca Raton, Florida, 1984, p. 1.
112. Atkinson, M. M., and Sheridan, J.: *J. Cell Biol.* **99**, 401a (1984).
113. Azarnia, R., and Loewenstein, W. R.: *J. Membr. Biol.* **82**, 213 (1984).
114. Chang, C. C., Trosko, J. E., Kung, H. J., Bombick, D., and Matsumura, F.: *Proc. Natl. Acad. Sci. U.S.A.* **82**, 5360 (1985).
115. Chang, C. C., Gibson-D'Ambrosio, R. E., Trosko, J. E., and D'Ambrosio, S. M.: *Cancer Res.* **46**, 6360 (1986).
116. El-Fouly, M. H., Trosko, J. E., Chang, C. C., and Warren, S. T.: *Molec. Carcinogenesis* **2**, 131 (1989).
117. Dotto, G. P., El-Fouly, M. H., Nelson, C., and Trosko, J. E.: *Oncogene* **4**, 637 (1989).
118. Azarnia, R., Reddy, S., Kimiecki, T. E., Shalloway, D., and Loewenstein, W. R.: *Science* **239**, 398 (1988).
119. Azarnia, R., and Loewenstein, W. R.: *Molec. Cell. Biol.* **7**, 946 (1987).
120. Reynolds, S. H., Stowers, S. T., Patterson, R. M., Maronpot, R. R., Aaronson, S. A., and Anderson, M. W.: *Science* **237**, 1309 (1987).
121. Wilson, D. M., Goldsworthy, T. L., Popp, J. A., and Butterworth, B. E.: *Proc. Am. Assoc. Cancer Res.* **31**, 103 (1990).
122. Brookes, P.: *Molec. Carcinogenesis* **2**, 305 (1989).
123. Mass, M. J. and Austin, S. J.: *Biochem. Biophys. Res. Commun.* **65**, 1319 (1989).
124. Fox, T. R., Schuman, A. M., Watanabe, P. C., Yano, B. V., Maker, V. M., and McCormick, J. J.: *Cancer Res.* **50**, 4014 (1990).
125. Kumar, R., Sukumar, S., and Barbacid, M.: *Science* **248**, 1101 (1990).
126. de Feijter, A. W., Ray, J. S., Weghorst, C. M., Klaunig, J. E., Goodman, J. I., Chang, C. C., Ruch, R. J., and Trosko, J. E.: *Mol. Carcino.* **3**, 54 (1990).
127. Kalimi, G. H., Trosko, J. E., Hampton, L. L., and Thorgeirsson, S. S.: *Proc. Am. Assoc. Cancer Res.* **31**, 132 (1990).
128. Koi, M., and Barrett, J. C.: *Proc. Natl. Acad. Sci. U.S.A.* **83**, 5992 (1986).
129. Geiser, A. G., Anderson, M. J., and Stanbridge, E. J.: *Cancer Res.* **49**, 1572 (1989).
130. Ruch, R. J., Trosko, J. E., Madhukar, B. V., Somani, P., and Klaunig, J. E.: *Toxicologist* **10**, 76 (1990).
131. Dotto, G. P., Parada, L. F., and Weinberg, R. A.: *Nature* **318**, 472 (1985).
132. Chester, J. F., Gaissert, H. A., Ross, J. S., and Malt, R. A.: *Cancer Res.* **46**, 2954 (1986).
133. Rose, S. P., Stahn, R., Passovoy, D. S., and Herschman, H.: *Experientia* **32**, 913 (1976).
134. Stoscheck, C. M., and King, L. E.: *Cancer Res.* **46**, 1030 (1986).
135. Takizawa, S., and Hirose, F.: *Gann* **69**, 723 (1978).
136. Yager, J. D., and Yager, R.: *Cancer Res.* **40**, 3680, (1980).

137. Yoshida, H., Fukunishi, R., Kato, Y., and Matsumoto, K.: *J. Natl. Cancer. Inst.* **65**, 823 (1980).
138. Lipton, A., Kepner, N., Rogers, C., Witkoski, E., and Leitzel, K.: A Mitogenic Factor for Transformed Cells from Human Platelets. *In* "Interactions of Platelets and Tumor Cells" (G. A. Jamieson. ed.). Alan Liss, New York, 1982, p. 233.
139. Harrison, J., and Auersperg, N.: *Science* **213**, 218 (1981).
140. Gansler, T., and Kopelovich, L.: *Cancer Lett.* **13**, 315 (1981).
141. Boutwell, R. K., Verma, A. K., Ashendel, C. L., and Astrup, E.: Mouse Skin: A Useful Model System for Studying the Mechanism of Chemical Carcinogenesis. *In* "Carcinogenesis" (E. Hecker, N. E. Fusenig, W. Kunz, F. Marks, and H. W. Thielmann, eds.). Raven Press, New York, 1982, p. 1.
142. Spray, D. C., and Bennett, M. V. L.: *Annu. Rev. Physiol.* **47**, 281 (1985).
143. Nishizuka, Y.: *Science* **233**, 305 (1986).
144. Trosko, J. E., and Chang, C. C.: Chemical and Oncogene Modulation of Gap Junctional Intercellular Communication. *In* "Tumor Promoters: Biological Approaches for Mechanistic Studies and Assay Systems" (R. Langenbach, J. C. Barrett, and E. Elmore, eds.). Raven Press, New York, 1988, p. 97.
145. Takeda, A., Hashimoto, E., Yamura, H., and Shimazu, T.: *FEBS Lett.* **210**, 169 (1987).
146. Wiener, E. C., and Loewenstein, W. R.: *Nature* **305**, 433 (1983).
147. Saez, J. C., Spray, D. C., Nairn, A. C., Hertzberg, E., Greengard, P., and Bennett, M. V. L.: *Proc. Natl. Acad. Sci. U.S.A.* **83**, 2473 (1986).
148. Azarnia, R., and Russell, T. R.: *J. Cell Biol.* **100**, 265 (1985).
149. Flagg-Newton, J. L., Dahl, G., and Loewenstein, W. R.: *J. Membr. Biol.* **63**, 105 (1981).
150. Mehta, P. P., Bertram, J. S., and Loewenstein, W. R.: *Cell* **44**, 187 (1986).
151. Demaziere, A. M. G. L., and Scheuerman, D. W.: *Cell Tissue Res.* **239**, 651 (1985).
152. Veld, P. I., Schuit, F., and Pipeleers, D.: *Eur. J. Cell Biol.* **36**, 269 (1985).
153. Saez, J. C., Bennett, M. V. L., and Spray, D. C.: *Science* **236**, 967 (1987).
154. Warngard, L., Flodstrom, S., Ljungquist, S., and Ahlborg, U. G.: *Carcinogenesis* **8**, 1201 (1987).
155. Aylsworth, C. F., Trosko, J. E., Chang, C. C., Benjamin, K., and Lockwood, E.: *Cell Biol. Toxicol.* **5**, 27 (1989).
156. Cerutti, P. A.: *Science* **227**, 375 (1985).
157. Hasler, C. M., Frick, M. A., Bennink, M. R., and Trosko, J. E.: *Tox. Appl. Pharmacol.* **103**, 389 (1990).
158. Saez, J. C., Spray, D. C., and Hertzberg, E. L.: *In Vitro Toxicol.* **3**, 69 (1990).
159. Blalock, J. E.: *J. Immunol.* **132**, 1067 (1984).
160. Grossman, C. J.: *Science* **227**, 257 (1985).
161. Marx, J. L.: *Science* **227**, 1190 (1985).
162. Roth, J., Roith, D. L., Shiloach, J., and Rubinovitz, C.: *Clin. Res.* **31**, 354 (1983).
163. Field, L. J.: *Science* **239**, 1029 (1988).
164. Trosko, J. E.: *Eur. J. Cancer Clin. Oncol.* **23**, 599 (1987).
165. Vitkauskas, B. V., and Canellakis, E. S.: *Biochim. Biophys. Acta* **823**, 19 (1985).
166. Knudson, A. G.: *Cancer Res.* **45**, 1437 (1985).
167. Klein, G.: *Science* **238**, 1539 (1987).
168. Harris, H.: *Cancer Res.* **48**, 3302 (1988).

APPENDIX TO PART 1

Chemical Cancerogenesis: Definitions of Frequently Used Terms[1,2]

K. E. Appel, G. Fürstenberger, H. J. Hapke, E. Hecker,
A. G. Hildebrandt, W. Koransky, F. Marks, H. G. Neumann,
F. K. Ohnesorge, and R. Schulte-Hermann

I. INTRODUCTION

Chemical substances and mixtures of substances that, owing to a possible cancerogenic effect, are likely to endanger human health are referred to as chemical risk factors of cancer. The health risk originating from them must be determined and evaluated for severity, to provide a basis for adequate preventive measures. The information required for a weighted risk assessment is provided by a systematic analysis of chemical and biological characteristics of a substance and thorough research into its mechanisms of action. Although present-day knowledge of chemical cancerogenesis is largely incomplete and cannot supply all the necessary information, numerous findings from experimental research on chemical cancerogenesis can be arranged into a classification scheme that will be helpful in evaluating the risk posed by chemical risk factors of cancer, even though it is certainly incomplete and, in part, hypothetical in nature.

The object of this work is to contribute to a standardization of the way terms are used, and thus to prevent terminological confusion in the future.

II. DEFINITIONS

A. Chemical Cancerogenesis

Chemical cancerogenesis is understood as a process in which, as a consequence of the impact of chemical risk factors of cancer, an uncontrolled and irregular *de novo* forma-

---

[1]The authors of this Appendix are members of an ad hoc group of experts, engaged in cancer research and/or governmental regulation, set up jointly by the Senate Commission on "Plant Treatment, Protection, and Storage Products" of the Deutsche Forschungsgemeinschaft and by the Bundesgesundheitsamt (Federal Health Office). Chaired by A. G. Hildebrandt, the ad hoc group attempted to define and classify the terms that are frequently used in the context of chemical cancerogenesis (Table 1) and to explain them with reference to our present knowledge.
[2]This article originally appeared as a Guest Editorial in the *Journal of Cancer Research and Clinical Oncology*, Vol. 116, pp. 232–236, © 1990 Springer-Verlag. Reprinted by permission.

tion of tissue (neoplasia) takes place. The term *neoplasia* refers to benign as well as to malignant tumors (cancer).

In German the term *Karzinogenese* (or *Carcinogenese*) is used interchangeably with *Kanzerogenese*. The former term should be avoided, even though it is more closely related to the English term *carcinogenesis*, because in its strict sense it signifies the development of an epithelial tumor only (a carcinoma). In view of the problems associated with the generalization of the English term *carcinogenesis*, the authors have used the term *cancerogenesis* (see footnote to Table 1) in preference. The terms *tumorigenesis* and *oncogenesis* are also used indiscriminately to mean processes leading to benign or malignant tumors. Frequently, however, these terms are used to denote the development of benign tumors only. Such a limitation is problematic, because the degeneration of benign tumors to malignant ones cannot be excluded.

B. Chemical Risk Factors of Cancer

Substances and mixtures of substances contributing to the development of cancer in man and/or in suitable animal models are referred to as chemical risk factors of cancer. Their action may become evident in an elevated cancer incidence, a reduced latency period

TABLE 1. **Overview of Terms Used Frequently in the Context of Chemical Cancerogenesis and Defined in the Text, Together with the Corresponding Terms in German[a,b]**

English	German
A. Chemical cancerogenesis	A. Chemische Kanzerogenese
B. Chemical risk factors of cancer	B. Chemische Krebsrisikofaktoren
C. Solitary cancerogens (synonyms: cancerogens, complete cancerogens)	C. Solitärkanzerogene (syn. Kanzerogene, komplette Kanzerogene)
Direct cancerogens	Direkte Kanzerogene
Indirect cancerogens (synonym: procancerogens)	Indirekte Kanzerogene (syn. Prokanzerogene)
Ultimate cancerogens	Ultimale Kanzerogene
D. Conditional cancerogens (conditionally cancer-generating factors)	D. Bedingt krebsauslösende Faktoren
E. Multistage model of cancerogenesis	E. Mehrstufen-Modell der Kanzerogenese
Initiation, initiators	Initiation, Initiatoren
Promotion, promoters	Promotion, Promotoren
F. Progression	F. Progression
G. Cocancerogenesis	G. Kokanzerogenese
H. Syncancerogenesis	H. Synkanzerogenese
I. Anticancerogenesis	I. Antikanzerogenese
J. Synpromotion	J. Synpromotion
K. Antipromotion	K. Antipromotion
L. Genotoxicity	L. Gentoxizität
Substances with immediate genotoxicity	Unmittelbar gentoxische Stoffe
Substances with mediated genotoxicity	Mittelbar gentoxische Stoffe
M. Threshold values for chemical risk factors of cancer	M. Schwellenwerte für chemische Krebsrisikofaktoren
Solitary cancerogens	Solitärkanzerogene
Conditional cancerogens	Bedingt krebsauslösende Faktoren

[a]In English, the term carcinogenesis is frequently used. Because of the problems associated with the generalization of this term, the authors propose to replace the term carcinogenesis by cancerogenesis also in English (see text).

[b]The capital letters preceding the terms refer to the subsections in Section II (Definitions).

for tumor development, the occurrence of forms of cancer not observed among the corresponding controls, and shifts in the spectrum of cancer forms. *The chemical risk factors of cancer are defined by the processes of cancerogenesis that they cause* according to present-day knowledge (*see* Sections II.B and II.C).

Examples. Asbestos, zinc chromate, 2-naphthylamine, *N*-nitrosodimethylamine, diterpene esters, 2,3,7,8-tetrachlorodibenzo-*p*-dioxin, phenobarbital, tobacco smoke, beechwood dust.

C. Solitary Cancerogens (Synonyms: Cancerogens, Complete Cancerogens)

Solitary cancerogens are chemical risk factors of cancer that produce cancer either per se or after metabolic transformation. This effect is irreversible and at least additive. Solitary cancerogens often exhibit a pronounced organotropic action (*e.g.,* aromatic amines, *N*-nitrosamines). In the present state of knowledge, it must remain an open question whether or not additional effects produced by solitary cancerogens (*e.g.,* promotional effects) are essential for their activity. At least in animal experiments, a single exposure to a solitary cancerogen can be sufficient to produce tumors in the organism exposed to it. No additional action of further *exogenous* risk factors of cancer is required. As a rule, solitary cancerogens are mutagenic and show covalent binding to DNA. They often trigger DNA repair processes. In this sense, they are also referred to as having genotoxic activity. In the multistage model of cancerogenesis (see Section II.E), solitary cancerogens act as initiators.

Examples. Certain natural and anthropogenic, inorganic, and organic substances.

Direct Cancerogens. Direct cancerogens do not require metabolic activation to be effective.
Examples. *N*-Nitroso-*N*-methylurea, methylmethanesulfonate.

Indirect Cancerogens (Synonym: Procancerogens). Indirect cancerogens are transformed to their active molecular forms (ultimate cancerogens) by metabolism.
Examples. Benzo[*a*]pyrene, vinylchloride, *N*-nitrosodimethylamine.

Ultimate Cancerogens. Ultimate cancerogens are the metabolically produced active molecular forms of indirect cancerogens.
Examples. Possibly 7,8-dihydroxy-9,10-epoxy-7,8,9,10-tetrahydrobenzo[*a*]pyrene from benzo[*a*]pyrene, *N*-acetoxy-*N*-acetylaminofluorene from *N*-acetylaminofluorene.

D. Conditional Cancerogens (Conditionally Cancer-Generating Factors)

This heading subsumes those chemical risk factors of cancer whose cancer-producing action, according to present-day knowledge, involves types of activities different from those of solitary cancerogens. In cases where an initiating activity cannot be detected, the following criteria may be used for the evaluation and classification of a risk factor of cancer of this type as a "conditional cancerogen":

Nonlinear log/log dose–response relationship
Reversibility of demonstrable primary effects
Promoting activity in the multistage model
Necessity (as a rule) of long-term action to produce tumors

Hormone action on target organs or regulating systems
Chronic proliferation stimulus in the target tissue

Furthermore, this category may include substances that, beyond a certain dose limit, produce alterations of metabolic turnover rates; when such acceleration of reactions result in the formation of cancer risk factors they take on an increased importance.
Examples. Certain hormones, promoters, nitrilotriacetic acid, thiourea.

E. Multistage Model of Cancerogenesis (Initiation, Promotion)

Initiation. In the multistage model of cancerogenesis, the term *initiation* is used to designate a persistent cell change that is transmitted to subsequent cell generations. It enables the affected cell to respond preferentially to a promoter by multiplication (tumor formation). *Initiation is an operationally defined stage of cancerogenesis;* at the low dosage chosen, initiation alone will not lead to tumor formation. In contrast to promotion, initiation is assumed to take place rapidly; it is probably the result of genotoxic effects.

Initiators. In the multistage model of cancerogenesis, initiators are defined by their ability to induce at a subcancerogenic dose level, persistent changes (probably due to genotoxic effects) in the cell (initiation). In the case of subsequent promotion these changes may result in tumor formation. Solitary cancerogens have an initiating effect, which therefore may exhibit organotropy.
Examples. 2-Acetylaminofluorene, 7,12-dimethylbenz[*a*]anthracene, *N*-nitrosodiethylamine.

Promotion. In the multistage model of cancerogenesis, the term *promotion* designates the accelerated formation of tumors induced by certain chemical risk factors of cancer (promoters), probably by way of a preferential multiplication of the cells changed by initiation. Promotion does not immediately or necessarily lead to the generation of *malignant* cells. However, by a multiplication of cells changed by initiation, it increases the risk of progression toward a malignant tumor. *Promotion is an operationally defined stage of cancerogenesis.* Promotion takes place *after* initiation. Unlike initiation, it is a slowly progressing process. It requires the long-term action of a promoter and may take weeks, months, or even years. Promotion is frequently associated with enzyme induction, hyperplasia, and/or tissue damage. The essential primary effects of promotion are considered reversible. An immediate genotoxic action is probably not required for the process of promotion.

Promoters. In the multistage model of cancerogenesis, promoters are considered to be chemical risk factors of cancer that are capable of triggering preferential multiplication of cells changed by initiation. Often, following initiation, a long-term action on the target tissue is necessary. Promoters often cause enzyme induction, hyperplasia, and/or tissue damage. The essential primary effects are considered reversible. As a rule, promoters do not bind covalently to cell components and do not exert an immediate genotoxic activity. (The absence of such effects should not be considered as a necessary characteristic of promoters; generally speaking, the absence of particular effects cannot be proven conclusively.) Promoters often show organotropic activity.
Examples. Liver, phenobarbital; lung, butylhydroxytoluene; bladder, saccharine; colon, bile acids; mammary gland, prolactin; skin, 12-*O*-tetradecanoylphorbol-13-acetate.

F. Progression

Phenotypic and genotypic cellular changes do not reach a fixed end point in the process of cancerogenesis. "Progression" is used to mean an increase in autonomous growth and malignancy, and in particular, to describe the transition from benign to malignant tumors and the advance of malignancy. There are probably numerous stages of progression during neoplastic development. The process of progression plays a leading role in the general model of cancerogenesis as well as in the multistage model.

G. Cocancerogenesis

The term *cocancerogenesis* is used to describe processes that augment the initiating action of a substance. These processes take place before and during the initiation process and may favor the formation and availability of the ultimate cancerogens (the immediate initiating agents) in the target cell. Alternatively, cocancerogenic factors may produce changes in the target cells that increase their susceptibility to initiators. For example, stimulation of DNA synthesis in the target cells and simultaneous administration of an initiator or solitary cancerogen may result in intensified initiation manifesting in increased tumor incidence.

Examples. Pyrocatechol, hydroquinone, and pyrogallol are cocancerogens for mouse skin. Increased availability of an ultimate cancerogen due to simultaneous administration of ethanol and *N*-nitrosamines causes a change in organotropism and leads to an increased tumor incidence in the target organ. Increased susceptibility of the target cell, due to partial hepatectomy followed by administration of *N*-nitrosomethylurea, leads to an increased incidence of preneoplasia in rat liver.

H. Syncancerogenesis

The term *syncancerogenesis* is used to describe the joint action of several solitary cancerogens. The effects of the individual components can be additive or overadditive. Exposure can be simultaneous or staggered; the time sequence of exposure appears to be of no importance for the appearance of a synergistic effect. It can, however, be important for the extent of the synergistic augmentation.

Example. Increased tumor incidence in rat liver following consecutive administration of *N*-nitrosodiethylamine, *N*-nitrosopyrrolidine, and *N*-nitrosodiethanolamine or consecutive administration of *N*-nitrosodiethanolamine and 4-dimethylaminoazobenzene.

I. Anticancerogenesis

The term *anticancerogenesis* is used for all processes in which cancerogenesis is inhibited by the action of chemical factors. There is a distinct difference between anticancerogenesis and chemotherapy. Anticancerogenesis refers to influencing the process of cancer development and entails the possibility of tumor prevention, whereas chemotherapy refers to a curative effect on clinically manifest tumors.

Examples. Chemoprevention by inhibition of the metabolism of an indirect cancerogen if the inhibitory substance is administered before or at the same time as the cancerogen. Disulfiram inhibits the cancerogenic effect of 1,2-dimethylhydrazine in the colon.

J. Synpromotion

So far, no reliable experimental data have become available on the joint action of several promoters. Nevertheless, a synergism of several promoters with the same type of action when administered simultaneously cannot be ruled out.

K. Antipromotion

A number of chemical factors are known to inhibit cancerogenesis if administered during the promotion stage. Such antipromoters do not necessarily annul initiation, or exhibit a cytotoxic effect on initiated cells.

Examples. Retinoids, corticosteroids, antioxidants, protease inhibitors, inhibitors of the metabolism of arachidonic acid, cyclosporins.

L. Genotoxicity

Chemical risk factors of cancer can induce toxic effects on genes. These effects are characterized by processes that alter the genetic information, as a rule irreversibly. Such alterations involve an elevated error rate in reduplication of the genome and an increase in mutations beyond the level of spontaneous incidence. In this context, the term *mutation* comprises stable changes of the genome, *i.e.,* changes transmitted to the daughter cells, such as exchange, addition and deletion of bases (gene mutations), sequence and number of genes, and structure (chromosome mutations) and number (genome mutations) of chromosomes.

In the present state of knowledge, it remains an open question whether or not effects — such as changes in the methylation pattern of the DNA or in the tertiary structure of the chromosome (conversion to heterochromatin) and sister chromatid exchange — contribute to an irreversible change in the cellular genotype, *i.e.,* represent genotoxicity.

Substances with Immediate Genotoxicity. These are substances which, in their original molecular form or after metabolic conversion, cause an irreversible change in the cellular genotype and exert an immediate toxic action on genes (*see also* Section IIC, Direct Cancerogens and Indirect Cancerogens).

Substances with Mediated Genotoxicity. A mediated toxic action on genes is exerted by substances causing an irreversible change in the genotype by an indirect route, such as a modification of cellular reactions (*e.g.,* influence on DNA repair, generation of nucleotide imbalance, formation of reactive metabolites in the endogenous metabolism or of activated oxygen).

M. Threshold Values for Chemical Risk Factors of Cancer (Non-Observed-Effect Level, No-Effect Level, Threshold Value)

The term *non-observed-effect level* is used to denote the highest dosage of a substance at which no statistically demonstrable alteration of a defined parameter (*e.g.,* number of tumors or precursor lesions) compared with controls is observed during the experimental period.

Solitary Cancerogens (Chemical Risk Factors of Cancer with Initiating Action). With regard to the chemical risk factors of cancer that are capable of irreversibly altering the genetic information, experimental studies, in particular those examining the relationships between dose, exposure time, and effect, as well as theoretical considerations concerning the mechanism of action of chemical cancerogens indicate an irreversible and thus an additive effect of even minute doses. It follows that, theoretically, there is no finite dose (threshold value) for solitary cancerogens below which an effect cannot be expected. Thus, for solitary cancerogens a no-effect level or threshold value practically does not exist. For this reason, low doses of solitary cancerogens constitute a low yet distinct risk. As a rule, contemporary experimental methods permit an estimation but not a determination of the level of risk.

Conditional Cancerogens (Chemical Risk Factors of Cancer without Initiating Action). Theoretical considerations concerning the mechanism of action of conditional cancerogens (*e.g.,* receptor-mediated, chronic proliferation stimulus) and preliminary experimental approaches indicate that for such substances there are dose ranges over which, by analogy with known pharmacological principles, no biological effects (tumor formation) are induced. This has become evident in particular from quantitative analyses of dose–time–effect relationships for tumor promoters of the diterpene ester type. It seems that in this connection, the reversibility of the effects of the promoter, which can be demonstrated in certain model situations, plays the essential part.

It appears that these principles could also be valid for other conditional cancerogens. Such substances probably have a no-effect level and a threshold value. Thus, correspondingly low doses of conditional cancerogens should not constitute a risk of cancer.

Exogenous Factors and Endogenous Biological Parameters That Modulate Chemical Carcinogenesis

CHAPTER 8

Immunotoxicology of Chemical Carcinogens[1]

Karen A. Sullivan and John E. Salvaggio

I. INTRODUCTION

The immune system constitutes the first and primary defense against the environment. It provides defense against foreign substances and organisms such as bacteria and viruses. It is also a surveillance system for protection against the development of malignant disease. When the immune system is severely compromised there are life-threatening consequences. The devastating consequences of the acquired immune deficiency syndrome (AIDS) exemplifies the importance of a healthy immune system.

There are a number of structural classes of chemicals which are carcinogenic in humans and animals. Many of these chemicals are also immunotoxic, *i.e.*, have a selective adverse effect on the immune system in moderate doses. Some studies indicate that carcinogenicity and immunotoxicity appear to be related toxicological endpoints.

Since the intent of this chapter is to review the immunotoxic effects of carcinogenic chemicals and to give background information for the analysis of perturbations in the functioning of the immune system brought about by exposure to these chemicals, it is necessary to provide a brief perspective on the components, development, and function of the immune system in vertebrate organisms.

II. THE IMMUNE SYSTEM

The immune system is a highly complex regulatory system that requires cooperative interaction between a variety of immunocompetent cells and their products. These cells reside in the lymphoid system which consists of lymphoreticular tissues and organs distributed throughout the body. The primary lymphoid organs are the thymus and the bone marrow; the secondary lymphoid organs are the spleen, the lymph nodes usually at junctions of lymphatic vessels, and the Peyer's patches which are unencapsulated small masses of lymphoid tissue in the small intestine. The various immunocompetent cells interact with virtually all organs, including the endocrine, cardiovascular, and central nervous systems.

---

[1]Abbreviations used are listed on p. 268.

The immune system is capable of generating a great diversity of genetically distinct lymphocyte clonal populations with multiple specificities. Individual lymphocytes are programmed to respond to a limited number of structurally related antigens, prior to contact of the immune system with any given antigen. This programming is defined by the expression, on the surface membrane of the lymphocyte, of receptors that are specific for structural determinants on particular antigens. A clone of lymphocytes will differ from another clone in its receptor population (the combining sites). Therefore, each clone differs in the range of antigens to which it can respond. Because of the very large number of different lymphocyte clones and receptors, humans and other vertebrate organisms have the capacity to respond to virtually any antigen. Other cells of the immune system are not endowed with such specificity, but either depend on the lymphocytes to orchestrate their responsiveness or act nonspecifically.

There are two major lineages of lymphocytes, T cells and B cells, which are morphologically indistinguishable from each other in the resting stage. Although all cells of the immune system arise from pluripotent stem cells found in the bone marrow (1), T cells and B cells mature and differentiate at different anatomic locations. T cells mature in the thymus and B cells mature in the bone marrow and fetal liver (Figure 1). From these primary lymphoid organs, mature cells travel through the blood and lymphatic system to seed secondary lymphoid organs.

A. T Cells

T lymphocytes mature in the thymus. Stem cells or T cell precursors from bone marrow migrate to the thymus where, influenced by various growth and maturational factors (thymic hormones) produced by local epithelial cells, they undergo an ordered process of differentiation and division. During this process, T cells acquire a unique series of glycoproteins expressed on their cell surface (are membrane bound), called differentiation antigens. These cell surface molecules of the T cells are recognized by groups of monoclonal antibodies. Monoclonal antibodies appearing to detect related antigens allowed the delineation of "Clusters of Differentiation" (CD). The stages of differentiation of T cells can thus be defined through a "CD nomenclature". The number of CD designations continue to expand rapidly. The CD designations, refined through four international workshops, are shown in Table 1 (2). The differentiation of thymocytes to mature T cells can be followed by analysis of the expression of these molecules, some of which are retained by the T cells upon entering the peripheral circulation (3). The CD3 complex, for example, is present on only a very small percentage of thymocytes, but is present on all mature T cells in the peripheral blood. Additionally, the most immature thymocytes fail to express either the CD4 or CD8 antigen. These "double negative cells" mature into "double positive" cells, expressing both CD4 and CD8 antigen. Double positive cells acquire CD3, and further mature into exportable subpopulations of mature cells that enter the circulation and express either CD4 or CD8 (Figure 1).

T cells are of major importance in cellular immunity, including delayed-type hypersensitivity (DTH) reactions, allograft rejection, graft *versus* host reactions, reactions to obligate intracellular microorganisms, immune responses to tumors, and in providing help to B cells to develop into antibody producing cells. Depending on the differentiation

---

FIGURE 1.   Maturation of T cells and B cells. The CD1 and CD2 antigens expressed by early thymocytes are continuously expressed throughout thymocyte maturation and by mature T cells in the peripheral circulation. [Adapted from B. E. Bozelka and J. E. Salvaggio: *Environ. Carcino. Rev.* **C3**, 1 (1985).]

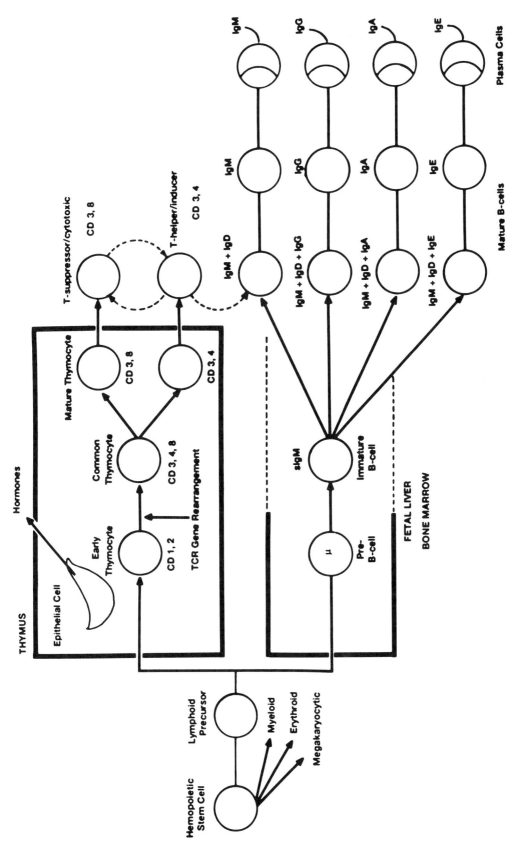

239

TABLE 1.   **Designations of Human Leukocyte Differentiation Antigens[a]**

CD designation	Defining set of monoclonal antibodies	Main cellular distribution
CD1a	NA1/34;T6;VIT6;Leu6	Thy, DC, B subset
CD1b	WM-25;4A76;NUT2	Thy, DC, B subset
CD1c	L161;M241;7C6;PHM3	Thy, DC, B subset
CD2	9.6;T11;35.1	T
CD2R	T11.3;VIT13;D66	Activated T
CD3	T3;UCHT1;38.1;Leu4	T
CD4	T4;Leu3a;91.D6	T subset
CD5	T1;UCHT2;T101;HH9;AMG4	T, B subset
CD6	T12;T411	T, B subset
CD7	3A1;4A;CL1.3;G3-7	T
CD8	αchain:T8;Leu2a;M236;UCHT4; T811βchain:T8/2T8-5H7	T subset
CD9	CLB-thromb/8;PHN200	Pre-B, M, Plt
CD10	J5;VILA1;BA-3	Lymph. Prog., cALL, Germ Ctr. B, G
CD11a	MHM24;2F12; CRIS-3	Leukocytes, broad
CD11b	Mol;5A4.C5;LPM19C	M, G, NK
CD11c	B-LY6;L29;BL-4H4	M, G, NK, B sub
CDw12	M67	M, G, Plt
CD13	MY7, MCS-2, TUKI, MOU28	M, G
CD14	Mo2, UCHM1, VIM13, MoP15	M, (G), LHC
CD15	My1, VIM-D5	G, (M)
CD16	BW209/2;HUNK2;VEP13; Leu11c	NK, G, Mac.
CDw17	GO35, Huly-ml3	G, M, Plt
CD18	MHM23;M232;11H6;CLB54	Leukocytes, broad
CD19	B4;HD37	B
CD20	B1;1F5	B
CD21	B2;HB5	B subset
CD22	HD39;S-HCL1;To15	Cytopl. B/surface B subset
CD23	Blast-2, MHM6	B subset, act. M, Eo
CD24	VIBE3;BA-1	B, G
CD25	TAC;7G7/B6;2A3	Activated T, B, M
CD26	134-2C2;TS145	Activated T
CD27	VIT14;S152;OKT18A;CLB-9F4	T subset
CD28	9.3;KOLT2	T subset
CD29	K20;4B4;A-IA5	Broad, T subset
CD30	Ki-1;Ber-H2;HSR4	Activated T, B, Sternberg–Reed cells
CD31	SG134;TM3	Plt, M, G, B, (T)
CDw32	CIKM5;41H16;IV.3	M, G, B
CD33	My9;H153;L4F3	M, Prog., AML
CD34	My10, B1-3C5, ICH-3	Prog.
CD35	TO5, CBO4, J3D3	G, M, B
CD36	5F1, CIMeg1	M, P, (B)
CD37	HD28;HH1;G28-1	B, (T, M)
CD38	HB7, T16	Lymph. Prog., PC., Act. T
CD39	AC2;G28-2	B subset, (M)
CD40	G28-5	B, carcinomas
CD41	LO-PL3b;PBM 6.4;CLB-thromb/7	Plt
CD42a	FMC25;BL-H6;GR-P	Plt
CD42b	PHN89;PHN103;GN287	Plt
CD43	OTH 71C5;G19-1;MEM-59	T, G, brain
CD44	GRHL1;F10-44-2;33-383;BRIC35	T, G, brain, RBC

TABLE 1. (continued)

CD designation	Defining set of monoclonal antibodies	Main cellular distribution
CD45	T29/33;BMAC 1;AB187	Leukocytes
CD45RA	G1-15;FB-11-13;73.5	T subset, B, G, M
CD45RB	PT17/26/16	T subset, B, G, M
CF45RO	UCHL1	T subset, B, G, M
CD46	HULYM5;122-2;J4B	Leukocytes, broad
CD47	BRIC 126;C1KM1;BRIC 125	Broad distribution
CD48	WM68;LO-MN25;J4-57	Leukocytes
CDw49b	CLB-thromb/4;Gil4	Plt, Activated T, Thy
CDw49d	B5G10;HP2/1;HP1/3	M, T, B, LHC, Thy
CDw49f	GoH3	Plt, (T)
CD50	101-1D2;140-11	Leukocytes, broad
CD51	13C2;23C6;NK1-M7;NK1-M9	Plt, (B)
CDw52	097;YTH66.9;Campath-1	Leukocytes
CD53	H129;H136;MEM-53;HD77	Leukocytes
CD54	7F7;WEH1-CAM1	Broad distribution
CD55	143-30;BRIC 110;BRIC 128; F2B-7.2	Broad distribution
CD56	Leu19;NKH1;FP2-11.14;L185	NK, Activated lymphocytes
CD57	Leu7;L183;L187	NK, T, B sub, Brain
CD58	G26;BRIC 5;TS2/9	Leukocytes, Epithel
CD59	Y53.1;MEM-43	Broad distribution
CDw60	M-T32;M-T21;M-T41;UM4D4	T sub
CD61	Y2/51;CLB-thromb/1;V1-PL2; BL-E6	P, (B)
CD62	CLB-thromb/6;CLB-thromb/5; RUU-SP1.18.1	Plt activ.
CD63	RUU-SP2.28;CLB-gran/12	Plt activ., M, G, T, B
CD64	Mab32.2;Mab22	M
CDw65	VIM2;HE10;CF4;VIM8	G, M
CD66	CLB gran/10;YTH71.3	G
CD67	B13.9;G10F5;JML-H16	G
CD68	EBM11;Y2/131;Y-1/82A;Ki-M7; Ki-M6	Macrophages
CD69	MLR3;L78;BL-Ac/p26;FN50	Activated B, T
CDw70	Ki-24;HNE 51;HNC 142	Activated B,-T, Sternberg-Reed cells
CD71	138-18;120-2A3;MEM-75; VIP-1;Nu-TIR2	Proliferating cells, Mac
CD72	S-HCL2;J3-109;BU-40;BU-41	B
CD73	IE9.28.1;7G2.2.11;AD2	B subset, T subset
CD74	LN2;BU-43;BU-45	B, M
CDw75	LN1;HH2;EBU-141	Mature B, (T subset)
CD76	HD66;CRIS-4	Mature B, T subset
CD77	38.13 (BLA);424/4A11; 424/3D9	Restr. B
CDw78	Anti Ba;LO-panB-a;1588	B, (M)

Abbreviations used: AML, acute myeloid leukemia; B, B cells; cALL, common acute lymphocytic leukemia; CD, clusters of differentiation; Cytopl, cytoplasmic; DC, dendritic cells; Eo, eosinophils; Epithel, epithelial cells; G, granulocytes; Germ Ctr B, germinal center B cells; LHC, epidermal Langerhans cells; M, monocytes; Mac, macrophages; NK, natural killer (cells); PC, plasma cells; Plt, platelets; Prog, progenitor cells; RBC, red blood cells; T, T cells; Thy, thymocytes.

[a]Adapted from Nomenclature Committee [*J. Immunol.***143**, 758 (1989)].

antigens expressed, T cells can be grouped into subpopulations with regulatory and/or effector functions (4). Circulating T cells can be divided into two main groups based on their mutually exclusive expression of CD4 or CD8. In general, CD4$^+$ T cells express helper or regulatory functions for all T–T and T–B interactions and account for 45 to 70% of peripheral T cells. CD8$^+$ T cells, which make up the remaining 30 to 55% of peripheral T cells, are cytotoxic effector cells (killer cells) and also exert suppressive effects on immune responses. Although the immune functions associated with each of these major subsets are generally uniform, some CD4 expressing cells can be cytotoxic or suppressive whereas some CD8 expressing cells may interact directly with other T cells.

The functions of CD4$^+$ T cells and CD8$^+$ T cells are restricted by the products of the genes of the major histocompatibility complex (MHC).[2] In the human, MHC is located on chromosome 6 and is called "human leukocyte antigens" (HLA) (5). CD8$^+$ cells recognize antigen(s) as products of the MHC subregions A, B, C, etc., *i.e.*, the HLA-A, HLA-B, and HLA-C antigens; these are called class I antigens. Thus, individuals who are immune to a particular virus, such as mumps or measles, will have specific cytotoxic T lymphocytes (CTL) capable of killing virus-infected cells of the same HLA type. In addition to performing effector functions, the CD8$^+$ T cell population contains regulator T cells, *i.e.*, the T suppressor cell (T$_S$). These cells negatively regulate the immune response, most likely by down-regulating T helper cell activity (6), and are also MHC class I restricted. T$_S$ cells secrete soluble suppressor factors (lymphokines) and may be important in developing immunologic tolerance.

CD4$^+$ cells recognizes MHC-encoded class II antigens (*i.e.*, HLA-DR antigens). These cells also have effector and regulatory functions. CD4$^+$ effector cells carry out DTH reactions (so-called type IV hypersensitivity). Their inflammatory reactions are facilitated through the production of lymphokines such as the interleukins (IL). The regulatory function of helper T (T$_H$) cells is required for B cells to produce antibody; T$_H$ cells are also involved in activating other T cells. The production of lymphokines by these cells is a mediator of their function. The correlation between CD4 expression and requirement for class II corecognition is stronger than the correlation between CD4 expression and helper function. Similarly, the association of CD8 expression and class I corecognition is stronger than CD8 expression and effector/suppression function (7). Thus, for example, in allograft rejection if the host and graft show only MHC class II differences, CD4$^+$ T cell effectors account for graft rejection. Conversely, if only MHC class I differences are present, then CD8$^+$ T cell effectors are responsible for rejection (8–10).

There are additional multiple subsets of T cells. Both CD4 and CD8 populations can be subdivided on the basis of their expression of isoforms of the common leukocyte antigen, CD45 (Tables 2 and 3). The CD4$^+$CD45RA$^+$ T cell subset appears to include a population of naive or virgin T, CD45RA$^+$/RO$^-$ cells (in mice, called T$_H$1). These cells produce the lymphokine IL-2 and provide help in T–T interactions for the production of CTL and T$_S$ cells. The CD4$^+$CD45RA$^-$/RO$^+$ T cell population produces, in addition to IL-2, preferentially the lymphokines IL-4, IL-6, and γ-IFN. These cells are *memory cells* which respond to soluble recall antigens. They provide help to B cells in antibody production and are called T$_H$2 cells in mice. The CD8$^+$ subsets are less well characterized. Nonetheless, CD8$^+$CD45RA$^+$ T cells exhibit mixed lymphocyte reaction (MLR)[3]-

---

[2]The MHC is a cluster of genes that encode cell surface antigens which are polymorphic within a species, leading to graft rejection if these loci differ. MHC class I and class II antigens are encoded in this region.
[3]In mixed culture allogeneic lymphocytes mutually induce eath other's proliferation (MLR) proportionally to the disparity of their MHCs.

TABLE 2. CD4$^+$ T Cell Subsets and CD45 Isoforms[a]

Parameter	CD4$^+$CD45RA$^+$ RO$^-$	CD4$^+$CD45RA$^-$ RO$^+$
Allogeneic mixed lymphocyte culture (MLC)	+++	+++
Autologous MLC	+++	+
PYHA stimulation	+++	+
Cytokine sensitivity on activation (Il-1)(IL-1, IL-2, IL-4, IL-6)	+++	+
Anti-CD3 stimulation (low dose)	++	+++
Response to soluble "memory" recall antigens	−	+++
B cell help in antibody production	−	+++
	(Naive, virgin)	(Memory)
T–T help (CTL generation)	+	+
IL-2 production	+++	+
T–T suppression inducer (T$_S$ generation)	+	
Direct suppression (neonates)	+	−
γ-IFN, IL-4, IL-6 production	±	+++
Increased expression of IL-2R, Class II MHC	No	Yes
Increased expression of adhesion molecules [LFA-1(CD18/CD11a), LFA-3 (CD58), CD2, ICAM-1 (CD54), CD29 VLA integrin family)]	No	Yes
Endothelial venule adhesion molecules (Leu-8, TQ1, LAM-1)	Yes	No

Abbreviations used: CD, clusters of differentiation; CTL, cytotoxic T lymphocytes; ICAM, intercellular adhesion molecules; IFN, interferon; IL, interleukin; LAM, lymphocyte associated molecule; LFA, leukocyte function antigens; MLC, mixed lymphocyte culture; PYHA, phytohemagglutinin; TQ1, (antigen complementary to the anti-TQ1 monoclonal antibody); VLA, very late antigens.
[a]Summarized from L.T. Clement [*J. Clin. Immunol.* **12**,1 (1992)].

TABLE 3. CD8$^+$ T Cell Subsets and CD45 Isoforms[a]

Parameter	CD8$^+$CD45RA$^+$	CD8$^+$CD45RA$^-$
CTL precursors	Yes	Yes
CTL effectors (helper cell dependent)	No	Yes
MLR-induced suppressors	Yes	No
Suppress B-cell differentiation	Yes	Yes
Helper cell independent CTL generation	Yes	No

Abbreviations used: CTL, cytotoxic T lymphocytes; MLR, mixed lymphocyte response.
[a]Summarized from L. T. Clement [*J. Clin. Immunol.* **12**,1 (1992)].

induced suppressor activity and helper cell independent CTL generation (natural killer [NK]-like activity) while CD8$^+$CD45RA$^-$ T cells contain helper cell dependent CTL effectors. Both RA$^+$ and RA$^-$CD8$^+$ T cells suppress B cell differentiation (11).

B. B Cells

B lymphocytes represent the antigen-specific arm of acquired humoral immunity. B cells synthesize and secrete antibodies. Immunoglobulin (Ig) is the collective term for all antibody molecules. Ig units are composed of two heavy (H) chains and two light (L) chains and contain two antibody-binding sites. There are five major classes of Igs: IgM, IgG, IgA, IgE, and IgD, distinguished by differences in their H chains.

B cell development begins between the eighth and ninth weeks of gestation and continues throughout the lifetime of the host. Pre-B cells express IgM heavy (μ) chains in their cytoplasm following genomic DNA rearrangement that involves the *V* (Variable), *D*

(Diversity), and *J* (Joining) genes of the μ chain. Following further genomic rearrangement of DNA (the *V* and *J* chains) for light chains, immature B cells express the monomeric form of IgM on their cell surface. Although this surface IgM (sIgM) can recognize antigen (*i.e.*, act as a receptor), contact with antigen at this stage usually leads to deletion of these cells instead of proliferation. Mature B cells express both IgM and IgD. All of these changes occur in the absence of antigen (12). Maturation of B cells continues outside the bone marrow environment. Within peripheral lymphoid organs, certain B cells undergo the phenomenon of "class switching" and change from expression of sIgM to one of the other Ig isotypes, *i.e.*, IgG, IgA, or IgE (13). Ultimately, interaction of B cells with antigen or with antigen and T_H cells induces the B cells to enter their final stage of maturation. Those B cells that selectively interact with a specific antigen are triggered to proliferate (clonal expansion) and differentiate into antibody-secreting plasma cells. All progeny of a particular clone have the same specificity for antigen. A proportion of the cells resulting from clonal expansion become memory B cells. Terminal differentiation into plasma cells also requires non-antigen-specific T cell factors. Long-lived memory B cells ensure the ability of a host to mount a subsequent and more rapid response upon reexposure to antigen.

Mature B cells are characterized by the presence of Ig molecules on their cell surface. In addition, B cells express other cell surface markers such as receptor for the Fc segment[4] of IgG (CD16), or CD19 and CD20, some of which are receptors for hormones or T cell products, and which appear or disappear at different stages of B cell development. B cells, beginning at the pre-B cell stage, also express the products of the class II genes of the MHC which are integral to the presentation of antigens for T cell help in the activation of B cells.

C. Natural Killer Cells (NK Cells)

These cells are large granular lymphocytes (LGLs) with a lower nuclear/cytoplasmic ratio and azurophilic cytoplasmic granules which contain up to 20% of circulating lymphocytes (14). NK cells lack the surface antigen receptors of T and B cells (*i.e.*, CD3 complex, T cell receptors, [T_{CR}], surface immunoglobulins [sIg]). However, NK cells usually express the cell surface antigens CD16 and NKH-1 (CD56) as well as the Fc receptors[5] and the alpha (α) chain of the IL-2 receptor. The cell lineage of NK cells is probably separate from that of either T or B cells. Functionally, these cells are not MHC restricted and have the ability to kill certain neoplastic cells, virus-infected cells, and other target cells coated with antibodies (antibody-dependent cellular cytotoxicity [ADCC]). In addition, by direct stimulation with IL-2, NK cells can be activated into so-called lymphokine-activated killer (LAK) cells capable of lysing fresh tumor cells (15,16).

D. Monocytes and Antigen Processing

Cells of the mononuclear monocyte/macrophage series derive from the bone marrow. Macrophage precursors undergo limited replication and, upon termination of DNA synthesis, enter the blood to become monocytes. Monocytes have endocytic activity, circulate in the blood for approximately 24 hours and then migrate into different tissues. Monocytes are exposed to differentiation signals unique to the site of their migration.

---

[4]The Fc segment of antibody molecules contains the C terminal domains of the H chains. It does not bind antigen, but mediates the biological role of the antibody once antigen has been bound to the antigen-binding Fab segments. Differences in the Fc segment is the basis of the existence of classes of antibodies (isotypes).

[5]Receptors on the cell surface with binding specificity to the Fc segment of antibody molecules. Many types of cells contain Fc receptors.

These tissue factors ultimately determine the characteristics of the resident, terminally-differentiated macrophages which form the reticuloendothelial system established in many organs (17). Depending on the tissues in which they reside, macrophages vary in their extent of surface receptors, oxidative metabolism, arachidonate products, and expression of MHC class II antigens (18,19). Such macrophages actively phagocytize particulate material *in vitro* and adhere strongly to glass and plastic. They possess a well-developed Golgi complex and many intracytoplasmic lysosomes containing a variety of hydrolases and peroxidases. These in turn are important in killing microorganisms ingested by macrophages and in tumor lysis by macrophages.

An important immunologic function for cells of the monocyte/macrophage lineage is processing and presentation of antigen to specific lymphocytes (1). While B cells can recognize structural determinants (epitopes) on native soluble or particulate antigens and be triggered to secrete antibody, T cells require that antigen be processed and presented in the context of MHC molecules for recognition (Figure 2). "Antigen-presenting" or "antigen-processing" cells (APCs) consist of a heterogeneous cell population, including macrophages, which possess immunostimulatory capacity. Among the classic APCs besides monocytes/macrophages are Langerhans cells of the skin, follicular dendritic cells, endothelial cells, and even B cells. Most APCs are found primarily in lymph nodes, skin, spleen, and thymus, but are not limited to these organs.

Because macrophages release enhancing and suppressive modulatory cytokines and because they have receptors for lymphokines, macrophages also participate in the immune response as regulatory cells and effector cells (7). Macrophage-derived cytokines can increase B cell growth and T cell reactivity (IL-1), promote NK cells to release γ-interferon (γ-INF), and enhance tissue inflammation, among other properties. Macrophages can also secrete interferons. Macrophages possess receptors for and respond to IL-1, tumor necrosis factor (TNF) and IL-4, as well as to γ-INF, and this results in their activation.

E. Lymphocyte Activation

1. Role of the T Cell Receptor (T_{CR})

The definitive cell surface marker for T cells is the T_{CR}. The T_{CR} molecule is a disulfide-linked heterodimer that occurs in two major forms, $T_{CR}\alpha\beta$ and $T_{CR}\gamma\delta$, and has similarity to the Ig molecule. The T_{CR} molecule is associated on the cell surface with the CD3 molecular complex (20–23). The majority of T cells express the alpha (α) and beta (β) chain form, while a minority population expresses the gamma (γ) and delta (δ) form. T_{CR}'s, like Ig genes, are encoded by distinct *V*, *D*, *J*, and *C* (Constant) genes which, also like Ig, undergo gene rearrangements to yield the mature molecules, a process resulting in the enormous diversity of T_{CR}'s (24–28).

The T_{CR}/CD3 complex is central to the specific activation of T cells. T cells, through their T_{CR}'s, recognize antigen on the surface of other cells, called antigen-presenting cells (APCs). T_{CR}'s do not recognize free antigenic determinants (29–31), but instead recognize a cleaved peptide fragment in association with an MHC class I or class II protein (32,33). Two methods of antigen processing that form the appropriate MHC–peptide complex have been recognized—an exogenous pathway and an endogenous pathway (34,35). In the exogenous pathway, antigen is endocytosed by APCs, fragmented inside vesicles, associated with MHC class II molecules, and expressed on the cell surface. In the endogenous pathway, antigens that are synthesized within a cell, *e.g.*, viral antigens, are fragmented in the cytoplasm and associated with MHC class I molecules. The complex is then expressed on the cell surface. $CD4^+$ T cells recognize MHC–peptide complex produced by the exogenous pathway and $CD8^+$ T cells recognize MHC–peptide complex produced by the endogenous pathway.

When antigen is presented to a T cell that has a specific T_{CR} for that particular peptide–MHC complex, the T cell is activated. At the same time, IL-1 is released by the APC and contributes to the activation and proliferation of the activated T cell. In addition to specific antigen–MHC complex, T cells can also be nonspecifically activated by polyclonal activators, such as the plant lectins concanavalin-A (Con-A) and phytohemagglutinin (PYHA), or by monoclonal antibody, *e.g.*, anti-CD3. These lectins and monoclonal antibodies are mitogenic and interact with T cell surface receptors that are different from the T_{CR}. Unlike specific T_{CR}–antigen interaction which results in a clonal T cell response, the response to lectin (or monoclonal antibody) activation is polyclonal in nature.

2. Cytokines/Lymphokines/Monokines

Specific interaction with antigen leads to the production of growth and differentiation factors by APCs and T cells. These factors, known as cytokines, are responsible for the rapid expansion and differentiation of the small numbers of antigen-specific lymphocytes present in a previously unexposed host. Cytokines are a subset of low-molecular-weight peptide regulatory factors with specific high-affinity cell surface receptors and a short to intermediate range of action (36). Cytokines, which include lymphokines and monokines, *i.e.*, peptides produced by lymphocytes and monocytes, respectively, represent a group of usually glycosylated, immunoregulatory polypeptides which act locally on adjacent cells (paracrines) or on the same cells that secrete them (autocrines). An illustrative partial list of some cytokines and related lymphokines including ILs, IFNs and colony-stimulating factors (CSFs) produced by macrophages, monocytes, and related cell types, together with a list of their targets and activities, is given in Tables 4 and 5.

The large diverse group of cell-derived mediators can have wide-ranging effects on most organ systems of the body. Three general types of lymphokine-mediated effects have been recognized: (i) costimulant effects, where more than one lymphokine is necessary to produce an effect; (ii) inductive/quantitative effects, where one lymphokine induces the production of another; and (iii) cascading type of mediator release, where a lymphokine may either amplify the effect(s) of the original stimulus or inhibit the primary mediator in a feedback inhibition fashion.

3. Interleukins

The complexity of the cytokine/lymphokine system is illustrated by the family of IL molecules which mediate many of the effects of T cells and B cells. At least eleven ILs have been described, of which eight have been best characterized. The number of characterized ILs continues to expand.

One of the best characterized is IL-1. IL-1 is produced by many cell types in response to damage by environmental agents, infections, or other antigens, and induces production of acute phase proteins (38). IL-1 has multiple functional properties, including stimulation of thymocyte proliferation, activation of certain T cells, activation of B cells, NK cells, and macrophages. IL-1 acts either directly or indirectly in order to increase the activity of sensitized cells or potentiate their responses to other lymphokines. For example, proliferation of murine $T_H 2$ cell lines which produce IL-4 and IL-6 requires, or

FIGURE 2.   Activation of immune responses. [Adapted from B. E. Bozelka and J. E. Salvaggio: *Environ. Carcino. Rev.* **C3**, 1 (1985).]

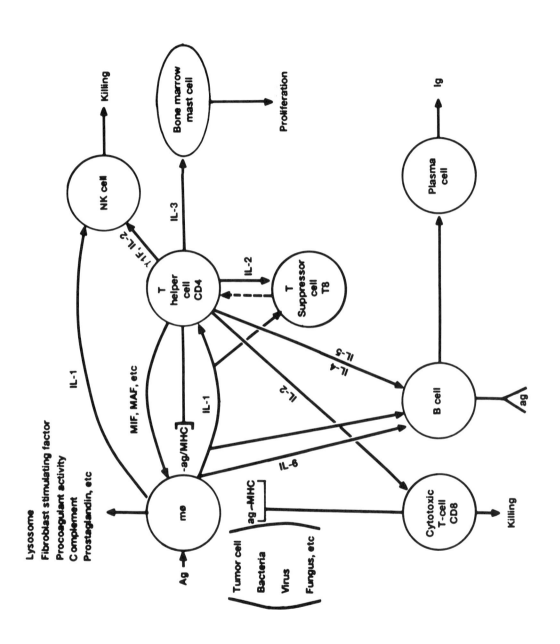

TABLE 4. Biological Response Modifiers: Interferons and Other Cytokines[a]

Cytokine	Abbreviation	Biologic activity
α- or β-Interferon	α- or β-IFN	Exerts antiviral activity; induces MHC class I antigen expression; augments NK cell activity; has fever-inducing and antiproliferative properties
γ-Interferon	γ-IFN	Induces MHC class I and class II antigens; activates macrophages and endothelial cells; augments NK cell activity; exerts antiviral activity; augments or inhibits other cytokine activities
Tumor necrosis factor α or β	TNF α or β	Is cytotoxic to some tumor cells; induces fever, sleep, and other systemic acute-phase responses; activates endothelial cells and macrophages; mediates inflammation, catabolic processes, and septic shock; stimulates synthesis of other cytokines
Granulocyte colony-stimulating factor	G-CSF	Stimulates growth of granulocyte colonies and activates mature granulocytes; increases antibody-dependent, neutrophil-mediated cytotoxicity; induces *in vitro* differentiation of leukemia cell lines; stimulates proliferation of leukemic progenitors
Granulocyte-macrophage colony-stimulating factor	GM-CSF	Stimulates growth of granulocyte, monocyte, early erythrocyte and megakaryocyte progenitors; activates mature granulocytes and monocytes; enhances antibody-dependent, cell-mediated cytotoxicity
Macrophage colony-stimulating factor	M-CSF	Stimulates growth of monocyte colonies; supports *in vitro* survival of monocytes; activates mature monocytes; enhances antibody-dependent, monocyte-mediated cytotoxicity

Other abbreviations used: MHC, major histocompatibility complex; NK, natural killer (cells).
[a]Adapted from H. F. Oettgen, and L. J. Old: *In* "Biologic Therapy of Cancer" (V. T. De Vita, Jr., S. Hellman, and S. A. Rosenberg, eds.), Lippincott, Philadelphia, 1991, p. 87.

is enhanced by IL-1, whereas $T_H 1$ cells which produce IL-2 and γ-IFN are insensitive to IL-1 (37). This selective effect of IL-1 may result in a humoral antibody response rather than a cellular response (38). IL-1 also increases IL-2 receptor (IL-2R) expression and functions as an endogenous pyrogen. IL-1 has been found to be increased or decreased in a variety of diseases (39–41) and can be inhibited by naturally occurring inhibitors (42).

IL-2, originally described as T cell growth factor (43,44), is transiently secreted (2–3 days) by T cells after their activation by antigen or mitogen and has a proliferating effect on mature T cells and thymocytes. IL-2 induces T cell cytotoxicity and stimulates NK cell activity. IL-2 can also activate B cells to become antibody-secreting cells, depending on the quantity of IL-2 and on the ability of the B cells to express the IL-2R β chain on the cell surface (38). This B cell effect of IL-2 may be enhanced by γ-IFN. The level of IL-2 production has been measured in a variety of immunodeficiency, autoimmune, and related diseases. Marked increases in IL-2 have been noted in certain autoimmune and related inflammatory diseases and its production is decreased in a variety of immunodeficiency states (45–47).

The IL-2R consists of two polypeptide chains α and β, each containing an IL-2 binding site (38). IL-2Rs are not detectable on resting T cells, which appear to have small numbers of α chains on their surface and no β chains. Following activation, β chains are synthesized and expressed and within 3 days all activated T cells express IL-2Rs. The interaction of IL-2 with both chains of the receptor results in "high-affinity" binding. Soluble IL-2R (sIL-2R), detected by monoclonal antibody to the β chain (or "TAC

TABLE 5. **Biological Response Modifiers: Interleukins[a]**

Cytokine	Abbreviation	Biologic activity
Interleukin-1 α or β	IL-α or β	Activates resting T cells; makes early hemato-poietic progenitors more sensitive to later acting factors (hematopoietic 1 activity); induces CSF production by accessory cells; induces fever, sleep, ACTH release, neutrophilia, and other acute-phase responses; activates endothelial cells and macrophages; mediates inflammation catabolic process, and nonspecific resistance to infection; stimulates synthesis of other cytokines
Interleukin-2	IL-2	Is a cofactor for growth and differentiation of T and B cells; augments lymphocyte killer activity; induces production of other cytokines
Interleukin-3	IL-3	Stimulates early growth of granulocyte, monocyte, erythrocyte, and megakaryocyte progenitor cells; supports mast cell growth; induces acute nonlymphocytic leukemia blasts to proliferate
Interleukin-4	IL-4	Is growth factor for activated B cells; induces MHC class II antigens on B cells; promotes IgG secretion; is growth factor for resting T cells; enhances cytolytic activity of cytotoxic T cells; supports mast cell growth; synergizes with other growth factors to promote colony growth
Interleukin-5	IL-5	Induces proliferation and differentiation of eosinophil progenitors
Interleukin-6	IL-6	Induces B cell differentiation; enhances Ig secretion by B cells; synergizes with other growth factors to promote colony growth; synergizes with IL-1 in stimulating T cell proliferation
Interleukin-7	IL-7	Supports the growth of B cell precursors
Interleukin-8	IL-8	Neutrophil activating protein; T cell chemotactic factor

[a]Adapted from H. F. Oettgen, and L. J. Old: *In* "Biologic Therapy of Cancer" (V. T. De Vita, Jr., S. Hellman, and S. A. Rosenberg, eds.), Lippincott, Philadelphia, 1991, p. 87.

peptide"), is released by activated T cells during many immunologically mediated inflammatory responses, including autoimmune diseases, graft *versus* host reactions, infectious and parasitic diseases, lymphoreticular malignancies, multiple sclerosis, and AIDS, among others (48–51). In autoimmune diseases such as systemic lupus erythematosus and rheumatoid arthritis (RA), high serum levels of IL-2 and IL-2R have shown correlation with disease activity (47). In addition, plasma and urine levels of IL-2R are increased during renal and heart allograft rejection.

IL-3 is a potent CSF that regulates hematopoietic and lymphoid progenitor cells (52). It is produced by activated T cells and may affect the growth of pre-B cells (38). IL-3 has not been extensively studied in human disease, but it may play an important role in allergic and hematologic diseases.

IL-4 is a costimulator of B cell proliferation. It induces increased expression of class II MHC molecules and low-affinity receptors for the Fc portion of IgE on B cells. IL-4 induces high levels of IgE *in vivo* (38,54). IL-4 also stimulates the proliferation of T_H and of CTLs, it induces the proliferation of thymocytes in combination with phorbol ester, and can induce the expression of CD8 on CD4$^+$ T cells. In addition to its positive effects, IL-4 inhibits B cell proliferation induced by IL-2 as well as IL-2–induced generation of NK cells. IL-4 is produced by T cells, mainly by the T_H 2 subset, which in mice contains the most efficient helper activity for B cells. IL-4 has not been extensively studied in human disease. However, because of its effects on IgE production *in vivo*, studies of the effects of this molecule in patients with common IgE allergic disease, as well as of methods to prevent its activity, are of increasing interest.

IL-5 has several effects on B cells, including induction of IgM and IgA production. It may act as an isotype switch factor (38,55). It is also a growth factor for eosinophils and has been reported to be elevated in diseases associated with eosinophilia.

IL-6 is produced by T cells (preferentially by $T_H 2$ cells) and affects both T cell and B cell function. IL-6 induces B cell differentiation and induces secretion of Igs from B cells without B cell proliferation. It is a myeloid growth factor, stimulating bone marrow progenitor cells into granulocyte and macrophage colony formation. It also acts as a costimulator in the mitogen-induced IL-2–independent proliferation of T cells, induces thymocyte proliferation, and, like IL-1, induces the production of acute phase proteins (38,56,57). IL-6 has been reported to be elevated in certain infectious diseases and associated with hypergammaglobulinemia and autoantibody production (56–58). It has also been found to be increased in synovial fluid and in the serum of patients with RA (59).

IL-7 appears to be a developmental factor for both T and B cells. It is a costimulus for mitogen activation of T cells, a growth stimulus for pre-B cells, and induces proliferation of immature and mature thymocytes (38,60). The effect(s) of IL-7 on human disease has not yet been substantially studied.

IL-8, previously known as neutrophil activating protein and T cell chemotactic factor, is produced by a variety of cells. As indicated by its synonyms, IL-8 plays an important role in the activation and chemotaxis of neutrophils and T cells (61).

IFN was originally described as a factor produced following a viral infection and which protects other cells from viral attack (62). Three types of IFN are now known — α-IFN, β-IFN, and γ-IFN. γ-IFN has a more central role in regulating immune responses than the other two types (38,63). γ-IFN is produced by antigen-specific T cells and by IL-2–recruited NK cells. Its immunoregulatory effects include activation of macrophages (enhancing tumor cytolysis and phagocytosis), activation and proliferation of cytolytic T cells and NK cells, induction of MHC class II antigen expression on various cells, induction of Fcγ receptor expression on different cell types, induction of Ig secretion by IL-2–activated B cells, potentiation of IL-4–induced B cell proliferation, and induction of high levels of IgG_{2a} complement fixing antibody. In addition to its inductive and potentiating effects, γ-IFN inhibits some of the action of IL-4. For example, γ-IFN inhibits IL-4–induced expression of MHC class II antigens as well as the IL-4–enhanced IgE synthesis in lipopolysaccharide-stimulated B cells. Studies of the effects of γ-IFN in human disease indicate that this molecule can modulate resistance to some microbial infections and may increase vaccine effectiveness (63). In addition, it has been useful in chronic granulomatous disease, restoring granulocyte bactericidal activity. It has not proven useful in the treatment of solid tumors and may even contribute to the pathophysiology of disease [*e.g.*, in one study, multiple sclerosis patients who were treated with γ-IFN had an increased relapse rate (64)].

The remaining ILs are still in the process of being characterized (61,65). In general, however, ILs affect the functions of many cell types and are produced by lymphocytes, monocytes, and multiple other cells. They modulate immune responses by regulating differentiation, growth, and function of lymphoid and other accessory cells as well as by regulating their own production. They may also be subject to naturally occurring inhibitors. The ability to monitor levels of ILs and their receptors is becoming very important in the diagnosis and treatment of autoimmune, allergic, neoplastic, and infectious diseases that are suspected to occur as a result of exposure to immunotoxins.

4. B Cell Activation

Specific activation of B cells involves binding of antigen that is complementary to Ig expressed on the B cell surface. Following activation, B cells divide and differentiate into specific antibody-secreting plasma cells. Lymphokines such as IL-1 and IL-6 are essential for B cell differentiation into plasma cells. Response by B cells to certain antigens are T cell dependent, whereas response to others, *e.g.*, polysaccharide antigens, are T cell independent. In a T cell–dependent response, APCs present antigen to a T cell which is thereby activated and secretes lymphokines; the lymphokines, in the context of specific antigen, enable B cells to transform into plasma cells (Figure 2). In the T cell–independent pathway, B cells are triggered directly to become plasma cells by antigen without T cell help. In general, T cell–independent antigens induce weak IgM responses and poor immunological memory.

F. Regulation of Immune Response

Immunosuppression and hypersensitivity responses are normal activities of the immune system. Suppressive activity is a normal regulatory component of immunity that "down"-regulates responses. DTH responses protect against certain infections with viruses, fungi, and parasites and are involved in allograft rejection, contact dermatitis, immune surveillance against tumors, and some autoimmune responses involving solid organ tissues. Immediate hypersensitivity responses protect against parasitic diseases and are involved in the pathogenesis of common respiratory allergic diseases (asthma and rhinitis), anaphylaxis, and some gastrointestinal and skin diseases (urticaria, food allergy). The intensity of any immune response reflects a particular balance of external and internal factors that either amplify or depress the response. All immune responses are regulated in this manner and aberrations of immune regulation are believed to play important roles in the development of autoimmunity, allergic hypersensitivity, immune deficiency, tolerance, and probably in the aging process.

Jerne's network theory (66) holds that all antigen receptors (idiotopes) on T and B cells can induce complementary (anti-idiotype) T cells or B cells which by themselves or through their products can down-regulate production of the original idiotope. In the case of B cells, an antibody and the B cells that produce it bear an idiotope which can stimulate another B cell clone to make antibody directed against this particular antigen receptor (anti-idiotypic antibody). B cell and T cell activity is also regulated by lymphokines produced by themselves or other cells. For example, IL-4 and/or IL-5 induce B cells to produce certain Igs (IgE, IgG_1, and/or IgA), whereas γ-IFN induces production of IgG_{2a} and inhibits other IgG subclasses (67). Additionally, IL-4 increases the density of MHC class II molecules on B cells, presumably making them better antigen presenters, while immune IFN blocks class II up-regulation in B cells, but induces expression of the class II molecules in macrophages.

Genetic factors also play a key role in determining immune responsiveness. In mice and other animals, failure to respond to certain antigens has been linked to the specific MHC genes expressed by the animal. In some cases, the unresponsiveness may be due to an inability to produce the appropriate T cell or B cell receptor(s). In other cases, stimulation of T_S cells rather than T_H or effector cells may occur, resulting in tolerance. In humans, certain diseases (usually with an autoimmune component) such as Reiter's syndrome, ankylosing spondylitis, myasthenia gravis, coeliac disease, Addison's disease, and insulin-dependent diabetes mellitus are associated with MHC class I or class II haplotypes (68). In addition, patients with common atopic or IgE-mediated allergic respiratory disease have a familial (*i.e.*, ill-defined genetic) basis for their responsiveness predisposing them to inappropriately overproduce IgE antibody against common inhalant allergens.

III. IMMUNE SURVEILLANCE AND CARCINOGENESIS

The immune surveillance theory of carcinogenesis (69) holds that one of the major functions of the immune system is to protect the host from development and growth of cancer. The immune system is thought to recognize and destroy occasional abnormal and possibly malignant cells which may arise as a result of mutations occurring during the normal replacement of cells. If a malignant cell escapes this surveillance, then neoplasia occurs. The theory correctly predicts an increased incidence of malignancies in immuno-deficient or immunosuppressed individuals. However, the theory remains controversial. For example, it can be argued that the incidence of all cancers should be increased in immunosuppressed individuals rather than the particular malignancies (usually of the immune system itself) that have been described (70). Another argument against the immune surveillance theory is the observation that athymic or thymectomized mice without functional T cells do not have an abnormally high incidence of neoplasms. Moreover, spontaneously or certain nonvirally induced tumors appear to lack detectable tumor-associated antigens on their cell surface and, therefore, are poorly immunogenic and may not be detected by a specific cellular immunologic response. On the other hand, virally induced neoplasms and tumors induced in animals by high doses of carcinogenic chemicals (*e.g.*, 3-methylcholanthrene [3-MC]) express tumor-associated antigens (not found in normal untransformed cells) or viral proteins unique to the virus or chemical agent which are strongly immunogenic and readily induce specific CTL responses.

Lymphoid cells of the immune system other than T_H and CTL cells, such as NK cells and LAK cells, do not require MHC antigen presentation (71–74); interference with their function or numbers may enhance tumorigenesis. The accumulation of NK cells and tumor infiltrating lymphocytes (TILs) can reduce growth and metastatic potential (75,76). TILs are isolated from solid tumors; they comprise a heterogenous population of lymphocytes in which $CD8^+$ cells are often predominant and which express markers of T cell activation not normally expressed on circulating T cells (*e.g.*, MHC class II antigen and IL-2R) (77). Some TILs, NK, and LAK cells are capable of lysing a variety of neoplastic cell types that are refractory to CTLs. It should be noted in this regard that some chemical carcinogens have been shown to reduce NK cell functions.

In Sections V.A through V.G below, the variety of immunotoxic effects of some major classes of environmentally occurring chemical carcinogens, as well as selected illustrative examples of other immunotoxins, are reviewed. The suppression of or injury to relevant effector mechanisms of the immune system may increase the incidence of tumors. Conversely, the enhancement or stimulation of appropriate arms of the effector mechanism could result in a decreased incidence.

IV. IMMUNOTOXICOLOGY

Immunotoxicity is defined by the Office of Technology Assessment (OTA) "as an adverse or inappropriate change in the structure or function of the immune system after exposure to a foreign substance. Adverse effects can be manifest as immunosuppression, hypersensitivity, or autoimmunity". The OTA further defines an immunotoxicant as "a substance that leads to undesired effects on the immune system" (78). Immunotoxicology, then, might be defined as a study of the immune system and its components as targets for detection of general and selective chemically induced toxicity (79). A variety of environmental agents, chemicals, and drugs have been found through clinical experience, occupational exposure, and industrial accidents to act collectively or individually on components of the immune system, resulting in autoimmunity, hypersensitivity, immune deficiency, or decreased tumor "immune surveillance". Such immunotoxins can potentially affect the immune system exclusively as a primary target, or they can act on a secondary target such as the skin, lungs, thyroid, or nervous system, or they can simultaneously act on both the primary and secondary targets. The magnitude and type of effect on the immune system is also influenced by other factors, such as the host's immune status, nutritional status, and/or the presence of concurrent diseases. An immunotoxin may simultaneously act as an antigen, sensitizing the host to future exposures; *e.g.*, beryllium, which is profoundly toxic at high doses, induces hypersensitivity at lower doses. An immunotoxin may also act as an immune response modifier either inhibiting or amplifying reactivity. For example, IgE antibody production to common inhalant allergens is increased with cigarette smoking and exposure to diesel exhaust (80–82).

V. CHEMICAL CARCINOGENS AND OTHER IMMUNESUPPRESSANTS: EFFECTS ON THE IMMUNE SYSTEM

Most human cancers result from complex interactions between a variety of environmental factors, and genetic and other endogenous host factors. Animals, more specifically mice, rats, and hamsters, are the species in which the greatest amount of data were, and continue to be, obtained on the carcinogenicity of chemical agents. In general, considerably higher doses are used than those to which humans would normally be exposed. The doses used in experimental animals can vary by as much as 10^5 to 10^6 in order of magnitude. For example, aflatoxin B_1, a mycotoxin contaminant in food, induces tumors in 50% of rats at daily microgram dose levels; on the other hand, 10 to 100 mg benzidine is required for tumor induction (83). Moreover, the species, strain, sex, age, and route of administration very significantly affect the manifest potency of a carcinogen and, in addition, target organs can differ. For example, aromatic amines induce bladder cancer in humans, but predominantly liver or other tumors in rodents (83).

In a similar manner, chemical carcinogens in the environment exert a variety of effects on the immune system. Once again, most data regarding the effects of these agents on the immune system have been obtained from animal studies in which the route of exposure, dose, genetics (species, strain), sex, and age all affect the results obtained. Environmental agents that are potentially carcinogenic may induce specific immunity, allergic hypersensitivity, and autoimmunity. They may enhance immune responses nonspecifically and inhibit, suppress, or modulate immunoresponsiveness. An environmental agent may be selective in its target, and can affect the functionality or even the detectability of only one particular immune response component. For example, NK cells or NK activity may be inhibited or potentiated and B cell differentiation may be inhibited, resulting in arrested development and panimmunoglobulin suppression. Furthermore, the inhibition or stimulation of cytokines such as IL-1 or γ -IFN and/or their receptors can lead to dysfunction of T cells, B cells, and monocytes/macrophages.

Various rodent species are used most often for investigating the potential immunotoxic effects of chemicals. This is because (a) the dose, route of administration, sex, age, genetic background, nutrition, and general experimental environment can be controlled; and (b) animals can be exposed to a putative toxic substance and subsequently be challenged with an infectious agent or tumor cells, followed by sacrifice and direct examination of organs and tissues. Impairment of the ability to fight infection or reject tumors following exposure to an agent is a good measure of the overall toxicity of the agent toward the immune system. A substance which significantly increases the incidence of morbidity and mortality rate, as compared to nonexposed animals, would be considered a likely immunotoxin. In humans this type of analysis can only be obtained following industrial accidents or prolonged occupational exposure, and requires good epidemiological, clinical, and laboratory assessment.

In humans, tests evaluating possible immunotoxic effects on the immune system are usually carried out employing *in vitro* assays using peripheral blood, bronchoalveolar lavage fluid, or nasal lavage fluid. Hypersensitivity skin testing and pulmonary function tests can be carried out on both animals and humans to determine the allergenicity of an agent. In humans, skin testing and exposure by inhalation with pulmonary function testing must be done under carefully controlled clinical conditions. Measurement of specific IgE levels for a particular antigen in blood or lavage fluids can also be performed for certain organic and inorganic chemicals of low molecular weight and for high-molecular-weight proteins. Table 6 lists many of the common tests for the assessment of immune function.

In general, significant deviations from "normal" reference ranges or expected activity established for each assay and cell population evaluated would indicate a possible toxic

TABLE 6.   **Common Tests for the Assessment of Immune Function**

Test	Stimulant/Reagent	Measure
Lymphocyte quantitation	Mab to specific CD molecules and fluorescence-activated cell analysis	Enumeration of T cells, T cell phenotypic subsets, B cells, NK cells, monocytes, etc.
Lymphocyte activation by mitogens	PYHA, Con-A, PWM, protein A	T cell polyclonal proliferation, B cell polyclonal proliferation, cytokine production
by specific antigen	Candida, tetanus	Recall responses, cytokine production
Mixed lymphocyte response (MLR)	MHC disparate lymphocytes	T cell proliferation, allograft response, cytokine production
Cytotoxic T cell assay	MHC disparate or viral protein expressing cells	MHC-restricted, specific T cell lysis of target cells
NK cell assay	Certain cell lines	MHC-unrestricted nonspecific lysis of target cells
Ig levels in serum	Anti-Ig class reagents	Ig levels proportional to number of B cells which secrete antibodies
RAST	Allergen	Antigen-specific and/or total IgE levels
PFC assay	T-independent antigen and/or T-dependent antigen	Number of B cells which produce antibodies and/or T helper function
Skin test		
(a) Immediate	Specific antigen or substance	Immediate hypersensitivity reactions
(b) Delayed	Recall antigens (e.g., candida, mumps)	Delayed-type (cell-mediated) hypersensitivity

Abbreviations used: CD, clusters of differentiation; Con-A, concanavalin-A; Mab, monoclonal antibody; MHC, major histocompatibility complex; MLR, mixed lymphocyte response; NK, natural killer (cells); PFC, plaque-forming cells; Protein A, (protein obtained from *S. aureus*); PWM, pokeweed mitogen; PYHA, phytohemagglutinin; RAST, radioallergosorbent test.

effect. Interpretation, particularly in humans, can be difficult, however, because of many confounding variables. In assays of cellular functions the variables can include contamination of cultures, dose of agent employed, time of incubation, cell concentrations, cell harvesting techniques, and regulatory influences present in cultures. In the case of mitogen assays employing Con-A, for example, T_S cells can be activated by this plant lectin, which may significantly reduce the proliferative response. Dose and time kinetics are also important in lymphocyte activation. Altered function can lead to shifts to the right or left of optimal dose– and time–response curves. Multiple factors in human serum can also suppress or activate lymphocyte proliferation. Other variables that can affect the quantity and function of lymphocyte populations include the wide range of "normal" values, age, cigarette smoking, concomitant viral infections, drugs or medications, underlying disease states, and even the time of day (because of circadian rhythm) when a sample is obtained. As one example, the number of CD4$^+$ T cells normally decrease from 8 a.m. to 12 noon in association with the normal diurnal changes in androgenic corticosteroid production. Each of the above factors can have an activating or suppressive effect on results. It is important to differentiate these effects from intrinsic suppression or activation.

With regard to delayed skin test responses, most antigens used for eliciting recall responses *in vitro* are those used for hypersensitivity skin test responses. Normal subjects usually show good correlation between lymphocyte activation *in vitro* and delayed hypersensitivity skin test responses.

The National Toxicology Program has recommended a 2-tiered approach for determining the immunotoxic effects of chemicals in rodents. This is outlined in Table 7.

Limitation of space within the scope of this chapter precludes the discussion of every carcinogenic chemical agent reported to be immune suppressive in experimental animals. Therefore, the discussion is limited to the immunotoxic effects of representative examples of widely recognized carcinogens to which individuals are exposed in their daily environment through pollution, medication, and agricultural or industrial occupations.

A. Polycyclic Aromatic Hydrocarbons

Polycyclic aromatic hydrocarbons (PAHs) are widespread in the environment. They are the result of forest fires, decay of organic matter, burning refuse, and burning fossil fuels (petroleum products and coal). Exposure to PAHs occurs from breathing, consuming contaminated food and water, and also from tobacco smoke, *i.e.*, from common exposures in daily living. Many of these compounds, beginning with benzo[*a*]pyrene (BaP) present in coal tar (84,85) (besides many other pyrogenated materials) have been shown to be carcinogenic (86). In general, the carcinogenic compounds among the PAHs have demonstrated toxic effects on the immune system in experimental animals. Many carcinogenic PAHs have been shown to be immune suppressive both *in vitro* and *in vivo*, but their noncarcinogenic analogs have no immune suppressive effects (87,88). As with most environmental pollutants, little data are available on the immunotoxic effects of these compounds in humans.

PAHs suppress both cell-mediated and humoral immunity and may also have suppressive effects on macrophages and other cellular components of the immune system. The ability and degree to which PAHs induce immune suppressive effects depend on their route of administration, dose, duration of exposure, and, in mice, the strain used.

The PAH most extensively studied for its effects on cell-mediated immunity is 7,12-dimethylbenz[*a*]anthracene (DMBA). DMBA is a potent carcinogen. Following *in vivo* exposure of mice, DMBA exerts both immediate and persistent (from weeks to

TABLE 7.   Procedures for Detecting Immune Alterations Following Chemical or Drug Exposure[a]

Parameter	Procedures
	Screen (Tier I)
Immunopathology	Hematology—complete blood count and differential Weights—body, spleen, thymus, kidney, liver Cellularity—spleen Histology—spleen, thymus, lymph node
Humoral-mediated immunity	Enumerate IgM antibody plaque-forming cells to T-dependent antigen (sheep red blood cells [SRBC]) Response to lipopolysaccharide (LPS) endotoxin mitogen
Cell-mediated immunity	Lymphocyte blastogenesis to mitogens (concanavalin-A) and mixed leukocyte response (MLR) against allogeneic leukocytes
Nonspecific immunity	Natural killer (NK) cell activity
	Comprehensive (Tier II)
Immunopathology	Quantitation of splenic B and T cell numbers
Humoral-mediated immunity	Enumeration of IgG antibody response to SRBC
Cell-mediated immunity	Cytotoxic T lymphocyte (CTL) cytolysis Delayed-type hypersensitivity (DTH) response
Nonspecific immunity	Macrophage function–quantitation of resident peritoneal cells, and phagocytic ability (basal, and activated by macrophage-activating factor [MAF])
Host resistance challenge models (endpoints)[b]	Syngeneic tumor cells PYB6 sarcoma (tumor incidence) B16F10 melanoma (lung burden) Bacterial models *Listeria monocytogenes* (mortality) *Streptococcus* species (mortality) Viral models Influenza (mortality) Parasite models *Plasmodium yoelii* (Parasitemia)

[a]Adapted from M. I., Luster, A. E., Munson P. T., Thomas, M. P., Holsapple, J. D., Fenters, K. L. White, Jr., L. D., Lauer, D. R., Germolec, G. J., Rosenthal, and J. H. Dean [*Fundam. Appl. Toxicol.* **10**, 2 (1988)].

[b]For any particular chemical tested two or three host resistance models were selected for examination.

months) suppression of Con-A and PYHA responses, MLR, cytotoxic T lymphocyte generation and activity, cutaneous DTH reactions, allograft rejection of skin and hearts, NK cell activity, and production of all forms of IFN (87–90). In addition, susceptibility to infection and tumorigenesis was increased. DMBA also has profound suppressive effects on humoral immunity as measured by serum antibody titers, plaque-forming cell (PFC) assays, antibody-dependent cellular cytotoxicity (ADCC), and resistance to bacterial infections. Suppression of the humoral immune response by DMBA is persistent and, following *neonatal* injection, has been reported to be permanent. Both T cell–dependent and T cell–independent antibody responses are affected. Studies by various investigators have suggested that B cells and B cell precursors, APCs, or T_H cells which synthesize IL-2 are the primary targets (87,88,90).

Recently, Ladics and co-workers (91) presented studies in which the 3,4-diol metabolite of DMBA exerted a 65-fold more potent suppression on the *in vitro* PFC response to sheep red blood cells (SRBC) in splenocyte cultures, than DMBA itself. Addition of α-naphthoflavone, an inhibitor of cytochrome P-450 isozymes, reversed or attenuated the suppression induced by DMBA. These investigators suggested that the immune suppressive effects of PAHs are due to cytochrome P-450–generated metabolites similar to the metabolites responsible for their carcinogenic effects (diol epoxides) (91,92). However, Ladics et al. (91) also reported that BaP, a PAH less carcinogenic than DMBA, exerts stronger *in vitro* effects on the PFC response to SRBC than DMBA, which conflicts with the *in vivo* findings. Therefore, DMBA metabolites generated in the spleen may be only partially responsible for immune suppression in the whole animal.

The comparative immune suppressive effects of 3-MC and BaP (highly potent and potent carcinogens, respectively) have also been studied (87,88). Once again, the effects of these PAHs are dependent on dose, strain, route, and duration of exposure, and can be selective for a particular arm of the immune response. Ward et al. (87) and White (88) found that while 3-MC affects both cell-mediated and humoral parameters of immunity similarly to DMBA, BaP has less effect on cell-mediated immunity than on humoral immunity. Selectivity of effect on the immune response is illustrated by the finding of increased tumor susceptibility following subchronic exposure of mice to BaP, at the same time that susceptibility to *Listeria monocytogenes* was unaltered. As earlier indicated, PAH suppression of humoral immunity includes T cell–dependent and T cell–independent responses. However, exposure to BaP resulted in suppression of response to TNP–ficoll (a T cell–independent antigen that stimulates mature B cells), but not to TNP–LPS (a T cell–independent antigen that stimulates immature B cells), suggesting that BaP acts on mature B cells. Conversely, DMBA exposure resulted in a persistent suppression of responsiveness to both hapten conjugates, implicating a B cell precursor effect (87). The ability of PAHs to exert suppressive effects of humoral immunity is not limited to direct exposure. For example, mice exposed to BaP *in utero* (*i.e.*, maternal exposure) demonstrated suppression of their PFC response to SRBC into adulthood (87,93). Lastly, PAHs have not been found to affect the complement system.

PAHs are environmental contaminants that humans encounter daily. They have, in general, profound suppressive effects on various immune response parameters (*see* Table 8 for summary); however, the mechanisms through which PAHs exert these effects have not been fully elucidated. The mechanisms of metabolic activation of the PAHs are,

TABLE 8.   Effects of Polycyclic Aromatic Hydrocarbons on Immune Response Parameters

Parameter	PAH		
	DMBA	3-MC	BaP
Allograft survival[a]	↑	↑	—
DTH (skin)	↓	↓	None
Mitogen response	↓ PYHA, ↓ LPS	↓ PYHA, ↓LPS	↓ PYHA, ↓ LPS
MLR	↓ (Persistent)	—	None
CTL generation	↓	↓	None
CTL activity	↓	↓	↓ (Transient)
Host resistance			
Infection	↓	—	None
Tumor challenge	↓	—	None to ↓[c]
Serum antibody titers[b]	↓	↓	↓
PFC number[b]	↓	↓	↓

Abbreviations used: BaP, benzo[a]pyrene; CTL, cytotoxic T lymphocytes; DMBA, 7,12-dimethylbenz[a]anthracene; DTH, delayed-type hypersensitivity; LPS, lipopolysaccharide (endotoxin); MLR, mixed lymphocyte response; PFC, plaque-forming cells; PYHA, phytohemagglutinin; 3-MC, 3-methylcholanthrene.
[a]Across minor histocompatibility differences only.
[b]T cell-dependent and T cell-independent responses.
[c]Subchronic exposure.

however, well known. This includes (a) cytochrome P-450–mediated two-electron oxidation to vicinal diol-epoxides or one-electron oxidation to radical cations (depending on the PAH), which form DNA adducts and (b) binding to *Ah* receptors, inducing *Ah* gene complex activation (87,94).

B. Asbestos

Asbestos is one of the few carcinogens for which the immunotoxic effects in humans have been well established. Exposure to asbestos occurs primarily through the respiratory tract. Chronic, prolonged inhalation of its fibers can result in the interstitial fibrotic lung disease, asbestosis. A high incidence of bronchogenic carcinoma and malignant mesothelioma occurs in occupationally exposed individuals as compared to nonexposed individuals (95,96).

Asbestos fibers are divided into two groups, serpentine and amphibole. Chrysotile asbestos is obtained from serpentine rock and accounts for more than 95 percent of asbestos used worldwide. The amphibole fibers include crocidolite, amosite, and anthophyllite. Because of their heat resistance and strength, asbestos fibers are widely employed in industry, particularly in construction. Therefore, materials containing asbestos, including cement, tile, insulation, molding, plastic, brake linings, and corrugated sheeting, are widely disseminated in our environment and contact with asbestos-containing materials is common.

A number of immunological effects have been reported subsequent to asbestos inhalation by man and animals. Cell-mediated immune response abnormalities associated with asbestos exposure include cutaneous anergy, decreased circulating T cells and T cell subsets, modulated T cell proliferative responses to mitogens, and decreased bone marrow precursor cells (95,97,98). The aberrations of cell-mediated immunity, however, do not necessarily parallel the severity of the disease (99,100). In one study of occupationally exposed workers, decreased T cell subsets correlated with interstitial lung disease. In another, no correlation between the severity of lung disease and decreased peripheral blood lymphocyte (PBL) T cells and B cells was found.

While most evaluations involving cellular immunity show a suppressed effect, asbestos exposure appears to have a polyclonal activating effect on B cells. In occupationally exposed individuals, all serum Ig levels are elevated as is secretory IgA. In addition, these individuals have an increased prevalence of rheumatoid factor, antinuclear antibodies (ANA), cold reactive lymphocytotoxic antibodies, and immune complexes. These abnormalities do not necessarily correlate with the severity of pulmonary disease. *In vitro* studies have shown asbestos fibers to be directly cytotoxic to macrophages, to stimulate immature B cell lines, and to suppress PYHA-induced proliferation. Different types of asbestos may have different effects; for example, chrysotile fibers suppress PYHA-induced proliferation, but augment both the Con-A and PWM proliferative responses, while amosite fibers cause suppression.

Macrophages are also affected by asbestos fibers. When incubated *in vitro* with asbestos fibers, alveolar macrophages release a number of factors, including prostaglandins, fibroblast growth factors, neutrophil chemotactic factor, and cytokines. Cultures of splenocytes with alveolar macrophages from mice exposed *in vivo* to crocidolite or chrysotile fibers contain increased levels of IL-1 and IL-2, and the macrophages showed increased class II (Ia) antigen expression. T cells proliferated when cocultured with alveolar macrophages obtained from animals exposed to crocidolite fibers *in vivo*. Furthermore, mice exposed to chrysolite maintain elevated serum Ig levels, ANAs, and splenic PFC, all prior to developing pulmonary fibrosis or tumors.

C. Therapeutic Drugs

Therapeutic drugs that suppress the immune system are used to prevent or treat allograft rejection in organ and tissue transplantation. They are also employed in the treatment of cancer, autoimmune diseases, and chronic inflammatory diseases. These agents can be considered to be immunotoxins due to their well-documented immune suppressive effects. Because of their prevalent use, more information on their effects on the human immune system is available than for most other carcinogenic chemicals. The most frequently used agents include glucocorticosteroids, antimetabolites, alkylating agents, natural products, polyclonal antibodies, and monoclonal antibodies (Table 9). Although the details are still being investigated, each type of immune suppressive drug exerts its effects through a different mechanism.

Prednisone, prednisolone, and methylprednisolone are glucocorticosteroids that have been shown to interfere with cell proliferation, alter phagocytosis, and depress T cell and B cell functions. They also interfere with the activity of cytokines on cell surface receptors. Side effects associated with steroid treatment include: increased susceptibility to infections, hypertension, hyperglycemia, hyperkalemia, osteoporosis, increased capillary fragility, weight gain, acne, cataracts, avascular necrosis, elevated cholesterol, and growth suppression in children. Steroids act by binding to segments of nuclear DNA and, thus, affect mRNA production. Specifically, corticosteroids inhibit mRNA transcription of IL-1, block IL-6 gene activation, and inhibit the production of γ-IFN. They also indirectly block IL-2 release which requires IL-1 stimulated IL-6 release and thus, interfere with T cell proliferation (101).

Corticosteroids can induce lymphopenia with decreased monocytes and eosinophils, but with increased neutrophils. In humans, this effect is transient (a few hours) and due to an alteration in "cell trafficking". Mononuclear cells, especially T cells, are redistrib-

TABLE 9.   Effects of Therapeutic Drugs on the Immune Response Parameters

Agent	Targets	Mechanism	Effect
Gluco-corticosteroids	$T_{H/I}$ cells; macrophages; B cells (indirect)	Inhibit IL-1, IL-6, γ-IFN production	Suppresses CD4$^+$T helper cells and activation of immune response
Azathioprine antimetabolite	$T_{H/I}$ cells	Inhibits DNA and RNA synthesis	Inhibits primary immune responses
Cyclosporin macrolide	$T_{H/I}$ cells; B cells (indirect)	Inhibits expression of IL-2, IL-3, IL-4, GM-CSF, TNF-α, IL-2Rα, IL-1R	Inhibits primary immune response
Cyclophosphamide alkylating agent	T_S precursors; B cells; other T cells	Disrupts mitosis	Inhibits primary immune responses
ALG, ALS polyclonal antibodies	Lymphocytes	Opsonization, complement-mediated lysis	Induces suppressor cells; primary and secondary responses affected
OKT3 monoclonal antibody	CD3$^+$T cells	Blocks T cell functions	Inhibits all T cell functions; primary and secondary responses affected

Abbreviations used: ALG, antilymphocyte globulin; ALS, antilymphocyte serum; CD, clusters of differentiation; GM-CSF, granulocyte macrophage colony stimulating factor; IFN, interferon; IL, interleukin; IL-2R, interleukin-2 receptor; $T_{H/I}$, helper/inducer T cells; T_S, T suppressor cells; TNF, tumor necrosis factor.

uted into peripheral lymphoid organs and their reentry into the circulation is reduced. The primary targets of corticosteroids are T cells. Although all T cell functions have been shown to be affected, certain subsets are more affected than others. Most available data indicate that $CD4^+$ helper/inducer T cells ($T_{H/I}$) are the more sensitive target. This is consistent with the observation that steroids exhibit their greatest effects at the time of initial antigen exposure. In addition, the generation of $CD8^+$ CTLs or T_S can be inhibited by therapeutic doses of steroids, although the functions of mature CTLs or T_S are resistant except at suprapharmacological concentrations. A second important target of steroids is the monocyte/macrophage lineage of cells. Steroids have been shown to reduce monocyte/macrophage recruitment into inflammatory sites, tumors, and infectious lesions, probably by altering their response to chemotactic factors. Steroids have also been shown to reduce monocyte/macrophage fungicidal and microbicidal activity, the expression of Fc receptors and thus ADCC activity,[6] the ability to function as APCs, probably to reduced MHC class II antigen density, the response to γ-IFN, and the number of epidermal Langerhan's cells.

Most data suggest that B cells are less sensitive to steroids than T cells or monocyte/macrophages. In steroid-sensitive experimental animals, Ig levels and antibody production are reported to be reduced. In man, results have been equivocal and discordant. Some reduction in Ig levels has been reported, while stimulation *in vitro* with antigen or mitogens has resulted in increased, decreased, or no change in Ig production, dependent on the species, methodology employed, and possibly some unspecified fine details of the investigation(s). It is possible that steroid effects on B cells are indirect and are the result of T cell impairment.

Azathioprine is an example of an antimetabolite with immune suppressive effects. Along with steroids, it was the primary form of treatment in allograft rejection for 20 years. As an antimetabolite, azathioprine inhibits protein synthesis, is active against all rapidly proliferating cell populations, and is an anti-inflammatory agent. Its side effects include bone marrow suppression (and thus, severe lymphopenia, thrombocytopenia and granulocytopenia, hepatotoxicity, gastrointestinal disturbances, fever, susceptibility to infection, and induction of malignancy). Azathioprine is a purine analog, an imidazole derivative of 6-mercaptopurine. Upon being catabolized to 6-mercaptopurine and other antimetabolites, it prevents gene replication by inhibiting DNA and RNA synthesis. Azathioprine inhibits primary immune responses, but has little effect on established responses and none on secondary responses. Its primary targets are T cells, blocking their activation (although at a later stage than steroids or macrolides) and inhibiting their proliferation. B cells are less sensitive and are relatively spared. Like steroids, azathioprine affects T cell subsets differently. Since the primary immune response is affected by azathioprine, it is not surprising that its primary target is the $CD4^+T_{H/I}$ cell subset. Studies in man and experimental animals have demonstrated that azathioprine inhibits the generation of $CD8^+$ CTL cells, but has no effect on mature CTL function. In addition, $CD8^+T_S$ suppressor activity in patients did not change with azathioprine treatment. Mitogen-induced *in vitro* generation of T_S cells is less sensitive, requiring higher doses than does T cell help for antibody synthesis. Thus, azathioprine has its greatest effect on the afferent (generation) arm of the immune response while the efferent (effector) arm is resistant. Some reduction in NK cell activity and monocyte/macrophage function has also been reported.

Cyclosporin A (CSA) is a macrolide and an example of a natural immune suppressive compound. A small cyclic peptide, CSA is derived from the fermentation of two species

---

[6]ADCC activity depends on coating cells with antibodies that allows targeting those cells by killer cells (which bear Fc receptors).

of fungi. CSA suppresses T cell function, but generally spares B cell, NK cell, and monocyte/macrophage functions. Although its predominant use has been in transplantation to prevent rejection (cadaveric renal allograft survival increased to 80 to 85% at 1 year), CSA is also effective in the treatment of autoimmune diseases like psoriasis, Behçt's disease, and insulin-dependent diabetes (102). Side effects of CSA treatment include increased infections, increase in non-Hodgkins lymphoma, nephrotoxicity, hepatotoxicity, hypertension, altered glucose metabolism, and others.

CSA suppresses T cell function by blocking activation of IL-2 and other lymphokine genes. CSA binds to cyclophillin, which prevents IL-2 mRNA transcription. IL-2 is not secreted and, in the absence of IL-2, T cells do not proliferate, γ-IFN is not released, B cell and other cell activating factors (*e.g.*, IL-3, IL-4, granulocyte–macrophage [GM]-CSF) are not released, and T cell activation is curtailed. CSA also inhibits the expression of IL-2R and IL-1R on T cells. A reduction in IL-1 has been found which may be indirectly responsible for the lack of IL-2 and GM-CSF (101,102).

CSA exerts its inhibitory effects on T cell–dependent immune responses at the time of initial antigen exposure. Already established immune responses are not affected; therefore, the value of CSA treatment is limited to acute allograft rejection episodes. *In vitro* responses to mitogen or allogeneic cells (MLR) are inhibited only when CSA is present at initial establishment of cell culture. There is also little effect on proliferation induced by the addition of exogenous IL-2 or IL-4. The CSA effects on B cells are indirect, as CSA does not inhibit non-T cell mitogen proliferative responses, most T cell–independent antigen responses, or *in vitro* Ig production induced by Epstein-Barr virus. However, there is some suggestion that T cell–independent responses to soluble polysaccharides are as sensitive to CSA as T cell mitogen responses (103). In general, NK cells and monocytes/macrophages are relatively resistant to CSA. The effects of CSA on APCs is controversial. Various reports indicate no effect to some impairment of antigen uptake and processing. In recent studies (103,104), CSA inhibited alloantigen presentation by murine macrophages without affecting expression of MHC class II antigen. This inhibitory activity required higher CSA doses than needed for IL-2 inhibition. Thus, similarly to azathioprine, the primary targets of CSA are $T_{H/I}$ cells and the afferent arm of an immune response.

Cyclophosphamide (CYC) is an example of an immunotoxic alkylating agent. It is used in bone marrow transplantation as a cytoreductive pretreatment to prevent graft rejection. It is also used in the treatment of cancer and autoimmune diseases. Alkylating agents disrupt cell functions, especially mitosis, and are highly toxic to proliferating cells. CYC is biologically inactive, but is rapidly converted by liver microsomal oxidases to active metabolites that alkylate nucleic acids. CYC causes immune suppression or immunoaugmentation, depending on the dose. At certain dosages in man, CYC causes bone marrow suppression and depletion of lymphocytes from peripheral lymphoid organs, resulting in B cell, T cell, and monocyte deficiencies (105,106). CYC exerts its immune suppressive effects most effectively at the time of immunization. Humoral immune responses are suppressed by effects of CYC on both T cells and B cells. T cell–independent antigen responses as well as T cell–dependent antigen responses are inhibited by CYC. Cell-mediated immune responses such as DTH, GVH, and allograft rejection are also inhibited by CYC action on $T_{H/I}$ cells and the generation of CTL and T_S cells. Lymphocytes, however, exhibit a differential sensitivity to CYC which is concentration dependent. Studies have shown that B cells are more sensitive to CYC than T cells involved in DTH responses. *In vitro* generation of T_S cells for anti-SRBC DTH is more sensitive to CYC than are T_H cells for anti-SRBC antibody response or generation of T_C cells. Mature CTL and T_S cells are the least sensitive to CYC. NK cell numbers and functions are also suppressed by CYC. Monocyte/macrophage functions are resistant, although monocytopenia can be seen with persistent treatment and accompany the effect of CYC on the bone marrow.

Immunoaugmentation by CYC is apparently due to its effects on the regulatory T_S cell subset. For example, increased DTH response has been reported after CYC treatment at doses not affecting antibody response. Also, in both animal and human studies it is possible to selectively eliminate suppressor cells *in vitro* and leave other subsets unaffected. Additionally, clinical studies have shown that B cell responses to KLH (keyhole limpet hemocyanine) in patients with advanced cancer were suppressed by high doses of CYC, while T cell response (DTH) was augmented at either high or low doses. Patients with renal cell carcinoma and metastatic melanoma have also shown clinical responsiveness following administration of low dose CYC and autologous cancer cell vaccines. Furthermore, some melanoma patients exhibited augmented responses following CYC and exogenous IL-2 administration (103,104).

D. "Immunotoxic" Polyclonal and Monoclonal Antibodies

Antilymphocyte antibodies, generally produced by immunizing horses, were the first attempt to selectively target cells of the immune system in allograft rejection therapy. The most commonly used xenogeneic antibodies for immune suppression are ALS (antilymphocyte serum), ALG (antilymphocyte globulin), and ATS (antithymocyte serum). Serum sickness and systemic anaphylaxis are two of the serious side effects from the use of these reagents. ALS, ALG, and ATS are thought to exert their immune suppressive effects through opsonization, expansion of suppressor cell populations, complement-dependent lysis, and, perhaps, blindfolding of active sites. Upon administration, a rapid and profound lymphopenia is induced which soon abates with a gradual increase in the number of circulating T cells when treatment is stopped. Proliferative responses remain, however, impaired longer, due possibly to suppressor cells. These therapeutic drugs affect both T and B cells. Although they have been used prophylactically, these agents are most commonly used as "salvage therapy" to rescue an allograft from a rejection episode. Besides the high incidence of serious side effects, ALS, ALG, or ATS are frequently unavailable and lack standardization. Because of the lack of standardization, there are variations in constituent antibodies and therefore variable efficacy. The newer and more specific monoclonal antibodies are better reagents for these purposes.

Although a number of monoclonal antibodies specific for various components of the immune response (*e. g.*, to IL-2R) are under investigation, only OKT3 is available for therapeutic use. OKT3 is a monoclonal antibody that binds to the CD3 complex found on all T_{CR} expressing T cells. OKT3-treated T cells shed or internalize the T_{CR}–CD3 complex and become unable to recognize or bind antigen. OKT3 can also fix complement and cause T cell lysis. Because OKT3 inhibits all T cell functions, including CTLs, by either blinding T cells to antigen or eliminating them, it is an effective form of "rescue therapy" for allograft rejection. OKT3 has also been used to purge bone marrow of mature T cells before bone marrow transplantation and as a prophylactic therapy in organ transplantation. Because OKT3 is a murine product, its use is limited; some patients can develop anti-mouse neutralizing antibody. OKT3 is also mitogenic and its use has been associated with an increased incidence of lymphomas in transplant patients (70,105).

E. Halogenated Aromatic Hydrocarbons

Halogenated aromatic hydrocarbons (HAH), as here defined, are structurally related industrial compounds or byproducts that include the polychlorinated biphenyls (PCB), the polybrominated biphenyls (PBB), the polychlorinated dibenzo-*p*-dioxins (PCDD), and the polychlorinated dibenzofurans (PCDF). PCB, which are now banned, have been used as plasticizers and as heat transfer medium. PBB have been used as fire retardant. PCDD and PCDF are contaminant byproducts in commercial substances such as chlorinated phenolic pesticides, *e.g.*, pentachlorophenol (PCP). These environmental contaminants are lipophilic, stable, and resistant to metabolism and therefore persist in the environment (78).

The most toxic and most studied of these chemicals is 2,3,7,8-tetrachlorodibenzo-*p*-dioxin (TCDD). TCDD and related HAH induce similar toxic and biochemical effects in laboratory animals, including weight loss, carcinogenesis, thymic and peripheral lymphoid organ atrophy, and profound immunotoxicity. The immunotoxic effects of HAH include suppression of both cellular and humoral immune responses in laboratory animals (Table 10).

In doses of TCDD that do not affect thymic or spleen cellularity, humoral responses in mice to T-dependent or T-independent antigens are dramatically reduced. Current data suggest that the immunotoxic and possibly carcinogenic effects of HAH are partially mediated by the ability of HAH to bind the *Ah* receptor protein (94,107–109). This binding induces pleiotropic responses, including activation of aryl hydrocarbon hydroxylase (a P-450–associated monooxygenase) and results in toxic responses. Backcrosses between (C57BL/6 × DBA/2)F_1 mice and the C57BL/6-sensitive parent or the DBA/2-resistant parent show that the immunotoxic response segregates with the *Ah* locus located on chromosome 17 (94,107,108).

The ability of HAH to suppress immune responses correlates with their ability to bind to the *Ah* receptor. The thymus may also contribute to the immunotoxicity of HAH, depending on the immune response parameter measured. Although in adult thymectomized animals TCDD did not induce antibody suppression, other studies suggest HAH may act through thymic epithelium in the induction of T cells that suppress CTL activity. Macrophage function and NK cell activity are not appreciably affected by TCDD.

TABLE 10. Immunotoxicity of TCDD and Halogenated Biphenyls

Halogenated aromatics	Reported effects
TCDD	Induces thymic and lymphoid organ atrophy ↓ DTH ↓ T cell mitogen responses ↓ Generation of alloreactive T_c cells ↓ Ig levels ↓ PFC responses ↓ Antibody titers in primary and secondary responses ↑ Susceptibility to infections ↑ Susceptibility to tumors
PBB	Induces thymic and lymphoid organ atrophy ↓ Antibody responses ↓ Mitogen responses ↓ DTH ↑ Sensitivity to endotoxin
PCB	Induces thymic and lymphoid organ atrophy ↓ DTH ↓ Antibody responses ↑ Susceptibility to infections

Abbreviations used: CTL, cytotoxic T lymphocytes; DTH, delayed-type hypersensitivity; PBB, polybrominated biphenyls; PCB, polychlorinated biphenyls; PFC, plaque-forming cells; TCDD, 2,3,7,8-tetrachlorodibenzo-*p*-dioxin.

In neonates and perinatally exposed animals the immune defects induced by TCDD exposure are the same, since TCDD and other HAH cross the placenta and accumulate in mother's milk. However, lower doses of TCDD resulted in more prolonged suppressive effects in perinatally exposed animals than in adults (94,107,108).

The immunotoxic effects of HAH on humans have been controversial and difficult to assess. In two industrial accidents, one involving exposure to PBB and one involving exposure to PCB—when immunological parameters including Ig levels, mitogen responses, and total T and B cells were evaluated—conflicting results were obtained (78,110). Individuals exposed to milk products containing PBB were reported to have decreased T cell numbers, reduced responses to T cell and B cell mitogens, and elevated Ig levels. Others reported these values to be normal in exposed individuals. Exposure to rice bran oil containing PCB (contaminated with TCDD-related chlorinated dibenzofurans) resulted in enhanced responses by mitogens and increased skin DTH to tuberculin and streptococcal antigens, but decreased T_H cells. Although clinical symptoms such as general malaise, arthralgias, headache, fatigue, and neurological disturbances were reported, in neither exposure case has there been an increased incidence of infections or malignancy over a 12- to 18-year follow-up. In another study, individuals who had been exposed for a period of 14 years to TCDD which had been sprayed on a dirt road by their homes were evaluated for immunotoxic effects. Investigators reported essentially normal T cell subsets, but an increased incidence of anergy as assessed by DTH skin tests with recall antigens. However, only a few subjects demonstrated decreased PYHA, Con-A, and tetanus toxoid responses consistent with their DTH skin test results. On the other hand, PWM responses and the absolute numbers of non-T cells were elevated. As in the previous studies, no increased susceptibility to infections or malignancy was noted (110,111). More recently, a retrospective study has been conducted on mortality in chemical workers who were exposed to substances contaminated with TCDD (112). They found that overall mortality was essentially the same as that for the U.S. population as a whole. However, the frequency of deaths to all cancers was elevated by 102 to 130% of the expected value. In workers with ≥1-year exposure to TCDD and a ≥20-year latency period, mortality from soft-tissue sarcomas and cancers of the respiratory system was significantly increased. Although duration of exposure or employment did not show significant trends, mortality for all forms of cancer increased with increasing latency.

F. Pesticides

Immune dysfunction or suppression by pesticides and related byproducts has been reported in experimental animal studies by many investigators as a result of acute or subacute high-dose exposure (78,107,113–115). Human exposure to toxic (high) doses (*e.g.*, from accidental spills) has resulted in a variety of severe *acute* effects involving multiple organ systems, including the immune system, dependent on the agent and the exposure level involved. Regarding *chronic* impairment of immune function, in the authors' view definitive evidence is lacking that occupational pesticide exposure or casual contact with pesticides results in significant immunological impairment in humans.

A number of types of pesticides have been studied, including organochlorines, organophosphates, carbonates, organotins, and captans. Lead and arsenic compounds used as insecticides will be discussed in the next section. Organochlorine pesticides which include chlorinated ethane derivatives (*e.g.*, DDT) and chlorinated cyclodienes (*e.g.*, chlordane, dieldrin, endrin, aldrin, heptachlor) are promoters of carcinogenesis in experimental animals (Chapter 5). No evidence exists indicating carcinogenic effects in man, although increased numbers of chromosome breaks in human cells exposed *in vitro* to dieldrin have been reported (107,115). In experimental animals, different organochlorine pesticides reportedly affect one arm of the immune response more than another (*see* Table 11). For example, DDT has been reported to cause suppression of the humoral immune response, but to have no effect on cell-mediated immunity. On the other hand, chlordane has immunomodulatory effects on cell-mediated immunity, but no apparent effects on humoral immunity. Chlordane has been found to suppress DTH responses in mice, but to augment T cell mitogen responses and MLR. Mice exposed to chlordane *in utero* exhibited decreased DTH, but increased antibody responses and resistance to influenza virus as adults. It is possible that the different organochlorine pesticides affect different subsets of T cells, inhibiting T_H cells involved in DTH responses, or T_S cells that modulate antibody and other T cell responses. They may also affect accessory APCs. For example, dieldrin has been reported to decrease the phagocytic activity of monocytes/macrophages.

In general, the carbamate pesticides have not been shown to be carcinogenic. Urethan (ethyl carbamate), a nonpesticide carbamate previously used as a veterinary anesthetic and a contaminant in certain foods, is, however, a potent carcinogen in animals. This agent has been shown to reduce antibody responses to T cell–independent and to T cell–dependent antigens, as well as to suppress NK cell activity. DTH and T cell mitogen responses have variously been reported to be decreased or unaffected (107,116). No effects on MLR, on macrophage function, or on cell-mediated cytotoxicity (except perhaps allograft rejection) have been reported. In addition, tumor incidence has been

TABLE 11. Immunomodulatory Effects of Pesticides

Pesticides	Reported effects
Organochlorines	
DDT	May or may not depress humoral immunity
Chlordane	↓ DTH
	↑ T cell mitogen response
	↑ MLR
Dieldrin	↓ Antibody titers
	↓ Macrophage phagocytosis
	↑ Susceptibility to infections
	↑ Chromosome breaks *in vitro*
Organophosphates	
Malathion	Impairs neutrophil chemotaxis
	↑ DTH
	↑ Upper respiratory tract infections
	↑ IgE-mediated asthma?
Carbamates	
Urethan	↓ Humoral immune responses
	↓ NK cell activity
	↑ Incidence of tumor
Aldicarb	↓ Macrophage accessory cell function in mitogen responses
	↓ IL-1 production
	↓ Macrophage chemiluminescence
	↓ PFC response and hemolysin titers
	↑ Chromosomal breaks *in vitro*
Carbofuran	Variable Ig subclass levels
	↓ Mitogen response
	↓ Lymphocytes and bone marrow
	↑ Susceptibility to lethal infections

Abbreviations used: DTH, delayed-type hypersensitivity; IL, interleukin; MLR, mixed lymphocyte response; NK, natural killer (cells); PFC, plaque-forming cells.

reported to correlate with the degree of NK cell suppression (107). It appears then that the primary targets of urethan are NK cells, B cells, and subsets of $T_{H/I}$ cells.

Aldicarb, another carbamate, has the highest toxicity of any pesticide registered for use in the United States. It is found predominantly as a contaminant of ground water, is rapidly metabolized, and does not persist in body tissues. Aldicarb inhibits acetyl-cholinesterase activity, causing muscular paralysis and inhibition of respiration. Although not known to be a carcinogen or teratogen, it has been found to cause an increase in the number of chromosome breaks (113). Its immunotoxic effects include suppression of murine antibody responses to SRBC and spleen cell responses to PYHA, Con-A, and the mitogenic monoclonal antibody to CD3 antigen (OKT3). In recent studies, Aldicarb was found to produce its effects on mitogen responses by affecting macrophages (113). The suppressive effect of Aldicarb on mitogen responses of isolated T cells was seen only in the presence of macrophages from Aldicarb-treated mice. In addition, IL-1 production was decreased and IL-1–dependent responses could be restored by addition of exogenous IL-1. Other reported effects of various carbamate pesticides are given in Table 11. Carbamate pesticides were shown to induce hepatic monooxygenase activities. Their toxic effects may involve the *Ah* locus.

The organophosphates, *e.g.*, malathion, as compared to other pesticides, are strong contact sensitizers. They induce DTH in humans as well as in experimental animals. In some instances, these effects may be due to contaminants; if, for example, the level of the contaminant diethyl fumarate is reduced, "malathion sensitivity" decreases. Besides contact sensitivity, workers exposed to organophosphates were found to have impaired neutrophil chemotaxis, and in one study increased respiratory infections (117). Asthmatic responses to organophosphates have also been noted. However, most investigators feel that these agents are irritants, and there is no evidence that these agents can act as allergens to induce IgE-mediated allergic responses. Individuals with underlying allergy may show increased symptoms temporarily after exposure to pesticides. Such individuals, who have hyperirritable airways secondary to chronic mucosal inflammation, are well known to have temporary respiratory symptoms following exposure to many irritants, including exhaust fumes, cooking odors, and perfumes, among many others.

G. Metals and Metalloids

Metals/metalloids and their compounds are widely distributed in the environment: in air, water, soil, and many commercial products. Many of these are essential trace elements (*e.g.*, Cu, Fe, Zn, Cr). Metals/metalloids found to be carcinogenic in experimental animals include beryllium (Be), cadmium (Cd), cobalt (Co), chromium (Cr), nickel (Ni), lead (Pb), and antimony (Sb). Metals/metalloids for which epidemiological data exist to support carcinogenicity in humans are Be, Cd, Cr, Ni, Sb, and arsenic (As). A number of these have been studied for their effect on the immune system.

Arsenic is a component of some herbicides and pesticides. Limited and conflicting results have been obtained with regard to As as an immunotoxin. Sodium arsenite has been reported to inhibit IFN production, inhibit primary and secondary antibody responses, and potentiate or suppress the *in vitro* T cell response to PYHA at low or high doses, respectively (107).

Lead is released into the environment through combustion products, varnishes, paints, grease, batteries, and pesticides. There is no epidemiological evidence that lead is a carcinogen in humans, although it is associated with the induction of renal tumors in experimental animals. Studies on lead-exposed children have shown no significant effects on major serum Ig levels or immune responses to protein antigens. On the other hand, lead workers have been shown to have lower serum Ig and complement protein C3, as well as lower salivary IgA levels. In addition, there is a higher incidence of arthritis, renal disease, cardiovascular disease, and senility in lead-exposed workers (79,107,118). Recent studies using human lymphocytes exposed *in vitro* to lead chloride (at concentrations equivalent to the range found in the blood of occupationally exposed workers) resulted in increased Ig synthesis in resting and PWM-activated lymphocytes. The effect of $PbCl_2$ was additive to that of PWM, dose dependent, and correlated with lead content in the nuclear fraction of cells (119).

In experimental animals the effects of lead on immune responses vary, depending on dose, molecular form, route of administration, length of exposure (acute *vs.* chronic), and species and strain of animal studied. In one report (118), mice inoculated with lead exhibited increased mortality from *Listeria* infection, while mice exposed by ingestion (drinking water for a year) demonstrated no increased mortality nor any effect on antibody response, MLR, generation of CTLs, or T cell response to Con-A. Lead acetate has been reported to simultaneously augment IgM and suppress IgG antibody responses to T cell–dependent, but not to T cell–independent antigens in adult mice. In doses that suppressed PYHA and PWM responses, lead acetate augmented DTH response. Lead carbonate, lead nitrate, and lead oxide, on the other hand, depressed DTH response. Exposure to lead has also been reported to induce autoimmunity, enhance B cell activation and proliferation, and to inhibit T cell suppressors. Phagocytosis, antigen presentation, cytokine production, and O_2 consumption by macrophages are also affected, depending on dose, strain, and route of administration. Lead modulates cAMP and cGMP effects on B cells and alters the intracellular levels of nucleotides in cells. All these effects may contribute to its modulation of the immune responses.

Cadmium, a human and animal carcinogen, is present in cigarettes and in the food chain (especially shellfish and liver, where it can be concentrated) and in various industrial applications (in particular, the electrical and electronics industry, space technology, and weapons manufacture). Cadmium displaces other metals in metalloenzyme complexes, rendering them nonfunctional; for example, carboxypeptidases and aminopeptidases, enzymes required to break down Ig light chains, are affected. Cadmium workers were found to excrete up to 900 mg of light chains per day (normal = 5 mg) (95). In experimental animals, Cd exposure increases susceptibility to infections and induces tumors of the lung, testes, and the prostate. Both potentation, but more often suppression of humoral immunity have been reported as a result of exposure to cadmium. Some investigators have found that either oral or i.p. administration of cadmium chloride suppressed the IgM and IgG PFC responses. The effect was long term, with no IgG PFC response on challenge with the antigen 40 days after exposure. In other studies, i.p. exposure augmented IgM and IgG PFC responses, while oral exposure suppressed these responses (95,120). The reported effects of Cd on cell-mediated immune responses are less consistent. MLR and mitogen responses are either increased, decreased, or not affected. This variability may also be attributed to the route of exposure, dose, and strain of experimental animal studied. The effects of exposure of monocytes/macrophages to $CdCl_2$ also varied. *In vitro* exposure inhibited ATPase and oxidative phosphorylation, depressed oxygen consumption by activated alveolar macrophages, and decreased phagocytosis, bactericidal effects, and tumor cell killing. Conversely, phagocytosis, oxidative metabolism in alveolar macrophages, and bactericidal capacity have been reported to be elevated in experimental animals following *in vivo* exposure (95,121).

Mercury is a heavy metal that induces DTH contact sensitivity, autoantibody to glomerular basement membrane, polyclonal activation of B cells, increased susceptibility to infections, and augmentation of anaphylaxis by enhancing IgE production. Some of its effects may be due to alteration of T cell activation as a result of interference with presentation of MHC and antigen (115).

Beryllium is another known carcinogen in humans and experimental animals. Beryllium compounds, usually as Be oxide, induce berylliosis, a form of generalized and pulmonary granulomatous hypersensitivity in factory workers. Beryllium sulfate can either inhibit or stimulate lymphocyte metabolism and has been found to induce DTH skin reactivity and lymphokine production by sensitized T cells (122–124).

Nickel, chromium, and platinum fumes or compounds can induce IgE-mediated hypersensitivity, whereas zinc, vanadium, and cobalt are causative agents of asthma in humans (125–129). Beryllium, chromium, and nickel salts appear to act as haptens, combining with host proteins to elicit DTH hypersensitivity or other T cell–dependent responses. It is also possible that some metals may result in "neoantigen formation", inducing carrier or hapten–carrier-specific immune responses as has been demonstrated in the case of toluene diisocyanate and trimellitic anhydride sensitivity.

Abbreviations Used: ADCC, antibody-dependent cellular cytotoxicity; ALG, antilymphocyte globulin; ALS, antilymphocyte serum; ANA, antinuclear antibodies; APC, antigen-presenting or antigen-processing cells; ATS, antithymocyte serum; B cells, lymphocytes maturing in bone marrow; BaP, benzo[*a*]pyrene; CD, clusters of differentiation; Con-A, concanavalin-A; CSA, cyclosporin A; CSF, colony-stimulating factor; CTL, cytotoxic T lymphocytes (MHC-restricted killers); CYC, cyclophosphamide; DMBA, 7,12-dimethylbenz[*a*]anthracene; DTH, delayed-type hypersensitivity; GM, granulocyte-macrophage; GVH, graft *versus* host reaction; HAH, halogenated aromatic hydrocarbons; HLA, human leukocyte antigens; Ig, immunoglobulin; IFN, interferon; IL, interleukin; IL-2R, IL-2 receptor; LAK, lymphokine-activated killer (cells); LGL, large granular lymphocytes; 3-MC, 3-methylcholanthrene; MHC, major histocompatibility complex; MLR, mixed lymphocyte response (against allogeneic leukocytes); NK, natural killer cells (MHC-nonrestricted); PAH, polycyclic aromatic hydrocarbon; PBB, polybrominated biphenyls; PBL, peripheral blood lymphocyte; PCB, polychlorinated biphenyls; PCDD, polychlorinated dibenzo-*p*-dioxins; PCDF, polychlorinated dibenzofurans; PFC, plaque-forming cells; PYHA, phytohemagglutinin; PWM, pokeweed mitogen; RA, rheumatoid arthritis; sIg, surface immunoglobulin; SRBC, sheep red blood cells; T cells, lymphocytes maturing in thymus; T_{CR}, T cell receptors; T_H, helper T cells; $T_{H/I}$, helper/inducer T cells; T_C, antigen-specific MHC-restricted CTL; T_S, T suppressor cells; TILs, tumor-infiltrating lymphocytes; TCDD, 2,3,7,8-tetrachlorodibenzo-*p*-dioxin; TNF, tumor necrosis factor; *V*, *D*, *J* genes, the genes coding for IgM μ chain.

REFERENCES

1. Roitt, I., Brostoff, J., and Male, D.: "Immunology". Gower, London, England, 1989, pp. 2.13–2.14.
2. Nomenclature Committee: *J. Immunol.* **143,** 758 (1989).
3. Jackson, A., and Warner, H.: Preparation Stainings and Analysis by Flow Cytometry of Peripheral Blood Leukocytes. *In* "Manual of Clinical Laboratory Immunology" (N. Rose, H. Friedman, and J. Fahey, eds.). Am. Soc. Microbiol., Washington, D.C., 1986, p. 226.
4. Reinherz, E. L., and Schlossman, S.: *Cell* **19,** 821 (1980).
5. Zinkernagel, R., and Doherty, P.: *Adv. Immunol.* **27,** 51 (1979).
6. Dorf, M., and Benacerraf, B.: *Annu. Rev. Immunol.* **2,** 127 (1984).
7. Paul, W. E.: The Immune System: An Introduction. *In* "Fundamental Immunology" (W. E. Paul, ed.), 2nd ed. Raven Press, New York, 1989, p. 3.
8. Sprent, J., Schaefer, M., Lo, D., and Korngold, R.: *J. Exp. Med.* **163,** 998 (1986).
9. Cobbold, S., and Waldman, H.: *Transplantation* **41,** 634 (1986).
10. Rosenberg, A. S., Mizuochi, T., Sharrow, S. O., and Singer, A.: *J. Exp. Med.* **165,** 1296 (1987).
11. Clement, L. T.: *J. Clin. Immunol.* **12,** 1 (1992).

12. Kincade, P. W.: *Adv. Immunol.* **31**, 177 (1981).
13. Kuritani, T., and Cooper, M.: *J. Exp. Med.* **155**, 389 (1982).
14. Ritz, J., Schmidt, R. E., Michon, J., Hercend, T., and Schlossman, S. F.: *Adv. Immunol.* **42**, 181 (1988).
15. Phillips, J. H., and Lanier, L. L.: *J. Exp. Med.* **164**, 814 (1986).
16. Berke, G.: Functions and Mechanisms of Lysis Induced by Cytotoxic T Lymphocytes and Natural Killer Cells. *In* "Fundamental Immunology" (W. E. Paul, ed.), 2nd ed. Raven Press, New York, 1989, p. 735.
17. van Furth, R.: Cells of the Mononuclear Phagocyte System. Nomenclature in Terms of Sites and Conditions. *In* "Mononuclear Phagocytes, Functional Aspects" (R. van Furth, ed.). Martinus-Nijhoff, The Hague, Netherlands, 1980, p. 1.
18. Unanue, E. R.: Macrophages, Antigen-Presenting Cells, and the Phenomena of Antigen Handling and Presentation. *In* "Fundamental Immunology" (W. E. Paul, ed.), 2nd ed. Raven Press, New York, 1989, p. 95.
19. Meltzer, M. S., and Nacy, C. A.: Delayed-Type Hypersensitivity and the Induction of Activated Cytotoxic Macrophages. *In* "Fundamental Immunology" (W. E. Paul, ed.), 2nd ed. Raven Press, New York, 1986, p. 765.
20. Allison, J. P., McIntyre, B. W., and Bloch, D.: *J. Immunol.* **129**, 2293 (1982).
21. Meuer, S. C., Fitzgerald, K. A., Hussey, R. E., Hodgson, J. C., Schlossman, S. F., and Reinherz, E. L.: *J. Exp. Med.* **157**, 705 (1983).
22. Haskins, K., Kubo, R., White, J., Pigeon, M., Kappler, J., and Marrack, P.: *J. Exp. Med.* **157**, 1149 (1983).
23. Samelson, L. E., Harford, H. B., and Klausner, R. D.: *Cell* **43**, 223 (1985).
24. Chien, Y., Becker, D. M., Lindsten, T., Okamura, M., Cohen, D. I., and Davis, M. M.: *Nature* **312**, 31 (1984).
25. Saito, H., Kranz, D., Takagaki, Y., Hayday, A., Eisen, H., and Tonegawa, S.: *Nature* **312**, 36 (1984).
26. Hedrick, S. M., Cohen, D. I., Nielsen, E. A., and Davis, M. M.: *Nature* **308**, 149 (1984).
27. Yanagi, Y., Yoshikai, Y., Leggett, K., Clark, S. P., Aleksander, I., and Mak, T. W.: *Nature* **308**, 145 (1984).
28. Hedrick, S. M., Nielsen, E. A., Kavaler, J., Cohen, D. I., and Davis, M. M.: *Nature* **308**, 153 (1984).
29. Meuer, S. C., Schlossman, S. F., and Reinherz, E.: *Proc. Natl. Acad. Sci. U.S.A.* **79**, 4395 (1982).
30. Spits, H., Borst, J., Terhorst, C., and de Vries, J. E.: *J. Immunol.* **129**, 1563 (1982).
31. Krensky, A. M., Reiss, C. S., Nier, J. W., Strominger, J. L., and Burakoff, S. J.: *Proc. Natl. Acad. Sci. U.S.A.* **79**, 2365 (1982).
32. Babbit, B. P., Allen, P. M., Matsueda, G., Haber, E., and Unanue, E. R.: *Nature* **317**, 359 (1985).
33. Buus, A., Sette, A., Colon, S. M., Janis, D. M., and Grey, H. M.: *Cell* **47**, 1071 (1986).
34. Germain, R. N.: *Nature* **322**, 687 (1986).
35. Morrison, L. A., Lukacher, A. E., Braciale, V. L., Fan, D. P., and Braciale, T. J.: *J. Exp. Med.* **163**, 903 (1986).
36. Green, A. R.: *Lancet* **1**, 705 (1989).
37. Kurt-Jones, E. A., Biller, D. I., Mizel, S. B., and Unanue, E. R.: *Proc. Natl. Acad. Sci. U.S.A.* **82**, 1204 (1985).
38. O'Garra, A. O.: *Lancet* **1**, 1003 (1989).
39. Miyasaki, N., Sato, K., Goto, M., Sasano, M., Natsuyama, M., Inoue, K., and Nishioka, K.: *Arthritis Rheumatol.* **31**, 480 (1988).
40. Buchan, G., Barrett, K., Turner, M., Chantry, D., Maini, R. N., and Feldmann, M.: *Clin. Exp. Immunol.* **73**, 449 (1988).
41. Maury, C. P. J., Salo, E., and Pelkonen, P.: *New Engl. J. Med.* **319**, 1670 (1988).
42. Seckinger, P., and Dayer, J. M.: *Ann. Inst. Pasteur Immunol.* **138**, 486 (1987).
43. Morgan, D. A., Ruscetti, F. W., and Gallo, R.: *Science* **193**, 1007 (1976).
44. Gillis, S., Ferm, M. M., Ou, W., and Smith, K. A.: *J. Immunol.* **120**, 2027 (1978).
45. Malkovsky, M., Sondel, P. M., Strober, W., and Dalgleish, A. G.: *Clin. Exp. Immunol.* **74**, 151 (1988).
46. Dinarrello, C. A., and Mier, J. W.: *New Engl. J. Med.* **317**, 940 (1987).
47. Warrington, R. J.: *J. Rheumatol.* **15**, 616 (1988).
48. Campen, D. H., Horwitz, D. A., Quismorio, F. P., Jr., Ehresmann, G. R., and Martin, W. J.: *Arthritis Rheumatol.* **31**, 1358 (1988).
49. Josimovic-Alasevic, O., Feldmeier, H. J., Zwingenberger, K., Harms, G., Hahn, H., Shrisuphanunt, M., and Diamantstein, I.: *Clin. Exp. Immunol.* **72**, 249 (1988).
50. Sethi, K. K., and Naher, H.: *Immunol. Lett.* **13**, 179 (1986).
51. Manoussakis, M. N., Papadopoulos, G. K., Drosos, A. A., and Moutsopoulos, H. M.: *Clin. Immunol. Immunopathol.* **50**, 321 (1989).
52. Schrader, J. W.: *Annu. Rev. Immunol.* **4**, 205 (1986).
53. Oettgen, H. F., and Old, L. J.: The History of Cancer Immunotherapy. *In*: "Biologic Therapy of Cancer" (V. T. De Vita, Jr., S. Hellman, and S. A. Rosenberg, eds.). Lippincott, Philadelphia, 1991, p. 87.

54. Vercelli, D., Jabara, H. H., Arai, K. -I., and Geha, R. S.: *J. Exp. Med.* **169**, 1295 (1989).
55. Harriman, G. R., and Strober, W.: *J. Immunol.* **139**, 3553 (1987).
56. Hirano, T., Taga, T., Yasukawa, K., Nakajima, K., Nakano, N., Takatsuki, F., Shimizu, M., Murashima, A., Tsunasawa, S., Sakiyama, F., and Kishimoto, T.: *Proc. Natl. Acad. Sci. U.S.A.* **84**, 228 (1987).
57. Freeman, G. J., Freedman, A. S., Rabinowe, S. N., Segil, J. M., Horowitz, J., Rosen, K., Whitman, J. F., and Nadler, L. M.: *J. Clin. Invest.* **83**, 1512 (1989).
58. Sutton, M. G. S. J., Mercier, L., Giulliani, E. R., and Lie, J. T.: *Mayo Clin. Proc.* **55**, 371 (1980).
59. Wasge, A., Kaufmann, C., Espevik, T., and Husby, G.: *Clin. Immunol. Immunopathol.* **50**, 394 (1989).
60. Morrissey, P. J., Goodwin, R. G., Nordan, R. P., Anderson, D., Grabstein, K. H., Cosman, D., Sims, J., Lupton, S., Acres, B., Reed, S. G., Mochizuki, D., Eisenman, J., Conlon, P. J., and Namen, A. E.: *J. Exp. Med.* **169**, 707 (1989).
61. Larsen, C. G., Anderson, A. O., Appella, E., Oppenheim, J. J., and Matsushima, K.: *Science* **243**, 1464 (1989).
62. Isaacs, A., and Lindeman, J.: *Proc. Roy. Soc. Lond. (Biol.)* **259**, 67 (1957).
63. Balkwill, F. R.: *Lancet* **1**, 1060 (1989).
64. Panitch, H. S., Hirsch, R. L., Hally, A. S., and Johnson, K. P.: *Lancet* **1**, 893 (1987).
65. Westwick, J., Li, S. W., and Camp, R. D.: *Immunol. Today* **10**, 146, (1989).
66. Jerne, N. K.: *Immunol. Rev.* **79**, 193 (1983).
67. Hodes, R. J.: T-Cell-Mediated Regulation: Help and Suppression. *In* "Fundamental Immunology" (W. E. Paul, ed.), 2nd ed. Raven Press, New York. 1989, p. 587.
68. Svejgaard, A., Plotz, P., and Ryder, L.: *Immunol. Rev.* **70**, 193 (1983).
69. Burnet, F. M.: *Progr. Exp. Tumor Res.* **13**, 1 (1970).
70. Penn, I.: "Principles of Tumor Immunity: Immuno-competence and Cancer." *In* "Biologic Therapy of Cancer" (V. T. De Vita, Jr., S. Hellman, and S. A. Rosenberg, eds.). Lippincott, Philadelphia, 1991, p. 53.
71. Ettinghausen, S. E., and Rosenberg, S. A.: *Springer Semin. Immunopathol.* **9**, 51 (1986).
72. Rosenberg, S. A., Spiess, P., and Lafrelniere, R.: *Science* **233**, 131 (1986).
73. Herberman, R. B.: "NK Cells and Other Natural Effector Cells." Academic Press, New York, 1982.
74. Volkman, A.: "Mononuclear Phagocyte Function". Dekker, New York, 1984.
75. Topalain, S. L., Soloman, D., and Rosenberg, S. A.: *Immunology* **142**, 3714 (1989).
76. Rosenberg, S. A., Packard, B. S., Aebersold, P. M., Solomon, D., Topalian, S. L., Toy, S. T., Simon, P., Lotze, M. T., Yang, J. C., Seipp, C. A., Simpson, C., Carter, C., Bock, S., Schwartzentruber, D., Wei, J. P., and White, D. E.: *N. Engl. J. Med.* **319**, 1676 (1988).
77. Topalian, S. L., and Rosenberg, S. A.: Adaptive Cellular Therapy: Basic Principles. *In* "Biologic Therapy of Cancer" (V. T. De Vita, Jr., S. Hellman, and S. A. Rosenberg, eds.). Lippincott, Philadelphia, 1991, p. 178.
78. Office of Technology Assessment: "Identifying and Controlling Immunotoxic Substances" (Background paper). OTA, *United States Congress*, Washington, D.C., 1991.
79. Salvaggio, J. E., and Sullivan, K. A.: Environmental Chemicals and the Immune System. *In* "Environmental and Occupational Medicine" (W. N. Rom, ed.), 2nd ed. Little, Brown, Boston, 1992, p. 69.
80. Zetterstrom, O., Nordvall, S. L., Bjorksten, B., Ahlstedt, S., and Stelander, M.: *J. Allergy Clin. Immunol.* **75**, 594 (1985).
81. Kjellman, N.-I. M.: *Lancet* **1**, 993 (1981).
82. Muranaka, M., Suzuki, S., Koizumi, K., Takafuji, S., Miyamoto, T., Ikemori, R., and Tokiwa, H.: *J. Allergy Clin. Immunol.* **77**, 616 (1986).
83. World Health Organization: "Cancer—Causes, Occurrence and Control", *IARC Sci. Publ.* **100**, IARC Lyon France, 1990.
84. Woo, Y.-t., and Arcos, J. C.: Environmental Chemicals. *In* "Carcinogens in Industry and the Environment" (J. M. Sontag, ed.). Dekker, New York, 1981, p. 168.
85. Harvey, R. G.: *Am. Scientist* **70**, 386 (1982).
86. Zedeck, M. S. J.: *Environ. Pathol. Toxicol.* **3**, 537 (1980).
87. Ward, E. C., Murray, M. J., and Dean, J. H.: Immunotoxicity of Nonhalogenated Polycyclic Aromatic Hydrocarbons. *In* "Immunotoxicology and Immunopharmacology" (J. H. Dean, M. I. Luster, A. E. Munson, and H. Amos, eds.). Raven Press, New York, 1985, p. 291.
88. White, K. L., Jr.: *Environ. Carcino. Rev.* **C4**, 163 (1986).
89. Medina, D., Stockman, G., and Griswold, D.: *Cancer Res.* **34**, 2663 (1974).
90. Yamashita, U., and Hamaoka, T.: *Gann* **73**, 773 (1982).
91. Ladics, G. S., Kawabata, T. T., and White, K. L.: *Toxicol. Appl. Pharmacol.* **110**, 31 (1991).
92. DiGiovanni, G., and Juchau, M. R.: *Metab. Rev.* **11**, 61 (1980).
93. Urso, P., and Gengozian, N.: *J. Toxicol. Environ. Health* **6**, 569 (1980).

94. Davis, D., and Safe, S.: *Toxicology* **63**, 97 (1990).

95. Bozelka, B. E., and Salvaggio, J. E.: *Environ. Carcino. Rev.* **3**, 1 (1985).

96. Selikoff, I. J., Hammond, E. C., and Seildman, H.: *Ann. N.Y. Acad. Sci.* **330**, 91 (1979).

97. Miller, K., and Brown, R. C.: The Immune System and Asbestos-Associated Disease. *In* "Immunotoxicology and Immunopharmacology" (J. H. Dean, M. I. Luster, A. E. Munson, and H. Amos, eds.). New York, Raven Press, 1985, p. 429.

98. Boorman, G. A., Dean, J. H., Luster, M. I., Adkins, B., Brody, A., and Hong, H. L.: *Toxicol. Appl. Pharmacol.* **72**, 148 (1984).

99. de Shazo, R. D., Hendrick, D. J., Diem, J. E., Nordberg, J., Baser, Y., Bevier, D., Jones, R. N., Barkman, H. W., Salvaggio, J. E. and Weill, H.: *J. Allergy Clin. Immunol.* **72**, 454 (1983).

100. Miller, L. G., Sparrow, D., and Ginns, L. C.: *Clin. Exp. Immunol.* **51**, 110 (1983).

101. Strom, T. B.: Immunosuppression in Tissue and Organ Transplantation. *In* "Organ Transplantation— Current Clinical and Immunological Concepts" (L. Brent and R. A. Sills, eds.). Bailliere Tindall, London, 1989, p. 39.

102. Sigal, N. H., and Dumont, F. J.: *Annu. Rev. Immunol.* **10**, 519 (1992).

103. Mihich, E., and Ehrke, M. J.: Immunomodulation by Anticancer Drugs. *In* "Biologic Therapy of Cancer" (V. T. De Vita, Jr., S. Hellman, and S. A. Rosenberg, eds.). Lippincott, Philadelphia, 1991, p. 776.

104. Ehrke, M. J., Mihich, E., Berd, D., and Mastrangelo, M. J.: *Semin. Oncol.* **16**, 230 (1989).

105. Penn, I.: Neoplastic Consequences of Immunosuppression. *In* "Immunotoxicology and Immunopharmacology" (J. H. Dean, M. I. Luster, A. E., Munson, and H. Amos, eds.). Raven Press, New York, 1985, p. 79.

106. Spreafico, F., Allegrucci, M., Merendino, A., and Luini, W.: Chemical Immunodepressive Drugs: Their Action on the Cells of the Immune System and Immune Mediators. *In* "Immunotoxicology and Immunopharmacology" (J. H. Dean, M. I. Luster, A. E. Munson, and H. Amos, eds.). Raven Press, New York, 1985, p. 179.

107. Exon, J. H., Kerkvliet, N. I., and Talcott, P. A.: *Environ. Carcino. Rev.* **C5**, 73 (1987).

108. Thomas, P. T., and Faith, R. E.: Adult and Perinatal Immunotoxicity Induced by Halogenated Aromatic Hydrocarbons. *In* "Immunotoxicology and Immunopharmacology" (J. H. Dean, M. I. Luster, A. E. Munson, and H. Amos, eds.). Raven Press, New York, 1985, p. 305.

109. Silkworth, J. B., and Vecchi, A.: Role of the Ah Receptor in Halogenated Aromatic Hydrocarbon Immunotoxicity. *In* "Immunotoxicology and Immunopharmacology" (J. H. Dean, M. I. Luster, A. E. Munson, and H. Amos, eds.). Raven Press, New York, 1985, p. 263.

110. Bekesi, J. G., Roboz, J., Fischbein, A., Roboz, J. P., Salomon, S. and Greaves, J.: Immunological, Biochemical, and Clinical Consequences of Exposure to Polybrominated Biphenyls. *In* "Immunotoxicology and Immunopharmacology" (J. H. Dean, M. I. Luster, A. E. Munson, and H. Amos, eds.). Raven Press, New York, 1985, p. 393.

111. Hoffman, R. E., Stehr-Green, P. A., Webb, K. B., Evans, R. G., Knutsen, A. P., Schramm, W. F., Staake, J. L., Gibson, B. B., and Steinberg, K. K.: *JAMA* **255**, 2031 (1986).

112. Fingerhut, M. A., Halperin, W. E., Marlow, D. A., Piacetelli, L. A., Honchar, P. A., Sweeney, M. H., Greife, A. L., Dill, P. A., Steenland, K., and Suruda, A. J.: *New Engl. J. Med.* **324**, 212 (1991).

113. Dean, T. N., Kakkanaiah, V. N., Nagarkatti, M., and Nagarkatti, P. S.: *Toxicol. Appl. Pharmacol.* **106**, 408 (1990).

114. Lee, T. P., and Chang, K. J.: Health Effects of Polychlorinated Biphenyls. *In* "Immunotoxicology and Immunopharmacology" (J. H. Dean, M. I. Luster, A. E. Munson, and H. Amos, eds.). Raven Press, New York, 1985, p. 415.

115. Olson, L. J., Erickson, B. J., Hinsdell, R. D., Wyman, J. A., Porter, W. P., Binning, L. K., Bidgood, R. C., and Nordheim, E. V.: *Arch. Environ. Contam. Toxicol.* **16**, 433 (1987).

116. Luebke, R. W., Rogers, R. R., Riddle, M. M., Rowe, D. G., and Smialowicz, R.: *Immunopharmacology.* **13**, 1 (1987).

117. Hermanowicz, A., and Kossman, S.: *Clin. Immunol. Immunopathol.* **33**, 13 (1984).

118. Lawrence, D. A.: Immunotoxicity of Heavy Metals. *In* "Immunotoxicology and Immunopharmacology" (J. H. Dean, M. I. Luster, A. E. Munson, and H. Amos, eds.). Raven Press, New York, 1985, p. 341.

119. Borella, P., and Giordina, A.: *Environ. Res.* **55**, 165. (1991).

120. Bozelka, B. E., Burkholder, P. M., and Chang, L. W.: *Environ. Res.* **17**, 390 (1978).

121. Bozelka, B. E., and Burkholder, P. E.: *Environ. Res.* **27**, 421 (1982).

122. Sakaguchi, S., Sakaguchi, T., Nakamura, I., and Kudo, Y.: *Pharmacol. Toxicol.* **61**, 325 (1987).

123. Williams, W. R., and Williams, W. J.: *Arch. Allergy Appl. Immunol.* **67**, 175 (1982).

124. Price, C. D., Jones Williams, W., Pugh, A., and Joynson, D. H.: *J. Clin. Pathol.* **30**, 24 (1977).

125. Pepys, J.: *Clin. Immunol. Allergy* **4**, 131 (1984).

126. Joules, H.: *Lancet* **2**, 1348 (1932).

127. Dolvich, J., Evans, S. L., and Niebore, E.: *Br. J. Ind. Med.* **41**, 51 (1984).
128. Malo, J. L., and Cartier, A.: *J. Allergy Clin. Immunol.* **79**, 117 (1987).
129. Salvaggio, J. E.: *J. Allergy Clin. Immunol.* **85**, 689 (1990).
130. Luster, M. I., Munson, A. E., Thomas, P. T., Holsapple, M. P., Fenters, J. D., White, Jr., K. L., Lauer, L. D., Germolec, D. R., Rosenthal, G. J., and Dean, J. H.: *Fundam. Appl. Toxicol.* **10**, 2 (1988).

SOURCE BOOKS AND REVIEWS

1. Alberts, B., Bray, D., Lewis, J., Raff, M., Roberts, K., and Watson, J. D.: "Molecular Biology of the Cell", 3rd ed., *see* Chapter 23: "The Immune System". Garland Publishing, New York, 1994.
2. Benjamini, E., and Leskowitz, S.: "Immunology—A Short Course", 2nd ed. Wiley, New York, 1991.
3. Sell, S.: "Basic Immunology: Immune Mechanisms in Health and Disease". Elsevier, New York, 1987.
4. Berkow, R., and Fletcher, A. J., Eds.: "The Merck Manual of Diagnosis and Therapy", 16th ed., *see* Chapter 2: "Immunology—Allergic Disorders". Merck Res. Labs. publishers, Rahway, New Jersey, 1992.
5. Descotes, J.: "Immunotoxicology of Drugs and Chemicals". Elsevier, Amsterdam, 1986.
6. Burger, E. J., Tardiff, R. G., and Bellanti, J. A., Eds.: "Environmental Chemical Exposures and Immune System Integrity". Princeton Publishing, Princeton, New Jersey, 1990.
7. Dean, J. H., Cornacoff, J. B., and Luster, M. I.: Toxicity to the Immune System: A Review. *In* "Immunopharmacology Reviews", Vol. I (J. W. Hadden and A. Szentivanyi, eds.). Plenum Press, New York, 1990.
8. Gleichmann, E., Kimber, I., and Purchase, I. F. H.: "Immunotoxicology: Suppressive and Stimulatory Effects of Drugs on the Immune System". *Arch. Toxicol.* **63**, 257 (1989).
9. Dean, J. H., and Padarathsingh, M., Eds.: "Biological Relevance of Immune Suppression As Induced by Genetic, Therapeutic and Environmental Factors". Van Nostrand Reinhold, New York, 1981.
10. Bigazzi, P. E.: "Autoimmunity Induced by Chemicals". *Clin. Toxicol.* **26**, 125 (1988).
11. Thomas, P. T., Busse, W. W., Kerkvliet, N. I., *et al.*: Immunological Effects of Pesticides. *In* "The Effects of Pesticides on Human Health" (S. R. Baker and C. F. Wilkinson, eds.). Princeton Publishing, Princeton, New Jersey, 1990.
12. Gershwin, M. E.: "Nutrition and Immunity". Academic Press, Orlando, 1985.

CHAPTER **9**

The Effect of Diet on Tumor Induction

Whoever gives these things (food) no consider-
ation, and is ignorant of them, how can he
understand the diseases of man?
Hippocrates, 400 B.C.

Contents: **Section I:** Effect of Caloric (Energy) Restriction. **Section II:** Modulation by Protein and Individual Amino Acids. **Section III:** Modulation by Vitamins. **Section IV:** Modulation by Minerals. **Section V:** Dietary Fiber and Its Effect on Cancer Incidence. **Editors' Note I:** Indirect Modification of Chemical Carcinogenesis by Nutritional Factors Through Regulation of the Mixed-Function Oxidase System. **Editors' Note II:** On Evidence for Preventive Significance of Dietary Supplementation.

SECTION **I**

Effect of Caloric (Energy) Restriction

David Kritchevsky

I. CALORIC RESTRICTION EFFECTS ON TUMORIGENESIS: HISTORICAL BEGINNINGS

The earliest example of the influence of caloric restriction on tumorigenesis was recorded in 1909 by Moreschi (1), who found that the growth of transplanted tumors was inhibited in underfed mice (Table 1). Rous (2) examined the influence of diet in both transplanted and spontaneous mouse tumors and found growth of both types to be reduced when the animals were underfed. Sugiura and Benedict (3) excised spontaneous tumors from mice and then determined the effect of full feeding or underfeeding on recurrence of the tumors. Total recurrence of tumors was observed in 82% of mice fed fully (3 g/day) in contrast to 27% recurrence incidence in mice fed 1 g/day. The underfed

TABLE 1.   Effect of Underfeeding on Growth of Transplanted Sarcoma 7 in Mice[a]

Group	Number	Feed intake (g/day)	Weight change (g)	Tumor weight (g)
1	13	1.0	−4.2	1.3±0.2
2	7	1.5	−1.9	3.6±0.5
3	8	2.0	−2.4	5.2±0.5
4	8	Ad libitum	+1.8	7.6±0.8

[a]After C. Moreschi [Z. *Immunitätsforsch.* **2**, 651 (1909)].

mice lived an average of 142 days after the operation as compared to 96 days for the full-fed controls. Bischoff *et al.* (4) examined the influence of varying the level of caloric restriction on the growth of Sarcoma 180 in mice. Restriction of intake by only 20% had no inhibitory effect on tumor growth; 33% restriction reduced tumor growth, but the findings were of questionable significance; at 50% restriction of intake there was a marked inhibition of tumor growth. A later experiment (5) in which the commercial diet used was replaced in part by fat or starch purported to show that the observed effects were due to caloric restriction rather than to absence or presence of a specific nutrient.

Sivertsen and Hastings (6), working with mice bearing spontaneous mammary tumors, showed that feeding only enough diet to maintain weight (about one half of that ingested *ad libitum*) reduced tumor incidence from 88 to 16% and delayed significantly the age at which the tumors have appeared. Dietary restriction increased average life span from 358 ± 8 days to 482 ± 6 days (25.7%). Visscher and coworkers (7,8) showed that a 33% reduction in caloric intake prevents the emergence of spontaneous mammary tumors in C3H mice and suggested that the mechanism of inhibition involve a reduced level of ovarian secretion. Lavik and Baumann (9) examined the effects of dietary fat content and total caloric intake on 3-methylcholanthrene (3-MC)-induced tumorigenesis in mice (summarized in Table 2). Mice received, per 25 g body weight, 12 cal/day ("high" cal. regimen) or were restricted to 8 cal/day ("low" cal. regimen); at each caloric level fat intake was adjusted to 60 mg ("low" fat) or 240 mg ("high" fat) per day. Table 2 shows that regardless of the level of fat the tumor incidence was much higher on the high caloric than on the low caloric diet, but at each caloric intake level the incidence was higher on the high fat diet than on the corresponding low fat diet. Almost a half century later, Albanes (10) reviewed data on 82 published experiments involving caloric restriction and tumorigenesis in mice. The findings are strikingly similar to the observations made by Lavik and Baumann (9). In 23 studies involving a low-fat, low-calorie diet, tumor incidence was 34.4 ± 4.3%; low-fat, high-calorie regimen (18 studies) gave an average incidence of 52.4 ± 4.7%; high-fat, low-calorie diets (19 experiments) resulted in average tumor incidence of 23.1 ± 4.7%; and in the 22 studies in which the diets were high in both fat and calories average tumor incidence was 54.4 ± 3.4%. Caloric restriction in

TABLE 2.   Effects of Fat and Calories on Incidence of 3-MC-Induced Skin Tumors in Mice[a]

Regimen		Tumor incidence (%)
Fat	Calories	
Low	Low	0
High	Low	28
Low	High	54
High	High	66

[a]After P. S. Lavik, and C. A. Baumann [*Cancer Res*, **3**, 749 (1943)].

the ranges 7–20%, 21–30%, 31–40%, and 41–58% gave reductions in tumor incidence of 20, 50, 53, and 62%, respectively.

II. MODALITIES OF CALORIC RESTRICTION

Caloric restriction can be brought about in one of two ways. The simplest is direct underfeeding. In this mode the restricted animals are fed less of the same diet which is being offered to the controls. The early studies of caloric restriction and cancer were indeed carried out in this manner. The criticism of this experimental design is that the test animals may be ingesting less of a critical mineral or vitamin which is influencing metabolic outcome as well as growth. In the second experimental protocol, the diet of the test animals is designed to specifically contain levels of micronutrient equal to those of the control diet, but the restriction is due to specific reduction in levels of macronutrient. Both methods of feeding have been used with similar results.

III. THE EARLY WORK OF ALBERT TANNENBAUM

The greatest early impact in the area of dietary effects on experimental or spontaneous tumorigenesis was made by Albert Tannenbaum, who worked in the 1940s. In his early studies he examined the effects of underfeeding on the incidence of spontaneous and induced tumors in mice. The basal diet consisted of 64.4% cracked wheat, 17.8% dog chow, 11.1% flour, and 6.7% skim milk powder (11). The restricted animals were fed sufficient diet to maintain weight at 18–20 g. Tannenbaum studied the effects of underfeeding on both spontaneous and induced tumors and found that it consistently inhibited tumorigenesis (Table 3). Subsequently Tannenbaum (12) formulated a diet the calories of which he could estimate and began to study caloric restriction. The basal diet consisted of 1.2 g dog chow, 0.8 g skim milk powder, and 1.4 g corn starch. Caloric restriction was brought about by totally removing or restricting the amount of corn starch. Using this diet he found that about 32% caloric restriction inhibited benzo[a]pyrene (BaP)-induced skin tumorigenesis by 69% in DBA male mice and inhibited the emergence of sarcomas by 43% in C57 black female mice. The appearance of primary lung tumors was inhibited by about 50% in ABC mice and by about 80% in Swiss mice. Tannenbaum (13) also showed that caloric restriction is most effective during the promotion phase of tumorigenesis. Thus, mice fed *ad libitum* throughout the study exhibited a 69% incidence of BaP-induced tumors; those fed *ad libitum* during initiation, but restricted during promotion, had a 34% incidence; caloric restriction during initiation, but *ad libitum* feeding during promotion, resulted in a 55% incidence; and when calories were restricted throughout the study, tumor incidence was only 24%. The degree of caloric restriction was also shown to influence the emergence of spontaneous tumors (14). Thus, in DBA virgin female mice spontaneous mammary tumor incidence

TABLE 3. Underfeeding and Tumorigenesis in Mice[a]

Tumor type	Group	Tumor incidence (percent)
Spontaneous (mammary)	Control	40
	Underfed	2
Induced (BaP–skin)	Control	16
	Underfed	4

[a]After A. Tannenbaum [*Am. J. Cancer* **38**, 335 (1940)].

was 54% in those fed 11 cal/day, 12% in those fed 8 cal/day, and 0% in those fed 7 cal/day. In DBA parous female mice, reduction of caloric intake from 11.7 to 8.1 cal/day reduced the incidence of mammary tumors from 85 to 35%. Dietary composition also played a role. Large (six- to ninefold) increases in the percentage of fat in the diet led to increased tumor incidence despite caloric restriction (15); incidence of 3-MC-induced skin tumors in mice fed 8.5 cal/day went from 15 to 20 to 29% as the level of dietary fat rose from 2 to 3 to 18%. Spontaneous mammary tumor incidence in C3H virgin female mice given 10.0 cal/day and 2% fat was 40% and it rose to 67% when the diet contained 18% fat. Boutwell et al. (16) fed BaP-treated mice semi-purified diets varying in fat and calorie content, and examined the effects on skin tumorigenesis. They confirmed the earlier findings relative to caloric restriction. Isocaloric diets containing 2 or 61% fat exerted similar effects, showing an incidence of 64 or 78% of BaP-induced skin tumors. Over the next few decades there was little work in the area of caloric effects on tumorigenesis, but enough data had been accumulated to permit White (17) to review the area in 1961.

IV. CALORIC RESTRICTION *VERSUS* DIETARY FAT CONTENT

Interest in this area was renewed early in the 1980s. Giovanella et al. (18) reported that underfeeding reduced the growth of human tumors transplanted into nude mice. Kritchevsky et al. (19) showed that 7,12-dimethylbenz[a]anthracene (DMBA)-induced mammary tumor growth was totally inhibited in female Sprague-Dawley rats whose caloric intake was 40% lower than that of the controls. The dietary fat was coconut oil (13%) plus enough corn oil (1%) for essential fatty acid repletion. The control diet contained 4% corn oil. The calorically-restricted rats exhibited no tumors even though their daily fat intake was twice that of the controls. The results of their experiments relating to caloric restriction and chemically induced colon or mammary tumors in rats are detailed in Table 4. In a similar study, Boissoneault et al. (20) administered DMBA to three groups of female F344 rats. One group was fed a high-fat diet (30% corn oil) *ad libitum*, one was fed a low-fat diet (5% corn oil), and the third was given the high-fat diet,

TABLE 4. Influence of 40% Caloric Restriction and Type of Fat on Colonic and Mammary Tumors in Rats

Regimen	Fat (percent)[a]	Tumor incidence (percent)
	Colonic Tumors[b]	
Ad libitum	Butter oil (3.9)	85
Restricted	Butter oil (8.4)	35
Ad libitum	Corn oil (3.9)	100
Restricted	Corn oil (8.4)	53
	Mammary Tumors[c]	
Ad libitum	Coconut oil (3.9)	58
Restricted	Coconut oil (8.4)	0
Ad libitum	Corn oil (3.9)	80
Restricted	Corn oil (8.4)	20

[a]Butter oil and coconut oil diets also contained 1 percent corn oil.
[b]Induced by 1,2-dimethylhydrazine in male F344 rats.
[c]Induced by 7,12-dimethylbenz[a]anthracene in female Sprague-Dawley rats.

TABLE 5. **Influence of Fat and Calories on DMBA-Induced Mammary Tumors in Rats**[a]

	Diet		
	High fat **(ad libitum)**	**Low fat** **(ad libitum)**	**High fat** **(restricted)**
Fat (corn oil) percent of diet	30	5	30
Fat intake (g/rat/day)	2.7	0.6	2.2
Tumor incidence (percent)	73	43	7

[a]After G. A. Boissonneault, C. E. Elson, and M. W. Pariza [*J. Natl. Cancer Inst.* **76**, 335 (1986)].

pair-fed to the low-fat diet in terms of net energy. Table 5 shows that whereas the low-fat diet reduced tumor incidence by 41%, the high-fat, energy-restricted diet reduced tumor incidence by 92%. Pollard *et al.* (21) showed that 25% caloric restriction inhibited methylazoxymethanol (MAM)-induced colon tumorigenesis in rats. Pollard and Luckert (22) have also provided evidence that while caloric restriction reduces the incidence of colon tumors caused by MAM, an indirect-acting carcinogen, caloric restriction has no such effect on *N*-nitroso-*N*-methylurea (NMU), a direct-acting carcinogen. However, there were very few rats (ten per group) used in this study, and the work requires confirmation using larger numbers of test animals. This interesting dichotomy, which has not been investigated further so far, may reflect a property specific to NMU. Caloric restriction or underfeeding have been shown to inhibit osteosarcomas induced by ^{45}Ca treatment (23), or tumors induced by ultraviolet (24) or gamma ray irradiation (25,26). The incidence of colon tumors caused by feeding of 1,2-dimethylhydrazine (DMH) (27) or subcutaneous injection of azoxymethane (28) is reduced significantly by caloric restriction of 40 or 30%, respectively. In the former study the actual fat intake of the calorie-restricted group was almost double that of the *ad libitum*-fed controls. Tucker (29) studied long-term food restriction (by 20%) in mice and rats. *Ad libitum*-fed male rats showed 72% survival at 2 years, whereas restricted rats exhibited 88% survival. In female rats the 24-month survival was 68% for those fed *ad libitum* and 90% for the calorie-restricted ones. In male mice fed *ad libitum*, survival was 4% at 3 years compared to 36% in food-restricted mice. Survival in female mice was 8% in the *ad libitum* group compared to 36% in the calorie-restricted group. Spontaneous tumorigenicity was significantly reduced in calorie-restricted mice of either gender (Table 6). In male rats there were significantly fewer tumors of the pituitary and skin, and in female rats there were significantly fewer mammary and pituitary tumors. In mice,

TABLE 6. **Incidence of Spontaneous Tumors in Calorie-Restricted (20 Percent) Rats and Mice**[a, b]

	Incidence (percent)[a]		
	Ad libitum	**Restricted**	**p <**
Rats			
Male	66	24	0.001
Female	82	56	0.005
Mice			
Male	80	52	0.01
Female	82	46	0.001

[a]After M. J. Tucker [*Int. J. Cancer* **23**, 803 (1979)].
[b]Fifty animals per group.

significant differences were observed in liver tumors in males and in pituitary tumors in females.

The influence of restriction of dietary components other than fat has been studied by Shimokawa *et al.* (30). They reviewed the effects of restriction of fat, protein, minerals, or calories in male F344 rats. Restriction of fat, protein, or minerals *versus ad libitum* feeding had little effect on either leukemia or pituitary adenoma, but dietary restriction resulted in significantly lower incidence of both tumors (Table 7).

The data suggested that caloric restriction may override the tumor-enhancing effect of high-fat diets. To test this possibility, in a study on DMBA-induced mammary tumorigenesis, Klurfeld *et al.* (31) fed female Sprague-Dawley rats *ad libitum* diets containing 5,15, or 20% corn oil or placed them on 25% caloric restriction on diets containing 20 or 26.7% corn oil. Thus, the restricted animals ingested exactly as much fat daily as did the controls, receiving either 15 or 20% fat. Restriction of calories by 25% was chosen because other studies had shown that a significant reduction in tumor incidence takes place between 20 and 30% restriction (32). As Table 8 shows, tumor incidence was lower in the two restricted groups (fed 20 or 26.7% fat) than in the *ad libitum*–fed control groups whose diet contained only 5% fat. Plasma insulin levels are reduced significantly by caloric restriction (31,32). Beth *et al.* (33) showed that 30% caloric restriction inhibited NMU-induced mammary carcinogenesis, whereas fat content or fat composition had much less influence on tumorigenesis.

TABLE 7. Onset Rates of Leukemia and Pituitary Adenoma in Rats Deprived of Various Nutrients[a]

Dietary group	Leukemia[b]	Pituitary adenoma[b]
Fat restricted	1.16[c]	0.84[c]
Protein restricted	1.04[c]	0.70[c]
Minerals restricted	0.79[c]	0.99[c]
Diet restricted	0.80[d]	0.41[e]

[a]After I. Shimokawa, B. P. Yu, and E. J. Masoro [*J. Gerontol. Biol. Sci.* **46**, B228 (1991)].
[b]Observed/expected.
[c]Not significant ($p > 0.05$).
[d]$p = 0.002$.
[e]$p < 0.0001$.

TABLE 8. Effects of Dietary Fat Level and 25 Percent Caloric Restriction on DMBA-Induced Mammary Tumors in Rats[a]

Regimen	Tumor		
	Incidence (percent)	Multiplicity	Weight (g)
Ad libitum			
5 percent corn oil	65	2.9 ± 0.3	2.0 ± 0.7
15 percent corn oil	85	3.0 ± 0.6	2.3 ± 0.7
20 percent corn oil	80	4.1 ± 0.6	2.9 ± 0.5
Restricted			
20 percent corn oil	60	1.9 ± 0.4	0.8 ± 0.2
26.7 percent corn oil	30	1.5 ± 0.3	1.4 ± 1.0

[a]After D. M. Klurfeld, C. B. Welch, L. M. Lloyd, and D. Kritchevsky [*Int. J. Cancer* **43**, 922 (1989)].

V. INFLUENCE OF THE TIMING OF CALORIC RESTRICTION

Does the time of institution of caloric restriction influence eventual outcome? Tannenbaum (11) found that the appearance of spontaneous breast tumors in DBA mice (determined at 20 months of age) was completely inhibited when caloric restriction was started at 2 months of age, 95% inhibited when restriction commenced at 5 months of age, and 80% inhibited when restriction was begun at 9 months of age. Weindruch and Walford (34) found inhibition of the appearance of spontaneous tumors in mice calorie-restricted from 1 year of age on. Ross and Bras (35) showed that lifelong dietary restriction (by 60%) greatly increases the life-span of rats and reduces spontaneous tumor incidence by 90%. In a third group of rats, restriction was maintained for 7 weeks (immediately after weaning) and they were then returned to the *ad libitum* diet. This relatively short period of restriction did not influence life span, but decreased spontaneous tumor incidence by almost 40%. However, instituting caloric restriction relatively late in the tumorigenic process affects both body weight and tumor incidence. The effect appears to be related to feed efficiency (36).

Tannenbaum and Silverstone (37) reported that the proportion of protein (casein) in the diet does not influence spontaneous mammary tumorigenesis in C3H female mice. Ross and coworkers (38,39) found that high-protein intake shortly after weaning definitely increases the risk of tumorigenesis. Other factors leading to increased risk were high feed efficiency, high food intake, and rapid growth rate.

VI. CALORIC INTAKE *VERSUS* CALORIC EXPENDITURE

If reduction of caloric intake inhibits tumorigenesis, what does increased caloric expenditure bring about? Rusch and Kline (40) found that vigorous exercise inhibited the growth of a transplanted tumor in rats. Moore and Tittle (41) administered DMBA to control rats, to rats exercised vigorously, or to rats underfed to keep their body weight similar to that of the exercised rats. After 28 weeks the control rats exhibited a 55% incidence of tumors, whereas both test groups were free of tumors. Exercise has been shown to inhibit NMU-induced mammary carcinogenesis (42), pancreatic carcinogenesis induced by azaserine (43), or DMH-induced colon carcinogenesis (44,45) in rats (Table 9). On the other hand, Thompson *et al.* (46,47) reported that exercise actually increases the incidence of DMBA-induced mammary tumors in rats. Their data seem to indicate that a determining factor is whether or not the exercise reduces carcass fat. It should be noted in this regard that their exercised rats ingested 13% *more energy* than the sedentary controls.

TABLE 9. Influence of Treadmill Exercise and Caloric Restriction on Incidence of DMH-induced Colon Tumors in Rats[a]

Diet[b]	Exercise[c]	Tumor incidence (percent)	Tumors per tumor-bearing rat
AL	−	75	2.1 ± 0.4
AL	+	36	1.3 ± 0.2
CR (25%)	−	35	1.3 ± 0.2
CR (25%)	+	29	1.1 ± 0.1
CR (40%)	−	21	1.2 ± 0.2

[a]After D. M. Klurfeld, C. B. Welch, E. Einhorn, and D. Kritchevsky [*FASEB J.* **2**, A433 (1988)].
[b]AL, *Ad libitum;* CR, calorie restricted; AL exercised were pair fed to AL sedentary.
[c]Treadmill speed 24 meters/min at 7° angle incline; 60 min/day, 5 days/week.

VII. MECHANISM OF ACTION OF CALORIC RESTRICTION

What is the mechanism by which caloric restriction affects tumorigenesis? Ruggeri (48) has summarized and reviewed the potential mechanisms of tumor inhibition by caloric restriction (Table 10). Albanes and Winick (49) and others (50,51) have proposed that cancer risk is proportional to the number of proliferating cells which is a function of the number of cells (in a tissue/organ) and the rate of cell division. Caloric restriction has been shown to reduce proliferative activity in the mammary gland (52), intestine (53), urinary bladder (54), and skin (55). Calorie restriction also reduces total cell number (56,57). Bullough and Eisa (55) suggested that the mitotic activity of carcinogen-activated cells is decreased by caloric restriction and increased by caloric excess.

Boutwell *et al.* (58) have investigated the physiological effects of 40% caloric restriction in mice. They suggested that energy restriction causes the pituitary to elaborate essential adrenocorticotropin at the expense of less critical hormones. Caloric restriction has been shown to decrease the levels of circulating insulin (31,32), of pituitary hormones (59), and of hypothalamic catecholamines (60), while increasing the levels of ACTH (61), corticosterone (62), testosterone (63), and adrenal norepinephrine (64).

Prevention of mammary tumor formation in mice by low-calorie diets has been attributed to low levels of circulating prolactin and reduction of mammary tumor virus expression (65). Aflatoxin B is bound less readily to DNA, is cleared more rapidly, and is excreted to a greater extent in calorie-restricted rats (66). Proto-oncogene (*myc*) expression is significantly reduced in mice whose caloric intake is restricted by 40% (67). Increasing caloric restriction lowers the ratio of large (over 100 mg) to small (under 100 mg) mammary tumors in DMBA-treated rats. Study of enzymes of carbohydrate metabolism in these tissues indicates increased activity in the smaller tumors. The data suggest an adaptive, more efficient substrate utilization in the smaller tumors (68). However, with a more sparing substrate utilization, but working against a decreasing availability of substrate (due to energy restriction), the tumors cannot develop.

Caloric restriction decreases plasma insulin and IGF-1 levels (31,32,69). Insulin is a growth factor for both normal and neoplastic tissues (70) and is also a growth factor for cell culture (71). It may also regulate IGF-1 (somatomedin C) activity (72). Heuson and Legros (73) found that when DMBA-treated rats were made alloxan diabetic, tumor emergence was inhibited and established tumors regressed. The effect was somewhat more pronounced in diabetes than in caloric restriction. Boissonneault (74) has discussed the possible interplay of insulin, IGF-1, and growth hormone in man as well as in other species. Food restriction reduces the levels of prostaglandin metabolites in rats (75). It has been suggested (76) that prostaglandins may be necessary to stimulate tumor growth and, in fact, inhibition of cyclooxygenase by indomethacin has been shown to inhibit tumor

TABLE 10. Mechanisms by Which Caloric Restriction Might Inhibit Tumorigenesis[a]

1. Elevated glucocorticoid levels leading to growth inhibition
2. Reduction of mitotic activity and cell proliferation
3. Prolonged and/or increased immune response
4. "Starvation" of preneoplastic cells
5. Influence on specific hormones (mammotrophic hormones in the case of mammary tumors)
6. Influence on peptide growth factors or receptors
7. Modulation and repair of DNA damage
8. Influence on oncogene or proto-oncogene expression

[a]After B. A. Ruggeri [*In* "Human Nutrition: A Comprehensive Treatise", Cancer and Nutrition Ser. (R. B. Alfin-Slater and D. Kritchevsky, eds.), Vol. 7. Plenum, New York, 1991, p. 187].

induction in several tissues (77–79). Studies of the mechanisms underlying the effects of caloric restriction on tumorigenesis are just beginning. Eventually they may provide important clues to biochemical steps governing tumor emergence and progression.

VIII. OVERNUTRITION-RELATED FACTORS AND LACK OF MUSCULAR ACTIVITY *VERSUS* CANCER RISK

Excess weight, due to excess caloric intake, has been implicated in increased tumorigenesis in rats and mice (38,80–82). Dogs which were thin as juveniles have a significantly reduced risk of breast cancer (83).

Almost 80 years ago, Hoffman (84,85) suggested that the increase of the frequency of cancer world wide (already noticed at that time) might be due to overnutrition. This suggestion was echoed by Berg (86) in 1975. The epidemiology of breast cancer suggests that early menarche puts women at risk (87,88). Albanes and Taylor (89) reviewed data from 24 populations and found that all-sites cancer incidence has a high correlation with height in both men and women. Positively associated with height in men were cancers of the central nervous system, prostate, bladder, pancreas, lung, and colon. In women, positive correlations were seen with cancers of the rectum, pancreas, ovary, central nervous system, breast, uterus, and bladder. Body mass index (BMI) correlates positively with breast cancer in women (90,91) and with colon cancer in men (92). It is probable that weight, height, or BMI at various stages of life may play an important role in defining risk (93–95). These factors are influenced by nutrition. Lew and Garfinkel (96) showed a relationship between overweight and cancer mortality in a cohort of 750,000 men and women. Overweight (by 40% or more) increased the cancer mortality ratio in men and women by 33 and 55%, respectively (97). Excess calorie (energy) intake has been implicated in increased risk of colon cancer in several epidemiological studies (98–101).

Another aspect of the calorie equation is energy expenditure. In 1921, Sivertsen and Dahlstrom (102) suggested that lack of muscular activity could present a positive risk for cancer in men. Generally, increased levels of physical activity decrease the risk of cancers of the breast and reproductive system in women (103) and of the colon in men (104,105). Lifelong strenuous occupational activity has been shown to reduce the risk of colon (106–108) or prostate (109) cancer in men.

The effect of reduction of energy flux on carcinogenesis has been known for some time. As we increasingly explore the metabolic basis for this effect we should soon understand the underlying mechanism(s), which would point toward the directions for prevention and possibly treatment. It is noteworthy that in 1945 Potter (110) recommended reduced caloric intake and exercise as a means of cancer prevention.

REFERENCES

1. Moreschi, C.: *Z. Immunitätsforsch.* **2,** 651 (1909).
2. Rous, P.: *J. Exp. Med.* **20,** 433 (1914).
3. Sugiura, K., and Benedict, S. R. *J. Cancer Res.* **10,** 309 (1926).
4. Bischoff, F., Long, M. L. and Maxwell, L. C.: *Am. J. Cancer* **24,** 549 (1935).
5. Bischoff, F., and Long, M. L.: *Am. J. Cancer* **32,** 418 (1938).
6. Sivertsen, I., and Hastings, W. H. *Minn. Med.* **21,** 873 (1938).
7. Visscher, M. D., Ball, Z. B., Barnes, R. H., and Sivertsen, I.: *Surgery* **11,** 48 (1942).
8. Huseby, R. A., Ball, Z. B., and Visscher, M. B.: *Cancer Res.* **5,** 40 (1945)
9. Lavik, P. S., and Baumann, C. A.: *Cancer Res.* **3,** 749 (1943).
10. Albanes, D.: *Cancer Res.* **47,** 1987 (1987)

11. Tannenbaum, A.: *Am. J. Cancer* **38**, 335 (1940).
12. Tannenbaum, A.: *Cancer Res.* **2**, 460 (1942).
13. Tannenbaum, A.: *Cancer Res.* **4**, 673 (1944).
14. Tannenbaum, A.: *Cancer Res.* **5**, 609 (1945).
15. Tannenbaum, A.: *Cancer Res.* **5**, 616 (1945).
16. Boutwell, R. K., Brush, M. K., and Rusch, H. P.: *Cancer Res.* **9**, 741 (1949).
17. White, F. R.: *Cancer Res.* **21**, 281 (1961).
18. Giovanella, B. C., Shepard, R. C., Stehlen, J. S., Venditti, J. M., and Abbott, B. J.: *J. Natl. Cancer Inst.* **68**, 249 (1982).
19. Kritchevsky, D., Weber, M. M., and Klurfeld, D. M.: *Cancer Res.* **44**, 3174 (1984).
20. Boissonneault, G. A., Elson, C. E., and Pariza, M. W.: *J. Natl. Cancer Inst.* **76**, 335 (1986).
21. Pollard, M., Luckert, P. H., and Pan, G. Y.: *Cancer Treatment Rep.* **68**, 405 (1984).
22. Pollard, M., and Luckert, P. H.: *J. Natl. Cancer Inst.* **74**, 1347 (1985).
23. Brown, C. E., Barnes, L. L., Sperling, G., and McCoy, C. M. *Cancer Res.* **20**, 329 (1960).
24. Rusch, H. P., Kline, B. E., and Baumann, C. A.: *Cancer Res.* **5**, 431 (1945).
25. Gross, L., and Dreyfuss, Y.: *Proc. Natl. Acad. Sci. U.S.A.* **81**, 7596 (1984).
26. Gross, L., and Dreyfuss, Y.: *Proc. Natl. Acad. Sci. U.S.A.* **83**, 7928 (1986).
27. Klurfeld, D. M., Weber, M. M., and Kritchevsky, D.: *Cancer Res.* **47**, 2759 (1987).
28. Reddy, B. S., Wang, C. X., and Maruyama, H.: *Cancer Res.* **47**, 1226 (1987).
29. Tucker, M. J.: *Int. J. Cancer* **23**, 803 (1979).
30. Shimokawa, I., Yu, B. P., and Masoro, E. J.: *J. Gerontol. Biol. Sci.* **46**, B228 (1991).
31. Klurfeld, D. M., Welch, C. B., Lloyd, L. M., and Kritchevsky, D.: *Int. J. Cancer* **43**, 922 (1989).
32. Klurfeld, D. M., Welch, C. B., Davis M. J., and Kritchevsky, D.: *J. Nutr.* **199**, 286 (1989).
33. Beth, M., Berger, M. R., Aksoy, M., and Schmähl, D.: *Int. J. Cancer* **39**, 737 (1987).
34. Weindruch, R., and Walford, R. L.: *Science* **215**, 1415 (1982).
35. Ross, M. H., and Bras, G.: *J. Natl. Cancer Inst.* **47**, 1095 (1971).
36. Kritchevsky, D., Welch, C. B., and Klurfeld, D. M.: *Nutr. Cancer* **12**, 259 (1989).
37. Tannenbaum, A., and Silverstone, H.: *Cancer Res.* **9**, 162 (1949).
38. Ross, M. H., and Bras, G.: *J. Nutr.* **103**, 944 (1973).
39. Ross, M. H., Lustbader, E. D., and Bras, G.: *Nutr. Cancer* **3**, 150 (1982).
40. Rusch, H. P., and Kline, B. E.: *Cancer Res.* **4**, 116 (1944).
41. Moore, C., and Tittle, P. W.: *Surgery* **73**, 329 (1973).
42. Cohen, L. A., Choi, K., and Wang C. X.: *Cancer Res.* **48**, 4276 (1988).
43. Roebuck, B. D., McCaffrey, J., and Baumgartner, K. J.: *Cancer Res.* **50**, 6811 (1990).
44. Klurfeld, D. M., Welch, C. B., Einhorn, E., and Kritchevsky, D.: *FASEB J.* **2**, A433 (1988).
45. Kritchevsky, D.: *Proc. Soc. Exp. Biol. Med.* **193**, 35 (1990).
46. Thompson, H. J., Ronan, A. M., Ritacco, K. A., Tagliaferro, A. R., and Meeker, L. D.: *Cancer Res.* **48**, 2720 (1988).
47. Thompson, H. J., Ronan, A. M., Ritacco, K. A., and Tagliaferro, A. R.: *Cancer Res.* **49**, 1904 (1989).
48. Ruggeri, B. A.: The Effect of Caloric Restriction on Neoplasia and Age-Related Degenerative Processes. *In* "Human Nutrition: A Comprehensive Treatise", Cancer and Nutrition Ser. (R. B. Alfin-Slater and D. Kritchevsky, eds.), Vol. 7. Plenum, New York, 1991, p. 187.
49. Albanes, D., and Winick, M.: *J. Natl. Cancer Inst.* **80**, 772 (1988).
50. Craddock, V. M., and Frei, J. V.: *Br. J. Cancer* **30**, 503 (1974).
51. Clayson, D. B.: *Mutat. Res.* **185**, 243 (1987)
52. Welsch, C. W., Dehoog, J. V., O'Connor, D. H., and Scheffield, L. G.: *Cancer Res.* **45**, 6147 (1985).
53. Koga, A., and Kimura, S.: *J. Nutr Sci. Vitaminol.* **25**, 265 (1979).
54. Lok, E., Nera, E. A., Iverson, F., Scott, F., So, Y., and Clayson, D. B.: *Cancer Lett.* **38**, 249 (1988).
55. Bullough, W. S., and Eisa, E. A.: *Br. J. Cancer* **4**, 321 (1950).
56. Winnick, M., and Noble, A.: *J. Nutr.* **89**, 300 (1966).
57. Merry, B. J., and Holehan, A. M.: *Exp. Gerontol.* **20**, 15 (1985).
58. Boutwell, R. K., Brush, M. K., and Rusch, H. P.: *Am. J. Physiol.* **154**, 517 (1949).
59. Campbell, G. A., Kurcz, M., Marshall, S., and Meites, J.: *Endocrinology* **100**, 580 (1977).
60. Wurtman, R. J., and Wurtman J. J.: "Nutrition and Brain", Vol. 2. Raven Press, New York, 1977, p. 171.
61. Mulinov, M. G., and Pomerantz, L.: *J. Nutr.* **19**, 493 (1940).
62. Riegle, G., and Hess, G.: *Neuroendocrinology* **9**, 175 (1972).
63. Snyder, D. L., and Towne, B.: The Effect of Dietary Restriction on Serum Hormone and Blood Chemistry Changes in Aging Lobund-Wistar Rats. *In* "Dietary Restriction and Aging" (D. L. Snyder, ed.). Alan Liss, New York, 1989, p. 135.
64. Nekvasil, N. P., and Kingsley, T. R.: Age-Related Changes in Adrenal Catecholamine Levels and

Medullary Structure in Male Lobund-Wistar Rats. *In* "Dietary Restriction and Aging" (D. L. Snyder, ed.). Alan Liss, New York, 1989, p. 147.

65. Sarkar, N. H., Fernandes, G., Telang, N. T., Kourides, I. A., and Good, R. A.: *Proc. Natl. Acad. Sci. U.S.A.* **79**, 7758 (1982).
66. Pegram, R. A., Allaben, W. T., and Chou, M. W.: *Mech. Aging Dev.* **48**, 167 (1989)
67. Nakamura, K. D., Duffy, P. H., Lu, M. H., Turturro, A., and Hart, R. W.: *Mech. Aging Dev.* **48**, 199 (1989).
68. Ruggeri, B. A., Klurfeld, D. M., and Kritchevsky, D.: *Biochim. Biophys. Acta* **929**, 239 (1987).
69. Ruggeri, B. A., Klurfeld, D. M., Kritchevsky, D., and Furlanetto, R. W.: *Cancer Res.* **49**, 4130 (1989).
70. Harmon, J. T., and Hilf, R.: Insulin and Mammary Cancer. *In* "Influence of Hormones in Tumor Development" (J. A. Kellen and R. Hilf, eds.), Vol. 2. CRC Press, Boca Raton, Florida, 1979, p. 111.
71. Shamay, A., and Gerther, A.: *Cell. Biol. Int. Rep.* **10**, 923 (1986).
72. Grant, D., Hambly, J., Becker, D., and Pimstone, B.: *Arch. Dis. Childhood* **45**, 596 (1973).
73. Heuson, J. C., and Legros, N.: *Cancer Res.* **32**, 226 (1972).
74. Boissonneault, G. A.: Calories and Carcinogenesis — Modulation by Growth Factors. *In* "Nutrition, Toxicity and Cancer" (I. R. Rowland, ed.). CRC Press, Boca Raton, Florida, 1991, p. 413.
75. Browning, J. D., Reeves, P. G., and O'Dell, B. L.: *J. Nutr.* **113**, 755 (1983).
76. Levine, L.: *Adv. Cancer Res.* **35**, 49 (1981).
77. Carter, C. A., Milholland, R. J., Shea, W., and Ip, M. M.: *Cancer Res.* **43**, 3559 (1983).
78. Pillard, M., and Luckert, P. H.: *J. Natl. Cancer Inst.* **70**, 1103 (1983).
79. Rubio, C. A.: *J. Natl. Cancer Inst.* **72**, 705 (1984).
80. Loeb, L., Suntzeff, V., Blumenthal, H. T., and Kirtz, M. M.: *Arch. Pathol.* **33**, 845 (1942).
81. Waxler, S. H., Tabar, P., and Melcher, L. R.: *Cancer Res.* **13**, 276 (1953).
82. Waxler, S. H.: *J. Natl. Cancer Inst.* **14**, 1253 (1954).
83. Sonnenschein, E. G., Glickman, L. T., Goldschmidt, M. H., and McKee, L. J.: *Am. J. Epidemiol.* **133**, 694 (1991).
84. Hoffman, F. L.: "The Mortality from Cancer Throughout the World". Prudential, Newark, New Jersey, 1915.
85. Hoffman, F. L.: "Cancer Increase and Overnutrition". Prudential, Newark, New Jersey, 1927.
86. Berg, J. W.: *Cancer Res.* **35**, 3345 (1975).
87. Staszewski, J.: *J. Natl. Cancer Inst.* **47**, 935 (1971).
88. Apter, D., and Vihko, R.: *J. Clin. Endocrinol. Metab.* **57**, 82 (1983).
89. Albanes, D., and Taylor, P. R.: *Nutr. Cancer* **14**, 69 (1990).
90. Albanes, D.: *Nutr. Cancer* **9**, 1997 (1987).
91. DeWaard, F.: *Cancer Res.* **35**, 3351 (1975).
92. Nomura, A., Heilbrun, L. K., and Stemmerman, G. N.: *J. Natl. Cancer Inst.* **74**, 319 (1985).
93. Hebert, J. R., Augustine, A., Barone, J., Kabat, G. C., Kinne, D. W., and Wynder, E. L.: *Int. J. Cancer* **42**, 315 (1988).
94. Le Marchand, L., Kolonel, L. N., Earle, M. J., and Mi, M-P.: *Am. J. Epidemiol.* **128**, 137 (1988).
95. Vatten, L. J., and Kvinnsland, S.: *Br. J. Cancer* **61**, 881 (1990).
96. Lew, E. A., and Garfinkel, L.: *J. Chronic Dis.* **32**, 563 (1979).
97. Garfinkel, L.: *Ann. Intern. Med.* **103**, 1034 (1985).
98. Jain, M., Cook, G. M., Davis, F. G., Grace, M. G., Howe, G. R., and Miller, A. B.: *Int. J. Cancer* **26**, 757 (1980)
99. Bristol, J. B., Emmett, P. M. Heaton, K. W., and Williamson, R. C. N.: *Br. Med. J.* **291**, 1467 (1985).
100. McMichael, A. J., and Potter, J. D.: *Natl. Cancer Inst. Monogr.* **69**, 223 (1985).
101. Lyon, J. L., Mahoney, A. W., West, D. W., Gardner, J. W., Smith, K. R., Sorenson, A. W., and Stanish, W.: *J. Natl. Cancer Inst.* **78**, 853 (1987).
102. Sivertsen, I., and Dahlstrom, A. W.: *Am. J. Cancer* **6**, 365 (1921).
103. Frisch, R. E., Wyshak, G., Albright, N. L., Albright, T. E., Schiff, I., Jones, K. P., Witschi, J., Shiang, E., Koff, E., and Marguglio, M.: *Br. J. Cancer* **52**, 885 (1985).
104. Gerhardsson, M., Floderus, B., and Norell, S. E.: *Int. J. Epidemiol.* **17**, 743 (1988).
105. Ballard-Barbash, R., Schatzkin, A., Albanes, D., Schiffman, M. H., Kreger, B. E., Kannel, W. B., Anderson, K. M., and Helsel, W. E.: *Cancer Res.* **50**, 3610 (1990).
106. Garabrant, D. H., Peters, J. M., Mack, T. M., and Bernstein, L.: *Am. J. Epidemiol.* **119**, 1005 (1984).
107. Vena, J. E., Graham, S., Zielezny, M., Swanson, M. K., Barnes, R. E., and Nolan, J.: *Am J. Epidemiol.* **122**, 357 (1985).
108. Fredriksson, M., Bengtsson, N. O., Hardell, L., and Axelson, O.: *Cancer* **63**, 1838 (1989).
109. Le Marchand, L., Kolonel, L. N., and Yoshizawa, C. N.: *Am. J. Epidemiol.* **133**, 103 (1991).
110. Potter, V. R.: *Science* **101**, 105 (1945).

Modulation by Protein and Individual Amino Acids[1]

Erwin J. Hawrylewicz

I. INTRODUCTION

W. Roger Williams, commenting in 1908 on the relationship between excess dietary protein and growth of malignant tumors, wrote (1):

> Malignant tumors in mankind and animals consist mainly of albuminous or protein substances; and it seems not unreasonable to suppose that they may be the outcome of excess of these substances in the body and especially of such of them as serve for nuclear pabulum. When excessive quantities of such highlight stimulating forms of nutrient are ingested, by beings whose cellular metabolism is defective, I believe there may thus be excited in those parts of the body where vital processes are most active, such excessive and disorderly proliferation as may eventuate in cancer.

The relationship between protein in foods and carcinogenesis has been studied for the past half century. In 1982, the Committee on Diet, Nutrition and Cancer of the National Research Council (NRC) reviewed the literature of the relationship of nutrition and cancer and concluded (2) that

> evidence from both epidemiological and laboratory studies suggests that high protein intake may be associated with an increased risk of cancer at certain sites. Because of the relative paucity of data on protein compared to fat, and the strong correlation between the intakes of fat and protein in the U.S. diet, the committee is unable to arrive at a firm conclusion about an independent effect of protein.

The difficulty of determining a relationship between dietary protein and carcinogenesis is due to the: (a) inability of epidemiologic studies to isolate the effect of protein in a food (such as meat) from the effect of fat or from a synergistic relationship between the two; (b) limited number of animal experiments specifically designed to determine the effect of dietary protein on carcinogenesis; and (c) complexity of evaluating human protein requirements as compared to actual daily protein consumption in its relationship to carcinogenesis.

---

[1]Abbreviations used in this section are given on p. 311.

II. SOME BACKGROUND CONCEPTS

A. Dietary Protein Requirement

Magendie (3) demonstrated in France, in 1816, that dogs fed only carbohydrates and fat would die. Subsequently, Boussingault in 1830 established the nutrient value of feed materials in growing farm animals. He concluded that "the nutritious principles of plants reside in their nitrogen-containing principles" and that the nutrient value is directly related to the nitrogen concentration (4).

Von Liebig (5) concluded in 1845 that nitrogenous plant materials were not only required for muscle growth, but also through their breakdown provided energy for muscle contraction. Other organic components in foods were considered of little nutritional value. In the 1890s Atwater and Woods (6) in the U.S. Department of Agriculture (USDA) continued to advocate the utilization of protein foods as an energy source. They recommended a daily protein intake of 112 to 150 g. Based on this assumption, high levels of protein foods were consumed in the United States since the early 1900s. Gortner (7) summarized the USDA's statistics on per capita nutrient availability in the United States since 1909 (Table 1).

Klurfeld and Kritchevsky (8) noted that the average fat intake available in the U.S. diet increased by 25%, with an appropriate decrease in carbohydrate during the period from 1907 to 1974. They also noted that in the early 1900s the major carbohydrate source was complex carbohydrates derived from cereal products and potatoes, in contrast to refined sugars in the 1970s. Their analysis also revealed that protein availability did not change. However, in 1909 only 50% of dietary protein was derived from animal sources, in contrast to an estimated 66% presently. Apparently the source and type of dietary protein have changed, which could influence essential amino acid availability.

In addition to the change of source of dietary protein, the recommended requirement for dietary protein to achieve optimal growth has also changed. In 1948, the NRC (in ref. 9) recommended consumption of 3.3 g protein/kg body weight for children, which represents 13.2% of total energy intake. This number has been gradually reduced by the Food and Agriculture Organization/World Health Organization (FAO/WHO) and the NRC; in 1974 the recommendation stood at 1.35 g/kg body weight, representing 5.4% of total energy. Current recommendations for protein intake for infant formula during the postnatal period is a minimum intake of 2 g/kg/day (10,11). Current infant formulas contain a minimum of 15 g protein/l. Based on a consumption of 170 ml/kg/day it is estimated that 2.7 g of protein per kilogram per day would be consumed. Jarvenpaa *et al.* (12,13) indicated that these formulas provide significantly more protein than is required.

TABLE 1. Daily Per Capita Nutrient Availability: 1909–1974[a]

Year	Energy (kcal)	Carbohydrate (g)	Protein (g)	Fat (g)
1909	3,530	497	104	127
1920	3,290	457	93	123
1930	3,440	474	93	134
1940	3,350	429	93	143
1950	3,260	402	94	145
1960	3,140	375	95	143
1970	3,300	380	100	157
1974	3,350	388	101	158

[a]Based on U.S. Department of Agriculture statistics as summarized by W. A. Gortner [*Cancer Res.* **35**, 3246 (1975)].

Raiha (14) recommended "that current estimates for dietary protein requirement for normal term infants should be re-evaluated."

Current NRC (15) recommendation for young male adults is based on nitrogen balance studies. Short-term studies proposed a mean requirement of 0.61 g/kg/day for reference protein. A coefficient of variation was estimated to be 12.5%; accordingly, a value of 25% (2 SD) above the average requirement should meet the requirements of 97.5% of the population. Based on this assumption it is recommended that 0.75 g/kg/day (*i.e.*, 52.5 g per 70-kg person) of reference protein be consumed. Since, on the basis of protein availability information (8), the ingestion of 100 g of protein by a young male is conceivable, this would constitute large excess consumption. Thus, it appears, in retrospect, that since the turn of the century Americans have been consuming an excess of protein. Therefore, the recommendations for growing infants and adolescents need to be re-evaluated.

In the light of the NRC statement that "high protein intake may be associated with an increased cancer risk" (2), it is important to assess the significance of the epidemiologic and experimental data on dietary protein intake for cancer risk.

B. Tumor Protein Requirement

Warburg (16,17) reported in 1956 that animal and human tumors have a high rate of anaerobic glycolysis. He noted, furthermore, that the rate of anaerobic glycolysis of tumor cells is approximately identical for all tumors. However, the rate of *aerobic* glycolysis increases with the rate of growth, which is a parameter of the degree of malignancy of cancer cells.

Tessitore *et al.* (18,19) studied overall protein metabolism in the gastrocnemius muscle and liver in rats into which a fast-growing ascites hepatoma (Yoshida AH-130) has been transplanted. Early progressive atrophy developed in the muscle which was primarily due to an elevated rate of protein degradation; there was no change in anabolism. Protein synthetic rates were noted to increase in the liver, but not sufficiently to overcome the increased rate of degradation. The overall outcome was rapid body-weight loss and tissue-wasting cachexia. In contrast to the surrounding normal host tissue, tumor protein synthesis and degradation rates were increased, and they maintained a balance in spite of increased protein degradation.

Tayek *et al.* (20) have discussed protein utilization in tumors and concluded that tumors act as "nitrogen traps". Tumors have an increased requirement for protein nitrogen which may be provided by muscle wasting or diet. Many studies suggest, in fact, that hyperalimentation of tumor-bearing animals results in larger tumors and does not prolong survival as compared to protein-depleted animals (21,22).

Tumor cells grown in culture with amino acid mixtures have been used to determine the individual amino acids required for tumor growth. In addition to an increased requirement for essential amino acids, tumor cells may display an enhanced requirement for a specific amino acid, for example, the amino acid asparagine; this specific feature is important for the growth of lymphoid malignancies. It has been shown that infusion of exogeneous L-asparaginase affects T cells differently than B cells, and this feature has been exploited with some success for the therapy of leukemia.

Conversely, excess of and deprivation from methionine have been studied extensively. Relevant studies are reviewed in Section V.A.

III. EPIDEMIOLOGY

A. Breast Cancer

Carroll and Khor (23) correlated the availability of fat with breast cancer incidence in countries around the world. These results have frequently been cited as evidence that increasing dietary fat positively correlates with increasing breast cancer incidence. A related set of data has shown that a positive correlation also exists between increased dietary protein availability and increased breast cancer incidence. It was noted in the 1982 NRC report (2) that, while many epidemiologic studies exist which correlate dietary fat with cancer risk, fewer studies have examined the role of dietary protein. This difficulty is attributable in part to the complex nature of protein foods, such as meat, and to the difficulty of accurately establishing the protein content–associated cancer risk.

In 1979, Gaskill *et al.* (24) conducted a food consumption survey in four regions of the United States. Based on these data they concluded that, within the United States, age-adjusted breast cancer mortality is positively associated with the consumption of milk, butter, and total milk fat. They suggested a possibly special role for dairy products in the etiology of breast cancer. They also observed that breast cancer had only a weakly positive association with the intake of protein and total calories.

Utilizing the FAO/WHO annual estimates of food availability per person, per day, in 38 countries, Drasar and Irving (25) reported that cancer of the breast and colon are highly correlatable with the consumption of animal protein and fat. The authors suggested that the stimulation of estrogen biosynthesis, owing to high consumption of animal protein and fat, may be the basis for the elevated rate of breast cancer.

In 1987, utilizing the Japanese Vital Statistics and National Nutritional Survey Report, Kato *et al.* (26) demonstrated that a relationship exists between westernization of dietary habits and mortality from breast and ovarian cancers. Twelve geographic districts in Japan were surveyed. The data showed that with increasing population size and urbanization, the age-adjusted death rates for breast and ovarian cancer increased with increasing consumption of animal protein, fat, and western-style foods. The association of age-adjusted death rates was stronger after age 45 to 54 for both breast and ovarian cancer. These authors concluded from chronological correlation analyses that the correlation coefficients for some foods were highest when the time-lag between food intake and cancer mortality was assumed to be about 10 years. In the period from 1949 to 1984, per capita intake of meat increased 13.2 times and dairy products 30.2 times. During the same period the age-adjusted death rates for breast cancer increased 1.5 times and ovarian cancer increased 3.6 times.

In 1992, Hawrylewicz and Huang (27) completed a survey, using food balance questionnaires from Taiwan, covering the period of 1950 to 1985. These data indicate that, during this 35-year period, the availability of total protein increased by 280% to reach a level of more than 30 grams/day per individual; the major increase in dietary protein was derived however from animal products and this amounted to 400%. During this same period the availability of total dietary fat increased by 293% (currently 35% of calories) and total calories increased by 37%. These major shifts to a westernized diet occurred *after* 1975, paralleling the increased affluence of the Taiwan society. Comparing the ten most frequent types of cancers in the period 1979–1985, data from the Taiwan Department of Health indicated the greatest increase in the breast cancer rates, paralleling the increased availability of dietary animal protein and fat (Figure 1).

Among the scant studies that found no significant difference in the mean intake of animal protein and fat between cases and controls is the one by Hirohata *et al.* (28) in 1987, who conducted a case-control study in Hawaii with 183 sets (case and control) of Japanese and 161 sets of Caucasian women. There was a lack of strong association between dietary protein and fat *versus* breast cancer risk in both ethnic groups.

However, most case-control studies have documented a positive correlation between animal protein consumption and breast cancer rates. Hems (29) utilized the FAO/WHO estimates of per capita consumption of protein, fat, carbohydrates, and calories in 41 countries in the period 1964–1966. He found a positive correlation with animal protein,

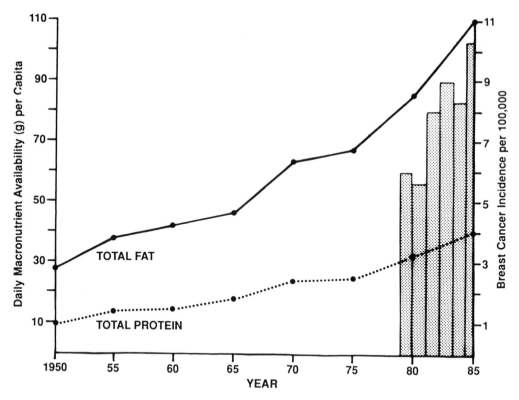

FIGURE 1.   Breast cancer incidence in Taiwan for the years 1979 through 1984, relative to macronutrient availability. *Note:* The increase in total dietary protein shown in the graph was, however, due mainly to increase in protein derived from animal products, which increase was 400% from 1950 to 1985. Adapted from E. J. Hawrylewicz and H. H. Huang [*In* "Dietary Proteins in Health and Disease" (G. Liepa, ed.), American Oil Chem. Soc., Champaign, Illinois, p. 123].

total fat, and calories *versus* breast cancer mortality rates for women during the period 1970–1971. The three components also correlate with one another very closely, and it was not possible to establish an independent or interactive role for any component. Hems (30) subsequently reported that breast cancer mortality for all women in England is associated with changes in the level of animal protein, sugar, and fat consumption that occurred 1 to 2 decades earlier. Lubin *et al.* (31) reported on 577 women with breast cancer and 826 appropriate matched controls in the period 1976–1977 in Alberta (Canada). Based on relative risks, breast cancer mortality increased with increasing consumption of animal protein (beef) and animal fat, and the relative risk was twofold higher in the high-consumption group than in the low-consumption group. Cancer incidence rates show wide variations among ethnic groups in Hawaii (Caucasians, Japanese, Chinese, Filipinos, and Hawaiians). Kolonel *et al.* (32) suggested that diet contributes to differences in cancer incidence. Utilizing an aggregate correlational analysis, they found significant positive association between dietary animal protein and saturated fat intake *versus* breast cancer incidence in postmenopausal women. Case-control studies in Israel also indicated a strong positive correlation between meat and milk consumption and breast cancer incidence (33). Recently, Toniolo *et al.* (34) reported a case-control study in Italy using data on 250 women with breast cancer and 499 controls. With the use of a dietary history questionnaire and a multivariate analysis, it was found that the relative risk for breast cancer in the highest quintile of consumption of animal protein was 2.9 and saturated fat 3.0. Differences in protein consumption were mainly due to an increased consumption of meat proteins (*not* vegetable proteins) compared to controls. A reduced risk was found for women who derived less than 9.6% of their calories from animal protein. Lubin *et al.* (35) conducted a case-control study with 818 breast cancer cases in Israel. They concluded that women in the highest quartile of animal protein and fat consumption had a risk which was about twice as high as that of women in the lowest quartile.

Case-control studies by Richardson *et al.* (36) examined the role of fat, protein, and vitamin consumption on breast cancer risk in 924 patients in France. A dietary history questionnaire, which included inquiry on 55 food items as well as on portion sizes, was used. Multivariate analysis of their data suggested that dietary fat, but not animal protein, was a risk for breast cancer.

Analyzing data on 14, 500 Norwegian women in a prospective study, Vatten *et al.* (37) found 152 cases of breast cancer in an 11- to 14-year follow-up study. A positive association was observed between the frequency of overall meat intake and breast cancer risk.

Although the very great majority of epidemiologic reports suggest an association between increased breast cancer risk and increased consumption of animal protein and fat, in the writer's view the data reported so far do not allow the identification of a clearly conclusive role for dietary protein or protein–fat interaction in the emergence of breast cancer.

B. Colon Cancer

Early nutritional surveys (25,38,39) have noted a positive correlation between the per capita consumption of animal protein and the incidence and death rate from colon cancer. Armstrong and Doll (39) determined that meat and animal protein consumption was the variable which most highly correlated with colon cancer. The excess consumption of protein and fat has its consequences on cancer incidence and on other degenerative diseases — dubbed the "diseases of affluence". Affluence seems to bring changes in the diet which include the consumption of excess animal protein. Leveille (40) calculated that protein intake in the United States — more than double the recommended dietary allowance — is clearly in excess.

The positive association of excess animal protein intake with the incidence and mortality of colon cancer is supported by case-control studies. Howell (41) noted in 1974 that beef stood out as the food item most consistently associated with colon cancer. Her correlation studies showed a positive association between colorectal cancer and animal protein and fat intake. Manousos *et al.* (42) reported the results of a case-control study consisting of 100 cases (with appropriate controls). Dietary histories on the frequency of consumption of 80 food items were obtained. On this basis they determined that the risk for developing colon cancer increases about eightfold when comparing the high-vegetable:low-meat diet *versus* high-meat:low-vegetable diet study data.

Recently, Potter and McMichael (43) conducted a case-control study in Australia on 419 patients with colon and rectal cancer, and 732 controls. They found that the most consistent risk factor for colorectal cancer was increased dietary protein, which was associated with a two- to threefold relative risk for colon cancer. Moreover, the increased risk associated with high protein and high caloric intake was confined to those consuming a low-fiber diet. The studies of Reddy *et al.* (44) and Wise *et al.* (45) showed that increased dietary protein levels are associated with elevated bacterial enzyme activities in the gastrointestinal tract, involved in the transformation of bile acids into mutagens. This may in part explain the increased risk for colon cancer associated with a high–animal protein diet.

C. Other Cancers

A limited number of case-control studies were conducted on the specific role of dietary protein as compared to a number of other food items and their relationship to other cancers. Byers *et al.* (46) concluded that there was no significant risk associated with increased consumption of total dietary protein and epithelial carcinoma of the ovary. The study included 249 cases and 505 controls. Jedrychowski *et al.* (47) reported the results from a case-control study on stomach cancer in Poland, where the risk of this disease is among the highest reported worldwide. After controlling for the effect of vegetables, salads, and fruits, they observed a positive association of increasing level of protein consumption and incidence of stomach cancer. Heshmat *et al.* (48) reported one of the first case-control studies in Afro-Americans, relating dietary protein intake to the risk of prostate cancer. They found a risk enhancement associated with increased intake of protein. They proposed that the increased dietary protein accelerated growth rates, which could affect endocrine metabolism, which in turn affects the evolution of hormone-dependent prostate cancers.

These epidemiologic studies provide strong suggestive evidence that consumption of excess dietary animal protein and protein–fat-containing or -derived products are associated with increased risk for certain cancers—namely breast, colon, and prostate cancer.

IV. ANIMAL STUDIES WITH WHOLE PROTEINS

A. Mammary Tumors

Protein synthetic rates in tumors are generally elevated compared to those of the tissue of origin. It is logical, therefore, to assume that the protein intake of the host is a significant modulating factor in tumor growth. Yet, early studies by Tannenbaum and Silverstone (49) revealed no noteworthy differences in the incidence of spontaneous mammary carcinomas in mice despite the fact that the dietary protein level varied fivefold in the study. These investigators utilized a semipurified diet, substituting vitamin-free casein for some of the cornstarch to achieve the desired protein levels. Initially, diets containing 18 or 32% casein were given *ad libitum* to young adult mice (age 9 to 16 weeks). In the preliminary phase of this study, in which a limited number of mice were used, fewer animals died with spontaneous mammary tumors in the 32% casein group than in the 18% group. The experiments were then continued with a larger number of animals per group (50 mice). The diets (9, 18, 27, 36, and 45% casein) were commenced after body growth rate decreased (13 to 14 weeks old). From the latter experiments, Tannenbaum and Silverstone concluded that the level of protein does not affect the time of appearance of the mammary tumors or the incidence. Furthermore, there appeared to be no relationship between the level of dietary protein and the incidence of lung metastases originating from the mammary tumors.

Studies conducted by Engel and Copeland (50) appeared to support *in part* the results of Tannenbaum and Silverstone (49). Engel and Copeland incorporated the carcinogen, 2-acetylaminofluorene, into base diets containing casein concentrations of 9, 20, 27, 40, and 60% which were fed to rats starting at 3 weeks of age and continued until death. Confirming the preliminary reports (51,52), the results (50) led these authors to the interpretation that a high concentration of dietary protein (60%) was protective against the induction of mammary tumors by 2-acetylaminofluorene. However, it is important to note that 8 rats among those which consumed the high-protein diet showed a 15% *loss in body weight* after as little as 16 weeks and *none* of these animals developed tumors. Among the other rats which consumed the 60% protein diet and yet *maintained a normal body weight*, the mammary tumor incidence was 83%.

In contrast to the conclusions drawn in the above studies by their respective authors, Shay *et al.* (53) found that rats fed either a 27 or 64% casein diet from 5 weeks of age on developed a slightly higher (although not significant) incidence of mammary tumors at 48 weeks of age compared to those fed a commercial cereal–fish meal diet. After a single gastric instillation of 3-methylcholanthrene, rats fed the 64% casein diet had a 19% tumor incidence compared to 9% in those fed the cereal–fish meal diet. But diets containing either 64% lactalbumin or ovalbumin caused no enhancement of 3-methylcholanthrene induction of mammary carcinomas. Hence, the authors concluded that "casein contains some factors which accelerate carcinogenesis in the breast induced with a polycyclic hydrocarbon."

Also, Nakagawa *et al.* (54) observed a positive association between increased casein intake and mammary cancer development. These investigators fed to rats diets containing casein at 10, 18, 27, and 36%, commencing 1 week after weaning. The diet with the highest protein concentration accelerated the body growth rate. At death (110 weeks) the number of spontaneous mammary tumors present and the incidence as a function of time were positively related to the level of dietary protein. This relationship was apparent in both Sprague–Dawley and Donryu rats.

Similarly, a positive association between casein intake and mammary tumor development was found by Tannenbaum and Silverstone (55) in contrast to their above-discussed earlier report (49). When mice were fed 10, 22, 34, or 46% casein diets and *food consumption was controlled to maintain equal body weights*, spontaneous mammary tumor incidence at 110 weeks of age was positively related to dietary casein levels; the tumor incidences were 45, 62, 73, and 73%, respectively.

These conflicting results and conclusions arose from the fact that the importance of several variables was not perceived in these early studies, such as: the relative amount of food consumed, the variability of natural ingredients in the diet, the extremes of dietary protein concentration, and the age at which the diet was initiated. For this reason it is difficult to interpret from these studies the role of dietary protein and its influence on chemical carcinogenesis or on the incidence of spontaneous mammary tumors.

Epidemiologic data discussed in Section III.A indicate that dietary protein, alone or in combination with fat in the form of meat or dairy products, is positively associated with increased mammary cancer incidence. Thus, to establish the role of these macronutrients also in an experimental context, Clinton *et al.* (56) attempted to determine the effects of dietary protein, and fat, and of their combination, on the initiation and progression of 7,12-dimethylbenz[*a*]anthracene (DMBA)-induced mammary cancer in the rat.

The diets were designed so that each successive increment of corn oil or casein doubled the percentage of dietary kilocalories derived from that source. Dextrin and sucrose calories were adjusted to compensate for the increased calories from protein and fat. Consequently, within a series of varying fat concentrations at a given protein concentration, the total caloric value of the diet increased by 23%. Casein, a protein complete in the essential amino acids, was used. However, since in AIN-76 diet (20% casein) the methionine concentration (0.5 g/100g diet) is marginal (57), it was supplemented with L-methionine. It is important to note that in the Clinton *et al.* (56) study, the exogenous L-methionine added to the diet (ranging from 0.15 to 0.74 g/100g diet) was directly *proportional to the casein concentration*. Thus, the total L-methionine concentration in the high-protein diet (36.9% protein) was approximately 1.92 g/100g diet (far beyond the required 0.61 g/100 g). Administration of the test diets was initiated shortly after weaning and continued throughout the experiment (30 weeks).

These feeding experiments yielded results suggesting that the concentration of dietary protein has no significant effect on the mammary tumor incidence, tumor weight, or tumor histopathology. On the other hand, the study did indicate that the incidence of mammary adenocarcinoma and adenoma is positively related to the concentration of fat (*i.e.*, corn oil) in the diet. However, data of Thompson *et al.* (58) and Kritchevsky *et al.* (59) indicate that additional calories in the high-fat diets may be as important as the fat itself for the stimulation of mammary carcinogenesis.

In order to distinguish whether or not the protein/fat diets affect mammary tumorigenesis during the initiation phase or promotion phase, Clinton *et al.* (60,61) have undertaken additional studies. In the context of the same experimental design, rats were fed the test diets from weaning until 7 weeks of age (60). At 7 weeks the rats were administered DMBA (initiation) after which all rats were switched to a standard diet, containing 16% of calories from protein and 24% from fat, for an additional 22 weeks. The results indicate that dietary protein and fat do have a significant effect on the tumor incidence. Tumor incidence was positively associated with the fat content of the diet fed during the initiation phase; diets containing 12, 24, and 48% of the calories from fat resulted in 116, 153, and 231 total number of tumors, respectively. In contrast, both the tumor incidence and the total number of palpable mammary tumors were inversely related to the protein concentration in the diet. As an example, the total number of tumors decreased from 69 to 63 to 39 in rats fed a diet with 8, 16, and 32% of calories derived from protein, respectively. In conclusion, these studies indicated that rats consuming diets with increased fat prior to carcinogen exposure (initiation) cause enhanced tumor growth, whereas increased protein in the same animal model decreased tumor load and incidence.

Subsequently, Clinton *et al.* (61) have investigated the effect of increasing dietary protein and fat *after* administration of the carcinogen—that is, in the tumorigenesis promotion phase. Using the animal model and test diets previously described—but reversing the sequence of test diet and standard diet administration—Clinton and associates have shown that at a given constant protein concentration increase of dietary fat positively affects both the tumor incidence and the total number of tumors. However, increase of dietary protein at a given constant fat concentration has no effect on these parameters. Neither was the histologic type of the tumors affected by the diet protein or fat concentration.

A mechanistic rationale for the decrease of tumor load and incidence with increased protein at the initiation stage may be derived from earlier results of Clinton *et al.* (62) that arylhydrocarbon hydroxylase activity in the liver increases with increasing dietary protein content. Based on this observation, Clinton *et al.* (60) concluded that with high-protein diet DMBA is rapidly metabolized in the liver and less of the potential carcinogen reaches the mammary gland, accounting for the decreased tumor incidence in those rats fed a high-protein diet.

At variance with the observations of Clinton and coworkers, Hawrylewicz and associates (63–67) have found a positive correlation between protein concentration in the diet and enhancement of mammary tumorigenesis (as characterized by tumor incidence and tumor histopathology). At this point it should be noted that important differences exist between the two study designs. In the studies of Hawrylewicz and his group the following experimental conditions were maintained: (a) fat concentration in the diet was fixed at 10% and protein concentration was varied; (b) all diets were isoenergetic; (c) test diets were initiated with the mother and continued with the pups, *i.e.*, a two-generation model in contrast to the postlactation, one-generation model; (d) exogenous DL-methionine was added in a fixed amount (0.3 g/100g diet) for *all* dietary protein concentrations (the importance of this aspect is further discussed in this section, below);

and (e) both an indirect-acting carcinogen (DMBA) and a direct-acting carcinogen, nitrosomethylurea (NMU), were studied.

Hawrylewicz *et al.* (63) hypothesized that increased dietary protein fed to the mother may affect neurotransmitter synthesis in the brain, causing altered hypothalamic function and pituitary regulation. Changes in pituitary hormone release may alter serum steroid hormone concentrations in the pups and influence, consequently, mammary tumor growth. To test this hypothesis, Hawrylewicz *et al.* (63) fed isoenergetic test diets containing either 8, 19.5, or 31% casein, together with 0.3% DL-methionine and 10% corn oil, to young adult female rats. The diets were continued throughout pregnancy and lactation. The female pups were continued on the same diet that was fed to their mothers (two-generation model). At 30 weeks of age, animals fed the 8% casein diet had a 28% reduction of body weight, compared to animals fed either the 19.5% or 31% casein diet. Twenty-five weeks after DMBA administration the number of mammary tumors directly correlated with the concentration of protein in the diet (Table 2). Furthermore, as Table 2 also shows, histologic examination of the tumors revealed a direct correlation between tumor grade and increased consumption of protein.

It is interesting to note that the rats fed the low-protein diet required a significantly longer period of time to reach sexual maturation, 68.6 days compared to 37.0 days for the normal protein diet (19.5% casein) group. In contrast, animals fed the high-protein diet reached sexual maturation at a significantly younger age, 30.5 days.

Low-protein diet during the development of the rat appears to affect the time of appearance of systemic regulatory mechanisms. Huang *et al.* (64) demonstrated that the development of neuroendocrine and gonadal regulation was significantly delayed in rats fed the low-protein diet. The concentration of serum prolactin and ovarian steroid hormones was significantly depressed 3 weeks after vaginal opening compared to the normal or high-protein diet groups. No significant differences in hormone concentrations were observed between the normal and high-protein diet groups.

The mammary gland is an integral part of the female reproductive system and, as such, is subject to regulation by hormones from the pituitary, gonads, and adrenal glands, in various phases of development. Following DMBA initiation the development of mammary tumors is dependent on hormone stimulation (68). Removal of ovarian

TABLE 2. **Mammary Tumor Incidence and Histopathologic Grade as a Function of Percent of Protein in Diet Fed to Rats Administered DMBA[a]**

Dietary protein	Total no. of tumors	No. of fibro-adenomas (% of total)	No. of adeno-carcinomas (% of total)	No. of Grade 1 adeno-carcinomas (% of total adeno-carcinomas)	No. of Grade 2 adeno-carcinomas (% of total adeno-carcinomas)	No. of Grade 3 adeno-carcinomas (% of total adeno-carcinomas)
8%	27	11 (41%)[b]	16 (59%)[d]	6 (38%)	8 (50%)	2 (12%)
19.5%	46	0 (0%)[c]	46 (100%)	12 (26%)	19 (41%)	15 (33%)[f]
31%	57	8 (14%)	49 (86%)	0 (0%)[e]	22 (45%)	27 (55%)[g]

[a]Adapted from E. J., Hawrylewicz, H. H., Huang, J. Q., Kissane, and E. A. Drab, [*Nutr. Rep. Int.* **26**, 793 (1982)].
[b]Significantly different from 19.5 and 31% protein diet ($p < 0.005$, $p < 0.01$, respectively).
[c]Significantly different from 31% protein diet ($p < 0.025$).
[d]Significantly different from 19.5 and 31% protein diet ($p < 0.01$, $p < 0.05$, respectively).
[e]Significantly different from 8 and 19.5% protein diet ($p < 0.01$, $p < 0.001$, respectively).
[f]Significantly different from 8% protein diet ($p < 0.05$).
[g]Significantly different from 8 and 19.5% protein diet ($p < 0.005$, $p < 0.01$, respectively).

hormones from rats by ovariectomy, *immediately after* administration of the carcinogen, inhibits the incidence of mammary tumors. However, excision of the ovaries 7 days following DMBA treatment does not prevent mammary tumor development. This would suggest that the low incidence of tumors in the low-protein group is associated in part with decreased hormonal activity. The increased incidence in the high-protein group is not explained, however, by altered neuroendocrine regulation or hormonal activity.

During the adolescent growth period the morphologic development of the mammary duct tissue is affected by the concentration of protein in the diet. Sanz *et al.* (65) showed that at 3 weeks following the age of sexual maturation, the number of terminal end buds in the developing mammary epithelial ducts was significantly reduced in the low-protein group, compared to the normal or high-protein diet groups (Figure 2). In contrast, the number of alveolar buds and lobules in the normal and high-protein groups were similar, but significantly higher than in the low-protein group. These data support the concept that hormone availability during the adolescent growth phase markedly influences the growth of mammary duct structures.

With the direct-acting carcinogen, NMU, rats maintained on high-protein–high-fat diets (two-generation model) showed an increased mammary tumor load compared to rats fed a normal-protein–high-fat diet (66). The increased tumor load was directly related to the increased level of protein in the diet, stimulated by the high fat level.

To further delineate the effect of the high-protein and normal-protein diet on the development of the mammary duct epithelium, the activity of the enzyme ornithine decarboxylase (ODC) was determined before and after exposure to NMU. Hawrylewicz *et al.* (67) reported that in the two-generation animal model a high-protein diet enhances ODC activity in the mammary epithelial tissue at 7 weeks of age, compared to those fed a normal-protein diet.

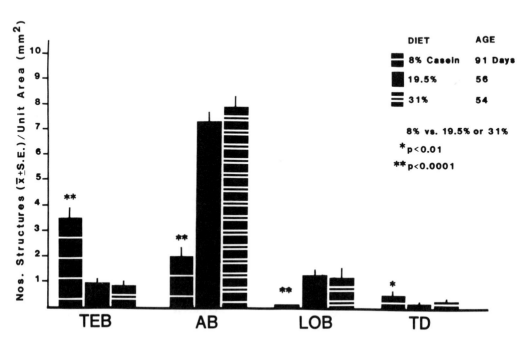

FIGURE 2.   Relative levels of morphologic structures in mammary duct tissue as a function of dietary protein in rats at sexual maturity plus 3 days. TEB = terminal end buds; AB = alveolar buds; LOB = lobules; TD = terminal ducts. Adapted from M. C. A. Sanz, J. M. Liu, H. H. Huang, and E. J. Hawrylewicz [*J. Natl. Cancer Inst.* **77,** 477 (1986)].

ODC activity in the normal protein group is increased 8 weeks following exposure to NMU, but prior to the detection of palpable tumors. Importantly, the high-protein group showed a *very marked increase* in ODC activity, significantly higher than the activity in the control group. Changing the diet from a high- to a normal-protein diet 4 weeks after exposure to NMU significantly reduces the increased level of ODC activity resulting from exposure to the carcinogen. In contrast to findings in mammary epithelial tissue, ODC activity in the liver is not affected by NMU exposure, nor did liver tumors develop under the conditions of the experiment.

Russell (69) implicated increased ODC activity as an invariant component of polyamine biosynthesis and cell proliferation. Several investigators (70–72) demonstrated that either fasting or feeding a protein-free diet, followed by refeeding casein or casein hydrolysate, caused a significant increase in ODC activity in the liver, kidney, and small intestine. These studies support the concept that the nutritional status of the animals appears to be an important factor in the regulation of ODC synthesis and cell proliferation. Specifically, the studies of Hawrylewicz *et al.* (67) would indicate that the enhanced sensitivity to a carcinogen, in response to feeding a high-protein diet during the adolescent growth phase, is related to increased mammary epithelial cell proliferation.

Casein, a protein complete in the essential amino acids, has been used extensively in dietary cancer studies. However, as has been already pointed out above in this section, in the AIN-76 (20% casein) diet, methionine concentration (0.5 g/100g diet) is marginal (57). Consequently, as discussed earlier, the AIN-76 diet should be supplemented with L-methionine, to bring the total methionine level to approximately 0.65 g L-methionine/100g diet. In the studies conducted by Hawrylewicz and coworkers (63,67), 0.15 g L-methionine per 100 g was customarily added to the normal (20%) casein and high (32%) casein diets, bringing the total L-methionine concentration to 0.65 g and 0.87 g/100g diet, respectively. This is slightly above the required 0.61 g/100 g level, but significantly less than the toxic level of 1.50 g/100g diet, as per the findings of Benevenga and Steele (73) and Harper *et al.* (74) on the toxic effects of excess methionine.

Thus, the critical difference between the experimental protocol used by the Hawrylewicz model and that used by Clinton *et al.* (56,60–62) is *the amount of methionine added to the diet*. In the Hawrylewicz protocol, a fixed amount of L-methionine (0.15 g), based on the casein level in the control diet, is added to 100 g of the test diet. In the Clinton protocol, L-methionine is increased *proportionally with* the increased amount of casein in the diet. Thus, in the high-protein diet (42%) of the Clinton protocol, supplementation of the diet with 0.74 g of L-methionine brings up the total L-methionine to the very high level of 2.01 g/100g diet.

Methionine and its metabolic derivatives are essential components in protein synthesis, polyamine synthesis, and in transmethylation reactions (75). The primary derivative of L-methionine metabolism is *S*-adenosylmethionine (Ado Met). Kramer *et al.* (76) provided substantive evidence that Ado Met is a pivotal molecule which has a determining role in cellular processes associated with initiation, maintenance, and cessation of cell growth and/or differentiation. Ado Met is the obligatory methyl donor in almost all transmethylation reactions and also has a critical role as a propylamino group donor in polyamine synthesis.

Hawrylewicz and associates have initiated studies (published in a preliminary form in 1992, *see* ref. 77) to evaluate the effects of high-protein, high-methionine diets on NMU-induced mammary tumorigenesis and on ODC and *S*-adenosylmethionine decarboxylase activities in mammary epithelial tissue and in liver. Preliminary results indicate that the tumor incidence in the high-protein diet (34%) group is significantly higher than in the normal-protein diet (19%) group: 74 and 37%, respectively. If the total L-methionine is increased in the high-protein group from 0.87 g to 1.2 g/100 g of diet, tumor incidence was decreased to 20%. In the two-generation model, excess dietary methionine repressed ODC activity in the mammary epithelial tissue and *S*-adenosylmethionine decarboxylase activity in the liver (Figures 3 and 4).

These preliminary data support the possibility that the high (probably borderline toxic) concentration of methionine in the high-protein diets used by Clinton and coworkers (56,60–62) may have contributed to the observed repression of tumor growth.

B. Colon Tumors

Several previously cited epidemiology studies (25,38–43) have shown a positive association between consumption of high-meat diets (or diets high in protein content) and the risk of developing colorectal cancer. Manousos *et al.* (42) reported that individuals consuming a high-protein, low-vegetable diet had an eightfold increase of risk of developing colon cancer, compared to individuals consuming a low-protein, high-vegetable diet.

In spite of these epidemiologic data, very few animal studies have been carried out to verify the epidemiologic observations and to provide insight into the possible metabolic basis for these findings. Visek and Clinton (78) reviewed recently the literature on the association between dietary protein and colon cancer.

Topping and Visek (79) addressed this issue experimentally with 1,2-dimethyl-hydrazine (DMH)-induced colon cancer in rats. Weanling rats were fed isocaloric diets containing either 7.5, 15, or 22.5% casein. Groups of animals were also fed identical diets which were supplemented with 2.5% urea (urea was added to the diets to provide a

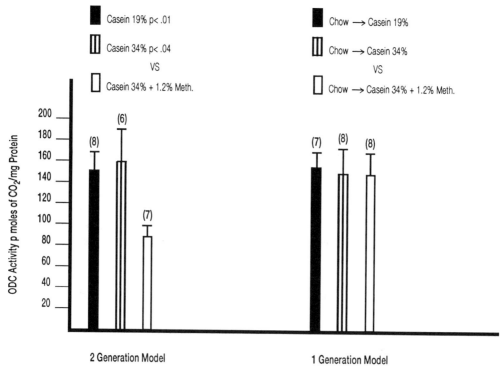

FIGURE 3. Ornithine decarboxylase (ODC) activity in mammary epithelial tissue of rats maintained on normal protein (19% casein) diet and high-protein (34% casein) diet with and without excess dietary methionine (meth.). The number of animals is given in ( ); T = S.E.

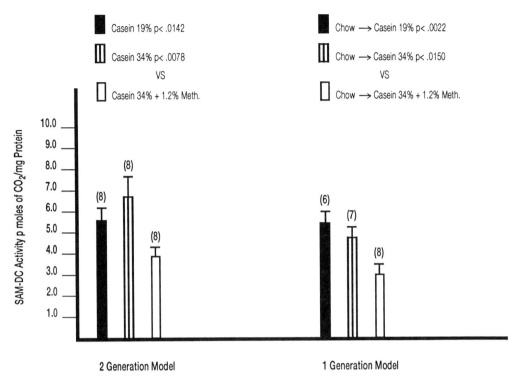

FIGURE 4.   *S*-Adenosylmethionine decarboxylase (SAM-DC) activity in the liver of rats maintained on normal protein (19% casein) diet and high-protein (34% casein) diet with or without excess dietary methionine (meth.). The number of animals is given in ( ); **T** = S.E.

substrate for release of ammonia in the colon). The rationale for urea incorporation into the diet was based on the observation of Weisburger *et al.* (80), which implicated intracellular ammonia as a carcinogenesis-enhancing chemical. Animals were given weekly intraperitoneal injections of DMH (15 mg/kg body weight) for 24 weeks. After 28 weeks, the animals fed the 15 and 22.5% protein diets had a greater number of tumors classified as adenocarcinoma in the small and large intestines, compared to those fed a 7.5% protein diet. In addition, it was observed that keratin-producing papillomas of the sebaceous glands of the external ear arose in some rats in all DMH-treated groups; the number of ear tumor–bearers was highest in the 22.5% protein group.

Animals fed the 7.5% protein diet gained less weight and, consequently, the dose of DMH received was less (by 15%) after 24 weeks of DMH injections. Nonetheless, Topping and Visek (79) concluded that the differences in the number and size of tumors between the low and higher protein groups is too great to be based solely on DMH dosage.

Addition of urea to the diet does not change the pH, urease activity, and ammonia concentration in the cecum and the colon. It was documented that supplementation of diets with urea has no effect on tumor incidence. Yet a significant increase in cecal and (to a lesser degree) colon ammonia concentration was measured as dietary protein concentration was increased. The study of Weisburger *et al.* (80) suggests that the association of increased intestinal tumors with increased dietary protein might be ascribed to increased ammonia in the intestinal mucosa. However, Topping and Visek (79) expressed reservations regarding the possible role of the nitrogen pool, in this form, in the enhancement of carcinogenesis.

To elucidate the mechanism by which increased dietary protein content enhances DMH tumorigenesis in the rat colon, Kari *et al.* (81) studied the metabolic activation of

DMH. DMH is a procarcinogen which yields the active metabolic intermediate, methyl-carbonium ion. The postulated pathway involves the formation, successively, of azomethane (AM), azoxymethane (AOM) and methylazoxymethanol (MAM). Mice (C57Bl/6 × C3H)F1 were placed on the test diets (2.5, 5, 10, 20, and 40% protein) at 21 to 24 days of age and the diet was continued for an additional 14 days. Two independent methods were used to determine the *in vivo* metabolism of DMH as a function of dietary protein concentration. One measured AM and carbon dioxide derived from DMH via the AOM pathway and the other measured host-mediated mutagenic activity. Mice fed the low-protein diet (2.5% casein) and given [^{14}C]DMH expired more $^{14}CO_2$ from labeled DMH than animals fed the 40% protein diet. Retained metabolites were two- to threefold greater in the 10 and 40% protein groups compared with the low-protein group. The mutagenicity assay also showed a greater loss of the AM and CO_2 in the low-protein group. It was hypothesized that low-protein diets decreased the conversion of AOM to MAM, accounting for the observed decrease of mutagenicity and tumorigenicity at low protein concentrations.

Siegler and Kazarinoff (82,83) investigated whether or not ODC activity was altered in the colon as a consequence of a change in protein level in the diet. ODC catalyzes the rate-limiting step in the biosynthesis of polyamines (84), which is important in tissue proliferation (85). Increase in ODC activity has been associated with tumorigenesis, especially with the promotional phase (86).

In the experimental protocol of Siegler and Kazarinoff (82,83), rats were acutely deprived of dietary protein. Acute deprivation was achieved in rats by feeding either 1 or 5% casein diet or 20% casein diet pair-fed to the 1% group. Animals were sacrificed on day 0 and every 2 days thereafter. Surprisingly, the animals fed the 1% casein diet had significantly greater ODC activity in the colon than either animals from the 20% casein diet pair-fed groups or from the 20 or 5% groups fed *ad libitum*. Feeding either 5 or 20% casein diet for 10 days to adult male rats had no effect on the basal level of colonic ODC activity. Sodium deoxycholate, a promoter of colon carcinogenesis, was used to induce colonic ODC. Induced colonic ODC activity was significantly greater in the 5% protein group compared to the 20% protein group.

Reddy *et al.* (87) studied the effect of protein- and fat-enriched diets on DMH-induced colon carcinogenesis in the rat. The high-protein, high-fat diets were composed of either 40% soybean protein and 20% corn oil or 40% beef protein and 5% corn oil plus beef fat. The control diets contained either 20% soybean protein and 5% corn oil or 25% beef protein and no additional oil. Animals were injected weekly for 20 weeks and sacrificed 10 weeks later. Animals fed diets with a high level of soybean or beef protein and fat had a significantly higher incidence and total tumor load of colonic tumors (classified as adenocarcinomas) compared to those animals fed the lower protein and fat control diets. Tumor multiplicity for adenomas was similar in all groups. The authors concluded from these studies that diets with high levels of protein and fat enhanced DMH colon carcinogenesis, and furthermore, that the source of protein (vegetable or meat) had no major influence on the incidence of colon tumors. Reddy *et al.* (88) also reported that increasing either corn oil or lard content in the diet from 5 to 20% enhanced colon tumor incidence.

In a similar study, Clinton *et al.* (89) compared the effect of diets containing either 20% soybean protein plus methionine, 20% raw beef protein, or charcoal-broiled beef protein on the growth of DMH-induced colon tumors. All three diets contained a high level of beef tallow (20%). Tumor incidence and total tumor load was similar in all three groups. Clinton *et al.* (89) concluded that the source of protein or the added risk from carcinogens in charcoal-broiled beef did not modify DMH-induced colon cancer incidence. These conclusions are similar to those of Reddy summarized above.

The studies by Reddy *et al.* (87) and Clinton *et al.* (89) were designed to assess the effect of protein concentration and source on colon carcinogenesis; however, these diets were formulated at a high fat concentration of 20%. The enhanced effect on DMH-induced colon carcinogenesis resulting from an enriched fat diet could obviate any effect from the enriched protein diet or source of protein. Similarly, the effect of increased dietary fat and protein on NMU-induced mammary carcinogenesis in rats was studied by Hawrylewicz and associates. These investigators found that rats fed a 20% corn oil diet containing either 19 or 33% casein had similar tumor incidences. In contrast, rats fed diets containing 5% corn oil had significantly increased mammary tumor incidence and number of tumors per tumor-bearing animal when the protein content was increased from 19 to 33% casein (90). Additional studies varying only the protein (and not the fat) will be needed before conclusions can be reached on the effect of either the source of protein or the quantity of protein on DMH-induced colon carcinogenesis.

The colonic ODC activity data stand in marked contrast to the induction of this activity in mammary epithelial tissue. From the results of Hawrylewicz *et al.*, (67), an enriched protein diet (32%) increases ODC activity in the mammary epithelial tissue of young female rats, compared to rats fed a 20% protein diet. Treatment with NMU caused, in the high-protein group, a marked increase of ODC activity in the mammary epithelium prior to the appearance of tumors. Increased ODC activity directly paralleled the increased mammary tumor incidence.

C. Liver Tumors

The effect of dietary protein on liver carcinogenesis has been primarily focused on the hepatotoxin, aflatoxin. In many areas of the world, aflatoxins cause liver injury and have been associated with human liver cancer (91,92). Madhavan *et al.* (93) suggested that individuals in many areas of the world affected by *Aspergillus flavus* contamination are also at high risk for malnutrition, principally protein deficiency.

Subsequently, Madhavan and Gopalan (94) examined the relationship between dietary protein intake and the susceptibility of monkeys to aflatoxin injury. Young rhesus monkeys, male and female, were fed either a 1 or 16% casein diet which also contained wheat flour. Aflatoxin was administered at either 500 or 100 μg/day. Significant liver injury (fatty livers and biliary fibrosis) was induced in the monkeys subsisting on the low-protein diet and exposed to the low dose of aflatoxin for 2 to 4 weeks. Monkeys consuming the high-protein diet and exposed to the low dose of aflatoxin remained apparently healthy.

At the higher dose of 500μg, monkeys in both dietary groups died within 4 weeks. The authors estimated that 2 ppm would be sufficient to produce liver damage. Madhavan and Gopalan (95) further investigated the toxic and hepatocarcinogenic properties of aflatoxin in the rat. As reported in the studies on monkeys, rats maintained on a low 4% protein diet plus 50 μg of aflatoxin per day developed extensive liver abnormalities after as little as 20 days of feeding. The lesions included heavy fatty infiltration, bile duct proliferation, and periductal fibrosis. The histologic appearance of livers in the high-protein (20%) diet group was markedly different. The vast majority of liver cells were swollen and exhibited a peculiar vacuolation. The nuclei appeared pycnotic. Atypical liver cells with large nuclei, which were vesicular and occasionally contained prominent nuclei, were also present. These cells were considered as possibly precancerous. It was concluded that the rat liver is increasingly susceptible to the hepatotoxic effect of aflatoxin in protein deficiency.

Regarding the question of the relationship between carcinogenesis and aflatoxin exposure *versus* the amount of protein consumed, Madhavan and Gopalan (95) determined that 50% of the rats fed the 20% casein diet and exposed to aflatoxin developed hepatomas or tumors in other organs. The remaining animals showed only precancerous lesions. In contrast, none of the animals fed the 5% casein diet developed tumors or precancerous lesions in the liver. The results of these experiments indicate that increased protein consumption increased the formation of hepatocarcinoma.

Studies by Wells *et al.* (96) support the above data on the increased tumorigenic response to aflatoxin as a function of increased dietary protein. These investigators fed weanling rats diets containing either 8, 22, or 30% casein with aflatoxin B$_1$ at 1.7 ppm. In addition, half of the animals also received supplemental cystine (0.6%) in the diet. The aflatoxin regimen continued for 3 months and the animals were observed for an additional 9 months. Weight gain was markedly decreased and liver weights increased in response to aflatoxin in all groups except the low-protein group. No tumors were found in the livers of the low-protein group. In the other groups the extent of liver involvement increased with increasing protein concentration in the diet. Of significance is the observation that cystine supplementation accelerated the emergence of liver tumors. The incidence was higher in the high-protein than in the low-protein group. This effect of the sulfur amino acid–deficient diet further supports the observations described for unsupplemented soybean protein and its effect on mammary tumorigenesis.

Prince and Campbell (97) observed that the risk of aflatoxin-induced hepatocarcinoma is greater in males than in females. They also confirmed that the incidence of hepatocarcinomas was higher in the high-protein than in the low-protein diet groups. For elucidating the biological mechanism which might explain these differences in tumorigenicity, male and female rats were fed either a 5 or 20% casein diet for 6 weeks, then injected with [^{3}H]aflatoxin B$_1$ and killed 2 h later. The authors found that sex difference and protein intake altered several parameters of aflatoxin binding to the histone and nonhistone fractions extracted from liver chromatin, in a manner consistent with their effect on tumor incidence. The binding of aflatoxin to chromatin proteins was more influenced by the level of dietary protein than by the sex of the animal.

Further studies by Appleton and Campbell (98) support the positive relationship between increased dietary protein intake during the tumor promotion phase and aflatoxin-induced tumorigenesis. Increased γ-glutamyl transferase (GGT)-positive areas in liver sections have been associated with preneoplastic nodules and hepatocarcinoma in aflatoxin-treated rats (99). These studies found that the number of GGT lesions in the liver was decreased by 75% in the rats fed 5% casein diet during the promotional phase (following the aflatoxin exposure), compared to the 20% casein group. However, there was no further increase in GGT foci when the dietary protein level was increased from 20 to 40%. Changing from a 5 to a 20% protein diet in the mid/post-dosing period caused an increase in the number of GGT foci from the 5% up to the 20% casein group (100). The data show that the development of the preneoplastic GGT foci in the liver is modulated by dietary protein levels.

Appleton and Campbell (101) have also established that rats fed the low-protein (5% casein) diet during the aflatoxin dosing period developed a characteristic spectrum of hepatotoxicities, including hepatomegaly, severe bile duct proliferation, and cholangiofibrosis. Conversely, animals fed the 20% diet experienced only mild bile duct proliferation. In the post-dosing period, increased consumption of dietary protein significantly increased (sixfold) the number of GGT foci, regardless of the level of dietary protein fed during the initiation period. Increased dietary protein in the post-initiation period positively increased the number of precancerous GGT lesions.

Continuing these studies, Dunaif and Campbell (102) administered by oral gavage aflatoxin B$_1$ in daily doses of 235, 250, 270, 300, and 350 μg/kg/day for ten doses. Dietary protein levels of 4, 8, 12, 16, and 20% casein were fed in the post-dosing period. Based on the number of GGT foci developed, it was concluded that the nutrient intake during the post-dosing GGT foci development period is more rate limiting than is the carcinogen dose. A decreased number of foci developed in the low-protein group, even with an increased caloric consumption per 100 g body weight (103).

The growth sensitivity of the GGT foci as a function of dietary protein levels during the post-dosing period was also shown by the continuing studies of Youngman and Campbell (104). Following dosing with aflatoxin the rats were fed either a 5 or a 20% casein diet. Diets were switched every 3 weeks for a total of 12 weeks. Switching from 20 to 5% casein resulted in marked remodeling (regression) of the growing lesions to a response level similar to that in animals not receiving the initial promotional stimulus from the high-protein feeding. Refeeding the high protein caused the appearance of a significant number of additional foci. These studies uniquely illustrate the extreme sensitivity and positive response of developing precancerous GGT foci in the liver to increasing levels of dietary protein.

D. Pancreatic Tumors

As noted by Pour *et al.* (105), the pancreas is a dynamic organ actively involved in the synthesis of large amounts of protein (digestive enzyme), which is secreted through the pancreatic juice that can amount to a liter per day (106). Wynder *et al.* (107) reported a positive association between meat consumption and pancreatic cancer. However, from this study it is difficult to establish the independent contribution of fat or protein to the development of pancreatic cancer.

Since there is a significant reduction of nuclear DNA level in dietary protein deficiency, the hypothesis may be advanced that since decreased DNA concentration is expected to correlate positively with decreased incidence of cancer, dietary protein deficiency would delay/inhibit the emergence of pancreatic cancer. To test this hypothesis, Pour *et al.* (105) conducted studies to determine the effect of a purified protein-free diet on the development of N-nitrosobis(2-oxopropyl)amine (BOP)-induced pancreatic cancer in hamsters. The effect of feeding the protein-free diet for 4 weeks before, during, or after treatment with the carcinogen, BOP, was studied. After 4 weeks on the protein-free diet all animals were fed commercial chow for approximately 1 year. Regardless of when the protein-free diet was fed during the initiation period, there was a significant decrease in the incidence and number of pancreatic tumors (adenomas and carcinomas) at termination.

To gain further insight into the nature of the association between the level of dietary protein and induction of pancreatic cancer, Pour and Birt (108) fed three different levels of protein prior to or following BOP injection. Hamsters were fed either a 9% (low) or 36% (high) casein diet from 3 to 7 weeks of age, followed by BOP treatment at 8 weeks of age. The hamsters were then fed either a low- or a high-protein diet until termination. It was found that the high-protein diet enhanced, but the low-protein diet inhibited the development of pancreatic tumors in female hamsters. The tumor incidence was not, however, significantly affected by dietary protein levels in males. The data provide additional support for the thesis that the level of dietary protein influences tumor initiation and development. However, the reason for the sex difference in response between female and male hamsters was not apparent.

2-Hydroxypropyl-2-oxopropylnitrosamine (HPOP), a common metabolite of the pancreatic carcinogen, BOP, was evaluated for the induction of pancreatic lesions using the constant infusion procedure of Kokkinakis and Scarpelli (109). They found that a continuous infusion of HPOP for 1 week (total dose of 220–250 mg/kg) into Syrian hamsters induced ductal adenocarcinomas (41%) in the pancreas and cholangiomas (18%) and cholangiocarcinomas (18%) in the liver 25 weeks after the initiation of treatment. To determine the effect of dietary protein as a modifying factor in HPOP-induced pancreatic carcinogenesis, animals were fed either a high-protein (20% casein) or a low-protein (8% casein) diet. The diet was fed for a period of 10 to 15 days until the hamsters reached a body weight of 85 to 90 g. The animals were then treated with HPOP, by the method stated above, and the diet continued for an additional 10 days. All the animals were fed regular chow for the remaining 25 weeks. As in the experiments of Pour and coworkers (105,108), the animals on the high-protein diet developed ductal adenocarcinomas more frequently and had three times as many pancreatic preneoplastic lesions than the animals fed the low-protein diet prior to and post-treatment with HPOP. In the animals fed the low-protein diet, hepatic cytochrome P-450 activity dropped sharply. Glucuronidation of HPOP increased as the levels of dietary protein decreased, while sulfation followed an opposite pattern.

The basis for the increased carcinogenic effectiveness of HPOP in the high-protein group has not been elucidated. Changes in cytochrome P-450 activity in the liver and a pronounced effect on the pathways of detoxification, as a function of the dietary protein level, may contribute to the observed differences in tumor susceptibility.

E. Kidney Tumors

Early studies by Magee and Barnes (110) demonstrated that a single dose (30 mg/kg) of dimethylnitrosamine (DMN) causes acute liver damage and leads to the development of kidney tumors in 20% of the surviving animals. Subsequently, McLean and McLean (111) found that feeding a protein-free diet protects against the lethal and hepatotoxic effects of carbon tetrachloride and of DMN. The decreased toxicity was correlated with a 60% reduction in DMN metabolism in liver slices from protein-deficient rats. In contrast, metabolism by kidney slices was unaffected by protein deficiency (112). They have also observed that, in the rats fed the protein-free diet, methylation of kidney DNA and RNA was three times higher. Magee and Swann (113) concluded that the possible mechanism of protection against liver damage is the decreased metabolic activation of DMN to a toxic alkylating intermediate, because of depressed enzyme systems in the liver of protein-deficient rats.

To test this hypothesis, rats were fed a protein-free diet for 7 days before, and 7 days after, treatment with a single dose of DMN followed by chow diet. Surviving rats had a significantly greater number of renal tumors compared to the saline-treated controls (114). The decreased metabolism by the liver rendered more carcinogen available to kidney tissue, which was unaffected by the protein diet. Consequently, an increased kidney tumor incidence resulted.

In a similar study by Hard and Butler (115), rats maintained on protein-free diet developed renal tumors in 89% of the animals, compared to 35% of the animals fed a protein-supplemented diet. The kidney tumors arose from mesenchymal elements within the cortical intertubular spaces near the glomeruli.

To elucidate the effect of the protein-free diet on the metabolism of DMN, Swann and McLean (116) fed either a protein-free diet or commercial chow diet for 7 days. As noted previously, metabolism of DMN was reduced by 55% in liver slices in the protein-free group, but kidney slices continued to metabolize the carcinogen at the same rate as kidney slices from rats fed chow diet. Importantly, methylation by DMN of the N-7 position in guanine in liver RNA and DNA in rats fed a protein-free diet was similar to the chow diet group. In contrast, the methylation of guanine in kidney nucleic acids was threefold greater in the protein-free group. The increased methylation of kidney RNA and DNA directly paralleled the increased kidney tumor incidence.

F. Pituitary Tumors

In an interesting series of experiments, Ross and associates (117) fed diets containing either 10, 22, or 51% casein diets to rats, from weaning until death. The animals were fed either *ad libitum* or received restricted, but isocaloric amounts. The three diets differed only in the protein–calorie ratio. The data were evaluated to determine the relationship of the dietary protein consumed, total calories consumed, and weight gained at various ages, to the incidence of spontaneous tumors of the pituitary gland.

Five times as many chromophobe adenomas were found in the *ad libitum*-fed rats compared to the same diets fed in restricted and isocaloric amounts. In the *ad libitum*-fed animals, the largest number of tumors occurred in the diet group containing 22% protein, and the smallest number in the low-protein group. In the restricted group the number of spontaneous tumors was positively related to the protein level in the diet. There was twice the number of tumors in the high-protein compared to the normal-protein group and a threefold increase over the low-protein group. In the *ad libitum*-fed group the tumor incidence was not related to the level of dietary protein, but rather to the amount of food consumed.

To determine the dietary condition associated with the spontaneous occurrence of anterior pituitary gland tumors, rats were permitted freedom of dietary choice throughout life. The animals were allowed to regulate their protein intake independently from calorie intake. Ross *et al.* (118) reported that an unusually high growth rate, together with a high level of conversion of the food consumed into body mass during early life, was conducive to a high probability of spontaneous pituitary tumor emergence. In addition, a high intake of protein relative to body weight during early adult life was also associated with increased tumor incidence. They concluded that protein overnutrition was a risk factor for developing spontaneous pituitary tumors. It would appear that a high protein intake over body weight ratio before 15 weeks of age, followed by a low protein intake, enhanced pituitary tumor development. This study emphasized the importance of diet during the period of rapid body growth on the development of tumors later in adult life.

G. Tumors in Other Organs

In the United States, lung cancer remains the most prevalent cancer in males and females. Comparing the period of 1955–57 to 1985–87, age-adjusted lung cancer death rate increased by 131 and 420% in males and females, respectively (119). The estimated total number of deaths from lung cancer in 1991 was 143,000. Epidemiologic studies suggest that ingestion of foods rich in β-carotene can reduce the risk for developing lung cancer. However, there appears to be no information on the association between the quality of macronutrients in general and their effect on lung cancer incidence or progression. A single animal study has examined the effect of the level of dietary protein consumed on the incidence of DMBA-induced lung cancer (120). Mice were injected with DMBA shortly after birth and were fed either a high-protein (25%) or a 15% (later lowered to 10%) casein diet. All of the animals in the high-protein group developed lung tumors, compared to a 36% lung cancer incidence in the low-protein group. The average number of tumors per tumor-bearing animal was similar. The authors stated that it was not possible to make a sharp distinction between benign and malignant tumors; the histological sections showed a gradation from one type to another.

No further studies are available in the literature since this early 1964 report. Considering the magnitude of the lung cancer problem, additional studies determining the relationship between macronutrient intake and lung cancer incidence and progression are emphatically warranted.

There is a significantly higher incidence of and mortality from cancer of the stomach in China compared to the United States. Hu *et al.* (121) conducted a case-control study on 241 patients, using an equal number of controls, in the northeastern province of Heilongjiang, in which they focused on the role of single food items and their possible association with stomach cancer. An inverse association between the consumption of vegetables and stomach cancer was observed. In contrast, high consumption of potatoes and of salted and fermented soy paste appeared to be high-risk factors. Chinese cabbage appears to play an important role in reducing the risk of developing stomach cancer. This epidemiologic study did not identify any macronutrient as a risk factor.

The effect of feeding a low-protein diet to rats on the incidence and number of gastric tumors induced by *N*-methyl-*N'*-nitro-*N*-nitrosoguanidine (MNNG) was investigated by Tatsuta *et al.* (122). The experiment was designed to study the effect of protein level on the promotion phase of carcinogenesis by MNNG. The test animals were given drinking water for 20 weeks containing MNNG. The animals were then given normal tap water and divided into three diet groups: 25% (normal), 10% (low), and 5% (very low) casein diet; the diet was continued for 32 weeks.

The animals that were fed the *very low* (5%) casein diet had a fourfold increase in the incidence of gastric cancer compared to either the low- or the high-protein groups. The latter two groups had essentially the same incidence. There was no significant difference in the histologic types of adenocarcinomas in the three groups. Tatsuta *et al.* (122) have stated on this basis that populations on poor diets high in carbohydrate and low in protein are at a high risk for developing stomach cancer.

Earlier studies by Tatsuta *et al.* (123) established that, following treatment with MNNG, prolonged administration of a monoamine oxidase inhibitor (nialamide) resulted in a significant increase in norepinephrine concentration in the gastric wall and in the incidence of gastric cancers in Wistar rats. On the basis of the suggestion made (124) that compounds which stimulate the sympathetic nervous system enhance carcinogenesis, Tatsuta and coworkers (122) concluded in their study that the very low-protein diet caused a stimulation of the sympathetic nervous system and this, in turn, led to an enhancement of gastric carcinogenesis.

V. EFFECT OF INDIVIDUAL DIETARY AMINO ACIDS ON CARCINOGENESIS

A. Methionine

The key role of Ado Met, the metabolically generated derivative of L-methionine, has been briefly pointed out above in Section IV, A.

When rats were maintained on a diet containing 1.9 g of L-methionine (an over 200% excess), increased concentrations of Ado Met, *S*-adenosylhomocysteine, and betaine were found in the liver (74,125). Feeding a casein diet with excess L-methionine (1.5 g/100 g) to adult rats for 14 days caused significant increase in Ado Met and *S*-adenosyl-homocysteine concentrations and in methionine adenosyltransferase activity in the liver (126). Excess amount of *S*-adenosylhomocysteine is known to be a potent inhibitor of most Ado Met–dependent transmethylation reactions (75) and, under the experimental conditions of Smith *et al.* (126), spermine synthetase activity in the liver was decreased. Thus, the results suggest that elevated dietary levels of L-methionine can adversely affect transmethylation reactions and polyamine synthesis. Conversely, the rapid depletion of Ado Met pools results in an immediate decrease in methyltransfer reactions involving nucleic acids, whereas biosynthesis of polyamines appears to be only minimally affected (due to increase in ODC activity). This is shown by the results of Kramer *et al.* (76) who, using a methionine-analog inhibitor of *S*-adenosylmethionine synthetase, found rapid depletion of Ado Met in cultured L-1210 cells. Under the same experimental conditions, putrescine pools increased threefold, accompanied by a two- to fourfold increase in ODC activity. These studies illustrate the importance of the level of dietary L-methionine on the synthesis of Ado Met and its effect on the interdependent transmethylation and polyamine metabolic pathways.

The data available at present allow no definitive conclusions regarding the effect of L-methionine on the rate of appearance and incidence of tumors. Depending on the experimental design, deficiency or excess of L-methionine may enhance or inhibit carcinogenesis. The review of the data below illustrates this point.

According to one perspective, since site-specific DNA methylation has a strong "silencing" effect on genes, disruption of this cellular process should activate or potentiate gene expression (127).

In accordance with this view are the observations of Bhave *et al.* (128), Feo *et al.* (129), and Hoffman (127) that diets deficient in methionine result in hypomethylation of DNA, and this leads to enhancement of hepatocarcinogenesis. Similarly, in the long-term (13 to 24 months) feeding studies of Ghoshal and Farber (130) with methionine-choline–deficient diets, a 100% incidence of putative preneoplastic hepatocyte nodules and a 51% incidence of true hepatocellular carcinomas were obtained. In line with these reports are the preliminary data of Anisimov *et al.* (131) that excess dietary methionine lowers the incidence of mammary tumors induced by either DMBA or NMU. Also, Huang *et al.* (77) have shown that ingestion of *excess methionine* delays the appearance of NMU-induced mammary tumors and lowers the tumor incidence. This study prompted the inclusion of 0.3% DL-methionine into the AIN-76 standard casein diet (containing 20% casein), so as to bring the total L-methionine concentration to the required level of 0.61 g/100 g diet. In this study (77) the AIN-76 was compared to either a protein-enriched diet (34% casein and 0.3% DL-methionine) or to a protein-enriched diet containing excess methionine (1.2% DL-methionine). These diets were fed to virgin female rats prior to mating and continued through the pregnancy and lactation periods. The female pups were continued on the diets fed to their mothers. Following injection of NMU (40 mg/kg body weight at 7 weeks of age) the animals were observed for 8 months. As previously noted (63,66), the enriched protein diet was associated with a significantly increased incidence of mammary tumors. But those animals that were fed the casein diets containing excess methionine experienced a marked reduction in tumor incidence. Food consumption and body weights of the animals in all three diet groups were similar.

The apparent protection provided by excess methionine against tumor emergence was also noted with certain spontaneously occurring tumors. Wainfran *et al.* (132) reported that chow diet fortified with 2% DL-methionine and 1% choline significantly increases the survival of AKRJ mice bearing spontaneous thymic lymphomas.

Another perspective is opened, however, by results contrasting with the observations reviewed above. The studies summarized below suggest that methionine fosters tumor emergence.

Firstly, studies by Tannenbaum and coworkers (*quoted in* ref. 133) on spontaneous benign hepatomas suggests that the emergence of tumors is dependent upon adequate amounts of methionine in the diet. Tannenbaum and coworkers have found that the incidence of benign hepatomas was about equal in mice given diets containing either 18 or 45% casein. However, if the mice were fed only a 9% casein diet, significantly fewer tumors developed. It was established that the difference in tumor incidence was not due to differences in caloric intake or body weight gain. It was further ascertained that the difference in tumor incidence was not solely due to differences in the amount of protein ingested. On a diet containing 9% gelatin (methionine *deficient*) plus 9% casein, the number of tumors remained significantly less than in those animals consuming an 18% casein diet. *However*, supplementation of the 9% casein diet with methionine and cysteine produced a tumor incidence similar to those animals fed an 18% casein diet.

Secondly, experiments with carcinogen-induced tumors in animals fed comparatively soy protein isolate diet or casein diet, and using methionine supplementation, provided an additional support for this latter perspective. Soybean protein isolate is a highly purified commercial protein (91.5% protein) prepared by a process involving heat treatment. Heat treatment significantly decreases the protease inhibitor activity which is an inhibitor of tumor growth (134). The methionine concentration in soybean protein is 1.3 g/100 g protein, about half that in casein (approximately 2.6 g/100 g protein). Methionine concentration in soybean protein is inadequate for maximal growth in young animals, but adequate for the adult (10,135).

Carroll (136) found that soy protein isolate diet compared to casein diet has no effect on DMBA-induced mammary carcinogenesis (the study was limited, however, to only ten rats per group). Hsueh and Park (137) confirmed this initial observation utilizing 30 animals per diet group; these investigators reported that the DMBA-induced mammary tumor incidence was 85 and 79% in the casein and soy protein isolate diet groups, respectively. Subsequently, studies by Hsueh and Pournayebzadeh (138) did show, however, the significance of methionine for tumor emergence. Rats fed soy protein diet supplemented with methionine developed 1.4 times the number of DMBA-induced mammary tumors than the rats fed either the unsupplemented soy protein diet or the casein diet. They also reported that 100% of the mammary tumors were classified as adenocarcinomas in the methionine-supplemented soy protein and casein diet groups. In contrast, only 20% of the tumors in the unsupplemented soy protein diet were classified as adenocarcinomas.

Hawrylewicz *et al.* (139) reported that feeding a soy protein isolate diet compared to casein diet delayed the appearance of NMU-induced mammary tumors and significantly reduced the incidence, tumor weight, and tumor multiplicity. All rats were fed casein diet from weaning on. Before mammary tumors became palpable (5 weeks post-treatment), one third of the rats were switched to the soy protein diet. The diet was continued during the tumor promotion phase until termination. A third group consisted of rats which were fed a soy protein isolate diet containing exogenous methionine at a concentration equivalent to the casein group. Addition of methionine to the soy protein diet increased the mammary tumor incidence from 42 to 64%. Although the increased tumor incidence did not reach the 80% level of the casein group, a positive response to methionine supplementation was observed.

The effect of soy protein diet on mammary tumor progression following excision of the primary tumor in NMU-treated rats was reported by Hawrylewicz *et al.* (140). Following excision of the primary tumor, rats were switched from casein (AIN-76) diet to either a 19 or 33% soy protein diet. The latency period (disease-free interval) for the first recurrent mammary tumor was significantly prolonged in the 19% soy protein group. The 33% soy protein diet had an intermittent latency period, approaching that of the casein diet group. The average tumor multiplicity was also significantly reduced from 5.1 in the casein diet group to 2.3 in the 19% soy protein diet group.

Similar conclusions were reached in a different tumor system by Breillout *et al.* (141), who studied the effect of diets deficient in methionine on metastatic rhabdomyosarcoma in Wistar Ag rats. Diets contained casein as a protein source, or were substituted with either soy protein or soy protein with added methionine. The study showed that the diet unsupplemented with methionine significantly reduces the mean number of lung metastases without affecting the growth of the primary tumor.

The requirement of methionine for tumor emergence and tumor growth could also be demonstrated in cell culture. Breillout *et al.* (142) have also shown the effect of a methionine-deficient culture medium on the growth of normal cells and tumor cells. When homocysteine replaced methionine in the culture medium, normal cells and fibroblasts proliferated normally, but tumor cells did not grow, or grew only slowly. Interestingly, methionine dependency was acquired simultaneously with cell transformation as noted with a human mammary epithelial cell line (HBL 100) that became more malignant as the number of passages increased. They further observed that a positive relationship exists between metastatic potential and methionine dependency in a series of cell lines derived from RMS-0, a rat rhabdomyosarcoma cell line. The higher the metastatic potential of a cell line, the higher the concentration of methionine required to maintain cell proliferation. Methionine-independent cells (derived from RMS-0 line by growing them in culture media with gradually decreasing concentrations of methionine) lost their ability to "take" and grow into established tumors when injected into rats fed a methionine-deficient diet.

The requirement of tumor cells for methionine was also demonstrated by Breillout *et al.* (142) by following tumor growth and metastatic spread in rats bearing the metastatic tumor line RMS-J1 (derived from the RMS-0 rhabdomyosarcoma original line). These investigators found significant decrease in tumor growth and metastatic spread when the rats were maintained on a diet containing an amino acid mixture reproducing casein composition, but in which homocysteine was substituted for methionine. The suggestion was made by them that the methionine requirement for tumor growth and metastatic spread may be exploited for therapeutic purposes.

It is of interest to compare the data from the animal studies to the epidemiology results obtained by Lee *et al.* (143). These authors examined 200 Chinese women from Singapore with histologically confirmed breast cancers, using 420 matched controls. In the premenopausal women, a high level of consumption of animal protein and red meat was associated with increased risk for breast cancer. Decreased risk was associated with the consumption of soy protein and total soy products and with a high proportion of soy to total protein. The suggestion of these authors was that soy products protect against breast cancer in younger women, because of the phytoestrogens in these foods. Alternatively, the results from the studies by Hawrylewicz *et al.* (139,140) and Breillout *et al.* (141,142) lend credence to the view that diets rich in soy protein products are relatively deficient in methionine, and this inhibits the progression of tumor growth.

B. Tryptophan

Early studies of Dunning *et al.* (144) explored the effects of dietary tryptophan on diethylstilbestrol induction of mammary tumors in rats. The report showed that addition of 1.4% DL-tryptophan to a synthetic diet containing 25% tryptophan-free casein hydrolysate increased the number and incidence of tumors and significantly reduced the average latency period, compared to the control group fed 26% casein diet. Decreasing the dietary tryptophan concentration to 0.14% resulted in a decreased number of mammary tumors and a significantly prolonged latency period.

Using Fischer 344 rats and the carcinogen, 2-acetylaminofluorene, Dunning *et al.* (145) determined the effect of 1.4 and 4.3% dietary tryptophan on the development of malignant hepatomas. The tryptophan-free control group was fed 2-acetylamino-fluorene in a 26% casein diet. Increasing the casein level from 26 to 45% increased the incidence of malignant hepatomas from 37 to 92% (while maintaining similar body weight). No bladder tumors were observed in either of these groups. Rats fed either of the diets containing excess tryptophan had double the incidence (74%) of hepatomas seen in the 26% casein control group (37%). Most importantly, however, the tryptophan diets were also associated with a gross papillary and squamous-cell bladder cancer incidence of over 90%. The increased susceptibility occurred in these rats in spite of a 20 and 40% decrease in body weight in the animals fed 1.4 and 4.3% excess tryptophan, respectively.

These findings were later substantiated by the work of Sidransky *et al.* (146). Partial hepatectomy was performed in rats, and 18 hours later they were treated with diethylnitrosamine. Subsequently, the rats were fed a diet containing an excess of L-tryptophan (2%) and either adequate or inadequate amounts of choline. Hepatic GGT–positive foci were markedly elevated in the livers of those rats fed the excess tryptophan and choline-deficient diet. These experiments indicate that excess dietary tryptophan increases the incidence of bladder, mammary, and liver cancer and has, in general, a promoting effect on liver carcinogenesis.

Birt *et al.* (147) further explored the relationship between dietary tryptophan and the incidence of bladder tumors in rats. Price *et al.* (148) already noted much earlier that a number of tryptophan metabolites, such as kynurenine and anthranilic acid and their corresponding *o*-aminophenols, are aromatic amines and are present at elevated levels in the urine of bladder cancer patients. In Birt's experiments, Fisher 344 rats were treated with the bladder carcinogen, *N*-[4-(5-nitro-2-furyl)-2-thiazolyl] formamide (FANFT), and fed semipurified diets containing an excess amount of tryptophan. Urinary tryptophan metabolites were influenced by the treatment, but the results did not correlate with tumor yields. Excess dietary tryptophan did not increase urinary bladder cancer when the diet had adequate amounts of pyridoxine (vitamin B_6, which functions as a cofactor for several enzymes involved in the metabolism of tryptophan to niacin). Deficiency of vitamin B6 could alter this metabolic pathway area, resulting in an increased synthesis of metabolites that are suspected to be bladder carcinogens. Bladder cancer patients with abnormal tryptophan metabolite excretion show a high recurrence rate of bladder tumors (149).

Similarly, DeGeorge and Brown (150) examined the levels of tryptophan metabolites excreted in the urine of breast cancer patients before and after tryptophan loading. Patients with advanced disease and metastatic spread excreted increased amounts of tryptophan metabolites compared to patients with localized disease. Results from comparisons of male bladder cancer cases having Grades III and IV lesions with those having Grades I and II lesions were also found to positively correlate with excreted tryptophan metabolite concentrations.

Consistent with the possible enhancement of various tumors resulting from excess dietary tryptophan, a tryptophan-free diet appears to decrease the mammary tumor incidence and tumor weight in diethylstilbestrol-treated rats (151). However, regression of already established mammary adenocarcinomas in C3H mice did not occur when moderate tryptophan restriction was introduced into an otherwise balanced diet (152). Just as with dietary methionine, an excess or deficiency of dietary tryptophan, deviating from the optimal concentration, can significantly affect tumor initiation and progression.

C. Tyrosine and Phenylalanine

Early studies by Hui *et al.* (153–155) demonstrated that diets deficient in phenylala-nine inhibit the development of spontaneous mammary hyperplastic alveolar nodules and of tumors in C3H female mice. Mice fed diets containing 0.075 and 0.090% phenylalanine did not develop tumors; however, mice fed diets containing 0.135, 0.150, and 0.300% phenylalanine displayed a 100% tumor incidence after 10 months. The authors concluded that the repressed nodule formation in the animals fed phenylalanine-deficient diets was related to a disturbed hormonal milieu, caused by the absence of estrus cycles and the presence of poorly developed mammary glands and atrophic ovaries lacking corpora lutea.

In a series of investigations, Meadows and coworkers (156–159) have found that modification of the host nutritional status, by restricting dietary intake of tyrosine and phenylalanine, exerts a significant antimetastatic effect. Dietary restriction of tyrosine-phenylalanine, alone or in combination with experimental chemotherapy, inhibits the growth of BL6 melanoma. Tyrosine–phenylalanine restriction alone inhibits tumor growth and prolongs survival of tumor-bearing mice up to 42%. Inhibition of tumor growth by diet was most effective as an enhancer of levodopa methylester chemotherapy; these two together brought about a doubling of the median survival time of mice bearing primary subcutaneous tumors.

These authors suggested that since tyrosine and/or phenylalanine limitation is known to affect host immunity, an immunologic mechanism may be involved in the observed antitumor effect. To test this hypothesis, they have determined the effect of dietary tyrosine and phenylalanine restriction on the metastasizing ability of three rodent tumors, BL6 melanoma, 3LL carcinoma, and RT7-4bs hepatocarcinoma. Dietary limitation in these two amino acids was found to inhibit outgrowth of pulmonary tumor colonies in a lung and colon assay, and also to block spontaneous hematogenous metastasis. Thus, it appears that restriction in these amino acids may starve the tumor and this results in decreased tumor growth rate. However, restriction of dietary intake of phenylalanine and tyrosine reduced the plasma levels of these amino acids by only about 30%; therefore, an additional mechanism must be involved. It was noted that phenylalanine-restricted animals needed two to three times higher doses of whole-body radiation than normal mice for immunosuppression. The authors interpreted this as an indication of the increased participation of radiation-resistant cells, such as natural killer cells or macrophages.

D. Leucine and Isoleucine

Kakizoe *et al.* (160) noted that isolated bladder cells from rats that have been treated with various bladder carcinogens, such as *N*-butyl-*N*-(4-hydroxybutyl)nitrosamine (BHBN) or FANFT, show increased agglutinability with concanavalin A. This agglutinability disappears within 3 to 6 weeks after discontinuation of treatment with BHBN or FANFT. After discontinuation of treatment with the carcinogens, the animals were treated with known bladder tumor promoters, such as tryptophan or saccharin. The bladder cells in the culture retained their agglutination properties for at least 20 weeks (161). Utilizing the concanavalin A agglutination as a test for bladder tumor promoters, these investigators (162) tested 21 amino acids. The results indicate that leucine, isoleucine, and valine are effective in the agglutination test to a similar degree as saccharin and tryptophan. Following these *in vitro* tests they assayed the potential enhancing effect of a diet containing 2% L-leucine or isoleucine, following treatment with the carcinogen

BHBN (163). In contrast to the animals treated with the carcinogen alone, leucine- or isoleucine-fed and carcinogen-treated animals had a significant increase in bladder carcinomas, but no difference in the incidence of papillomas or degree of hyperplasia. Additional experiments confirmed that these branched-chain amino acids (BCAA) were, in fact, tumor-promoting agents for bladder cancer. The number of carcinomas positively correlated with the concentration of leucine or isoleucine in the diet. From these studies the authors concluded that excess amino acids (in the form of meat) consumed in the western countries may be an etiologic factor in the high incidence of bladder cancer in these areas.

The BCAA, leucine and isoleucine, also play an important role serving as metabolic fuel to muscle tissue and possibly to the tumor itself. Paxton *et al.* (164) demonstrated in rats, bearing Morris hepatoma, that the rate of $^{14}CO_2$ production from [1-^{14}C] leucine was significantly increased in tumor-bearing rats. Skeletal muscle is quantitatively the most important site of BCAA oxidation (165). The carbon moiety arising from the transamination of BCAA provides a major source of energy for muscle tissue and possibly for tumor tissue in the tumor-bearing individual (166). The amino groups are utilized in the synthesis of the gluconeogenic amino acids, alanine and glutamine (167). Paxton *et al.* (164) determined in liver, kidney, skeletal muscle, and liver tumor tissue the activity of the first two enzymes in the metabolic sequence for leucine (leucine aminotransferase and 2-oxoisocaproate dehydrogenase [OADH]). The results indicated a 4.5-fold increase in OADH activity (rate-limiting enzyme for leucine catabolism) in skeletal muscle. The tumor and kidney tissue also showed an increased OADH activity. The pathophysiological importance of tumor-enhanced leucine oxidation is uncertain (164). The results clearly indicate, however, the profound effect of the presence of a tumor-load upon the amino acid metabolism of the host.

The results of Kakizoe and coworkers (160–162) and Nishio *et al.* (163) that exogenous leucine and isoleucine can function as promoters for bladder carcinogenesis, together with the finding of Paxton *et al.* (164) that BCAA have probably an important role as metabolic fuel in tumor-bearing rats, suggest that these amino acids may be more rapidly catabolized in the bladder of tumor-bearing animals. Thus, their promoter activity may be grounded in providing energy to facilitate the growth of bladder tumors.

VI. CLOSING NOTE

The NRC report (2) stated that, based on evidence from both epidemiologic and laboratory studies, high-protein diets are probably associated with an increased risk for cancer at certain sites. Carefully controlled animal studies indicate that increased dietary protein with a balanced amino acid composition is, indeed, consistently associated with an enhanced response to chemical carcinogens resulting in an increased mammary tumor incidence.

It should be noted that virtually all recent studies on the effect of dietary protein on chemically induced tumorigenesis used the AIN-76, 20% casein diet. This basic diet is fed for 6 months or longer. Although the growth of the rat reaches a plateau by this age, the animal still consumes a diet rich in protein. It is conceivable, therefore, that in the young adult rat a 20% casein diet may represent a moderately high protein intake. This circumstance may blur the true stimulatory effect of a high-protein diet. It would be important to evaluate a diet with a lower protein content in the control group.

This has significant public health implications for the diet of young humans. In the

United States many children and adolescents probably consume an excess amount of protein. Based on animal studies it is conceivable that the enriched protein diet stimulates proliferation of normal epithelial cells in the developing mammary ducts and possibly increase the risk of cancer. In association with a high-fat diet, an enriched protein diet may also stimulate tumor growth during the tumor promotion growth phase.

In animal studies the correct age of the beginning of a test diet should be further studied; in this, the adolescent growth phase may be of special concern. The composition of the diet, the duration of consumption of the test diet prior to carcinogen exposure, and the age at which the diet is initiated are all critically important elements that must be considered, aside from the effect of the test diet on tumor initiation and growth.

There were some reports that high-protein diets inhibit tumor growth in animals. However, critical evaluation of these studies invariably indicates that diets exceeding 40 to 60% protein were used. It is probable that prolonged feeding of these diets may affect renal function and cause other metabolic malfunctions. It is essential, therefore, to define an enriched or high-protein diet as one that has no detectable adverse effect on body growth or on physiologic function.

Certain studies utilizing a "low-protein" diet suffer from other shortcomings. Examination of the protocol and data indicates that the protein in some of these diets was so low that wasting occurred with significant impairment of the metabolic system. Thus, the interpretation of the *actual effect* of protein level on tumor growth is severely restricted by these unphysiologic levels of protein in the basal diet.

Surprisingly, very few studies have been carried out that compare the effect of *different sources* of protein on tumor initiation and growth. Yet, variation in the amino acid levels of a protein may markedly influence the growth of tumors. To a limited extent this has been demonstrated in animal studies with soybean protein diets, which are methionine deficient.

The protein source of human diet is milk, meats, and grains. Soybeans constitute a major source of dietary protein in vast areas of the world. The deficiency of methionine in soybean protein may influence tumor development. In contrast, excess methionine inhibits mammary tumor development in animal models.

Excess dietary intake of tryptophan appears to have a promoting effect on liver carcinogenesis. Additionally, several studies have shown that inadequate metabolism of tryptophan is associated with increased bladder cancer and mammary cancer. Bladder cancer is also positively correlated with the concentration of leucine or isoleucine in the diet.

The enrichment of experimental diets with various amino acids significantly alters tumor incidence at various tissue sites. Whether or not this is relevant to humans has not been determined. Therefore, it is necessary to further study diets, which utilize proteins with amino acid compositions other than that found in casein, before a definitive conclusion can be drawn on the effect of dietary protein on human cancer.

Abbreviations Used: Ado Met, S-adenosylmethionine; AM, azomethane; AOM, azoxymethane; BCAA, branched-chain amino acids; BHBN, N-butyl-N-(4-hydroxybutyl) nitrosamine; BOP, N-nitrosobis(2-oxopropyl)amine; DMBA, 7,12-dimethylbenz[a]-anthracene; DMH, 1,2-dimethylhydrazine; DMN, dimethylnitrosamine; FANFT, N-[4-(5-nitro-2-furyl)-2-thiazolyl]formamide; FAO/WHO, Food and Agriculture Organization/World Health Organization; GGT, γ-glutamyl transferase; HPOP, 2-hydroxypropyl-2-oxopropylnitrosamine; MAM, methylazoxymethanol; MNNG, N-methyl-N'-nitro-N-nitrosoguanidine; NMU, N-nitroso-N-methylurea; NRC, National Research Council; OADH, 2-oxoisocaproate dehydrogenase; ODC, ornithine decarboxylase; USDA, U.S. Department of Agriculture.

REFERENCES

1 Williams, W. R.: "The Natural History of Cancer with Special Reference to Its Causation and Prevention". Royal College of Surgeons, London, 1908.
2. National Research Council: "Diet, Nutrition and Cancer". National Academy Press, Washington, D.C., 1982.
3. Magendie, F.: *Ann. Chem. Phys.* **3**, 66 (1816).
4. Boussingault, J. B.: "Rural Economy". Orange Judd, New York, 1843, p. 387.
5. von Liebig, J.: "Animal Chemistry", 3rd ed. Taylor and Walton, London, 1846.
6. Atwater, W. O., and Woods, C. D.: U.S. Department of Agriculture Office of Experimental Stations Bull. No. 32 (1896).
7. Gortner, W. A.: *Cancer Res.* **35**, 3246 (1975).
8. Klurfeld, D. M., and Kritchevsky, D.: *J. Am. College Nutr.* **5**, 477 (1986).
9. Carpenter, K. J.: *J. Nutr.* **116**, 1364 (1986).
10. European Society for Pediatric Gastroenterology and Nutrition, Committee on Nutrition: Guidelines for Infant Nutrition. *Acta Pediatr. Scand. Suppl.* **262**, 1 (1977).
11. Committee on Medical Aspects of Food Policy. Department of Health and Social Subjects, vol. 18, Her Majesty's Stationery Office, London, 17 (1982).
12. Jarvenpaa, A. L., Raiha, N. C. R., and Rassin, D. K.: *Pediatrics* **70**, 214 (1982).
13. Jarvenpaa, A. L., Rassin, D. K., Raiha, N. C., and Gaull, G. E.: *Pediatrics* **70**, 221 (1982).
14. Raiha, N. C.: *Pediatrics* **75**, 136 (1985).
15. National Research Council, Committee on Dietary Allowances, Food and Nutrition Board: "Recommended Dietary Allowances", 9th ed. Natl. Acad. Sci., Washington, D. C., 1980.
16. Warburg, O. (ed.): "The Metabolism of Tumors". A. Smith, New York, 1931.
17. Warburg, O.: *Science* **123**, 309 (1956).
18. Tessitore, L., Bonelli, G., and Baccino, F. M.: *Biochem. J.* **241**, 153 (1987).
19. Tessitore, L., Bonelli, G., Cecchini, G., Amenta, J., and Baccino, F. M.: *Arch. Biochem. Biophys.* **225**, 372 (1987).
20. Tayek, J. A., Istfon, N. W., Jones, C. T., Hamawy, K. J., Bristrian, B. R., and Blackburn, G. L.: *Cancer Res.* **46**, 5649 (1986).
21. Gerry, K. L., Witt, B. H., Track, N. S., McDonnell, M., Makowka, L., and Falk, R. E.: *J. Surg. Res.* **33**, 332 (1982).
22. Thomas, R. J., and Chan, H.: *Proc. Aust. Symp. Nutr. and Cancer*, Adelaide, Australia (1978).
23. Carroll, K. K., and Khor, H. T.: *Progr. Biochem. Pharmacol.* **10**, 308 (1975).
24. Gaskill, S. P., McGuire, W. L., Osborne, C. K., and Stern, M. P.: *Cancer Res.* **39**, 3628 (1979).
25. Drasar, B. S., and Irving, D.: *Br. J. Cancer* **27**, 176 (1973).
26. Kato, I., Tominaga, S., and Kuroishi, T.: *Jpn. J. Cancer Res.* **78**, 349 (1987).
27. Hawrylewicz, E. J., and Huang, H. H.: Effect of Dietary Protein and Methionine Supplementation on Mammary Tumorigenesis. *In* "Dietary Proteins in Health and Disease" (G. Liepa, ed.) Am. Oil Chem. Soc., Champaign, Illinois, 1992, p. 123.
28. Hirohata, T., Nomura, A. M., Hankin, J. H., Kolonel, L. N., and Lee, J.: *J. Natl. Cancer Inst.* **78**, 595 (1987).
29. Hems, G.: *Br. J. Cancer* **37**, 974 (1978).
30. Hems, G.: *Br. J. Cancer* **41**, 429 (1980).
31. Lubin, J. H., Burns, P. E., Blot, W. J., Ziegler, R. G., Lees, A. W., and Fraumeni, J. F.: *Int. J. Cancer* **28**, 685 (1981).
32. Kolonel, L. N., Nomura, A. M., Hinds, M. W., Hirohata, T., Hankin, J. H., and Lee, J.: *Cancer Res.* **43**, 2397s (1983).
33. Rose, D. P., Boyar, A. P., and Wynder, E. L.: *Cancer* **58**, 2363 (1986).
34. Toniolo, P., Riboli, E., Protta, F., Charrel, M., and Cappa, A. P.: *J. Natl. Cancer Inst.* **81**, 278 (1989).
35. Lubin, F., Wax, Y., and Modan, B.: *J. Natl. Cancer Inst.* **77**, 605 (1986).
36. Richardson, S., Gerber, M., and Cenée, S.: *Int. J. Cancer* **48**, 1 (1991).
37. Vatten, L. J., Solvoll, K., and Loken, E. B.: *Int. J. Cancer* **46**, 12 (1990).
38. Correa, P.: *Cancer Res.* **41**, 3685 (1981).
39. Armstrong, B., and Doll, R.: *Int. J. Cancer* **15**, 617 (1975).
40. Leveille, G. A.: *J. Anim. Sci.* **41**, 723 (1975).
41. Howell, M. A.: *J. Chronic Dis.* **28**, 67 (1975).
42. Manousos, O., Day, N. E., Trichopoulos, D., Gerovassilis, F., Tzonou, A., and Polychronopoulou, A.: *Int. J. Cancer* **32**, 1 (1983).
43. Potter, J. D., and McMichael, A. J.: *J. Natl. Cancer Inst.* **76**, 557 (1986).

44. Reddy, B. S., Mangat, S., and Weisburger, J. H.: *Cancer Res.* **37**, 3533 (1977).
45. Wise, A., Mallett, A. K., and Rowland, I. R.: *Nutr. Cancer* **4**, 267 1983).
46. Byers, T., Marshall J., Graham, S., Mettlin, C., and Swanson, M.: *J. Natl. Cancer Inst.* **71**, 681 (1983).
47. Jedrychowski, W., Wahrendorf, J., Popiela, T., and Rachtan, J.: *Int. J. Cancer* **37**, 837 (1986).
48. Heshmat, M. Y., Kaul, L., Kovi, J., Jackson, M. A., Jackson, A. G., Jones, G. W., Edson, M., Enterline, J. P., Worrell, R. G., and Perry, S. L.: *Prostate* **6**, 7 (1985).
49. Tannenbaum, A., and Silverstone, H.: *Cancer Res* **9**, 162 (1949).
50. Engel, R. W., and Copeland, D. H.: *Cancer Res.* **12**, 905 (1952).
51. Engel, R. W., and Copeland, D. H.: *Cancer Res.* **8**, 336 (1948).
52. Engel, R. W., and Copeland, D. H: *Cancer Res.* **9**, 608 (1949).
53. Shay, H., Gruenstein, M., and Shimkin, M. B.: *J. Natl. Cancer Inst.* **33**, 243 (1964).
54. Nakagawa, I., Sasaki, A., Kajimoto, M., Fukuyama, T., Suzuki, T., and Yamada, E.: *J. Nutr.* **104**, 1576 (1974).
55. Tannenbaum, A., and Silverstone, H.: *Cancer Res.* **13**, 56 (1953).
56. Clinton, S. K., Imrey, P. B., Alster, J. M., Simon, J., Truex, C. R., and Visek, W. J.: *J. Nutr.* **114**, 1213 (1984).
57. National Research Council, Subcommittee on Laboratory Animal Nutrition: "Nutritional Requirement of Laboratory Animals", 3rd ed., National Academy of Sciences, Washington, D.C. 1978.
58. Thompson, H. J., Meeker, L. D., Tagliaferro, A. R., and Roberts, J. S.: *Nutr. Cancer* **7**, 37 (1985).
59. Kritchevsky, D., Weber, M. M., Buck, C. L., and Klurfeld, D. M.: *Lipids* **21**, 272 (1986).
60. Clinton, S. K., Alster, J. M., Imrey, P. B., Nandkumar, S., Truex, R. C., and Visek, W. J.: *J. Nutr.* **116**, 2290 (1986).
61. Clinton, S. K., Alster, J. M., Imrey, P. B., Simon, J., and Visek, W. J.: *J. Nutr.* **118**, 1577 (1988).
62. Clinton, S. K., Truex, C. R. and Visek, W. J.: *J. Nutr.* **109**, 55 (1979).
63. Hawrylewicz, E. J., Huang H. H., Kissane, J. Q., and Drab, E. A.: *Nutr. Rep. Int.* **26**, 793 (1982).
64. Huang, H. H., Hawrylewicz, E. J., Kissane, J. Q., and Drab, E. A.: *Nutr. Rep. Int.* **26**, 807 (1982).
65. Alvarez-Sanz, M. C., Liu, J. M., Huang, H. H., and Hawrylewicz, E. J.: *J. Natl. Cancer Inst.* **77**, 477 (1986).
66. Hawrylewicz, E. J., Huang, H. H., and Liu, J. M.: *Cancer Res.* **46**, 4395 (1986).
67. Hawrylewicz, E. J., Moshovitis, C. K., Reger, C., and Madell, J: *J. Nutr.* **119**, 547 (1989).
68. Dao, T. L.: *Cancer Res.* **22**, 973 (1962).
69. Russell, D. H.: *Drug Metab. Rev.* **16**, 1 (1985).
70. Fausto, N.: *Biochim. Biophys. Acta* **190**, 193 (1969).
71. Farwell, D. C., Miguez, J. B., and Herbst, E. J.: *Biochem. J.* **168**, 49 (1977).
72. Moore, P., and Swendseid, M. E.: *J. Nutr.* **113**, 1927 (1983).
73. Benevenga, N. J., and Steele, R. D.: *Annu. Rev. Nutr.* **4**, 157 (1984).
74. Harper, A. E., Benevenga, N. J., and Wohlhueter, R. M.: *Physiol. Rev.* **50**, 428 (1970).
75. Finkelstein, J. D., Kyle, W. E., Harris, B. J. and Martin, J. J.: *J. Nutr.* **112**, 1011 (1982).
76. Kramer, D. L., Sufrin, J. R. and Porter, C. W.: *Biochem. J.* **247**, 259 (1987).
77. Huang, H. H., Zapata, J. J., and Hawrylewicz, E. J.: *Proc. Am. Assoc. Cancer Res.* **33**, 134 (1992).
78. Visek, W. J. and Clinton, S. K.: Dietary Protein and Cancer. *In* "Cancer and Nutrition" (R. B. Alfin-Slater, and D. Kritchevsky, eds.). Plenum Press, New York, 1991, p. 103.
79. Topping, D. C., and Visek, W. J.: *J. Nutr.* **106**, 1583 (1976).
80. Weisburger, J. H., Yamamoto, R. S., Glass, R. M., and Frankel, H. H.: *Toxicol. Appl. Pharmacol.* **14**, 163 (1969).
81. Kari, F. W., Johnston, J. B., Truex, C. R., and Visek, W. J.: *Cancer Res.* **43**, 3674 (1983).
82. Siegler, J. M., and Kazarinoff, M. N.: *Nutr. Cancer* **4**, 176 (1983).
83. Siegler, J. M., and Kazarinoff, M. N.: *J. Nutr.* **114**, 574 (1984).
84. Russell, D., and Snyder, S. H.: *Proc. Natl. Acad. Sci. U.S.A.* **60**, 1420 (1968).
85. Tabor, C. W., and Tabor, H: *Annu. Rev. Biochem.* **45**, 285 (1976).
86. O'Brien, T. S., Sumsiman, P. C., and Boutwell, R. K.: *Cancer Res.* **35**, 1662 (1975).
87. Reddy, B. S., Narisawa, T., and Weisburger, J. H.: *J. Natl. Cancer Inst.* **57**, 567 (1976).
88. Reddy, B. S., Narisawa, T., Maronpot, R., Weisburger, J., and Wynder, E.: *Cancer Res.* **35**, 342 (1975).
89. Clinton, S. K., Destree, R. J., Anderson, D. B., Truex, C. R., Imrey, P. B., and Visek, W. J.: *Nutr. Rep. Int.* **20**, 335 (1979).
90. Hawrylewicz, E. J., Huang, H. H., and Liu, J. M.: *Proc. Am. Assoc. Cancer Res.* **26**, 125, (1985).
91. Peers, F. G., Gilman, G. A., and Linsell, C. A.: *Int. J. Cancer*, **17**, 167 (1976).
92. Peers, F. G., and Linsell, C. A.: *Ann. Nutr. Aliment.* **31**, 1005 (1977).
93. Madhavan, T. V., Suryanarayana, K. R., and Tulpule, P. G.: *Ind. J. Med. Res.* **53**, 984 (1965).
94. Madhavan, T. V., and Gopalan, C.: *Arch. Pathol.* **80**, 123 (1965).

95. Madhavan, T. V., and Gopalan, C.: *Arch. Pathol.* **85**, 133 (1968).
96. Wells, P., Aftergood, L., and Alfin-Slater, R. B.: *J. Am. Oil Chemists* **53**, 559 (1975).
97. Prince, L. O., and Campbell, T. C.: *Cancer Res.* **42**, 5053 (1982).
98. Appleton, B. S., and Campbell, T. C.: *Nutr. Cancer* **3**, 200 (1982).
99. Kalengayi, M. M. R., Gilli, J., and Desmet, V. J.: Tissular Dynamics of the Oncofetal Markers α_1 Fetoprotein and γ-Glutamyl Transpeptidase in Rat Liver During Aflatoxin B$_1$ Induced Carcinogenesis. *In* "Prevention and Detection of Cancer 3" (H. E. Nieburgs, ed.). Dekker, New York, 1978, p. 246.
100. Appleton, B. S., and Campbell, T. C.: *J. Natl. Cancer Inst.* **70**, 547 (1983).
101. Appleton, B. S., and Campbell, T. C.: *Cancer Res* **43**, 2150 (1983).
102. Dunaif, G. E., and Campbell, T. C.: *J. Natl. Cancer Inst.* **78**, 365 (1987)
103. Horio, F., Youngman, L. D., Bell, R. C., and Campbell, T. C.: *Nutr. Cancer* **16**, 31 (1991).
104. Youngman, L. D., and Campbell, T. C.: *J. Nutr.* **121**, 1454 (1991).
105. Pour, P. M., Birt, D. F., Salmasi, S. Z., and Gotz, U.: *J. Natl. Cancer Inst.* **70**, 141 (1983).
106. Guyton, A.: "Textbook of Medical Physiology", 5th ed. Saunders, Philadelphia, 1976.
107. Wynder, E. L., Mabuchi, K., Maruchi, N., and Fortner, J. G.: *J. Natl. Cancer Inst.* **50**, 645 (1973).
108. Pour, P. M., and Birt, D. F.: *J. Natl. Cancer Inst.* **71**, 347 (1983).
109. Kokkinakis, D. M., and Scarpelli, D. G.: *Carcinogenesis* **10**, 699 1989).
110. Magee, P. N., and Barnes, J. M.: *J. Pathol. Bacteriol* **84**, 19 (1962).
111. McLean, A. E. M., and McLean, E. K.: *Br. Med. Bull.* **25**, 278 (1969).
112. Swann, P. F., and McLean, A. E. M.: *Biochem. J.* **107**, 14 (1968).
113. Magee, P. N., and Swann, P. F.: *Br. Med. Bull.* **25**, 240 (1969).
114. McLean, A. E. M., and Magee, P. N.: *Br. J. Exp. Pathol* **51**, 587 (1970).
115. Hard, G. C., and Butler, W. H.: *Cancer Res.* **30**, 2796 (1970).
116. Swann, P. F., and McLean, A. E. M.: *Biochem. J.* **124**, 283 (1971).
117. Ross, M. H., Bras, G., and Ragbeer, M. S.: *J. Nutr.* **100**, 177 (1970).
118. Ross, M. H., Lustbader, E. D., and Bras, G.: *J. Natl. Cancer Inst.* **70**, 1119 (1983).
119. American Cancer Society: "Cancer Facts and Figures". Am. Cancer Soc., New York, 1991.
120. Walters, M. A., and Roe, F. J. C.: *Br. J. Cancer* **18**, 312 (1964).
121. Hu, J., Zhang, S., Jia, E., Wang, Q., Liu, S., Liu, Y., Wu, Y., and Cheng, Y.: *Int. J. Cancer* **41**, 331 (1988).
122. Tatsuta, M., Iishi, H., Baba, M., Uehara, G. H., Nakaizumi, A., and Taniguchi, H.: *Cancer Res.* **51**, 3493 (1991).
123. Tatsuta, M., Iishi, H., Baba, M., and Taniguchi, H.: *Jpn. J. Cancer Res.* **80**, 521 (1989).
124. Gurkalo, V. K., and Volfson, N. I.: *Arch. Geschwülstforsch.* **52**, 259 (1982).
125. Finkelstein, J. D., and Martin, J. J.: *J. Biol. Chem.* **261**, 1582 (1986).
126. Smith, T. K., Hyvonen, T., Pajula, R. L., and Eloranta, T. O.: *Ann. Nutr. Metab.* **31**, 133 (1987).
127. Hoffman, R. M.: *Biochim. Biophys. Acta* **738**, 49 (1984).
128. Bhave, M., Wilson, M. J., and Poirier, L. A.: *Carcinogenesis* **9**, 343 (1988).
129. Feo, F., Garcea, R., Daino, R., Frasetto, S., Cozzolino, P., Vannini, M. G., Ruggiu, M. E., Simile, M., and Puddu, M.: S-Adenosylmethionine Antipromotion and Antiprogression Effects in Hepatocarcinogenesis: Its Association With Inhibition of Gene Expression. *In* "Chemical Carcinogenesis: Models and Mechanisms" (F. Feo, P. Pani, A. Columbano, and R. Garcea, eds.). Plenum Press, New York, 1988, p. 407.
130. Ghoshal, A. K., and Farber, E.: *Carcinogenesis* **5**, 1367 (1984).
131. Anisimov, V. N., Miretskii, G. I., Danetskaya, E. V., Troitskaya, M. N., and Ramzaev, P. V.: *Bull. Eksp. Biol. Med. USSR* **92**, 480 (1981).
132. Wainfran, E., Dizik, M., Kilkenny, M., and O'Callaghan, J. P.: *Carcinogenesis* **11**, 361 (1990).
133. Tannenbaum, A.: Nutrition and Cancer. *In* "The Pathophysiology of Cancer" (F., Homburger, ed.). Hoeber-Harper, New York, 1959.
134. Witschi, H., and Kennedy, A. R.: *Carcinogenesis* **10**, 2275 (1989).
135. Scrimshaw, N. S., and Young, V. R.: Soy Protein in Adult Human Nutrition: A Review with New Data. *In* "Soy Protein and Human Nutrition" (H. L. Wilcke, D. T. Hopkins, and D. H., Waggle, eds.). Academic Press, New York, 1979, p. 121.
136. Carroll, K. K.: *Cancer Res.* **35**, 3374 (1975).
137. Hsueh, A. M., and Park, H. S.: *1990 Meet. Am. Oil Chemists Soc.*, Baltimore, Maryland, Abstracts.
138. Hsueh, A. M., Pournayebzadeh, H., Inrham, V., and Turya-Mureeba, P.: *1991 Meet. Am. Oil Chemists Soc.*, Chicago, Illinois Abstracts.
139. Hawrylewicz, E. J., Huang, H. H., and Blair, W. H.: *J. Nutr.* **121**, 1692 (1993).
140. Hawrylewicz, E. J., Zapata, J. J., and Blair, W. H.: Soy and Experimental Cancer: Animal Studies. *In* "Proc. 1st Internat. Symp. of Soy in Preventing and Treating Chronic Disease" (M. J. Messina, V. Persky, S. Barnes, and K. D. R. Setchell, eds.). *J. Nutr.* (Suppl.), in press, 1995.

141. Breillout, F., Hadida, F., Echinard-Garvin, P., Lascaux, V., and Poupon, M. F.: *Anticancer Res.* **7**, 861 (1987).
142. Breillout, F., Antoine, E., and Poupon, M. F.: *J. Natl. Cancer Inst.* **82**, 1628 (1990).
143. Lee, H. P., Gourley, L., Duffy, S. W., Esteve, J., Lee, J., and Day, N. E.: *Lancet* **337**, 1197 (1991).
144. Dunning, W. F., Curtis, M. R., and Maun, M. E.: *Cancer Res.* **10**, 319 (1950).
145. Dunning, W. F., Curtis, M. R., and Maun, M. E.: *Cancer Res.* **10**, 454 (1950).
146. Sidransky, H., Garrett, C. J., Murty, C. N., Verey, E., and Robinson, E. S.: *Cancer Res.* **45**, 4844 (1985).
147. Birt, D. F., Julius, A. D., Hasegawa, R., St. John, M., and Cohen, S.: *Cancer Res.* **47**, 1244 (1987).
148. Price, J. M., Wear, J. B., Brown, R. R., Satter, E. J., and Olson, C.: *J. Urol.* **83**, 376 (1960).
149. Yoshida, O., Brown, R. R., and Bryan, G. T.: *Cancer* **25**, 773 (1970).
150. DeGeorge, F. V., and Brown, R. R.: *Cancer* **26**, 767 (1970).
151. Dunning, W. F., and Curtis, M. R.: *Cancer Res.* **14**, 299 (1954).
152. Kamath, S. K., Conrad, N. C., Olson, R. E., Kohrs, M. B., and Ghosh, L.: *J. Nutr.* **118**, 1137 (1988).
153. Hui, Y. H., DeOme, K. B., and Briggs, G. M.: *J. Natl. Cancer Inst.* **46**, 929 (1971).
154. Hui, Y. H., DeOme, K. B., and Briggs, G. M.: *J. Natl. Cancer Inst.* **47**, 245 (1971).
155. Hui, Y. H., DeOme, K. B., and Briggs, G. M.: *J. Natl. Cancer Inst.* **47**, 687 (1971).
156. Meadows, G. G., Pierson, H. F., and Abdallah, R. A.: *Cancer Res.* **42**, 3056 (1982).
157. Meadows, G. G., Abdallah, R. M., and Starkey, J. R.: *Cancer Chemother. Pharmacol.* **16**, 229 (1986).
158. Pierson, H. F., and Meadows, G. G.: *Cancer Res.* **43**, 2047 (1983).
159. Meadows, G. G., and Oeser, D. E.: *Nutr. Rep. Int.* **28**, 1073 (1983).
160. Kakizoe, T., Kawachi, T., and Sugimura, T.: *Cancer Res.* **40**, 2006 1980).
161. Kakizoe, T., Kawachi, T. and Sugimura, T.: *Cancer Res.* **41**,4702 (1981).
162. Kakizoe, T., Komatsu, H., Honma, Y., Niijima, T., and Sugimura, T.: *Gann* **73**, 870 (1982).
163. Nishio, Y., Kakizoe, T., Ohtani, M., Sato, S., Sugimura, T., and Fukushima, S.: *Science* **231**, 843 (1986).
164. Paxton, K., Ward, L. C., and Wilce, P. A.: *Cancer Biochem. Biophys.* **9**, 343 (1988).
165. Smith, R., and Elia, M.: *Proc. Nutr. Soc.* **42**, 473 (1983).
166. Lundholm, K. G.: Energy and Substrate Metabolism in the Cancer-Bearing Host. *In* "Nutrition in Cancer and Trauma Sepsis" (F. Bozzetti and R. Dionigi, eds.). Karger, Basel, 1985, p. 78.
167. Walser, M.: *Clin. Sci.* **66**, 1 (1984).

SECTION III

Modulation by Vitamins[1]

Edgar Petru, Yin-tak Woo, and Martin R. Berger

I. INTRODUCTION

Vitamins have long been known to be essential for the normal physiological functions of humans and animals (*rev.* in 1). Evidence has been accruing for some years that vitamins also have an important influence on carcinogenesis. Dietary deficiency in certain vitamins and quasi-vitamins[2] was found to be associated with increased susceptibility to, whereas dietary supplementation with a variety of vitamins showed protective effect against, carcinogenesis. When given in large amounts, however, some vitamins may enhance the effects of chemical carcinogens. This section presents a brief overview of the physiological and biochemical roles of vitamins with emphasis on their modulation of chemical carcinogenesis in experimental animals.

II. PHYSIOLOGICAL AND BIOCHEMICAL ROLES OF VITAMINS WITH SPECIAL EMPHASIS ON RELATIONSHIP TO CARCINOGENESIS

Vitamins are required for a variety of physiological and biochemical functions that are crucial for the normal growth and health of animals (*rev.* in 1). A number of physiological functions are particularly relevant to the process of carcinogenesis. Vitamin deficiency or overdosing may modulate chemical carcinogenesis at various stages which include: (a) *in vivo* formation of carcinogens from precursors, (b) uptake and/or transport of carcinogens across cell membranes, (c) metabolic activation/detoxification of carcinogens, (d) generation or scavenging of free-radicals or reactive intermediates from carcinogens, (e) interference/promotion of cell differentiation/proliferation, gene

---

[1]For the Abbreviations Used in this section see p. 329.
[2]The term "quasi-vitamins" has been used to denote compounds which appear to satisfy the criteria of vitamin status, but for only a few species or under only certain conditions. The list of quasi-vitamins includes such compounds as *choline, carnitine,* and *myo-inositol* which are required for optimal growth of certain poultry, insects, and fishes, respectively. A number of other compounds (*pyrroloquinoline quinone, ubiquinones, orotic acid, bioflavonoids, p-amino-benzoic acid, lipoic acid*) have also yielded some evidence for nutritional essentiality and are loosely considered as quasi-vitamins (*see* ref. 1).

316

expression and signal transduction, and (f) enhancement/suppression of immune surveillance.

Vitamin A has at least two key roles in affecting carcinogenesis: control of cell differentiation and maintenance of immunocompetence[3]. It is well documented (*rev.* in 1) that vitamin A deficiency characteristically results in a failure of differentiation of epithelial cells without impairment of proliferation. Vitamin A deficiency brings about, in humans and animals, replacement of normal mucus-secreting cells by cells producing keratin, particularly in the conjunctiva and cornea of the eye, the trachea, the skin, and other ectodermal tissues. The squamous metaplastic changes seen in vitamin A deficiency are indeed morphologically similar to experimentally induced precancerous lesions. This observation led to the insight and suggestion that vitamin A has a modifying role in the emergence of epithelial cell tumors. This is supported by the apparent protective effect of vitamin A against chemically induced carcinogenesis (*see* Subsection IV below). A family of nuclear receptors with high affinity for retinoic acid has recently been discovered and the role of these receptors in gene regulation is being investigated. The maintenance of a competent immune system is a vital defense against infectious agents and provides for surveillance against and rejection of certain immunogenic tumors in carcinogenesis (*see* Chapter 8). Accordingly, vitamin A deficiency has been frequently associated with increased susceptibility to infection (1), and recent studies clearly showed impairment of the immune system by vitamin A deficiency (*rev.* in 2). There is also some evidence that the carcinogenic action of some polyhalogenated aromatic compounds (*e.g.*, TCDD, PCB) may be due, at least in part, to their dysregulation of vitamin A homeostasis which leads to severe depletion of the vitamin (*rev.* in 3), culminating in impairment of the immune system.

Vitamins B_1 (thiamin), B_2 (riboflavin), B_6 (pyridoxine), B_{12} (cobalamin), niacin, folic acid, pantothenic acid, and biotin are all involved as coenzymes or as components of coenzymes. Thus, their possible modifying effect on chemical carcinogenesis is expectably related to their involvement in the metabolic activation or detoxification of specific types of carcinogens (*see* ref. 4 for an overview of enzyme systems involved in activation/detoxification of chemical carcinogens). For example, riboflavin is known to be a component of the coenzyme in the azo reductase system that detoxifies amino azo dyes. Consistent with this finding, the carcinogenic effect of certain amino azo dyes in rats can only be shown if the animals are maintained on a diet low in riboflavin but still compatible with the minimum requirement for near-normal growth rate; on the other hand, diets rich in riboflavin protect rats against amino azo dye carcinogenesis (*see* ref. 5, Vol. IIB, Section 5.1.4.1.5). In addition to direct modifying effects on chemical carcinogens through effect on metabolic activation/detoxification enzyme pathways, some of the B vitamins (and related compounds) may have indirect modifying effects on carcinogenesis. For example, folic acid deficiency may lead to lipotrope and methyl deficiency (*see* discussion below) as well as to disturbance of purine synthesis, which may all affect carcinogenesis.

Vitamin C (ascorbic acid) modulates carcinogenesis probably in a number of ways: (a) It is well documented that ascorbic acid can inhibit or prevent the formation of carcinogenic nitrosamines by blocking the reaction of secondary amines with nitrosating agents (*e.g.*, nitrite) under acidic conditions (*see* ref. 5, Vol. IIIA, Section 5.2.1.2.5.1.5).

---

[3]In this section, the term "vitamin A" is used to denote all compounds that exhibit vitamin A-like activity. These include the two major subgroups—the retinoids and the carotenoids. Although metabolically interconvertible, the serum levels of β-carotene are responsive to dietary intake, whereas those of vitamin A are regulated/maintained by supplies in the liver and are therefore less influenced by dietary intake.

Since humans are exposed to a variety of secondary amines (*e.g.*, pharmaceuticals, fish and seafoods, cheeses) and nitrosating agent (*e.g.*, nitrite in saliva and in processed meat products, nitrogen dioxide in air), ascorbic acid has been repeatedly proposed as a prophylactic agent against *in vivo* formation of carcinogenic nitroso compounds. (b) Ascorbic acid is involved in microsomal hydroxylation reactions catalyzed by mixed-function oxidases (MFO); thus, depending on the type of carcinogen involved, modification of the activity of MFO by ascorbic acid may affect activation or detoxification (1,6). (c) As an effective antioxidant at optimal physiological concentrations, ascorbic acid can act as a free-radical and active oxygen species scavenger and has a protective effect against damage to the genetic material (1,7). (d) However, at very high, supra-optimal concentrations ascorbic acid may act as a pro-oxidant since it can generate superoxide radical anions and hydroxyl radicals *if catalyzed* by the presence of free ferric or cupric ions; the *in vivo* significance of this reaction is not clear, however. (e) Ascorbic acid enhances various immune functions (1,8,9).

Vitamin D plays a critical role in the hormonal control network of the homeostasis of calcium. There is evidence that calcium plays a crucial role, as a "second messenger", in signal transduction of the control of cell proliferation, which is essential for the promotion of tumorigenesis (9,10). The activated form of vitamin D (1,25-dihydroxycholecalciferol) was reported to inhibit the proliferation of neoplastic cells in culture through a receptor-mediated process (9). There is also evidence that 1,25-dihydroxycholecalciferol binds to receptors localized in intestinal mucosal epithelial cells of rats and chicks. The receptor has been characterized and found to have substantial sequence homology with steroid and thyroid hormones and retinoic acid. The binding has been shown to trigger synthesis of mRNA that codes for calcium-binding proteins (1). Decreased levels of ornithine decarboxylase were reported in human and rodent colon mucosa exposed to increasing levels of calcium (11). Ornithine decarboxylase induction by vitamin D in intestinal cells may indicate the involvement of vitamin D in the polyamine biosynthesis pathways. The role of 1,25-dihydroxycholecalciferol in the regulation of calcium homeostasis is discussed in some detail in Chapter 11, Section 1.

Vitamin E (tocopherol) has antioxidant properties and, similarly to ascorbic acid, can act as a free-radical scavenger. Consistent with its lipophilic character, its principal focus of activity is the cell membrane, which it can protect from oxidative damage (7). In addition, tocopherol can increase the production of humoral antibodies (12) as well as enhance cell-mediated immunity (13,14). Tocopherol also increases the ability to repair DNA (15). Like ascorbic acid, tocopherol can inhibit the formation of carcinogenic nitrosamines from their precursors (16). It can potentiate the inhibitory effects of selenium on promotion and on subsequent proliferative stages in carcinogenesis (8).

Relatively little is known about the possible modifying role of vitamin K in carcinogenesis. Vitamin K is structurally related to potent cytostatic agents, such as doxorubicin, and, by virtue of its quinone structure, can act as an electron scavenger (*rev.* in 17). However, the same quinone structure may also generate oxidative stress when given at unphysiologically high doses. The oxidative stress includes the production of active oxygen species as well as depletion of the protective cellular nucleophile glutathione (GSH) (1). Thus, vitamin K may be expected to have an ambivalent effect on carcinogenesis, dependent upon the dose.

Among the quasi-vitamins several are known or may be expected to effect carcinogenesis; these include choline, inositol, bioflavonoids, and orotic acid. Choline, in phosphorylated form, is an important structural element of biological membranes. It is a lipotropic agent (*i.e.*, it promotes lipid transport) and is a source of labile methyl groups. Choline deficiency leads to fatty liver which is a predisposing condition to carcinogenesis.

Severe choline deficiency by itself can lead to hepatocarcinogenesis in rodent species; this is discussed in some detail in Subsection III. F below. Choline deficiency brings about methyl deficiency, which may lead to hypomethylation of DNA, thus causing changes in the expression of proto-oncogenes that play key roles in the regulation of growth (*e.g.*, c-*myc*, c-*fos*, and c-Ha-*ras*) as shown in the rodent liver (18). Alteration of DNA, nuclear membrane lipid peroxidation, and cell proliferation have also been observed in animals fed diets deficient in both choline and methionine (19). Phosphatidylinositol, a membrane constituent, is believed to have an important role in regulation of membrane-associated enzymes (*e.g.*, Na,K-ATPase) and membrane transport (*e.g.*, Ca^{++} mobilization) systems. It is a source of releasable arachidonic acid for synthesis of prostaglandins. Upon binding to various types of cell membrane receptors, phosphatidylinositol releases diacylglycerol as a second messenger which activates protein kinase C, a key enzyme involved in the promotion of tumorigenesis. Bioflavonoids may be expected to be anticarcinogenic at low doses through their antioxidant activity (1) and potentially carcinogenic at high doses (*see* ref. 5, Vol. IIIC, Section 5.3.2.6.3). Orotic acid is a precursor in the biosynthesis of pyrimidine (1); excess orotic acid can create an imbalance of the pyrimidine pool, characterized by an increase in uridine nucleotides and a decrease in adenosine nucleotides, leading to disturbance of the homeostasis of the cell through genetic as well as metabolic disorders (20).

III. VITAMIN DEFICIENCY AND CARCINOGENESIS

A. Vitamin A Deficiency and Carcinogenesis

A number of epidemiological studies have indicated a possible inverse relationship between vitamin A intake and the incidence of a variety of cancers at several organ sites, particularly cancers of the epithelial surfaces (*e.g.*, respiratory, urinary, skin) which require the vitamin for their integrity (9,21,22). In most of these studies, however, the estimates of vitamin A intake were based primarily on the frequency of ingestion of green and yellow vegetables (known to be a rich source of vitamin A) and not on the actual estimation of carotenoids (23). Clinical trials initiated in the late 1980s should provide a clue for the role of vitamin A deficiency in high-risk populations (24,25).

The serum level of vitamin A in animals is known to be under stringent homeostatic control. Recent studies (*rev.* in 3) indicate that a variety of polyhalogenated aromatic compounds (*e.g.*, TCDD, PCB) cause severe disturbances in vitamin A metabolism leading to its systemic depletion. As has already been stated above in subsection II, vitamin A deficiency-like symptoms have been frequently associated with TCDD and PCB intoxication. Both TCDD and PCB are known to be carcinogens (*see* ref. 5, Vol. IIIB) and it is probable that the mechanism of carcinogenic action of these compounds may at least in part involve depletion of vitamin A; this, in turn, could lead to enhancement of carcinogenesis through the impairment of immune surveillance.

Studies on the influence of vitamin A deficiency on the induction of cancer by a variety of chemical carcinogens has been conducted in rodents. The results are often inconclusive and appear to depend on the structure (and metabolism) of the chemical carcinogen, the animal species, and the target organ(s) involved. Thus, vitamin A deficiency significantly enhances liver carcinogenesis by aflatoxin B_1 (26) and lung tumorigenesis by 3-methylcholanthrene (3-MC) (27–29) or benzo[*a*]pyrene (BaP) (30) in rats. On the other hand, vitamin A deficiency has no effect on the induction of cancer in the lung, liver, and forestomach by N'-nitrosonornicotine (NNN) and 4-(methylnitrosamino)-1-(3-pyridyl)-1-butanone in mice (31); however, it reduces NNN-induced (32), but not methylbenzylnitrosamine (MBN)-induced esophageal carcinogenesis in rats (33). Skin tumorigenesis by 7.12-dimethylbenz[a]anthracene (DMBA) was reported to be significantly reduced in mice receiving a vitamin A deficient diet in one study (34), but enhanced in another (35). Vitamin A deficiency was found to reduce DMBA-induced mammary tumor induction in rats (36). The carcinogenic effect of N-[4-(5-nitro-2-furyl)-2-thiazolyl]formamide (FANFT) toward bladder was not influenced by vitamin A deficiency (37).

B. Deficiency in B Vitamins and Related Compounds

Animals maintained on diets deficient or low in riboflavin (B_2) showed greater susceptibility to DMBA-induced skin carcinogenesis (38), MBN-induced esophageal carcinogenesis (39), and azo dye–induced liver carcinogenesis (40; *see* also ref. 5, Vol. IIB, Section 5.1.4.1.5). However, the modifying effect may be dependent on the degree of severity of riboflavin deficiency; severe deficiencies may reduce rather than enhance tumor induction (9). There is some epidemiologic evidence of a possible association of increased esophageal cancer with riboflavin deficiency (22). Contradictory results have been reported from studies on vitamin B_6 (pyridoxine) deficiency, which enhances 2-acetylaminofluorene (AAF)–induced bladder carcinogenesis (41), reduces FANFT-induced bladder carcinogenesis (42), and has no significant effect on AAF–induced liver carcinogenesis (43). There is a possible association between vitamin B_6 deficiency and increased susceptibility to tumors and hyperplastic nodules in the kidney of humans (9). Folate deficiency has been associated with increased hepatocarcinogenesis; this topic will be further discussed under "Lipotrope Deficiency and Carcinogenesis" below.

C. Vitamin C Deficiency and Carcinogenesis

Since vitamin C has been considered to have anticarcinogenic effect (*rev.* in 1), low dietary intake of vitamin C has been suspected to have the opposite effect on carcinogenesis. Although the protective role of vitamin C in carcinogenesis has been extensively studied (*see* Subsection IV below), there appear to be very few systematic studies on the effect of vitamin C deficiency. An ascorbic acid–free diet was reported to have no significant effect on 3-MC–induced sarcoma development (44) and carcinogenesis by AAF (45) in the guinea pig.

D. Vitamin D Deficiency and Carcinogenesis

Decreasing vitamin D levels were found to promote DMBA-induced mammary carcinomas in rats fed a high-fat diet (46). However, vitamin D-deficiency did not alter development of colon tumors in rats induced by 1,2-dimethylhydrazine (DMH) (47).

E. Vitamin E Deficiency and Carcinogenesis

Epidemiologic evidence shows no significant evidence linking vitamin E deficiency to cancer susceptibility (9,21,48); nonetheless, data from some prospective studies suggest an association of lower plasma α-tocopherol levels with an increased risk of cancers of the lung, breast, and digestive tract (48). Other prospective studies may shed light on the role of vitamin E in cancer prevention (49). There are only a few studies on the influence of tocopherol deficiency on experimental chemical carcinogenesis. Tocopherol deficiency has been found to increase the incidence of DMBA-induced mammary cancer in rodents (50–52); the enhancing effect is particularly prominent in rats with high intake of polyunsaturated fat (52).

F. Lipotrope Deficiency and Carcinogenesis

Lipotropes are agents which help to regulate the metabolism of fat and cholesterol in the livers of animals. The principal lipotropic agents are choline and its precursor methyl group donors, methionine and folate. Copeland and Salmon (53) were the first to show that dietary deficiency in lipotropes has a hepatocarcinogenic effect in rodents. These investigators found that feeding bentonite (a kaolin-like adsorbent clay) to rats induces liver cirrhosis and tumors. This was traced to the adsorption and binding of choline from the diet to the clay, thus preventing the absorption of choline from the gut. The hepatocarcinogenicity of lipotrope deficiency has subsequently been confirmed in several species (19,54,55). In addition, there is also some suggestive evidence that borderline intake of folate combined with low intake of vitamin A may enhance the emergence of cervical cancer (22). Mechanistic studies indicate that lipotrope deficiency can cause lipid peroxidation in the nuclear membrane to generate free radicals which cause DNA damage (19). Fatty liver, increased cell proliferation, and DNA hypomethylation are all conducive to carcinogenesis.

Beyond being hepatocarcinogenic per se, lipotrope deficiency has also been shown to enhance or act synergistically with other chemical carcinogens. Rats fed diets deficient in choline, folate, and methionine showed consistent enhancement of chemically induced cancer of the liver, and to a lesser degree cancers of the pancreas and colon (*e.g.*, 56–59). The carcinogens whose activity can be enhanced by lipotrope deficiency include aflatoxin B_1, 2-AAF, DEN, DBN, azaserine, and ethionine. The enhancing effect appears to operate in both the tumorigenesis initiating as well as promoting phases of the carcinogenesis process (*rev.* in 18,58).

IV. MODULATION OF CARCINOGENESIS BY VITAMIN SUPPLEMENTATION

A. Influence of Vitamin A on Chemical Carcinogenesis

Several epidemiologic studies have indicated an inverse relationship between vitamin A and a variety of cancers at various organ sites, particularly those of epithelial surfaces (*e.g.*, respiratory, urinary, skin) which require the vitamin for their integrity (9,21,22). In all these studies, however, the estimates of vitamin A intake were based primarily on the frequency of ingestion of green and yellow vegetables (known to be a rich source of this vitamin) and not on the actual estimation of carotenoids (23). Some representative studies on the influence of vitamin A and related compounds on chemical carcinogenesis are summarized in Table 1. In the majority of studies involving the skin and the mammary gland, vitamin A exhibited protective effect against carcinogenesis induced by DMBA, BaP, *N*-nitroso-*N*-methylurea (NMU), and 17α-ethinylestradiol (17α-EE). However, this anticarcinogenic effect is not consistently uniform. In a number of experiments, promoting effects were observed. In one study, vitamin A derivatives were administered at maximum tolerated dose levels (61), while in another study (72) rats were given vitamin A only prior to the administration of the carcinogen. Contradictory results, or the lack of an influence of vitamin A on carcinogenesis, were reported for the lung, oral cavity,

TABLE 1.   Influence of Vitamin A and β-Carotene on Chemical Carcinogenesis in Rodents

Species	Carcinogen[a]	Organ site	Vitamin dosage	Route	Effect[b]	Ref.
			(A) Vitamin A and derivatives			
Mouse	DMBA	Skin	200 mg/kg 1×/2wk	p.o.	↓	60
			17–30 nmol 2×/wk	Topical	↑ or 0	61,62
			40–391 mg/kg diet	p.o.	↑	61
Mouse		Mammary gland	27×1 mmol/wk	p.o.	0	63
Mouse	DMBA + anthralin	Skin	170 nmol 2×/wk	Topical	0	64
Mouse	DMBA + TPA	Skin	200–700 IU/g diet for 5 wk	p.o.	↓	65
			(a) retinyl palmitate		↓	
			(b) 13-*cis*-retinoic acid		0	66
Mouse	DMBA + CO	Skin	0.009–0.015% sol'n. 5×/wk for 16–18wk	Topical	↓	66
Mouse	DMBA + phenol	Skin	0.009% sol'n. 5×/wk for 16 wk	Topical	↓	66
Rat	DMBA	Skin	12× 50,000 IU/day	i.m.	↓	67
		Mammary gland	Various doses	p.o.	↓	68–73
			0.03–0.08% diet	p.o.	↑ or 0	72
		Salivary gland	20–100 IU/g	p.o.	0	74
Hamster	DMBA	Oral cavity	2–15% sol'n.	Topical	↓	75
			10% sol'n.	Topical	↓	76
Rat	BaP	Mammary gland	250 ppm diet	p.o.	↑	77
Hamster	BaP	Lung	0.6–100 IU/g	p.o.	0	78
			2.4–3.3 mg/wk	i.g.	↑	79
Rat	3-MC	Lung	0.03–31 mmol/wk	p.o.	↓	80
Mouse	DEN	Liver	0.1–1 mmol/kg diet	p.o.	↑	81
Mouse	HBBN	Urinary bladder	0.02% diet	p.o.	↓	82
Mouse	ENU	Lymphoreticular system	170,000 IU/kg/day for 3 months	p.o.	↓	83
Rat	HBBN	Urinary bladder	0.024% diet	p.o.	↓	84,85
			8–32 mg/kg body wt	i.g.	0	86
			0.052% diet	p.o.	↑	87

Species	Carcinogen	Organ	Dose	Route	Effect[b]	Ref.
Rat	Methylbenzylnitrosamine	Esophagus	2.2–30 mg/kg diet	p.o.	0	33
Rat	MNNG	Stomach	150 IU/g diet	p.o.	0	88
Rat	NMU	Mammary gland	1–2 mmol/kg diet	p.o.	↓	72,73,89,90
Hamster	2,6-Di-Me-NO-morpholine	Colon	2 mmol/kg diet	p.o.	0	91
Hamster	BOPN	Liver	160 mg/kg	p.o.	↑	92
		Pancreas	0.4–1 mmol/kg diet	p.o.	↑	93
		Pancreas	0.25–0.5 mmol/kg or 100 IU/g diet	p.o.	0	94,95
Rat	DMH	Colon	2 mmol/kg diet	p.o.	0	86,91
Rat	FANFT	Urinary bladder	0.1–0.7 g/kg diet	p.o.	0	96
Rat	3'-Me-DAB	Liver	930–2500 IU/kg diet	p.o.	↓	97
Mouse	Estrone + progesterone	Mammary gland	1000 IU/kg diet	p.o.	↓	98
Rat	17α-EE	Mammary gland	82 mg/kg diet	p.o.	↓	99
Rat	Azaserine	Pancreas	412 IU/g diet	p.o.	↓	100
Rat	Azaserine	Pancreas	0.5–2 mmol/kg diet	p.o.	↓ or 0	101
Rat	BHA	Forestomach	0.25% diet	p.o.	↑	102
(B) β-Carotene						
Mouse	DMBA + CO	Skin	0.015% sol'n. 5×/wk for 18 wk	Topical	↑	66
Mouse	DMBA + phenol	Skin	0.015% sol'n. 5×/wk for 16 wk	Topical	↑	66
Mouse	DMBA + TPA	Skin	3% diet	p.o.	↓	103
Rat	DMBA	Salivary gland	290–1430 IU/kg/day	p.o.	0	104
Hamster	DMBA	Oral cavity	0.025% diet	p.o.	0	74
Rat	DMBA	Colon	190 ng/ml oil 3×/wk	Topical	↓	105
Rat	DMH	Colon	1% diet	p.o.	0	106

aFor the abbreviations used in this table, see p. 329.

b"↑" indicates significant enhancing effect on carcinogenicity. "↓" indicates significant inhibitory effect on carcinogenicity. "0" indicates no significant effect on carcinogenicity.

esophagus, stomach, colon, liver, pancreas, and urinary bladder. In most studies, vitamin A was not toxic. However, in some experiments, vitamin A was reported to cause significant decrease of body weight, enhance mortality, cause hair loss or peeling of the skin, limb paralysis, or testicular atrophy (79,86,91–93,95,97,101,102). Toxic effects occurred in studies revealing an enhancing or inhibiting effect of vitamin A on carcinogenesis. The influence of β-carotene on chemical carcinogenesis has not been as extensively studied; available data appear to be inconclusive with respect to its modulating effect on chemical carcinogenesis of the skin, oral cavity, and colon (*see* Table 1).

In addition to modulating effects on chemical carcinogenesis, there is some evidence that when given at high doses, vitamin A per se may be potentially carcinogenic under special experimental conditions. March and Biely (107) showed that white leghorn cockerels given diets containing high doses (11,000 or 20,000 IU/kg) of vitamin A (retinol) had significantly higher incidence of tumors of the reticuloendothelial system than control animals.

B. Influence of Vitamin B on Chemical Carcinogenesis

Thiamine exhibits no influence on skin tumorigenesis by DMBA or BaP (108). As discussed in Subsections II and III above, riboflavin is required for the functioning of the azo reductase system involved in the detoxification of azo dyes. Dietary supplementation with riboflavin has indeed been shown to inhibit hepatocarcinogenesis by different aminoazo dyes (109). This inhibitory effect appears to be specific for azo dyes; for example, riboflavin has no effect on diethylnitrosamine (DEN)-induced hepatocarcinogenesis (110). However, riboflavin also inhibits 3-MC–induced skin carcinogenesis (111), but has no effect on carcinogenesis by BaP or DMBA at this target (108). Nicotinamide exhibited inhibitory effect on skin carcinogenesis by DMBA in one study (112), but had no effect in another (108). Streptozotocin-induced diabetes significantly inhibits the induction of pancreatic carcinomas initiated by bis(2-oxopropyl)nitrosamine (BOPN) in hamsters. In these animals, nicotinamide restored the incidence of pancreatic carcinomas to that occurring in nondiabetic controls (113). In two studies, pyridoxine revealed a protective or enhancing effect on carcinogenesis (108,114). Cobalamin was found to enhance hepatocarcinogenesis induced by aflatoxin (115) or *p*-dimethylaminoazobenzene (116); however, these studies are not conclusive because of the use of high-protein or lipotrope-deficient diet, respectively. Two derivatives of cobalamin showed opposite modulatory effect on urethan-induced lung carcinogenesis (117).

C. Influence of Vitamin C on Chemical Carcinogenesis

Two epidemiologic studies, in Iran (118) and in New York (119), showed an inverse association between ascorbic acid intake and incidence of esophageal cancer or uterine/cervical dysplasia. Vitamin C has been shown to lower the incidence of ultraviolet-induced skin cancer through unknown mechanisms (22). Table 2 summarizes the results of representative studies on the modulation of chemical carcinogenesis by vitamin C. Skin tumorigenesis was inhibited in all studies cited. In all experiments involving administration of precursors of *N*-nitroso compounds (*i.e.,* nitrite + amine or urea compounds), vitamin C exhibits protective effects. The experiments on the modulation of carcinogenesis by *N*-nitroso compounds and other carcinogens in all other organs — in particular the lung, mammary gland, colon, urinary bladder, and subcutaneous tissue — did not reveal any protective effect of vitamin C. Ip (158) reported a negative influence of dietary ascorbic acid on the protective effect of selenium against DMBA-induced rat mammary carcinoma development. Some studies reported a promoting influence of vitamin C on carcinogenesis. This can in part be explained on the basis of the chemical behavior of the compounds (132), differences in the urinary pH (136,137,148), differences in urinary ion concentrations (136,148), and the dosage of the vitamin (131). In a few studies significant toxicity in terms of body weight loss was reported (124,136,137,140,147). Similarly to vitamin A, toxicity was observed in studies independently of the effect of vitamin C on carcinogenesis.

D. Influence of Vitamin D on Chemical Carcinogenesis

Recent epidemiologic studies suggest a protective role for vitamin D and calcium in colorectal cancer (159,160). Dietary calcium was reported to decrease colonic epithelial cell proliferation in individuals with genetic susceptibility to colon cancer (161). Newmark and Lipkin (11) recently suggested that a daily dietary calcium intake of 1500 mg/day for women and 1800 mg/day for men (three times higher than the current dietary calcium intake in western societies) may confer protection. Few studies have been conducted to investigate the effect of vitamin D on experimental chemical carcinogenesis. Dietary supplementation with 1,25-dihydroxycholecalciferol was reported to inhibit skin carcinogenesis initiated by DMBA and promoted by 12-*O*-tetradecanoylphorbol-13-acetate (TPA) (162,163) and colon carcinogenesis initiated by NMU and promoted by lithocholic acid (164); skin carcinogenesis induced by DMBA alone, however, was unaffected by this vitamin (165).

E. Influence of Vitamin E on Chemical Carcinogenesis

Vitamin E is expected to have a protective effect against chemical carcinogenesis because of its well-known antioxidant properties. Epidemiological studies around 1986 began to shed light on the potential usefulness of vitamin E in cancer prevention (166). Table 3 summarizes animal studies on the influence of vitamin E (tocopherol) in chemical carcinogenesis. The available data indicate that the induction of tumors in the ear ducts of rats and in the oral cavity of hamsters is successfully inhibited by tocopherol (Table 3). The data for all other organs appear to be inconclusive. For example, in five studies on the effect of tocopherol on DMH-induced colorectal carcinogenesis, two were inhibitory while the other three showed enhancement. Although tocopherol was reported to have no effect on DMBA-induced mammary carcinogenesis, its modulating effect was found to depend on the amount of dietary fat consumption (170). (*See also* Editors' Note II on p. 370.)

F. Influence of Other Vitamins, Lipotropes, and Other Quasi-Vitamins on Chemical Carcinogenesis

There is only one study on the effect of vitamin K and its derivatives. Vitamin K_1 (phylloquinone) increases the mortality rate of mice dying from BaP-induced tumors, whereas its synthetic derivative, 2-methyl-1,4-naphthoquinone (vitamin K_3), was found to reduce tumor development (186).

Since lipotrope deficiency is known to induce or promote carcinogenesis, the opposite effect may be expected from dietary supplementation with lipotropes. Dietary supplementation with choline and methionine has indeed been shown to suppress carcinogenesis by a variety of carcinogens, including ethionine (187), AAF (188), DEN (189), and a

TABLE 2.   Influence of Vitamin C on Chemical Carcinogenesis in Rodents

Species	Carcinogen[a]	Organ site	Vitamin dosage	Route	Effect[b]	Ref.
Mouse	DMBA	Skin	10 mg/kg/day	p.o.	↓	120
Mouse	DMBA + CO	Skin	2% diet	p.o.	↓	121
Mouse	DMBA + TPA	Skin	1 mg	Topical	↓	122
Mouse	TPA	Skin	20 × 12–56μmol/wk	Topical	↓	123
Rat	DMBA	Ear duct, mammary gland	5% diet	p.o.	0	124,125
Rat	DMBA	Mammary gland	1.3–3.7 g/kg body wt	p.o.	↓	68
Rat	BaP	s.c. tissue	2.5% in H_2O	p.o.	↓	126
Mouse	3-MC	s.c. tissue	20 × 30–175 mg/wk	p.o.	↓	127
Guinea pig	3-MC	s.c. tissue	0.3–10 mg/kg/day	p.o.	↓ or 0	128,129
			100 mg/kg/day	i.m.	↑	130
Mouse	Mononitrosopiperazine	Lung	2.3% diet	p.o.	↑	131
Mouse	Nitrosomorpholine	Lung	0.58–2.3%	p.o.	↑ or 0	131
Mouse	NMU	Lung	0.58–2.3% diet	p.o.	↑ or 0	131
Mouse	Dibutylamine + sodium nitrite	Liver	500 ppm diet	p.o.	↓	132
Mouse	Piperazine + sodium nitrite	Lung	0.58–2.3% diet	p.o.	↓	131
Mouse	Morpholine + sodium nitrite	Lung	0.58–2.3% diet	p.o.	↓	131
Mouse	Methylurea + sodium nitrite	Lung	0.58–2.3% diet	p.o.	↓	131
Rat	DEN	Liver	22 × 0.3 g/wk	p.o.	0	133
Rat	BHPN	Lung	5% diet	p.o.	0	134
Rat	DBN	Esophagus, forestomach	5% diet	p.o.	0	135
Rat	HBBN	Urinary bladder	5% diet (as Na ascorbate)	p.o.	↑	136–138
			5% (as ascorbic acid and three other salts[c])	p.o.	0	137,139,140
			1% diet (as Na ascorbate)	p.o.	0	137
Rat	N-Ethyl-N-(4-hydroxybutyl)-nitrosamine	Urinary bladder	20 × 0.5–0.6 mol/wk	p.o.	0	140
Rat	N-Nitrososarcosine ethyl ester	Forestomach	2% diet	p.o.	0	141
Rat	Nitrosomorpholine	Liver	2.3% diet	p.o.	↑	142
Rat	NMU	Thyroid gland, forestomach	5% diet	p.o.	0	125,143

Species	Compound	Organ	Dose	Route	Effect	Reference
Rat	NMU	Colon	1% diet	p.o.	0	144
Rat	ENU	Urinary bladder	5% diet	p.o.	↑	143
Rat	MNNG	Nervous system	0.2 g/kg on gestation day 22	p.o.	0	145
Rat		Stomach	0.04% in drinking H_2O	p.o.	↓	146
Rat	Ethylurea + sodium nitrite	Nervous system	0.2 g/kg on gestation day 22	p.o.	0	145
Rat	Nitrosamine mixture[d]	Liver	5% diet	p.o.	↓	147
		Thyroid			0	
		Kidney			↑ or 0	
		Urinary bladder			↑	
Hamster	Ethylurea + sodium nitrite	Nervous system	0.2 g/kg on gestation day 15	i.g.	↓	130
Rat	FANFT	Urinary bladder	4.4% diet or 0.25% in H_2O (as ascorbic acid)	p.o.	0	148,149
			5% diet (as Na ascorbate)	p.o.	↑	148
Mouse	DMH	Uterus	0.3% in drinking H_2O (a) as ascorbic acid (b) as Na ascorbate	p.o.	↓ / 0	150,151 / 150
Rat	DMH	Colon	7% diet	p.o.	↓	152,153
			50 mg/kg/day or 1%	p.o.	0	144,154
			5% diet	p.o.	↑	125,155
Hamster	DES	Kidney	1–2.5% diet	p.o.	↓	156
Hamster	17β-Estradiol	Kidney	1% in drinking H_2O	p.o.	↓	157

[a] For abbreviations used in this table, see p. 329.

[b] "↑" indicates significant enhancing effect on carcinogenicity. "↓" indicates significant inhibitory effect on carcinogenicity. "0" indicates no significant effect on carcinogenicity.

[c] Calcium L-ascorbate, L-ascorbate, L-ascorbic dipalmitate, L-ascorbic stearate.

[d] Mixture of HBBN, BHPN, and 2-hydroxyethylethylnitrosamine.

327

TABLE 3. Influence of α-Tocopherol (Vitamin E) on Chemical Carcinogenesis in Rodents

Species	Carcinogen[a]	Organ site	Vitamin dosage	Route	Effect[b]	Ref.
Mouse	DMBA	Forestomach	0.3 g 3×/wk	p.o.	0	167
Mouse	DMBA + TPA	Skin	20 × 80 μmol/wk	Topical	0	168
			1 mg/mouse	Topical	↓	122
Rat	DMBA	Ear duct	1.5% diet	p.o.	↓	124,125
		Mammary gland	1.5–2% diet	p.o.	0	125,169,170
Hamster	DMBA	Oral cavity	10 mg 2×/wk	p.o.	↓	171,172
			0.14 mg 3×/wk	Topical	↓	171
Mouse	3-MC	s.c. tissue	0.07–0.7% diet	p.o.	↓	173
Rat	DEN	Liver	0.05–0.72% diet for 6–47 wk	p.o.	0	174,175
			1.5% for 6 wk	p.o.	↓	174
Rat	BHPN	Lung	1% diet	p.o.	↓	135
Rat	HBBN	Urinary bladder	0.4–1.5% diet for 32 wk	p.o.	0	176
Rat	N-Nitrososarcosine	Forestomach	0.06% diet for 32 wk	p.o.	↓	141
Rat	NMU	Mammary gland	11.25 IU/day or 2% diet	p.o.	0	177,178
Rat	MNNG	Stomach	1% diet for 36 wk	p.o.	0	179
Rat	3'-Me-DAB	Liver	0.1–0.16% diet	p.o.	0	180
Mouse	DMH	Colon	0.02% diet for 31 days	p.o.	↑	181
Rat	DMH	Colon, rectum	0.06–1% or 1.75 IU/g diet	p.o.	0	153,182,183
		Colon, rectum, duodenum	4% diet for life	p.o.	↑	184
Rat	Azoxymethane	Colon	0.075% diet for 35 wk	p.o.	0	185

[a]For abbreviations used in this table, see p. 329.
[b]"↑" indicates significant enhancing effect on carcinogenicity. "↓" indicates significant inhibitory effect on carcinogenicity. "0" indicates no significant effect on carcinogenicity.

combination of DEN as initiator and DDT or phenobarbital as promoter (190). Wainfan *et al.* (191) showed that the survival of female AKR mice—known to have a high spontaneous incidence of leukemia—can be significantly prolonged by feeding diets supplemented with choline and methionine even though the time of onset of leukemia was not delayed or prevented.

Dietary supplementation with orotic acid enhances azoxymethane-induced carcinogenesis in the duodenum (192), DMBA-induced mammary tumorigenesis (193), the emergence of 2-hydroxypropyl-2-oxopropylnitrosamine–induced renal and pulmonary adenomas (194), and DEN-induced hepatocarcinogenesis (195). Since orotic acid is a normal cellular constituent, it has been suggested to be a potential multiorgan promoter (20). It is interesting to note that uracil, a close analog of orotic acid, has also been shown to be a promoter in 4-hydroxybutylbutylnitrosamine (HBBN)–induced urinary bladder carcinogenesis (196). At a high dose (3 percent diet), which induces urinary bladder stones, uracil alone can cause carcinoma development in the urinary bladder (197).

The influence of bioflavonoids on chemical carcinogenesis is not clearly understood. Being synergistic with vitamin C (*see* ref. 1), bioflavonoids are expected to inhibit chemical carcinogenesis. This has, in fact, been shown for certain bioflavonoids, such as quercetin, which clearly suppresses DMBA-induced skin carcinogenesis (198–201). However, other bioflavonoids such as myricetin and kaempferol, were found to promote DMBA-induced skin carcinogenesis (201). The picture is further complicated by the fact that many bioflavonoids are mutagenic (*see* ref. 5, Vol. IIIC, Section 5.3.2.6.3) and suspected to be carcinogenic at high doses. A recent bioassay by the National Toxicology Program (202) has shown that quercetin induces renal tubule cell tumors (predominantly adenomas) in male F344/N rats fed diets containing 1 or 4 percent (maximum tolerated dose) of quercetin.

Another quasi-vitamin which may be of potential concern if given at high doses is pyrroloquinoline quinone (PQQ). PQQ, also called "methoxatin", has protective effects in preventing skin lesions in mice. However, it is a tricarboxylic acid with a fused heterocyclic *o*-quinone ring system (*rev.* in 1) and has structural similarity to the heterocyclic aromatic amine compounds shown to be potent carcinogens by Sugimura and coworkers (203). The quinone moiety of PQQ is reactive toward nucleophilic moieties, such as sulfhydryl and amino groups (1). The possibility that PQQ may be genotoxic should be investigated.

V. CLOSING NOTE

Although the majority of experimental studies suggest protective effects of vitamins A, B, C, D, E, and K against chemical carcinogenesis, a number of investigations report lack of protective effect or, in some instances, even an enhancing influence on chemical carcinogenesis. Thus, existing data on the influence of vitamins on experimental carcinogenesis are not conclusive. The picture is complex because the induction of various types of tumors has been studied with different carcinogens at different doses, with different routes of administration, and with different species of animals. In addition, doses, routes, and times of administration of vitamins differed from experiment to experiment. Large doses of carcinogens may overwhelm the protective effect of vitamins. The use of commercially available animal diets, which may contain traces of carcinogens and anticarcinogens, can lead to different results than studies using purified diets (204).

Abbreviations Used: AAF, 2-acetylaminofluorene; AFB$_1$, aflatoxin B$_1$; BaP, benzo[*a*]pyrene; BHA, butylated hydroxyanisole; BHPN, bis(2-hydroxypropyl)nitrosamine; BOPN, bis(2-oxopropyl)nitrosamine; CO, croton oil; DBN, di-*n*-butylnitrosamine; DEN, diethylnitrosamine; DES, diethylstilbestrol; DMBA, 7,12-dimethylbenz[*a*]anthracene; DMH, 1,2-dimethylhydrazine; ENU, *N*-ethyl-*N*-nitrosourea; 17α-EE, 17α-ethinylestradiol; FANFT, *N*-[4-(5-nitro-2-furyl)-2-thiazolyl]formamide; GSH, glutathione; HBBN, 4-hydroxybutylbutylnitrosamine; MBN, methylbenzylnitrosamine; 3-MC, 3-methylcholanthrene; 3'-Me-DAB, 3'-methyl-4-dimethylaminoazobenzene; MFO, mixed-function oxidases; MNNG, *N*-methyl-*N'*-nitro-*N*-nitrosoguanidine; NMU, *N*-nitroso-*N*-methylurea; NNN, *N'*-nitrosonornicotine; PCB, polychlorinated biphenyls; PQQ, pyrroloquinoline quinone; TCDD, 2,3,7,8-tetrachlorodibenzo-*p*-dioxin; TPA, 12-*O*-tetradecanoylphorbol-13-acetate.

REFERENCES

1. Combs, G. F., Jr.: "The Vitamins: Fundamental Aspects in Nutrition and Health". Academic Press, San Diego, 1992.
2. Ross, A. C.: *Proc. Soc. Exp. Biol. Med.* **200,** 303 (1992).
3. Zile, M. H.: *Proc. Soc. Exp. Biol. Med.* **201,** 141 (1992).
4. Woo, Y.-T., Arcos, J. C., and Lai, D. Y.: Metabolic and Chemical Activation of Carcinogens: An Overview. *In* "Chemical Carcinogens: Activation Mechanisms, Structural and Electronic Factors, and Reactivity" (P. Politzer and F. J. Martin, Jr., eds.). Elsevier, Amsterdam, 1988, Chapter 1, p.1.
5. Arcos, J. C., Argus, M. F., Lai, D. Y., and Woo, Y.-T.: "Chemical Induction of Cancer", monograph series: Vol. I, 1968; Vol. IIA, 1974; Vol. IIB, 1974; Vol. IIIA, 1982; Vol. IIIB, 1985; Vol. IIIC, 1988. Academic Press, New York/Orlando/San Diego.
6. Newberne, P., and Suphakarn, V.: Influence of the Antioxidants Vitamins C and E and of Selenium on Cancer. *In* "Vitamins, Nutrition and Cancer" (K. Prasad, ed.). Karger, Basel, 1984, p. 46.
7. Shamberger R.: *Cancer Bull.* **34,** 150 (1982).
8. Milner, J. A.: Mechanism for Nutrition Inhibition of Carcinogenesis. *In* "Nutrition and Cancer Prevention" (T. E. Moon and M. S. Micozzi, eds.). Dekker, New York, 1989, p.13.
9. Newberne, P. M., and Locniskar, M.: *Recent Prog. Res. Nutr. Cancer* **346,** 119 (1990).
10. Rozengurt, E.: *Br. Med. Bull.* **45,** 55 (1989).
11. Newmark, H. L., and Lipkin, M.: *Cancer Res.* **52,** 2067s (1992).
12. Tengerdy, R., Mathias, M., and Nockels, C.: Effect of Vitamin E on Immunity and Disease Resistance. *In* "Vitamins, Nutrition and Cancer" (K. Prasad, ed.). Karger, Basel, 1984, p. 123.
13. Prasad, K., ed.: "Vitamins, Nutrition and Cancer". Karger, Basel, 1984.
14. Yasunaga, T., Ohgaki, T., Inamoto, T., and Hikasa, Y.: *Nippon. Gan Chiryo Gakkai Shi.* **17,** 2074 (1982).
15. Beckman, C., Roy, R., and Sproule, A.: *Mutat. Res.* **105,** 73 (1982).
16. Mirvish, S.: *Cancer* **58,** 1842 (1986).
17. Olson, R. E.: *Nutr. Rev.* **4,** 281 (1984).
18. Wainfan, E., and Poirier, L. A.: *Cancer Res.* **52,** 2071s (1992).
19. Ghosphal, A., Rushmore, T., and Farber, E.: Induction of Cancer by Dietary Deficiency without Added Carcinogens. *In* "Nongenotoxic Mechanisms in Carcinogenesis" (B. E. Butterworth, and T. J. Slaga, eds.), Banbury Report No. 25. Cold Spring Harbor Laboratory, Cold Spring Harbor, New York, 1987, p.179.
20. Manjeshwar, S., Sheikh, A., Pichiri-Coni, G., Coni, P., Rao, P. M., Rajalakshmi, S., Pediaditakis, P., Michalopoulos, G., and Sarma, D. S. R.: *Cancer Res.* **52,** 2078s (1992).
21. NRC: "Diet and Health: Implications for Reducing Chronic Disease Risk", National Research Council (NRC) Committee on Diet and Health, Food and Nutrition Board. National Academy Press, Washington, D.C., 1989.
22. Weisburger, J.: *Am. J. Clin. Nutr.* **53,** 226s (1991).
23. Newberne, P. M., Schrager, T. F., and Conner, M. W.: Experimental Evidence on the Nutritional Prevention of Cancer. *In* "Nutrition and Cancer Prevention" (T. E. Moon and M. S. Micozzi, eds.). Dekker, New York, 1989, p.33.
24. Clifford, C. K., Butrum, R. R., Greenwald, P., and Yates, J. N.: Clinical Trials of Low Fat Diets and Breast Cancer Prevention. *In* "Dietary Fat and Cancer" (C.Ip, ed.). Alan Liss, New York, 1986, p. 93
25. Lippman, S. M., and Meyskens, J. L., Jr.: Retinoids for the Prevention of Cancer. *In* "Nutrition and Cancer Prevention", (T. E. Moon and M. S. Micozzi, eds.). Dekker, New York, 1989, p. 101.
26. Suphakarn, V., Newberne, P., and Goldman, M.: *Nutr. Cancer* **5,** 41 (1983).
27. Nettesheim, P., Cone, M., and Snyder, C.: *Cancer Res.* **36,** 996 (1976).

28. Nettesheim, P., Snyder, C., and Kim, J.: *Environ. Health Persp.* **29**, 89 (1979).
29. Dogra, S., Khanduja, K., and Gupta, M.: *Br. J. Cancer* **52**, 931 (1985).
30. Gupta, M., Khanduja, K., Koul, L., and Sharma, R.: *Cancer Lett.* **55**, 83 (1990).
31. Padma, P., Lalitha, V., Amonkar, A., and Bhide, S.: *Carcinogenesis* **10**, 1997 (1989).
32. Raineri, R., Hecht, S., Maronpot, R., and Weisburger, J.: *Federation Proc.* **34**, 811 (1975).
33. Nauss, K., Bueche, D., and Newberne, P.: *J. Natl. Cancer Inst.* **79**, 145 (1987).
34. DeLuca, L., Shores, R., Spangler, E., and Wenk, M.: *Cancer Res.* **49**, 5400 (1989).
35. Davies, R.: *Cancer Res.* **27**, 237 (1967).
36. Zile, M., Cullum, M., Roltsch, I., DeHoog, J., and Welsch, C.: *Cancer Res.* **46**, 3495 (1986).
37. Cohen, S., Wittenberg, J., and Bryan, G.: *Cancer Res.* **36**, 2334 (1976).
38. Wynder, E., and Chan, P.: *Cancer* **26**, 1221 (1970).
39. Newberne, P., Charnley, G., Adams, K., Cantor, M., Roth, D., and Supharkarn, V.: *Food. Chem. Toxicol.* **24**, 1111 (1986).
40. Rivlin, R.: *Cancer Res.* **33**, 1977 (1973).
41. Melicow, M., Uson, A., and Price, D.: *J. Urol.* **91**, 520 (1964).
42. Birt, D., Julius, A., Hasegawa, R., John, M., and Cohen, S.: *Cancer Res.* **47**, 1244 (1987).
43. Morris, H., Sidransky, H., and Wagner, B.: *Tumori* **49**, 159 (1963).
44. Russell, W., Ortega, L., and Wynne, E.: *Cancer Res.* **12**, 216 (1952).
45. Breidenbach, A. W., and Argus, M. F.: *Q. J. Fl. Acad. Sci.* **19**, 68 (1956).
46. Jacobson, A., James, K., Newmark, H., and Carroll, K.: *Cancer Res.* **49**, 6300 (1989).
47. Sitrin, M., Halline, A., Abrahams, C., and Brasitus, T.: *Cancer Res.* **51**, 5608 (1991).
48. Mergens, W. J., and Bhagavan, H. N.: α-Tocopherol (Vitamin E). *In* "Nutrition and Cancer Prevention" (T. E. Moon and M. S. Micozzi, eds.). Dekker, New York, 1989, p. 305.
49. DeWys, W. D., Malone, W. F., Butrum, R. R., and Sestilli, M.: *Cancer* **58**, 1954 (1986).
50. Lee, C., and Chen, C.: *Proc. Am. Assoc. Cancer Res.* **20**, 132 (1979).
51. Newmark, H., and Mergens, W.: α-Tocopherol and Its Relationship to Tumor Induction and Development. *In* "Inhibition of Tumor Induction and Development" (M. Zedeck, ed.). Plenum Press, New York, 1981, p. 127.
52. Ip, C.: *Carcinogenesis* **3**, 1453 (1982).
53. Copeland, D. H., and Salmon, W. D.: *Am. J. Pathol.* **22**, 1059 (1946).
54. Buckley, G. F., and Hartroft, W. S.: *AMA Arch. Pathol.* **59**, 185 (1955).
55. Salmon, W. D., Copeland, D. H., and Burns, M. J.: *J. Natl. Cancer Inst.* **15**, 1549 (1955).
56. Lombardi, B., and Shinozuka, H.: *Int. J. Cancer* **23**, 565 (1979).
57. Yokoyama, S., Sells, M. A., Reddy, T. V., and Lombardi, B.: *Cancer Res.* **45**, 2834 (1985).
58. Newberne, P. M., and Rogers, A. E.: *Annu. Rev. Nutr.* **6**, 407 (1986).
59. Shinozuka, H., Katyai, S. L., and Lombardi, B.: *Int. J. Cancer* **22**, 36 (1978).
60. Bollag, W.: *Eur. J. Cancer* **8**, 689 (1972).
61. McCormick, D., Bagg, B., and Hultin, T.: *Cancer Res.* **47**, 5989 (1987).
62. Verma, A., Conrad, E., and Boutwell, R.: *Cancer Res.* **42**, 3519 (1982).
63. Welsch, C., DeHoog, J., and Moon, R.: *Carcinogenesis* **5**, 1301 (1984).
64. Dawson, M., Chao, W., and Helmes, T.: *Cancer Res.* **47**, 6210 (1987).
65. Gensler, H., Watson, R., Moriguchi, S., and Bowden, T.: *Cancer Res.* **47**, 967 (1987).
66. Shamberger, R.: *J. Natl. Cancer Inst.* **47**, 667 (1971).
67. Brown, I., Lane, B., and Pearson, J.: *J. Natl. Cancer Inst.* **58**, 1347 (1977).
68. Rao, A. R. N., Rao. A. R., Jannu, L., and Hussain, S.: *Jpn. J. Cancer Res.* **81**, 1239 (1990).
69. Welsch, C., and DeHoog, J.: *Cancer Res.* **43**, 585 (1983).
70. Moon, R., Grubbs, C., and Sporn, M.: *Cancer Res.* **36**, 2626 (1976).
71. Aylsworth, C., Cullum, M., Zile, M., and Welsch, C.: *J. Natl. Cancer Inst.* **76**, 339 (1986).
72. Grubbs, C., Eto, I., Juliana, M., Hardin, M., and Whitaker, L.: *Anticancer Res.* **10**, 661 (1990).
73. McCormick, D., Mehta, R., Thompson, C., Dinger, N., Caldwell, J., and Moon, R.: *Cancer Res.* **42**, 509 (1982).
74. Alam, B., Alam, S., and Weir, J.: *Nutr. Cancer* **11**, 233 (1988).
75. Kandarkar, S., Potdar, P., and Sirsat, S.: *Neoplasma* **31**, 415 (1984).
76. Polliack, A., and Levij, I.: *Cancer Res.* **29**, 327 (1969).
77. McCormick, D., Burns, F., and Albert, R.: *J. Natl. Cancer Inst.* **66**, 559 (1981).
78. Beems, R.: *Carcinogenesis* **5**, 1057 (1984).
79. Smith, D., Rogers, A., Herndon, B., and Newberne, P.: *Cancer Res.* **35**, 11 (1975).
80. Nettesheim, P., and Williams, M.: *Int. J. Cancer* **17**, 351 (1976).
81. McCormick, D., Hollister, J., Bagg, B., and Long, R.: *Carcinogenesis* **11**, 1605 (1990).
82. Becci, P., Thompson, H., Grubbs, C., Squire, R., Brown, C., Sporn, M., and Moon, R.: *Cancer Res.* **38**, 4463 (1978)
83. Wrba, H., Dutter, A., and Hacker-Rieder, A.: *Arch. Geschwülstforsch.* **53**, 89 (1983).

84. Becci, P., Thompson, H., Grubbs, C., Brown, C., and Moon, R.: *Cancer Res.* **39**, 3141 (1979).
85. Grubbs, C., Moon, R., Sporn, M., and Newton, D.: *Cancer Res.* **37**, 599 (1977).
86. Schmähl, D., and Habs, M.: *Arzneim.-Forsch.* **28**, 49 (1978).
87. Quander, R., Leary, S., Strandberg, J., Yarbrough, B., and Squire, R.: *Cancer Res.* **45**, 5235 (1985).
88. Kim, J., Park, J., Lee, M., Han, M., Park, S., Lee, B., and Jung, S.: *Jpn. J. Surg.* **15**, 427 (1985).
89. Moon, R., McCormick, D., and Mehta R.: *Cancer Res.* **43** (Suppl.), 2469s (1983).
90. Welsch, C., Brown, C, Goodrich-Smith, M., Chuisano, J., and Moon, R.: *Cancer Res.* **40**, 3095 (1980).
91. Silverman, J., Katayama, S., Zelenakas, K., Lauber, J., Musser, T., Reddy, M., Levenstein, M., and Weisburger, H.: *Carcinogenesis* **11**, 1167 (1981).
92. Stinson, S., Reznik, G., and Levitt, M.: *Proc. Am. Assoc. Cancer Res.* **23**, 225 (1982).
93. Birt, D., Davies, M., Pour, P., and Salmasi, S.: *Carcinogenesis* **4**, 1215 (1983).
94. Woutersen, R., and van Gardneren-Hoetmer, A.: *Cancer Lett.* **41**, 179 (1988).
95. Longnecker, D., Kuhlmann, E., and Curphey, T.: *Cancer Res.* **43**, 3226 (1983).
96. Croft, W., Croft, M., Paulus, K., Williams, J., Wang, C., and Lower, G.: *Carcinogenesis* **2**, 515 (1981).
97. Cohen, S., Wittenberg, J., and Bryan, G.: *Cancer Res.* **36**, 2334 (1976).
98. Mack, D., Reed, V., and Smith, L.: *Int. J. Biochem.* **22**, 359 (1990).
99. Welsch, C., Goodrich-Smith, M., Brown, C., and Crowe, N.: *J. Natl. Cancer Inst.* **67**, 935 (1981).
100. Holtzman, S.: *Carcinogenesis* **9**, 305 (1988).
101. Longnecker, D., Kuhlmann, E., and Curphey, T.: *Cancer Res.* **43**, 3219 (1983).
102. Hasegawa, R., Takahashi, M., Furukawa, F., Toyoda, K., Sato, H., and Hayashi, Y.: *Jpn. J. Cancer Res.* **79**, 320 (1988).
103. Lambert, L., Koch, W., Wamer, W., and Kornhauser, A.: *Nutr. Cancer* **13**, 213 (1990).
104. Steinel, H., and Baker, R.: *Cancer Lett.* **51**, 163 (1990).
105. Suda, D., Schwartz, J., and Shklar, G.: *Carcinogenesis* **7**, 711 (1986).
106. Colacchio, T., and Memoli, V.: *Arch. Surg.* **121**, 1421 (1986).
107. March, B. E., and Biely, J.: *Nature* **214**, 287 (1967).
108. Roe, F.: *Br. J. Cancer* **16**, 252 (1962).
109. Lambooy, J.: *Proc. Soc. Exp. Biol. Med.* **134**, 192 (1970).
110. Schmähl, D., and von Stackelberg, S.: *Arzneim.-Forsch.* **18**, 318 (1968).
111. Ohkoshi, M., Ohta, H., and Ito, M.: *Gann* **73**, 105 (1982).
112. Ludwig, A., Dietel, M., Schäfer, G., Müller, K., and Hilz, H.: *Cancer Res.* **50**, 2470 (1990).
113. Bell, R., McCullough, P., and Pour, P.: *Am. J. Surg.* **155**, 159 (1988).
114. Draudin-Krylenko, V., Bukin, I., and Nikonova, T.: *Vopr. Onkol.* **35**, 34 (1989).
115. Temcharoen, P., Anukarahanonta, T., and Bhamarapravati, N.: *Cancer Res.* **38**, 2185 (1978).
116. Day, P., Payne, L., and Dinning, J.: *Proc. Soc. Exp. Biol. Med.* **74**, 854 (1950).
117. McCully, K., and Vezeridis, M.: *Proc. Soc. Exp. Biol. Med.* **191**, 346 (1989).
118. Cook-Mozaffari, P.: *Nutr. Cancer* **1**, 51 (1979).
119. Wassertheil-Smoller, S., Romney, S. L., Wylie-Rosett, J., Slugle, S., Miller, G., Lucido, D., Duttagupta, C., and Palan, P. R.: *Am. J. Epidemiol.* **114**, 714 (1981).
120. Sadek, I., and Abdelmegid, N.: *Oncology* **39**, 399 (1982).
121. Shamberger, R.: *J. Natl. Cancer Inst.* **48**, 1491 (1972).
122. Slaga, T., and Bracken, W.: *Cancer Res.* **37**, 1631 (1977).
123. Smart, R., Huang, M., Han, Z., Kaplan, M., Focella, A., and Conney, A.: *Cancer Res.* **47**, 6633 (1987).
124. Hirose, M., Masuda, A., Inoue, T., Fukushima, S., and Ito, N.: *Carcinogenesis* **7**, 1155 (1986).
125. Ito, N., Hirose, M., Fukushima, S., Tsuda, H., Tatematsu, M., and Asamoto, M.: *Toxicol. Pathol.* **14**, 315 (1986).
126. Kallistratos, G., and Fasske, E.: *J. Cancer Res. Clin. Oncol.* **97**, 91 (1980).
127. Abdel-Galil, A.: *Oncology* **43**, 335 (1986).
128. Migliozzi, J.: *Br. J. Cancer* **35**, 448 (1977).
129. Rustia, M.: *J. Natl. Cancer Inst.* **55**, 1389 (1975).
130. Banic, S.: *Cancer Lett.* **11**, 239 (1981).
131. Mirvish, S., Cardesa, A., Wallcave, L., and Shubik, P.: *J. Natl. Cancer Inst.* **55**, 633 (1975).
132. Mokhtar, N., El-Aaser, A., El-Bolkainy, M., Ibrahim, H., El-Din, N., and Moharram, N.: *Eur. J. Cancer Clin. Oncol.* **24**, 403 (1988).
133. Wagner, W., Kessler, H., and Husemann, B.: *Zentralbl. Chirurg.* **113**, 1501 (1988).
134. Hasegawa, R., Furukawa, F., Toyoda, K., Takahashi, M., Hayashi, Y., Hirose, M., and Ito, N.: *Jpn. J. Cancer Res.* **81**, 871 (1990).
135. Fukushima, S., Sakata, Y., Tagawa, M., Shibata, M., Hirose, M., and Ito, N.: *Cancer Res.* **47**, 2113 (1987).
136. Fukushima, S., Shibata, M., Shirai, T., Kurata, Y., Tamano, S., and Imaida, K.: *Cancer Res.* **47**, 4821 (1987).

137. Fukushima, S., Uwagawa, S., Shirai, T., Hasegawa, R., and Ogawa, K.: *Cancer Res.* **50**, 4195 (1990).
138. Mori, S., Kurata, Y., Takeuchi, Y., Toyama, M., Makino, S., and Fukushima, S.: *Cancer Res.* **47**, 3492 (1987).
139. Fukushima, S., Ogiso, T., Kurata, Y., Shibata, M., and Kakizoe, T.: *Cancer Lett.* **35**, 17 (1987).
140. Inoue, T., Imaida, K., Suzuki, E., Okada, M., and Fukushima, S.: *Cancer Lett.* **40**, 265 (1988).
141. Bespalov, V., Trojan, D., Petrov, A., and Aleksandrov, V.: *Vopr. Onkol.* **35**, 1332 (1989).
142. Mirvish, S., Pelfrene, A., Garcia, H., and Shubik, P.: *Cancer Lett.* **2**, 101 (1976).
143. Imaida, K., Fukushima, S., Shirai, T., Masui, T., Ogiso, T., and Ito, N.: *Gann* **75**, 769 (1984).
144. Reddy, B., Hirota, N., and Katayama, S.: *Carcinogenesis* **3**, 1097 (1982).
145. Ivankovic, S., Zeller, J., Schmähl, D., and Preussmann, R.: *Naturwissenschaften* **60**, 525 (1973).
146. Balansky, R., Blagoeva, P., Mircheva, Z., Stoitchev, I., and Chernozemski, I.: *J. Cancer Res. Clin. Oncol.* **112**, 272 (1986).
147. Thamavit, W., Fukushima, S., Kurata, Y., Asamoto, M., and Ito, N.: *Cancer Lett.* **45**, 93 (1989).
148. Cohen, S., Ellwein, L., Okamura, T., Masui, T., Johansson, S., Smith, R., Wehner, J., Khachab, M., Chappel, C., Schoenig, G., Emerson, J., and Garland, E.: *Cancer Res.* **51**, 1766 (1991).
149. Soloway, M., Cohen, S., Dekernion, J., and Persky, L.: *J. Urol.* **113**, 483 (1975).
150. Turusov, V., Trukhanova, L., and Parfenov, Y.: *Cancer Lett.* **56**, 29 (1991).
151. Trukhanova, L., Parfenov, Y., and Turusov, V.: *Vopr. Onkol.* **36**, 563 (1990).
152. Colacchio, T., and Memoli, V.: *Arch. Surg.* **121**, 1421 (1986).
153. Colacchio, T., Memoli, V., and Hildebrandt, L.: *Arch. Surg.* **124**, 217 (1989).
154. Jones, F., Komorowski, R., and Condon, R.: *J. Surg. Oncol.* **25**, 54 (1984).
155. Shirai, T., Ikawa, E., Hirose, M., Thamavit, W., and Ito, N.: *Carcinogenesis* **6**, 637 (1985).
156. Liehr, J., and Wheeler, W.: *Cancer Res.* **43**, 4638 (1983).
157. Liehr, J., Roy, D., and Gladek, A.: *Carcinogenesis* **10**, 1983 (1989).
158. Ip, C.: *J. Natl. Cancer Inst.* **77**, 299 (1986).
159. Wargovich, M. J., Bear, A. R., Hu, P. J., and Sumiyoshi, H.: *Gastroenterol. Clin. North Am.* **17**, 727 (1988).
160. Sorenson, A. W., Slattery, M. L., and Ford, M. H.: *Nutr. Cancer* **11**, 135 (1988).
161. Lipkin, M., Friedman, E., Winawer, S. J., and Newmark, H.: *Cancer Res.* **49**, 248 (1989).
162. Wood, A., Chang, R., Huang, M., Uskokovic, M, and Conney, A.: *Biochem. Biophys. Res. Commun.* **116**, 131 (1983).
163. Chida, K., Hashiba, H., Fukushima, M., Suda, T., and Kuroki, T.: *Cancer Res.* **45**, 5426 (1985).
164. Kawaura, A., Tanida, N., Sawada, K., Oda, M., and Shimoyama, T.: *Carcinogenesis* **10**, 647 (1989).
165. Wood, A., Chang, R., Huang, M., Baggiolini, E., Partridge, J., Uskokovic, M., and Conney, A.: *Biochem. Biophys. Res. Commun.* **130**, 924 (1985).
166. DeWys, W. D., Malone, W. F., Butrus, R. R., and Sestilli, M.: *Cancer* **58**, 1954 (1986).
167. Wattenberg, L.: *J. Natl. Cancer Inst.* **48**, 1425 (1972).
168. Perchellet, J., Abney, N., Thomas, R., Guislain, Y., and Perchellet, E.: *Cancer Res.* **47**, 477 (1987).
169. Rao, A., Hussain, S., Jannu, L., Kumari, M., and Aradhana, M.: *Indian J. Exp. Biol.* **28**, 409 (1990).
170. McCay, P., King, M., and Pitha, J.: *Cancer Res.* **41**, 3745 (1981).
171. Shklar, G., Schwartz, J., Trickler, D., and Reid, S.: *J. Oral Pathol. Med.* **19**, 60 (1990).
172. Trickler, D., and Shklar, G.: *J. Natl. Cancer Inst.* **78**, 165 (1987).
173. Haber, S., and Wissler, R.: *Proc. Soc. Exp. Biol. Med.* **111**, 774 (1962).
174. Ura, H., Denda, A., Yokose, Y., Tsutsumi, M., and Konishi, Y.: *Carcinogenesis* **8**, 1595 (1987).
175. Hendrich, S., Duitsman, P., Krüger, S., Jackson, A., and Myers, R.: *Nutr. Cancer* **15**, 53 (1991).
176. Tamano, S., Fukushima, S., Shirai, T., Hirose, M., and Ito, N.: *Cancer Lett.* **35**, 39 (1987).
177. Beth, M., Berger, M., Aksoy, M., and Schmähl, D.: *Int. J. Cancer* **56**, 445 (1987).
178. King, R., and McCay, P.: *Cancer Res.* **43**, 2435 (1983).
179. Takahashi, M., Furukawa, F., Toyoda, K., Sato, H., Hasegawa, R., and Hayashi, Y.: *Cancer Lett.* **30**, 161 (1986).
180. Swick, R., and Bauman, C.: *Cancer Res.* **11**, 948 (1951).
181. Temple, N., and El-Khatib, S.: *Cancer Lett.* **35**, 71 (1987).
182. Cook, N., and McNamara, P.: *Cancer Res.* **40**, 1329 (1980).
183. Chester, J., Gaissert, H., Ross, J., Malt, R., and Weitzman, S.: *J. Natl. Cancer Inst.* **76**, 939 (1986).
184. Toth, B., and Patil, K.: *J. Natl. Cancer Inst.* **70**, 1107 (1983).
185. Reddy, B., and Tanaka, T.: *J. Natl. Cancer Inst.* **76**, 1157 (1986).
186. Israels, L, Walls, G., Ollmann, D., Friesen, E., and Israels, E.: *J. Clin. Invest.* **71**, 1130 (1983).
187. Brada, Z., Altman, N. H., Hill, M., and Bulba, S.: *Res. Commun. Chem. Pathol. Pharmacol.* **38**, 157 (1982).
188. Brada, Z., Altman, N. H., Hill, M., and Bulba, S.: *Federation Proc.* **43**, 591 (1984).
189. Rogers, A. E.: *Cancer Res.* **37**, 194 (1977).

190. Shivaparkar, N., Hoover, K. L., and Poirier, L. A.: *Carcinogenesis* **7**, 547 (1986),

191. Wainfan, E., Dizik, M., Kilkenny, M., and O'Callaghan, J. P.: *Carcinogenesis* **11**, 361 (1990).

192. Rao, P. M., Laconi, E., Vasudevan, S., Denda, A., Rajagopal, S., Rajalakshmi, S., and Sarma, D. S. R.: *Toxicol. Pathol.* **15**, 190 (1987).

193. Elliott, T. S., and Visek, W. J.: *FASEB J.* **3**, A474 (1989).

194. Kokkinakis, D. M., Scarpelli, D. G., and Oyasu, R.: *Carcinogenesis* **12**, 181 (1991).

195. Laconi, E., Vasudevan, S., Rao, P. M., Rajalakshmi, S., and Sarma, D. S. R.: *Proc. Am. Assoc. Cancer Res.* **27**, 142 (1986).

196. Shirai, T., Tagawa, Y., Fukushima, S., Imaida, K., and Ito, N.: *Cancer Res.* **47**, 6726 (1987).

197. Okumura, M., Shirai, S., Tamano, S., Ito, M., Yamada, S., and Fukushima, S.: *Carcinogenesis* **12**, 35 (1991).

198. Van Duuren, B. L., and Goldschmidt, B. M.: *J. Natl. Cancer Inst.* **56**, 1237 (1976).

199. Nishino, H., Iwashima, A., Fujiki, H., and Sugimura, T.: *Jpn. J. Cancer Res.* **75**, 113 (1984).

200. Kato, R., Nishidate, T., Yamamoto, S., and Sugimura, T.: *Carcinogenesis* **4**, 1301 (1983).

201. DiGiovanni, J., Slaga, T. J., Viaje, A., Berry, D. L., Harvey, R. G., and Juchau, M. R.: *J. Natl. Cancer Inst.* **61**, 135 (1978).

202. Dunnick, J., and Hailey, J. R.: *Fundam. Appl. Toxicol.* **19**, 423 (1992).

203. Sugimura, T., Sato, S., and Wakabayashi, K.: Mutagens/Carcinogens in Pyrolysates of Amino Acids and Proteins and in Cooked Foods: Heterocyclic Aromatic Amines. *In* "Chemical Induction of Cancer," Vol. IIIC (by Y.-T. Woo, D. Y. Lai, J. C. Arcos, and M. F. Argus). Academic Press, San Diego, 1988, Appendix III, p. 681.

204. Chen, L., Boissoneault, G., and Glauert, H.: *Anticancer Res.* **8**, 739 (1988).

Modulation by Minerals[1]

Maryce M. Jacobs and Roman J. Pienta

I. INTRODUCTION

In recent decades a large volume of literature has evolved that addresses the modulation of chemical induction of cancer by minerals in the diet. Prior to this, research was directed more toward the general toxicity and in particular the potential carcinogenicity of metals. Inorganic salts and/or organic forms of selenium, nickel, chromium, cobalt, titanium, lead, manganese, and other metals were reported to cause tumors, and mercury, arsenic, and beryllium compounds to cause genetic damage, but not always tumors (1–5). Research then turned toward the therapeutic attributes of minerals, when platinum coordination complexes and selenium compounds were found to be effective in cancer therapy and prevention (1, 6). Contemporary research has emphasized chemoprevention of cancer by minerals with the aim to elucidate the mechanisms by which minerals modulate chemical carcinogenesis in experimental animals (1, 2, 7–25). It is interesting to note that while many minerals inhibit chemical carcinogenesis, mineral supplementation often increases the growth of established experimental tumors. Furthermore, it is not uncommon for deficiencies in many minerals to result in increased neoplasia.

The preponderance of data concerning mineral effects is on the dietary selenium modulation of carcinogenesis. These results, which have established the anticarcinogenic properties of selenium, have been extensively reviewed (1, 2, 7, 9–22, 26, 27). Chemoprevention and modulation of carcinogenesis with other trace elements and metals have also been reviewed (1, 2, 5, 7, 28). Table 1 identifies experimental animal studies on the effects of dietary selenium supplementation on chemical carcinogenesis. The majority of studies concern selenium effects on colon, liver, and mammary gland carcinogenesis. Effects of selenium at other organ sites are also discussed. Table 2 addresses the effect of selenium-deficient diets and of very low level selenium diets on carcinogenesis. Table 3 summarizes reports on modulation of chemical induction of tumors by copper and Table 4 summarizes reports on zinc. The important issue of nutrient interactions in carcinogenesis, particularly selenium interactions with fats, vitamins, and other metals, is addressed, although the data are scarce on this topic. Representative studies from the large number of references cited in the tables are described. Throughout this section proposed mechanisms by which minerals influence the carcinogenic process are discussed. Many of the mechanisms are speculative, at best, due to the lack of confirmatory data and the wide range of carcinogens, mineral salts, diets, animals, dosing regimens, and other experimental conditions employed.

---

[1]Abbreviations used in this section are given on p. 352.

II. SELENIUM MODULATION OF CHEMICAL CARCINOGENESIS

Selenium is an element in subgroup VIA of the periodic chart and closely resembles sulfur in its chemical properties. It is widely distributed in soil, plants, and tissues and is an integral component of glutathione peroxidase, an enzyme involved in the catabolism of hydrogen and hydrogen peroxide (29). Historically, selenium has climbed the path from poison to potion. In the 1930s selenium was primarily considered to be a toxicant (30), and in the 1940s selenium was reported to be hepatocarcinogenic (31). In the 1950s and 1960s selenium was recognized as an essential nutrient that is effective in preventing exudative diathesis in chicks, unthriftiness in cattle, and white muscle disease in sheep (32–34).

Clayton and Baumann (35), in their 1949 landmark study, demonstrated the anticarcinogenic properties of selenium. They observed a 50% reduction in liver tumor incidence in rats that were fed 5 ppm selenium (as sodium selenite) in an intermediate period during feeding the potent azo dye, 3'-methyl-4-dimethylaminoazobenzene (3'-Me-DAB). This early observation was neither noticed nor confirmed for nearly 3 decades, when it was reported that provision of either a drinking water supplement of inorganic sodium selenite or a dietary supplement of organic selenium from a *Saccharomyces cerevisiae* yeast inhibits 3'-Me-DAB-induced hepatocarcinogenesis (36, 37). The supplements given during the first few weeks of feeding this azo dye were more effective than when given with this carcinogen in the last half of the study.

Meanwhile, Kubota *et al.* (38) mapped the selenium content of forage crops, Allaway *et al.* (39) showed the geographic trends of relationships between selenium levels in forage crops and in human blood, and Shamberger and Frost (40) suggested an inverse relationship between selenium status and cancer rates. Subsequently, in skin tumor promotion studies, Shamberger (41) found that topical application of sodium selenide markedly reduces the number of tumors induced by 7,12-dimethylbenz[*a*]anthracene (DMBA) and croton oil. The above sequence of observations sparked the curiosity of many investigators to explore the anticarcinogenic potential of selenium. The surge of research is evidenced by the tremendous expansion of literature on selenium modulation of carcinogenesis in the 1970s and 1980s.

A. Selenium Modulation of Colon Carcinogenesis

Table 1 highlights reports on the modulation by selenium supplements of colon cancer induced primarily by 1,2-dimethylhydrazine (DMH) and also by azoxymethane (AOM), methylazoxymethanol acetate (MAMAC), and *N*-nitrosobis(2-oxopropyl)amine (BOP) (13, 42–49). Both dietary and drinking water supplements of selenium effectively inhibit colon carcinogenesis. The efficacy of selenium is dependent on: (a) the dose of carcinogen administered, (b) whether selenium is provided before, during, or after the carcinogen, (c) the amount of selenium, (d) the level of selenium supplement relative to the dose of carcinogen, (e) the inorganic or organic form of selenium, and (f) the presence of other dietary constituents.

In the first report by Jacobs *et al.* (42), that selenium inhibits colon carcinogenesis, Sprague-Dawley rats were injected weekly for 20 weeks with either DMH or MAMAC. Addition of 4 ppm selenium (Na selenite) in the drinking water reduced the number of rats developing DMH-induced colon tumors from 13 to 6 in groups of 15 each; also the total number of tumors observed in these two groups was reduced from 39 in the DMH-only treated group to 11 in the DMH-treated plus selenium-supplemented group. The incidence of MAMAC-induced colon tumors was high in both groups, 93% (14/15) with selenium supplement and 100% (14/14) without selenium supplement; this is because the dose of

TABLE 1. Modulation of Chemical Carcinogenesis by Selenium Supplementation

Organ site	Animal species	Carcinogen	Effect[a]	References
Colon	Rat	DMH	I	42–44
Colon	Rat	DMH	None	43,44
Colon	Rat	MAMAC	I	42
Colon	Rat	AOM	I	45,49
Colon	Rat	AOM	E	46
Colon	Rat	BOP	I	48
Liver	Rat	3'-Me-DAB	I	35–37
Liver	Rat	AAF	I	57–59
Liver	Rat	AAF	E	57
Liver	Rat	AAF	None	57,60
Liver	Rat	AOM	I	61
Liver	Rat	AFB	I	62–65
Liver	Rat	DEN	I	66
Liver	Rat	DEN	None	67
Mammary	Mouse	DMBA	I	77–80,82,83
Mammary	Rat	DMBA	I	73–75,81,84–87,95
Mammary	Rat	DMBA	None	74
Mammary	Rat	NMU	I	84,88–90
Mammary	Rat	AAF	I	57,59

[a]The effect of selenium may be to inhibit (I), enhance (E), or have no apparent influence (None) on chemical carcinogenesis. In studies where only one selenium dose was tested, if the incidence or multiplicity of tumors was lower than in the carcinogen-only treated control, the effect is recorded as inhibition. In studies where low, medium, and high selenium doses were tested, if the incidence or multiplicity of tumors was higher, equal to, or lower than the carcinogen-only treated control, the effect is recorded as enhancement, none, or inhibition, respectively.

MAMAC was so high that it obscured a possible protective effect of selenium. Even so, the supplement of selenium was sufficiently high to decrease the total number of colon tumors induced by MAMAC to 42 compared with a total of 73 tumors in rats receiving only MAMAC. Both carcinogens, DMH and MAMAC, induced tumors with a higher frequency in the transverse colon than in the proximal or distal colon. The 4 ppm selenium supplement was not toxic as evidenced by the lack of adverse effects on both weight gain and survival of the animals. In subsequent studies, Jacobs *et al.* (43, 44) confirmed the protective role of supplemental selenium against DMH-induced carcinogenesis using doses of 20 and 10 mg/kg body weight of DMH for 20 weeks. They also found (43) that the selenium-treated rats had increased glutathione *S*-transferase activity. Therefore, inhibition of DMH carcinogenesis by selenium is, at least in part, attributable to an enhancement of detoxification by this enzyme and, thus, a decreased presence of carcinogenic electrophiles. These latter studies demonstrate the importance of the level of selenium supplementation, of the dose of the carcinogen, and of the timing of exposures to both carcinogen and anticarcinogen, in order to elicit optimal short-term and long-term protection (44). In the short term, rats given selenium supplementation before DMH exposure were best protected. In the long term (*e.g.*, 20 weeks after DMH treatments), the most effective method for preventing colon tumor induction was continuous exposure to selenium before, during, and after DMH treatment.

Selenium occurs predominantly in organic form (*e.g.*, selenomethionine) in cereals, grains, and vegetables. On one hand, selenomethionine has reportedly inhibited mammary carcinogenesis; however, on the other hand, it has caused liver necrosis and fibrosis. In an effort to identify organic selenium compounds that are chemopreventive, Reddy *et al.* (49) studied the influence of benzylselenocyanate (BSC) on AOM-induced colon carcinogenesis. When fed during the initiation stage of carcinogenesis, BSC inhibited both the incidence of colon adenocarcinomas and multiplicity of small-intestinal adenocarcinomas. Selenium-dependent glutathione peroxidase activity was increased in both tissues, suggesting that tumor inhibition was in part due to increased enzyme-dependent detoxification of AOM.

The critical steps in the metabolic activation of DMH,

$$DMH \longrightarrow azomethane \longrightarrow AOM \longrightarrow methylazoxymethanol\ (MAM)$$
$$\longrightarrow methylazoxyformaldehyde\ (MOF),$$

to a reactive species that can alkylate DNA, are (a) the hydroxylation of AOM to MAM and (b) the oxidation of MAM to MOF (50–52). The hydroxylation occurs predominantly in the liver, probably by a cytochrome P-450–dependent pathway, and to a limited degree in the colon mucosa (53). The oxidation of MAM is affected by liver and colon microsomes (51) as well as by cytosol alcohol dehydrogenase from these tissues (52). The unstable compound, MAM, readily yields the methyldiazonium ion, which can alkylate macromolecules by enzymatic and nonenzymatic processes in the liver and colon (50–52). Alternatively, MAM has been found to be a substrate for NAD^+-dependent dehydrogenase present in the colon and liver, suggesting that the active metabolite of MAM may be the corresponding aldehyde (54). Speculation is that BSC inhibition of colon carcinogenesis may be attributed to alterations in the activation and detoxification of AOM and to BSC induction of glutathione peroxidase activity (49).

Induction of colon cancer with another carcinogen, BOP, was inhibited by dietary sodium selenite. Accompanying this inhibition was an apparent increase in the repair of BOP-induced DNA damage in colon tissue (48).

The combined effects of dietary factors is of utmost relevance to the real world and yet is infrequently studied. Two examples that contrast the combined effects on colon carcinogenesis are selenium and fat *versus* selenium and vitamin C. Most experiments to assess the effects of selenium are carried out with animals fed normal fat diets. A high-fat diet can double the number of tumors in rats induced with DMH (55). Nigro and coworkers (45) reported that rats fed 30% beef fat diets with concurrent selenium supplements had an average of 3.1 AOM-induced intestinal tumors, whereas animals fed this high-fat diet and no selenium supplement had an average of 6.5 intestinal tumors. Mechanisms of selenium-altered carcinogen metabolism and selenium related protection against oxidative damage via the selenoenzyme glutathione peroxidase are postulated, but unsubstantiated in this study.

The influence of concurrent selenium and vitamin C supplementation on DMH-induced colon carcinogenesis was presented by Jacobs and Griffin (7, 56). Sprague-Dawley rats receiving DMH and given selenium in the drinking water and vitamin C in the diet had an 83% colon tumor incidence compared to a lower 64% incidence in the unsupplemented DMH-only control. This increased tumor incidence with the concurrent supplement of two antioxidants was not anticipated by the gross observations of normal weight gain, good survival, and good health of the animals. No studies were carried out to detect antagonistic or interactive mechanisms relating the influence of the combined antioxidant supplements on DMH-induced colon carcinogenesis.

B. Selenium Modulation of Liver Carcinogenesis

Hepatocarcinogenesis by a variety of agents was shown to be inhibited by selenium in animal models, and numerous mechanisms have been postulated for the selenium effects. The liver carcinogenesis studies cited in Table 1 include selenium modulation of hepatocarcinogenesis induced by the azo dye, 3'-Me-DAB (35–37), by 2-acetylamino-fluorene (AAF) (57–60), AOM (61), aflatoxin B$_1$ (AFB) (62–65), and *N,N*-diethyl-nitrosamine (DEN) (66, 67). As noted earlier, Clayton and Baumann (35) reported a reduced liver tumor incidence in rats fed diets that *alternated* selenium supplementation and 3'-Me-DAB supplementation. In their study, albino rats were maintained on semisynthetic diets and were given 0.065% 3'-Me-DAB for 2 weeks. Subsequently, the animals were placed on dye-free diet supplemented with 5 ppm selenium as sodium selenite. Finally, the rats were provided with a selenium-free but dye-containing diet for an additional 4 weeks. The liver tumor incidence was reduced approximately 50% as compared to control animals receiving basal diet during the intermediate period. This study is considered to be the earliest report of an inhibition by selenium of chemical carcinogenesis.

In 1977, Griffin and Jacobs (36) confirmed this early report. They provided male Sprague-Dawley rats organic and inorganic selenium supplements and exposed the animals to the azo dye in the diet. They observed that both forms of this selenium supplement reduced the hepatic tumor incidence. 3'-Me-DAB (0.05%) was incorporated into the diet for a period of 8 weeks and then removed. During carcinogen administration, and for an additional 4 weeks prior to sacrifice, the rats were maintained on 6 ppm selenium supplements. The selenium was provided as either sodium selenite in the drinking water or as an organic form in yeast (*S. cerevisiae*) containing 118 mg selenium/g yeast. The inorganic selenium reduced the tumor incidence from 92 to 46% and the organic selenium reduced the incidence from 92 to 64%. At 6 ppm selenium, neither the organic nor inorganic forms elicited toxic effects evidenced by expected weight gain and survival.

In another study with male Sprague-Dawley rats, Grant *et al.* (62) noted a protective effect of dietary sodium selenite on lesions induced by AFB. Animals were administered 25 mg AFB *per os* 5 days a week for 4 weeks and selenium (0.03–5 ppm) in the diet. After 17 months, a low (20%) incidence of hepatocarcinomas was observed in the 1 ppm selenium-treated rats. Changes in dietary selenium gave rise to variations in glutathione peroxidase activities and tissue selenium levels. The authors observed that dietary selenium, together with repeated AFB, results in the formation of large bizarre renal tubule cells.

Investigations using another hepatocarcinogen, AAF, show inhibition by selenium and implicate a mechanism for reduced carcinogenesis by the trace element. Adult male Sprague-Dawley rats were provided 0.03% AAF in the diet for 14 weeks followed by AAF-free diet. The basal diet was Purina laboratory chow. Simultaneous administration of a 4-ppm selenium supplement (Na$_2$SeO$_3$) in the drinking water reduced the hepatic tumor incidence by 50% (58). Metabolic activation of AAF proceeds through *N*-hydroxy-AAF to several proposed metabolites, including *N*-hydroxyaminofluorene. Further investigation indicated that selenium inhibits AAF activation with apparent specificity for inhibiting hydroxylation at certain positions on the AAF molecule (58, 68). The *N*-hydroxylase activity was reduced, with a corresponding reduction in the anticipated *N*-OH-AAF metabolite, but there was an increase in the ring-hydroxylated intermediate, 3-OH-AAF. The observed antitumorigenic effect of selenium may very well reflect the reduction in the formation of the highly carcinogenic metabolite, *N*-OH-AAF, and the production of the noncarcinogenic metabolite, 3-OH-AAF.

In earlier studies by Harr *et al.* (57, 59), selenium reduced the number of tumors in rats given AAF. The group of rats receiving 0.03% AAF in the diet and 4 ppm selenium (Na$_2$SeO$_3$) in the drinking water for 14 weeks had a final tumor incidence of 4/14 rats. The control group receiving dietary AAF and no additional selenium had a tumor incidence of 9/13 rats. Harr *et al.* (59) also reported hepatic toxicity, neoplasia, and tumor induction at extrahepatic sites, including the mammary gland. It is important to distinguish their experimental model from that used in the above-discussed studies by Marshall *et al.* (58). Harr *et al.* (59) employed young female OSU-Brown rats fed a low selenium ration supplemented with 60 ppm vitamin E. To this formula diet 0.015% AAF was added. Either 0, 0.1, 0.5, or 2.5 ppm selenium supplements were provided in the drinking water. Differences in selenium-to-carcinogen ratios, rat strains, age, and basal diets each contribute to different effects of selenium. Harr *et al.* (59) proposed that the selenite was either preventing carcinogenesis or modifying the rate of induction, but provided no mechanistic support data.

Other studies with AAF and the hepatocarcinogen, DEN, have demonstrated inhibition by high (6 ppm), but not low (0.1 ppm) levels of selenium, of cell proliferation as a mechanism of inhibition or delaying liver tumor induction (67). With DEN a high-level selenium supplement of 6 ppm, but not 0.1 or 3 ppm selenium, significantly reduced the number of rats with foci, the numbers of foci per animal, and the mean volume of foci. With AAF the 6-ppm level (but not the 0.1 or 3 ppm levels) of selenium significantly reduced the number of nodules per liver and mean volume of nodules, but did not inhibit induction of hepatocellular carcinoma (67).

A dose–response study in which rats were dosed intraperitoneally with 80 mg/kg DEN and provided 1, 5, and 10 ppm selenium (sodium selenite) supplements in the diet revealed no inhibition at the lower 1 and 5 ppm selenium levels, but significant inhibition at 10 ppm selenium (66). However, simultaneous supplementation with four antioxidants in the diet (vitamin C, vitamin E, butylated hydroxytoluene, and selenium) had no effect on DEN hepatocarcinogenesis even when selenium was at the 10 ppm level (66). An earlier report indicated *enhancement* of DMH-induced colon carcinogenesis by vitamin C plus selenium (56).

An interesting report addresses the question of what is the mechanism by which selenium inhibits AAF-induced hepatic tumors and MAM-induced colon tumors (69). In these studies, Sprague-Dawley rats were either given 4 ppm selenium in the drinking water for 1 week or injected intraperitoneally with 1 mg/kg selenium prior to carcinogen treatment. Selenium by either route afforded no protection against AAF- and MAM-induced acute inhibition of RNA and DNA synthesis. The authors proposed that the tumor prevention by selenium probably occurs via a mechanism other than interference with carcinogen activation and interaction with cellular macromolecules (69). Clearly, this hypothesis is in sharp contrast with the above discussed selenium inhibition of carcinogen activation, and formation of DNA adducts.

The combined effects of dietary fat and selenium on AFB-induced hepatocarcinogenesis have been studied by Baldwin and Parker (64, 65). Their data implicate an interaction between dietary fat and selenium during initiation, but not during early promotion (64). Like Harr *et al.* (57), they proposed that selenium influences promotion independently from the fat effect. Furthermore, dietary fat and selenium appear to function by different mechanisms at different stages of carcinogenesis. Provision of high dietary fat (20%) with low (0.02–0.15 ppm) selenium during initiation yielded increases in both the number and size of γ-glutamyl transferase (GGT)-positive liver foci compared with low-fat groups (64). Feeding both high fat and high selenium during initiation decreased preneoplastic development compared with low-fat groups. Feeding high selenium during promotion did not afford greater protection. Early after AFB treatment they observed transient increases in hepatic lipid content and modifications of lipid metabolism, glutathione peroxidase activity, and hepatic glutathione, none of which correlated directly with foci development (64). In a study designed to center on initiation, Milks *et al.* (63) noted that dietary selenium influences initiation. Levels of 2.0 to 5.0 ppm selenium decreased AFB-induced, GGT-positive foci as well as hepatic necrosis. Addressing the mechanisms of selenium action, Chen *et al.* (70) observed that both a selenium excess and a selenium deficiency reduces the *in vivo* covalent binding of AFB to RNA, DNA, and to protein in rats. In later studies, Burk and Lane (71) reported that selenium deficiency protects against AFB hepatotoxicity and suggested that the mechanism of this protection is related to more rapid glutathione synthesis and higher glutathione *S*-transferase activity in selenium-deficient livers. This suggestion is, however, in sharp contrast with the finding of Jacobs (43) of increased glutathione *S*-transferase activity in selenium-*treated* rats.

Tanaka *et al.* (61) synthesized an organic selenium compound, *p*-methoxybenzeneselenol (MBS), to test its chemopreventive effects against AOM-induced hepatocarcinogenesis in F344 rats. Dietary MBS reduced liver tumor incidence and multiplicity and liver foci incidence nearly fourfold. The effective dose (5 ppm) of this organoselenium compound did not cause adverse toxicological effects such as decreased weight gain, low survival, or poor condition. This study supports the concept that foci are precursors of hepatocellular neoplasms (72). This is an important issue, since many studies on potential antihepatocarcinogens are carried out with liver foci models rather than hepatocellular carcinoma models.

C. Selenium Modulation of Mammary Gland Carcinogenesis

Many studies in the 1980s explored the mechanisms by which dietary selenium might inhibit or otherwise modulate mammary gland carcinogenesis induced with DMBA (41, 73–87), with *N*-nitroso-*N*-methylurea (NMU), (84, 88–90), or with AAF (57–59).

Perhaps more investigations have been carried out with DMBA-induced mammary gland carcinogenesis in rats to elucidate the degree of protection, and mechanism of action of selenium, than with any other model. Most of the studies have used inorganic selenium, usually as selenate or selenite, and sometimes as selenium dioxide. A few experiments have compared the protective effects of inorganic with organic selenium compounds, such as selenomethionine. Together, these studies illustrate: (a) dose–response effects of selenium supplementation, (b) the stage(s) of carcinogenesis influenced by selenium, (c) the effect of selenium on DNA-adduct formation, (d) host systemic functions, and (e) the effect of other dietary factors on the anticarcinogenic efficacy of selenium. Several reviews of the extensive literature on selenium modulation of mammary gland carcinogenesis are available (9, 13, 15, 20, 22, 26, 91).

It is appropriate to note that one of the earliest reports of selenium inhibition of mammary cancer is the observation of Schrauzer (17) and Schrauzer and Ishmael (92) in the mid 1970s that drinking water supplementation with subtoxic doses of selenite lowers the incidence of spontaneous mammary tumors in female C3H mice. Although C3H mice have been extensively used as a model to study human cancer development, these reports on spontaneous rather than chemical carcinogenesis are not within the purview of this section.

As evidenced in Table 1, numerous studies have shown selenium inhibition of DMBA-induced mammary carcinogenesis in rats and mice. The degree of selenium inhibition is generally proportional to the dose of selenium up to 5 ppm. The anticarcinogenic effect of selenium is reported to be diminished by high doses of the carcinogen. The response of DMBA-induced tumorigenesis to selenium is highly dependent on the level and type of dietary fat, and probably other dietary components. A high level of unsaturated fat in the diet appears to exacerbate the tumorigenicity of DMBA, and this effect can be reversed by selenium (85, 86, 93, 94). Evidence for this is that rats fed a diet deficient in selenium and containing a high level of unsaturated fat (*e.g.*, 25% corn oil) had a higher incidence of DMBA-induced mammary tumors than rats given the same high-fat diet supplemented with 0.1 ppm selenium. When the dietary fat was lowered to either 1–5% corn oil or changed to 1% corn oil plus 24% of saturated coconut oil, selenium had no effect on the mammary tumor incidence. Selenium reduced the number of tumors in rats fed unsaturated fat, but not saturated-fat diets.

In an effort to assess the influence of selenium on initiation and promotion, rats were provided supplemental selenium before, during, or after DMBA treatment (95). Selenium appeared to inhibit both initiation and promotion, with the greatest inhibition of tumorigenesis resulting from continuous selenium supplementation. Provision of the selenium supplements up to 24 weeks, following DMBA treatment, still inhibited mammary gland tumorigenesis. Similar observations of selenium inhibition of NMU-induced mammary carcinogenesis (88) have been made, although NMU is less potent as a carcinogen than DMBA.

Selenium has been reported to increase rat liver aryl hydrocarbon hydroxylase (AHH) activity (96). Selenium causes increased DNA adduct formation 6 hours after DMBA treatment, but causes significantly less adduct formation 24 hours after DMBA treatment, suggesting that this trace element can enhance DNA repair (97).

Lastly, Medina (22) has proposed that the antitumorigenic effect of selenium might be the result of the effect of selenium on the endocrine or immune systems. No evidence exists showing selenium modulation of sex hormone levels. There is, however, evidence that dietary selenium can enhance the cell-mediated immune response (98, 99).

D. Selenium Modulation of Carcinogenesis at Other Sites

Trachea

Thompson and Becci (100) administered 0.5% NMU to hamsters weekly for 12 weeks beginning at 7 weeks of age. The hamsters were fed 1 and 5 ppm selenium throughout NMU treatment and for an additional 16 weeks. No inhibition of tracheal carcinogenesis was observed. NMU is a direct-acting carcinogen. Had there been a selenium effect, it would have occurred in the post-initiation phase of carcinogenesis. The lack of effect may have been due to treatment with a relatively high dose of carcinogen relative to the level of selenium supplement.

Tongue

Goodwin *et al.* (101, 102) painted hamster tongues with 0.5% DMBA while feeding formula yeast-based diets supplemented with 3 and 6 ppm selenium. A 2- to 3-week delay in the onset of leukoplakia and inhibition of the development of DMBA-induced squamous cell carcinomas of the tongue were observed in selenium-treated groups. They also reported that retinoic acid, although toxic, was a stronger inhibitor than selenium, but the combined selenium and retinoic acid inhibitory effect was no greater than with retinoic acid alone.

Esophagus

Bogden *et al.* (103) reported an interesting study on the effects of selenium on methylbenzylnitrosamine (MBN)-induced esophageal carcinogenesis. Although MBN is extensively metabolized by both hepatic and esophageal microsomes, it induces cancer in the esophagus, but not the liver. When MBN was administered intragastrically to rats twice weekly for 5 weeks, followed by a 12-week period for tumor promotion, and a 4-ppm selenium supplement in the drinking water was provided throughout, the incidence of esophageal carcinomas was significantly reduced. At sacrifice, many tissues were analyzed for various metals. Selenium-treated rats had higher levels of iron in head, kidney, and spleen and higher urinary excretion of manganese and iron than unsupplemented controls. The authors proposed that the antitumor activity of selenium might be related to its effects on the delivery of zinc, copper, and other trace elements to tumor cells or the utilization and metabolism of these trace elements by tumor cells.

Pancreas

The combined effects of dietary selenium and fat on BOP-induced pancreatic carcinogenesis in hamsters was studied by Birt *et al.* (104). Selenium was fed beginning 4 weeks before BOP and continuing until sacrifice at 70 weeks. Because different BOP doses and types of selenium, low- and high-fat diets, and two BOP dosing regimens were used, the interpretation of the selenium-induced effects independent of other variables is questionable. Even so, the implications of the data are that (a) on a low-fat diet, increasing selenium from 0.1 to 2.5 ppm appears to decrease the incidence of pancreatic tumors, although this was not statistically significant; (b) on a high-fat diet, an increase in selenium significantly increases pancreatic ductal carcinoma; and (c) repair of BOP-induced single-strand DNA breaks is not affected by selenium in ductal cells, but was enhanced in acinar cells. In another multivariant study, increased dietary selenium inhibited pancreatic ductular adenoma, but not pancreatic carcinoma (105).

E. Modulation of Carcinogenesis by Selenium Restriction/Deficiency

Most of the animal studies demonstrating inhibition of tumor induction utilize high-level, presumably subtoxic, dose exposure to selenium compounds, especially sodium selenite. Selenium supplements to diet and drinking water used to demonstrate antitumorigenicity are generally in the range of 2 to 6 ppm and have been as high as 10 ppm. The dietary requirement for selenium in most species is in the range of 0.1 to 0.2 ppm (and for humans probably 50–60 μg/day) (13). Selenium-deficient diets contain less than 0.02 ppm selenium. Because selenium salts, including sodium selenite, can be toxic (106–109), many studies have tested the influence on chemical carcinogenesis of nutritionally limiting or deficient levels of selenium in the diet. Table 2 highlights these studies and indicates a frequent lack of protection and lack of consistency in the effect of these low levels of selenium on chemical carcinogenesis in colon, liver, and mammary gland (13). In several studies, selenium deficiency enhanced mammary gland carcinogenesis (73, 74, 86, 93, 110) and in one report the selenium deficiency enhanced AOM-induced colon carcinogenesis (111). The average number of mammary tumors induced by NMU in rats fed torula yeast diets with either restricted (0.01 ppm) or adequate (1.0 ppm) selenium levels were increased from 1.49 to 2.11 tumors per rat by the selenium restriction (88). In contrast, restriction of selenium decreased the AAF-induced liver tumor incidence in rats in another study (59). Pence and Buddingh (112) observed that diets deficient in selenium, provided either as an organic yeast supplement or as sodium selenite, neither inhibited nor enhanced DMH-induced colon carcinogenesis. Ip and Daniel (73) reported that neither selenium deficiency nor an excess had any significant effect on the levels of DMBA–DNA adducts in liver and mammary gland.

TABLE 2. **Modulation of Chemical Carcinogenesis by Selenium Restriction/Deficiency**

Organ site	Animal species	Carcinogen	Effect[a]	References
Colon	Rat	DMH	None	112
Colon	Rat	AOM	E	111
Liver	Rat	AAF	None	73
Liver	Rat	AAF	I	57,59
Mammary	Rat	DMBA	None	73,89
Mammary	Rat	DMBA	E	73,74,86
Mammary	Rat	NMU	I	127
Mammary	Rat	NMU	E	88
Mammary	Rat	AAF	None	57

[a]E = Enhancement; I = Inhibition.

III. COPPER MODULATION OF CHEMICAL CARCINOGENESIS

Copper is an essential trace element for animals and plays a critical role in a number of oxidative enzyme systems. Supplements of copper salts in the diet or drinking water of rats and mice inhibit the effects of a variety of chemical carcinogens (Table 3). Changes in enzyme activities affecting the metabolism of the carcinogens and observations on retention of copper in the liver accompany a number of reports. The inhibitory effects of dietary supplementation with copper salts on hepatic tumorigenicity have been reviewed (24, 113–120). Dietary supplementation with copper was protective for some extrahepatic tumors (120), but not for others (121, 122).

Sharpless (113) reported that increases of 0.15, 0.3, and 0.5% in dietary copper did not prevent the emergence of hepatic tumors induced by 4-dimethylaminobenzene (DAB) in rats, but did prolong the induction time by 25 to 50%. Pedrero and Kozelka (114) confirmed his results using the more potent carcinogen, 3'-Me-DAB. The incidence of hepatomas in rats supplemented with 0.25% copper was 66.6% compared to 86.3% in animals fed 3'-Me-DAB alone. The mortality rate after 90–100 days was 62.5% with the carcinogenic diet alone and 40% with the copper-supplemented diet. Hepatic copper levels were subnormal, indicating that the presence of neoplasms can significantly decrease copper concentration in the liver. King *et al.* (115) confirmed the results of Sharpless (113) and Pedrero and Kozelka (114) in that a high level of copper (300 ppm in the diet as $CuSO_4$) inhibited development of liver tumors in rats fed 3'-Me-DAB. The

TABLE 3. **Effect of Dietary Copper Supplementation on Chemically Induced Experimental Tumors**

Tumor site	Animal species	Carcinogen	Effect[a]	References
Liver	Rat	DAB	R	113
Liver	Rat	3'-Me-DAB	I	114,115,126
Liver	Rat	DAB	R	116
Liver	Rat	MeOAB	I	24,117,118
Liver	Rat	AAF	None	127
Liver	Rat	Ethionine	I	119
Liver	Rat	DMN	None	120
Skin	Rat	3-methoxy-DAB	None	121
Ovary	Mouse	DMBA	I	122
Lung	Mouse	DMBA	None	122
Lymphomas	Mouse	DMBA	None	122
Extrahepatic (lungs, spleen, skin)	Rat	AAF	I	120

[a]I = Inhibition (reduced tumor incidence); R = Retardation (extended latent period).

incidence of tumors was reduced from 84 to 22% in one experiment and from 50 to 0% in another experiment. Howell (116) reported that 0.5% copper acetate in the diet retarded hepatic tumorigenesis in rats fed DAB (incidence of 1/16 with copper supplementation diet *versus* 8/8 without copper supplementation). Liver damage and cirrhosis as well as splenic damage was always less in copper-supplemented rats than in rats receiving 3'-Me-DAB alone.

Many reports on antitumorigenic properties of copper compounds also describe changes in enzyme activities affecting metabolism of the carcinogen and observations on the retention of copper. Fare (24), Fare and Woodhouse (118), and Fare and Howell (117) administered to albino rats 0.09% dietary levels of azo dye carcinogens in corn diets. Addition of 0.5% copper as cupric oxyacetate hexahydrate to the diets reduced the incidence of liver tumors induced by 3-methoxy-4-aminoazobenzene (MeOAB) from 5/10 in control animals to 0/10 in copper-supplemented animals (117); under the same conditions of copper administration, but using the parent dye, DAB, the amount of azo dye bound to liver proteins rose to a maximum after 150 days and then progressively decreased (24). The amount of copper in the liver increased 40% after 315 days in the groups tested with carcinogen and copper. The copper content increased 40-fold after 330 days in rats fed copper only. The mean serum optical rotations in rats fed corn diet only, corn diet plus DAB, and corn diet plus DAB plus copper were 46.2, 43.1, and 39.0, respectively (123). In further studies these authors noted a decrease in liver succinoxidase activity and a concomitant change in the distribution of subcellular fractions of protein, RNA, and DNA in rats treated with DAB alone, as compared to controls and copper-treated animals (118).

Yamane and Sakai (23) and Yamane *et al.* (124, 125) investigated biochemical changes in livers of Wistar rats fed DAB and copper acetate. DAB alone decreased the total lactate dehydrogenase (LDH) activity with the appearance of the LDH isozyme 3. Neither change was seen in rats fed DAB and copper (125). In another study these authors reported that azo reductase activity in the liver was enhanced by copper. The level of *N*-demethylase activity in rats fed DAB was reduced by copper. Although the total DAB-metabolizing activity was increased in rats fed DAB together with copper and phenobarbital (23), the increase of ring hydroxylation was most significant. These authors also reported that adding 3-methylcholanthrene (3-MC) to the diets of rats, treated with DAB and copper, elevated both the azo reductase and *N*-demethylase activities. The increases in ring hydroxylase and azo reductase levels were seen primarily in microsomal fractions and were paralleled by increased microsomal copper levels.

Yamane and Sakai (126) examined the effect of concurrent administration of salts of heavy metals such as copper, manganese, zinc, and nickel in suppressing hepatocarcinogenesis by 0.06% 3'-Me-DAB in Wistar rats. The effect of these metals on the formation of protein-bound dye in the liver and on the hepatic metabolism of DAB was examined in an effort to elucidate the mechanism of their suppression of hepatocarcinogenesis. Carcinogenesis by 3'-Me-DAB was inhibited most markedly by 0.05% of copper acetate followed by 0.5% manganese acetate and nickel acetate. Zinc acetate was ineffective. Suppression of azo dye carcinogenesis by these metals appeared to parallel their capacity to reduce the level of protein-bound azo dye and to enhance hepatic azo reductase activity. No correlation was found between the anticarcinogenicity of these metal acetates and their effect on other enzymatic activities related to aminoazo dye metabolism (*e.g.*, *N*-demethylation and ring hydroxylation).

In contrast to the experiment with orally administered azo dye carcinogens, Wistar rats given cupric oxyacetate hexahydrate (0.1%) in their drinking water were not protected from either liver injury or hepatoma induction when 2-aminofluorene was administered percutaneously by skin painting; there was no inhibition or retardation of the carcinogenic response (127). The author concluded that the aboved-discussed inhibition of azo dye hepatocarcinogenesis by excess copper was not a general phenomenon common with other carcinogens, but might be due to some feature of metabolism of the azo dye carcinogens, DAB or 3'-Me-DAB. This appears to be supported by the finding of Fare and Orr (121) that 0.5% cupric oxyacetate hexahydrate in the diet offers no protection against multiple skin tumors in rats painted with 0.2% 3-methoxy-4-dimethylaminoazobenzene, just as was found in a previous study with the extrahepatic (skin and earduct) neoplasms induced by MeOAB and its *N*-monomethyl derivative, 3-methoxy-4-monomethylamino-azobenzene (117).

Brada *et al.* (128, 129) reported an increase in *S*-adenosylethionine in the liver of rats fed a mixture of ethionine (0.3%) plus cupric acetate (0.3%) in comparison to rats fed ethionine only. Liver analyses are confounded by the fact that only about 70% of the ethionine is absorbed during passage through the gastrointestinal tract. Analysis of the soluble part of the lumen content showed a rise in ethionine metabolites during passage. The presence of copper acetate prevented the formation of the new metabolites. Kamamoto *et al.* (119) demonstrated that hepatoma induction in rats fed diets containing 0.25% ethionine for 24 weeks could be completely prevented by the addition of 0.25% cupric acetate for 12, 16, or 20 weeks, but not by copper supplementation for only 4 or 8 weeks. Biochemical examination of the livers suggested that copper was bound to ethionine and deposited in the nuclei, thus providing a mechanism for the protective effect of copper against ethionine carcinogenesis.

Copper sulfate was administered in the drinking water of 3- to 6-month old C57BL/6J and virgin and pseudopregnant strain A mice. The mice received DMBA either as a single i.v. injection or by repeated skin paintings to induce tumors of the breast and ovary, and lymphomas in C57BL/6J mice and lung tumors in strain A mice (122). Copper sulfate supplementation appeared to reduce the incidence of ovarian tumors in C57BL/6J mice. However, all ovaries in mice treated with DMBA and copper sulfate showed precancerous changes, indicating that copper had no effect on the initiation step of DMBA tumorigenesis, but may have delayed the development of granulosa cell tumors. Copper supplementation had no effect on the incidence of DMBA-induced adenomas of the lung or lymphomas.

Carlton and Price (120) studied the effects of copper-deficient (1 ppm) and copper-supplemented (800 ppm) diets on the induction of neoplasms by AAF and *N,N*-dimethylnitrosamine (DMN). Excess of copper was toxic as shown by reduced body weight gains and increased mortality. The incidence of liver tumors was similar in DMN-treated rats fed either copper-deficient or excess copper diets. The incidence of kidney tumors in these DMN-treated rats was 57% in the group receiving the copper-deficient diet and 0% in the copper-supplemented group. In AAF-fed rats the incidence of extrahepatic neoplasms (occurring in the lungs, spleen, skin, intestine, pancreas, and muscle) was 40% in the copper-deficient rats, but only 17% in the copper-supplemented animals.

IV. ZINC MODULATION OF CHEMICAL CARCINOGENESIS

Zinc is a trace element that is essential to the normal growth and development of tissues and cells in a variety of species. Zinc deficiency affects the activity of zinc-dependent enzymes necessary for cell replication. Dietary zinc deficiency as well as zinc supplementation can both increase the incidence of certain tumors and decrease the incidence of others (Table 4). The mechanisms by which zinc alters carcinogenesis is not

TABLE 4. Effect of Dietary Zinc on Chemically Induced Experimental Tumors

Tumor site	Animal species	Carcinogen	Zinc level[a]	Effect[b]	References
Skin	Mouse	3-MC	S	I	136
Skin	Mouse	3-MC	D	I	136
Cheek pouch	Hamster	DMBA	S	I	138
Cheek pouch	Hamster	DMBA	S	None	139
Submandibular gland	Rat	DMBA	S	I	140
Esophagus	Rat	MBN	D	E	141–145
Forestomach	Rat	MBN precursors	D	E	144
Oral cavity	Rat	4NQO	S	E	146
Oral cavity	Rat	4NQO	D	I	146
Oral cavity	Rat	4NQO	S	R	147
Oral cavity	Rat	4NQO	D	E	147
Brain	Rat	ENU	S	E	148
Hepatoma	Rat	3'-Me-DAB	S	I	137
Hepatoma	Rat	3'-Me-DAB	D	I	137
Sarcoma	Mouse	3-MC	S	I	149

[a]D = Deficient; S = Supplement.
[b]I = Inhibition (reduced tumor incidence); E = Enhancement (increased tumor incidence); R = Retardation (extended latent period).

fully understood. The role of zinc in the epidemiology, biochemistry, nutrition, and the inhibition and enhancement of carcinogenesis has been comprehensively reviewed (44, 130–135).

Duncan and Droesti (136) reported a reduction in tumor DNA synthesis and tumor growth in both rats and mice fed high and low zinc diets. In one experiment (137), female Wistar rats received implants of hepatoma induced by 3'-Me-DAB. Test groups were given a semisynthetic diet containing 0.4 to 2500 μg Zn/g diet. Control animals received the same diet containing 60 μg Zn/g diet. The growth of transplanted hepatoma was significantly ($p < 0.001$) reduced in rats maintained on the test diets either low in zinc (0.4 μg/g) or high in zinc (500 μg/g), compared to the controls. Greater inhibition of tumor growth was not achieved at toxic levels (2500 μg/g) of zinc in the diet. In another experiment by Duncan and Droesti (136), rats bearing 3'-Me-DAB-induced hepatomas were maintained on the same diet regimen. After 3 weeks labeled thymidine was injected i.p. and tumors were excised. DNA synthesis was significantly reduced in rats maintained on low-zinc (0.4 μg/g) and high-zinc (500 μg/g) diets when compared with controls receiving 60 μg zinc/g diet. To evaluate the effect of zinc intake on carcinogenesis, female Swiss mice were administered the same experimental levels of dietary zinc for 10 weeks and skin painted with 0.5% 3-MC. Papilloma development and incidence of malignancy were considerably reduced in mice receiving the same low or high zinc diets during the induction period. The authors suggested that the reduced DNA synthesis observed in tumors transplanted to rats supports an earlier proposal that decreased tumor growth arises from a block in cell division cycle at the level of DNA replication.

Poswillo and Cohen (138) demonstrated zinc inhibition of DMBA-induced carcinogenesis in hamsters. Young Syrian golden hamsters received 21.9 ppm zinc sulfate supplement in the diet and also 100 ppm of this supplement in the drinking water. After 4 days, painting with 0.5% solution DMBA on the cheek pouch was begun. DMBA treatments were three times weekly for 4 weeks. Zinc supplementation inhibited the emergence of tumors based on an up to 10 months observational period. In a similar experiment, Edwards (139) applied 0.5% DMBA to the hamster cheek pouch three times weekly for 4 weeks. Drinking water was supplemented with 100 ppm zinc. A distinct inhibitory effect on tumorigenesis was not observed. Premalignant changes were noted in almost all animals, and malignant changes ensued in two thirds of them. The latent period for malignant change was slightly extended by zinc supplementation, but the overall differences were not statistically significant.

Supplemental zinc in the drinking water retards the growth of DMBA-induced tumors in 4- to 5-month old Wistar rats, given 50-, 100-, and 250-ppm zinc supplements in their drinking water (140). DMBA pellets were implanted in the submandibular gland and the glands were dissected and examined histologically 3 months later. Control rats, receiving deionized water and no added zinc, developed well-differentiated squamous carcinomas. Increasing concentrations of zinc progressively decreased the amount of squamous epithelium, while an inflammatory response became more marked. The authors (140) suggested that the increase in lymphatic tissue in tumors from rats on high zinc could indicate an immune response to the developing carcinoma.

Several studies (141–145) showed that a zinc-deficient diet (3–7 ppm) significantly enhances esophageal tumor incidence in rats exposed to MBN. Depending upon the total MBN dosage (8–48 mg/kg body weight) and the severity of the zinc deficiency, esophageal tumor incidence was increased from about 30% in control-diet rats to 60 to 100% in zinc-deficient rats.

Schrager *et al.* (132) reported that a zinc-deficient diet significantly increased [^{3}H]-thymidine incorporation into esophageal epithelium DNA, but not into liver DNA. The findings suggested to the authors that the enhancement of MBN-induced esophageal tumorigenesis by zinc deficiency is due in part to the increased proliferation of target cells and greater accessibility of the cellular DNA to the carcinogen. Fong *et al.* (144) demonstrated an increased incidence of forestomach tumors induced by precursors of MBN in the zinc-deficient rat.

In a study of Wallenius *et al.* (146), groups of 4-week-old female Sprague-Dawley rats were fed either a 0.23 (zinc deficient), 0.77 (zinc adequate), or 3.06 (zinc supplemented) mmol zinc/kg diet, and oral cancer was induced by repeated applications of 4-nitro-quinoline *N*-oxide (4NQO). In rats fed the zinc-supplemented diet, oral cancer appeared earlier and survival time was shorter than in either of the other groups. Rats on the zinc-deficient diet exhibited some oral cancers as well as transient, presumably benign changes in the palatal mucosa, and survived longer. Development of oral cancer in zinc-deficient rats was slower than in the other groups. In another study (147), 3-week-old female rats were fed 0.09 (zinc deficient), 0.77 (zinc adequate), or 3.98 (zinc supplemented) mmol zinc/kg diet and the palatal mucosa was painted with 4NQO three times a week for 20 weeks. The zinc-supplemented diet delayed the onset of carcinogenesis, whereas dysplastic changes in the palatal mucosa were noted earlier in the zinc-deficient group than in the other two groups. However, once the initial changes had been induced, the supplementary zinc accelerated their further advancement to malignancy.

Rath and Enke (148) investigated the effect of zinc supplementation on the incidence of *N*-ethyl-*N*-nitrosourea (ENU)-induced brain tumors in BD IX rats. Rats, which received drinking water containing 22.8 mmol/l zinc acetate from the fourth week until 180 days, developed three times more brain tumors than rats of the control groups treated with ENU alone. The incidence of brain tumors in rats that received the zinc supplement from the 150th day corresponded to that of the control group treated with ENU alone.

Verma *et al.* (149) reported that the incidence of 3-MC-induced sarcomas in mice was reduced from 45 to 15% when the standard mouse diet was supplemented with zinc sulfate at the rate of 10 mg/kg body weight. However, the latent period was increased from 10.9 weeks to 20 weeks and the average tumor size was reduced from 41.0 cm^3 to 6.6 cm^3. The incidence of splenic amyloidosis was also diminished in zinc-supplemented mice.

V. MODULATION OF CHEMICAL CARCINOGENESIS BY OTHER MINERALS

A. Magnesium

The role of magnesium on the induction of neoplasia under various experimental conditions have been reviewed by Durlach *et al.* (150, 151) and Kasprzak and Waalkes (152). It has been established that magnesium deficiency inhibits the growth of transplanted tumors and chemically induced or spontaneous tumors in the rat (153–155). The influence of magnesium on the growth of transplanted or chemically-induced tumors is not consistent in that inhibition or enhancement may occur (155, 156).

Bazikyan and Akimov (157) reported on the effect of elevated magnesium levels on chemically-induced carcinogenesis. Mature male mice received 15 mg/kg magnesium chloride in their drinking water prior to and concurrent with the skin painting with DMBA. A significantly lower percentage of tumors and deaths were observed in magnesium-supplemented mice. Other mice in the same study were injected with dibenz-[*a,h*]anthracene. After 200 days, the incidence of tumors was 37% in mice receiving supplemental magnesium compared to 83% in the unsupplemented controls.

Galt *et al.* (158) reported that deprivation of magnesium restricted the growth of established renal cortical tumors induced in rats by lead subacetate. Of 18 rats in the magnesium-deficient diet (3 mg%), 2 had small carcinomas and no large adenomas of the adrenal cortex. Of 18 rats fed excess magnesium (65 mg%), 7 had eight carcinomas and five large adenomas of the renal cortex.

Poirier *et al.* (159) reported that calcium or magnesium acetate, administered as 3% dietary supplements, do not significantly affect the yields of tumors in rats induced at the injection site (subcutaneous fibrosarcomas) or distantly from the site (testicular tumors) by the subcutaneous injection of cadmium chloride. Simultaneous injection of magnesium chloride at the same site completely prevented the injection-site tumors, but had no effect on the yield of distant testicular tumors. Similar results were seen with muscle tumors induced by nickel subsulfide, in that 3% dietary magnesium acetate or calcium acetate failed to inhibit tumor response induced at the injection site.

B. Calcium

To investigate the effect of dietary calcium supplementation on thyroid follicular carcinogenesis, newborn rats were given either 5 or 10 μCi^{131}I, then placed on diets containing 2000, 500, or 100 mg% calcium (160). The 500 mg% calcium is the normal nutritional requirement. The incidence of thyroid follicular tumors was 29% in the low calcium diet group, 33% in the normal control diet, and 41% in the high calcium diet. These differences were statistically significant.

Karkare *et al.* (161) supplemented 5% fat diets of rats with calcium above (1.0 or 2.0%) or below (0.2%) the U. S. National Academy of Science, National Research Council (NAS/NRC) recommended dose of 0.5%. All calcium doses were administered during the promotion phase of colon cancer induced by DMH and reduced the incidence of distal colon tumors and benign adenomatous polyps. The role of calcium in neoplasia has been comprehensively reviewed (162).

C. Lead

Kasprzak *et al.* (163) reported that calcium acetate enhances the renal carcinogenicity of lead subacetate in Sprague-Dawley rats. The rats were fed a diet with or without a 1%

admixture of lead subacetate and 0, 0.3, 1, 3, and 6% calcium acetate. Kidney tumors developed in 45% of the rats fed lead subacetate only, with a latent period of 58 weeks. Addition of calcium acetate to the lead subacetate–containing diet increased the incidence of kidney tumors to 71%. Primary nonrenal tumors were found only occasionally in rats fed the lead subacetate plus calcium acetate diet. Lead subacetate was found to promote renal carcinogenesis induced by *N*-ethyl-*N*-hydroxyethylnitrosamine (164, 165) and to enhance the carcinogenicity of AAF (166). In one study (166), Wistar rats were fed a standard diet, or diets supplemented with 0.06% AAF, or 0.06% AAF plus 1% lead subacetate, or 1% lead acetate alone. In rats fed lead subacetate alone, cortical epithelial tumors appeared after 6 months. In the group fed AAF plus lead acetate, the greatest incidence of tumors consisted of hepatic and renal carcinomas with metastases to the lung. A high incidence of cancer of the urinary bladder and ear duct, as well as cerebral gliomas and leukemia, also developed. Oyasu *et al.* (167) reported the induction of cerebral gliomas in rats by dietary lead subacetate and AAF. The highest incidence (8.6%) occurred in animals ingesting lead subacetate alone. In animals given AAF the incidence (2.5%) of gliomas was lower and the latency period was delayed. The incidence of gliomas was not increased by combining lead subacetate with AAF.

D. Iron

Webster (168a) studied the effect of dietary iron deficiency on the induction of tumors in rats by DMBA or 3-MC. Test animals were fed an iron-deficient, semisynthetic diet containing 2 mg/kg of ferrous iron. Control animals were fed an identical diet supplemented with 180 mg/kg of ferrous aluminum sulfate. There was no difference between control animals and animals fed the iron-deficient diet for induction time, tumor size, total number of tumors, histological characteristics, or incidence of metastases.

Thompson *et al.* (168b) investigated the effect of iron deficiency or iron excess on the induction of mammary carcinogenesis by NMU in Sprague-Dawley rats. Rats were fed a diet with an iron content that was deficient (2 ppm), adequate (120 ppm), or in excess (1200 ppm) of a standard diet. The latent period of tumor induction was markedly increased in the iron-deficient group compared to those given an adequate or excess level of iron. However, the final tumor incidence was elevated (70%) in the rats given an excess of iron compared to tumor incidences of 53 and 52% in the groups receiving the iron-deficient or iron-adequate diets, respectively.

Siegers *et al.* (169) reported that feeding NMRI mice a diet enriched with iron fumarate increased after 20 weeks the rate of DMH-induced colorectal tumors to four times that of the control group. The total number of tumors was increased fivefold in the iron-supplemented group over the control. Vitale *et al.* (170) studied the effect of iron deficiency as well as of the quality of fat on DMH-induced colon cancer in the rat. The quality of the fat was found to alter the incidence of colon tumors. Highly unsaturated-fat diets promoted colon carcinogenesis, whereas highly saturated-fat diets reduced the risk of colon cancer. Iron deficiency not only redirected the site localization of DMH-induced tumorigenesis from colon to liver, but decreased the induction time 245 days in nondeficient rats to 126 days for iron-deficient rats. Nelson *et al.* (171) reported that dietary iron supplementation augments the incidence of colorectal tumors induced by DMH in Sprague-Dawley rats. The tumor incidence was 20% in rats fed a basal diet (35 mg iron/kg diet) and 63% in rats fed the iron-supplemented diet (580 mg/kg). These studies suggest that iron might enhance both initiation and promotion.

E. Potassium

In a preliminary report, Jacobs (172) showed that supplementation of the drinking water with potassium chloride inhibits the incidence of gastrointestinal tumors induced by DMH in Sprague-Dawley rats. Male rats were injected weekly with 20 mg DMH/kg body weight for 20 weeks. Potassium was provided in the drinking water from 1 week before initiation of DMH treatment and was continued until the animals were sacrificed 14 weeks after the last treatment. Rats in the KCl-supplemented group ingested approximately 288 mg potassium per day, compared to approximately 180 mg per day in the unsupplemented group. The incidence of DMH-induced tumors of the small intestine was significantly ($p < 0.05$) reduced from 46% (6/13) in the unsupplemented group to 6% (1/17) in the KCl-supplemented group. The incidences of tumors of the colon and of the Zymbal gland were also reduced, however, to a lesser extent and not statistically significantly. Liver glutathione S-transferase activity was increased in KCl-supplemented animals, suggesting that inhibition of DMH-induced carcinogenesis by potassium may be attributed in part to the enhancement of a detoxification pathway.

F. Sodium

Takahashi and Hasegawa (173) reported that only a relatively short term of treatment (8 weeks) with 100 mg/l of N-methyl-N'-nitro-N-nitrosoguanidine (MNNG) in the drinking water of rats was needed to adequately initiate gastric carcinogenesis when 10% NaCl was concurrently administered in the diet. Supplementation of the diet with 10% NaCl for 32 weeks in a two-step promotion protocol enhanced the rate of tumor emergence in the glandular stomach of MNNG-initiated rats. The data suggest that high levels of NaCl enhance both the initiation and promotion phases of gastric carcinogenesis, and the effects are possibly related to the damage by NaCl to the gastric mucosa. Previously, Tatematsu *et al.* (174) demonstrated in rats that exceedingly high doses of NaCl given concurrently with carcinogen increases the incidence of tumors in the forestomach induced by 4NQO and in the glandular stomach induced by MNNG. Fine *et al.* (175) injected B16 melanoma cells into hybrid mice maintained on sodium-restricted diets and observed that sodium restriction significantly reduces the tumor growth rates.

G. Arsenic

Data presently existing suggest that dietary arsenic has a strain-dependent effect on mouse skin tumorigenesis by polycyclic hydrocarbons. Milner (176) reported that arsenic trioxide fed to CxC3H hybrid mice has an inhibitory effect on the development of papillomas induced by topical application of 3-MC. However, in DBA mice, dietary arsenic appeared to slightly increase the number of papillomas, although the latter observation was not statistically significant. In humans, arsenic intake correlates inversely with male lung cancer mortality (8).

H. Iodine

The role of dietary iodine in thyroid cancer has been reviewed by Franceschi *et al.* (177) and Ward and Ohshima (178). Eskin (179) reviewed the role of iodine in mammary cancer. In several studies, iodine deficiency was shown to enhance the carcinogenic activity of DMBA in rat mammary tissue (180–182).

I. Germanium and Other Minerals

Germanium supplementation of the drinking water of Swiss mice was found to reduce the spontaneous tumor incidence from 32%, in the unsupplemented controls, to 19% (183). In a second study, Kanisawa and Schroeder (184) reported a reduction of spontaneous tumor incidence in germanium-fed Long-Evans rats. Studies on the effects of various other metals/metalloids—arsenic, tin, chromium, and lead (as salts)—on spontaneous tumorigenesis have also been reported by Kanisawa and Schroeder (184). The influence of a variety of trace metals on the hydroxylation of benzo[*a*]pyrene (BaP) was studied by Calop *et al.* (185). Swiss mice were treated with 3-MC to induce microsomal mixed-function oxidases, sacrificed 2 days later, and the livers isolated. The AHH activity toward BaP was measured in *in vivo* liver cultures containing 0.01 to 100 ppm concentrations of each trace element. The investigators report AHH inhibition by zinc, copper, nickel, chromium, vanadium, manganese, and cadmium salts.

Thompson *et al.* (186) demonstrated that dietary vanadium inhibits murine mammary carcinogenesis induced by NMU in Sprague-Dawley rats. Feeding of a purified diet, supplemented with 25 ppm vanadium as vanadyl(IV) sulfate during the post-initiation phases of NMU carcinogenesis, reduces both the cancer incidence and the average number of tumors per rat and prolongs the latent period (without inhibiting, however, the overall growth of the animals).

Komada *et al.* (187) examined the effect of dietary molybdenum on esophageal carcinogenesis induced in F344 rats by MBN (2.5 mg/kg body weight s.c., once a week for 20 weeks). The rats were fed a low-molybdenum diet (0.032 ppm) or a high-molybdenum diet (2 ppm). The incidence and development of tumors in the esophagus were significantly lower in the high-molybdenum group (44%) than in the low-molybdenum group (73%). Xanthine oxidase activity in the esophagus and forestomach was significantly higher in the high-molybdenum group, whereas in the liver and serum this activity was not significantly different from the low- to the high-Mo groups. The authors (187) concluded that xanthine oxidase in the esophagus plays a significant role in the inhibitory effect of molybdenum on esophageal carcinogenesis.

Luo *et al.* (188) described the inhibitory effects of molybdenum on esophageal and forestomach carcinogenesis in Sprague-Dawley rats induced by gastric intubation with *N*-nitrososarcosine ethyl ester (NSEE). Rats were given either 2 or 20 ppm molybdenum or 100 or 200 ppm tungsten in the drinking water. The addition of molybdenum at both levels significantly inhibited NSEE-induced esophageal and forestomach carcinogenesis. The high-level tungsten inhibited NSEE-induced esophageal and forestomach carcinogenesis less effectively than the low-level molybdenum supplementation.

Abbreviations Used: AAF, 2-acetylaminofluorene; AFB, aflatoxin B_1; AHH, aryl hydrocarbon hydroxylase; AOM, azoxymethane; BOP, *N*-nitrosobis(2-oxopropyl) amine; BaP, benzo[*a*]pyrene; BSC, benzylselenocyanate; DAB, 4-dimethylaminoazobenzene; DEN, *N,N*-diethylnitrosamine; DMBA, 7,12-dimethylbenz[*a*]anthracene; DMH, 1,2-dimethylhydrazine; DMN, *N,N*-dimethylnitrosamine; ENU, *N*-ethyl-*N*-nitrosourea; GGT, γ-glutamyl transferase; LDH, lactate dehydrogenase; MAMAC, methylazoxymethanol acetate; MBN, methylbenzylnitrosamine; MBS, *p*-methoxybenzeneselenol; 3-MC, 3-methylcholanthrene; 3′-Me-DAB, 3′-methyl-4-dimethylaminoazobenzene; MeOAB, 3-methoxy-4-aminoazobenzene; MNNG, *N*-methyl-*N'*-nitro-*N*-nitro-soguanidine; NMU, *N*-nitroso-*N*-methylurea; MOF, methylazoxyformaldehyde; 4NQO, 4-nitroquinoline-*N*-oxide; NSEE, *N*-nitrososarcosine ethyl ester.

REFERENCES

1. Kazantzis, G.: *Environ. Health Perspect.* **40**, 143 (1981).
2. Issaq, H. J.: The Role of Metals in Tumor Development and Inhibition. *In* "Metal Ions in Biological Systems" (H. Sigel, ed.). Marcel Dekker, New York 1980, p. 56.
3. Fishbein, L.: Toxicology of Selenium and Tellurium. In "Toxicology of Trace Elements" (R. A. Goyer and M. A. Mehlman, eds.). Wiley, New York, 1977, p. 191.
4. Furst, A.: Inorganic Agents as Carcinogens. *In* "Advances in Modern Toxicology, Environmental Cancer" (H. F. Kraybill and M. A. Mehlman, eds.). Wiley, New York, 1977, p. 209.
5. Sunderman, W. F., Jr.: *Biol. Trace Element Res.* **1**, 63 (1979).
6. Weisburger, A. S., and Suhrland, L. G.: *Blood* **10**, 19 (1955).
7. Jacobs, M. M., and Griffin, A. C.: Trace Elements and Metals as Anticarcinogens. *In* "Inhibition of Tumor Induction and Development" (M. S. Zedeck and M. Lipkin, eds.). Plenum, New York, 1981, p. 169.
8. Schrauzer, G. N., White, D. A., and Schneider, C. J.: *Bioinorg. Chem.* **7**, 35 (1977).
9. Milner, J. A.: *Adv. Exp. Med. Biol.* **206**, 449 (1986).
10. Griffin, A. C.: *Adv. Cancer Res.* **29**, 419 (1979).
11. Combs, G. F., Jr., and Combs, S. B.: Selenium and Cancer. *In* "The Role of Selenium in Nutrition". Academic Press, New York, 1986, p. 413.
12. Vernie, L. N.: *Biochim. Biophys. Acta* **738**, 203 (1984).
13. Combs, G. F., Jr.: Selenium. *In* "Nutrition and Cancer Prevention — Investigating the Role of Micronutrients" (T. E. Moon and M. S. Micozzi, eds.). Marcel Dekker, New York, 1989, p. 389.
14. Ip, C.: *Biol. Trace Elements Res.* **5**, 317 (1983).
15. Whanger, P. D.: *Fundam. Appl. Toxicol.* **3**, 424 (1983).
16. Diplock, A. T.: *Curr. Top. Environ. Toxicol. Chem.* **8**, 433 (1985).
17. Schrauzer, G. N.: *Bioinorg. Chem.* **5**, 275 (1976).
18. Ip, C.: The Chemopreventive Role of Selenium in Carcinogenesis. *In* "Essential Nutrients in Carcinogenesis, Advances in Experimental Medicine and Biology" (L. A. Poirier, P. M. Newberne, and M. W. Pariza, eds.). Plenum, New York, 1986, p. 431.
19. Hocman, G.: *Int. J. Biochem.* **20**, 123 (1988).
20. Milner, J. A.: Rationale and Possible Mechanisms by Which Selenium Inhibits Mammary Cancer. *In* "Vitamins and Minerals in the Prevention and Treatment of Cancer" (M. M. Jacobs, ed.). CRC Press, Boca Raton, Florida, 1991, p. 95.
21. Combs, G. F., Jr., and Clark, L. C.: *Nutr. Rev.* **43**, 325 (1985).
22. Medina, D.: *J. Am. Coll. Toxicol.* **5**, 21 (1986).
23. Yamane, Y., and Sakai, K.: *Chem. Pharm. Bull.* **22**, 1126 (1974).
24. Fare, G.: *Biochem J.* **91**, 473 (1964).
25. Jacobs, M. M., and Pienta, R. J.: Relationships Between Potassium and Cancer. *In* "Vitamins and Minerals in the Prevention and Treatment of Cancer" (M. M. Jacobs, ed.). CRC Press, Boca Raton, Florida, 1991, p. 227.
26. Medina, D.: Selenium and Murine Mammary Tumorigenesis. *In* "Diet, Nutrition and Cancer: A Critical Evaluation" (B. S. Reddy and L. A. Cohen, eds.). CRC Press, Boca Raton, Florida, 1985, p. 23.
27. Birt, D. F.: *Proc. Soc. Exp. Biol. Med.* **183**, 311 (1986).
28. Birt, D. F.: *Magnesium* **8**, 17 (1989).
29. Rotruck, J. T., Pope, A. L., Ganther, H. E., Swanson, A. B., Hafeman, D. G., and Hoekstra, W. G.: *Science* **179**, 588 (1973).
30. Franke, K. W., and Painter, E. P.: *Cereal Chem.* **15**, 1 (1938).
31. Nelson, A. A., Fitzhugh, D. G., and Calvery, H. O.: *Cancer Res.* **3**, 230 (1943).
32. Schwartz, K. A., and Foltz, C. M.: *J. Am. Chem. Soc.* **79**, 3292 (1957).
33. McCoy, K. E. M., and Weswig, P. H.: *J. Nutr.* **98**, 383 (1969).
34. Underwood, E. J. "Trace Elements in Human and Animal Nutrition" 4th ed. Academic Press, New York, 1977, p. 311.
35. Clayton, C. C., and Baumann, C. A.: *Cancer Res.* **9**, 575 (1949).
36. Griffin, A. C., and Jacobs, M. M.: *Cancer Lett.* **3**, 177 (1977).

37. Daoud, A. H., and Griffin, A. C.: *Cancer Lett.* **9**, 299 (1980).
38. Kubota, J., Allaway, W. H., Carter, D. L., Cary, E. E., and Lazar, U. A.: *J. Agr. Food Chem.* **15**, 448 (1967).
39. Allaway, W. H., Kubota, J., Losee, F., and Roth, M.: *Arch. Environ. Health* **16**, 342 (1968).
40. Shamberger, R. J., and Frost, D. V.: *Can. Med. Assoc. J.* **100**, 682 (1969).
41. Shamberger, R. J.: *J. Natl. Cancer Inst.* **44**, 931 (1970).
42. Jacobs, M. M., Jansson, B., and Griffin, A. C.: *Cancer Lett.* **2**, 133 (1977).
43. Jacobs, M. M.: *Cancer Res.* **43**,, 1646 (1983).
44. Jacobs, M. M., Forst, C. F., and Beams, F. A.: *Cancer Res.* **41**, 4458 (1981).
45. Soullier, B. K., Wilson, P. S., and Nigro, N. D.: *Cancer Lett.* **12**, 343 (1981).
46. Nigro, N. D., Bull, A. W., Wilson, P. S., Soullier, B. K., and Alousi, M. A.: *J. Natl Cancer Inst.* **69**, 103 (1983).
47. Jacobs, M. M.: *Cancer* **40**, 2557 (1977).
48. Birt, D. F., Lawson, T. A., Julius, A. D., Runice, C. E., and Salmasi, S.: *Cancer Res.* **42**, 4455 (1982).
49. Reddy, B. S., Sugie, S., Maruyama, H., El-Bayoumy, K., and Marra, P.: *Cancer Res.* **47**, 5901 (1987).
50. Fiala, E. S.: *Cancer* **40**, 2436 (1977).
51. Fiala, E. S., Kulakis, C., Christiansen, G., and Weisburger, J. H.: *Cancer Res.* **38**, 4515 (1978).
52. Fiala, E. S., Caswell, N., Sohn, O. S., Felder, M. R., McCoy, G. D., and Weisburger, J. H.: *Cancer Res.* **44**, 2885 (1984).
53. Oravec, C. T., Jones, C. A., and Huberman, E.: *Cancer Res.* **46**, 5068 (1986).
54. Zedeck, M. S., Frank, N., and Wiessler, M.: Metabolism of the Colon Carcinogen Methylazoxymethanol Acetate. *In* "Frontiers of Gastrointestinal Research" (L. van der Reis, ed.). Karger, Basel, 1979, p. 32.
55. Bull, A. W., Soullier, B. K., Wilson, P. W., Hayden, M. T., and Nigro, N. D.: *Cancer Res.* **39**, 4956 (1979).
56. Jacobs, M. M., and Griffin, A. C.: *Biol. Trace Element Res.* **1**, 1 (1979).
57. Harr, J. R., Exon, J. H., Whanger, P. D., and Weswig, P. H.: *Clin. Toxicol.* **5**, 187 (1972).
58. Marshall, M. V., Arnott, M. S., Jacobs, M. M., and Griffin, A. C.: *Cancer Lett.* **7**, 331 (1979).
59. Harr, J. R., Exon, J. H., Weswig, P. H., and Whanger, P. D.: *Clin. Toxicol.* **6**, 487 (1973).
60. LeBoeuf, R. A., Laishes, B. A., and Hoekstra, W. G.: *Cancer Res.* **45**, 5489 (1985).
61. Tanaka, T., Reddy, B. S., and El-Bayoumy, K.: *Jpn. J. Cancer Res. (Gann)* **76**, 462 (1985).
62. Grant, K. E., Conner, M. W., and Newberne, P. M.: *Toxicol. Appl. Pharmacol.* **41**, 166 (1977).
63. Milks, M. M., Witt, S. R., Ali, I. I., and Couri, D.: *Fundam. Appl. Toxicol.* **5**, 320 (1985).
64. Baldwin, S., and Parker, R. S.: *Carcinogenesis* **8**, 101 (1987).
65. Baldwin, S. and Parker, R. S.: *Nutr. Cancer* **8**, 273 (1986).
66. Balansky, R. M., Blagoeva, P. M., and Mirtcheva, Z.: *Biol. Trace Element Res.* **5**, 331 (1983).
67. Dorado, R. D., Porta, E. A., and Aquino, T. M.: *Hepatology* **5**, 1201 (1985).
68. Marshall, M. V., Jacobs, M. M., and Griffin, A. C.: *Proc. Am. Assoc. Cancer Res.* **19**, 75 (1978).
69. Banner, W. P., Tan, Q. H., and Zedeck, M. S.: *Cancer Res.* **42**, 2985 (1982).
70. Chen, J., Goethchius, M. P., Campbell, T. C., and Combs, G. F.: *J. Nutr.* **112**, 324 (1982).
71. Burk, R. F., and Lane, J. M.: *Fundam. Appl. Toxicol.* **3**, 218 (1983).
72. Williams, G. M.: *Biochim. Biophys. Acta* **605**, 167 (1980).
73. Ip, C., and Daniel, F. B.: *Cancer Res.* **45**, 61 (1985).
74. Thompson, H. J., Meeker, L. D., Becci, P. J., and Kokoska, S.: *Cancer Res.* **42**, 4954 (1982).
75. Liu, J. Z., Gilbert, K., Parker, H. M., Haschek, W. M., and Milner, J. A.: *Cancer Res.* **51**, 4613 1991.
76. Ip, C.: *J. Natl. Cancer Inst.* **80**, 258 (1988).
77. Medina, D., Lane, H. W., and Tracey, C. M.: *Cancer Res. (Suppl.)* **43**, 2460 (1983).
78. Medina, D. and Shepherd, F.: *Carcinogenesis* **2**, 451 (1981).
79. Medina, D., Lane, H., and Shepherd, F.: *Anticancer Res.* **1**, 377 (1981).
80. Medina, D., and Shepherd, F. S.: *Cancer Lett.* **24**, 227 (1984).
81. Welsch, C. W., Goodrich-Smith, M., Brown, C. K., Greene, H. D., and Hamel, E. J.: *Carcinogenesis* **2**, 519 (1981).
82. Lane, H. W. and Medina, D.: *J. Natl. Cancer Inst.* **75**, 675 (1985).
83. O'Connor, T. P., Youngman, L. D., and Campbell, T. C.:*Federation Proc.* **42**, 670 (1983).
84. Thompson, H. J., Meeker, L. D., and Kokoska, S.: *Cancer Res.* **44**, 2803 (1984).
85. Ip, C., and Sinha, D. K.: *Carcinogenesis* **2**, 435 (1981).
86. Ip, C.: *Cancer Res.* **41**, 2683 (1981).
87. Ip, C., and Ip, M. M.: *Carcinogenesis* **2**, 915 (1981).
88. Thompson, M. J., and Becci, P. J.: *J. Natl. Cancer Inst.* **65**, 1299 (1980).
89. Thompson, M. S., Meeker, L. D., and Becci, P. J.: *Cancer Res.* **41**, 1413 (1981).
90. Ip, C.: *Carcinogenesis* **2**, 915 (1981).
91. Ip, C.: *J. Am. Coll. Toxicol.* **5**, 7 (1986).

92. Schrauzer, G. N., and Ishmael, D.: *Ann. Clin. Lab. Sci.* **2**, 441 (1974).
93. Ip, C., and Sinha, D. K.: *Cancer Res.***41**, 31 (1981).
94. Ip, C.: *Nutr. Cancer* **2**, 136 (1981).
95. Ip, C.: *Cancer Res.* **41**, 4386 (1981).
96. Capel, I. D., Jenner, M., Darrell, H. M. and Williams, D. C.: *IRCS Med. Sci. Libr. Compend.* **8**, 382 (1980).
97. Thompson, H. J.: *J. Agr. Food Chem.* **32**, 422 (1984).
98. Spallholz, J. E., Martin, J. L., Gerlach, M. L., and Henizerling, R. H.: *Proc. Soc. Exp. Biol. Med.* **143**, 685 (1973).
99. Spallholz, J. E., Martin, J. L., Gerlach, M. L., and Henizerling, R. H.: *Infect. Immunol.* **8**, 841 (1973).
100. Thompson, H. J., and Becci, P. J.: *Cancer Lett.* **7**, 215 (1979).
101. Goodwin, W. J., Jr., Huijing, F., Bordash, G. D., and Altman, N.: *Ann. Otol. Rhinol. Laryngol.* **95**, 162 (1986).
102. Goodwin, W. J., Bordash, G. D., Xue, J. W., Huijing, F., and Altman, N.: *Otolaryngol. Head Neck Surg.* **93**, 373 (1985).
103. Bogden, J. D., Chung, H. B., Kemp, F. W., Holding, K., Bruening, K. S., and Naveh, Y.: *J. Nutr.* **116**, 2432 (1986).
104. Birt, D. F., Julius, A. D., Runice, C. E., White, L. T., Lawson, T., and Pour, P. M.: *Nutr. Cancer* **11**, 21 (1988).
105. Birt, D. F., Julius, A. D., Runice, C. E., and Salmasi, S.: *J. Natl. Cancer Inst.* **77**, 1281 (1986).
106. Jacobs, M. M., and Forst, C.: *J. Toxicol. Environ. Health* **8**, 575 (1981).
107. Jacobs, M. M., and Forst, C.: *J. Toxicol Environ. Health* **8**, 587 (1981).
108. Schroeder, H. A., and Mitchener, M.: *J. Nutr.* **101**, 1531 (1971).
109. Schroeder, H. A., and Mitchener, M.: *Arch. Environ. Health* **24**, 66 (1972).
110. Thompson, H. J., Herbst, E. J., and Meeker, L. D.: *J. Natl. Cancer Inst.* **77**, 595 (1986).
111. Reddy, B. S., and Tanaka, T.: *J. Natl. Cancer Inst.* **76**, 1157 (1986).
112. Pence, B. C., and Buddingh, F.: *J. Nutr.* **115**, 1196 (1985).
113. Sharpless, G. R.: *Federation Proc.* **5**, 239 (1946).
114. Pedrero, E., Jr., and Kozelka, F. L.: *Arch. Pathol.* **52**, 455 (1951).
115. King, H. J., Spain, J. D., and Clayton, C. D.: *J. Nutr.* **63**, 301 (1957).
116. Howell, J. S.: *Br. J. Cancer* **12**, 594 (1958).
117. Fare, G., and Howell, J. S.: *Cancer Res.* **24**, 1279 (1964).
118. Fare, G., and Woodhouse, D. L.: *Br. J. Cancer* **17**, 512 (1963).
119. Kamamoto, Y., Makiura, S., Sugihara, S., Hiasa, Y., Arai, M., and Ito, N.: *Cancer Res* **33**, 1129 (1973).
120. Carlton, W. W., and Price, P. S.: *Fd. Cosmet. Toxicol.* **11**, 827 (1973).
121. Fare, G., and Orr, J. W.: *Cancer Res.* **25**, 1784 (1965).
122. Burki, H. R., and Okita, Y.: *Br. J. Cancer* **23**, 591 (1973).
123. Fare, G.: *Nature* **200**, 481 (1963).
124. Yamane, Y., Sakai, K., Uchiyama, I., Tabata, M., Taga, N., and Hanaki, A.: *Chem. Pharm. Bull.* **17**, 2488 (1969).
125. Yamane, Y., Sakai, K., Hayashi, M., Matsuzaki, M., and Hanaki, A.: *Chem. Pharm. Bull* **18**, 1050 (1970).
126. Yamane, Y., and Sakai, K.: *Gann* **64**, 563 (1973).
127. Goodall, C. M.: *Br. J. Cancer* **18**, 777 (1964).
128. Brada, Z., Altman, N. H., and Bulba, S.: *Proc. Am. Assoc. Cancer Res.* **15**, 145 (1974).
129. Brada, Z., and Altman, N. H.: *Adv. Exp. Med. Biol.* **91**, 193 (1978).
130. van Rensburg, S. J.: *J. Natl. Cancer Inst.* **67**, 243 (1981).
131. Schrauzer, G. N.: *Adv. Exp. Med. Biol.* **91**, 323 (1978).
132. Schrager, T. F., Busby, W. F., Jr., Goldman, M. E., and Newberne, P. M.: *Carcinogenesis* **7**, 1121 (1986).
133. Petering, H. G.: *Adv. Exp. Med. Biol.* **91**, 207 (1978).
134a. Nordberg, G. F., and Andersen, O.: *Environ. Health Perspect.* **40**, 65 (1981).
134b. Barch, D. H., and Iannaccone, M.: *Adv. Exp. Med. Biol.* **206**, 517 (1986).
135. Vallee, B. L.: Zinc Biochemistry in Normal and Neoplastic Growth Processes. *In* "Cancer Enzymology" (M. Schultz and F. Ahmad, eds.), Vol. 12. Academic Press, New York, 1976, p. 159.
136. Duncan, J. R., and Dreosti, I. E.: *J. Natl. Cancer Inst.* **55**, 195 (1975).
137. Duncan, J. R., Dreosti, I. E., and Albrecht, C. F.: *J. Natl. Cancer Inst.* **53**, 277 (1974).
138. Poswillo, D. E., and Cohen, B.: *Nature* **231**, 447 (1971).
139. Edwards, M. B.: *Arch. Oral Biol.* **21**, 133 (1976).
140. Ciapparelli, L., Retief, D. H., and Fatti, L. P.: *So. Afr. J. Med. Sci.* **37**, 85 (1972).
141. Fong, L. Y. Y., Sivak, A., and Newberne, P. M.: *J. Natl. Cancer Inst.* **61**, 145 (1978).

142. Gabrial, G. N., and Newberne, P. M.: Zinc Deficiency, Alcohol and Esophageal Cancer. *In* "Trace Substances in Environmental Health" (D. D. Hemphill, ed.). University of Missouri Press, Columbia, Missouri, 1979, p. 184.

143. Gabrial, G. N., Schrager, T. F., and Newberne, P. M.: *J. Natl. Cancer Inst* **68**, 785 (1982).

144. Fong, L. Y. Y., Lee, J. S. K., Chan, W. C., and Newberne, P. M.: *J. Natl. Cancer Inst.* **72**, 419 (1984).

145. van Rensburg, S. J., duBruyn, D. B., and van Schalkwyk, D. J.: *Nutr. Rep. Int.* **22**, 891 (1980).

146. Wallenius, K., Mathur, A., and Abdulla, M.: *Int. J. Oral Surg.* **8**, 56 (1979).

147. Mathur, A., Wallenius, K., and Abdulla, M.: *Acta Odontol. Scand.* **37**, 277 (1979).

148. Rath, F-W., and Enke, H.: *Arch. Geschwülstforsch.* **54**, 201 (1984).

149. Verma, R., Jain, S., Arora, H. L., Sareen, P. M., Kalra, V. B., and Lodha, S. K.: *Indian J. Cancer* **19**, 126 (1982).

150. Durlach, J., Larvor, P., Augusti, Y., and Albengres-Moineau, E.: *Concours Med.* **95**, 6295 (1973).

151. Durlach, J., Bara, M., Guiet-Bara, A., and Collery, P.: *Anticancer Res.* **6**, 1353 (1986).

152. Kasprzak, K. S., and Waalkes, M.: *Adv. Exp. Med. Biol.* **206**, 497 (1986).

153. Young, G. A., and Parsons, F. M.: *Eur. J. Cancer* **13**, 103 (1977).

154. Hass, G., Laing, G., Galt, R., and MacCreary, P.: *Magnesium Bull.* **3**, 5 (1981).

155. Seelig, M. S.: *Biol. Trace Element Res.* **1**, 273 (1979).

156. Blondell, J. M.: *Med. Hypotheses* **6**, 863 (1980).

157. Bazikyan, K. A., and Akimov, A. A.: *Vopr. Onkol.* **14**, 57 (1968).

158. Galt, R. M., Laing, G. H., and Hass, G. M.: *Trace Subst. Environ. Health* **16**, 205 (1982).

159. Poirier, L. A., Kasprzak, K. S., Hoover, K. L., and Wenk, M. L.: *Cancer Res.* **43**, 4575 (1983).

160. Triggs, S. M., and Williams, E. D.: *Acta Endocrinol.* **85**, 84 (1977).

161. Karkare, M. R., Clark, T. D., and Glauert, H. P.: *J. Nutr.* **121**, 568 (1991).

162. Mikkelsen, R. B.: *Prog. Exp. Tumor Res.* **22**, 123 (1978).

163. Kasprzak, K. S., Hoover, K. L., and Poirier, L. A.: *Carcinogenesis* **6**, 279 (1985).

164. Hiasa, Y., Ohshima, M., Kitahori, Y., Fujita, T., Yuasa, T., and Miyashiro, A.: *J. Natl. Cancer Inst.* **70**, 761 (1983).

165. Shirai, T., Ohshima, M., Masuda, A., Tamano, S., and Ito, N.: *J. Natl. Cancer Inst.* **72**, 477 (1984).

166. Shakerin, M., Paloucek, J., Oyasy, R., and Hass, G. M.: *Federation Proc.* **24**, 684 (1965).

167. Oyasu, R., Battifora, H. A., Clasen, R. A., McDonald, J. H., and Hass, G. M.: *Cancer Res.* **30**, 1248 (1970).

168a. Webster, D. J. T.: *Anticancer Res.* **1**, 293 (1981).

168b. Thompson, H. J., Kennedy, K., Witt, M., and Juzefk, J.: *Carcinogenesis* **12**, 111 (1991).

169. Siegers, C. P., Bumann, D., Baretton, G., and Younes, M.: *Cancer Lett.* **41**, 251 (1988).

170. Vitale, V. J., Broitman, S. A., Vaurousek-Jakuba, E., Rodday, P. W., and Gottlieb, L. S.: *Adv. Exp. Med. Biol.* **91**, 229 (1978).

171. Nelson, R. L., Yoo, S. L., Tanure, J. C., Andrianopoulos, G., and Misumi, A.: *Anticancer Res.* **9**, 1477 (1989).

172. Jacobs, M. M.: *Nutr. Cancer* **14**, 95 (1990).

173. Takahashi, M., and Hasegawa, R.: Enhancing Effects of Dietary Salt on Both Initiation and Promotion Stages of Rat Gastric Carcinogenesis. In "Diet, Nutrition, and Cancer" (Y. Hayashi, M. Nagao, T. Sugimura, S. Takayama, L. Tomatis, L. W. Wattenberg, and G. N. Wogan, eds.) Japan Sci. Soc. Press, Tokyo/VNU Sci. Press, Utrecht, 1986, p. 169.

174. Tatematsu, M., Takahashi, M., Fukushima, S., and Shirai, T.: *J. Natl. Cancer Inst.* **55**, 101 (1975).

175. Fine, B. P., Ponzio, N. M., Denny, T. N., Maher, E., and Walters, T. R.: *Cancer Res.* **48**, 3445 (1988).

176. Milner, J. A.: *Arch. Environ. Health* **18**, 7 (1969).

177. Franceschi, S., Talamini, R., Fassina, A., and Bidoli, E.: *Tumori* **76**, 331 (1990).

178. Ward, J. M., and Ohshima, M.: *Adv. Exp. Med. Biol.* **206**, 529 (1986).

179. Eskin, B. A.: *Adv. Exp. Med. Biol.* **91**, 293 (1978).

180. Eskin, B. A., Murphey, S. A., and Dunn, M. R.: *Nature* **218**, 1162 (1968).

181. Jabara, A. G., and Maritz, J. S.: *Br. J. Cancer* **28**, 161 (1973).

182. Kellen, J. A.: *J. Natl. Cancer Inst.* **48**, 1901 (1972).

183. Kanisawa, M., and Schroeder, H. A.: *Cancer Res.* **27**, 1192 (1967).

184. Kanisawa, M., and Schroeder, H. A.: *Cancer Res.* **29**, 892 (1969).

185. Calop, J., Burckhart, M. F., and Fontanges, R.: *Eur. J. Toxicol.* **9**, 271 (1977).

186. Thompson, H. J., Chasteen, N. D., and Meeker, L. D.: *Carcinogenesis* **5**, 849 (1984).

187. Komada, H., Kise, Y., Nakagawa, M., Yamamura, M., Hioki, K., and Yamamoto, M.: *Cancer Res.* **50**, 2418 (1990).

188. Luo, X-M., Wei, H. J., and Yang, S. P.: *J. Natl. Cancer Inst.* **71**, 75 (1983).

Dietary Fiber and Its Effect on Cancer Incidence

David Kritchevsky

I. DIETARY FIBERS: SOURCES, CLASSIFICATION, DEFINITIONS

Dietary fiber has been defined as plant cell wall material which is not degraded by human endogenous intestinal secretions. Hipsley (1) coined the term dietary fiber to describe the unavailable carbohydrate present in plant foods. However, the number of substances which are described as fiber keeps increasing. The cell wall components of plants are cellulose, hemicellulose, pectin, and lignin. The last of these is the only one which is not a carbohydrate. We now regard nonstructural cell wall contents such as carrageenans as fiber, and this designation has been extended to include other nonstructural components such as mucilages (guar gum, locust bean gum) and exudates (gum arabic, gum ghatti, gum karaya). Other materials which could come under the designation of fiber are naturally occurring substances such as resistant starch, Maillard products, cutins, waxes, and tannins and manufactured materials like lactulose or polydextrose. Fiber is also loosely classified as insoluble (cellulose, lignin, some hemicelluloses) and soluble (pectins, gums, mucilages, algae polysaccharides, some hemicelluloses). Insoluble fibers are poorly fermented by the gut microflora, whereas soluble fibers are highly fermented. Fermentation of fiber yields water, carbon dioxide, methane, hydrogen, and short-chain fatty acids (SCFA), principally acetic, propionic, and butyric acids. The SCFA may be reabsorbed and are of physiologic import. In 1982 the definitions and terminology of dietary fibers were summarized by Southgate (2a).

The dietary fiber hypothesis suggests that diets high in fiber may be protective against some of the noninfectious diseases endemic in industrialized countries. However, the analysis of dietary fibers is not yet standardized and as of 1990 we still did not have generally accepted methods based on universally accepted definitions (2b). Thus, while we talk about fiber content of foods we rarely discuss the spectrum of fibers present in any particular food. When one discusses foods rather than isolated fibers, the other materials present in the food must also be considered.

Spiller and Jenkins (3) have suggested four broad categories of dietary fibers:

1. Whole foods high in fiber.
2. A high-fiber fraction (wheat bran, for example) which is extracted/produced without affecting the structure or composition of that fraction as it exists in whole food.

3. Concentrated fibers which are altered in the course of extraction and purification (cellulose and pectin are examples).
4. Fiber-enriched foods.

II. METHODOLOGICAL CONCEPTS AND LIMITATIONS OF THE ASSESSMENT OF FIBER EFFECTS

The assessment of fiber effects in disease must consider all of the vagaries of the current state of the technology and health effects of fibers.

Nutritional effects on cancer can be investigated by way of direct experiments in animals or retrospective studies in humans. In animal experiments the subject (almost always from a rodent species) is usually treated with a chemical carcinogen and observed for a period of time, the duration of which is determined more by convention than by science; in some instances spontaneous or transplanted tumors have been studied. Such animal/tumor models have been used to study the effect of fiber in terms of some parameter(s) of tumor induction or tumor progression. The positive aspect of these studies is that the investigator has total control in choosing the conditions (number of animals, type and dose of carcinogen, diet, and duration of treatment). The negative aspects are the arbitrary nature of the experiment and the absence of any universally accepted protocol. Thus, different investigators use rats of different strains and gender, use different carcinogens or the same one, but administered by different routes, and vary the type and dosage of fiber (4,5). The sole thread of consistency is that wheat bran is the only dietary fiber additive that most consistently inhibits chemically induced colon cancer. Cohen *et al.* (6) have recently reported inhibition by wheat bran of chemically induced mammary tumors in rats.

Human studies are either ecological (intra- or international comparisons of populations) or else they examine differences between cases and controls. The diets being compared are usually recent types, which is a distinct weakness when we consider a disease condition that has developed over decades. In both types of study the dietary data relate to fiber-rich foods which can contain any number of other materials (vitamins, minerals, carotenoids, flavonoids, etc.) which may affect the course of tumorigenesis. In general, a diet high in plant materials is low in fat and calories and this, too, may influence tumorigenesis. The influence of caloric content of a diet on potential carcinogenicity has been commented on in the course of some epidemiological studies (7,8) and is discussed in greater detail in Section I of this chapter.

III. PROTECTION BY DIETARY FIBER AGAINST COLORECTAL CANCER

More than 30 years ago, Higginson and Oettle (9) suggested that some aspect of the diet, probably the fiber, was responsible for the very low incidence of colon cancer among black Africans. Burkitt (10) also attributed differences in colon cancer between Western and African populations to differences in dietary fiber intake. Several reviews in the 1980s summarized the findings relative to fiber intake and cancer risk. A review volume edited by Pilch (11) examined data from 18 ecological and 22 case-control studies and found fiber to be protective in two-thirds of the former and one-third of the latter. Jacobs (12) reviewed data from 24 ecological and 27 case-control studies and found fiber to be protective in 40–50% of them. The findings from these two reviews are shown in Table 1.

TABLE 1. Association Between Fiber Intake and Colon Cancer Risk

	Reviewers	
	Pilch et al. (11)	Jacobs (12)
Ecological studies		
Number	18	24
% Protective	66.7	54.2
% Enhancing	5.6	4.2
% No effect	27.8	41.6
Case-Control studies		
Number	22	27
% Protective	36.4	44.4
% Enhancing	22.7	14.8
% No effect	40.9	40.7

Note: Some studies reported separately on fiber, cereals, vegetables, etc.

Bingham (13) studied the outcomes of 30 case-control studies, conducted between 1969 and 1989, as they related to the levels of intake of fiber, vegetables, cereals, and starch. The ratios, protection to nonprotection, were different for the different components. Thus, the percentages of protection and nonprotection were: fiber — 50 and 41; cereals — 23 and 54; starch — 50 and 50; and vegetables — 63 and 32.

The data are provocative, but still equivocal at the time of this writing. A committee of the U.S. National Academy of Sciences (14) concluded in 1982: "The committee found no conclusive evidence to indicate that dietary fiber (such as that present in fruits, vegetables, grains and cereals) exerts a protective effect against colorectal cancer in humans." In 1988, Rogers and Longnecker (15) concluded, "Most epidemiologic studies of fiber and fiber-containing food intake in relation to risk of colorectal cancer are consistent with a very small inverse association or no association." A probable reason for these conclusions is that fiber-rich foods contain many substances which may influence carcinogenicity and that interactions among dietary components are seldom considered. Two Australian studies highlight the problems of considering single dietary components. Potter and McMichael (7) examined 121 male cases and 241 male controls and 99 female cases and 197 female controls in Adelaide. They found increasing risk with increasing fiber intake. Increasing dietary protein and total energy intake were also associated positively with risk. About 400 miles away, in Melbourne, Kune et al. (16) compared 388 male and 327 female cases with 398 male and 329 female controls. Relative risk was halved in the third, fourth, and fifth quintiles of fiber intake. Kune et al. (16) suggested that a multifactorial hypothesis could best resolve the findings.

TABLE 2. Incidence Rate of Colorectal Cancer and Fiber Intake in Finnish and Danish Men[a]

	Incidence rate (per 10⁶)		Fiber intake (mg/g diet)[b]
Country	Colon	Rectum	
Denmark (1968–1972)			
Copenhagen	22.8	39.3	13.2
Them	12.9	15.0	18.0
Finland (1970–1975)			
Helsinki	17.0	8.7	14.5
Parikkala	6.7	7.5	18.4

[a]After O. M. Jensen, R. MacLennon, and J. Wahrendorf, *Nutr. Cancer* **4**, 5 (1982).
[b]Measured in 50- to 59-year-old men.

TABLE 3. Variables Relating to Trend of Large-Bowel Cancer in Denmark and Finland[a]

Negative	Positive	Not significant[b]	
Carbohydrates	Alcohol	Cellulose	Stool wt.
Cereals	Fecal bile acids (mg/g)	Cheese	Transit time
Protein		Meats	Total fat
Saturated fatty acids		Milk	Vegetables
Starch		Total calories	Vitamin A
Total fiber		Fecal bile acids (g/day)	Vitamin C

[a]After O. M. Jensen, R. MacLennon, and J. Wahrendorf, *Nutr. Cancer* **4**, 5 (1982).

[b]Other variables found not to be significant were coffee, eggs, fats and oils, fish, fruits and berries, hexose (fiber), milk products, pentose (fiber), rye, wheat, unsaturated fat, as well as body weight and height.

Jensen *et al.* (17) studied colorectal cancer and diet in Finland and Denmark. They studied populations in large and small cities in both countries—Copenhagen and Them in Denmark, and Helsinki and Parikkala in Finland (Table 2). Only alcohol intake and fecal bile acid concentration were found to correlate positively with large-bowel cancer trends, whereas starch, refined carbohydrates, cereals, protein, saturated fatty acids, and total fiber intake correlated negatively. They found no correlation between colon cancer and more than thirty other variables (Table 3).

Slattery *et al.* (18) studied aspects of fiber-rich diets and colon cancer risk in 231 cases and 391 controls in Utah. Highest quartiles of intake of vegetables and fruits were associated with decreased risk of colon cancer. The third quartile of intake of fiber and starch seemed to be more protective than the fourth quartile, suggesting that at highest intake some other protective substance is reduced (Table 4).

TABLE 4. Colon Cancer Risk Associated with Dietary Factors[a]

	Quartile (OR)[b]			
	Lowest	2	3	Highest
NDF[c]				
Males	1.0	0.7	0.8	0.9
Females	1.0	1.3	1.0	0.7
Grains				
Males	1.0	1.1	1.6	1.0
Females	1.0	0.7	0.6	1.1
Vegetables				
Males	1.0	0.6	0.4	0.6
Females	1.0	1.0	0.8	0.3
Fruits				
Males	1.0	0.4	0.5	0.3
Females	1.0	0.8	0.8	0.6
Starch				
Males	1.0	1.5	0.9	1.7
Females	1.0	0.4	0.7	1.2

[a]After M. L. Slattery, A. W. Sorensen, A. W. Mahoney, T. K. French, D. Kritchevsky, and J. C. Street, *J. Natl. Cancer Inst.* **80**, 1474 (1988).

[b]OR = Odds ratio.

[c]NDF = Neutral detergent fiber.

TABLE 5.   **Age-Adjusted Relative Risks of Colon Cancer in American–Japanese in Hawaii. Given by Quintile of Dietary fiber and Total Fat Intake[a]**

Dietary fiber (g/day)	Fat intake (g/day)[b]	
	<61.0	>61.0
<7.50	2.28	0.82
7.50–10.39	1.36	0.52
10.40–13.09	1.53	0.61
13.10–14.79	0.79	0.91
>14.80	1.00	1.00
p value	0.042	0.237

[a]After L. K. Heilbrun, A. Nomura, J. H. Hankin, and G. N. Stemmermann *Int. J. Cancer* **44**, 1 (1989).

[b]51 subjects in each group.

The importance of dietary interactions can be adduced from recent studies in Hawaii and Singapore. Heilbrun *et al.* (19) carried out a case-control study of 8006 Japanese Americans in Hawaii. They found a significant negative association between dietary fiber and colon cancer risk in men consuming less than 61 g of fat per day (Table 5). Lee *et al.* (20) studied diet and colorectal cancer in Singapore Chinese. They found no consistent trends for either fat or fiber intake, but there was a protective role associated with high intake of cruciferous vegetables. A high ratio of meat/vegetable intake was associated positively with risk of colon cancer. (Table 6)

Graham *et al.* (21) reviewed 225 male and 223 female confirmed cases of colon cancer. Fiber alone exhibited no correlation with risk, but they found an association when fiber intake was analyzed in conjunction with other nutrients. They concluded that dietary fiber was only equivocally associated with risk. After their study of colon and rectal cancer by this same group (21) and reassessment of earlier results, these investigators concluded that fiber from grain or vegetables or fruit was associated with reduced risk in men, but only fiber from grain was associated with reduced risk in women. Willett *et al.* (24) related fiber intake to colon cancer risk in a prospective study of 88,751 women and found increasing intake of fiber from fruit to be associated with a trend toward reduced risk. Fiber from other sources (vegetables, cereals) was not associated with significant changes in risk of colon cancer. A recent study from China (25) reported that colon cancer mortality ranged from 0 to 6.7/1000. In this study no correlation was observed between mortality from colon cancer and total dietary fiber or any of its components.

TABLE 6.   **Relative Risk of Colon Cancer Associated with Highest and Lowest Quintiles of Dietary Variables[a]**

Quintile	Relative risk	p <
Cruciferous vegetables		
Lowest	1.67	
Highest	0.74	0.05
Meat/vegetables		
Lowest	0.91	
Highest	1.86	0.05

[a]After H. P. Lee, L. Gourley, S. W. Duffy, J. Esteve, J. Lee, and N. E. Day, *Int. J. Cancer* **43**, 1007 (1989).

IV. MECHANISM OF FIBER PROTECTION AGAINST COLORECTAL CANCER

What aspects of fiber intake might affect colon cancer risk? Table 7 lists the major effects of dietary fiber in the human colon. Fecal weight and transit time have not been associated with colon cancer risk in Scandinavian (17) or Hawaiian–Japanese (26) populations.

Bile acids can be promoters of chemically induced colon cancer (27), and any substance which might bind them could, theoretically, reduce their effectiveness as promoters. Dietary fibers do indeed have an affinity for bile acids and bile salts, the extent of binding being dependent on both the nature of the fiber and the substrate (28,29). Fibers also bind steroid hormones which might be involved in tumor promotion (30). Surprisingly, however, when cholestyramine (an ion-exchange resin that binds bile acids most avidly) was fed to groups of rats, each of which had been treated with one of three different chemical carcinogens, the number of tumors in the proximal colon was increased from two to four-fold and from four to twenty-nine-fold in the distal colon (31).

Dietary fiber increases fecal bulk, which is regarded to represent the dilution of fecal chemicals. Concentration of fecal bile acids correlates with colon cancer incidence. Hill *et al.* (32) reported results of a study on fecal steroid concentrations in countries with high (England, Scotland, United States) or low (Uganda, Japan, India) incidence of colon cancer. The concentration of fecal bile acids was 6.15 ± 0.66 mg/g in the countries with high colon cancer incidence and 0.61 ± 0.13 mg/g in those with low incidence. Crowther *et al.* (33) studied diet and cancer in three socioeconomic groups in Hong Kong. As income increased, so did incidence of colon cancer. Concentration of fecal bile acids also rose with increasing income. If the incidence of colon cancer in the low-income group (11.7/100,000) is taken as unity (1.00), then the incidences in the middle- and high-income groups are 1.50 and 2.28, respectively. Fecal bile acid excretion (mg/g) is 2.2 in the low-income group. If that value is taken as 1.00, then the fecal excretion levels in the middle- and high-income groups are 1.41 and 2.14, respectively.

Residents of Kuopio, Finland are at low risk of colon cancer. They excrete an average of 60.3 g of feces daily which contain 277 mg of bile acids. New York City residents are at higher risk of colon cancer. They excrete 22.3 g of feces daily which contain 275 mg of bile acids. Although the excretion of bile acids in the two population groups is identical, *the concentration* of fecal bile acids is 4.59 mg/g feces/day in the Finns and 12.33 mg/g feces/day in the Americans (34). The Scandinavian study cited earlier (17) found rural Finns to have a 27% higher concentration of fecal bile acids than rural Danes, and urban Finns to have a 23% higher concentration than urban Danes.

TABLE 7.   Major Effects of Dietary Fiber in the Human Colon

Increases fecal weight
Increases frequency of defecation
Decreases transit time
Dilutes colonic contents
Increases microbial growth
Alters energy metabolism
Decreases bile acid dehydroxylation
Produces hydrogen, methane, carbon dioxide
Produces short-chain fatty acids

The primary bile acids are those produced by the liver, namely, cholic (3a,7a,12a-trihydroxycholanoic) and chenodeoxycholic (3a,7a-dihydroxycholanoic) acids. These bile acids are dehydroxylated at the 7 position to yield deoxycholic acid (3a,12a-dihydroxycholanoic acid) and lithocholic acid (3a-hydroxycholanoic acid). The secondary bile acids possess comutagenic or cocarcinogenic activity (35). The ratios of fecal primary to secondary bile acids are similar throughout populations which exhibit different incidences of colon cancer (36,37). However, Owen *et al.* (38) have reported a higher lithocholic/deoxycholic ratio in feces of cancer patients than in controls. The foregoing suggests a role for the intestinal microflora which can possibly be influenced by type and amount of dietary fiber.

Except for lignin, dietary fibers are fermented by the colonic microflora to yield, among other products, SCFA, principally acetic, propionic, and butyric acids. SCFA are the predominant anions present in human feces and are present at concentrations of 60 to 170 mmol/l. The molar ratio of acetate:propionate:butyrate is approximately 3:1:1. Sakata (39) reported that SCFA infusions increase proliferation at all levels of the gastrointestinal tract. Presence of SCFA would tend to reduce colonic pH which, according to Thornton (40), may inhibit carcinogenesis. MacDonald *et al.* (41) have shown that individuals with bowel cancer have higher fecal pH than controls. Walker *et al.* (42) reported that the colon cancer incidence of different racial groups in South Africa was reflected in their fecal pH levels, whereas their fiber intake was similar (Table 8).

Butyrate has been shown to suppress cellular proliferation (43) and to induce differentiation of colorectal cancer cells *in vitro* (44). In animal studies, Freeman (45) found that sodium butyrate (1–2% in drinking water) increases colonic tumor incidence, but Deschner *et al.* (46) reported that 5% tributyrin does not affect tumorigenesis in mice. The eventual levels of butyric acid in the colon would be different since the substrates would be metabolized differently. Studies on fiber fermentation *in vitro* could identify those fibers that would yield the greatest proportion of butyrate.

The effects of energy restriction on carcinogenesis are discussed in Section I of this chapter. Dietary fiber has been shown to enhance fecal energy loss (47,48), which could affect tumorigenesis.

The data relating dietary fiber intake to colon cancer risk provide an inconsistent perspective. This may be due to the effects of other plant components which may vary from one fiber source to another, and these components could further influence the course of carcinogenesis. Thus, it is this writer's view that at the present time the earlier conclusions regarding fiber and colon cancer risk (14,15) still remain valid.

TABLE 8. Fiber Intake and Colon Cancer in South African Populations[a]

	Population				
	Rural Black	Urban Black	Indian	Colored	White
Proneness to colon cancer	0	±	+	+	+ + +
Energy (cal/day)	2045	2220	2330	2393	2010
Protein (g/day)	68	72	79	78	73
Fat (g/day)	38	66	99	85	82
Fiber (g/day)	25.2	18.1	20.5	21.3	22.6
Fecal pH	6.12	6.15	6.21	6.29	6.88

[a]After A. R. P. Walker, B. F. Walker, and A. J. Walker: *Br. J. Cancer* **53**, 489 (1986).

V. DIETARY FIBER EFFECT ON CANCER OF THE BREAST AND PANCREAS: EPIDEMIOLOGICAL STUDIES

Dietary fiber may also exert a protective effect against breast cancer. Rose (49) reviewed the data commenting on the effects of phytoestrogens and lignans. He asserted that the finding that vegetarians excrete more fecal estrogen and less urinary estrogen than omnivores suggests limited enterohepatic circulation of these hormones. Adlerkreutz *et al.* (50) reported that subjects with breast cancer exhibit high plasma estrogen levels, high levels of urinary estrogen, low levels of fecal estrogen, and low levels of urinary phytoestrogens and lignans. They attributed the findings to a low intake of fiber. However, in a Finnish study estrogen and lignan excretion patterns were similar in the cases and the controls (51).

There are several recently published case–control studies relating fiber intake to risk of breast cancer. Rohan *et al.* (52) found a statistically not significant reduction of risk at the upper quintiles of fiber intake. Katsouyanni *et al.* (53) found no evidence of a protective effect of dietary fiber. Pryor *et al.* (54) studied the relation of adolescent diet to eventual breast cancer. The findings are somewhat confusing. In premenopausal women, all sources of fiber are related to decreased risk, whereas in postmenopausal women risk is slightly reduced with increasing intake of grains, but rises markedly with intake of crude fiber. Van't Veer *et al.* (55) studied 133 cases and 238 controls. Fiber intake was lower in the cases (25.4 ± 6.7 g/day) than in controls (27.7 ± 7.4 g/day). The trend toward a protective effect of cereals was, however, not significant.

Howe *et al.* (56) reported on 249 cases of pancreatic cancer and 505 controls in Canada. An inverse correlation was found between risk and intake of fiber from fruits, vegetables, or cereals. There was a strong positive correlation with total caloric intake.

In summary, the epidemiologic data relating dietary fiber intake to reduction of cancer risk are suggestive, but have not been confirmed unequivocally. One major difficulty in attempting to clarify this problem is that fiber is part of a diet rich in plant foods which contain carotenes, vitamins A and C, and other substances known to affect the cancer incidence. There are good reasons for ingesting a diet high in fiber, mainly because a high-fiber diet provides bulk and is generally low in fat content. There is no particular problem with eating fat, except that it provides excess calories to a population which is becoming increasingly sedentary. Thus, a high-fiber diet carries with it the advantage of reduction of caloric intake. One other admonition with regard to fiber: a high-fiber diet is not a low-fiber diet supplemented with fiber. That is, fiber should be obtained at the grocery store, not at the pharmacy.

REFERENCES

1. Hipsley, E. H.: *Br. Med. J.* **2**, 420 (1953).
2a. Southgate, D. A. T.: Definitions and terminology of dietary fiber. *In* "Dietary Fiber in Health and Disease". (G. V. Vahouny and D. Kritchevsky, eds.). Plenum Press, New York, 1982, p. 1.
2b. Marlett, J. A.: *Adv. Exp. Biol. Med.* **270**, 183 (1990).
3. Spiller, G. A., and Jenkins, D. J. A.: "Proceedings of the XIII International Congress of Nutrition" (T. G. Taylor, and N. K. Jenkins, eds.). John Libbey, London, 1986, p. 184.
4. Kritchevsky, D.: *Cancer Res.* **43**, 2991s (1983).
5. Kritchevsky, D.: *Nutr. Cancer* **6**, 213 (1985).
6. Cohen, L. A., Kendall, M. E., Zang, E., Meschter, C., and Rose, D. P.: *J. Natl. Cancer Inst.* **83**, 496 (1991).
7. Potter, J. D., and McMichael, A. J.: *J. Natl. Cancer Inst* **76**, 557 (1986).
8. Lyon, J. L., Mahoney, A. W., West, D. W., Gardner, J. W., Smith, K. R., Sorenson, A. W., and Stanish, W.: *J. Natl. Cancer Inst.* **78**, 853 (1987).

9. Higginson, J., and Oettle, A. G.: *J. Natl. Cancer Inst.* 24, 589 (1960).
10. Burkitt, D. P.: *Cancer* **28**, 3 (1971).
11. Pilch, S. M. (ed.).: "Review of Physiological Effects and Health Consequences of Dietary Fiber." FASEB, Bethesda, Maryland, 1987.
12. Jacobs, L. R.: *Gastroenterol. Clin. North Am.* **17**, 747 (1988).
13. Bingham, S. A.: *Proc. Nutr. Soc.* **49**, 153 (1990).
14. Committee on Diet and Cancer, National Research Council: "Diet Nutrition and Cancer." Natl. Academy Press, Washington, D.C., 1982.
15. Rogers, A. E., and Longnecker, M. P.: *Lab. Invest.* **59**, 729 (1988).
16. Kune, S., Kune, G. A., and Watson L. F.: *Nutr. Cancer* **9**, 21 (1987).
17. Jensen, O. M., MacLennon, R., and Wahrendorf, J.: *Nutr. Cancer* **4**, 5 (1982).
18. Slattery, M. L., Sorensen, A. W., Mahoney, A. W., French, T. K., Kritchevsky, D., and Street, J. C.: *J. Natl. Cancer Inst.* **80**, 1474 (1988).
19. Heilbrun, L. K., Nomura, A., Hankin, J. H., and Stemmermann, G. N.: *Int. J. Cancer* **44**, 1 (1989).
20. Lee, H. P., Gourley, L., Duffy, S. W., Esteve, J., Lee, J., and Day, N. E.: *Int. J. Cancer* **43**, 1007 (1989).
21. Graham, S., Marshall, J., Haughey, B., Mittelman, A., Swanson, M., Zielezny, M., Byers, T., Wilkinson, G., and West, D.: *Am. J. Epidemiol.* **128**, 490 (1988).
22. Freudenheim, J. L., Graham, S., Marshall, J. R., Haughey, B. P., and Wilkinson, G.: *Am. J. Epidemiol.* **131**, 612 (1990).
23. Freudenheim, J. L., Graham, S., Horvath, P. J., Marshall, J. R., Haughey, B. P., and Wilkinson, G.: *Cancer Res.* **50**, 3295 (1990).
24. Willett, W. C., Stampfer, M. J., Colditz, G. P., Posner, B. A., and Speizer, F. E.: *N. Engl. J. Med.* **323**, 1664 (1990).
25. Chen, J., Campbell, T. C., Li, J., and Peto, R.: "Diet, Life-Style and Mortality in China." Oxford Univ. Press, Oxford England, 1990.
26. Glober, G. A., Nomura, A., Kamiyama, S., Shimoda, A., and Abba, B. C.: *Lancet* **2**, 110 (1977).
27. Narisawa, L. F., Magadea, N. E., Weisburger, J. H., and Wynder, E. L.: *J. Natl. Cancer Inst.* **55**, 1093 (1975).
28. Eastwood, M. A., and Hamilton, D.: *Biochim. Biophys. Acta* **152**, 165 (1968).
29. Story, J. A., and Kritchevsky, D.: *J. Nutr.* **106**, 1292 (1976).
30. Shultz, T. D., and Howie, B. J.: *Nutr. Cancer* **8**, 141 (1986).
31. Nigro, N. D., Bhadrochari, N., and Chomchai, C.: *Dis. Colon Rectum* **16**, 438 (1973).
32. Hill, M. J., Drasar, B. S., Aries, V. C., Crowther, J. S., Hawksworth, G., and Williams, R. E. O.: *Lancet* **1**, 95 (1971).
33. Crowther, J. S., Drasar, B. S., Hill, M. J., MacLennan, R., Magnin, D., Pech, S., and Teah-Chan, C. H.: *Br. J. Cancer* **34**, 191 (1976).
34. Reddy, B. S., Hedges, A. R., Laakso, K., and Wynder, E. L.: *Cancer* **42**, 2832 (1978).
35. Hill, M. J.: Bile Acids and Human Colorectal Cancer. *In* "Dietary Fiber in Health and Disease" (G. V. Vahouny and D. Kritchevsky, eds.). Plenum Press, New York, 1982, p. 299.
36. Mower, H. F., Ray, R. M., Shoff, R., Stemmermann, G. N., Nomura, A., Glober, G. A., Kamiyama, S., Shimada, A., and Yamakawa, H.: *Cancer Res.* **39**, 328 (1979).
37. Kritchevsky, D., and Klurfeld, D. M.: Fat and Cancer. *In* "Nutrition and Cancer: Etiology and Treatment" (G. R. Newell and N. M. Ellison, eds.). Raven Press, New York, 1981, p. 173.
38. Owen, R. W., Dodo, M., Thompson, M. H., and Hill, M. J.: *Biochem. Soc. Trans.* **12**, 861 (1984).
39. Sakata, T.: *Br. J. Nutr.* **58**, 95 (1987).
40. Thornton, J. R.: *Lancet* **1**, 1081 (1981).
41. MacDonald, I. A., Webb, G. R., and Mahony, D. E.: *Am. J. Clin. Nutr.* **31**, s233 (1978).
42. Walker, A. R. P., Walker, B. F., and Walker, A. J.: *Br. J. Cancer* **53**, 489 (1986).
43. Hagopian, H. K., Riggs, M. G., Swartz, L. A., and Ingram, V. M.: *Cell* **12**, 855 (1977).
44. Kim, Y. S., Tsao, D., Siddiqui, B., Whitehead, J. S., Arnstein, P., Bennett, J., and Hicks, J.: *Cancer* **45**, 1185 (1981).
45. Freeman, H. J.: *Gastroenterology* **91**, 596 (1986).
46. Deschner, E. E., Ruperto, J. F., Lupton, J. R., and Newmark, H. L.: *Cancer Lett.* **52**, 79 (1990).
47. Southgate, D. A. T., and Durnin, J. V. G. A.: *Br. J. Nutr.* **24**, 517 (1970).
48. Kelsay, J. L., Behall, K. M., and Prather, E. S.: *Am. J. Clin. Nutr.* **31**, 1149 (1978).
49. Rose, D. P.: *Nutr. Cancer* **13**, 1 (1990).
50. Adlerkreutz, H., Hamalainen, E., Gorbach, S. R., Goldin, B. R., Woods, M. N., and Dwyer, J. T.: *Am. J. Clin. Nutr.* **49**, 433 (1989).
51. Adlercreutz, H., Hockerstedt, K., Baunwart, C., Bloigu, S., Hamalainen, E., Fotsis, T., and Ollus, A.: *J. Steroid Biochem.* **27**, 1135 (1987).
52. Rohan, T. E., McMichael, A. J., and Baghurst, P. A.: *Am. J. Epidemiol.* **128**, 478 (1988).

53. Katsouyanni, K., Willett, W., Trichopoulos, D., Boyle, P., Trichopoulou, A., Vasilaros, S., Papadia-mantes, J., and MacMahon, B.: *Cancer* **61**, 181 (1988).
54. Pryor, M., Slattery, M. L., Robison, L. M., and Egger, M.: *Cancer Res.* **49**, 2161 (1989).
55. Van't Veer, P., Kobb, C. M., Verhoef, P., Kok, F. J., Schonten, E. G., Hermus, R. J. J., and Sturmans, F.: *Int. J. Cancer* **45**, 825 (1990).
56. Howe, G. R., Jain, M., and Miller A. B.: *Int. J. Cancer* **45**, 604 (1990).

Indirect Modification of Chemical Carcinogenesis by Nutritional Factors Through Regulation of the Mixed-Function Oxidase System

The nutritional status of the host may significantly affect chemical carcinogenesis through modification of its microsomal mixed-function oxidase (MFO) system in the target tissue(s). The MFO system, a multifunction monooxygenase enzyme system—consisting of cytochrome P-450 (as the terminal oxidase) and cytochrome P-450 reductase—is the key enzyme system involved in the activation and/or detoxification of most, if not all, chemical carcinogens. The overall effect of nutritional modification of chemical carcinogenesis via MFO is dependent on: (i) the type of nutritional factor, (ii) the metabolic activation/detoxification profile of the chemical carcinogen, (iii) the specific enzymic form of cytochrome P-450 affected, and (iv) the specific target tissue involved.

Nutritional factors that have been shown to modify MFO may be loosely classified as general nutritional status (e. g., starvation), macronutrients (e.g., dietary protein, lipid), micronutrients (e.g., vitamins), and other dietary factors (e.g., certain nonessential dietary constituents). The effect of starvation is rather complex. Fasting usually leads to increase in MFO activities in animals; however, the opposite effect has also been reported. In general, males appear to be more responsive than females to the effect of starvation (1). The effects of dietary protein and lipid on the MFO system have been reviewed by Hayes and Campbell (2). Compared to a control diet with 20% casein, animals fed a low-protein (5% casein) diet for 8 to 14 days had substantially lower (75–80%) MFO activity, with concomitant decreases in the cytochrome P-450 content and cytochrome P-450 reductase activity. Protein deficiency not only decreased the basal MFO activity, but also decreased the extent of MFO induction by typical inducers such as phenobarbital and 3-methylcholanthrene. Although less extensively studied, dietary fat may also modify MFO activity. For instance, diet deficient in essential fatty acids depresses hepatic microsomal MFO activity (3). A specific direct role of carbohydrate in the modification of the MFO system does not appear to have been demonstrated (1). However, high dietary glucose lowers rodent MFO activity involved in the demethylation of dimethylnitrosamine (4) and in the azoreduction of dimethylaminoazobenzene (5). There is some evidence that humans given a low-carbohydrate–high-protein diet had higher drug metabolizing (MFO) activity than those given a high-carbohydrate–low-protein diet (6).

The effect of micronutrient deficiencies on MFO activity has been extensively reviewed by Campbell and Hayes (1). Vitamin A deficiency has been associated with depression of hepatic N-hydroxylase and N-demethylase in rodents with concomitant decrease in cytochrome P-450 level; in contrast, nitroreductase activity was unaffected (7). Among the B vitamins, thiamine appears to be required for the induction of a specific form of cytochrome P-450, riboflavin availability may affect azoreductase activity, and niacin deficiency may lead to the depletion of NADPH in the MFO system. Dietary deficiency of vitamin C or E has been reported to reduce MFO activity in rodents. Deficiencies in dietary calcium, magnesium, iron, iodine, zinc, selenium, and copper may affect, to various degrees, the MFO system. Certain specific nonessential dietary constituents may also have profound effects. For instance, dietary indole, flavonoid and safrole compounds, alcohols, polycyclic aromatics, are all well-known inducers of MFO (*e.g.*, 8,9). On the other hand, some dietary constituents (*e.g.*, turmeric, dietary fiber) are inhibitors/repressors of MFO (*e.g.*, 10,11).

Since the MFO system includes a variety of enzymic activities which can — depending on the carcinogen substrate involved — be either activating or detoxifying, the outcome of nutritional modification of MFO on tumor induction must be a function of the metabolic activation/detoxification profile of the chemical. For instance, epoxide hydrase is a detoxifying enzyme for aliphatic epoxides; on the other hand, for epoxides of polynuclear compounds, such as benzo[*a*]pyrene-7,8-oxide, epoxide hydrase is an activating enzyme that generates the dihydrodiol proximate carcinogen. There is presently abundant evidence that the term "cytochrome P-450" covers actually a supergene family of diverse oxidases with different catalytic activities and substrate specificities (*revs.* 12–14). The effect of nutritional modification of MFO on chemical carcinogenesis is dependent on the specific enzymic form of cytochrome P-450 involved and its substrate specificity toward the chemical.

Another important factor is the organ-specificity of the nutritional modification of MFO. For instance, the small intestine is by far the most sensitive tissue/organ to the induction of MFO by cabbage, a cruciferous vegetable (8). The MFO systems in the skin and the colon mucosa appear to be more sensitive than the one in liver to the MFO-depressing effect of dietary deficiencies in essential fatty acids (2). The effect of dietary protein deficiency affects MFO in liver and lung to a much greater extent than MFO in kidney and is believed to be a determining factor in the dimethylnitrosamine target organ shift from liver to kidney in rodents maintained on a low-protein diet (15).

From the mechanistic point of view, nutritional factors may modify MFO system at the transcriptional, translational, as well as posttranslational level. It is now well documented that there are at least five subfamilies of cytochrome P-450 (14). The induction and/or repression of MFO is under multiple transcriptional regulatory control. At least three types of receptors involved in the modification of MFO activity — aromatic hydrocarbons (Ah) receptor, mouse peroxisome proliferator-activated receptor (mP-PAR), and nuclear steroid hormone receptor — have been identified. There is some evidence that Ah and mPPAR may belong to the same steroid hormone receptor superfamily, but require accessory proteins for these differing specificities (*rev.* 16). Nutritional factors may conceivably affect induction/repression by acting as agonists/antagonists for the receptors and/or by regulating the adaptive synthesis of the receptor molecules. There is some evidence that the starvation-induced enhancement of dimethyl-nitrosamine demethylase synthesis is the consequence of enhanced transcription or greater stabilization of messenger template (4). Dietary fiber has been shown to reduce the induction of cytochrome P-450IAI in rat colon by 3-methylcholanthrene; however, the mechanism is still unknown (11). Dietary indole-3-carbinol and 5,6-benzoflavone induce cytochrome P-450IAI in rat colon and liver by expression of the P-450IAI gene, as evidenced by increase in P-450IAI mRNAs (17).

Even less is known about possible modification at the translational level. There is some evidence that the repression of rat liver 4-dimethylaminoazobenzene reductase (5) and dimethylnitrosamine demethylase (4) by dietary glucose may be at the translational level. Glucose appears to bring about a cessation of serine dehydratase synthesis in animal tissues (18) and may affect the availability of the amino acid for protein synthesis.

At the posttranslational level, nutritional factors may affect MFO by affecting the structure and fluidity of the endoplasmic reticulum membranes in which the MFO system is embedded, or by limiting the availability of cofactors for MFO activity. Lang (19) reported that rats maintained on a diet rich in unsaturated fatty acids showed alterations of microsomal membrane and depressed MFO activities. Conversely, diet rich in cholesterol was found to increase hepatic microsomal MFO activity in the rat (20). These differing effects of dietary unsaturated fatty acids and cholesterol on MFO activities are likely to be mediated through the effect of these lipoidic substances on phase transitions in the endoplasmic reticulum membrane. There is indeed substantial evidence that conformation-dependent coupling/uncoupling between cytochrome P-450 and cytochrome P-450 reductase is a membrane-governed MFO regulatory function modulated by the composition of membrane lipids (*e.g.*, 21–23).

Evidence for MFO activity modification through cofactor limitation has been provided by Levy and DiPalma (24), who showed that niacin deficiency causes partial depletion of NADPH with concomitant decrease in drug-metabolizing activity.

REFERENCES

1. Campbell, T. C., and Hayes, J. R.: *Pharmacol. Rev.* **26**, 171 (1974).
2. Hayes, J. R., and Campbell, T. C.: Nutrition as a Modifier of Chemical Carcinogenesis. *In* "Modifiers of Chemical Carcinogenesis" (T. J. Slaga, ed.), Carcinogenesis — A Comprehensive Survey, Vol. 5. Raven Press, New York, 1980, p. 207.
3. Norred, W. P., and Wade, A. E.: *Biochem. Pharmacol.* **21**, 2887 (1972).
4. Venkatesan, N., Arcos, J. C., and Argus, M. F.: *Cancer Res.* **30**, 2563 (1970).
5. Jervell, K. F., Christoffersen, T., and Morland, J.: *Arch. Biochem.* **111**, 15 (1965).
6. Alvares, A. P., Kappas, A., Anderson, K. E., Pantuck, E. J., and Conney, A. H.: Nutritional Factors Regulating Drug Biotransformation in Man. *In* "Drug Action Modification — Comparative Pharmacology" (G. Olive, ed.), Vol. 8 *Adv. Pharmacol. Therap.* (Proc. 7th Int. Congr. Pharmacol., Paris, 1978). Pergamon, Oxford, 1979, p. 43.
7. Becking, G. C.: *Can. J. Physiol. Pharmacol.* **51**, 6 (1973).
8. Wattenberg, L. W.: *J. Natl. Cancer Inst.* **60**, 11 (1978).
9. Woo, Y.-T., Lai, D. Y., Arcos, J. C., and Argus, M. F.: "Chemical Induction of Cancer," Vol. IIIC. Academic Press, Orlando, Florida, 1988.
10. Azuine, M. A., and Bhide, S. V.: *Nutr. Cancer* **17**, 77 (1992).
11. Kawata, S., Tamura, S., Matsuda, Y., Ito, N., and Matsuzawa, Y.: *Carcinogenesis* **13**, 2121 (1992).
12. Guengerich, F. P.: *Cancer Res.* **48**, 2946 (1988).
13. Gonzalez, F. J.: *Pharmacol. Ther.* **45**, 1 (1990).
14. Nebert, D. E., Nelson, D. R., Coon, M. J., Estabrook, R. W., Feyercisen, R., Fuji-Kuriyama, Y., Gonzalez, F. J., Guengerich, F. J., Gonsalus, I. C., Johnson, E. F., Lopez, J. C., Sato, R., Waterman, M. R., and Waxman, D. J.: *DNA Cell Biol.* **10**, 1 (1991).
15. Swann, P. F., and McLean, A. E. M.: *Biochem. J.* **124**, 283 (1972).
16. Mile, J. S., and Wolf, C. R.: *Carcinogenesis* **12**, 2195 (1991).
17. Vang, O., Jensen, M. B., and Autrup, H.: *Carcinogenesis* **11**, 259 (1990).
18. Jost, J. P., Khairallah, E. A., and Pitot, H. C.: *J. Biol. Chem.* **243**, 3057 (1968).
19. Lang, M.: *Gen. Pharmacol.* **7**, 416 (1976).
20. Lang, M.: *Biochim. Biophys. Acta* **455**, 947 (1976).
21. Stier, A.: *Biochem. Pharmacol.* **25**, 109 (1976).
22. Duppel, W., and Ullrich, V.: *Biochim. Biophys. Acta* **426**, 399 (1976).
23. Murphy, M. G.: *J. Nutr. Biochem.* **1**, 68 (1990).
24. Levy, H. A., and DiPalma, J. R.: *J. Pharmacol. Expt. Therap.* **109**, 377 (1953).

EDITORS' NOTE II

On Evidence for Preventive Significance of Dietary Supplementation

Chapter 4 and Sections III and IV of the present chapter review the tumor inhibitory and/or carcinogenesis chemopreventive effects in experimental animals of certain vitamins and minerals, in particular vitamin A-like compounds (retinoids and carotenoids), vitamin C, vitamin E, vitamin D_3 (as 1,25-dihydroxycholecalciferol), selenium, calcium, and copper.

Although dietary supplementation has been used in the treatment of human malignancies for a long time, mainly on an empirical basis, formal clinical and epidemiological evidence gathering in recent years increasingly lend credence to claims of the cancer preventive and therapeutic efficacy of dietary supplementation. The use of retinoids was probably the earliest instance of formal exploration of the cancer therapeutic efficacy of a dietary supplement (vitamin A)-related substance. Although retinoids have been studied primarily for cancer chemoprevention (*see* Chapter 4), considerable experimental and clinical evidence justify now their use as anticancer chemotherapeutic agents (*e.g., revs. in* 1,2). The cancer preventive efficacy of dietary supplementation is consistent with the repeatedly confirmed epidemiological finding that elevated intake of fresh fruits and vegetables is associated with reduced risk of stomach, esophageal, and lung cancer, and combined cancer incidence at all sites (*e.g.,* 3,4, *see also* ref. 5). These studies are also consistent with the protective effect of carotenoid intake against lung cancer in particular (6).

A major nutritional intervention trial conducted from 1986 to 1991 on 29,000 participating rural residents (40 to 69 years of age) in the Linxian County in China indicated that daily vitamin and mineral supplementation, particularly with the combination of β-carotene, vitamin E, and selenium, reduces the cancer risk in this population (7,8). Linxian, a county in the Henan Province of north-central China, has one of the world's highest rates of esophageal squamous cell carcinomas (and gastric cardia region adenocarcinomas) of the world (9). The rates of these cancers, considered as a single clinical entity, exceed the Chinese national average by 10-fold and the American average for whites by 100-fold (10). The very high cancer rates at these sites coexisted with consistently low levels (by Western standards) of retinol, β-carotene, riboflavin, vitamin C, and vitamin E in Linxian residents, established in sampling surveys between about 1982 and 1987 (*cited in* ref. 7). The trial revealed (7) a 21% reduction of mortality from stomach cancer, a 20% reduction of mortality from all cancer sites combined, and a 4% reduction of mortality from esophageal cancer (taken as a single entity); this is consistent with other findings (*see* Chapter 2) that the effect of systemically administered anticarcinogenic factors may vary by site and/or cell type.

REFERENCES

1. Lupulescu, A.: "Hormones and Vitamins in Cancer Tretrment". CRC Press, Boca Raton, Florida, 1990.
2. Merrill, A. H., Foltz, A. T., and McCormick, D. B.: Vitamins and Cancer. *In* "Cancer and Nutrition" (R. B. Alfin-Slater and D. Kritchevsky, eds.). Plenum Press, New York, 1991, p. 262.

3. Steinmetz, K. A., and Potter, J. D.: *Cancer Causes Control* **3**, 325 (1991).

4. Le Marchand, L., Yoshizawa, C. N., Kolonel, L. N., Hankin, J. H., and Goodman, M. T.: *J. Natl. Cancer Inst.* **81,** 1158 (1989).

5. National Research Council: "Diet and Health: Implications for Reducing Chronic Disease Risk". National Academy Press, Washington, D.C., 1989.

6. Le Marchand, L., Hankin, J. H., Kolonel, L. N., Beecher, G. R., Wilkens, L. R., and Zhao, L. P.: *Cancer Epidemiol. Biomarkers Prevention* **2,** 183 (1993).

7. Blot, W. J., Li, J.-Y., Taylor, P.R., *et al.*: *J. Natl. Cancer Inst.* **85,** 1483 (1993).

8. Li, J.-Y., Taylor, P.R., Li, B., *et al.*: *J. Natl. Cancer Inst.* **85,** 1492 (1993).

9. Li, J.-Y.: *Natl. Cancer Inst. Monogr.* **62,** 113 (1982).

10. Blot, W. J., and Li, J.-Y.: *Natl. Cancer Inst. Monogr.* **69,** 29 (1985).

CHAPTER 10

The Effect of Animal Age
on Tumor Induction

Yvonne Leutzinger and John P. Richie, Jr.

I. INTRODUCTION

One of the major factors that affects the induction of cancer by chemical compounds, and which has not yet been thoroughly investigated, is the age of the host. As a number of significant metabolic changes occur throughout the life span of an organism, host age is likely to have an impact on the manifested potency of cancer-causing agents. Since humans can be exposed to carcinogens at any point throughout their lifetime, it is important to understand the risks associated with exposure at all stages of the life span.

Cancer is primarily a disease of old age, as the incidence and mortality rates of most cancers increase exponentially over this later portion of the life span (1–3). The term "aging" refers specifically to changes occurring during the later segment of the life span and is synonymous with "senescence". The term "age", on the other hand, refers simply to the passage of time and is synonymous with "chronological age". While changes occurring earlier in the life span may be important for the study of childhood and multigenerational cancers and have been the subject of review elsewhere (4, 5), there is a distinct need for a comprehensive and critical review of the literature focusing on chemical carcinogenesis specifically during senescence.

Before examining the literature in this area, it is important to assess the current state of knowledge on the biology of the aging process. Therefore, this chapter begins with a brief overview of aging research and an outline of the established and potential relationships between the aging process and chemical carcinogenesis. This is followed by a description of the basic research approaches which have been used in the field. The background information is followed by a critical review of the literature on both experimental animal and human studies, arranged by specific carcinogens or classes of carcinogens. Finally, the changes in the host which occur as a result of aging and are likely to affect the carcinogenic process are discussed.

II. BACKGROUND

A. The Aging Process

The biological aging process or senescence is a phenomenon associated with a progressive deterioration of functional capacity and overall health, and leads eventually to death. Aging represents a normal phase of the life cycle which naturally follows the periods of growth, development, and maturity. Although this process is associated with increased incidence of disease and eventual death, it is not considered a disease process itself. Nevertheless, the relationship between aging and disease represents an important aspect of this phase of life.

For each animal species there appears to be a specific maximum life span or life span potential (6). For example, the life span potential for mice is about 30 months, whereas for humans it is about 100 years. It is believed that differences in the rate of aging between species result in the observed differences in species-specific life span. It is this relationship between longevity and aging which defines senescence as the portion of the life span associated with an exponential increase in mortality. According to this definition, aging can be quantitated by examining death rates from cohort survival data.

At the population level, the inevitable final outcome of aging is death. Accordingly, it would appear that information on the causes of death in old age would provide important clues on the biological mechanisms of senescence. In humans, where the most accurate and detailed information exists on causes of death, a variety of causes can be identified, ranging from specific chronic disease states, such as heart diseases and cancers, to a variety of different infections and accidents (7). Perhaps the strongest conclusion which can be drawn from examination of these data is the association of aging with an increased susceptibility to diseases and environmental insults. This association is the basis for the classical definition of senescence as an "increased vulnerability which occurs with advanced age" (8). However, this generalized concept provides little insight into the mechanisms responsible for aging impairments.

Another important observation of senescence is the apparent deterioration of function and physical health. A great deal of research over the past 50 years has been aimed at identifying those physical processes which are affected by aging. In the course of this research it became evident that the increased incidence of disease observed during aging was a major confounding factor (9). As this factor was not appreciated in a majority of earlier studies, disease-specific effects were often confused with changes due to aging, and this led to a number of misconceptions regarding the overall decline in general health during aging. It was not until the work of Nathan Shock in the 1950s that this important fact was recognized and an effort was set forth to focus gerontological studies on "normative aging" using only healthy individuals in order to weed out apparent aging changes that are actually secondary to disease (10, 11).

Human research on the physiology of aging was also hampered by the inherent limitation of *cross-sectional studies* (10). In these studies, measurements are made once on a population of subjects covering a wide range of ages, so that average differences between age groups are identified. Among the shortcomings of this experimental design are the unavoidable natural selection of only "surviving" subjects in the older age groups and cohort effects caused by factors other than age which differ between age groups. To avoid these limitations, *longitudinal study designs* have been used (10). In these studies, sequential measurements are made repeatedly on the same individuals over time so that aging changes can be identified in a self-controlled and more sensitive manner. However, this design poses practical problems such as high cost, difficulties with subject recruitment and attrition, maintenance of study uniformity and quality control, and the necessity for extremely long-term studies.

Over the past 30 years, using the data from both cross-sectional and longitudinal studies, a number of physiological parameters which are markedly altered during the natural course of aging have been identified. These aging changes have been extensively reviewed (12–14). It has also become clear that aging is not associated with a general decline in all aspects of physical health, as was commonly thought. In fact, the observed impairments are, in most cases, quite small and occur progressively over the latter part of the life span (13). Indeed, the progressive nature of these changes often makes their detection difficult.

Despite the tremendous interest in this area of gerontological research, the biochemical mechanisms by which the aging process regulates life span remain unclear. While it appears unlikely that there is a single cause of aging, the homogeneity of life span characteristics among species suggests that this process is tightly controlled. Over the years, a number of theories have been developed to explain the aging process (15). Early theories were based on the imprecise notion of the body "wearing out" with time, whereas others suggested that aging was based on the rate at which a "metabolic pool" was used up and its exhaustion was leading to death. The "error theory" of aging proposed that errors in protein synthesis accumulate in older organisms, leading to defective enzymes and structural proteins. More recent theories include the "free radical theory", which suggests that aging is due to an accumulation of damage caused by highly reactive free radicals formed during metabolism, predominant among these being oxygen free radical species; one early formulation of this theory is the "cross-linking theory", which attributes aging to the cumulative cross-linking and, hence, gradual functional impairment of enzymes, structural proteins, and synthetic template macromolecules by reactive byproducts of metabolism ("metabolic clinkers"). Finally, a variety of genetic theories (based on the "genetic clock" notion) suggest that aging is preprogrammed in the genome of every cell. While all of these theories have epistemologically attractive features, there is insufficient experimental evidence to establish the *exclusive* validity of any of them. It is also possible that aging is a process with a multifactorial etiology and that certain aspects of all these theories together are involved in what is the "mechanism of aging".

Human studies have played an important role in gerontological research. However, a number of problems limit their utility. These include the heterogeneous genetic and environmental backgrounds of human subjects, the lack of availability of most tissues and organ systems, and the prohibitively long observation periods required for longitudinal studies. Therefore, the use of animal models is an essential aspect of the study of aging and longevity.

Regrettably, the use of inappropriate models has been and still remains a major problem in gerontology (16). Many studies have been flawed by the use of animals that were too young, so that growth instead of senescent changes were determined. Thus, the development and characterization of experimental animal models has been a primary consideration in gerontological research. In general, the ideal animal models should be well characterized and validated, biochemically similar to man, easy and inexpensive to grow and maintain, and short-lived so that life span studies are feasible. A further discussion of appropriate animal models for research on cancer and aging, along with information on their proper use, is provided below in Section II.C.

B. Relationship Between Aging and Cancer

It is well documented that the incidence and mortality rates from cancer increase progressively with age in humans (1–3). A similar aging-related pattern in tumor incidence is also observed in experimental animals (17, 18). With the exception of those cancers that occur predominantly in children and young adults, such as nephroblastomas, retinoblastomas, bone and testicular tumors, and lymphoid leukemia, the incidence of most neoplasms increases exponentially with age, reaching a maximum between 50 and 70 years of age. The magnitude of this problem is likely to grow as the percentage of elderly is expected to increase from about 11 percent of the current population to nearly 20 percent by the year 2000 (7).

The nature of the relationship between the biological aging process and the development of neoplasms remains unknown (19). It has been suggested that the underlying mechanisms of aging and carcinogenesis are closely related. Indeed, theories of aging based on an accumulation of nonrepairable lesions which occur in cells over time, such as the free radical theory (20, 21), are analogous to theories developed to explain the occurrence of cryptogenic tumors (22).

Others have argued that there is no relationship between aging and cancer and cite inconsistencies such as the loss of replicative capacity of senescent cells (23–25). This view attributes the aging-associated increase in cancer to cumulative carcinogen doses and increased exposure to carcinogen action with time. However, spontaneous tumor incidence does not correlate with life span among different species despite widely differing life span potentials (26–29). Although the dose and time of exposure relationship may be an important factor in the aging-related increase in cancer incidence, it seems likely that other factors are also involved.

Another hypothesis to explain the relationship between aging and cancer proposes that specific changes which occur in the host during natural aging result in an increased susceptibility to neoplasia. Indeed, this notion is consistent with the definition of senescence as "an increased vulnerability occurring with advanced age" (8). Based on current knowledge of the mechanisms of chemical carcinogenesis, there are a number of factors which, if altered in senescence, could result in an increase in susceptibility to carcinogens. These include enhancement of carcinogen activation, DNA susceptibility to chemical damage, and cell proliferation or impairments in carcinogen detoxification, DNA repair, and immunological surveillance. However, there is only limited experimental evidence to suggest which of these factors might play an important role in carcinogenesis during aging.

C. Research Approaches

Perhaps the most straightforward approach to examining the effects of aging on chemical carcinogenesis is to simultaneously administer a carcinogen to mature and old animals and to observe the resulting emergence of tumors. However, this simple research design is complicated by a number of technical problems and questions which must be addressed regarding the chemical carcinogens, animal models, and bioassay conditions to be used.

A number of parameters must be considered in the selection of the carcinogen. Different types of carcinogens exist; each type is metabolized, activated, or detoxified differently. As the testing in "old" animals precludes the use of long-term bioassays, the carcinogen and its associated dosage regimen should be relatively fast acting. If a specific change in systemic metabolism during aging is being examined in terms of its effect on carcinogenesis, then a carcinogen should be chosen which primarily targets the particular organ/tissue involved in the pertinent aspect of systemic metabolism. It must also be realized that the carcinogenicity of compounds that is actually expressed is regulated by a number of factors such as absorption, metabolism, disposition, immune function, DNA repair, and cell turnover. Finally, the use of promoters should be carefully considered, since aging changes that may influence promoter efficacy can confound bioassay results.

The appropriate choice of experimental animal is of major importance. In the design and interpretation of results from studies using aging animal models, it is necessary to have information on the animals' survival characteristics in order to establish the biological stages of the life span (Table 1) that are associated with each age group under study. Inbred mice and rats are the most commonly used models in aging and cancer research, and there exists a wide variation in life span amongst the different inbred strains

TABLE 1.   **Biological Stages of the Life Span**

Prenatal
Neonatal
Growth and development
Mature adult
Old
Very old

and substrains (30). The survival characteristics of three common strains of inbred mice representing a range of life span potentials are given in Figure 1. From these data it is clear that ages which are considered old for one strain may not be old for another. For example, a 400-day old C3H/HeJ mouse in this experiment would represent a very old animal (< 10% survival), while a 400-day old C57BL/6J mouse would be considered mature, but not old (>98% survival). In general, the longer-lived strains have been utilized for studies on aging, since most short-lived strains are unusually sensitive to specific diseases such as cancer. A number of excellent reviews have been written comparing survival information on the most commonly used inbred strains of mice and rats (30–32).

It should also be recognized that the survival characteristics of each strain or substrain may vary with local laboratory conditions (32). In reviewing data from different laboratories, it is often observed that the survival of control animals is substantially lower than the known life span for that particular strain. In this event, it is likely that suboptimal conditions in animal care existed, making interpretation of any experimental change difficult. Therefore, it is important that the survival data of control animals be provided when experimental animals are aging in specific local laboratories. Finally, in order to detect the progressive changes which can occur during aging and to distinguish them from growth or developmental changes, the animals should be sampled systematically at several age points throughout the progression of the entire life span.

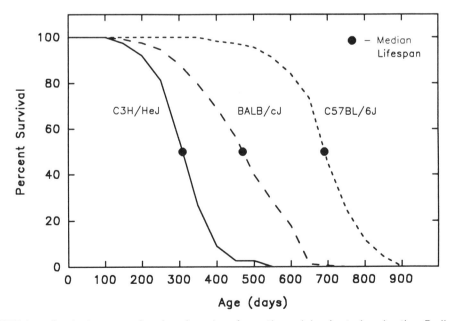

FIGURE 1.   Survival curves for female mice from three inbred strains in the Pedigreed Expansion Stocks, The Jackson Laboratory. (Adapted from E. S. Russell: *In "Biology of the Laboratory Mouse"* (E. L. Green, ed). Dover, New York, 1968, p. 511, with permission.)

TABLE 2. Protocol Differences in Studies on Chemical Carcinogenesis During Aging

---

Experimental animal model
    Species, strain, substrain, gender, virgin *versus* bred
    Local environment, single or multiple housing
    Diet
    AGE
Carcinogen
    Type
    Mechanism of action (initiator, promoter)
    Metabolism (activation, detoxification)
    Administration
        (a) size and number of doses
        (b) route of administration
        (c) period of administration (short or long compared to life span)
Bioassay of carcinogen effect
    Different types of cancers or tumors
    Method of monitoring tumors (by their appearance or threshold size)
    Period of observation (short-term, limited term, or lifetime)

Moreover, the large variation in protocols of the studies reported makes it difficult to compare the results obtained (33). The classification of adult animals as being "old" is an often encountered major problem. Another problem is that very diverse bioassay experimental designs are used, so that even with the same species and carcinogens, valid comparisons between studies cannot always be made. Some of the major parameters which differ in protocol design are summarized in Table 2. Problems also arise with the analysis of experimental results. It is not infrequent for important data to be missing from a report, making interpretation difficult.

Scheduled terminations throughout the life span sometimes give rise to different tumor yields than necropsies on animals found dead or moribund. In the latter case there are two ways to express tumor incidence (34, 35). One way is to express the frequency of lesions found in dead animals as a percentage of the number of animals that died in that particular time interval. The other way is to express it as a percentage of those that were alive at the beginning of the particular time period (equivalent to the incidence in the population at risk). The first method assumes that the incidence in dead animals is the same as that in animals that are alive. This is true for "incidental" lesions, *i.e.*, for those that are not related to death. The second method reflects the incidence for lesions that develop rapidly and are life threatening, that is, for "fatal lesions".

According to Peto *et al.* (34), comparison of the number of animals with tumors is more appropriate than the number of tumors per animal. These investigators stress the importance of recording the context of observation (incidental, fatal, and mortality-independent) and of calculating the expected (in the absence of treatment) numbers of tumor-bearing animals, corrected for longevity.

III. STUDIES ON CHEMICAL CARCINOGENESIS IN AGING ANIMALS

The majority of the literature dealing with carcinogenesis and aging contains studies that compare the effects of chemical carcinogens between very young and adult, but not truly old animals (33). In experiments where old animals are actually used, they are often compared to young growing animals rather than mature adults. Thus, any differences that may be observed in the effects of carcinogens cannot be separated as either growth or aging related. There are significantly fewer studies comparing mature adult to truly old animals. These studies, and also some others in this section, although they do not meet the proper age criteria, may still shed some light on the effects of aging. A few studies are discussed with the aim of illustrating the variety of details that must be considered in interpreting data and the wide range of methodologies from which the data derive.

A. Polycyclic Aromatic Hydrocarbons

Polycyclic aromatic hydrocarbons (PAHs) are activation-dependent genotoxic chemicals found in many environmental products such as coal, tobacco smoke, or petroleum (36, 37). They include benzo[*a*]pyrene (BaP), a strong carcinogen formed from incomplete combustion of carbon compounds, and 7,12-dimethylbenz[*a*]anthracene (DMBA), a powerful synthetic carcinogen. The metabolic activation of a number of PAHs, such as BaP, consists in oxidation of a segment of the molecule termed bay region, resulting in the formation of highly reactive intermediates, the diol epoxides. These reactive metabolites of PAHs are the form in which they bind to DNA; however, the overwhelming portion of these metabolites is rapidly conjugated and detoxified. Rodents are particularly sensitive to PAHs; their target organs include the skin, the breast, and the lung.

1. In Skin

A series of studies in two-stage carcinogenesis was carried out using DMBA as the initiating agent in skin carcinogenesis. These studies examined the relationship between tumorigenesis and the time elapsed between initiation and promotion or the age of the animals at the time of initiation and promotion. An overall decrease in tumor incidence was found both with increasing age and increasing time interval between initiation and promotion.

Two basic types of treatment schedules were used in these experiments. In one type of experiment, initiation occurred at the same time in all animal groups, but the *time interval to promotion was varied* (Figure 2, part A). It should be noted that with this design, the longer the interval, the older the animals were at the time of promotion. Thus, the effect of interval length on tumor incidence cannot be separated from the effect of age on promotion. In the second type of treatment schedule, the *time interval between initiation and promotion was kept constant* in all animal groups, but the *treatments occurred at different periods in the life span* (Figure 2, part B). While the intent of these experiments was to examine the effect of age on promotion, it must be recognized in interpreting the results that both initiation and promotion can be affected by age.

In one study, the experimental protocol consisted of a single dose of DMBA followed by phorbol myristate acetate (PMA) three times weekly for 365 days (38). This gave rise to papillomas in 100% of the female ICR/Ha Swiss mice. To *investigate the effect of age*, the interval between initiation with DMBA (20 µg in 0.1 ml acetone) and promotion with PMA (2.5 µg in 0.1 ml acetone) was kept constant so that initiation/promotion occurred at 6/8, 44/46, or 56/58 weeks. Papillomas measuring 1 mm that persisted for more than 30 days were counted (39, 40). It was found that the rate of appearance of papillomas decreased with age, as did the number of tumors per mouse (9.4, 8.7, and 4.2 tumors/ mouse, respectively).

To *examine the effect of interval* between initiation and promotion the animal groups that received treatments at 6/8 or 6/62 weeks were compared: in the latter group the rate of tumor appearance was slower and the tumor number per mouse was decreased (from 9.4 to 3.2, respectively). Clearly, the effect of initiation persisted even when promotion occurred a year later. These results suggested that tumor yield decreased as a

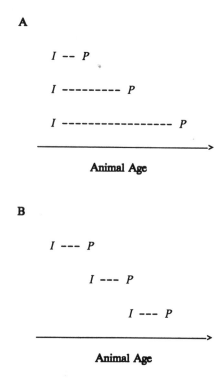

FIGURE 2. Protocols used for determining the effect of age and interval between initiation (I) and the start of promotion (P) in two-stage carcinogenesis.

result of an increase in either the interval between initiation and promotion or the age of the animals at promotion. Also, tumor yield decreased as the age of animals at initiation and promotion increased.

In another study that examined initiation and promotion of skin tumors at different ages, similar conclusions to those above were reached (41, 42). In this large study involving 2200 Swiss mice, the initiating carcinogen was again DMBA, while the promoter was the phorbol ester 12-O-tetradecanoyl-phorbol-13-acetate (TPA). To examine the effect of age, TPA (3.2 μg) was applied at a constant interval of 3 weeks after DMBA (10–300 μg) with initiation/promotion at 8/11, 48/51, or 69/71 weeks. The promoter was applied twice weekly for 15 weeks, and papillomas over 10 mm that appeared within 20 weeks of the start of promotion were counted. The effects of initiation/promotion were similar in the 8/11- and 48/51-week groups, but were significantly diminished in the 68/71-week group in terms of the number and size of papillomas as well as the number of malignant tumors. Thus, initiation/promotion appears less effective in older animals. However, it should be pointed out that in this study, as well as in the previous study, the comparison is being made between groups of young and mature adult animals and no "truly old" animals were included, based on survival characteristics for these strains of mice.

Different conclusions about the effect of age on promotion were reached in a later study (43). The animals were female NMRI mice, all initiated with DMBA at the same age of 12 weeks and then promoted with TPA for a period of 25 weeks starting 4, 8, 16, 24, 32, or 40 weeks after initiation. A key difference between this experiment and the one described above was that the administration of DMBA, which consisted of a single dose of 50 mg/kg body weight, was by intragastric route via stomach tube. This was done on the premise that skin irritation due to local administration of DMBA has an additional promoting effect, which is apparent especially when the interval between promotion and initiation is short. With this oral administration the effective dose at the skin is several orders of magnitude lower than that for topically applied DMBA.

The results of this study confirmed the persistence of the initiating effect of DMBA up to 40 weeks, but it was concluded that promotion was not affected by age. This conclusion was reached because in the animals which developed papillomas ($>90\%$), the tumor yield per animal was the same, irrespective of the age at promotion. However, there were no data provided on the size or persistence of the tumors that were counted. Further, other data were reported which demonstrated a decreasing incidence of squamous cell carcinoma with increasing age of promotion. Therefore, the experiments do not convincingly show a lack of effect of age on promotion, as concluded by the authors.

The above studies all concern the effects of age on two-stage skin carcinogenesis, requiring both initiation and promotion. There have also been a number of studies involving single carcinogens which did not require additional promotion. Although the results from this experimental design should be more straightforward, very few of the studies utilize appropriate animal ages for investigating chemical carcinogenesis in senescence.

In one experiment using male C57BL/Icrf mice, a single subcutaneous dose of 200 μg 3-methylcholanthrene (3-MC) was given, subcutaneous tumors at the site of injection were recorded weekly, and histologic examinations were performed at the time of autopsy (44). The age groups were 21 days, 6 months, and 20 months. The results demonstrated that only 75% of the weanling animals developed tumors at the injection site compared to 96 and 100% of the older groups; also, the tumors in the weanling animals developed more slowly. There was apparently no difference in tumor incidence between 6-month-old and 20-month-old animals, which—according to the life span characteristics of this long-lived strain of mice—represent growing and mature adults, respectively.

A study which utilized a better choice of age groups designed to shed light on adult/senescent differences in response to carcinogens involved the use of BALB/c mice. This is a relatively long-lived strain with a mean life span of approximately 575 days for virgin females and 539 days for males. In the first experiment, skin was grafted from 14-month-old and 2-month-old BALB/c mice onto 2-month-old syngeneic recipients (45). Twelve months later, DMBA (1 μg in 0.025 ml acetone) was applied once to the now 26- and 14-month-old grafts; 2 months later it was found that 60% of grafts from the older donors had papillomas *versus* 25% from the younger ones. That is, the senescent skin itself (26 months old) was more susceptible to initiation and growth of tumors than adult skin (14 months old), independently of other possible age-dependent changes in the animal.

This conclusion was supported by a further study in which DMBA was applied again 5 months after the original treatment (46). Three months later 5 out of 41 of the 22-month-old grafts had carcinomas, while 16 out of 41 had carcinomas in the 34-month-old grafts.

Not only were old grafts more susceptible than adult grafts, but in another experiment it was found that young mice (4 months old) were also more susceptible to DMBA than adult mice (20 months old) (47). It should be noted that in this experiment the dose of DMBA was much higher: 32 μg DMBA in 0.025 ml acetone was applied three times at 2-week intervals. When the susceptibility to DMBA of 4-month-old skin grafts was compared between 4- and 20-month-old recipients, the age of the recipient was found to be irrelevant. This result confirmed the previous conclusion (45,46) that the age of the skin itself is important, not the age of the recipient. Thus, in the development of some cancers, local organ-specific changes with aging may be more important than other influences.

An entirely different experimental situation arises when the protocol calls for lifetime administration of a chemical and the effects of age are due to the age of the animal when treatment was begun. Such a study design was used in an experiment examining the incidence of skin tumors in mice after applying BaP (24). The animals were female Swiss albino mice and the start of treatment spanned almost a year, starting when they were 10, 25, 45, or 55 weeks old. BaP (20 μg in 0.25 ml acetone) was applied to the skin twice weekly for the duration of the animals' life span. Epithelial tumors were recorded once every 2 weeks as being 2, 6, or 10 mm in diameter. They were prepared for histological examination either when a mouse died or was killed after a tumor exceeded 10 mm. For tumors that arose after the same length of treatment, their rate of growth from 2 mm to 10 mm was found to be the same, irrespective of the age of the mice at the start of treatment. Life table analyses of the percent of mice without tumors, plotted *versus* age or duration of exposure, showed that the incidence of malignant tumors was dependent on exposure duration, but not on the age of mice.

In this study (24), cancer incidence was found to be much more strongly dependent on the duration (length) of treatment than on the dose of the carcinogen. The authors also concluded that cancer incidence is a function of an exponent value of the *length of treatment* (the 3rd power for this particular experiment), rather than of the age of the animals at the start of treatment; that is, cancer incidence appeared to be independent of age. This is because, when in continuous application, the effect of a potent carcinogen has such a high power dependency on treatment length that it is likely to override any age-dependent effect. A better experimental design for revealing possible age differences is therefore to compare animals of different ages receiving equal lengths of treatment. One may conclude from these data that for certain carcinogen/organ combinations, differences in susceptibility with age may not be relevant when the animal is subject to prolonged exposure (compared to its life span).

Overall, the studies which have been described above for skin carcinogenesis give rise to three different conclusions. The results of experiments with DMBA initiation in the skin of adult Swiss mice suggest that later promotion leads to fewer tumors (40–42). In these experiments, a decrease in susceptibility to chemical carcinogens in adult skin was observed in animals that differed in age by only 3 or 4 months. In contrast, studies involving the chronic lifetime application of BaP to animals indicated that tumor incidence was not sensitive to the age of the animals at the start of treatment, but was dependent on its duration (24). Finally, from the skin graft experiments, "old" skin grafts were found to be more susceptible to initiation by DMBA than "mature" grafts (45).

In spite of the similarities (type of carcinogen, animal species, target organ), these three sets of results cannot be compared to one another as they involve two-stage *versus* one-stage carcinogenesis, a different duration of treatment and period of observation, and different animal ages. The most appropriate experimental conditions for discerning the effects of senescence on chemical carcinogenesis are those of the last set of experiments because of the relevant ages of the animals and the brief application of treatment.

2. In Cell Culture

In a study of the effects of donor age on the *in vitro* transformation of bladder epithelium, the epithelial cells from old donors were shown to be more susceptible to the carcinogen (48). In this experiment, explants from young (5–7-month-old) and old (28–30-month-old) C57BL/Icrf-a mice were established. On the second day in culture the cells were treated with DMBA [0.1 μg/ml in 0.05% dimethylsulfoxide (DMSO)] for 24 hours. Controls were treated with DMSO alone. Transformed foci appeared with a higher frequency (28%) in cultures from old mice than in cultures from young mice (0.9%), and they also appeared sooner (40–60 days *versus* 100 days). Also, the cultures from old donors had a low frequency (5%) of spontaneous transformation, whereas the younger cultures had none.

B. Aromatic Amines

Aromatic amines are synthetic compounds widely used in dye and drug manufacturing and as antioxidants (37). Many cause cancer of the liver or urinary tract in male rodents or of the breast in female rodents. Despite very substantial research interest in these important carcinogens, there have been few studies on aromatic amine–induced carcinogenesis during senescence.

In one study, 3,2'-dimethyl-4-aminobiphenyl (DMAB), a prostate carcinogen requiring metabolic activation (49), was used. The role of aging in prostate carcinogenesis is of special interest, as this cancer is found predominantly in the elderly population. In this study, male F344 rats were used and DMAB, in four doses of 150 mg/kg body weight, was given subcutaneously in four consecutive weekly injections starting at the age of 5 weeks or of 65 weeks. All animals were terminated 60 weeks after the beginning of treatment. No differences were observed when prostate carcinoma induction was compared in growing and adult animals. However, the conclusions from this work are limited by both the absence of control animals receiving no carcinogen for either age group and the overall very low tumor yield observed.

C. Nitrosamines Requiring Activation

Nitrosamines are synthetic compounds derived from secondary amines by nitrosation (37, 50). They undergo oxidative metabolism to reactive electrophiles. In rodents, symmetric dialkyl nitrosamines induce tumors in specific organs; for example, in the rat the principal target for diethylnitrosamine is the liver, for dibutylnitrosamine it is the urinary bladder, and for diamylnitrosamine it is the lung. The organotropism of nitrosamines is species specific and also dose dependent.

The age dependence of carcinogen activation in a particular tissue can be expected to have an important effect on the overall cancer incidence. For a meaningful examination of cancer susceptibility in aging tissues, the rate of metabolic activation in that tissue should be determined together with the tumor incidence. In most studies such determinations have not been made, however.

A study that examined the effect of age on tumor induction was carried out with nitrosobis(2-oxopropyl)amine (BOP) (51); (the experiments with nitrosomorpholine in the same study will not be discussed here, as they involved a comparison between growing, young animals). BOP was administered to male F344 rats by gavage in 0.2 ml corn oil twice weekly either for 29 weeks at high dose (348 mg total/animal) or for 35 weeks at low dose (175 mg total/animal). The experiments with BOP compared rats whose treatment started at 8 weeks (growing animals) to rats whose treatment started at 65 weeks (adult animals). The survival of the older animals was slightly better at the higher carcinogen dose, whereas the opposite was observed with the lower dose. The distribution of tumors was completely different between the two groups. Half the older animals developed liver tumors, whereas no tumors were observed in the liver of young rats. However, the young group developed substantially more lung, kidney, urinary bladder, and thyroid carcinomas than the old group.

Diethylnitrosamine (DEN), another metabolically activated carcinogen, was more extensively used. In one study, whose purpose was to determine whether or not tumor incidence and distribution would differ between young and old animals exposed to DEN, female BALB/c mice (2.5, 9.5, and 17 months old) were given DEN orally over a period of 11 weeks (52). Cumulative doses of carcinogen/kg body weight in each age group were recorded and varied from 397 to 309 to 283 mg, from the youngest to the oldest group, respectively. The major finding was that although the same type (forestomach, liver, and lung), size, and incidence of tumors were induced in all age groups, the median time of death after treatment was much shorter in the oldest group, in spite of this group receiving the smallest dose of carcinogen. Age-matched untreated mice died from different causes than the DEN-treated mice. These experiments clearly showed that old animals had a shorter time to tumor induction and shorter interval between DEN treatment and death.

Another investigation involving DEN examined the incidence of liver tumors in male Fischer rats (53). The animals were given 40 ppm DEN in the drinking water, *ad libitum*, for 10 weeks. Rats were 3, 6, 9, or 12 months old at the beginning of treatment and were sacrificed at the end of 10 weeks. Although the total intake of DEN varied between the groups (it was least for the 3-month-old rats and most for the 6-month-old rats), the youngest animals showed the highest tumor incidence with no significant differences between the other groups.

An extensive statistical study (54) on the dose and time relationships of various nitrosamines in Colworth rats included also DEN (which was the only nitrosamine studied regarding the aging aspect). DEN was fed at 16 different doses, given in constant ppm (v/v) in the drinking water *ad libitum*; the doses actually consumed were then recalculated to mg/day per kg *adult* body weight (ABWD) based on the approximation that adult males and females consumed about 41 and 72 ml/day drinking water per kg adult body weight, respectively. Treatment of the rats with DEN started at 3 or 6 or 20 weeks of age and continued for 2 years or at least up to the life span of surviving rats (if less than 2 years from the onset of treatment). Esophageal and liver tumors were observed. The tumor rate, evaluated at autopsy, depended on the dose and duration of treatment (in years or fraction thereof) and was expressed using the equation:

$$\text{Cumulative Incidence} = (\text{Weibull } b \text{ value}) (\text{treatment years})^7$$

The "*b* value" of the Weibull distribution depends on the dose rate. For esophageal tumors the *b* value is approximately proportional to the 3rd power of the dose-rate *d* of DEN (males $21 \cdot d^3$, where *d* is expressed in mg/kg ABWD; females $11 \cdot d^3$). For liver tumors induced by DEN, the *b* value is approximately proportional to the 4th power of the dose-rate + 0.04 in mg/kg ABWD [males $19(d + 0.04)^4$ and females $32(d + 0.04)^4$].

The data indicate that for esophageal tumors there was only a small, if any, difference in the tumor yield between animals in the different age groups. By contrast for liver tumors, the relative incidence of tumors, compared to rats started at the age of 6 weeks, was threefold higher in rats started earlier (at 3 weeks) and twofold lower in rats started later (at 20 weeks) — all determined after a fixed duration of treatment. These results show that the sensitivity of liver to neoplasia is highly dependent on the age of the animals when the nitrosamine treatment was begun during the first few weeks of life. However, beyond this early age susceptibility to tumorigenesis gradually decreases.

D. Direct-Acting Nitrosamines

Many nitroso derivatives of alkylureas, alkylamides, and esters do not require activation. They can cause leukemias, cancers of the gastrointestinal and respiratory tracts, and other tissues. An especially potent carcinogen in this class, *N*-methyl-*N*-nitrosourea (MNU), was at one time used in industrial applications (37). MNU can induce pancreatic tumors in animals 2 to 3 months following a single intraperitoneal dose and does not require activation or promotion (55). As pancreatic cancer is an important age-dependent neoplasia, which occurs in the human population mainly in people over age 40, MNU-induced pancreatic tumors in rodents provide a good model system for studying this aging-related cancer.

In a well-designed investigation comparing the development of MNU-induced pancreatic carcinomas in young, adult, and old animals, male C57BL/6J mice were given one intraperitoneal injection of MNU (12.5 or 37.5 μg/g body weight) at the age of 3, 12, or 24 months (55). The animals, whose normal life expectancy is 29 to 30 months, were sacrificed 5 months after the injection of MNU and autopsied for detailed examination. A variety of tumors were seen in young as well as old animals, although the number was always larger in the very old compared to adult animals. For example, intestinal carcinomas occurred in 13% of young, 14% of adult, and 60% of old animals, bronchiogenic carcinoma occurred in 3% of adult and 20% of old animals. Control mice in each age group received an injection of vehicle without MNU. In the old animals only, intestinal carcinomas, bronchiogenic carcinomas, and lymphosarcomas were seen in the controls. In contrast, pancreatic tumors were found only in the very old treatment group (in 15% of the animals) and none were seen in old controls or in the younger treatment groups ($p \leq 0.01$).

The importance of age in the development of this particular cancer was confirmed in an *in vitro* study of pancreatic cells obtained from young and old C57BL/6J mice treated with MNU (56). Cells were obtained from 8- and 24-month-old animals which had been injected with MNU (37.5 μg/g body weight) 6 weeks prior to sacrifice. Of old mice, 21% produced cell lines that proliferated longer than 30 days in culture. In contrast, young MNU-treated animals did not give rise to viable cell lines unless the potent tumor promoter TPA was added to the cultures. This suggests that MNU was able to initiate both young and old cells, but the young cells were resistant to transformation. With this *in vitro* approach, factors that may play a role in carcinogenesis with respect to aging *in vivo*, such as immunologic competence, were eliminated, pointing to some aging-related changes in the pancreatic cells themselves.

Based on these results, Zimmerman and Carter (33) proposed that pancreatic acinar cells in senescent C57BL/6J mice are effectively in a state of promotion. They suggested that cellular events associated with aging give rise to a growth potential that must be induced in younger cells by treatment with a promoter. Certainly, this particular *in vitro* system appears to be a good model for study of the biochemical events that are directly related to these aging changes.

Another study examined the carcinogenicity of MNU in female rats of different ages at the start of treatment (57). The biological characteristics of this rat strain were not given and its life span appears short (approximately 22 months, based on the survival of control animals in this study). Animals either 3 months or 15 months old were given a single intravenous injection of MNU (0, 10, 20, or 50 mg/kg of body weight). Animals that died before the end of the study were autopsied at that time. The remainder were terminated and autopsied 14 months after administration of the chemical. In both young and adult rats the 10-mg/kg dose did not alter survival characteristics of the rats, but with both the 20- and 50-mg/kg doses there was a reduction in survival. Within this experimental design, in young rats only, the incidence of some tumor types (renal, colon, ovary, and breast adenocarcinomas) was proportional to dose. In the older rats, no correlation was found between tumor incidence and dose. Overall, there was a higher incidence of mammary, intestinal, ovarian, and renal tumors in the young rats, whereas uterus and cervix were the more frequently affected tissues in the older rats.

In a related experiment with the same strain of rats, the animals were injected with MNU (100 mg/kg body weight in two i.v. injections of 50 mg/kg) either at 3 months or 14 months (58). The animals were palpated weekly for mammary tumors and the presence of other tumors was determined in autopsy. When the percentage tumor incidence was plotted against the time from carcinogen application onward, parallel lines were obtained for the growth period (approximately 3 to 15 months) and aging period (approximately 14 to 26 months), with the appearance of tumors in the younger rats being delayed by about 1 month. This dose–response relationship suggested a lack of significant age-related changes in overall cancer rates, although the incidences of tumors in individual organs were very different between the two age groups.

E. Halogenated Hydrocarbons

Halogenated hydrocarbons are often chemically stable compounds which can be found in many industrial and consumer products. Vinyl chloride (VC) or monochloroethylene is an important industrial chemical which is a human as well as a rodent genotoxic carcinogen, with liver being its main target organ (59).

A large study investigated the effects of duration of exposure to VC and the age at start of exposure on the development of tumors in rats, mice, and hamsters (60). The purpose of this work was to investigate the use of shorter and earlier inhalation exposures of animals to carcinogens in bioassays of carcinogenicity. Only female animals were used: Fischer F344 rats, Syrian golden hamsters, hybrid B6C3F1 mice (female C57BL/6N × male C3H/HIN), and CD-1 Swiss mice. The animals were in exposure chambers 6 hours/day, 5 days/week with VC concentrations of 100 ppm for rats, 50 ppm for mice, and 200 ppm for hamsters. The exposure periods were of 6 months duration and covered the life span: from birth to 6 months, from 6 to 12, from 12 to 18, or from 18 to 24 months of age; the 12-month-long exposure periods were applied from 0 to 12 months, from 6 to 18 months, or from 12 to 24 months of age. Animals were allowed to live out their life span and were necropsied when found dead or moribund. Only the data pertaining to adult and old animals will be discussed here.

The use of several animal species in the same study showed not only the different patterns of carcinogenesis, but also the different effects of age in each species. It should be noted that the survival of carcinogen-treated animals compared to controls decreased when exposure started at birth. The results are summarized below for those species that did not manifest extensive VC toxicity.

Rats — The incidence of hemangiosarcomas which resulted from VC exposures during different 6- or 12-month periods is provided in Table 3. It can be seen that for both the 6- and 12-month exposure times, the earliest treated animals had the highest tumor incidence. With 12-month exposures, a decrease in tumor incidence was observed during both the growth and aging periods. On the other hand, with 6-month exposures, only an early growth change was observed, as none of the animals exposed as adults developed tumors. In the mammary gland, adenocarcinomas were less in old *versus* adult exposed rats. No difference in the incidence of hepatocellular carcinoma between adult and old animals was seen.

Syrian golden hamsters — The frequency of hemangiosarcomas and skin carcinomas was again highest in young and growing animals. No tumors were found in either mature adult or old animals. Thus, the age-related decline in frequency occurred during growth and maturation and was not aging-specific. Adult animals did develop mammary gland

TABLE 3. Effect of Age on the Induction of Hemangiosarcomas by
Vinyl Chloride in Female Fischer 344 Rats[a,b]

Length of exposure (months)	Age at start (months)	Tumor Incidence (percent)
No exposure		1.8
6	0	5.3
6	6	3.8
6	12	0.0
6	18	0.0
12	0	21.4
12	6	9.1
12	12	4.0

[a]Animals were exposed to VC concentrations of 100 ppm for 6 hours/day, 5 days/week.

[b]Adapted from R. T. Drew, G. A. Boorman, J. K. Haseman, E. E. McConnell, W. M. Busey, and J. A. Moore, [*Toxicol. Appl. Pharmacol.* **68**, 120 (1983)].

carcinomas and stomach adenomas, while old animals developed significantly fewer of these tumors or none at all (depending on relative exposures).

Swiss mice — For all cancers related to VC exposure (hemangiosarcomas, mammary gland carcinomas, and lung carcinomas), incidence fell sharply between adult and older animals exposed for the same duration. For example, hemangiosarcoma incidence fell from 22.4 percent for the 6–12-month exposure to 9.4% for the 12–18-month exposure, and also fell from 37.0% for the 6–18-month exposure to 6.0% for the 12–24-month exposure.

In conclusion, in all three species, the older animals showed a decreased susceptibility to VC-induced carcinomas. However, that shorter and earlier exposures would suffice for carcinogenicity testing may be only valid for VC. It may not be excluded that other carcinogens may be more effective in older animals and therefore older animals should be included in the bioassay protocol.

Apparently opposite results to those above were obtained in another study which examined the induction of liver angiosarcomas in male and female Sprague–Dawley rats exposed to VC at different ages (61). However, these divergent results could be attributed to differences in experimental conditions. In this experiment, the dose of VC was higher, 948 ppm (*versus* 100 ppm), 7 hr/day, 5 days/week for 25 weeks, and the majority of animals were sacrificed as early as 3, 6, or 9 months after the start of exposure. Animals were 6, 17–18, 32–33, or 51–53 weeks old at the beginning of treatment. The highest incidence of angiosarcomas was observed in the 52-week age group followed by the 32-week group. No angiosarcomas were observed in animals in the younger two age groups. While these results demonstrate an apparent increased sensitivity in older rats, they could also be explained by the late developing nature of angiosarcomas. Because of the planned schedule of sacrifices, younger animals were not maintained long enough for optimal tumor development to be reached.

IV. STUDIES ON CHEMICAL CARCINOGENESIS IN AGING HUMANS

There have been very few studies examining the effect of aging on the susceptibility to chemically induced cancer in humans. This is due to the limited availability of information on carcinogen exposure in humans. However, a few laboratories have attempted to draw conclusions based on data resulting from either smoking or occupational exposure studies.

For lung cancer due to smoking there appears to be a 4th power relationship between the duration of exposure and incidence of the disease (62) or the death rate (24, 63). Although such a strong relationship points to the importance of duration of the exposure, it is difficult to extrapolate from these data whether or not age-specific changes in susceptibility to cancer do occur. To resolve this question, cohorts of individuals that have smoked for the same length of time in early adulthood and in late adulthood would have to be compared, but this is difficult since few people begin smoking late in life. Additional data on lung, as well as breast, cancer occurring after the atomic bombing of Hiroshima and Nagasaki indicate that the risk of these cancers is increased due to radiation (64). While the relative risk of cancer was found to be sharply increased for individuals who were adolescents at the time of irradiation, no differences were observed in individuals who were between 20 and 50 years old at the time of irradiation.

Also relevant to the issue of aging is a study in which the incidence of nasal sinus cancer in men employed in a nickel refinery in South Wales was examined with respect to age at exposure (65). In each of the five age groups examined, from less than 20 to over 35 years of age, a steady increase in susceptibility was observed. After combining the younger groups, there was a 69% increase in susceptibility between men exposed in adulthood (20 to 35 years) and those exposed later in life. Although a very significant increase in susceptibility, this represents less than a doubling in cancer incidence due to aging alone. Thus, it is likely that if exposure continued and the incidence of tumors was increasing as some power of duration (such as 4th), the effect of increased susceptibility due to age would be undetectable due to the effects of prolonged exposure.

Finally, in a case–control study of occupational bladder carcinogenesis (66), a decrease in cancer risk was observed with increasing age at start of employment in the high-risk occupation. Men first employed in a hazardous occupation by the age of 25 years or younger had a risk 2.4 times that of men never employed ($p < 0.02$), whereas no excess risk was observed for those first employed over the age of 25 years. While the authors suggest that this age effect may be due to an increased susceptibility in younger people, they also indicate that differences in the type of job to which younger and older persons were assigned may also be a factor. As this study also demonstrated a latent period of 41 to 50 years between first exposure and cancer diagnosis, it seems likely that individuals who begin employment at older ages will die of other causes before reaching the age at which bladder cancer could be expected. Thus, although a decreased susceptibility with increasing age was suggested, certainly alternative explanations cannot be ruled out.

V. STUDIES ON CHEMICAL CARCINOGENESIS DURING OTHER PHASES OF THE LIFE SPAN

As was the case with the investigation of senescence, there have been few systematic studies of chemical carcinogenesis during periods of the life span other than senescence. While a number of studies have included animals of young ages, the nature of the experimental design often did not allow for changes, which might occur during specific periods of the life span, to be assessed.

One exception to this has been the area of perinatal carcinogenesis. Carcinogenic risk from perinatal exposures to environmental carcinogens is an important public health concern. Over the past 30 years, a number of investigations have systematically examined the carcinogenic process during the pre- and postnatal periods. This research has been the subject of a number of excellent reviews and monographs (4,67–69). Results from these studies provide ample evidence that exposure of pregnant animals to certain, but not all chemical carcinogens results in the occurrence of tumors in their progeny. This increase in tumor incidence may also occur *in more than one subsequent generation of descendents*. The types of tumors observed from prenatal exposure exhibit large quantitative and qualitative differences from those observed from postnatal exposure. For example, transplacental exposure of rats to the direct-acting alkylating agents MNU and *N*-ethyl-*N*-nitrosourea (ENU) results mainly in tumors of the nervous system and kidney, whereas tumors of these tissues are rarely induced after comparable postnatal exposures. On the other hand, hepatocellular and pulmonary tumors, which are the predominant tumors induced by postnatal exposures, are rarely, if ever, observed in animals exposed prenatally (4).

While perinatal animals exhibit unique sensitivity to carcinogenesis, little is known regarding the cancer risk related to perinatal exposures in humans. Investigations in this important field are continuing in four basic areas: biochemical/molecular mechanisms of tumorigenesis in the perinatal period; postnatal influences on prenatally initiated neoplasms; study of specific perinatal human exposure situations with animal models; and the epidemiology of childhood cancers (68).

VI. HOST FACTORS AFFECTING CHEMICAL CARCINOGENESIS IN AGING

The results and concepts discussed in the foregoing parts of this chapter lead to the conclusion that the actually observed effect of aging on carcinogenesis will depend on the particular chemical and animal model used and the specific organ under observation. This is because the overall response of an aging animal to a chemical carcinogen is regulated by a number of factors at the organism, target tissue, and molecular levels. Some of these factors include the overall absorption, metabolism, and distribution of the carcinogen, including its tissue-specific activation and detoxification, susceptibility of the target tissue DNA to chemical damage and its capacity for DNA repair and cell proliferation, and the potential for immunological surveillance. Dissecting these components through appropriate experimental design will help to shed light on the changes in susceptibility of aging tissues to chemical carcinogenesis.

A. Metabolism and Disposition of Carcinogens

The effectiveness of most chemical carcinogens depends on the balance between their pathways of metabolic activation and detoxification. The dominant mechanism for carcinogen activation involves the cytochrome P-450 components of the microsomal mixed-function oxidase system as well as other oxidative enzymes. Detoxification generally involves the reaction of activated metabolites of the carcinogen with water and with a variety of water-soluble, easily excreted compounds, as well as conjugation reactions prior to activation. Aging-specific changes in the activity of components of these enzyme systems could lead to changes in susceptibility to carcinogens.

1. Carcinogen Activation

The majority of chemical carcinogens are metabolically activated by the microsomal mixed-function oxidase system, also known as the Phase I metabolic pathway

(37). The major components of this system are the various cytochrome P-450 isozymes and their associated oxidoreductases. While the majority of mixed-function oxidase activity is localized in the liver, evidence is rapidly increasing on the importance of site-specific activation of carcinogens at the target organs/tissues.

A few studies have examined the effect of aging on cytochrome P-450 levels. While decrease in total P-450 content was observed in certain rodent models (70), no change was observed in other species and tissues (71). Before any conclusion can be drawn, more information is needed on the activity of specific P-450 isozymes directed at particular carcinogens in individual target tissues.

The activation of carcinogens can also be assessed by means of the Ames test following incubation with liver S9 homogenates, rather than measuring the activities of individual enzymes. For example, Baird and Birnbaum (72) measured the production of mutagenic metabolites of BaP and 2-aminofluorene (2-AF) in liver homogenates (S9) from adult (300-day) and old (over 700-day) male CFN rats and C57BL/6J mice. Quantitative estimates of mutagenicity were obtained from the reversion frequency in strains TA98 and TA100 of *Salmonella typhimurium*. For both animal species, mutagenicity was much higher with homogenates from the old animals.

One has to consider, therefore, the implication of possibly increased carcinogen activation in older animals in interpreting the results of such experiments as those of Ebbesen (45–47) or Van Duuren *et al.* (39, 40). The increased skin cancer incidence found by these investigators could possibly be explained by a more rapid metabolism of the chemicals as opposed to higher susceptibility of older skin per se. On the other hand, the above findings could be attributed to the fact that the animals had been pretreated with a polychlorinated biphenyl mixture, a potent inducer of drug-metabolizing enzymes. Without such pretreatment, Robertson and Birnbaum (73) found liver and kidney metabolism of aflatoxin B_1, of 2-AF, and of 2-acetylaminofluorene to be the same in adult and old female Long–Evans rats.

In another type of study, the metabolism of orally administered ^{14}C-benzene in male C57BL/6N mice, 3–4 months old or 18 months old, was investigated (74). By examining the excretion of radioactivity in urine, feces, and exhaled CO_2, they found considerable differences in the disposition of benzene between the two age groups, which was attributed to senescence. However, based on the survival characteristics of this strain of mice, the comparison which was actually made was between young, growing mice and mature, but not yet old mice. Thus, the differences observed could be more accurately ascribed to growth or maturation. With a similar study of benzene metabolism in 24 + months old mice, one might be able to determine whether or not equally large changes occur in aging animals. Even then, direct extrapolation to differences in carcinogenesis might be difficult because local tissue-specific changes in benzene metabolism are probably more relevant to tumorigenesis.

2. Carcinogen Detoxification

The metabolic detoxification of carcinogens by conjugation is an important determinant of carcinogenesis. The enzymes involved, often called the Phase II drug-detoxification pathway, catalyze the conjugation of carcinogens, either before or after activation, with various compounds such as glutathione (GSH), glucuronic acid, or sulfate, rendering them more water soluble and less toxic. While these reactions most often result in detoxification, for a few carcinogens and organs such as the bladder, carcinogenicity may actually be enhanced owing to the greater availability of the water-soluble carcinogen conjugates to the organ.

One of the most important detoxification systems involves the conjugation of xenobiotics with the cysteine-containing tripeptide, GSH, *via* glutathione-*S*-transferases (75). GSH is an endogenous antioxidant found in high concentrations (0.5 – 8.0 m*M*) in nearly all living cells. Studies by Lang and coworkers (76–82) on a variety of aging models indicate that GSH deficiency is a general phenomenon of aging tissues: lower GSH levels were found in a number of experimental aging organisms and tissues. Studies using the drug acetaminophen (APAP) – activated to a reactive electrophile by the mixed-function oxidase system and subsequently detoxified by conjugation with GSH – demonstrated that the detoxification capacity for APAP is reduced in very old compared to the mature adult *Aedes aegypti* mosquitoes and C57BL/6NIA mice (83–85). Furthermore, the observed aging-related loss in detoxification capacity highly correlates with the aging-specific decrease of GSH concentration and could be regained after the tissue GSH levels were replenished by administering GSH-monoethylester (86). Collectively, these results support the hypothesis that a GSH deficiency leading to a loss in detoxification capacity may be an important factor in carcinogenesis induced by those chemicals which are detoxified by GSH.

Little work has been carried out on glutathione-*S*-transferase activity in aging animals. The results vary, ranging from no change (87, 88) to lower specific activities with age (89–92). Two other common detoxification reactions involve conjugation of carcinogens with glucuronic acid or sulfate. These reactions are carried out by the enzymes UDP-glucuronyl transferase and sulfotransferase, respectively. As with GSH, these conjugation reactions increase the water solubility of carcinogens, allowing for ready excretion. Very little is known about the effects of aging on these enzyme systems. Both slight increases and decreases have been observed in UDP-glucuronyl transferase activity in aging F344 rats (90).

B. DNA Susceptibility to Chemical Damage

The interaction between chemical carcinogens and DNA is a complex process which may be altered as aging progresses. Few valid aging studies have addressed this aspect, however. Recent *in vitro* studies have demonstrated that cells from older humans are more susceptible to chromosomal damage by [^{3}H]-thymidine than those from younger subjects (93–95). These results suggest that old cells are more vulnerable to chromosome rearrangement and to the toxic effects of irradiation. Research is needed to determine the relationship of this age-related change to carcinogenesis.

C. DNA Repair

The DNA repair systems that eliminate carcinogen-induced damage in DNA structure are thought to play a critical role in maintaining gene integrity. An impairment in DNA repair may therefore contribute both to the mechanisms of aging and of carcinogenesis. Since the original studies of Hart and Setlow (96) describing a correlation between DNA excision repair capacity and aging, there have been a number of studies on the relationship between aging and DNA repair. These studies have been reviewed (1, 97). While both increases and decreases in DNA repair during aging have been reported, in the majority of studies no changes were found. This disparity is likely due to variation in methodological approaches in measuring DNA repair, as well as to differences in the animal models used (1).

The results of two studies involving a differentiated epithelial cell type, representative of an *in vivo* population, suggest that a decline in DNA repair activity is an important factor in the aging process. In hepatocytes isolated from 6- to 32-month-old F344 rats, Plesko and Richardson (98) observed that repair of UV-induced DNA damage was significantly impaired in cells from animals of more than 14 months of age. In a related study, UV-induced DNA repair synthesis in hepatocytes from five different mammalian species was found to positively correlate with life span potential (99). These investigations should be extended to other types of DNA damage.

D. Cell Proliferation

The level of proliferative activity of tissues is an important factor that determines susceptibility to chemical carcinogenesis. Enhancement of proliferation in tissues in which DNA damage has occurred will reduce the effectiveness of the DNA repair mechanisms. There are a number of processes that can repair damaged DNA, but if the cell divides before repair can take place, the damage is translated into a permanent change in the base sequence and mutation results. Thus, the actual success of DNA repair is an inverse function of the level of proliferative activity of the damaged tissue. While the data available indicate that the proliferative activity of the majority of growing and renewing tissues is decreased in senescence (100), more research is needed to determine the actual significance of this loss of proliferative capacity in tumor progression.

E. Immune Competence

Immunological function is an important factor involved in tumor promotion; thus, a decline in the effectiveness of the immune system may affect the incidence of cancer in older age groups. This notion is based on the immunological surveillance hypothesis of Burnet (101), which assumes that cancer cells carry surface antigens that differ from those of the host, and, thus, immunological defense mechanisms can be mobilized against the tumor cells. Indeed, a number of dramatic changes in immune structure and function have been described in aging organisms (102, 103). Central to these changes is the involution of the thymus, resulting in a loss of 90% of its cellular mass by the age of 50 years (104). As a result of this loss, a dramatic depletion of thymic hormone is observed between 30 and 60 years (105), as well as a redistribution of T-lymphocyte subpopulations in which the percentage of immature T cells in the blood greatly increases (106). Although the hypothesis of immunological surveillance was widely accepted at first, it has since been challenged (107–109). A particular point of importance is that nude mice, which have virtually no T-lymphocytes, have a very low incidence of cryptogenic tumors and do not exhibit increased sensitivity to chemical carcinogens (110).

VII. CLOSING NOTE

Animal age is an important factor in the process of carcinogenesis, particularly the period of senescence when the incidence of specific types of cancer increases exponentially. However, to date, little information is available regarding the influence of host age on chemical carcinogenesis. While a number of studies have attempted to provide data on this relationship, many of them are flawed by the use of improper experimental designs and the injudicious use of animal models and age groups.

There is a clear need for systematic investigations on chemical carcinogenesis during aging, as well as during other periods of the life span. These studies should include well-characterized aging models, sampled throughout their life span, to clearly delineate any aging-specific changes which might occur. In addition, standardized carcinogen bioassays which are suitable for studies on aging animals should be used. With the information gained from such studies, public health strategies for cancer prevention in the elderly can be developed. Further, this information could provide a better understanding of carcinogen bioassays as they relate to human cancer risk.

REFERENCES

1. Anisimov, V. N.: "Carcinogenesis and Aging". CRC Press, Boca Raton, Florida, 1987.
2. Newell, G. R.: Epidemiology of Cancer. *In* "Principles and Practice of Oncology" (T. DeVita, Jr., S. Hellman, and S. A. Rosenberg, eds.). Lippincott, Philadelphia, 1985, p. 169.
3. Yancic, R.: Frames of Reference: Old Age as the Context for Prevention and Treatment of Cancer. *In* "Perspectives on Prevention and Treatment of Cancer in the Elderly" (R. Yancic, ed.). Raven Press, New York, 1983, p.5.
4. Napalkov, N. P., Rice, J. M., Tomatis, L., and Yamasaki, H. (eds.): "Perinatal and Multigeneration Carcinogenesis", IARC Sci. Publ. 96. IARC, Lyon, France, 1989.
5. Likhachev, A., Anisimov, V., and Montesano, R. (eds.): "Age-Related Factors in Carcinogenesis", IARC Sci. Publ. 58. IARC, Lyon, France, 1985.
6. Kirkwood, T. B. C.: Comparative and Evolutionary Aspects of Longevity. *In* "Handbook of the Biology of Aging" (C. E. Finch and E. L. Schneider, eds.). Van Nostrand-Reinhold, New York, 1985, p. 27.
7. Brody, J. A., and Brock, D. B.: Epidemiologic and Statistical Characteristics of the United States Elderly Population. *In* "Handbook of the Biology of Aging" (C. E. Finch and E. L. Schneider, eds.). Van Nostrand-Reinhold, New York, 1985, p. 3.
8. Comfort, A.: "The Biology of Senescence", 3rd ed. Elsevier, New York, 1979.
9. Rowe, J. W., Andres, R., Tobin, J. D., Noris, A. H., and Shock, N. W.: *J. Gerontol.* **31**, 155 (1976).
10. Shock, N. W., Grevlich, R. C., Costa, P. T., Jr., Andres, R., Lakatta, E. G., Arenberg, P., and Tobin, J. D.: "Normal Human Aging: The Baltimore Longitudinal Study of Aging", NIH Publ. No. 84–2450. Washington, D. C., 1984.
11. Lang, C. A., and Richie, J. P., Jr.: *Exp. Gerontol.* **21**, 235 (1986).
12. Finch, C. E., and Schneider, E. L., (eds.): "Handbook of the Biology of Aging". Van Nostrand-Reinhold, New York, 1985.
13. Shock, N. W.: Longitudinal Studies of Aging in Humans. *In* "Handbook of the Biology of Aging" (C. E. Finch and E. L. Schneider, eds.). Van Nostrand-Reinhold, New York, 1985, p. 721.
14. Masoro, E. J. (ed.): "CRC Handbook on the Physiology of Aging". CRC Press, Boca Raton, Florida, 1981.
15. Warner, H. R., Butler, R. N., Sprott, R. L., and Schneider, E. L. (eds.): "Modern Biological Theories of Aging". Raven Press, New York, 1987.
16. Lang, C. A.: Research Strategies for the Study of Nutrition and Aging. *In* "Nutritional Aspects of Aging" (L. H. Chen, ed.), Vol. 1. CRC Press, Boca Raton, Florida, 1986, p. 3.
17. Tannenbaum, A.: *Cancer Res.* **2**, 460 (1942).
18. Sass, B., Rabstein, L. S., Madison, R., Nims, R. M., Peters, R. L., and Kelloff, G. J.: *J. Natl. Cancer Inst.* **54**, 1449 (1975).
19. Richie, J. P., Jr., and Williams, G. M.: Aging and Cancer. *In* "The Potential for Nutritional Modulation of Aging Processes" (D. K. Ingram, G. T. Baker III, and N. W. Shock, eds.). Food & Nutrition Press, Trumbull, Connecticut, 1991, p. 51.
20. Harman, D.: *Proc. Natl. Acad. Sci. U.S.A.* **78**, 7124 (1981).
21. Harman, D.: *Radiat. Res.* **16**, 753 (1962).
22. Anisimov, V. N.: *Adv. Cancer Res.* **40**, 265, (1983).
23. Doll, R.: Age. *In* "Host Environment Interactions in the Etiology of Cancer in Man", IARC Sci. Publ. No. 7 (R. Doll and I. Vodopija, eds.). IARC, Lyon, France, 1973.
24. Peto, R., Roe, F. J. C., Lee, P. N., Levy, L., and Clack, J.: *Br. J. Cancer* **32**, 411 (1975).
25. Peto, R., Parish, S. E., and Gray, R. G.: There Is No Such Thing as Aging, and Cancer Is Not Related to It. *In* "Age-Related Factors in Carcinogenesis", IARC Sci. Publ. 58 (A. Likhachev, V. Anisimov, and R. Montesano, eds.). IARC, Lyon, France, 1985, p. 43.
26. Anisimov, V. N.: *Vopr. Onkol.* **22**, 98 (1976).
27. Stukonis, M. K.: Cancer Cumulative Risk, IARC Int Tech. Rept. No. 79/004. IARC, Lyon, France, 1979.
28. Dix, D., Cohen, P., and Flannery, J.: *J. Theor. Biol.* **83**, 163 (1980).

29. Staats, J.: *Cancer Res.* **40**, 2083 (1980).
30. Gibson, D. C., Adelman, R. C., and Finch, C.: "Development of the Rodent as a Model System of Aging, Book II", NIH Publ. No. 79-161. 1982.
31. Zurcher, C., van Zwieten, M. J., Solleveld, H. A., and Hollander, C. F.: Aging Research. *In* "The Mouse in Biomedical Research, Vol. IV: Experimental Biology and Oncology" (H. L. Foster, J. D. Small, and J. G. Fox, eds.). Academic Press, New York, 1982, p. 11.
32. Russell, E. S.: Lifespan and Aging Patterns. *In* "Biology of the Laboratory Mouse" (E. L. Green, ed.). Dover, New York, 1968, p. 511.
33. Zimmerman, J. A., and Carter, T. H.: *J. Gerontol. Biol. Sci.* **44**, 19 (1989).
34. Peto, R., Pike, M. C., Day, N. E., Gray, R. S., Lee, P. N., Parish, S., Peto, J., Richards, S., and Wahrendorf, J.: "Guidelines for Simple Sensitive Significance Tests for Carcinogenic Effects in Long-Term Animal Experiments", Annex *in* Suppl. No.2, IARC Monographs. IARC, Lyon, France, 1980, p. 311.
35. Solleveld, H. A., and McConnell, E. E.: *Toxicol. Pathol.* **13**, 128 (1985).
36. Arcos, J. C., and Argus, M. F.: "Chemical Induction of Cancer", Vol. IIA. Academic Press, New York, 1974, p. 86.
37. Williams, G. M., and Weisburger, J. H.: Chemical Carcinogenesis. *In* "Toxicology, the Basic Science of Poisons" (M. O. Amdur, J. Doull, and C. D. Klaassen, eds.), 4th ed. Pergamon, New York, 1991, p. 127.
38. Van Duuren, B. L., Sivak, A., Segal, A., Seidman, I., and Katz, C.: *Cancer Res.* **33**, 2166 (1973).
39. Van Duuren, B. L., Sivak, A., Katz, C., Seidman, I., and Melchionne, S. M.: *Cancer Res.* **35**, 502 (1975).
40. Van Duuren, B. L., Smith, A. C., and Melchionne, S. M.: *Cancer Res.* **38**, 865 (1978).
41. Stenback, F., Peto, R., and Shubik, P.: *Br. J. Cancer* **44**, 1 (1981).
42. Stenback, F., Peto, R., and Shubik, P.: *Br. J. Cancer* **44**, 15 (1981).
43. Loehrke, H., Schweizer, J., Dederer, E., Hesse, B., Rosenkranz, G., and Goertler, K.: *Carcinogenesis* **4**, 771 (1983).
44. Franks, L. M. and Carbonell, A. W.: *J. Natl. Cancer Inst.* **52**, 565 (1974).
45. Ebbesen, P.: *Nature* **241**, 280 (1973).
46. Ebbesen, P.: *Science* **183**, 217 (1974).
47. Ebbesen, P.: *J. Natl. Cancer Inst.* **58**, 1057 (1977).
48. Summerhayes, I. C., and Franks L. M.: *J. Natl. Cancer Inst.* **62**, 1017 (1979).
49. Shirai, T., Nakamura, A., Fukushima, S., Takahashi, S., Ogawa, K., and Ito, N.: *Jpn. J. Cancer Res.* **80**, 312 (1989).
50. Arcos, J. C., Woo, Y. T., and Argus, M. F.: "Chemical Induction of Cancer", Vol. IIIA. Academic Press, New York, 1982, p. 148.
51. Lijinski, W., and Kovatch, R. M.: *Jpn. J. Cancer Res.* **77**, 1222 (1986).
52. Clapp, N. K., Perkins, E. H., Klima, W. C., and Cacheiro, L. H.: *J. Gerontol.* **36**, 158 (1981).
53. Mochizuki, Y., and Furukawa, K.: *Tumor Res.* **16**, 19 (1981).
54. Peto, R., Gray, R., Brantom, P., and Grasso, P.: *IARC Sci. Publ.* **57**, 627 (1984).
55. Zimmerman, J. A., Trombetta, L. D., Carter, T. H., and Wetsbroth, S. H.: *Gerontology* **28**, 114 (1982).
56. Zelinsky-Papez, K., Carter, T. H., and Zimmerman, J. A.: *In Vitro Cell. Develop. Biol.* **23**, 118 (1987).
57. Anisimov, V. N.: *Vopr. Onkol.* **33**, 65 (1987).
58. Anisimov, V. N.: *Exp. Pathol.* **19**, 81 (1981).
59. Woo, Y. T., Lai, D. Y., Arcos, J. C., and Argus, M. F.: "Chemical Induction of Cancer", Vol. IIIB. Academic Press, New York, 1985, p. 53.
60. Drew, R. T., Boorman, G. A., Haseman, J. K., McConnell, E. E., Busey, W. M., and Moore, J. A.: *Toxicol. Appl. Pharmacol.* **68**, 120 (1983).
61. Groth, D. H., Coate, W. B., Ulland, B. M., and Hornung, R. W.: *Env. Health Perspect.* **41**, 53 (1981).
62. Doll, R.: *Cancer Res.* **38**, 3573 (1978).
63. Kahn, H. A.: *NCI Monogr.* **19**, 1 (1966).
64. Shimizu, Y., Schull, W. J., and Kato, H.: *JAMA* **264**, 601 (1990).
65. Doll, R., Morgan, L. G., and Speizer, F. E.: *Br. J. Cancer* **24**, 624 (1970).
66. Hoover, R., and Cole, P.: *N. Engl. J. Med.* **288**, 1040 (1973).
67. National Cancer Institute: "Perinatal Carcinogenesis", NCI Monograph No. 51, NIH Publ. No. 79-1633, Bethesda, Maryland, 1979.
68. Vesselinovitch, S. D.: *Prog. Clin. Biol. Res.* **331**, 53 (1990).
69. Anderson, L. M., Jones, A. B., and Rice, J. M.: *Br. J. Cancer* **64**, 1025 (1991).
70. Schmucker, D. L., and Wang, R. K.: *Mech. Aging Dev.* **15**, 189 (1981).
71. Sun, J. Q., and Strobel, H. W.: *Exp. Gerontol.* **21**, 523 (1986).
72. Baird, M. B., and Birnbaum, L. S.: *Cancer Res.* **39**, 4752 (1979).
73. Robertson, G. C., and Birnbaum, L. S.: *Chem. Biol. Interact.* **38**, 243 (1982).
74. McMahon, T. F., and Birnbaum, L. S.: *Drug Metab. Dispos.* **19**, 1052 (1991).

75. Coles, B., and Ketterer, B.: *Critical Rev. Biochem. Mol. Biol.* **25,** 47 (1990).
76. Abraham, E. C., Taylor, J. F., and Lang, C. A.: *Biochem. J.* **174,** 819 (1978).
77. Hazelton, G. A., and Lang, C. A.: *Biochem. J.* **188,** 25 (1980).
78. Hazelton, G. A., and Lang, C. A.: *Biochem. J.* **210,** 289 (1983).
79. Hazelton, G. A., and Lang, C. A.: *Proc. Soc. Exp. Biol. Med.* **176,** 249 (1984).
80. Nanyshkin, S., Miller, L., Lindeman, R., and Lang, C. A.: *Federation Proc.* **40,** 3179 (1981).
81. Schneider, D., Naryshkin, S., and Lang, C. A.: *Federation Proc.* **41,** 7671 (1982).
82. Chen, T. S., Richie, J. P., Jr., and Lang, C. A.: *Proc. Soc. Exp. Biol. Med.* **190,** 399 (1989).
83. Richie, J. P., Jr., and Lang, C. A.: *Drug Metab. Dispos.* **13,** 14 (1985).
84. Chen, T. S., Richie, J. P., Jr., and Lang, C. A.: *Drug Metab. Dispos.* **18,** 882 (1990).
85. Richie, J. P., Jr., Lang, C. A., and Chen, T. S.: *Biochem. Pharmacol.* **44,** 129 (1992).
86. Chen, T. S., Richie, J. P., Jr., and Lang, C. A.: *Pharmacologist* **30,** A78 (1988).
87. Jenkinson, S. G., Duncan, C. A., Bryan, C. L., and Lawrence, R.A.: *Am. J. Med. Sci.* **302,** 347 (1991).
88. Birnbaum, L. S., and Baird, M. B.: *Chem. Biol. Interact.* **26,** 245 (1979).
89. Spearman, M. E., and Leibman, K. C.: *Biochem. Pharmacol.* **33,** 1309 (1984).
90. Kitahara, A., Ebina, T., Ishikawa, T., Soma, Y., Sato, K., and Kanai, S.: Changes in Activities and Molecular Forms of Rat Hepatic Drug Metabolizing Enzymes During Aging. *In* "Liver and Drugs" (K. Kitani, ed.). Elsevier, Amsterdam, 1982, p. 135.
91. Stohs, S. J., Al-Turk, W. A., Angle, L. R., and Heinicke, R.J.: *Gen. Pharmacol.* **13,** 519 (1982).
92. Fujita, S., Kitagawa, H., Ishizawa, H., Suzuki, T., and Kitani, K.: *Biochem. Pharmacol.* **34,** 3891 (1985).
93. Staiano-Coico, L., Darzynkiewicz, Z., Hefton, J. M., Dutkowski, R., Darlington, G. J., and Weksler, M. E.: *Science* **219,** 1335 (1983).
94. Staiano-Coico, L., Darzynkiewicz, Z., Melamed, M. R., and Weksler, M. E.: *Cytometry* **3,** 79 (1982).
95. Dutkowski, R. T., Lesh, R., Staiano-Coico, L., Thaler, H., Darlington, G. J., and Weksler, M. E.: *Mutat. Res.* **149,** 505 (1983).
96. Hart, R. W., and Setlow, R. D.: *Proc. Natl. Acad. Sci. U.S.A.* **71,** 2169 (1974).
97. Warner, H. R., and Price, A. R.: *J. Gerontol.* **44,** 45 (1989).
98. Plesko, M. M., and Richardson, A.: *Biochem. Biophys. Res. Commun.* **118,** 730 (1984).
99. Maslansky, C. J., and Williams, G. M.: *Mech. Aging Dev.* **29,** 191 (1985).
100. Cameron, I., and Thrasher, J. D.: *Interdiscip. Top. Gerontol.* **10,** 108 (1976).
101. Burnet, F. M.: *Transplant Rev.* **7,** 3 (1971).
102. Makinodan, T., and Hirayama, R.: *IARC Sci. Publ.* **58,** 55 (1985).
103. Kaesberg, P. R., and Ershler, N. B.: *J. Gerontol.* **44,** 63 (1989).
104. Boyd, E.: *Am. J. Dis. Child.* **43,** 1162 (1932).
105. Lewis, V. M., Twomey, J. J., Bealmear, P., Goldstein, G., and Good, R. A.: *J. Clin. Endocrinol. Metab.* **48,** 145 (1978).
106. Schwab, R., Staiano-Coico, L., and Weksler, M. E.: *Diagn. Immunol.* **1,** 195 (1983).
107. Baldwin, R. W.: *Adv. Cancer Res.* **18,** 1 (1973).
108. Kripke, M. C., and Borsos, T.: *J. Natl. Cancer Inst.* **52,** 1393 (1974).
109. Currie, G.: *Biochim. Biophys. Acta* **458,** 135 (1976).
110. Rygaard, J., and Poulsen, C. O.: *Transplant Rev.* **28,** 43 (1976).

CHAPTER 11

The Effect of Hormones on Tumor Induction

Jonathan J. Li and Sara A. Li

Contents: Introduction. **Section I:** Brief Overview of the Endocrine System. **Section II:** Hormonal Carcinogenesis. **Section III:** Effects of Hormones on Carcinogenesis by Nonhormone Chemical Agents.

Introduction

It has long been known that the endocrine status of the host has a critical influence on the induction of cancer by nonhormone chemical compounds and on the emergence of "spontaneous" tumors in a variety of mammalian species including the human. In the absence of the specific hormone the target gland atrophies, whereas if hormone is in excess the target tissue hypertrophies. The growth-promoting, anabolic properties of sex hormones toward their target tissues has been recognized as early as 1849 when Berthold (1) reported the regression of the comb of roosters following castration and restoration of the comb by testicular implants; since then the growth-promoting properties of sex hormones toward their different target organs has been confirmed in many species. The growth-promoting properties, their ability to elicit cell proliferation, largely but not solely underlie the fact that both pituitary and gonadal hormones are capable of enhancing tumor induction in various species. Conversely, some hormones, under different experimental conditions, were found to inhibit tumor induction by chemical agents. Administered alone—without the concurrent effect of a nonhormone chemical carcinogen—certain hormones by themselves can be tumorigenic through the creation of an excess hormonal stimulus; thereby the endocrine balance *appropriate for that organism* is shifted away from the "normal" steady-state. The concept of endocrine imbalance is indeed highly relevant to the etiology of endocrine-associated human malignancies emerging, in most instances, in the absence of any identifiable chemical or physical agent responsible; this is particularly true for such prevalent cancers as those of the breast, ovary, endometrium, cervix/vagina, prostate, the less common estrogen/androgen–associated liver neoplasms, and perhaps even for colon cancer.

The "normal" endocrine balance depends on the relative rates of production of hormones interacting in a complex feedback regulatory network: for example, the secretion of steroid hormones by both the adrenals and the gonads is stimulated by the levels of specific peptide hormones secreted by the hypophysis, and secretion of the hypophyseal hormones is, in turn, regulated by both the levels of adrenal and gonadal steroid hormones acting back upon the hypophysis and by hormone-releasing and release-inhibiting factors secreted by the hypothalamus; thus, hormones represent a major group of humoral signals of intercellular communication. Moreover, the secretion of hypothalamic hormones is modulated by neurological signals from the nervous system. Finally, the steady-state rates of production of individual hormones are set/modulated by genetic determinants and by a host of dietary, lifestyle, stress, and environmental factors and influences. Hence, the problem of hormonal carcinogenesis and of the modulation of nonhormone chemical carcinogenesis by hormones should be viewed as a piece of the complex mosaic of interactive influences which often determine the actual outcome of the tumorigenic process.

Because of the negative feedback relationships between the hypophysis and the target tissues of the trophic hormones, stoppage of secretion by a target gland leads to persistent overproduction of the respective pituitary trophic hormone. If this is maintained for a large part of the animal's life span, tumor will develop in either the overactive hypophysis or the overstimulated target gland. The place of tumor occurrence (whether the hypophysis or a particular hormone target gland) will depend on the target gland involved by the endocrine manipulation and on the species and strain used. Stoppage of secretion of a target gland may be brought about experimentally by gland ablation or irradiation or chemical blockage or by transplantation of glandular tissue into a site where its secreted hormone product is catabolized before it can reach the general circulation, precluding signaling back to the pituitary and the hypothalamus. Considerable experimental efforts during the years explored the tumorigenic and carcinogenesis-modifying effects of different types of artificially induced endocrine imbalances; these studies represent a quasi-dissection of the regulatory modalities existing in the endocrine system.

Consistent with the above is the general consensus that hormones—either amine, peptide, protein, or steroid—are capable of enhancing neoplastic processes in various animal systems. While hormones may have profound effects in altering the metabolism of nonhormonal chemical carcinogens, possibly the most relevant feature of hormones for enhancing tumorigenesis is their characteristic property to elicit and stimulate cell proliferation at any phase of the multistage process leading to neoplasia. This latter characteristic of hormones has received increasing attention in relation to the unknown etiology of prevalent endocrine-associated human cancers mentioned earlier in this Introduction. A primary role for hormone-driven cell proliferation for some of these endocrine-associated human neoplasms has been suggested (2, 3).

This chapter consists of three sections: Section I provides a brief refresher overview of the endocrine system; Section II reviews carcinogenesis by hormone administration and by artificially induced endocrine imbalance (both in the absence of any nonhormone chemical carcinogen); and Section III reviews the modifying effects of hormones and of induced endocrine imbalance upon carcinogenesis by nonhormone chemical agents, as well as of some known molecular mechanistic aspects of such effects.

REFERENCES

1. Berthold, A. A.: *Arch. Anat. Physiol. wiss. Med* **2**, 42 (1849).
2. Henderson, B. E., Ross, R. K., Pike, M. C., and Casagrande, J. T.: *Cancer Res.* **42**, 3232 (1982).
3. Henderson, B. E., Ross, R., and Bernstein, L.: *Cancer Res.* **48**, 246 (1988).

Brief Overview of the Endocrine System[1]

The endocrine system is involved in virtually all aspects of the mammalian organism, its biochemical, physiological, locomotor, reproductive, and psychologic functions. At the cellular level, hormones participate in gametogenesis, fertilization, implantation, organogenesis, and differentiation. In the total organism hormones mediate, for example, muscular activity, respiration, digestion, hematopoiesis, thought, mood, and behavior. There are few, if any, organs or tissues in mammalian systems that are not affected either directly or indirectly by the endocrine system. Therefore, the concept of specific target organs or tissues for hormones is probably only valid insofar as the degree of sensitivity and the extent at which organs or tissues are affected by a given hormone. The involvement and complexity of the endocrine system in mammalian organisms are astonishing, pervasive, and downright awesome.

The principal emphasis in this section is on the most centralized part of the endocrine system, the hypothalamic–pituitary axis, which controls through its output of trophic hormones the adrenal glands, the thyroid, and the gonads (and mammary glands), as well as through its growth hormone output many general aspects of overall systemic metabolism (the latter function not being distinctly linked to any particular target tissue). This emphasis is because the hypothalamic–pituitary axis and its peripheral target glands were the principal focus of research on hormonal carcinogenesis and on the modifying effect of hormones on tumor induction by nonhormone chemical carcinogens. To provide a more balanced perspective of the endocrine system, however, this section also summarizes the hormonal control of calcium homeostasis—proceeding through the interaction of parathormone (PTH), calcitonin (CT), and activated vitamin D with bone, the kidneys, and the intestinal tract—as well as the hormonal control of energy utilization and storage through the opposing effects of insulin (anabolic) and glucagon (catabolic). Finally, because the most useful classification of hormones as well as the basic understanding of hormone action along the principal dividing line between the two major categories (lipophilic and hydrophilic hormones) depends on the nature and localization of and interaction with hormone receptors, the section begins—in a seemingly unusual order—with a discussion of the mechanisms of action.

I. MECHANISMS OF HORMONE ACTION: INTERACTION WITH RECEPTORS

The chemical signaling function of hormones is expressed through interaction with cellular receptors. Thus, the ability of a cell to respond to a particular hormone depends upon the presence of cellular receptors specific for that hormone.

---

[1]Abbreviations used in this section are given on p. 427.

The receptors are proteins which may contain several structural domains. The particular amino acid sequences in the receptors provide for a very high degree of binding specificity; mutation in the amino acid sequence can lead to total loss of hormone binding. Binding brings about an allosteric change in the conformation of the receptor. This conformational change triggers a series of molecular events: interaction of the hormone–receptor complex with the genetic material *or* a cascade of enzymatic reactions, depending on whether the hormone is a hydrophobic molecule, such as a steroid hormone or thyroxine, or a hydrophilic amine/peptide/protein hormone, such as gonadotropin or insulin. This is because the steroid and thyroid hormones (themselves lipophilic) diffuse freely through the plasma membrane of the cell and thereby can interact with specific receptors that are primarily within the nucleus. Amine/peptide/protein hormones, that are water soluble, cannot enter the cell, but interact with specific receptors present *in the cell membrane*.

Whereas a nuclear receptor–hormone complex interacts directly with DNA, a membrane receptor–hormone complex triggers the synthesis/transport of a soluble intracellular "second messenger" which then transmits the information to the cell machinery ("signal transduction"), resulting in a biological response. The second messenger concept arose from the observation of Sutherland that epinephrine binds to the plasma membrane of pigeon erythrocytes (activating adenyl cyclase) and increases intracellular cAMP. Investigations that followed up this initial observation brought the realization that cAMP mediates many cellular effects of hormones (see, *e.g.*, Table 1).

A. Steroid Receptors: Structure and Function

Steroid hormones exert a long-term effect on their target cells; they stimulate cell growth and differentiation, and regulate the synthesis of specific proteins. The steroid receptor complex regulates the synthesis of specific proteins, primarily by altering the rate of transcription of specific genes. Using monoclonal antibodies specific for a number of receptors, and immunocytochemistry, it is now established that—contrary to earlier investigations—the steroid receptors, both free and occupied, as well as the receptors for triiodothyronine, T_3 (the metabolically activated form of thyroxine, T_4), for 1,25-dihydroxycholecalciferol (1,25-DHCC) (*see* Section III, B below), and for retinoic acid are located in the nucleus.

All steroid receptors have the same general structure as well as a high degree of homology in their hormone binding and DNA-binding domains (HBD, DBD). Steroid receptors have three regions that are highly conserved: a hydrophobic carboxy-terminal steroid-binding domain; an amino-terminal domain of unknown function; and a central DNA-binding domain which is of greatest homology. Mutations in the carboxy-terminus domain result in loss of steroid binding, and mutations in the central domain impair the ability of the receptor to bind to DNA. In the carboxy-terminus domain two conserved regions (near the carboxy end) constitute the HBD proper: HBD_1 and HBD_2 of 42 and 22 hydrophobic amino acids, respectively. The free, unbound carboxy-terminus inhibits binding of the central domain to DNA and it is this inhibition which is lifted by binding of the steroid. Thus, *if isolated*, the central polypeptide domain is independently capable of interacting with DNA without the mediation of a steroid; however, specifically in the progesterone receptor, the presence of the amino-terminal domain is required for interaction with DNA. It is believed that the general role of the amino-terminal domain is to enhance the specificity of binding to particular regions of DNA. The DBD, composed of 66 to 68 amino acids, contains 9 highly conserved cysteine residues. This domain contains two repeated units rich in the basic amino acids Lys and Arg. These repeated

TABLE 1. Some Known Effects of Cyclic AMP[a]

Enzyme or process affected	Tissues/cells/organisms	Change in activity or rate
Protein kinase[b]	Several	Increased
Phosphorylase	Several	Increased
Glycogen synthetase	Several	Decreased
Phosphofructokinase	Liver fluke	Increased
Lipolysis	Adipose	Increased
Clearing factor lipase	Adipose	Decreased
Amino acid uptake	Adipose	Decreased
Amino acid uptake	Liver and uterus	Increased
Synthesis of several enzymes	Liver	Increased
Net protein synthesis	Liver	Decreased
Gluconeogenesis	Liver	Increased
Ketogenesis	Liver	Increased
Steroidogenesis	Several	Increased
Water permeability	Epithelial	Increased
Ion permeability	Epithelial	Increased
Calcium resorption	Bone	Increased
Renin production	kidney	Increased
Discharge frequency	Cerebellar Purkinje	Decreased
Membrane potential	Smooth muscle	Increased
Tension	Smooth muscle	Decreased
Contractility	Cardiac muscle	Increased
HCl secretion	Gastric mucosa	Increased
Fluid secretion	Insect salivary glands	Increased
Amylase release	Parotid gland	Increased
Insulin release	Pancreas	Increased
Thyroid hormone release	Thyroid	Increased
Calcitonin release	Thyroid	Increased
Histamine release	Mast cells	Decreased
Melanin granule dispersion	Melanocytes	Increased
Aggregation	Platelets	Decreased
Aggregation	Slime mold	Increased
Messenger RNA synthesis	Bacteria	Increased
Synthesis of several enzymes	Bacteria	Increased
Proliferation	Thymocytes	Increased
Cell growth	Tumor cells	Decreased

[a]Adapted from Sutherland, E. W., *Science*, 177, 401 (1972).
[b]Stimulation of protein kinase mediates the effects of cyclic AMP on most systems.

units are folded into a finger structure containing four Cys groups that coordinate one zinc ion. The loop of the so-called "zinc finger" is made up of 12 to 13 amino acids. These DNA-binding fingers could have the capacity to insert into the grooves of DNA.

A free receptor is rather loosely associated with nuclear components and can be released to the soluble fraction (cytosol) upon homogenization of the tissue in low-salt buffers. The occupied receptor, on the other hand, is bound within the nucleus with high affinity and cannot be readily released to the cytosol upon tissue homogenization. In contrast to other types of steroid receptors, free glucocorticoid receptors appear to be present both in the cytoplasm and the nucleus.

A typical target cell can contain a minimum of 10,000 steroid receptor molecules, each of which can reversibly bind to one molecule of a steroid hormone. The pools of unoccupied steroid receptors exist as aggregates which dissociate upon steroid binding; the carboxy-terminus plays a role in receptor aggregation. Depending on the particular steroid receptor, phosphorylation appears to have different roles in the activation. For example, the progesterone receptor in the phosphorylated state does not bind to chromatin, only the dephosphorylated form does. On the other hand, there is no change in the total phosphorylation in glucocorticoid binding to its receptor. Steroid binding is reversible. If the hormone concentration falls, the receptors increasingly revert to the aggregated form.

Steroid hormones regulate different genes in different target cells. In different target cells the receptors are identical for a given steroid; however, different genes are regulated. The activated receptor–hormone complexes, through interaction with specific sequences in DNA, stimulate gene expression: the transcription of specific mRNAs. The specific DNA sequences to which the activated receptor–hormone complexes become bound are believed to be adjacent to the genes that are actually regulated by the hormone. The binding of the steroid receptor–hormone complex to these sites increases the rate of transcription of specific genes, resulting in the accumulation of mature mRNAs. The mRNAs enter the cytoplasm, bind to ribosomes, and are translated into specific proteins, thus modifying the metabolic functions of the cell.

Several mechanisms at the DNA level may account for the transcription-triggering effect of activated ligand–receptor complexes: (a) the establishment of a looped domain in which the receptor complex clamps two regions of DNA together by recognizing and binding to specific sequences at the base of each loop; (b) the binding sequence is a hormonally regulated "enhancer" (a short DNA sequence that can enhance transcription by driving the promoter sequence); (c) binding to a suppressor gene which is a negative regulatory element keeping a usually active gene unexpressed in the presence of a tissue-specific factor; (d) the receptor complex directly interacts with and increases the effectiveness of factor(s) required for transcription. *Alternately*, a steroid may trigger gene expression that represents negative control (*i.e.*, inhibition of transcription); this may result from binding to a "silencer" DNA sequence. An example for this is the inhibition of casein gene expression in the rat mammary gland by progesterone.

B. Amine and Peptide Hormone Receptors: Structure and Function

Because nonsteroid hormones (such as amine and peptide/protein hormones) are hydrophilic, they cannot translocate through the cell membrane; they act via the generation of intracellular "second messenger" molecule(s), which catalytically amplify the signal represented by the hormone, the "first messenger". The receptors for amine and peptide/protein hormones are distributed in the plasma membrane of target cells; because of the fluidity of the phospholipid bilayer of the membrane, membrane receptors have a high degree of mobility. These receptors are composed of: an extracellular domain with hormone-binding capability, a transmembrane segment, and an intracellular domain (which can generate the output, triggering the synthesis of a "second messenger"). The primary structure of several receptors such as for insulin, ANP, EGF, and PDGF have been determined.

For many cell membrane receptors, cAMP is the intracellular messenger. These receptors express the message of hormone binding through interaction with a guanine-nucleotide-binding protein (G protein). A G protein is an intermediate for interaction with adenylate cyclase which synthesizes cAMP from ATP + Mg^{2+}.

The sequence of events in the generation of cAMP via G protein triggered by a ligand-bound receptor may be represented as follows. Owing to the fluidity of the cell membrane the ligand-bound, activated receptor migrates randomly and activates a G protein. Because of this activation the G protein releases GDP and becomes bound to GTP; this binding brings about a conformational change in the G protein, which dissociates from the receptor and diffuses away with its bound GTP to associate with and provide free energy to adenylate cyclase for the synthesis of cAMP. Following hydrolysis of GTP, the G protein returns to its original, low-energy conformation and dissociates from adenylate cyclase and the cycle is repeated as long as the ligand maintains the activated conformation of the receptor. The cAMP generated is a source of high-energy phosphate for cAMP-dependent protein kinases. Thus, these kinases serve as catalysts for the transfer of high-energy phosphate from ATP, via cAMP, to the hydroxyl group of serine and, to a lesser extent, threonine moieties on cellular proteins. This is the major mechanism by which cAMP regulates a variety of cellular functions (*e.g.*, Table 1). Also, cAMP alters eukaryotic gene expression through a protein kinase–mediated phosphorylation of specific DNA-binding proteins that subsequently change the transcriptional activity of specific genes.

The level of cAMP is regulated by the balance of activities of adenylate cyclase (which generates cAMP) and of cyclic nucleotide phosphodiesterases (which hydrolyze cAMP to $5'$-AMP). Trophic hormones, which stimulate the release of other hormones, generally elevate cAMP level, whereas somatostatin, which represses the release of many hormones, decreases cAMP levels. The actions of a number of hormones, including insulin and catecholamines, are mediated, *in part*, by activation of cyclic nucleotide phosphodiesterases which bring about a decrease of cellular cAMP levels. Hormones that act through an adenylate cyclase–mediated mechanism, such as adrenocorticotropic hormone (ACTH), glucagon, luteinizing hormone (LH), follicle-stimulating hormone (FSH), and thyroid-stimulating hormone (TSH), bring about an increase of the cellular cAMP level. It is interesting to note that the two hormones involved in the balance of energy metabolism, glucagon and insulin, show a reciprocal relationship in their effects on cAMP level.

The activation of phosphodiesterases proceeds via a different signal transduction mechanism. The proposed mechanism of action involves the binding of a specific hormone to the receptor, resulting in the rapid activation of plasma membrane–associated phospholipase C, which catalyzes the hydrolysis of a specific inositol phospholipid within the plasma membrane, phosphatidylinositol 4,5-bis-phosphate (PIP_2), to form the second messengers diacylglycerol (DG) and inositol 1,4,5-triphosphate (IP_3). The hydrolysis of PIP_2 and the formation of IP_3 results in a profound increase in the levels of free cytosolic calcium ion (which may act directly or through calmodulin), whereas DG stimulates protein kinase C (which then activates other membrane-bound enzymes through phosphorylation). These then trigger the subsequent physiological responses important for the regulation of cell function. Hormone–receptor interactions that result in the formation of these second messengers include epinephrine and norepinephrine, vasopressin, and angiotensin II.

Another important category of receptors express the message of hormone binding at the extracellular domain through the increase of tyrosine kinase activity of the intracellular domain. In receptors with tyrosine kinase activity, the extracellular domain has the amino terminus and the cytoplasmic domain the carboxy-terminus; they are linked by a single α-helix transmembrane segment. The amino acid sequence of the extracellular domain is studded with cysteines; the pattern of distribution of the cysteines in the sequence is different with the different hormone-binding specificities. These cysteines may play a role in mediating the clustering of hormone-bound receptors in cell membrane invaginations. The cytoplasmic domain has phosphorylated sites; the role of these in the kinase activity is not clear, but appears to be different in various receptors. In addition, the extracellular domain is also glycosylated at several sites. An insulin receptor is a receptor with tyrosine kinase activity. Receptors for several locally acting growth factors, such as EGF, PDGF, and CSF, also act through tyrosine kinase activity. The receptors for growth hormone (GH) and prolactin (PRL) show sequence similarities with tyrosine kinase activity receptors.

The tyrosine kinase activity of these receptors is located in the intracellular domain. Binding of hormone to the extracellular domain receptor sites brings about an increase of enzyme activity, which increase may be several-fold. The basis of this increase appears to be exclusively an increase of the V_{max}, suggesting that the conformation of the tyrosine kinase–active site has not changed. The modality of transfer of molecular stimulus — generated by the binding of hormone to, and conformational change in, the extracellular domain — via the transmembrane helical segment is as yet unclear; it can represent conformational change of the helix or charge displacement along the peptide backbone.

A particularly interesting receptor discovered in the mid-1980s is the one for GH, the high-affinity GH-binding protein (GHBP). GHBP, a 238- to 246-amino acid glycoprotein, represents the extracellular domain of the complete plasma membrane GH receptor; hence GHBP has been termed a "circulating receptor". The carbohydrate moiety does not appear to be important for the binding function. Since there is a single gene that encodes the GH receptor, GHBP arises by proteolytic cleavage from the membrane receptor or is translated from an alternatively spliced mRNA encoding a shortened version of the GH receptor, or by both mechanisms. GHBP appears to be a key intermediary in the myriads of metabolic actions of GH, and there is suggestive evidence that ligand-bound GHBP may also have direct nuclear action on gene transcription.

Most of the types of receptors so far identified act conjointly with other receptor types; in particular, the family of tyrosine kinase receptors acts parallel with other receptor-controlled signal transduction pathways involving G proteins. The generation of more than one "second messenger" in the signal transduction triggered by certain hormones and the "cross activation" of other pathways by some of these messengers provide a rich branching of interactions. Superimposed is the great amplification of the original signal by the very nature of signal transduction, since each ligand-bound receptor can generate many messenger molecules. Some of the interactions may be additive or synergistic, whereas others may be antagonistic. The net result is the integrated control of cellular function, homeostasis, and growth.

II. CLASSIFICATION, BIOSYNTHESIS, RELEASE, AND DISPOSITION OF HORMONES

A. Classification of Hormones Based on Chemical Structure and Mechanism of Action

The chemical classification of hormones progressed throughout the 20th century, beginning with the elucidation of the structures of catecholamines, continuing with those of the steroid hormones, and then with the peptide and protein hormones. Hormones can be classified chemically as amines (catecholamines), iodo thyronine amines (*e.g.*, thyroxine), peptides (*e.g.*, vasopressin, oxytocin, and somatostatin), proteins (*e.g.*, insulin, glucagon, PRL, and GH), glycoproteins (*e.g.*, FSH, LH, and TSH), and steroids (*e.g.*, estrogens, progesterone, testosterone, and glucocorticoids). Another principle sets the dividing line between peptides and proteins at about 5 kDa or 40 amino acid residues; molecules below 5 kDa are termed peptides, those above are termed proteins. Following this terminology, glucagon (29 amino acids) is a peptide hormone, whereas insulin (51 amino acids) is a protein hormone.

However, another, perhaps more useful classification of hormones is based on the location of receptors and the nature of the signal(s) used to mediate hormonal action within the cell (Table 2). Except for the thyroid hormones (T_3 and T_4), the hormones in Group 1 are lipophilic and are derived from cholesterol. Group 1 hormones associate with

TABLE 2.   Classification of Hormones According to Mechanism of Action

Hormones That Bind to Intracellular Receptors

Group 1	Androgens	Mineralocorticoids	
	Estrogens	Calcitriol	
	Progestins	Thyroid hormones (T_3/T_4)	
	Glucocorticoids		

Hormones That Bind to Cell Surface Receptors

Cyclic AMP is the Second Messenger

Group 2A	Norepinephrine	ACTH	FSH
	Epinephrine	ADH	LPH
	Somatostatin	CG	LH
	Angiotensin II	CRH	MSH
	Calcitonin	TSH	PTH
	Glucagon		

Calcium and/or Phosphatidylinositol is the Second Messenger

Group 2B	Norepinephrine	Acetylcholine	ADH
	Epinephrine	Angiotensin II	GnRH
	Dopamine (PIF)	Glucagon	TRH

Unknown Intracellular Messenger

Group 2C	CS	Insulin	
	EGF	IGF-I, IGF-II	
	FGF	NGF	
	GH	PRL	
	PDGF	SRIF	

serum transport proteins, traverse the plasma membrane, and interact with nuclear receptors in target cells. The ligand–receptor complex *is* the intracellular messenger in this group. Group 2A consists of water-soluble hormones which bind to the plasma membrane of target cells. Such hormones regulate intracellular metabolic processes through intermediary molecules (second messenger), the hormone itself being the first messenger. In Group 2B, several hormones appear to use calcium or phosphatidylinositol metabolites (or both) as the intracellular signal. For Group 2C hormones, the intracellular messenger(s) have not as yet been definitely identified.

B. Biosynthesis and Release of Hormones

Peptide and protein hormones, such as insulin, are synthesized in the rough endoplasmic reticulum. The amino acid sequence of a protein hormone is determined by its specific mRNA which is synthesized in the nucleus and has a nucleotide sequence that has been coded by a specific gene. The specific mRNA sequence results in the synthesis of a protein larger than the mature hormone. The precursors of these hormones, the pre-pro-hormone and the pro-hormone, have an extended amino acid sequence, called leader or signal peptide. In addition, a pre-pro-hormone has internal cleavage sites that, upon enzymatic action, yield different bioactive peptides. In some instances, a peptide segment may act as a "spacer" between two bioactive peptides, or the pre-pro-hormone may contain peptide sequences that have no known biological activity (in such cases, these sequences are called "cryptic" peptides). The leader peptide sequence of both the pre-pro-hormones and pro-hormones allows the crossing of the newly synthesized protein through the endoplasmic reticulum membrane to the Golgi apparatus. During transport to the Golgi apparatus, and at this organelle, the hormone is processed by proteolytic enzymes, which remove the leader peptide and cleave the pro-hormone to yield mature hormone peptide chain(s). The hormone is then stored in granules that will fuse with the cell membrane during the release process and allow their contents to be released into the extracellular space. This process is called exocytosis and involves the participation of microtubules and the mobilization of calcium across the cell membrane.

Iodo thyronine amines and steroid hormones are synthesized from tyrosine and cholesterol, respectively. The precursors are either totally (tyrosine) or partially (cholesterol) transported to the cell of synthesis via the bloodstream. Once inside the cell, these precursor molecules are subjected to the sequential action of several enzymes, resulting in the formation of various intermediate products, several of which may be hormones. In contrast to protein hormones, thyroid and steroid hormones, once produced, can freely cross the cell membrane without having to be packaged in granules and actively exocytosed.

C. Patterns of Hormone Secretion

Regardless of their chemical nature, hormones are present in the bloodstream in very low concentrations (10^{-7} to 10^{-12} M). Their concentration in the circulation is generally regulated by control feedback mechanisms in response to physiologic needs. The basal secretion of most hormones is not a continuous process, but rather is pulsatile. Secretory pulses may proceed with different periodicities. For example, ACTH has a characteristic diurnal pattern of release with plasma levels rising sharply during the early morning hours, while the monthly preovulatory secretion of gonadotropins occurs approximately every 30 days. Other hormones, such as thyroxine, exhibit changes in plasma levels that occur over months. The secretion rate of most, if not all, hormones is regulated by negative and positive feedback mechanisms. Also, hormones act on different time scales: peptides act within seconds/minutes, proteins and glycoproteins within minutes/hours, steroids within hours, and iodo thyronine action requires days. If a peptide or protein hormone is continuously present, its effect may be exerted over a period of hours or even days.

D. Transport and Metabolism of Hormones

Once a hormone is released into the bloodstream it may circulate freely, if it is water soluble, or it may be bound to a carrier protein. In general, amines, peptides, and proteins circulate in free form, whereas steroids and thyroid hormones are bound to transport proteins. Some plasma proteins, such as albumin and prealbumin, can transport nonselectively a variety of low–molecular weight hormones. In contrast, some globulins act as specific transport proteins that have saturable, high-affinity binding sites for the hormones they carry. These proteins include thyroid hormone–binding globulin, testosterone-binding globulin, and cortisol-binding globulin. GH circulates in the blood through an intriguing transport modality. As discussed in Section I.B above, GH is transported by a high-affinity GHBP, which corresponds to the extracellular domain of the cell membrane GH receptor. In human plasma, a second GHBP has also been identified, which appears to be unrelated to the high-affinity GHBP or to the complete GH receptor.

Binding of hormones to carrier proteins has a significant impact on the hormone clearance rate from the circulation. The greater the binding capacity of the specific protein carrier, the slower the clearance rate of the hormone. Actually, only a small portion of the circulating hormones is absorbed and removed from the circulation by most target tissues. The majority of hormone clearance is carried out by the liver and the kidneys. This process includes enzymatic degradation involving hydrolysis, oxidation, hydroxylation, methylation, decarboxylation, sulfation, and glucuronidation.

There are several means of hormonal communication other than by way of the blood (*i.e.*, endocrine). Other important intercellular chemical signals (locally acting "parahormones" such as the eicosanoids and opiate peptides, the variety of tissue growth factors, and the neurotransmitters) are transmitted by diffusion. Locally acting chemical signals can be *autocrine*, *i.e.*, they influence phenotypically identical cells in the neighborhood, or they can be *paracrine*, *i.e.*, they influence phenotypically different cells close by, while neurotransmitters produced by neurons (*neurocrine* secretion) mediate synaptic transmission. *Solinocrine* secretion takes place when hormones are secreted into the lumen of the gut (*e.g.*, somatostatin, LHRH). The key roles of the variety of locally acting tissue growth factors in carcinogenesis are discussed in some detail in Chapter 5 on "Promotion and Cocarcinogenesis" and in Chapter 14 on "Mechanism of Viral Tumorigenesis and the Combination Effects of Viruses and Chemical Carcinogens".

The interaction of hormones with their target tissues is followed by intracellular degradation of the hormone. In the case of amine or peptide/protein hormones, degradation occurs after their binding to membrane receptors, internalization of the hormone–receptor complex, and dissociation of this complex into its two components. In the case of steroid or thyroid hormones, degradation occurs after binding of the hormone–receptor complex to its nuclear target.

III. PRINCIPAL COMPONENT SEGMENTS OF THE ENDOCRINE SYSTEM

A. The Hypothalamic–Pituitary Axis and Its Peripheral Gland Targets

The major known regulatory interrelationships of the hypothalamic–pituitary axis and its peripheral gland targets are schematically represented in Figure 1. The production of most, but not all, endocrine hormones is under direct or indirect hypothalamic–pituitary control. Anatomically, the hypothalamus is a segment of the diencephalon forming the floor of the median ventricle of the brain; it controls/modulates the hormonal outputs of the hypophysis (pituitary gland). The hypothalamus is, in turn, linked by neurons to the cortex, midbrain, hindbrain, and the spinal cord. This is the underlying anatomical basis of the fact that the hypothalamic modulation of endocrine balance via the pituitary is a reflection not only of the hormonal feedback from the pituitary and from the peripheral target glands upon the hypothalamus, but also of the totality of neurophysiological input received by the whole organism.

1. Hypophysis

The two lobes of the hypophysis are connected to the hypothalamus through a stalk (the infundibulum) that comprises the supraopticohypophyseal nerve tract "peptidergic neurons" leading to the posterior lobe (neurohypophysis) and the vasculature of the hypothalamo–hypophyseal portal system leading to the anterior lobe (adenohypophysis); the major anatomical segments of the mammalian hypophysis are listed in Table 3. In the human adult the pars distalis, the truly glandular part of the adenohypophysis, represents about 70% of the total weight of the hypophysis; the neurohypophysis represents about 20%; the remaining 10% consists of the tuberalis, the intermedia, and the capsule surrounding the gland. The pars tuberalis is a small

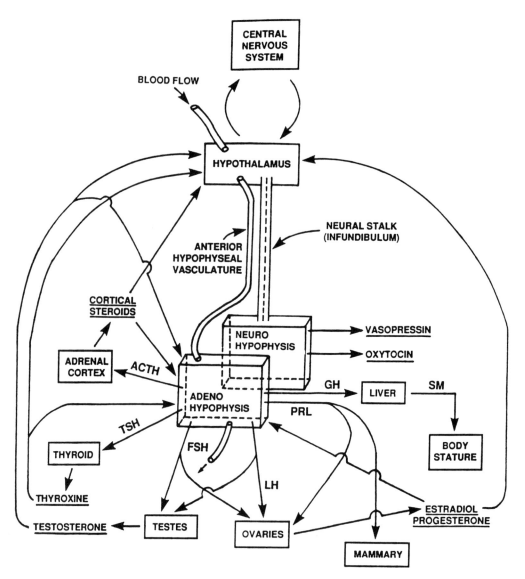

FIGURE 1.   Some major known regulatory interrelationships in the endocrine system. *Acronyms*: ACTH, adrenocorticotropic hormone; TSH, thyroid-stimulating hormone; FSH, follicle-stimulating hormone; LH, luteinizing hormone; PRL, prolactin; GH, growth hormone (somatotropin); SM, somatomedin.

structure consisting of a coarse network of cell cords surrounding in a collar-like fashion the neck of the infundibulum. The pars intermedia is a layer separating the pars distalis from the neurohypophysis. The pars tuberalis and intermedia are probably of little functional significance.

The adenohypophysis (which is overwhelmingly the pars distalis) and the neurohypophysis are in actuality two separate glands fused together, which have different developmental origins. During embryogenesis the neurohypophysis arises as an outgrowth from the floor of the median ventricle; keeping with its developmental origin, the pars neuralis remains connected to the ventricle by the infundibulum. On the other hand, the adenohypophysis arises in embryogenesis from an ectodermally lined invaginated structure, known as Rathke's pouch. The two lobes unite and fuse together toward the end stage of their individual embryonic developments.

TABLE 3.   Major Anatomical Segments of the Mammalian Hypophysis[a]

	Major Segments	Subdivisions	
Adenohypophysis	Lobus glandularis	• Pars distalis • Pars tuberalis • Pars intermedia	Anterior lobe
	Lobus nervosa (neural lobe)	• Pars nervosa (processus infundibuli)	Posterior lobe
Neurohypophysis	Infundibulum	• Pediculus infundibularis (stem) • Bulbus infundibularis • Labrum infundibularis (rim)/median eminence of the tuber cinereum	Neural stalk

[a]International Commission on Anatomical Nomenclature.

The two lobes are regulated differently and produce different classes of hormones. The neurohypophysis is directly regulated by the hypothalamus via the supraopticohypophyseal nerve tract. The neurohypophysis secretes two peptides (each composed of nine amino acids), vasopressin and oxytocin. The precursor of these (a "polyprotein") is synthesized in the peptidergic neurons of the hypothalamus. This polyprotein precursor is cleaved into three peptide fragments. The cleavage product, resulting from the central region, is neurophysin, a 10-kDa protein, a "spacer", which stabilizes the two other fragments for transport down to the neural lobe. The stabilized peptides are transported through the supraopticohypophyseal nerve tract axons in the infundibulum and are stored in the nerve endings of the neurohypophysis until release is triggered. The release-triggering stimuli are neurotransmitters; release is activated by cholinergic stimuli and inhibited by adrenergic stimuli. Hence these neurosecretory cells represent neuroendocrine transducers, converting neural stimulus to hormone release.

Vasopressin is an antidiuretic hormone. Hence its secretion is stimulated by conditions indicative of loss in the systemic economy of water, such as high blood osmolarity as well as substantial (10–25%) loss of blood volume; vasopressin release is also triggered by neural stimuli, such as response to stress. Oxytocin stimulates smooth-muscle contraction. An important function of oxytocin is in parturition; its secretion is linked in a positive feedback loop with uterine contractions, which linkage provides for gradually increasing strength of the contractions until the fetus is expelled.

The adenohypophysis is regulated by the hypothalamus through releasing and release-inhibiting hormones secreted into the bloodstream flowing through the hypothalamic–pituitary portal venous system and carried to the anterior lobe (Figure 1), where they bind to membrane receptors of specific hormone-secreting cells. Some hypothalamic regulatory hormones of known amino acid sequence are CRH (41 amino acids), GHRH (44 amino acids), GnRH (10 amino acids), SRIF (14 amino acids), and TRH (3 amino acids).

The hormone-secreting cells of the adenohypophysis are highly specialized. The acidophil-staining cells may be somatotrophs which secrete only GH, or mammotrophs which secrete only PRL. The basophil-staining cells secrete the trophic hormones which regulate the subordinated target glands: adrenals, thyroid, and the gonads. The respective trophic hormones are ACTH (or corticotropin), TSH (or thyrotropin), FSH, and LH.

GH (191 amino acids) and PRL (198 amino acids) are similar structures, each containing a large central disulfide loop. GH has both direct and indirect actions. The indirect action, schematically represented in Figure 1, involves the stimulation of the secretion in the liver of somatomedin C (also known as insulin-like growth factor I; IGF-I). While IGF-I does play a role in chondrocyte proliferation, sulfate uptake into the cartilage, and amino acid uptake and glucose uptake into muscle, GH has also a direct effect on the differentiation of chondrocytes. PRL secretion by the mammotroph cells is unique among adenohypophyseal hormones in that it is programmed to proceed without any release or stimulation by hypothalamic factors; it is subject only to inhibition by PIF (dopamine).

ACTH (39 amino acids) is synthesized as a part of a precursor polyprotein, pro-opiomelanocortin, which contains, in addition to ACTH, three segments representing melanocyte-stimulating hormones (MSH). ACTH stimulates the synthesis and secretion of adrenal steroids. TSH is a glycoprotein containing an α-chain (92 amino acids) and a β-chain (112 amino acids); it stimulates the synthesis in and release from the thyroid gland of thyroxine (T_4) and triiodothyronine (T_3). Both FSH and LH are also glycoproteins, having the same 92–amino acid α-chain subunit as TSH. Specificity of biological action resides in the sequences of their β-chains (FSH = 118 amino acids; LH = 115 amino acids).

2. Adrenal Glands

The adrenal glands consist of an outer layer, the cortex, that surrounds the inner part, the medulla. Like the hypophysis, these two parts of the gland are functionally different and have different embryogenetic origins. The cortex produces steroids (androgens, glucocorticoids, and mineralocorticoids), whereas the medulla synthesizes catecholamines, principally epinephrine. The cortex itself consists of three cell layers beneath the adrenal capsule: the zona glomerulosa, the zona fasciculata, and the zona reticularis next to the medulla. The only function of the outer layer, the zona glomerulosa, is the synthesis of aldosterone; the function of this mineralocorticoid is to promote transepithelial sodium transport. The zona fasciculata and reticularis synthesize androgens and glucocorticoids (cortisol or corticosterone). Dehydroepiandrosterone is the principal androgen produced by the adrenal gland (the major source of androgens in the human female). The major function of glucocorticoids is gluconeogenesis; these steroids are involved in virtually every metabolic step leading to gluconeogenesis (*e.g.*, protein degradation, amino acid deamination, lipolysis) and also have an anti-inflammatory function.

While the cortex develops from the mesothelium of the abdominal cavity during embryogenesis, the medulla develops from the neural crest and is in fact a sympathetic ganglion, part of the autonomic nervous system. It is, however, a modified sympathetic ganglion in that its neurotransmitter secretion, epinephrine, is secreted into the bloodstream rather than diffusing away toward some peripheral tissue. Consistent with their functional distinctness, the adrenal cortex and the medulla have their own separate blood supplies.

3. Thyroid Gland

The thyroid consists of two lateral lobes connected by an isthmus. Histologically, it is built from epithelial (follicular) cells arranged around colloid material. The sparse "C" cells, which synthesize CT, are adjacent to the follicular cell layers. The thyroid synthesizes T_3 and T_4. T_4 is generally regarded as the prohormone of T_3, since T_3 is responsible for most of the biological activities. Thus, T_3 deficiency produces hypothyroidism even though T_4 levels may be normal. Conversion of T_4 to T_3 is brought about by iodo thyronine deiodinase in the peripheral tissues.

Thyroid hormones exert a very great variety of effects, the principal effect being the stimulation of calorigenesis indicated by increased oxygen consumption. The tissue/organ systems most responsive to the effect of thyroid hormones are therefore those which normally handle large amounts of energy and transport volumes: the muscular, gastrointestinal (GI), and renal systems. T_3 does not actually appear to exert any specific effect, rather it potentiates the effects of many other hormones. Hence it has frequently been termed a "permissive hormone", the overall effect being to adjust the overall metabolic rate of the tissues to a higher level.

4. Gonads

a. Embryogenesis   The testes and the ovaries derive from the same embryologic structure; the undifferentiated fetal gonad has the potential of becoming either testis or ovary. The direction of sexual development depends on the chance of formation of an X-X (female) or an X-Y (male) pair of chromosomes during fertilization [in the human, the species-specific somatic chromosome number is 23 pairs of similar chromosomes plus a 24th balanced size X-X pair (in females) or dissimilar size (X-Y) pair (composed of a large X and small Y chromosome, in males)]. The chance occurrence of sex chromosome combination depends on whether the particular spermatozoa which will be successful in penetrating the ovum carries an X or a Y chromosome so as to establish in the zygote an X-X or X-Y combination.

The Y chromosome directs the development of an embryo along a morphogenetic pathway leading to a male. The specific locus on Y directing the male sexual development is termed the "testis-determining factor" (TDF) which has been characterized in 1990–91 as the *SRY* gene. All aspects of male sexual development follow from the presence of the TDF.

Should an X-Y combination result, the H-Y antigen, a product of the Y chromosome, interacts with cell membrane receptors, thereby inducing differentiation to Sertoli cells which then take over the directing of the sequence of cell migrations in the developing testis (in the *developed* testis the Sertoli cells lie at intervals in the wall of the seminiferous tubules). Once the fetal Leydig cells that arose mature, under the influence of the Y chromosome, they become responsive to stimulation by pituitary LH to secrete testosterone. This steroid causes differentiation to yield the external genital structures: the penis and scrotum, whereas its 5α-reduced metabolite, dihydrotestosterone (DHT), triggers differentiation that yields the internal genital structures: the epididymis, the vas deferens, the seminal vesicles, and the prostate. DHT is the active androgen; all adult tissues (except muscle) contain 5α-reductase which converts testosterone to DHT.

Contrary to the hormonal requirements for sexual development in male embryos, female embryos do not require the presence of estrogen or any other steroid for the development of the female genital structures. This is because female sexual development is genetically preprogrammed. Hence, castration of female embryos does not stop continued development of the genital structures during embryogenesis; moreover, congenital metabolic defect of normal estrogen production does not preclude morphologic normalcy at birth.

Whereas developed males and females secrete both androgens and estrogens, the systemic level of the former is dominant in males and of the latter in females. Moreover, the major organismic sources of these hormones are different in the two sexes, allowing for different endocrine control modalities of their respective levels. As mentioned above, in males the primary source of androgens are the Leydig cells of the testes, the testosterone secreted acting principally in the form of DHT. In the human male the source of estrogens is from the conversion of androgens by aromatase in peripheral tissues. In females the major source of estrogens are the ovaries. In the human female the major source of androgens is the adrenal cortex, which secretes dehydroepiandrosterone (as a by-product of the glucocorticoid pathway).

b. Testes   As mentioned above, the Leydig cells secrete testosterone, which acts at most sites (*e.g.*, prostate) in the form of DHT. Synthesis and release of testosterone is stimulated by LH. In many peripheral tissues, testosterone can also be converted to estradiol by aromatase.

Spermatogenesis is carried out in the seminiferous tubules, which contain the spermatogonia and the Sertoli cells. Spermatogenesis requires high levels of testosterone (supplied by the Leydig cells) as well as FSH, which induces the synthesis of an androgen-binding protein in the tubules. Spermatozoa arise as the result of a particular direction that spermatogonial cell division may take; it may cease dividing for a time, grow to a size markedly larger than the parent cell, and become differentiated as a primary spermatocyte. The future direction that the differentiation of such cells take is now irreversibly determined. They will pass through a stage known as secondary spermatocyte and then a stage known as spermatid, before becoming fully formed spermatozoa.

c. Ovaries and the Estrous Cycle   The functional role of the ovaries is to produce ova and to ensure cyclic, sequential production of estradiol (E_2) and progesterone in response to stimulation by the gonadotropins, FSH and LH. The precisely timed, synchronized release of these four hormones, together with the concomitant morphologic changes in the female reproductive system, is known as the estrus (menstrual) cycle.

In the human the menstrual cycle consists of four phases: the follicular, also known as the estrogenic or proliferative phase; ovulation; the luteal phase; and the menstrual phase. The follicular phase begins by FSH triggering and activating the maturation of 10 to 20 of these follicles in the ovaries [each of these follicles consists of an oocyte core surrounded by a squamous ("granulosa") cell layer coupled to the oocyte by gap junctions]; maturation begins by the proliferation of the cells in the granulosa cell layer. Through a series of precisely synchronized releases of FSH, LH, and E_2 pulses, primordial follicles undergo successive stages of maturation known as: "early" primary follicle (the oocyte being surrounded by a layer of cuboidal rather than squamous granulosa cells); "late" primary follicle (containing several stratified layers of granulosa cells); secondary follicle or antral follicle, a morphologically more diversified structure, that contains a fluid-filled cavity, the antrum; at this stage of maturation of the follicles the available FSH becomes a limiting factor so that most follicles degenerate and (in the human) usually only one persists – this surviving follicle, with a fully developed antrum, is known as the graafian follicle.

During the above stages of follicular development the primary oocytes (in the core of these competing follicles) themselves undergo meiosis and become arrested in metaphase; these are known as "secondary oocytes". At this point in the cycle, rising E_2 levels prepare the myometrium for sperm propagation and the endometrium for nidation of the fertilized ovum. Sudden increase of LH level, triggered by the rising E_2 level, brings about rupture of the graafian follicle to release the mature "secondary oocyte" with its granulosa cell layer. This completes the ovulation phase.

Following ovulation, the follicle now enters the luteal phase. The follicle collapses due to uncoupling, by the LH surge, of the follicle cells from the oocyte at the gap junctions and – under stimulation by LH – the empty follicle ("corpus luteum") produces large amounts of progesterone, cholesterol, and estrogens, conferring the yellow color (hence, the term "luteum"). The corpus luteum is LH dependent and, in the absence of fertilization, has a life span of 14 days (in the human). In the absence of fertilization, the production of progesterone and estradiol by the aging corpus decreases as the luteal phase progresses. This brings about a premenstrual rise of gonadotropins for recruiting a new set of follicles for maturation and ovulation in the next cycle.

If fertilization does occur, the corpus luteum – "rescued" by the chorionic gonadotropin secreted by the trophoblast (which will become the placenta) — supplies initially the high level of progesterone required throughout pregnancy [a function taken over by the trophoblast (at the 8th week in humans) when trophoblastic progesterone and estrogen production levels have become adequate]. Progesterone opposes the contractions of the myometrium (initially useful in aiding the progression of sperm, but which would endanger nidation), as well as brings about modifications of the endometrial surface to prepare the uterus for implantation and nourishment of the embryo.

If fertilization does not occur, there is a gradual decrease of estrogen and progesterone hormonal support for the endometrium, culminating in the spasm of the endometrial arteries, endometrial necrosis, desquamation, and bleeding.

B. Hormonal Regulation of Calcium Homeostasis

The maintenance of calcium concentration in the blood within narrow limits (2.2 to 2.55 mM) is critical because of the involvement of this ion in membrane transport and signal transduction at the cellular level, and in the functioning of muscles and nerves at the tissue level. The three regulatory hormones of calcium metabolism are PTH (84 amino acids), CT (32 amino acids), and an activated form of vitamin D, 1,25-DHCC. PTH is produced by the parathyroid glands, which represents functionally distinct segments of the posterior wall of each lateral lobe of the thyroid. CT is produced by specialized ("parafollicular") "C" cells in the thyroid follicles. Although the regulation of calcium proceeds via its level *in the blood*, virtually all calcium (>99%) is stored in bone and teeth. The role of PTH is to release calcium from bone and to increase its blood level; CT is an antagonist of PTH and blocks its effects on calcium disposition. The role of 1,25-DHCC in the disposition of calcium is twofold: in the GI tract it stimulates the production of a calmodulin-like (148 amino acid) peptide which is required for calcium absorption; in the bone it has a cooperative/enhancing effect on PTH action.

The cooperative action of these functional features of PTH, CT, and 1,25-DHCC in the regulation of extremes of calcium blood levels is illustrated as follows. In *hypercalcemia*, which depresses the secretion of PTH and stimulates the secretion of CT, the release of calcium from the bone will be reduced and the blockage by PTH of calcium excretion through the kidney will be lifted. At the same time, hypercalcemia shifts the hydroxylation pattern of cholecalciferol to 24,25-hydroxylation, yielding a functionally inactive derivative; thereby absorption of calcium from the intestinal tract will be reduced. The totality of these effects will thus compensate for the hypercalcemia. In *hypocalcemia* inhibition of PTH secretion is lifted, thereby calcium release from bone is promoted and calcium excretion through the kidneys is reduced. At the same time, both PTH and hypocalcemia induce cholecalciferol 1-hydroxylase activity and inhibit 24-hydroxylase activity. The shift of hydroxylated cholecalciferol from the inactive 24,25-form to the active 1,25-form will stimulate calcium absorption from the intestinal tract and will synergize the calcium release by PTH from bone. The resultant of these effects is to correct the low blood calcium level.

C. Hormonal Control of Energy Utilization and Storage

Two pancreatic hormones, insulin and glucagon, are the major regulators of energy utilization and storage. Insulin is an anabolic hormone, while glucagon is a catabolic hormone that antagonizes the effects of insulin. Some major regulatory interrelationships of insulin and glucagon are schematically illustrated in Figure 2.

Insulin is produced by the β-cells (core of the Langerhans islets). Actually, it is

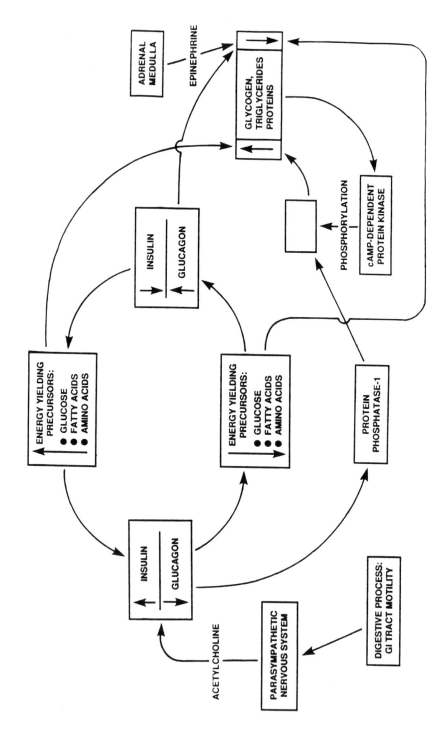

FIGURE 2. Some major regulatory interrelationships of insulin and glucagon.

originally synthesized in a precursor form, "proinsulin" (81 amino acids) which, following specific protease action, yields insulin. Insulin consists of two peptide chains (α-chain, 21 amino acids; β-chain, 30 amino acids) linked by disulfide bonds. Because of its primary anabolic function, elevated blood levels of glucose, fatty acids, and amino acids trigger insulin secretion. In addition, distal early signals of food intake provide anticipatory triggers for insulin release. For example, during the digestion of food, the motility of the GI tract is stimulated by the parasympathetic nervous system; acetylcholine, which is the neurotransmitter for the parasympathetic, also stimulates insulin release and thus provides advance readiness for the nutrients soon to appear in the circulation.

Beyond its direct anabolic functions to stimulate the conversion of free precursors in the blood to glycogen, triglycerides, and protein, the actions of insulin are manyfold and complex. Some of these consist in overriding the effects of other hormones. For example, insulin can override cAMP-dependent protein kinases involved in glycogenolysis and lipolysis by activating specific phosphatases that cleave the phosphate moieties from the kinases. These and other indirect effects of insulin are all consistent with its general anabolic function.

Glucagon is produced by the α-cells (the outermost rim of the Langerhans islets). It is a linear peptide chain consisting of 29 amino acids. Consistent with its primary catabolic function, low blood glucose levels will trigger the release of glucagon which, in turn, elevates the glucose level. Glucagon raises the blood glucose level by stimulating glycogenolysis in the liver and inhibiting glycolysis.

IV. FEEDBACK CONTROL IN THE ENDOCRINE SYSTEM: A SYNOPTIC OVERVIEW

In addition to perpetuating the species, a fundamental function of the endocrine system is to maintain homeostasis in the organism. This is possible through the intimate relationship existing between the endocrine and both the central and autonomic nervous systems. The maintenance of homeostasis requires continuous bidirectional flow of neural and endocrine information. *Positive feedback* occurs when a glandular structure is stimulated by the end product(s) to generate more hormone(s), whereas *negative feedback* occurs when the structure is inhibited by the end product(s) to yield less hormone(s).

Figure 1 and Table 2 together provide an overview of the hormones and of the major feedback relationships between the hypothalamic–pituitary and the regulated peripheral glands. To summarize these relationships, the adenohypophysis secretes the trophic hormones ACTH, TSH, FSH, and LH, which stimulate the production in and release of hormones from the adrenals, thyroid, and gonads (testes and ovaries), respectively; PRL is also a required input for the ovaries. Besides stimulating the production of hormones, FSH, LH, and PRL also stimulate the other glandular functions: production of sperm, ova, and milk secretion. GH has no specific target organ, but has many overall systemic roles in stimulating the growth of long bones, cartilage, and muscle mass; GH has both direct action, as well as indirect action through the production and release of somato-medin (IGF-I). At the hypothalamo–pituitary level the release of the trophic hormones is controlled by both releasing hormones and release-inhibiting hormones. The system-wide regulatory loops close by the feedback of the different peripheral gland hormones (adrenal steroids; T_3 and T_4; testosterone and DHT; and estradiol and progesterone) upon the hypothalamic–pituitary structures synthesizing the releasing and release-inhibiting hormones.

The feedback loops operative in the endocrine system are classified, in the cybernetic sense, as long, short, and ultrashort loops (Figure 3). These are, in this order, of

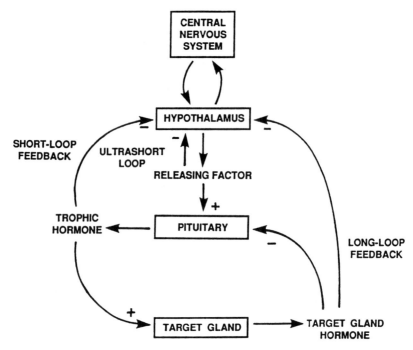

FIGURE 3. Schematic representation of the three types of feedback control loops in the endocrine system. Ultrashort-loop feedback occurs when a hormone acts in a paracrine manner on its own secretory cell type to limit its own secretion. "+" and "−" indicate enhancing or inhibiting effect on a gland.

decreasing importance for the functioning of the organism. Long-loop feedback is operative in most of the anterior pituitary hormone systems and becomes manifest when hormone synthesis or secretion in the end-target peripheral gland is reduced or abolished. An example of long-loop feedback system is when hypothalamic neurons release CRH into the hypophyseal portal system; ACTH is then released from pituitary corticotropes in response to CRH stimulation, which in turn stimulates the synthesis and secretion of cortisol from the adrenal cortex. Increasing cortisol output then acts to inhibit the secretion of ACTH from the pituitary and CRH secretion from the hypothalamus.

Testosterone, estrogen, and progesterone also mediate long-loop negative feedback on hypothalamus GnRH and pituitary LH. Conversely, during the late follicular phase of the menstrual cycle, high concentrations of unopposed E_2 progressively increase the secretion of LH; this is an example of long-loop positive feedback.

Short-loop feedback occurs largely in the regulation of hypophyseal hormones by anterior pituitary trophic hormones. For example, GH secreted by cells in the anterior pituitary stimulates the secretion of somatomedin C from the liver and other peripheral tissues. The somatomedins exhibit long-loop feedback on GH secretion. On the other hand, GH may also directly affect hypothalamic releasing and release-inhibiting hormones that regulate its secretion. This short-loop feedback can occur either by inhibition of the secretion of GHRH or by stimulation of the secretion of SRIF (the GH-release-inhibiting hormone).

It is an instance of ultra-short-loop feedback when a hormone acts on its own cell type in a paracrine manner to inhibit further secretion of itself. This is involved in the regulation of such hormones as oxytocin, vasopressin, and PRL.

Another type of the endocrine control system includes feed-forward loops, which can be negative or positive. Feed-forward loops are intrinsically unstable, since they do not function as closed loops; this is because they always form part of a large, more complex feedback circuit. A well-recognized example is the release of insulin by the β-cells of the islets of Langerhans in response to an increase in plasma glucose concentration. Upon stimulation of its secretion by the elevated glucose levels, insulin acts on the liver to enhance the uptake of glucose. When glucose levels fall to a basal level in plasma, insulin mobilization decreases and glucose uptake is reduced.

REFERENCE SOURCES

General

- Jones, T. C., Mohr, U., and Hunt, R. D., eds.: "Endocrine System". Springer-Verlag, Berlin, 1983.
- Slaunwhite, R.: "Fundamentals of Endocrinology". Dekker, New York, 1988.
- Alberts, B., Bray, D., Dewis, J., Raff, M., Roberts, R., and Watson, J. D.: "Molecular Biology of the Cell", 2nd ed. Garland Publ., New York, 1989. *See* Chapter 12: "Cell Signaling" and Chapter 15: "Germ Cells and Fertilization".

Classification of Hormones

- Tepperman, J., and Tepperman, H. M.: "Metabolic and Endocrine Physiology". Year Book Medical Publishers, Chicago/London, 1987.
- Bolander, F. F.: "Molecular Endocrinology", 2nd ed. Academic Press, San Diego, 1994.
- Granner, D. K.: Hormonal Action. *In* "Principles and Practice of Endocrinology and Metabolism" (K. L. Becker, ed.). Lippincott, New York, 1990, Chapter 4, p. 25.

Synthesis, Release, Transport, and Metabolism

- Tepperman, J., and Tepperman, H. M.: "Metabolic and Endocrine Physiology". Year Book Medical Publishers, Chicago/London, 1987.
- Bolander, F. F.: "Molecular Endocrinology", 2nd ed. Academic Press, San Diego, 1994.
- Ojeda, S. R., and Griffin, J. E.: Organization of the Endocrine System. *In* "Textbook of Endocrine Physiology" (J. E. Griffin and S. R. Ojeda, eds.). Oxford Univ. Press, New York/Oxford, 1992, Chapter 1, p. 3.

Receptors, Mechanisms of Action

- Conn, P. M., ed.: "The Receptors". Academic Press, Orlando, Florida, 1984.
- Posner, B. I., ed.: "Polypeptide Hormone Receptors". Dekker, New York, 1985.
- Tepperman, J., and Tepperman, H. M.: "Metabolic and Endocrine Physiology". Year Book Medical Publishers, Chicago/London, 1987.
- Bolander, F. F.: "Molecular Endocrinology", 2nd ed. Academic Press, San Diego, 1994.
- Mendelson, C. R.: Mechanisms of Hormone Action. *In* "Textbook of Endocrine Physiology" (J. E. Griffin and S. R. Ojeda, eds.). Oxford Univ. Press, New York/Oxford, 1992, Chapter 3, p. 28.
- Baumann, G.: Minireview—Growth Hormone-Binding Proteins. *Proc. Soc. Exp. Biol. Med.* **202**, 392 (1993).

Feedback Control Systems

- Bolander, F. F.: "Molecular Endocrinology", 2nd ed. Academic Press, San Diego, 1994.

- Darlington, D. N., and Dallman, M. F.: Feedback Control in Endocrine Systems. *In* "Principles and Practice of Endocrinology and Metabolism" (K. L. Becker, ed.). Lippincott, New York, 1990, Chapter 5, p. 38.

Genetics of Sex Determination

- Wachtel, S. S.: "Molecular Genetics of Sex Determination". Academic Press, San Diego, 1993.

Hormonal Carcinogenesis[1]

The dawn of hormonal carcinogenesis began with Beatson's (1) demonstration in 1898 that ovariectomy ameliorates the clinical course of breast cancer in women, carrying the implication that this cancer is due to/maintained by the continuous stimulus of ovarian hormone. This observation was confirmed in 1919 by Loeb in a rodent model (2). However, it was not until nearly 35 years later after Beatson's observation that Lacassagne (3) reported the induction of mammary tumors in mice by prolonged treatment with large doses of estrogen. This study launched the era of hormonal carcinogenesis. The initial observation was confirmed and extended by Gardner *et al.* (4-6), Nelson (7, 8), Shimkin and Grady (9), and many subsequent investigators.

The rapidly growing understanding in the early half of this century of the complex regulatory mechanisms operative in the endocrine system soon led to mechanistic studies in hormonal carcinogenesis. It was briefly mentioned in the Introduction that the artificial generation of an imbalance in the hypothalamic/pituitary–target glands axis brings about overproduction of hormone at some location of the endocrine system. If maintained long enough, such hormonal overstimulation will eventually bring about the emergence of tumors without the administration of exogenous hormones. This was first shown in the classical experiments of Biskind and Biskind (10, 11), who transplanted ovarian tissue into the spleen of gonadectomized female rats, resulting in a very high incidence of granulosa cell tumors in the grafted tissue. Since the estrogen produced by the graft tissue, because of its location, must pass via the portal circulation through the liver—where estrogen is destroyed (12)—little if any of the hormone reaches the pituitary to provide feedback; hence, the ovarian graft will be persistently overstimulated by the excessive pituitary secretion of gonadotropin, leading to the emergence of tumor from the graft. Consistent with the fact that the graft-produced estrogen does not reach the general circulation (and the pituitary), the graft-bearing rats showed castration atrophy of the uterus and vagina. In order to confirm this mechanism of tumor production in the splenic graft, in other experiments (11) ovarian transplants were made into the kidney or into spleen which, however, was provided with a vascularized connection to adjacent tissues, bypassing the liver and allowing transfer of estrogen to the general circulation; these rats remained tumor free as well as exhibited estrus.

The correctness of the general principle, that disruption of the hypothalamic/ pituitary–peripheral glands feedback leads to tumor induction, has subsequently been confirmed in a number of experiments involving other species and other glands. For

---

[1] Abbreviations and trade names used in this section are given on p. 427.

419

example, transplantation of ovarian tissue into the spleen of Strong A, C3H, and hybrid female and male mice yielded tumors, predominantly luteomas in females and granulosa cell tumors in males (13). Similarly, tumors are produced by extending the application of the ovary-into-spleen transplant technique to rabbits (14). Splenic transplantation of *testicular* tissue into castrated male rats leads to the development of interstitial tumors originating from the graft (15–17).

In the design of investigations exemplified in the foregoing, the gonadal tissue — although present in the animal body as a graft — was isolated from interaction with the hypophysis, and this led to overstimulation of and tumorigenesis in the graft. In other experimental designs, interruption of the feedback was brought about by outright removal of the gonads. The resulting uninhibited secretion of gonadotropin by the pituitary can lead to neoplastic transformation of the pituitary itself or to overstimulation of the adrenal cortex, leading ultimately to malignancy. For example, Little and Woolley and their coworkers observed malignant tumors of the adrenals in ovariectomized DBA mice (18), CE mice (19), and DBA × CE hybrid mice (20), as well as in castrated male mice (21). Finally, the induction of pituitary tumors by subcutaneous implantation of pituitary tissue into intact female mice has been reported (22).

It follows from the historical precedents (*e.g.*, 3–9), and is consistent with the carcinogenic effects of artificially induced endocrine imbalances exemplified above, that a variety of organ sites in different species are susceptible to induction of benign and malignant tumors by chronic administration of exogenous hormones. Hormonal carcinogenesis differs from carcinogenesis by nonhormone chemical agents in several aspects. Neoplastic transformation elicited solely by hormones is very highly tissue specific, it requires sustained and prolonged exposure to hormone at high levels, manifests long induction periods, and is preceded by cellular proliferation in the target tissue(s) during the latency period. However, similarly to nonhormone chemical carcinogens, hormone metabolism, as it affects cellular disposition, binding, and pharmacokinetic properties, has a determining effect on hormonal activity.

A synoptic tabulation of hormonal carcinogenesis in different animal models is given in Table 1. As the data in Table 1 show, the neoplasms produced by hormones occur characteristically in the hormone-responsive target tissues, and many are considered to be induced by the direct carcinogenic effect of the hormonal agent(s) involved. The results obtained in the major experimental systems are reviewed below.

I. KIDNEY

An extensively investigated experimental model in hormonal carcinogenesis is the hamster kidney tumor. The developmental basis why in hamsters tumors arise in the kidney, as a consequence of estrogen treatment, is that in hamsters the urogenital and reproductive tracts arise from the same embryonic germinal ridge (23, 24), and the kidney evidently carries genes that are expressed and responsive to estrogenic hormones. An illustration of this is the presence of estrogen receptor (ER) in the hamster kidney (which is increased by *in vivo* chronic estrogen exposure), as well as the concomitant induction of progesterone receptor (PR) as a result of prolonged (equal to or greater than 1 month) estrogen treatment (25, 26).

Multiple bilateral renal tumors are induced by both steroidal and stilbene estrogens in both intact and castrated male Syrian golden hamsters with an incidence approaching 100% (23, 25–28). Intact and ovariectomized female hamsters exhibit either low or no renal tumor incidence when exposed chronically to carcinogenic estrogens. Spontaneous

TABLE 1. **Tumors Induced by Hormones in Experimental Animals**

Hormone(s)[a]	Organ site	Species	% Incidence	Ref.
DES/E_2	Kidney	Hamster	90–100	23,25,27,28,31,35,38
DES	Liver	Rat	10–20	45,47–51,54–56
EE	Liver	Hamster	25–35	59
EE + ANF/DES + ANF	Liver	Hamster	80–100	57,58
P	Ovary	Mouse	—	105
E_1/E_3	Adrenal	Rat	20	106
E_1/E_2/DES/Equilin	Lymphoid	Mouse	35	6
DES + PRL/E_2 + PRL	Leydig cells	Mouse	29–71	74–77
DES/E_2	Epididymal head	Hamster	42	107
E_2/E_1/E_3/DES	Mammary gland	Mouse	12–92	3,5,8,9,86,87,108,109
E_1/E_2/DES	Mammary gland	Rat	70–80	8,90,110
Norethynodrel ± Mestranol	Mammary gland	Rat	40–50	8,88
Mestranol	Mammary gland	Dog	—	88,92
E_2/DES	Cervix/uterus	Mouse	20–60	4
DES	Uterus	Monkey	70	98
DES	Uterus	Mouse	—	99
DES	Pituitary, pars distalis	Mouse	5–75	5
DES	Pituitary, pars distalis	Rat	14–85	7,106,111
E_2	Pituitary, pars intermedia	Hamster	—	112
E_2	Pituitary, pars intermedia	Rat	—	106
P	Pituitary	Mouse	—	52
T + DES/T + E_2	Ductus deferens (smooth muscle)	Hamster	100	113
T + DES	Uterus (smooth muscle)	Hamster	100	114
T + DES	Scent gland	Hamster	83–100	115
E_2 + P/DES + P	Mammary gland	Rat	100	91
T or T + E_2	Prostate	Rat	20–100	61,64,65,73
E_2 + P	Ovary	Dog	—	116

[a] "/" means alternative treatments.

kidney tumor incidence has not been found in this species in numerous large colonies (23, 29, 30). A high incidence of estrogen-induced renal tumors has also been observed in male European hamsters (31), but not in Siberian hamsters (32). The differential susceptibility to the induction of renal tumors by estrogen is consistent with the genetic distinctness of the different species of hamsters. Estrogen-induced renal tumorigenesis is completely suppressed by concomitant administration of either androgen (23), progesterone (23, 33), or antiestrogen (33) and is, surprisingly, partially prevented by the synthetic estrogen, ethinylestradiol (EE) (28). With the exception of EE, which produces only a 10% renal tumor incidence, the potent estrogens, diethylstilbestrol (DES), Moxestrol (11β-methoxy-EE), 17β-estradiol (E_2), and hexestrol, induce high incidences of renal neoplasms compared to the relatively weak estrogens, estriol and 4-hydroxyestrone; no kidney tumors are induced by those estrogens which possess low or negligible hormonal activity (β-dienestrol, 17α-E_2, *d*-equilenin) (27, 34).

The classification of the estrogen-induced renal tumors is beset with considerable controversy. Based largely on histologic criteria, the kidney tumors have been classified as either adenocarcinoma (35) nephroblastoma variant (36), or mesenchymal tumor (37). Earlier studies have suggested that these hamster renal neoplasms arise either from the proximal convoluted tubule (35, 38), or from a combination of cortical tubular and interstitial stroma cells of the kidney (23). However, more recent reports indicate that the origin of the renal tumor is the juxtaglomerular apparatus (39) or the mesenchymal portion of the smooth muscle (37).

Since the kidney tumor exhibits tight junctions, and cilia, microvilli, and lumen formation (40)—which are cell characteristics in malignant epithelia—it is evident that the tumor develops from a cell committed to an epithelial developmental path. The presence of cytokeratin, an epithelial marker, clearly supports this view (40). Nevertheless, the hamster kidney tumor demonstrates features of renal embryogenesis and does not fit the usual characteristics of either renal adenocarcinomas or nephroblastomas described in humans. This is supported by the observation that the hamster renal neoplasm is unique in that it stains positive for all three intermediate filaments, namely desmin, vimentin, and cytokeratin (40). This finding clearly demonstrates its epithelial and mesenchymal characteristics. The sequence and relationships of some cytological events in estrogen-induced renal tumorigenesis in hamsters is illustrated in Figure 1.

A most unique feature of the hamster kidney is that it is an estrogen-responsive and estrogen-dependent organ. Estrogen treatment induces its own receptor as well as induces PR (25, 26)—a characteristic of many estrogen target tissues. The estrogen induction of renal PR in the hamster can be significantly reduced by concomitant treatment with either antiestrogens, androgens, or partially by synthetic progestins (25, 26, 41). That the steroid receptor system in the hamster kidney is functional is further supported by the finding that estrogen specifically induces proximal tubular cell proliferation in culture under serum-free, chemically defined conditions at physiological concentrations (42). Moreover, this estrogen-induced cell proliferation is inhibited by antiestrogen (42).

II. LIVER

Several studies have shown that prolonged administration of estrogens, both natural and synthetic, is essentially not carcinogenic in the liver of various rodent species (43–46). Moreover, no hepatic tumors have ever been associated with estrogen treatment in primates or dogs (45, 47). Small increases (1–21%) in hepatic adenomas have been described, however, in rodents treated with various estrogenic preparations (44, 47–50). More recently, Higashi *et al.* (51) indicated a low incidence (5.6%) of hepatocellular carcinomas in Wistar rats following oral administration of EE and norethindrone. Similar small increases in hepatic adenomas have been reported in rodents treated with various synthetic progestational agents (44, 52, 53). There is some controversy, however, whether or not these increases in liver tumor incidence consequent to sex hormone administration are significant, since spontaneous hepatic tumors have been shown to occur with low frequency in both mice and rats (45, 47).

Sumi *et al.* (54) reported a 44% incidence of liver tumors in a limited group of DES-treated, castrated male WF rats. Recently, Coe *et al.* (55, 56) described a high incidence of hepatocellular carcinomas following treatment of Armenian hamsters with DES. The induction of multinodular hepatocellular carcinomas in castrated male hamsters exposed to either EE or DES for 8–9 months and maintained on a diet containing 0.3–0.4% α-naphthoflavone (ANF) has been shown (57, 58). A low frequency of hepatic tumors arose under these conditions as early as 3.5–4 months after beginning of treatment. No liver tumors were observed in similar groups of animals treated with ANF alone for up to 13 months. A low, but significant incidence (≤35%) of the same liver tumors was observed with either EE or DES alone after 8–9 months of treatment in the absence of ANF (59). These data suggest that ANF may act as either a promoter or cocarcinogen in this liver tumor model, since the neoplasms can be induced by these

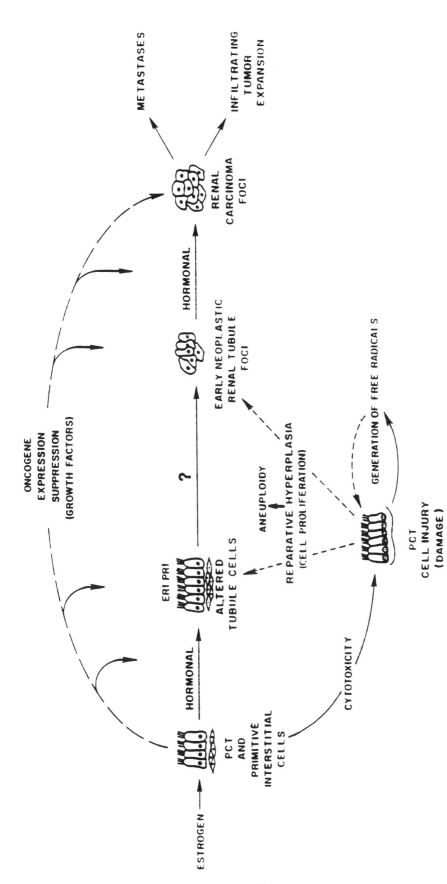

FIGURE 1. Proposed schematic representation of the sequence and relationships of some cytological events in estrogen-induced renal tumorigenesis in hamsters. [From J. J. Li, A. Gonzalez, S. Banerjee, S. K. Banerjee, and S. A. Li: *Environ. Health. Perspect.* **101** (Suppl. 5), 259 (1993), with permission].

423

synthetic estrogens in the absence of ANF. It is pertinent to note that E_2, estrone, and Moxestrol do not induce hepatic tumors in hamsters in the presence or absence of ANF (59). The incidence of hepatocellular carcinomas in the EE + ANF group was 80 to 100%. Neither progesterone, 5α-dihydrotestosterone (DHT), nor E_2 or estrone induced any neoplastic changes in hamster livers in the presence of continuous exposure to ANF. The observation that synthetic estrogen + ANF induces liver tumors is particularly significant, since the spontaneous liver tumor incidence in this species, unlike in other rodents, has been shown to be negligible (<0.01%) (29, 30, 44, 60). The presence of a small, but discrete, specific 8S ER in liver cytosols of castrated male hamsters has been demonstrated (57). Interestingly, the concentration of this cytosolic receptor is increased nearly threefold following 2–3 months of DES treatment and at least fivefold after DES + ANF administration, compared to levels found in livers of untreated castrated animals. It is pertinent that the increases in ER concentration following the above indicated treatments are reflected in corresponding elevations in nuclear ER levels.

III. PROSTATE

Long-term exposure of either Noble (Nb) or Lobund Wistar rats to testosterone (T) results in prostatic carcinomas (61, 62). Initially, Noble (63) observed a 20% incidence of grossly observable prostatic tumors when T was implanted in rats for 16 months. Subsequent studies showed a higher (50%) tumor incidence when treatment with T was applied for 13 months and estrone was substituted for 6 months (61). Maximum tumor yields, with an incidence approaching 90%, were obtained when T plus E_2 was given for 19 months (64). Recently, similar simultaneous exposure to T plus E_2 for 4 months resulted in consistent dysplastic lesions in the dorsolateral lobe of the prostate of Nb rats (65). Interestingly, when T is replaced by DHT (the active androgen in many species), prostatic tumors were not seen (66). These data suggest that E_2 may be involved in the etiology of these prostatic neoplasms, since T can be aromatized to E_2. This is further supported by the finding that treatment with T, in combination with E_2 or DES, produces a 75 to 100% incidence of dysplasia or preneoplastic lesions and a 20 to 100% incidence of carcinomas of the dorsolateral prostate (64, 65, 67). Moreover, nearly 20% of neonatally DES-treated mice also developed tumors in the dorsolateral prostate (68). In canine prostate, estrogen–androgen stimulation produces glandular hypertrophy, hyperplastic and metaplastic changes, organ weight gain, and an increase in DNA content (69–71). Similar hormonal exposure of Nb rats has also resulted in an increase in prostate weight and mitotic activity (72). Current evidence suggests that estrogen, acting on the androgen-supported prostate, is the inducer of cell proliferation in this tissue via a receptor-mediated process (73).

IV. TESTES

A variety of inbred mouse strains and their hybrids (74–76) are susceptible to the development of testicular tumor following prolonged estrogen treatment (≥10 months). There is a genetic component involved in the induction of these hormonally induced testicular tumors, since a number of mouse strains are resistant (76). Both DES and E_2 are equally effective in producing tumors at this site (76). Huseby and coworkers have demonstrated that the Leydig cells of the testes are target cells for estrogens (76). Estrogen probably triggers the appearance of these testicular tumors directly (77) through the modulation of steroid biosynthetic enzyme pathways as well as by altering nucleic acid metabolism, which has been noted in normal Leydig cells of hypophysectomized tumor-susceptible strain mice (78, 81). It has also been shown that ER proteins (82) are present in the Leydig cells and that, in strains of mice susceptible to Leydig cell tumor induction, treatment with estrogens induces a surge of DNA synthesis within the first few days of hormone exposure (83). After this DNA synthetic activity subsided, areas of Leydig cell hyperplasia developed several months later. This initial DNA synthetic activity was also noted in hypophysectomized mice, and it was concluded that this effect was a direct consequence of estrogen on Leydig cells (83).

Studies with BALB/c mice, implanted with E_2 pellet into the spleen, strongly suggest that the carcinogenic effect of E_2 results from the action of this estrogen directly upon the Leydig cells, rather than via the action of some systemic metabolite or alteration of the general endocrine status of the animals (84).

Pituitary hormones, particularly prolactin (PRL), play an obligatory role in estrogen-induced Leydig cell tumorigenesis in mice. This is concluded from the observation that testicular neoplasms cannot be induced in hypophysectomized BALB/c mice (76).

V. MAMMARY GLAND

In his pioneering study, Lacassagne (3) has demonstrated that injection of estrone into male mice induces mammary tumors within 6 months. Synthetic and natural estrogens, including estriol (85–87), can elicit tumorigenesis in the mammary gland of mice. However, a number of confounding factors limit the usefulness of the mouse mammary tumor model. First, the spontaneous tumor incidence in female mice varies between extreme limits (0 to 96%), depending on the susceptibility of the strain (88). Second, with the discovery of oncogenic viruses, such as the mammary tumor virus (MTV) present in this species, the role of sex hormones became obscured (88, 89). There are several viruses that are associated with the induction of mammary neoplasms in mice, and it is now generally held that hormones cannot produce a high incidence of mammary gland tumors in the absence of MTV. These oncogenic viruses are usually transmitted from one generation to the next through the milk of the nursing mother (hence, this was historically known as the "Bittner milk factor"). Genetic factors, operating independently of the virus, are also pertinent in mammary gland tumor induction by hormones. However, the nature of these genetic factors has, as yet, not been well described. In rats, the absence of a viral association indicates that in susceptible strains mammary tumor induction by estrogens may indeed be due to direct hormonal action. Nonetheless, a role of pituitary hormones, as well as unknown viral or other environmental factors, cannot as yet be ruled out. Although in many strains of rats the spontaneous incidence of *benign* mammary tumors (fibroadenomas) is very high (can be up to 90% in female animals), there is a very low incidence (0 to 7%) of mammary *carcinomas* in most rat strains (88, 89). The susceptibility to estrogens, either of the steroidal or stilbene type, in different rat strains is notable, and indicates that genetic factors may play a significant role in mammary gland tumor induction in this species. It is also probable that pituitary hormones act as synergists, because hypophysectomy abolishes the induction of these tumors (90). In intact rats that continuously receive estrogens, malignant tumors of the breast and adenomas of the pituitary frequently develop together. This is in contrast to mice and hamsters, in which there appears to be no correlation between the tendency to develop pituitary tumors and the susceptibility to mammary cancers. Moreover, in the induction of mammary carcinomas, progesterone has a synergistic effect in certain strains of rats (91). A few mammary tumors have been induced also in beagle dogs by several oral contraceptive agents (92).

VI. UTERUS

Endometrial tumors are readily induced by estrogen treatment in rabbits (93, 94). However, uterine adenocarcinoma preceded by cystic hyperplasia occurs spontaneously with a relatively high frequency (75%) in aging rabbits (93). Otherwise, endometrial cancer is infrequent in most animals (95, 96). Endometrial carcinomas in uterine horns may also be induced by either DES or E_2 in MTV^+ mice (97). Malignant mesotheliomas were also found in similar estrogen-treated mice. Interestingly, it is pertinent that the induction of uterine mesotheliomas in squirrel monkeys has been shown after prolonged treatment with DES or estradiol benzoate (98). Also, uterine cervical carcinomas have been induced in MTV^+ mice exposed to either nonsteroidal or natural estrogens (97).

Previous studies with neonatally estrogenized mice have not demonstrated high yields of malignant epithelial neoplasms in the reproductive tract. However, it has been reported recently that uterine adenocarcinoma is demonstrable in 90% of mice receiving DES for 5 days neonatally; the induction of these uterine epithelial lesions was age and dose related (99). Furthermore, the tumors were estrogen-dependent, since ovariectomy of tumor-bearing adult mice resulted in partial tumor regression, and these uterine tumors implanted in nude mice required estrogen for their continued growth and transplant-ability.

Estrogen appears to play two roles in murine uterine tumor induction. First, an induction role where exposure to an exogenous estrogen in the first week of life is apparently necessary for inducing the molecular defect that leads subsequently to tumor emergence (99). Secondly, an expression role where ovarian steroids (presumably endogenous estrogens at puberty), are required for the progression of the neonatally induced uterine lesions; animals treated with DES do not give rise to tumors if they are ovariectomized before puberty and the onset of ovarian function (99). Thus, in this model, estrogen is evidently involved in both the induction and the expression of growth and differentiation defects – giving rise, eventually, to the uterine tumor. Similarly, the neonatal hamster uterus appears to be very susceptible to neoplastic transformation by DES, since treatment of hamsters, when newborn, with DES results in hormone-dependent uterine carcinomas in nearly all animals that reach adulthood (100).

VII. NOTE ON THE MECHANISMS OF HORMONAL CARCINOGENESIS

In numerous laboratories the hypothesis was held that hormone metabolism plays a role in the processes of hormonally induced neoplastic transformation – particularly by estrogens – via the metabolic generation of reactive intermediates (25, 27, 101, 102). Moreover, the binding of a variety of putative reactive intermediates of hormones to cellular macromolecules, proteins, and nucleic acids have been proposed to be an early event during tumorigenesis, similar to the molecular events known to occur in carcinogenesis by nonhormone chemical agents. However, experimental data from other laboratories (*e.g.*, 28, 103) clearly indicate a number of critical inconsistencies, negating a significant role for metabolic activation in hormone-induced tumorigenesis. Therefore, the conclusion is compelling that hormones elicit the processes of tumorigenesis by nongenotoxic or epigenetic mechanisms. Accordingly, hormones are considered to be agents which do not have a direct interaction with the genetic material – in the sense as genotoxic carcinogens do – but are nevertheless capable of bringing about inheritable changes in the structure of the genetic material via a multistep process, leading eventually to the appearance of tumors.

Results obtained in numerous experimental models of hormonal carcinogenesis provide growing evidence that hormone-induced cell proliferation plays a critical role in hormone-initiated carcinogenesis (55, 65, 66, 72, 73, 83, 94, 99, 103, 104). For instance, estrogen-driven kidney or liver cell damage leads to estrogen-dependent regenerative or reparative hyperplasia (53, 103). A consequence of hormone-driven cytotoxicity and cell proliferation, at least in the hamster kidney, is aneuploidy and subsequent chromosomal abnormalities (104); this is schematically depicted in Figure 1. Alternatively, possibly in other experimental models, hormones may increase the frequency of cell replication and thus enhance the probability of error in DNA copying. All the above effects are generated by the multiple interactions of hormones with cellular receptors. The end result of interactions with receptors is influence upon DNA and upon the controls of gene expression. Moreover, it is even possible that direct modulating effects of steroid hormones on the signal transduction pathways of peptide hormones exist — all representing mechanistic modalities whereby the above cellular effects may be generated (*see* Section I above and Chapters 5 and 14 for pertinent discussion of cellular control systems).

Abbreviations and Trade Names Used in Sections I and II: ACTH, adrenocorticotropic hormone (corticotropin); ADH, antidiuretic hormone (also known as vasopressin, VP); ANF, α-naphthoflavone; ANP, atrial natriuretic peptide; 5'-AMP, adenosine monophosphate; cAMP, cyclic adenosine monophosphate; CG, chorionic gonadotropin; CRH, corticotropin (ACTH)-releasing hormone; CS, chorionic somatomammotropin; CSF, colony-stimulating factor; CT, calcitonin; DES, diethylstilbestrol; 1,25-DHCC, 1,25-dihydroxycholecalciferol; DHT, 5α-dihydrotestosterone; E_1, estrone; E_2, 17β-estradiol; E_3, estriol; EE, ethinylestradiol; EGF, epidermal growth factor; ER, estrogen receptor; FGF, fibroblast growth factor; FSH, follicle-stimulating hormone; GH, growth hormone (somatotropin); GHBP, growth hormone-binding protein; GHRH, growth hormone–releasing hormone; GnRH, gonadotropin-releasing hormone (also known as LHRH); IGF-I, II, insulin-like growth factors; LH, luteinizing hormone; LHRH, LH-releasing hormone (also known as GnRH); LPH, lipotropin; Moxestrol: 11β-methoxyethinylestradiol; MSH, melanocyte-stimulating hormone; MTV, mammary tumor virus; NGF, nerve growth factor; P, progesterone; PDGF, platelet-derived growth factor; PIF, prolactin-inhibiting factor (dopamine); PR, progesterone receptor; PRL, prolactin; PTH, parathyroid hormone ("parathormone"); SRIF, somatotropin (GH)-release-inhibiting factor (also known as somatostatin); T, testosterone; T_3, T_4, thyroid hormones; TSH, thyroid-stimulating hormone (thyrotropin); TRH, thyrotropin (TSH)-releasing hormone.

REFERENCES

1. Beatson, G. T.: *Lancet* **2**, 104 (1898).
2. Loeb, L.: *J. Med. Res.* **40**, 477 (1919).
3. Lacassagne, A.: *C. R. Acad. Sci.* **195**, 630 (1932).
4. Gardner, W. U., Allen, E., and Smith, G. M.: *JAMA* **110**, 1182 (1938).
5. Gardner, W. U.: *Cancer Res.* **1**, 345 (1941).
6. Gardner, W. U., Dougherty, T. F., and Williams, W. L.: *Cancer Res.* **4**, 73 (1944).
7. Nelson, W. O.: *Am. J. Physiol.* **133**, 398 (1941).
8. Nelson, W. O.: *Yale J. Biol. Med.* **17**, 217 (1944).
9. Shimkin, M. B., and Grady, H. G.: *J. Natl. Cancer Inst.* **2**, 55 (1941).
10. Biskind, M. S., and Biskind, G. S.: *Proc. Soc. Exptl. Biol. Med.* **55**, 176 (1944).
11. Biskind, G. S., and Biskind, M. S.: *Am. J. Clin. Pathol.* **19**, 501 (1949).
12. Zondek, B.: *Lancet* **227**, 356 (1934).
13. Li, M. H., and Gardner, W. U.: *Cancer Res.* **7**, 549 (1947).
14. Peckham, B. M., and Greene, R. R.: *Cancer Res.* **12**, 654 (1952).
15. Biskind, M. S., and Biskind, G. S.: *Proc. Soc. Exptl. Biol. Med.* **59**, 4 (1945).

16. Twombley, G. H., Meisel, D., and Stout, A. P.: *Cancer* **2**, 884 (1949).
17. Jones, A.: *Br. J. Cancer* **9**, 640 (1955).
18. Woolley, G. W., Fekete, E., and Little, C. C.: *Proc. Natl. Acad. Sci. U.S.A.* **25**, 277 (1939).
19. Woolley, G. W.: *Cancer Res.* **10**, 250 (1950).
20. Woolley, G. W., Dickie, M. M., and Little, C. C.: *Cancer Res.* **12**, 142 (1952).
21. Woolley, G. W., and Little, C. C.: *Cancer Res.* **5**, 211 (1945).
22. Mühlbock, O., and Boot, L. M.: The Mechanism of Hormonal Carcinogenesis. *In* "Carcinogenesis: Mechanisms of Action" (G. E. W. Wolstenholme and M. O'Connor, eds.). Churchill, London, 1959, p. 83.
23. Kirkman, H.: Estrogen-Induced Tumor of the Kidney in the Syrian Hamster. *Natl. Cancer Inst. Monogr.* **1**, 1 (1959).
24. Kirkman, H., and Algard, F. T.: Spontaneous and Nonviral-Induced Neoplasms. *In* "The Golden Hamster, Its Biology and Use in Medical Research" (R. A. Hoffman, R. Robinson, and H. Magalhaes, eds.), Chapt. 17. Iowa State Univ. Press, Ames, Iowa, 1968, p. 227.
25. Li, J. J., and Li, S. A.: *Arch. Toxicol.* **55**, 110 (1984).
26. Li, S. A., Li, J. J., and Villee, C. A.: *Ann. N.Y. Acad. Sci.* **286**, 369 (1977).
27. Li, J. J., and Li, S. A.: *Federation Proc.* **46**, 1858 (1987).
28. Li, J. J. and Li, S. A.: *Endocrine Rev.* **11**, 524 (1990).
29. Pour, P., Althoff, J., Salmasi, S. Z., and Stephen, K.: *J. Natl. Cancer Inst.* **56**, 949 (1976).
30. Pour, P., Althoff, J., Salmasi, S. Z., and Stephen, K.: *J. Natl. Cancer Inst.* **63**, 797 (1979).
31. Reznik-Schuler, H.: *J. Natl. Cancer Inst.* **62**, 1083 (1979).
32. Li, S. A., and Li, J. J.: Unpublished results.
33. Li, J. J., Cuthbertson, T. L., and Li, S. A.: *J. Natl. Cancer Inst.* **64**, 795 (1980).
34. Li, S. A., and Li, J. J.: Metabolism of Moxestrol in the Hamster Kidney: Significance for Estrogen Carcinogenesis. *In* "Hormonal Carcinogenesis" (J. J. Li, S. Nandi, and S. A. Li, eds.). Springer-Verlag, New York, 1992, p. 110.
35. Horning, E. S., and Whittick, J. W.: *Br. J. Cancer* **8**, 451 (1954).
36. Llombart-Bosch, A., and Peydro, A.: *Eur. J. Cancer* **11**, 403 (1975).
37. Hacker, H. J., Bannasch, P., and Liehr, J. G.: *Cancer Res.* **48**, 971 (1988).
38. Kirkman, H., and Bacon, R. L.: *Cancer Res.* **10**, 122 (1950).
39. Dodge, A. H., and Kirkman, H.: *Proc. Am. Assoc. Cancer Res.* **22**, 134 (1981).
40. Gonzalez, A., Oberley, T. D., and Li, J. J.: *Cancer Res.* **49**, 1020 (1989).
41. Li, J. J., and Li, S. A.: *Endocrinology* **108**, 1751 (1981).
42. Oberley, T. D., Pugh, T. D., Gonzalez, A., Goldfarb, S., Li, S. A., and Li, J. J.: *Proc. Natl. Acad. Sci. U.S.A.* **86**, 2107 (1989).
43. Gibson, J. P., Newberne, J. W., Kuhir, W. L., and Elsea, J. R.: *Toxicol. Appl. Pharmacol.* **11**, 489 (1967).
44. Schuppler, J., and Gunzel, P.: *Arch. Toxicol., Suppl.* **2**, 181 (1979).
45. Barrows, G. H., Christopherson, W. M., and Drill, V. A.: *J. Toxicol. Environ. Health* **3**, 219 (1977).
46. Heston, W. E., Vialraleis, G., and Desmukes, B.: *J. Natl. Cancer Inst.* **51**, 209 (1973).
47. El-Etreby, M. F.: Influence of Contraceptive Steroids on Tumor Development in Experimental Animals and Man: A Short Review. *In* "Pharmacological Modulation of Steroid Action" (E. Genazzani, F. Di Carlo, and W. I. P. Mainwaring, eds.). Raven Press, New York, 1980, p. 239.
48. Report by the Committee on Safety of Medicine: "Carcinogenicity Testing of Oral Contraceptives". Her Majesty's Stationery Office, London, 1972.
49. Schardein, J. L., Kaump, J. L., Woosley, E. T., and Jellems, M. M.: *Toxicol. Appl. Pharmacol.* **16**, 10 (1970).
50. Schardein, J. L.: *J. Toxicol. Environ. Health* **6**, 885 (1980).
51. Higashi, S., Tomita, T., Mizumoto, R., and Nakakaki, K.: *Gann* **71**, 576 (1980).
52. Poel, W. E.: *Science* **154**, 402 (1966).
53. Schardein, J. L.: *J. Toxicol. Environ. Health* **6**, 895 (1980).
54. Sumi, C., Yokoro, K., and Matsushima, R.: *J. Natl. Cancer Inst.* **70**, 937 (1983).
55. Coe, J. E., Ishak, K. G., and Ross, M. J.: *Hepatology* **11**, 570 (1990).
56. Coe, J. E., Ishak, K. G., Ward, J. M., and Ross, M. J.: *Proc. Natl. Acad. Sci. U.S.A.* **89**, 1085 (1992).
57. Li, S. A., and Li, J. J.: *J. Steroid Biochem.* **15**, 387 (1981).
58. Li, J. J., and Li, S. A.: *J. Natl. Cancer Inst.* **73**, 543 (1984).
59. Li, J. J., Kirkman, H., and Li, S. A.: Synthetic Estrogens and Liver Cancer: Risk Analysis of Animal and Human Data. *In* "Hormonal Carcinogenesis" (J. J. Li, S. Nandi, and S. A. Li, eds.). Springer-Verlag, New York, 1992, p. 227.
60. Pour, P., Knoch, N., Greiser, E., Mohr, U., Althoff, J., and Cardesa, A.: *J. Natl. Cancer Inst.* **56**, 931 (1976).
61. Noble, R. L.: *Int. Rev. Exp. Pathol.* **23**, 113 (1982).

62. Pollard, M., Snyder, D. L., and Lochert, P. H.: *Prostate* **10**, 325 (1987).
63. Noble, R. L.: *Cancer Res.* **40**, 3551 (1980).
64. Drago, J. R.: *Anticancer Res.* **4**, 255 (1984).
65. Leav, I., Ho, S.-M., Ofner, P., Merk, F. B., Kwan, P. W. L., and Damassa, D.: *J. Natl. Cancer Inst.* **80**, 1045 (1988).
66. Bruchovsky, N., and Lesser, B.: *Adv. Sex Hormone Res.* **2**, 1 (1976).
67. Ofner, P., Bosland, M. C., and Vena, R. L.: *Toxicol. Appl. Pharmacol.* **112**, 300 (1992).
68. Newbold, R. R., Bullock, B. C., and McLachlan, J. A.: *Proc. Am. Assoc. Cancer Res.* **29**, 239 (1988).
69. Leav, I., Merk, F. B., Ofner, P., Goodrich, G., Kwan, P. W. L., Stein, B. M., Sav, M., and Sten, W. E.: *Am. J. Pathol.* **93**, 69 (1978).
70. Mawhinney, M. G., and Neubauer, B. L.: *Invest. Urol.* **16**, 409 (1979).
71. Merk, F. B., Warhol, M. H., Kwan, P. W. L., Leav, I., Alroy, J., Ofner, P., and Pinkus, G. S.: *Lab. Invest.* **54**, 442 (1986).
72. Leav, I., Merk, F. B., Kwan, P. W. L., and Ho, S.-M.: *Prostate* **15**, 23 (1989).
73. Ho, S.-M., Yu, M., Leav, I., and Viccione, T.: The Conjoint Action of Androgens and Estrogens in the Induction of Proliferative Lesions in the Rat Prostate. *In* "Hormonal Carcinogenesis" (J. J. Li, S. Nandi, and S. A. Li, eds.). Springer-Verlag, New York, 1992, p. 18.
74. Andervont, H. B., Shimkin, M. B., and Canter, H. Y.: *J. Natl. Cancer Inst.* **18**, 1 (1957).
75. Andervont, H. B., Shimkin, M. B., and Canter, H. Y.: *J. Natl. Cancer Inst.* **25**, 1069 (1960).
76. Huseby, R. A.: *J. Toxicol. Environ. Health Suppl.* **1**, 177 (1976).
77. Huseby, R. A.: Hormonal Factors in Relation to Cancer. *In* "Environment and Cancer" (24th Symp. on Fundam. Cancer Res., M. D. Anderson Hosp. and Tumor Inst.). Williams & Wilkins, Baltimore, Maryland, 1972, p. 372.
78. Samuels, L. T., Short, J. G., and Huseby, R. A.: *Acta Endocrinol.* **45**, 487 (1964).
79. Samuels, L. T., Uchikawa, T., Zain-ul-Abedin, M., and Huseby, R. A.: *Endocrinology* **85**, 96 (1969).
80. Uchikawa, T., Huseby, R. A., Zain-ul-Abedin, M., and Samuels, L. T.: *J. Natl. Cancer Inst.* **45**, 525 (1970).
81. Kotoh, K., Huseby, R. A., Baldi, A., and Samuels, L. T.: *Cancer Res.* **33**, 1247 (1973).
82. Sato, B., Huseby, R. A., and Samuels, L. T.: Estrogen Receptor Systems in Testes of Strains of Mice with High and Low Incidence of Estrogen-Induced Leydig Cell Tumor. *Proc. Endocr. Soc. Abstr. No.* **205**, 1976.
83. Huseby, R. A., and Samuels, L. T.: *J. Natl. Cancer Inst.* **58**, 1047 (1977).
84. Huseby, R. A.: *Cancer Res.* **40**, 1006 (1980).
85. Lacassagne, A.: *Am. J. Cancer* **28**, 735 (1936).
86. Gass, G. H., Brown, J., and Okey, A. B.: *J. Natl. Cancer Inst.* **53**, 1363 (1974).
87. Rudali, G., Apiou, F., and Muel, B.: *Eur. J. Cancer* **11**, 39 (1975).
88. El-Etreby, M. F.: *Trends Pharmacol. Sci.* **1**, 362 (1980).
89. Li, J. J., and Nandi, S.: Hormones and Carcinogenesis: Laboratory Studies. *In* "Principles and Practice of Endocrinology and Metabolism" (K. L. Becker, ed.). Lippincott, New York, 1990, p. 1643.
90. Cutts, J. H., and Noble, R. L.: *Cancer Res.* **24**, 1116 (1964).
91. Riviere, M. -R., Chouroulinkov, I., and Guerin, M.: *C. R. Soc. Biol.* **155**, 2102 (1961).
92. Kwaplen, R. P., Giles, R. C., Gell, R. G., and Casey, H. W.: *J. Natl. Cancer Inst.* **65**, 137 (1980).
93. Griffiths, C. T.: *Surgical Forum* **14**, 399 (1963).
94. Hertz, R.: *J. Steroid Biochem.* **11**, 435 (1979).
95. Gardner, W. U.: *Adv. Cancer Res.* **1**, 173 (1953).
96. Lingemann, C. H.: Hormones and Hormonomimetic Compounds in the Etiology of Cancer. *In* "Carcinogenic Hormones" (C. H. Lingemann, ed.). Springer-Verlag, New York, 1978, p. 1.
97. Highman, B., Greeman, D. L., Norvell, M. J., Farmer, J., and Shellenberger, T. E.: *J. Environ. Pathol. Toxicol.* **4**, 81 (1980).
98. McClure, H. M., and Graham, C. E.: *Lab. Anim. Sci.* **23**, 493 (1973).
99. Newbold, R. R., Bullock, B. C., and McLachlan, J. A.: *Cancer Res.* **50**, 7677 (1990).
100. Leavitt, W. W., Evans, R. W., and Hendry, W. J. III.: Etiology of DES-Induced Uterine Tumors in Syrian Hamsters. *In* "Hormones and Cancer" (W. W. Leavitt, ed.). Plenum, New York, 1982, p. 63.
101. Metzler, M.: *Arch. Toxicol.* **55**, 104 (1984).
102. Gladek, A., and Liehr, J. G.: *J. Biol. Chem.* **264**, 16847 (1989).
103. Li, J. J. and Li, S. A.: Estrogen Carcinogenesis in the Hamster Kidney: A Hormone-Driven Multistep Process. *In* "Cellular and Molecular Mechanisms of Hormonal Carcinogenesis: Environmental Influences" (J. Huff, J. Boyd, and J. C. Barrett, eds.). Wiley-Liss, Philadelphia, 1994. In press.
104. Li, J. J., Gonzalez, A., Banerjee, S., Banerjee, S. K., and Li, S. A.: Estrogen Carcinogenesis in the Hamster Kidney. Role of Cytotoxicity and Cell Proliferation. *Environ. Health Perspect.* **101** (Suppl. 5), 259 (1993).
105. Lipschutz, A., Iglesias, R., Pamosevick, V., and Salinas, S.: *Br. J. Cancer* **21**, 153 (1967).

106. IARC: "Sex Hormones", IARC Monogr. Vol. 6. International Agency for Research on Cancer, Lyon, France, 1974.
107. Kirkman, H.: Tumors Induced by Estrogen and Androgen/Estrogen in the Syrian Hamster. Cold Spring Harbor Conferences on Cell Proliferation, Vol. 9: "Growth of Cells in Hormonally Defined Media". Cold Spring Harbor Laboratory, Cold Spring Harbor, New York, 1982, p. 3.
108. Jull, J. W.: *J. Pathol. Bacteriol.* **68**, 547 (1954).
109. Mühlbock, O.: *Neoplasma* **10**, 337 (1963).
110. Cutts, J. H.: *Cancer Res.* **24**, 1124 (1964).
111. Jacobi, J., Lloyd, H. M., and Mears, J. D.: *Hormone Metab. Res.* **7**, 228 (1975).
112. Vasquez-Lopez, E.: *J. Pathol. Bacteriol.* **56**, 1 (1944).
113. Kirkman, H., and Algard, F. T.: *Cancer Res.* **25**, 141 (1965).
114. Kirkman, H., and Algard, F. T.: *Cancer Res.* **30**, 794 (1970).
115. Kirkman, H., and Algard, F. T.: *Cancer Res.* **24**, 1569 (1964).
116. Jabara, A.: *Austral. J. Exptl. Biol. Med. Sci.* **40**, 139 (1962).

EDITORS' ADDITION

A timeless review on the role of endocrine imbalance

Crile, G., Jr.: "A Speculative Review on the Role of Endocrine Imbalances in the Genesis of Certain Cancers and Degenerative Diseases." *J. Natl. Cancer Inst.* **20**, 229–243 (1958).

Effect of Hormones on Carcinogenesis by Nonhormone Chemical Agents[1]

An early clue that the endocrine system has a significant influence on the induction of tumors by nonhormone chemical agents came from the study of Korteweg and Thomas (1) in 1939. They found that hypophysectomy increases the latent period of skin tumor induction in mice by epithelial application of benzo[a]pyrene (BaP) (108 to 184 days in operated mice *versus* 44 to 100 days in intact mice). However, Smith *et al.* (2) reported 3 years later that hypophysectomy has little or no effect on carcinogenesis by *subcutaneous* administration. Later results in the 1950s lent credence to the above divergent findings of Korteweg and Thomas (1) and Smith *et al.* (2). Thus, pituitary dwarf mice (which lack growth hormone [GH] and some other pituitary hormones) respond poorly to skin tumor induction by 3-methylcholanthrene (3-MC) (3), but respond normally to carcinogenesis by subcutaneous administration of this compound (4, 5).

Moreover, Shay *et al.* (6) noted in 1949 that, following gastric instillation of 3-MC to rats, the highest incidence of mammary adenocarcinomas occurred in intact females and the lowest in ovariectomized females as well as in males. Bielschowsky (7) observed as early as 1947 the opposite effects of gestation and lactation on 2-acetylaminofluorene (2-AAF)–induced mammary tumorigenesis in rats. In the early 1950s it was discovered that the rat mammary gland is a target tissue for polycyclic aromatic hydrocarbon-induced tumorigenesis, and E_2 was found to reduce the latency period and markedly increase the incidence of mammary tumors induced in the rat by intravenously given 7,12-dimethylbenz[a]anthracene (DMBA) (8). All these early findings led to an era of many investigations on the effects of hormonal status and endocrine manipulations — generating different hormonal steady-states or types of hormonal imbalance — on carcinogenesis by nonhormone chemical agents in different tissues.

I. ENHANCEMENT OF CHEMICAL CARCINOGENESIS BY HORMONES[2,3]

A. Mammary Gland

The emergence and growth of mammary tumors induced by the three carcinogens, 3-MC, DMBA, and *N*-methyl-*N*-nitrosourea (MNU) require both anterior pituitary and

---

[1] Abbreviations and trade names used in this section are given on p. 441.

[2] An overview of enhancement of chemical carcinogenesis by steroid and protein/peptide hormones is given in Table 1.

[3] *Editors' Note*: Although in the greater part of the recent literature on the modulation of chemical carcinogenesis by hormones the term "enhancement" as distinct from "promotion"

TABLE 1. **Enhancement of Chemical Carcinogenesis by Steroid and Protein Hormones**

Carcinogen	Hormone	Site	Species	Ref.
DBA	Estrone	Mammary gland	Mice	205,206
3-MC	Estrone	Mammary gland	Mice	207
	Progesterone	Mammary gland	Mice	207
	E_2 + progesterone	Mammary gland	Rat	208
2-AAF	Progesterone	Mammary gland	Rat	209
MNU	E_2 + progesterone	Mammary gland	Rat	13,210
DMBA	Insulin	Mammary gland	Rat	60–62
	E_2	Mammary gland	Rat	20,23
	Prolactin	Mammary gland	Rat	15,20,23–26
	Progesterone	Mammary gland	Rat	48–50
N-2-FDA	Progesterone	Liver	Rat	74
	Testosterone	Liver	Rat	71
	Thyroxine + testosterone	Liver	Rat	71
2-AAF	Testosterone	Liver	Rat	72
	E_2	Liver	Rat	211
DEN	EE, DES	Liver	Rat	78,79
Urethan	Testosterone (?)	Liver	Mice	212
DMBA	E_2	Liver	Mice	91
	E_2 (?)	Skin	Mice	98
3-MC	E_2	Skin	Mice	96
	Growth hormone	Skin	Mice	99
DBN, BHBN	DES	Bladder	Rat	108
BHBN	Testosterone	Bladder	Mice	102
DMAB	EE	Prostate	Rat	113
MNU	Testosterone	Prostate	Rat	111
3-MC	DES	Uterus	Mice	115
	Progesterone	Uterus	Mice	115
Hydrazine SO$_4$	Progesterone (?)	Lung	Mice	117
	E_2 (?)	Lung	Mice	117
DMBA	Testosterone	Salivary gland	Rat	118
Azaserine	Testosterone (?)	Pancreas	Rat	123

ovarian hormones. Early studies (9, 10) have shown that hypophysectomy inhibits the induction of both 3-MC- and DMBA-induced rat mammary carcinomas. The more recently discovered MNU-induced rat mammary tumors also exhibit endocrine dependence (11–13). The pituitary hormone most implicated in these hormone effects is prolactin (PRL) (14, 15). This has been clearly confirmed by numerous studies employing ergot alkaloids, which inhibit PRL secretion (16–19). Moreover, administration of this pituitary peptide stimulates tumor growth in intact, ovariectomized, adrenalectomized, and hypophysectomized rats as well as in rats subjected to any combination of these endocrine-depressing manipulations (20–24). Ovarian hormones appear to be necessary, however, to support mammary gland and tumor growth even when elevated serum PRL levels are evident (25, 26). A direct mitogenic effect of PRL in both normal mammary gland and in DMBA-induced rat mammary carcinoma has also been shown in organ and cell culture (27–30).

Consistent with the above, rat strains which are relatively refractory to DMBA-induced mammary gland carcinogenesis, such as the Long–Evans rat, exhibit indeed low serum PRL levels (31–33). Moreover, most Sprague–Dawley rat strains, which are

has been used, it is the Editors' view that this distinction is so far not clearly supported by molecular mechanistic evidence on endocrine hormone–induced cellular events mediated via the signal transduction pathways and steroid receptors [*cf.*, *e.g.*, Chapter 5 (Section I) and Chapter 14].

susceptible to these carcinogens, have high serum PRL levels. Yet although the mammary gland and carcinogen-induced rat mammary tumor possess specific membrane receptors for PRL (34), there is a poor correlation between the level of PRL binding and PRL-induced growth (35). In contrast to PRL, administration of growth hormone to rats bearing DMBA-induced mammary tumors has little or no effect on growth of these carcinomas (21, 36). While some other anterior pituitary hormones (*e.g.*, gonadotropins, TSH, ACTH) can affect growth and progression of rat mammary tumors in culture, there is little evidence for the direct effect of these pituitary hormones on tumor growth *in vivo*. However, they appear to elicit their effects by modulating the hormone secretion of their respective peripheral target glands (30).

Consistent with the early observations of Shay *et al.* (6) using 3-MC, Heimann *et al.* (37) found that ovariectomy of rats either prior to or shortly after single gastric instillation with DMBA dramatically suppresses the appearance of rat mammary tumors. It is clear that ovarian steroids are pertinent factors for carcinogen-induced mammary tumorigenesis. Stimulation of mammary tumorigenesis can be accomplished by even moderate doses of estrogen, either natural or synthetic (38, 39). However, the growth-promoting effects of estrogen on DMBA-induced rat mammary tumors is dependent upon a functional pituitary gland (40), suggesting that estrogen enhancement of tumor growth is in part mediated through estrogen-stimulated PRL secretion by the anterior pituitary.

Although it seems evident that not all estrogen effects on the mammary gland are a consequence of modulation of anterior pituitary secretion (such as in the case of PRL), it does remain puzzling that a stimulatory effect by estrogens is rarely detected *in vitro*, either in normal mammary gland or in carcinogen-induced mammary tumor, as assessed by the parameters of cell proliferation and/or DNA synthesis (41–43). It is well established that the mammary gland and carcinogen-induced mammary tumors exhibit significant quantities of estrogen receptors (44, 45). Moreover, there appears to be a good correlation between estrogen receptor levels of carcinogen-induced rat mammary tumors and neoplastic growth (23, 46, 47).

Another ovarian steroid, which appears pertinent to the emergence and growth of these carcinogen-induced rat mammary neoplasms, is progesterone. When moderate dose levels of progesterone are given at the time or after carcinogen exposure, mammary tumorigenesis is enhanced in either intact or ovariectomized rats (48–50). It has been observed that mammary tumor growth is most effectively stimulated when the tumor is exposed to progesterone and estrogen in combination (23, 51). Additionally, medroxyprogesterone acetate, the synthetic progestin, stimulates the growth of DMBA-induced mammary carcinomas in intact rats (52).

Progesterone is mitogenic in mammary gland cell and organ culture (27) and is capable of enhancing DNA synthesis in DMBA-induced rat mammary tumors (28, 48). The results of Yoshida *et al.* (53) suggest that it is unlikely that the progesterone-induced proliferative effects on the mammary gland are a consequence of its metabolic conversion to estrogen. Specific progesterone receptors in rodent mammary glands and carcinogen-induced mammary tumors have been widely described (*e.g.*, 51, 54–58). Administration of either PRL and/or estrogen restores tumors growth and progesterone receptor levels (23, 47). Therefore, the effect of estrogen on the murine mammary gland appears to be largely, although perhaps not entirely, indirect. Estrogen, by increasing PRL secretion in the anterior pituitary and progesterone receptor levels in the mammary gland, facilitates the availability of these two mitogenic agents for enhancing mammary gland cell proliferation. It should be borne in mind that estrogens may also have pertinent actions on the mammary gland stromal elements, not present in most *in vitro* culture systems. Unlike DMBA- or 3-MC-induced mammary tumors, MNU-induced mammary carcinomas appear to be more responsive to estrogen and growth hormone and relatively less responsive to PRL (59). The differential hormonal responses among these carcinogen-induced mammary neoplasms may serve to facilitate understanding of the role of estrogens in the enhancement of mammary tumorigenesis.

Insulin was found to have a direct growth-stimulating effect on DMBA-induced mammary tumor cells (60). Insulin given to intact rats enhances mammary tumor growth and is able to stimulate tumor growth in hypophysectomized rats (61, 62). Estrogen administration fails to prevent mammary tumor regression produced by alloxan diabetes (61).

B. Liver

Although the liver is generally not considered to be a target tissue for hormones, particularly for sex hormones, this view needs to be revised, since earlier and recent studies have amply shown that the liver exhibits considerable response to experimental endocrine manipulations (63–82).

It has been established that pituitary and/or gonadal steroids have a profound influence on liver tumorigenesis induced by a variety of potent carcinogens, including 2-AAF, 3'-methyl-4-dimethylaminoazobenzene (3'-Me-DAB), and diethylnitrosamine (DEN). Early studies indicated that certain carcinogenic azo dyes induce liver neoplasms more readily in female than in male mice. However, using 2-AAF, male rats were found markedly more susceptible to the development of hepatomas than females, exhibiting higher incidence and shorter latency periods (63). Around 1960, it was established that either hypophysectomy or adrenalectomy severely reduces liver tumor incidence induced by 2-AAF and related compounds (64, 66–70). Employing the Furth transplantable pituitary tumor, MtT/F_4, as a source of pituitary hormones, a number of reports clearly demonstrated that 2-AAF- or N-OH-2-AAF-induced hepatocarcinogenesis was potentiated (67–69). Since the MtT/F_4 tumor secretes ACTH, GH, and PRL, studies using individual hormones showed that GH, but not ACTH, promotes liver tumorigenesis by 2-AAF (66, 70). On the other hand, thyroidectomy was found to have an adverse effect on 2-AAF initiation of liver carcinogenesis, resulting in a strong inhibitory effect (71). Yet both thyroid hormones and testosterone were found to be necessary to restore the capacity for liver tumorigenesis in thyroidectomized rats exposed to 2-AAF (71).

Consistent with early studies that castration decreases liver tumor incidence in 2-AAF-fed male rats, it was subsequently shown that testosterone administration results in higher levels of hepatic tumor incidence. However, testosterone administered alone is ineffective in promoting hepatic carcinogenesis in either hypophysectomized or thyroidectomized animals receiving 2-AAF (72). On the other hand, adrenalectomy inhibits, whereas testosterone enhances liver tumorigenesis in rats fed N-2-fluorenyldiacetamide (N-2-FDA) (73). Progesterone, probably because of its anabolic–androgenic properties, increases the incidence of hepatocellular carcinomas in intact and castrated male as well as ovariectomized female rats when administered simultaneously with N-2-FDA (74). In intact male rats, cortisone also has a marked enhancing effect on 2-AAF hepatocarcinogenesis (73). Striking sex-dependent differences in hepatocarcinogenesis were also reported in mice and rats given dimethylnitrosamine (DMN) (75, 76), showing predominantly higher carcinogenicity in males.

More recent studies show a strong enhancing effect of estrogens, particularly the synthetic estrogen EE, in hepatocarcinogenesis. Treatment of ovariectomized rats with E_2 enhances the appearance of liver foci and nodules and of frank liver carcinomas in rats initiated with N-nitrosomorpholine (77). A subsequent investigation reported that EE or DES enhances the formation of hyperplastic nodules in rats exposed to DEN (78, 79). Consistent with this is the finding that DEN-initiated rats fed diets containing mestranol and norethynodrel have a higher frequency of liver γ-glutamyl transferase (GGT) foci, leading to the conclusion that these hormonal agents promote the appearance of preneoplastic hepatic foci (80). It is of interest that EE and mestranol do enhance DEN-induced hepatocarcinogenesis, whereas the naturally occurring estrogens, E_1, E_2, and estriol, do not when administered after the initiating agent (81). These results are similar to those found with EE/α-naphthoflavone–induced hepatocellular carcinomas in male Syrian hamsters which are unresponsive to tumor induction by E_1 and E_2 (82).

2,3,7,8-Tetrachlorodibenzo-*p*-dioxin (TCDD), which is a fairly potent hepatocarcinogen in intact Sprague–Dawley rats, is much less active in ovariectomized animals (83). That ovarian hormones have a promoting effect on the hepatocarcinogenic effect of TCDD is consistent with the earlier findings (84) that ovarian hormones enhance the TCDD-mediated increases in cell proliferation and preneoplastic foci in a two-stage model of hepatocarcinogenesis. Interestingly, in the lung, ovarian hormones appear to have the opposite effect. While spontaneous lung tumors are very rare in Sprague–Dawley rats, a 10% TCDD-induced lung tumor incidence was seen in ovariectomized rats against none in the controls (83).

C. Ovary

DMBA is the most potent carcinogen to induce granulosa cell ovarian tumors in mice (85–88). Overstimulation of the ovaries with gonadotrophic hormones appears necessary for ovarian tumorigenesis; tumorigenesis is supported by elevated levels of these hormones (89, 90). This view is further supported by the finding that when pregnant mice are given E_2 (and the offspring are thus neonatally exposed to the hormone) acceleration of ovarian granulosa cell tumor induction by DMBA is noted in the offspring (91). Under these circumstances, both plasma FSH and LH levels are significantly elevated.

Interestingly, both DHEA and testosterone significantly increase spontaneous ovarian tumor incidence in SWXJ-9 mice (92). In the same study, DHEA treatment was found to increase the FSH and PRL levels; therefore, it may be partially responsible for increasing the spontaneous ovarian tumor incidence in this strain. This finding, however, does not rule out a direct role of androgens in the ovary, since these male hormones are known to generate polycystic ovarian disease in rodents (93, 94).

D. Epidermis

A variety of endocrine manipulations can affect skin tumor induction by DMBA and 3-MC (alone or promoted with croton oil/phorbol esters) in male and female rodents (95–99). Female mice usually develop fewer skin papillomas than males (98). Ovariectomy increases the tumor incidence in female mice and the initiation of skin tumors in these rodents was found to be dependent on the stage of the estrous cycle; higher yields of skin papillomas were observed when DMBA was applied during diestrus. This suggested already a number of years ago that ovarian hormones are inhibitory toward the tumorigenic process. On the other hand, administration of estradiol benzoate to female mice was found to increase the incidence of epidermal tumors in female, but not in male, gonadectomized and intact mice initiated with 3-MC (96). GH administered prior to or after initiation with 3-MC enhances epidermal tumorigenesis in mice (99). The acceleration of tumor induction was attributed to the inflammatory response of the dermis to GH.

E. Bladder

Among the over 65 *N*-nitroso compounds tested, only dibutylnitrosamine (DBN) and its hydroxylated derivative, butyl-(4-hydroxybutyl)nitrosamine (BHBN), induce bladder tumors in BD strain rats (100, 101). The sex difference in susceptibility to induction of BHBN-induced bladder tumors may be abolished either by castration of males or by treating females with testosterone (102). Sex differences in response to bladder carcinogenesis have also been noted with N-[4-(5-nitro-2-furyl)-2-thiazolyl]formamide (FANFT), 4-ethylsulfonylnaphthalene-1-sulfonamide, and 2-AAF in rats and mice (103–105). Interestingly, the former two bladder carcinogens exhibit greater susceptibility to tumor induction in females (106, 107), whereas the latter bladder carcinogen, 2-AAF, is more effective in males (which is similar to the results obtained with DBN and BHBN). On the other hand, neonatal exposure of castrated male rats to DES increases the incidence of BHBN-induced urinary bladder tumors (108). However, when DES was administered to adult male rats concomitantly with or after BHBN treatment, this synthetic estrogen was found inhibitory (108). These conflicting data remain to be clarified.

F. Prostate

The most potent chemical carcinogens that induce prostatic adenocarcinomas in rats are 3,2'-dimethyl-4-aminobiphenyl (DMAB), DMBA, and MNU (109–111). Also, N-nitrosobis(2-oxopropyl)amine (NBOA) induces squamous cell carcinomas of the prostate in this species (112). A high incidence of prostatic carcinomas were induced in F344 rats exposed intermittently to EE and given DMAB after each treatment with EE (113). Following chemical castration with cyproterone acetate, testosterone was found to enhance MNU-induced, but not DMAB-induced prostatic carcinogenesis in Wistar rats (111). However, when Fischer rats were implanted with a testosterone-release source (silastic tubes containing the hormone) prior to and during DMAB administration, significant increases in prostatic carcinomas were seen in the dorsolateral prostate (113). Evidence has been presented that rats bearing MtT/F_4 tumor transplants, resulting in hyperprolactinemia and elevated GH secretion, may also promote DMAB-induced prostate carcinogenesis (114).

G. Other Organ Sites

The effect of modulation of the endocrine status upon chemical carcinogenesis induced at other organ sites such as the uterus (115), nasal cavity (116), lung (117), salivary gland (118), stomach (119), adrenal (120), thymus (121), and pancreas (122, 123) have been described.

As early as 1962, it was suggested that estrogens may potentiate the induction of uterine neoplasms by chemical carcinogens (115). In ovariectomized mice DES was found to act as a cocarcinogen with 3-MC and progesterone to increase the yield of uterine sarcomas induced by 3-MC. Ovarian steroids have also been shown to influence the induction of pulmonary tumors by hydrazine sulfate in BALB/c female mice (117). Moreover, the induction of malignant salivary gland neoplasms was increased in female rats given testosterone, in agreement with the view that hormonal determinants are involved in the relative incidences seen in males and females (118). A sex difference in gastric cancer was found in male and female rats given the carcinogen N-methyl-N'-nitro-N-nitrosoguanidine (MNNG) (119). Surprisingly, gonadectomy was observed to significantly increase the incidence of DMBA-induced adrenal cortical carcinomas in both sexes (120), suggesting the role of hormonal imbalance in tumorigenesis under these experimental conditions. Estrogens have been suggested to play a role in the development of N-nitroso-(2-hydroxypropyl)-(2-oxopropyl)amine (HPOP)-induced pancreatic ductal adenocarcinomas in hamsters (122), since a higher incidence of these tumors is found in females compared to males. On the other hand, there is evidence that E_2 may be an inhibitor and androgen a promoter in the early stage of pancreatic carcinogenesis in Fischer rats administered the carcinogen, azaserine (123).

II. INHIBITION OF CHEMICAL CARCINOGENESIS BY HORMONES[4]

The preceding discussion dealt largely with enhancement of chemical carcinogenesis by peptide/protein hormones and steroid hormones. Inherent in the concept of "hormone imbalance" as it brings about or affects the carcinogenic process is, however, the natural role of hormones to act — in certain circumstances — in opposition, so as to maintain homeostasis. It is not surprising, therefore, that some hormones are capable of suppressing carcinogen-induced tumorigenesis enhanced by other hormones as described above. In addition to hormone deprivation such as hypophysectomy or castration, other types of hormone manipulations may impede carcinogen-initiated tumorigenesis. For example, it has been broadly established that high dose levels of naturally occurring and certain synthetic estrogens inhibit the emergence and/or growth of 3-MC- or DMBA-induced rat mammary carcinomas (*e.g.*, 124–128). Similarly, when moderate or high doses of progesterone and estrogen were administered, inhibition of DMBA-induced rat mammary tumorigenesis and of the growth of the tumors was observed (124, 129). Mammary tumorigenesis is also inhibited when progesterone is given alone prior to carcinogen treatment (130, 131). Androgens, by opposing estrogen action, prevent DMBA- or 3-MC-induced mammary tumorigenesis (132–134). When 3-MC was given to either pregnant or lactating rats, a marked inhibition of mammary tumorigenesis was observed (135). The reduction in mammary tumorigenesis during lactation may be due to a loss of estrogen and/or progesterone or due to an increase in adrenocortical activity (136). The administration of moderately large amounts of glucocorticoid to rats leads to an inhibition of DMBA-induced rat mammary tumors (136, 137). The inhibition of tumorigenesis by glucocorticoids can be attributed to its anti-inflammatory properties. Neuroendocrine involvement in carcinogen-induced mammary tumorigenesis has been reported. Therefore, increasing hypothalamic dopaminergic or norepinephrine activity can reduce the growth of DMBA-induced mammary tumors (19, 138, 139). These effects are mediated mainly through the modulation of PRL secretion during carcinogen-initiated mammary tumorigenesis.

Since there is pronounced sex difference in 2-AAF-induced hepatic carcinogenesis, and since castration decreases liver tumor incidence using this hepatocarcinogen, it is expectable that ovarian hormones would have a protective role. Indeed, administration of the synthetic estrogen, DES, to either intact and castrated male rats receiving *N*-2-FDA markedly reduces both liver cirrhosis and tumor incidence (74). The opposite effect was observed with progesterone, which increases the incidence of hepatocellular carcinomas in castrated male as well as in ovariectomized female rats (74). In a study comparing the relative effectiveness of different estrogens to inhibit 4-dimethylaminoazobenzene (DAB)-induced hepatocarcinogenesis, estriol and EE produced the greatest inhibition (140).

Inhibition of DMBA-initiated and croton oil–promoted epidermal tumorigenesis in mice by glucocorticoids has been described (141). Hydrocortisone and cortisone also inhibit tumor induction by BaP, 3-MC, and DMBA, as well as tumor growth in mouse skin (95, 142–145). Similarly, induction by 3-MC of subcutaneous sarcomas in mice is also inhibited by glucocorticoids (146). On the other hand, the induction of lung tumors in rats

---

[4] A brief overview of inhibition of chemical carcinogenesis by steroid and other hormones is given in Table 2.

TABLE 2. Inhibition of Chemical Carcinogenesis by Steroid and Peptide Hormones

Carcinogen	Hormone	Site	Species	Ref.
3-MC	Thyroxine	Mammary gland	Rat	213,214
3-MC	E_1, E_2, DES	Mammary gland	Rat	124,133
DMBA	E_2 + progesterone	Mammary gland	Rat	124,129
DMBA	Enovid	Mammary gland	Rat	215,216
DMBA	Androgens	Mammary gland	Rat	132,134
MNU	Progesterone	Mammary gland	Rat	131
MNU	E_2 + progesterone	Mammary gland	Rat	210
DMBA	Glucocorticoids	Mammary gland	Rat	136
N-2-FDA	DES	Liver	Rat	74
DMBA/BaP/3-MC	Glucocorticoids	Skin	Mice	141–145
NQO	E_2	Lung	Rat	147

by 4-nitroquinoline-N-oxide (NQO) (147) is repressed by adrenalectomy or ovariectomy. In the salivary glands of male rats, low concentrations of DMBA induces twice as many sarcomas and carcinomas as in females (118); treatment with E_2 brings about a 50% reduction of these tumors in males only.

III. SOME MECHANISMS OF HORMONAL EFFECTS IN CHEMICAL CARCINOGENESIS

There are two major areas under study regarding the mechanisms involved in the enhancement (promotion) and inhibition of chemical carcinogenesis by hormones. First, hormones have a profound influence on gene expression/suppression, cell proliferation, differentiation, and growth. Second, hormones can dramatically modify the metabolism of chemical carcinogens, including the generation of reactive intermediates. It is not surprising, therefore, that hormones affect—sometimes profoundly—virtually all stages of carcinogenesis induced by nonhormone chemical agents (Figure 1).

The first category of mechanisms through which hormonal promoting effects may be mediated will not be touched upon in this chapter; however, relevant discussion may be found in Chapter 5 on "Promotion and Cocarcinogenesis". Regarding the second category, modification of the metabolism of xenobiotics by the hormonal milieu or imbalance has been abundantly established. Androgens, estrogens, progestational steroids, glucocorticoids, anabolic steroids, thyroid hormone, as well as insulin and other protein hormones, alter in various tissues the activity of mixed-function oxidase (MFO) to metabolize carcinogens and other xenobiotics (*e.g.*, 148–152 and revs. 153–156). It has been known for a number of years that a variety of MFO activities (*N*-dealkylation, *N*-oxidation, aromatic and steroid ring hydroxylation, azo linkage reduction, etc.) are higher in adult male than in adult female rats and are decreased by gonadectomy in both sexes (*e.g.*, 157–165). Consistent with this, the low MFO activity toward various substrates in sexually immature males can be increased by continuous administration of testosterone, whereas in adult males the high activity is decreased by castration (159) and then can be reestablished by testosterone administration (166); conversely, administration of testosterone to female rats increases the activity of the MFO system (157). In accord with this, in adult males estrogen administration brings about the opposite effect (157, 159, 167). Also, in contrast to testosterone, progesterone appears to manifest a differential effect, depending on the substrate studied (159, 168, 169). Booth and Gillette (170) found that the stimulation of MFO activity in female rats by testosterone derivatives parallels their anabolic activity more closely than their androgenic activity.

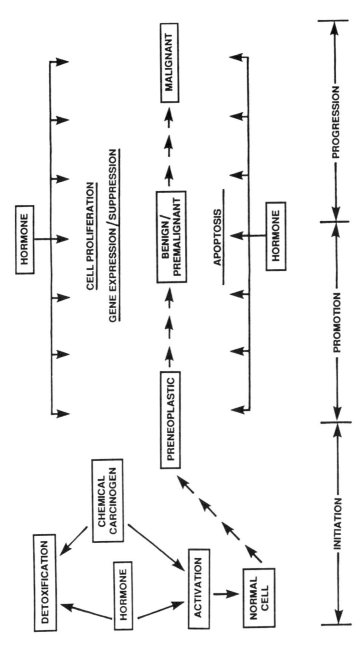

FIGURE 1. Schematic representation of the wide distribution of hormone effects in the multistage sequence of chemical carcinogenesis.

Adrenalectomy—another widely studied modification of the endocrine balance—generally lowers MFO activity toward different substrates in male as well as female rats (171, 172), and activity is restored by administration of cortisone or prednisolone (166, 171, 172). Studies by Bousquet *et al.* (173) and Driever *et al.* (174, 175) on adrenalectomized and hypophysectomized rats indicated already in the mid-1960s the regulatory function of the pituitary–adrenal axis in the control of MFO activities.

Chronic treatment with thyroxine was found to enhance or inhibit MFO activity, depending on the sex and the substrate studied (176–178). Thyroidectomy generally decreases MFO activity *in vivo*, but not *in vitro*, suggesting that the decreased body temperature in the thyroidectomized rats is responsible for the observed inhibition (179, 180).

The consequence of hormonal effects on MFO level and function is a change in the production of proximate/ultimate carcinogenic metabolite(s). This is exemplified by two instances. The first example comes from a series of studies which explored the endocrine effects on 2-AAF metabolism (69, 181–184). The earlier reports described differences between male and female rats in their ability to metabolize *N*-OH-2-AAF (181). The liver of female rats has only one fifth the level of sulfotransferase activity for *N*-OH-2-AAF compared to that of the more susceptible male rats (182). Moreover, female rats excrete more total metabolites and glucosiduronic acid conjugates than do males. Therefore, to explain the increased incidence of hepatocellular carcinomas in females when exposed to *N*-OH-2-AAF *together with* pituitary hormones (69, 183, 184) it was postulated that, as a consequence of the hormone administration, elevated amounts of *N*-OH-2-AAF is maintained because of lowered conversion to other metabolites through decreased dehydroxylation and deacylation.

The second example comes from the hormonal effects observed in DMBA-induced ovarian carcinogenesis. Activation of DMBA as well as of other polycyclic aromatic hydrocarbons (PAH) by ovarian arylhydrocarbon hydroxylase (AHH) is generally regarded to be the initial activating enzymatic step of key importance in the process of ovarian carcinogenesis (185, 186). It has been shown that DMBA hydroxylase activity in the rat ovary is increased by stimulation with gonadotropins (186). The DMBA hydroxylase is most probably under the control of the *Ah* locus, which is the regulatory gene for at least 20 monooxygenase activities, including BaP AHH (187). The major gene product of the *Ah* regulatory locus is known to be a 95-kDa cytosolic protein (188, 189), the receptor for PAH-type inducers of MFOs which translocates into the nucleus where induction-specific mRNA is transcribed from DNA and subsequently translated into induction-specific proteins (rev. in 190). The relationship of this cytosolic protein to the steroid receptors (191) appears to be unclear. Since the stimulation of DMBA-hydroxylase by gonadotropin (a peptide hormone) must pass through the second messenger pathway (*see* Section 1 of this chapter), this exemplifies that the regulation of this hydroxylase as well as of other MFOs are under the control of multiple regulating modalities.

Regarding the relationship of the *Ah*-product 95-kDa cytosolic receptor to the steroid receptors, it should be pointed out that the similarities between xenobiotic (such as PAH) and steroid hydroxylases suggested that PAH and steroids are substrates for the same hydroxylating MFOs (192, 193; *see also* rev. 154). For example, like a typical cytochrome P-450–dependent MFO which metabolizes xenobiotics, steroid hydroxylation is inhibited by carbon monoxide, which inhibitory effect can be prevented by 450 mμ monochromatic light (194). Furthermore, steroids have been reported to be potent competitive inhibitors of xenobiotic-metabolizing enzymes (195). The role of rat hepatic cytochrome P-450 in steroid metabolism has been extensively reviewed (*e.g.*, 196–198) and its sex-specific isoforms as determinants of sex difference in the metabolic disposition of xenobiotics has been documented (*e.g.*, 199, 200).

Finally, other investigations give additional insights into the variety of effects underlying hormonal promotion of chemical carcinogenesis. It has been shown that EE and mestranol promote the development of GGT-positive foci and hyperplastic nodules if preceded by DMN initiation (78, 201). Interestingly, testosterone, cortisone, and dexamethasone induced more foci than did DMN alone (202). Low doses of EE or mestranol were shown to rapidly stimulate liver DNA synthesis in a dose-dependent manner (81). Furthermore, when EE was added to hepatocyte cultures, EGF receptor levels were enhanced (203) and a decreased sensitivity of hepatocytes to the growth inhibitory actions of TGFβ was observed (204).

Abbreviations and Trade Names Used in Section III: 2-AAF, 2-acetylaminofluorene; AHH, arylhydrocarbon hydroxylase; ACTH, adrenocorticotropic hormone; BHBN, butyl-(4-hydroxybutyl)nitrosamine; BaP, benzo[*a*]pyrene; DAB, 4-dimethylaminoazobenzene; DBA, dibenz[*a,h*]anthracene; DBN, dibutylnitrosamine; DEN, diethylnitrosamine; DES, diethylstilbestrol; DHEA, dehydroepiandrosterone; DMAB, 3,2'-dimethyl-4-aminobiphenyl; DMBA, 7,12-dimethylbenz[*a*]anthracene; DMN, dimethylnitrosamine; E_1, estrone; E_2, 17β-estradiol; EE, ethinylestradiol; EGF, epidermal growth factor; Enovid: mestranol + norethynodrel; FANFT, *N*-[4-(5-nitro-2-furyl)-2-thiazolyl]formamide; FSH, follicle-stimulating hormone; GGT, γ-glutamyl transferase; GH, (somatotropin) growth hormone; HPOP, *N*-nitroso-(2-hydroxypropyl)-(2-oxopropyl) amine; LH, luteinizing hormone; 3-MC, 3-methylcholanthrene; 3'-Me-DAB, 3'-methyl-4-dimethylaminoazobenzene; MFO, mixed-function oxidase(s); MNNG, *N*-methyl-*N'*-nitro-*N*-nitrosoguanidine; MNU, *N*-methyl-*N*-nitrosourea; N-2-FDA, *N*-2-fluorenyldiacetamide; NBOA, *N*-nitrosobis(2-oxopropyl)amine; NQO, 4-nitroquinoline-*N*-oxide; PAH, polycyclic aromatic hydrocarbon(s); PRL, prolactin; TCDD, 2,3,7,8-tetrachlorodibenzo-*p*-dioxin; TGFβ, transforming growth factor β; TSH, thyroid-stimulating hormone

REFERENCES

1. Korteweg, R., and Thomas, F.: *Am. J. Cancer* **37**, 36 (1939).
2. Smith, D. L., Wells, J. A., and D'Amour, F. E.: *Cancer Res.* **2**, 40 (1942).
3. Bickis, I., Estwick, R. R., and Cambell, J. S.: *Cancer* **9**, 763 (1956).
4. Bielschowsky, F., and Hall, W. H.: *Br. J. Cancer* **7**, 358 (1953).
5. Bielschowsky, F., and Bielschowsky, M.: *Br. J. Cancer* **13**, 302 (1959).
6. Shay, H., Aegerter, E. A., Gruenstein, M., and Komaroo, S. A.: *J. Natl. Cancer Inst.* **10**, 255 (1949).
7. Bielschowsky, F.: *Br. Med. Bull.* **4**, 382 (1947).
8. Geyer, R. P., Bryant, J. E., Bleisel, V. R., Pierce, E. M., and Store, F. J.: *Cancer Res.* **13**, 503 (1953).
9. Moon, H. D., Simpson, M. E., and Evans, H. M.: *Science* **116**, 331 (1952).
10. Noble, R. L., and Walters, J. H.: *Proc. Am. Assoc. Cancer Res.* **1**, 35 (1954).
11. Gullino, P. M., Pettigrew, H. M., and Grantham, F. H.: *J. Natl. Cancer Inst.* **54**, 401 (1975).
12. Rose, D. P., and Noonan, J. J.: *Eur. J. Cancer Clin. Oncol.* **17**, 1357 (1981).
13. Arafah, B. M., Finegan, H. M., Roe, J., Manni, A., and Pearson, O. H.: *Endocrinology* **111**, 584 (1982).
14. Kim, U.: *Cancer Res.* **25**, 1146 (1965).
15. Welsch, C. W., and Nagasawa, H.: *Cancer Res.* **37**, 951 (1977).
16. Henson, J. C., Waelbroeck-Van Gaver, C., and Legros, N.: *Eur. J. Cancer* **6**, 353 (1970).
17. Cassell, E. E., Meites, J., and Welsch, C. W.: *Cancer Res.* **31**, 1051 (1971).
18. Clemens, J. A., and Shaar, C. J.: *Proc. Soc. Exp. Biol. Med.* **139**, 659 (1972),
19. Nagasawa, H., and Meites, J.: *Proc. Soc. Exp. Biol. Med.* **135**, 469 (1970).
20. Talwalker, P. K., Meites, J., and Mizuno, H.: *Proc. Soc. Exp. Biol. Med.* **116**, 531 (1964).
21. Nagasawa, H., and Yanai, R.: *Int. J. Cancer* **6**, 488 (1970).
22. Welsch, C. W., Louks, G., Fox, D., and Brooks, C.: *Br. J. Cancer* **32**, 427 (1975).
23. Asselin, J., Kelley, P. A., Caron, M. G., and Labrie, F.: *Endocrinology* **101**, 666 (1977).
24. Pearson, O. H., Llerena, O., Llerena, L., Molina, A., and Butler, T.: *Trans. Assoc. Am. Physicians* **82**, 225 (1969).

25. Leung, B. S., and Sasaki, G. H.: *Endocrinology* **97,** 564 (1975).
26. Leung, B. S., Sasaki, G. H., and Leung, J. S.: *Cancer Res.* **35,** 621 (1975).
27. Imagawa, W., Bandyopadhyay, G. K., and Nandi, S.: *Endocrine Rev.* **11,** 494 (1990).
28. Pasteels, J. L., Heuson, J. C., Henson-Stennon, J., and Legros, N.: *Cancer Res.* **36,** 2162 (1976).
29. Hallowes, R. C., Rudland, P. S., Hawkins, R. A., Lewis, D. J., Bennett, D., and Durbin, H.: *Cancer Res.* **37,** 2492 (1977).
30. Rudland, P. S., Hallowes, R. C., Durbin, H., and Lewis, D.: *J. Cell Biol.* **73,** 561 (1977).
31. Boyns, A. R., Buchan, R., Cole, E. N., Forrest, A. P. M., and Griffiths, K.: *Eur. J. Cancer* **9,** 169 (1973).
32. Brown, R. D., and Shellabarger, C. J.: *Cancer Res.* **34,** 2594 (1974).
33. Hawkins, R. A., Drewitt, D., Freedman, B., Killen, E., Jenner, D. A., and Cameron, E. H. D.: *Br. J. Cancer* **34,** 546 (1976).
34. Kelly, P. A., Bradley, C., Shiu, R. P. C., Meites, J., and Freisen, H. G.: *Proc. Soc. Exp. Biol. Med.* **146,** 816 (1974).
35. Holdaway, I. M., and Freisen, H. G.: *Cancer Res.* **36,** 1562 (1976).
36. Li, C. H., and Yang, W. H.: *Life Sci.* **15,** 761 (1974).
37. Heimann, R., Heuson, J. C., and Coune, A.: *Cancer Res.* **28,** 309 (1968).
38. Bradley, C. J., Kledzik, G. S., and Meites, J.: *Cancer Res.* **36,** 319 (1976).
39. Kiang, D. T., and Kennedy, B. J.: *Cancer* **28,** 1202 (1971).
40. Sterental, A., Dominguez, J. M., Weissman, C., and Pearson, O. H.: *Cancer Res.* **23,** 481 (1963).
41. Lewis, D., and Hallowes, R. C.: *J. Endocrinol.* **62,** 225 (1974).
42. Welsch, C. W., and Rivera, E. M.: *Proc. Soc. Exp. Biol. Med.* **139,** 623 (1972).
43. Chan, P. C., Tsuang, J., Head, J., and Cohen, L. A.: *Proc. Soc. Exp. Biol. Med.* **151,** 362 (1976).
44. Jensen, E. V.: *Can. Cancer Conf.* **6,** 143 (1966).
45. Mobbs, B. G.: *J. Endocrinol.* **36,** 409 (1966).
46. Mobbs, B. G., and Johnson, I. E.: *Eur. J. Cancer* **10,** 757 (1974).
47. Asselin, J., and Labrie, F.: *J. Steroid Biochem.* **9,** 1079 (1978).
48. Jabara, A. G.: *Br. J. Cancer* **21,** 418 (1967).
49. Jabara, A. G., and Harcourt, A. G.: *Pathology* **2,** 115 (1970).
50. Jabara, A. G., Toyne, P. H., and Harcourt, A. G.: *Br. J. Cancer* **27,** 63 (1973).
51. Horwitz, K. B., and McGuire, W. L.: *Cancer Res.* **37,** 1733 (1977).
52. Danguy, A., Legros, N., Develeeschouwer, N., Heuson-Stennon, J. A., and Heuson, J. C.: Effects of Medroxyprogesterone Acetate (MPA) on Growth of DMBA-Induced Rat Mammary Tumors: Histopathological and Endocrine Studies. *In* "Role of Medroxyprogesterone in Endocrine-Related Tumors" (S. Iacobelli and A. Di Marco, eds.). Raven Press, New York, 1980, p. 21.
53. Yoshida, H., Fukunishi, R., Kato, Y., and Matsumoto, K.: *J. Natl. Cancer Inst.* **65,** 823 (1980).
54. Terenius, L.: *Eur. J. Cancer* **9,** 291 (1973).
55. Asselin, J., Kelly, P. A., Caron, M. G., and Labrie, F.: *Endocrinology* **101,** 666 (1977).
56. Koenders, A. J., Geurts-Moespot, A., Zolingen, S. J., and Benraad, T. J.: Progesterone and Estradiol Receptors in DMBA-Induced Mammary Tumors Before and After Ovariectomy and After Subsequent Estradiol Administration. *In* "Progesterone Receptors in Normal and Neoplastic Tissues" (W. L. McGuire, J. D. Raymond, and E. E. Baulieu, eds.). Raven Press, New York, 1977, p. 71.
57. Allegra, J. C., Lippman, M. E., Thompson, E. B., Simon, R., Barlock, A., Green, L., Huff, K. K., Do, H. M. T., Aitken, S. C., and Warren, R.: *Cancer Res.* **39,** 1973 (1979).
58. Mobbs, B. G.: *Eur. J. Cancer Clin. Oncol.* **19,** 835 (1983).
59. Rose, D. P., and Noonan, J. J.: *Cancer Res.* **42,** 35 (1982).
60. Heuson, J. C., and Legros, N.: *Eur. J. Cancer* **6,** 349 (1970).
61. Heuson, J. C., and Legros, N.: *Cancer Res.* **32,** 226 (1972).
62. Heuson, J. C., Legros, N., and Heimann, R.: *Cancer Res.* **32,**233 (1972).
63. Sidransky, H., Wagner, B. P., and Morris, H. P.: *J. Natl. Cancer Inst.* **26,** 151 (1961).
64. Perry, D. J.: *Br. J. Cancer* **15,** 284 (1961).
65. Pai, S. R., Yamamoto, R. S., and Weisburger, J. H.: *Nature* **199,** 1299 (1963).
66. O'Neal, M. A., Hoffman, H. E., Dodge, B. G., and Griffin, A. C.: *J. Natl. Cancer Inst.* **21,** 1161 (1958).
67. Weisburger, J. H.: On Mechanisms of Liver Carcinogenesis—Effect of Pituitary Hormones and *N*-Hydroxy-*N*-2-Fluorenylacetamide. *In* "Cellular Control Mechanisms and Cancer" (P. Emmelot and O. Mühlbock, eds.). Elsevier, Amsterdam, 1964, p. 300.
68. Weisburger, J. H., Pai, S. R., Yamamoto, R. S., Korzis, J., and Weisburger, E. K.: *Isr. J. Med. Sci.* **4,** 1223 (1968).
69. Shirasu, Y., Grantham, P. H., and Weisburger, J. H.: *Int. J. Cancer,* **2,** 59 (1967).
70. Bielschowsky, F.: *Acta Unio Intern. contra Cancrum.* **17,** 121 (1961).
71. Reuber, M. D.: *J. Natl. Cancer Inst.* **36,** 775 (1966).
72. Toh, Y. C.: *J. Natl. Cancer Inst.* **48,** 113 (1972).

73. Goodall, C. M.: *New Zealand Med. J.* **67**, 32 (1968).
74. Reuber, M. D., and Firminger, H. I.: *J. Natl. Cancer Inst.* **29**, 933 (1962).
75. Vesselinovitch, S. D.: *Cancer Res.* **29**, 1024 (1969).
76. Engelse, L. D., Hollander, C. F., and Misdorp, W.: *Eur. J. Cancer* **10**, 129 (1974).
77. Taper, H. S.: *Cancer* **42**, 462 (1978).
78. Cameron, R., Imaida, K., and Ito, N.: *Gann* **72**, 339 (1981).
79. Wanless, I. R., and Medicine, A.: *Lab. Invest.* **46**, 313 (1982).
80. Yager, J. D., and Yager, R.: *Cancer Res.* **40**, 3680 (1980).
81. Yager, J. D., Campbell, H. A., Longnecker, D. S., Roebuck, B. D., and Benoit, M. C.: *Cancer Res.* **44**, 3862 (1984).
82. Li, J. J., and Li, S. A.: *J. Natl. Cancer Inst.* **73**, 543 (1984).
83. Lucier, G.: "Dose-Response Relationships for Dioxin". Presentation at the International Life Sciences Institute (ILSI), Washington, DC, March 19, 1992.
84. Lucier, G. W., Tritscher, A. M., Goldsworthy, T., Foley, J., Clark, G., Goldstein, G., and Maronpot, R.: *Cancer Res.* **51**, 1391 (1991).
85. Howell, J. S., Marchant, J., and Orr, J. W.: *Br. J. Cancer* **8**, 635 (1954).
86. Marchant, J.: *Br. J. Cancer* **13**, 652 (1959).
87. Kuwahara, I.: *Gann* **58**, 253 (1967).
88. Krarup, T.: *Br. J. Cancer* **24**, 168 (1970).
89. Jull, J. M.: *Methods Cancer Res.* **7**, 131 (1973).
90. Michael, S. D., Taguchi, O., and Nishizuka, Y.: *Endocrinology* **108**, 2375 (1981).
91. Taguchi, O., Michael, S. D., and Nishizuka, Y.: *Cancer Res.* **48**, 425 (1988).
92. Beamer, W. G., Shultz, K. L., and Tennent, B. J.: *Cancer Res.* **48**, 2788 (1988).
93. Familiari, G., Toscano, V., and Motta, P. M.: *Cell Tissue Res.* **240**, 519 (1985).
94. Ward, R. C., Costoff, A., and Mahest, V. B.: *Biol. Reprod.* **18**, 614 (1978).
95. Wolf, N. S. and Nishimura, E. T.: *Cancer Res.* **20**, 1299 (1960).
96. Gautieri, R. P. and Mann, D. E.: *J. Pharmacol. Sci.* **50**, 556 (1961).
97. Trainin, N.: *Cancer Res.* **23**, 415 (1963).
98. Bates, R. R.: *J. Natl. Cancer Inst.* **41**, 559 (1968).
99. Tipnis, U. V., and Sirsat, S. M.: *Indian J. Exp. Biol.* **7**, 197 (1969).
100. Druckrey, H., Preussmann, R., Ivankovic, S., and Schmähl, O.: *Z. Krebsforsch.* **69**, 103 (1967).
101. Druckrey, H., Preussmann, R., Ivankovic, S., Schmidt, C. H., Mennel, H. D., and Stahl, K. W.: *Z. Krebsforsch.* **66**, 280 (1964).
102. Bertram, J. S., and Craig, A. W.: *Eur. J. Cancer* **8**, 587 (1972).
103. Ertürk, E., Cohen, S. M., Price, J. M., and Bryan, G. T.: *Cancer Res.* **29**, 2219 (1969).
104. Clayson, D. B., Pringle, J. A. S., and Bonser, G. M.: *Biochem. Pharmacol.* **16**, 619 (1967).
105. Foulds, L.: *Br. J. Cancer* **1**, 172 (1947).
106. Yoshida, O., Ertürk, E., Bryan, G. T., and Lower, G. M.: *Invest. Urol.* **11**, 216 (1973).
107. Clayson, D. B., and Bonser, G. M.: *Br. J. Cancer* **19**, 311 (1965).
108. Ogiso, T., Arai, Y., Fukushima, S., Nishizuka, Y., and Ito, N.: *Gann* **73**, 862 (1982).
109. Katayama, S., Fiala, E., Reddy, B. S., Rivenson, A., Silverman, J., Williams, G. M., and Weisburger, J. H.: *J. Natl. Cancer Inst.* **68**, 867 (1982).
110. Shirai, T., Sakata, T., Fukushima, S., Ikawa, E., and Ito, N.: *Gann* **76**, 803 (1985).
111. Bosland, M. C., and Prinsen, M. K.: *Cancer Res.* **50**, 691 (1990).
112. Pour, P. M.: *Carcinogenesis* **4**, 49 (1983).
113. Shirai, T., Fukushima, S., Ikawa, E., Tagawa, Y., and Ito, N.: *Cancer Res.* **46**, 6423 (1986).
114. Nakamura, A., Shirari, T., and Ogawa, K.: *Cancer Lett.* **53**, 151 (1990).
115. Kaslaris, E., and Jull, J. W.: *Br. J. Cancer* **16**, 479 (1962).
116. Pour, P. M., and Gotz, U.: *J. Natl. Cancer Inst.* **70**, 353 (1983).
117. Biancifiori, C.: *J. Natl. Cancer Inst.* **45**, 965 (1970).
118. Glucksman, A., and Cherry, C. P.: *Br. J. Cancer* **25**, 212 (1971).
119. Furukawa, H., Iwanaga, T., Koyama, H., and Taniguchi, H.: *Cancer Res.* **42**, 5181 (1982).
120. Marchant, J.: *Br. J. Cancer* **21**, 750 (1967).
121. Ito, T., Hoshino, T., and Sawauchi, K.: *Gann* **57**, 201 (1966).
122. Kokkinakis, D. M.: *Carcinogenesis* **11**, 1909 (1990).
123. Sumi, C., Longnecker, D. S., Roebuck, B. D., and Brinck-Johnson, T.: *Cancer Res.* **49**, 2332 (1989).
124. Huggins, C., Moon, R. C., and Morii, S.: *Proc. Natl. Acad. Sci. U.S.A.* **48**, 379 (1962).
125. Lemon, H. M.: *Cancer Res.* **35**, 1341 (1975).
126. Quadri, S. K., Kledzik, G. S., and Meites, J.: *Cancer Res.* **34**, 499 (1974).
127. Fletcher, W. S., McSweeney, E. D., and Dunphy, J. E.: *Surg. Forum* **14**, 133 (1963).
128. Abul-Hajj, Y.: *Cancer Res.* **39**, 4882 (1979).

129. McCormick, G. M., and Moon, R. C.: *Eur. J. Cancer* **9**, 483 (1973).
130. Jabara, A. G., Toyne, P. H., and Harcourt, A. G.: *Br. J.Cancer* **27**, 63 (1973).
131. Gottardis, M., Ertürk, E., and Rose, D. P.: *Eur. J. Cancer Clin. Oncol.* **19**, 1479 (1983).
132. Griswold, D. P., and Green, C. H.: *Cancer Res.* **30**, 819 (1970).
133. Shay, H., Gruenstein, M., and Kessler, W. B.: *J. Natl. Cancer Inst.* **27**, 503 (1961).
134. Young, S., Baker, R. A., and Helfenstein, J. E.: *Br. J. Cancer* **19**, 155 (1965).
135. Dao, T. L., Bock, F. G., and Greiner, M. J.: *J. Natl. Cancer Inst.* **25**, 991 (1960).
136. Aylsworth, C. F., Hodson, C. A., Berg, G., Kledzik, G., and Meites, J.: *Cancer Res.* **39**, 2436 (1979).
137. Jull, J. W.: *Cancer Res.* **26**, 2368 (1966).
138. Kledzik, G. S., Bradley, C. J., and Meites, J.: *Cancer Res.* **34**, 2953 (1974).
139. Hodson, C. A., Mioduszewski, R., and Meites, J.: *IRCS J. Med. Sci.* **6**, 399 (1978).
140. Lacassagne, A., Jayle, M.-F., and Hurst, L.: *C. R. Acad. Sci.* **267**, 137 (1968).
141. Belman, S., and Troll, W.: *Cancer Res.* **32**, 450 (1972).
142. Boutwell, R. K., and Rusch, H. P.: *Proc. Am. Assoc. Cancer Res.* **1**, 5 (1953).
143. Baserga, R., and Shubik, P.: *Cancer Res.* **14**, 12 (1954).
144. Engelbreth-Holm, J., and Asboe-Hansen, G.: *Acta Pathol. Microbiol. Scand.* **32**, 560 (1953).
145. Ghadially, R. N., and Green, H. N.: *Br. J. Cancer* **8**, 291 (1954).
146. Nakai, T.: *Cancer Res.* **21**, 221 (1961).
147. Hisamatsu, T., Mori, K., and Okamoto, K.: *Gann* **57**, 299 (1966).
148. Schulte-Hermann, R., Ochs, H., Bursch, W., and Parzefall, W.: *Cancer Res.* **48**, 2462 (1988).
149. Mathis, J. M., Simpson, E. R., and Prough, R. A.: *Mol. Cell. Endocrinol.* **60**, 105 (1988).
150. Benrekassa, J., and Decloitre, F.: *Biochem. Pharmacol.* **32**, 347 (1983).
151. Pasleau, F., Kremers, P., and Gielen, J. E.: *Chem. Biol. Interact.* **34**, 279 (1981).
152. Hertzog, P. J., Ilacqua, V., Rustia, M., and Gingell, R.: *Toxicol. Appl. Pharmacol.* **54**, 340 (1980).
153. Conney, A. H., and Burns, J. J.: *Adv. Pharmacol.* **1**, 31 (1962).
154. Conney, A. H.: *Pharmacol. Rev.* **19**, 317 (1967).
155. Gillette, J. R., Davis, D. C., and Sasame, H. A.: *Annu. Rev. Pharmacol.* **12**, 57 (1972).
156. Remmer, H.: *Eur. J. Clin. Pharmacol.* **5**, 116 (1972).
157. Quinn, J. P., Axelrod, J., and Brodie, B. B.: *Biochem. Pharmacol.* **1**, 152 (1958).
158. Kato, R., and Gillette, J. R.: *J. Pharmacol. Exp. Therap.* **150**, 279 (1965).
159. Murphy, S. D., and DuBois, K. P.: *J. Pharmacol. Exp. Therap.* **124**, 194 (1958).
160. Meermann, J. H. N., Nijland C. and Mulder, G. J.: *Biochem. Pharmacol.* **36**, 2605 (1987).
161. Katayama, S., Ohmori, T., Maeura, Y., Croci, T. and Williams, G. M.: *J. Natl. Cancer Inst.* **73**, 141 (1984).
162. Waxman, D. J., Dannan, G. A. and Guengerich, F. P.: *Biochemistry* **24**, 4409 (1985).
163. Lamartiniere, C. A.: *Endocrinology* **117**, 523 (1985).
164. Colby, H. D.: Regulation of Hepatic Drug and Steroid Metabolism by Androgens and Estrogens. *In* "Advances in Sex Hormone Research" (J. A. Thomas and R. L. Singhal, eds.). Urban & Schwarzenberg, Baltimore, 1980, Vol. 4, p. 27.
165. Nulder, G. J.: *Chem.-Biol. Interact.* **57**, 367 (1979).
166. Ichii, S., and Yago, N.: *J. Biochem.* **65**, 597 (1969).
167. Inscoe, J. K., and Axelrod, J.: *J. Pharmacol. Exp. Therap.* **129**, 128 (1960).
168. Juchau, M. R., and Fouts, J. R.: *Biochem. Pharmacol.* **15**, 891 (1966).
169. DuBois, K. P., and Kinoshita, F.: *Arch. Int. Pharmacodyn. Therap.* **156**, 418 (1965).
170. Booth, J., and Gillette, J. R.: *J. Pharmacol. Exp. Therap.* **137**, 374 (1962).
171. Remmer, H.: *Arch. Exp. Pathol. Pharmakol.* **233**, 184 (1958).
172. Remmer, H.: *Naturwissenschaften* **45**, 522 (1958).
173. Bousquet, W. F., Rupe, B. D., and Miya, T. S.: *J. Pharmacol. Exp. Therap.* **147**, 376 (1965).
174. Driever, C. W., and Bousquet, W. F.: *Life Sci.* **4**, 1449 (1965).
175. Driever, C. W., Bousquet, W. F., and Miya, T. S.: *Int. J. Neuropharmacol.* **5**, 199 (1966).
176. Conney, A. H., and Garren, L.: *Biochem. Pharmacol.* **6**, 257 (1961).
177. Kato, R., and Gillette, J. R.: *J. Pharmacol. Exp. Therap.* **150**, 285 (1965).
178. Prange, A. J., Jr., Lipton, M. A., Shearin, R. B., and Love, G. N.: *Biochem. Pharmacol.* **15**, 237 (1966).
179. Gillette, J. R.: *Progr. Drug. Res.* **6**, 11 (1963).
180. Orrenius, S., Ericsson, J. L. E., and Ernster, L.: *J. Cell Biol.* **25**, 627 (1965).
181. Weisburger, E. K., Grantham, P. H., and Weisburger, J. H.: *Biochemistry* **3**, 808 (1964).
182. DeBaum, J. R., Rowley, J. Y., Miller, E. C., and Miller, J. A.: *Proc. Soc. Exp. Biol. Med.* **129**, 268 (1968).
183. Shirasu, Y., Grantham, P. H., Yamamoto, R. S., and Weisburger, J. H.: *Cancer Res.* **26**, 600 (1966).
184. Weisburger, E. K., Yamamoto, R. S., Glass, R. M., Grantham, P. H., and Weisburger, J. H.: *Endocrinology* **82**, 685 (1968).

185. Sims, P., and Grover, P. L.: *Adv. Cancer Res.* **20**, 165 (1974).
186. Bengston, M., and Rydstrom, J.: *Science* **219**, 1437 (1983).
187. Nebert, D. W.: Genetic Aspects of Enzyme Induction by Drugs and Chemical Carcinogens. In "The Induction of Drug Metabolism" (R. W. Estabrook and E. Lindenlaub, eds.), Schattauer Verl., Stuttgart, 1979, p. 419.
188. Poland, A., and Glover, E.: *Arch. Biochem. Biophys.* **261**, 103 (1988).
189. Fernandez, N., and Lesca, R. M.: *Eur. J. Biochem.* **172**, 585 (1988).
190. Nebert, D.: Mol. *Cell Biochem.* **27**, 27 (1979).
191. Bolander, F. F.: "Molecular Endocrinology". Academic. Press, San Diego, 1989, p. 78.
192. Kuntzman, R., Jacobson, M., Schneideman, K., and Conney, A. H.: *J. Pharmacol. Exp. Therap.* **146**, 280 (1964).
193. Kuntzman, R., Welch, R., and Conney, A. H.: *Adv. Enzyme Regul.* **4**, 149 (1966).
194. Conney, A. H., Ikeda, M., Levin, W., Cooper, D., Rosenthal, O., and Estabrook, R.: *Federation Proc.* **26**, 462 (1967).
195. Tephly, T. R., and Mannering, G. J.: *The Pharmacologist* **6**, 186 (1964).
196. Waxman, D. J.: *Biochem. Pharmacol.* **37**, 71 (1988),
197. Hanakoglu, I.: *J. Steroid. Biochem. Molec. Biol.* **43**, 745 (1992).
198. Schenkman, J. B.: *J. Steroid. Biochem. Molec. Biol.* **43**, 1023 (1992).
199. Kato, R., and Kamataki, T.: *Xenobiotica* **12**, 787 (1982).
200. Kobliakov, V., Popova, N., and Rossi, L.: *Eur. J. Biochem.* **195**, 585 (1991).
201. Yager, J. D., Jr. and Yager, R.: *Cancer Res.* **40**, 3680 (1980).
202. Cameron, R. G., Imaida, K., Tsuda, H., and Ito, N.: *Cancer Res.* **42**, 2426 (1982).
203. Shi, Y. E. and Yager, J. D.: *Cancer Res.* **49**, 3574 (1989).
204. Yager, J. D., Zurio, J., and Ni, N.: *Proc. Soc. Exp. Biol. Med.* **198**, 667 (1991).
205. Jull, J. W.: *Br. J. Cancer* **18**, 508 (1964).
206. Biancifiori, C., Caschera, F., Giornelli-Santilli, F. E., and Bucciarelli, E.: *Br. J. Cancer* **21**, 452 (1967).
207. Huggins, C., Briziarelli, G., and Sutton, H.: *J. Exp. Med.* **109**, 25 (1959).
208. Sydnor, K. L., and Cockrell, B.: *Endocrinology* **73**, 427 (1963).
209. Cantarow, A., Stasney, J., and Paschkis, K. E.: *Cancer Res.* **8**, 412 (1948).
210. Grubbs, C. J., Peckham, J. C., and McDonough, K. D.: *Carcinogenesis* **4**, 495 (1983).
211. Weisburger, J. H., Yamamoto, R. S., Korzis, J., and Weisburger, E. K.: *Science* **154**, 673 (1966).
212. Vesselinovitch, S. D., and Mihailovich, N.: *Cancer Res.* **27**, 1788 (1967).
213. Jull, J. W., and Huggins, C.: *Nature* **188**, 73 (1960).
214. Newman, W. C., and Moon, R. C.: *Cancer Res.* **28**, 864 (1968).
215. Weisburger, J. H., Weisburger, E. K., Griswold, D. P., and Casey, A. E.: *Life Sci.* **7**, 259 (1968).
216. Welsch, C. W., and Meites, J.: *Cancer* **23**, 601 (1969).

EDITORS' NOTE ADDED IN PROOF

On the Significance of Environmental Xenoestrogens

Because of the well-established connection between estrogens and neoplasia, a widely publicized 1993 epidemiological study [M. S. Wolff *et al.*: *J. Natl. Cancer Inst.* **85**, 648 (1993)] focused attention on the cancer risk of exposure to environmentally distributed chemical agents, which are either estrogenic themselves or affect estrogen production and metabolism (i.e., are *xenoestrogens*). This case-control study of 58 prospectively gathered cases from a cohort of 14,000 women found that women having the highest serum levels of DDE (a metabolite of the pesticide DDT) had a fourfold greater risk of breast cancer than women with the lowest levels. However, a second epidemiological study which revisited the topic one year later [N. Krieger *et al.*: *J. Natl. Cancer Inst.* **86**, 589 (1994)] came to a diametrically opposite conclusion and found no association between risk of breast cancer and serum levels of DDE in 150 women who developed breast cancer in an average of 14 years after the samples have been collected. Despite the overall inconclusive outcome of these two recent epidemiological studies, other results support the association between chlorinated organics and breast cancer. In one study the breast lipids of women with cancer at biopsy had about 40% more of certain chlorinated pesticides, such as metabolites of DDT and higher levels of PCBs [F. Falck, Jr., *et al.*: *Arch. Environ. Health* **47**, 143 (1992)]. In another study 50% more hexachlorocyclohexane was detected in pooled blood of breast cancer cases compared to a pooled reference group [H. Mussalo-Rauhamaa *et al.*: *Cancer* **66**, 2124 (1990)].

Concern about the use and widespread environmental distribution of estrogenic agents had been raised as early as 1980 [J. A. McLachlan, ed.: "Estrogens in the Environment". Elsevier, New York, 1980]. Many chemicals with widely different structures have been shown to have estrogenic activity. A representative list includes estradiol-17β, diethylstilbestrol (DES), coumestrol, equol, zearalenone, 3,9-dihydroxy-benz[*a*]anthracene, *o,p*-DDT, tetrahydrocannabinol [J. A. McLachlan *et al. in* M. V. Raloff and A. W. Wilson, eds.: "Human Risk Assessment: The Roles of Animal Selection and Extrapolation". Taylor & Francis, London, 1987, p. 187], DDT and its degradation products, di(2-ethylhexyl)phthalate, dicofol, hexachlorobenzene, kelthane, kepone, hexachlorocyclohexane stereoisomers, methoxychlor, octachlorostyrene, triazine herbicides, EBDC fungicides, certain PCB congeners, 2,3,7,8-TCDD and other dioxins, 2,3,7,8-TCDF and other polychlorodibenzofurans [Consensus Statement 1: "Chemically-Induced Alterations in Sexual Development: The Wildlife/Human Connection" *in Adv. Modern Environ. Toxicol.* **21**, 1 (1992)], bisphenol-A [A. V. Krishnan *et al.*: *Endocrinology* **132**, 2279 (1993)], and *p*-nonylphenol [A. M. Soto *et al.*: *Environ. Health Perspect.* **92**, 167 (1991)]. Because of the ubiquitousness of chemicals with estrogenic activity in the environment (some of which are bioaccumulative and highly persistent), it has been recommended that the study of xenoestrogenic potential of chemicals be made part of their toxicological evaluation [J. A. McLachlan: *Environ. Health Perspect.* **101**, 386 (1993)].

The total evidence available at the time of this writing supports the view that the massive release of xenoestrogens into the environment since World War II (*see* Appendix) likely underlies or is a key contributing factor to the worldwide rise of breast cancer incidence and various estrogen-associated dysfunctions [*cf.* Davis *et al.*: *Environ. Health Perspect.* **101**, 372 (1993) and McLachlan, 1993, *loc. cit.*]. Moreover, by disruption of the endocrine balance, xenoestrogens also produce profound developmental alterations in wildlife resulting in decrease of animal populations and a wide range of anatomical defects [*rev.* T. Colborn: *Environ. Health Perspect.* **101**, 378 (1993)]. In humans, the "DES syndrome" serves as a model for exposure to estrogenic environmental chemicals. DES was used from 1948 to 1971 to prevent spontaneous abortions. Female offspring, thus exposed *in utero* to DES, often display reproductive organ dysfunction, abnormal pregnancies, reduction in fertility, immune system disorders, and increased rates of vaginal adenocarcinomas [T. Colborn, 1993, *loc. cit.*]. Considerable literature has developed corroborating in experimental animals the deleterious effects of *in utero* exposure to DES during critical periods of organ differentation during embryogenesis[1].

Exposure to estrogens has also been associated with functional and morphologic abnormalities of and cancer in the male genital tract [*e.g.*, B. E. Henderson *et al.*: *Int. J. Cancer* **23**, 598 (1979); R. Santti *et al.*: *Int. J. Androl.* **13**, 77 (1990); R. Sharpe and N. E. Skakkebaek: *Lancet* **341**, 19392 (1993)]. Indeed, a gradual 50% decrease of average sperm

---

[1] A very readable popularized account of the noncancer health effects of xenoestrogens in wildlife and humans was given in two consecutive factually accurate articles [J. Raloff: *Sci. News* **145**, 24 and 56 (1994)]

density together with a 19% decrease of mean seminal volume (meaning that the total sperm count decreased even more than that indicated by the sperm density) occurred in the last half century [A. Giwercman *et al.*: *Environ. Health Perspect.* **101** (Supplement 2), 65 (1993)]. Also, the incidence of testicular cancer has increased 3- to 4-fold worldwide since the 1940s in countries with either a very high frequency of testicular neoplasia or a low frequency of this cancer, and there appears to be a link between semen quality and the incidence of testicular cancer [*rev.* A. Giwercman *et al.*, 1993, *loc.cit.*]. Male offspring of mothers exposed to DES during pregnancy have an increased risk of testicular abnormalities including cryptorchidism, testicular cancer, and an elevated percentage of morphologically abnormal sperm cells [*e.g.*, W. B. Gill *et al.*: *J. Urol.* **122**, 36 (1979)]; these clinical findings have been corroborated by animal studies [J. A. McLachlan *et al.*: *Science* **190**, 991 (1973); R. R. Newbold *et al.*: *J. Urol.* **137**, 1446 (1987)].

Another potential causal involvement of xenoestrogens in the male genital tract is with benign prostatic hypertrophy (BPH) and prostate cancer. The normal prostate is under androgen, estrogen, and progesterone control; receptors for all three are present in both the stromal and epithelial regions of the organ [J. A. Thomas and E. J. Keenan: *J. Androl.* **15**, 97 (1994)]. Distribution of the estrogen receptor populations vary among species and with age and endocrine status in the normal prostate. A number of studies have established that estrogen administration induces prostate gland hyperplasia in the rat, mouse, dog, and monkey [*rev.* J. A. Thomas and E. J. Keenan, 1994, *loc. cit.*; E. J. Keenan and J. A. Thomas: *Toxic Subst. J.* **13**, 29 (1994)] as well as in the guinea pig [A. Lipschütz *et al.*: *Cancer Res.* **5**, 515 (1945)]. Depending on species, age, and endocrine status, combined administration of estrogens with androgens may have a synergistic effect or may prevent estrogen-induced prostate gland hyperplasia [*rev.* J. A. Thomas and E. J. Keenan, 1994, *loc. cit.*; E. J. Keenan and J. A. Thomas, 1994, *loc. cit.*; A. Lipschütz *et al.*, 1945, *loc. cit.*].

Exposure to estrogen has also been implicated in the etiology of BPH in humans [F. S. von Saal *et al. in* E. Knobil *et al.*, eds.: "Physiology of Reproduction". Raven Press, New York, 1994, in press; R. Ghanadian, *in* R. Ghanadian, ed.: "The Endocrinology of Prostate Tumors". MTP Press, Lancaster (England), 1983, p. 59]. The role of estrogen in BPH in experimental animals and humans has been reviewed [M. F. El Etreby: *J. Steroid Biochem. Mol. Biol.* **44**, 565 (1993)]. The molecular mechanism of the combined effect of androgen, estrogen, and progesterone in governing prostate tissue homeostasis is not understood. Thomas and Keenan [1994, *loc. cit.*] reviewed the possible roles of estrogen in BPH. One of these was postulated to be the modification of metabolism by estrogen so as to result in excess dihydrotestosterone (the active form of testosterone) production [D. S. Coffey *et al. in* J. T. Hinman and F. Horton, eds.: "Benign Prostatic Hyperplasia II". NIH Publ. No. 87-2881 (1987), p. 1], which is consistent with the view that an estrogenic component is required for stimulation by androgen [D. S. Coffey *et al.*, 1987, *loc. cit.*].

The hypothesis is here advanced that *the direction* of the shift in the normal ratio of estrogen to androgen determines whether the outcome of persistent imbalance will be BPH or prostate cancer — excess estrogen favoring the former, whereas excess androgen the latter. It is important to stress that the direction of the shift is governed by a number of modulating factors in complex interaction with each other, such as: the hormone receptors' distribution and level, which are themselves regulated by genetic factors, endocrine status, dietary factors, and age, as well as by the levels of aromatase (estrogen synthetase) and testosterone 5α-reductase determining the levels of estrogen and androgen, respectively. Aromatase catalyzes the biosynthesis of C_{18} estrogens (aromatic) from C_{19} androgens containing the 3-ketone group; both aromatase and 5α-reductase are NADPH-dependent enzymes. Consistent with the above postulated role of estrogen in the etiology of BPH, treatment with antiestrogen [J. Geller and J. D. Albert *in* N. Bruchovsky *et al.*, eds.: "Regulation of Androgen Action", Congressdruck, Berlin, 1985, p. 51] as well as treatment with an aromatase inhibitory agent [M. F. El Etreby, 1993, *loc. cit.*] were found beneficial in the treatment of BPH. Conversely, a testosterone analog, finasteride, a competitive inhibitor of 5α-reductase is being explored for prostate cancer prevention [O. W. Brawley *et al.*: *Cancer Epidemiol. Biomarkers Prevent.* **3**, 177 (1994)]. For a 1982 but still useful review on aromatase, *see* H. A. Harvey *et al.*, eds.: *Cancer Res. Suppl.* **42**, 3261 (1982).

The estrogen to androgen ratio may, of course, also be shifted by induction or repression of the levels of aromatase and 5α-reductase. Many environmental chemicals, pertinently certain organochlorines, are well known to be inducers of typical mixed-function oxidases. Whether 5α-reductase (a nuclear membrane-bound enzyme) and aromatase are also induced by mixed-function oxidase inducers of the type encountered among the xenoestrogens does not appear to have been studied (Elizabeth Stoner, Merck Co., Rahway, New Jersey, May 11, 1994, personal communication). This needs to be investigated to gain further insight into the mechanism of xenoestrogen induction of sexual dysfunctions and pathology.

Finally, it should also be pointed out that the presence of xenoestrogens in the environment represents a selective pressure, and this may play a role in their putative induction of breast cancer. It has been known that selective pressure by mutagenic chemicals enhances the rate of development of genetically altered populations; this has been illustrated by studies on cultured cells [R. T. Schimke: *J. Biol. Chem.* **263**, 5989 (1988)]. Evolutionary processes will respond, however, to *any* selective environmental pressure exerted on any population, irrespective of the toxicological mechanism responsible for the selective pressure [G. A. LeBlanc: *Environ. Health Perspect.* **102**, 266 (1994)]. This has been dramatically shown by the emergence of a 500-fold increase of pesticide resistance in fish as a result of exposure to endrin, strobane and heptachlor [D. D. Culley and D. E. Ferguson: *J. Fish Res. Board Canada* **26**, 2395 (1969); D. E. Ferguson *et al.*: *Trans. Am. Fish Soc.* **95**, 335 (1966)]. Moreover, work ongoing since 1988 lends credence to the Lamarckian view of the inheritance of acquired characteristics. These studies [*e.g.*, J. Cairns *et al.*: *Nature* **335**, 142 (1988); R. S. Harris *et al.*: *Science* **264**, 258 (1994); *rev.* D. S. Thaler: *Science* **264**, 224 (1994)] suggest that contrary to the neodarwinian concept—that mutations arise irrespective of any advantage they may confer for the survival of organisms—selective environmental pressure can interact with an organism so as to generate precisely the variation selected. Such a mutation directed by selective pressure has been termed a "selection-induced" or "adaptive" mutation. Environmental factors representing selective pressure can interact with DNA through a variety of routes (*e.g.*, acting directly on DNA structure, on genes coding for DNA metabolism, on genetic change coupled to the organism's response to its environment); these routes also represent components of the feedback between cellular generators of genetic diversity and the environment that selects among the variants. The implications for ecosystem structure of inheritable characteristics (either acquired or selected in the neodarwinian sense) resulting from selective environmental pressure can be profound—whether the ecosystem is composed of whole organisms or of a multiplicity of cells coexisting in homeostatic balance in a tissue.

Appendix to Editors' Note: Prior to 1950, the production and use of pesticides were insignificant on today's scale. However, by 1970 the yearly U.S. aggregate use of "conventional pesticides" (defined as insecticides, herbicides, fungicides and plant growth regulators) grew to 740 million lb, and reached 1,175 million lb by 1980; pesticide use was virtually stationary through about 1987 (production levels closely parallel usage figures since the U.S. exportation of pesticides is only slightly higher than importation) [U.S. EPA: "Pesticides Industry Sales and Usage—1988 Market Estimates". Economic Analysis Branch, Office of Pesticide Programs. U.S. EPA, Washington, D.C., 1989, p. 11]. The growth of the production and use of pesticides—in terms of the potential presence of xenoestrogens in the environment—must be viewed, however, in the backdrop of the growth of the total number of chemicals in the Chemical Abstracts Service computerized registry as well as of the overall growth of the production of industrial chemicals. This is because chemical compounds other than those used as pesticides (the major use-category of organochlorines known to comprise xenoestrogens) may display hitherto undetected xenoestrogenic activity. In mid-1994 the registry had close to 13 million chemicals on file, and this number is growing by an annual rate of over 670 thousand. The annual growth rate was only 450 thousand about 8 years ago. So, in 8 years the growth rate itself has increased by about 50%. Consider, next, that the estimated aggregate U.S. production of synthetic organic chemicals was about 1 billion lb in the early 1940s and grew rapidly, spurred by the World War II era, to about 30 billion lb by 1950. Formal official records available from then on [U.S. International Trade Commission: "Synthetic Organic Chemicals" (Production Reports Published Yearly), U.S. ITC, Washington, D.C.] indicated production levels of over 100 billion lb in 1967, 150 billion lb in 1970, 210 billion lb in 1980, and over 290 billion lb in 1990.

CHAPTER 12

Effect of Genetic Susceptibility on Tumor Induction

Norman R. Drinkwater

I. INTRODUCTION

Phenomenal progress has been made during the last decade in the molecular identification of human "cancer genes", such as those resulting in the heritable development of retinoblastoma (1), Wilm's tumor (2), and familial adenomatous polyposis (3). These rare genetic diseases are inherited with very high penetrance, making cancer development in carriers of the mutant genes a virtual certainty. Because of this high penetrance and the rarity of the cancers (or extreme nature of the phenotype), it has been possible to identify these genes through formal genetic studies in affected families. In contrast, human genetic studies have been less effective in identifying "risk-modifier" genes that may influence the susceptibility of individuals to the development of more common malignancies. Even if such genes resulted in 5- to 50-fold increases in cancer risk, their recognition would be hampered by a relatively low penetrance and the large variation in environmental factors that influence cancer development in humans. In spite of these difficulties, King and coworkers (4, 5) have recently demonstrated the existence of a locus that increases the risk for breast cancer in humans by tenfold and have mapped the gene to human chromosome 17q21.

Animal models provide a powerful approach to the identification and characterization of risk-modifier genes that influence the development of cancer. There is substantial variation among inbred strains of rats and mice in their susceptibilities to spontaneous and chemically-induced carcinogenesis at a variety of tissue sites, and the genetic basis for this variation in risk can be studied under well-defined experimental conditions. This review will describe some of the genetic approaches to the analysis of modifier genes that control the susceptibility of rodents to carcinogenesis.

II. GENETIC APPROACHES TO STUDYING MECHANISMS OF CARCINOGENESIS

Two complementary approaches have been used to identify genetic factors that modulate susceptibility to spontaneous or chemically-induced carcinogenesis. First, the role of a specific gene product during carcinogenesis can be inferred from studies comparing tumor development in mice carrying a mutant allele with that in wild-type animals. Second, novel loci that modulate carcinogenesis may be identified through comparative studies of inbred strains of animals that differ in susceptibility to tumor induction. A pair of inbred strains may differ by more than 100-fold in the risk for tumor development. The genetic basis for this difference in susceptibility can be studied by analysis of the segregation of the phenotype in crosses between the two strains or in recombinant inbred strains derived from the inbred parental lines. Recent improvements in methods for mapping quantitative genetic traits and in molecular cloning based on positional information will facilitate the characterization of the gene products responsible for the high susceptibility of particular inbred strains to carcinogenesis.

A. Mutant and Congenic Strains

The mouse provides a rich genetic model with more than 1300 loci for which two or more alleles have been described (6). In a few cases, the identification of a locus has been based on its modulation of cancer susceptibility. A striking example is the Apc^{Min} mutation (7) (see Section IV.C, below), a chemically-induced mutation in the mouse homolog of the gene responsible for familial adenomatous polyposis in humans (3).

The role of a specific gene product in carcinogenesis may be determined by comparing a pair of congenic strains, which are genetically identical except that they carry different alleles at a single locus, for susceptibility to tumor induction. The two alleles may represent alternative forms of a polymorphic locus, or the wild type and a mutant gene for that locus. This approach has been used to investigate the importance of particular enzymatic pathways in the metabolic activation of chemical carcinogens (8, 9), the role of specific receptors in tumor promotion by halogenated aromatic hydrocarbons (10) or hormones (11), and the relevance of various immunological functions to the development of spontaneous and chemically-induced tumors (12). For example, *brachymorphic* (*bm*) mutant mice (see Section IV.E, below) are deficient in the production of 3′-phosphoadenosine-5′-phosphosulfate (PAPS), a required cofactor for sulfotransferase reactions. These mutant mice are resistant to the induction of liver tumors by *N*-hydroxy-2-acetylaminofluorene relative to wild-type littermates, demonstrating that this hepato-carcinogen is activated by metabolism to a reactive sulfuric acid ester (9). Similarly, comparative studies of the promotion of liver tumor induction by 3,4,5,3′,4′,5′-hexabromobiphenyl in mice congenic for the high-affinity or low-affinity forms of the *Ah* receptor (see Section IV.B, below) demonstrated that binding of this class of compounds to the *Ah* receptor is required for tumor promotion (10).

Mechanistic studies of this type are no longer restricted to genes for which naturally occurring polymorphisms or mutant alleles have been identified. Specific mutations may be introduced into embryonic stem cells by homologous recombination and these cells used to produce mutant animals (13). Thus, it is possible to study the role in carcino-genesis of any gene for which a DNA clone is available. While this method has been used to engineer null mutations by insertion into several cellular proto-oncogenes, including *c-src* (14) and *c-abl* (15), the observable phenotypes of the mutant animals have often been subtle, indicating a high degree of functional redundancy in the regulatory pathways influenced by the genes. However, Donehower *et al.* (16) have demonstrated that disruption of the *p53* tumor suppressor gene by homologous recombination results in a high frequency of spontaneous tumors at several sites in homozygous mutant animals.

B. Variation Among Inbred Strains

Inbred strains of mice or rats are constructed by brother–sister mating over the course of 20 or more generations, resulting in a population of genetically identical animals homozygous at each genetic locus. The genetic homogeneity within each inbred strain ensures that experimental results are reproducible both between laboratories and over periods of time (17). Of the over 200 inbred mouse and 100 inbred rat strains currently available, approximately a dozen strains of each species account for the large majority of the use of inbred strains in cancer research. Taken together, even these limited sets of inbred strains represent a wider spectrum of genetic variation than would be found in laboratory outbred or natural populations of mice (18).

Little developed the first inbred strains of mice early in the century with the aim of understanding the genetic basis for the development of cancer (*see in* ref. 19). Studies of both spontaneous and chemically-induced tumors in both mice and rats have demonstrated that there is considerable variation among inbred strains in their susceptibilities to carcinogenesis (see below, Section III). For a variety of tissue sites, including the lung, liver, mammary gland, and skin, it is possible to identify pairs of inbred strains that differ by up to 100-fold in their risk for tumor development. These differences provide a *prima facie* case for the importance of the genetic background of the host in determining cancer susceptibility.

After identifying a susceptible inbred mouse strain, a critical issue is the number of genes that play a role in determining the carcinogen-sensitive phenotype. One approach to answering that question is to study the segregation of susceptibility in crosses between the susceptible inbred strain and a second, resistant inbred strain. For example, in the case that an allelic difference at a single dominant locus was largely responsible for the difference in susceptibility between the two inbred strains, equal numbers of sensitive and resistant progeny would be expected among animals derived from a cross between F_1 hybrid and resistant inbred animals.

For a variety of tissues, including the lung, liver, and skin, multiple tumors induced by carcinogen treatment are enumerated readily, providing a more powerful approach to segregation analysis. The number of tumors observed in an individual animal is a random variable that reflects the intrinsic susceptibility to carcinogenesis for animals of that genotype. Thus, the distribution of tumor multiplicities obtained for animals in a segregating cross between susceptible and resistant parents may be analyzed as a quantitative genetic trait by the method of maximum likelihood (20). This approach is less useful for discriminating the effects of genes that contribute small amounts toward the susceptibility phenotype. However, the method is an efficient means for identifying those cases where one or two loci are largely responsible for a difference in carcinogen sensitivity between two inbred strains. It is in such cases that biological studies to determine the mechanism of action of the susceptibility genes are most appropriate.

Recombinant inbred (RI) strains of animals provide another approach to studying the inheritance of cancer susceptibility genes. The first set of RI mouse strains was constructed by Bailey (21) as an aid to linkage analysis and to study the genetics of disease incidence, which required analysis of populations of mice. A set of RI strains is constructed by the systematic inbreeding of independent lines derived from the F_2 cross between two genetically distinct inbred progenitor strains. After 20 or more generations of brother–sister inbreeding, each RI strain in the set has a replicable recombinant genotype in which one or the other parental alleles has been fixed for all loci that were dimorphic in the pair of progenitor strains. More than 20 different sets of RI strains of mice derived from various pairs of inbred parents are available, with each set consisting of from a few to 25 independent lines (22). In the last several years, particular sets of RI lines have been used in the analysis of susceptibility to lung (23), liver (20), intestinal (24), and skin carcinogenesis (25).

There are several important applications of RI strains to the analysis of susceptibility to carcinogenesis. Each line within an RI set may be typed for susceptibility to the induction of a particular neoplasm by treatment of groups of mice with an appropriate carcinogen, providing a strain distribution pattern (SDP) for the susceptibility phenotype. The distribution of susceptibility phenotypes within a set of RI strains provides information regarding the number of loci responsible for a difference in sensitivity to carcinogenesis between the inbred parental strains. When a single locus is largely responsible for sensitivity to carcinogen, pleiotropic effects of that locus can be discerned by comparison of the SDP for tumor susceptibility with that for other biochemical, physiological, or disease-related phenotypes. Finally, the comparison of the SDP for susceptibility to those for specific loci of known location can provide clues to the chromosomal location for the susceptibility gene (26). Such putative linkage relationships must be verified by analysis of an independent set of RI lines or by direct demonstration of cosegregation in a backcross or intercross experiment.

However, when multiple loci play important roles in determining susceptibility to carcinogenesis, the utility of RI strains is somewhat limited. Recently, Demant and Hart (27) have developed recombinant congenic strains to isolate the effects of specific sensitivity genes. The construction of these strains is analogous to that for RI strains, except that two generations of backcrossing to one of the parental strains are performed prior to brother–sister inbreeding. As a result, each strain in the set contains a small proportion (12.5%) of the genome of the parental strain not involved in the backcross. The applications of recombinant congenic strains to analysis of cancer susceptibility genes are similar to those described above for RI strains. Moen *et al.* (28) have derived recombinant congenic strains by backcrossing STS mice, which are susceptible to colon carcinogenesis, to resistant BALB/c mice. Analysis of these strains for susceptibility to 1,2-dimethylhydrazine (DMH)–induced colon cancer indicated that a small number of loci were responsible for the sensitivity of STS mice and that one of the relevant genes is located on chromosome 2(29).

III. GENETIC CONTROL OF CARCINOGENESIS IN INBRED STRAINS

The earliest observation demonstrating the genetic basis for cancer risk in experimental animals was made by Tyzzer (cited in ref. 30), who noted that the development of spontaneous lung tumors varied among "families" of mice. As inbred mouse strains were developed between 1910 and 1930, it was found that each inbred strain had a characteristic, tissue-specific pattern for the development of spontaneous tumors (30–34). For example, CBA and C3H male mice frequently develop spontaneous liver tumors (Table 1), with a lifetime incidence approaching 100% for some sublines of the latter strain. In contrast, while liver tumors are rare in A, RFM, and SWR mice, each of these strains has a high incidence of spontaneous lung tumors.

The susceptibilities of inbred strains to chemically-induced carcinogenesis at each site are well correlated with their spontaneous tumor incidences, revealing the same tissue specificity. Comparison of a series of inbred mouse strains for the induction of lung (35) and liver (M. Bennett, T. Poole, M. Winkler, N. Drinkwater, unpublished results) tumors (Table 2) reveals that the sensitivities to lung tumor induction follows the order

AKR ~ C3H ~ C57BR < DBA/2 < C57BL/6 < BALB/c < SWR < A/J

while that for hepatocarcinogenesis is

SWR ~ A/J ~ C57BL/6 < AKR ~ BALB/c < C57BR < DBA/2 < C3H

TABLE 1. Lifetime Incidences of Spontaneous Tumors in Inbred Mice

Strain	Number of mice	Median survival (months)	Tumor incidence (%)					Ref.
			Liver	Lung	Breast	Lymphoma	Other sites[b]	
A/WySn	61/60[a]	20/21	15/2	26/17	—[c]/—	13/10		31
CBA/BrARij	44/41	29/30	24/19	11/7	—/4	2/2	Testis (11/—) Ovary (—/83)	32
C3H/HeDiSn	61/60	22/21	51/3	10/3	—/43	5/7	Ovary (—/2)	31
C57BL/KaLw	105/44	24/22	5/—	3/—	—/—	9/16	Bone (1/7) Intestine (4/5) Thyroid (9/2)	32
C57BL/10Sn	59/58	32/28	2/—	3/2	—/—	29/36		31
DBA/2J	67/51	20/20	2/—	—/—	—/31	10/11	Sarcoma (3/—)	33
LP/J	77/51	25/24	6/2	5/4	3/14	1/8	Sarcoma (7/6)	33
NZB/Lac	50/44	18/14	2/—	—/2	—/2	6/14	Bone (6/—) Thyroid (6/—) Pituitary (—/5)	32
RFM/UnRij	42/47	20/20	—/—	24/19	—/—	17/21	Pituitary (—/9)	32
SWR/J	269/329	24/22	1/0.3	49/37	—/36	3/4	Uterus (—/15)	34
129/J	54/55	29/26	—/2	—/1	—/—	2/7	Sarcoma (2/1)	(33)

[a]For each entry in the table, the data given are male/female.
[b]Tumors at other sites, as noted by the authors. Note that the designation of these sites varied among the studies cited.
[c]The dash (—) indicates no tumors were reported at that site.

TABLE 2. Susceptibilities of Eight Inbred Mouse Strains to Chemically-Induced Lung and Liver Carcinogenesis

Strain	Lung[a]		Liver[b]	
	Number of mice	Tumor multiplicity (sd)[c]	Number of mice	Tumor multiplicity (sd)[c]
A/J	76	24 (1)	22	1.5 (1.9)
SWR/J	20	15 (2)	24	0.8 (1.3)
BALB/cByJ	30	1.8 (0.3)	23	9 (6)
C57BL/6J	21	0.86 (0.23)	23	1.4 (1.6)
DBA/2J	20	0.4 (0.21)	23	55 (20)
C3H/HeJ	15	0.07 (0.07)	22	78 (30)
AKR/J	11	0	18	7 (5)
C57BR/cdJ	10	0	32	37 (23)

[a]Data from Malkinson and Beer (35). Male and female mice were given a single injection of ethyl carbamate (1 mg) at 6–12 weeks of age and sacrificed 14–16 weeks after treatment.
[b]Data from unpublished experiments by M. Bennett, T. Poole, M. Winkler, and N. Drinkwater. Male mice were treated at 12 days of age with diethylnitrosamine (0.1 μmol/g body weight) and sacrificed at 32 weeks of age.
[c]Values in the table are mean tumor multiplicity (standard deviation).

Few studies of chemical carcinogenesis have compared directly a large number of inbred strains for their relative susceptibilities to tumor induction. Table 3 provides a compilation of studies that allow direct comparison of three or more inbred mouse or rat strains. Most of these studies have focused on tumor development in the lung, liver, skin, colon, breast, or connective tissue. A discussion of strain variation for the first five tissue sites is provided below; with the exception of rat mammary carcinogenesis, this section will focus on inbred mice. Strain variation in susceptibility to the induction of fibrosarcomas in mice is regulated primarily by the *Ah* locus, as described in the next section.

TABLE 3. Selected Studies of Strain Variation in Chemical Carcinogenesis

Carcinogenic treatment[a]	Species:strains	Target tissues[b]	Ref.
Ethyl carbamate (EC)	Mouse: A, CBA, C57BL, RIII, JU, KL	Lung	36
EC	Mouse: BALB/c, DBA, C3H	Lung	37
EC	Mouse: AKR/J, dd/I, A/J, SMA, CBA/H, C57BL/6	Lung, lymphoma, liver	38
EC	Mouse: CBA/J, A/J, C57BL/6J	Lung	39
Dimethylnitrosamine (DMN)	Mouse: C57BL/10, A/Wy, C3H/He	Lung	40
EC	Mouse: A/WySnJ, A/J, SWR/J, SS/IBG, BALB/cJ, LS/IBG, 129/J, BALB/cByJ, RIIIS/J, C57BL/6J, HS/IBG, C57BL/10ScN, DBA/2J, C3H/HeN, NZB/BINJ, C57BL/6By, C57BL/10SnJ, C57L/J, C3H/HeJ, AKR/J, C57BR/cdJ	Lung	35
EC	Mouse: A/J, SWR/J, BALB/cByJ, 129/J, RIIIS/J	Lung	41
EC	Mouse: C57BL/6J, A/J, AXB[c], BXA	Lung	23
N-Ethyl-N-nitrosourea (ENU)	Mouse: C57BL/6, C3H/He, DBA/2, AKR	Lung, lymphoma	42
2-Acetylaminofluorene	Rat: Marshall, BUFF, ACI, F344	Liver	43
Diethylnitrosamine (DEN), ENU	Mouse: C3H/HeJ, C57BL/6J, BXH	Liver	20
DEN/phenobarbital (PB)	Mouse: C3H/HeN, DBA/2N, C57BL/6N	Liver	44
ENU	Mouse: SWR/J, C57BL/6J, C57BR/cdJ, P/J, SM/J, CBA/J	Liver, lung	45
DEN/PB, clofibrate, estradiol	Mouse: BALB/c, C3H/HeN, C57BL/6N	Liver	46
3-Methylcholanthrene (3-MC)	Mouse: A, BALB/c, C57BL, C3H, DBA/2, I, RIII	Skin	47
7,12-Dimethylbenz[a]-anthracene (DMBA), benzo[a]pyrene/12-O-tetradecanoyl phorbol-13-acetate (TPA)	Mouse: LACA, BALB/c, C3H, AKR	Skin	48
15,16-Dihydro-11-methyl-cyclopenta[a]phen-anthren-17-one/TPA	Mouse: TO, C57BL, DBA/2	Skin	49
Ultraviolet light	Mouse: Sencar, BALB/c, C57BL/6	Skin	50
DMBA, MNNG/chry-sarobin, benzoyl peroxide	Mouse: Sencar, SSIN, DBA/2N, C57BL/6N	Skin	51
DMBA/TPA	Mouse: Sencar, DBA/2, C3H/He, C57BL/6, BXH, BXD	Skin	25
Methylazoxymethanol acetate	Mouse: SWR/J, C57BL/6J, AKR/J	Colon	52
1,2-Dimethylhydrazine (DMH)	Mouse: ICR/Ha, C57BL/Ha, DBA/2	Colon	53
DMH	Mouse: SWR/J, P/J, C57BL/6J, GR, AKR/J	Colon	54
DMH	Mouse: C57BL/6N, C57BL/6Ha, C57BL/6Ha, C57BL/6J	Colon	55
DMH	Mouse: C3H, CBA, C57BL/6J, BALB/c, DBA/2, AKR	Colon	56
DMH	Mouse: BXA, CXS	Colon	24
DMBA	Rat: W/Fu, F344, WxF344F₁	Breast	57
DMBA	Rat: NSD, WF, LEW, F344, ACI, COP	Breast	58

TABLE 3.   *(continued)*

Carcinogenic treatment[a]	Species:strains	Target tissues[b]	Ref.
DMBA	Rat: W/Fu, COP, F344	Breast	59
DMBA	Rat: OM, WF, NSD, LEW, BUFF, F344, AUG, ACI, WN, COP	Breast	60
Dehydroepiandrosterone	Mouse: SWR, SJL, SWXJ	Ovary	61
3,2'-dimethyl-4-aminobiphenyl	F344, ACI, LEW, CD, Wistar	Prostate, breast, skin	62
ENU	Rat: WF, LE, F344	Nervous system	63
3-MC	Mouse: C3H/HeJ, BALB/cBy, C57BL/6J, A/J, CBA/J, B6C3F1, C3B6F1, B6CF1, CD2F1	Fibrosarcoma	64
Dibenz[a,h]anthracene	Mouse: C3H/HeJ, C57BL/6J, AKR/J, DBA/2J	Fibrosarcoma	65

[a]For two-stage carcinogenesis protocols (*see* Chapter 5), the treatment is indicated as "initiating agents/promoters." Abbreviations used: EC, ethylcarbamate; DEN, diethylnitrosamine; DMN, dimethylnitrosamine; ENU, N-ethyl-N-nitrosourea; PB, phenobarbital; 3-MC, 3-methylcholanthrene; DMBA, 7,12-dimethylbenz[a]anthracene; TPA, 12-O-tetradecanoyl phorbol-13-acetate; DMH, 1,2-dimethylhydrazine.

[b]Tissues for which there were significant differences between strains in tumor response.

[c]AXB, BXA, BXD, BXH, CXS, SWXJ denote series of multiple recombinant inbred strains.

A. Lung Tumor Induction in Mice

The strain A mouse is extremely sensitive to the induction of lung adenomas by a wide variety of carcinogens and has provided an important model for studying both the genetics and biology of pulmonary carcinogenesis. As recently reviewed by Malkinson (66), the A mouse is at one extreme of a spectrum of sensitivities to spontaneous and chemically-induced lung tumors among inbred strains. Approximately 15 weeks after a single injection of ethyl carbamate (urethan) (1 mg/g body weight), A/J, GR, and SWR/J mice developed more than 15 lung tumors per mouse, MA/MyJ, BALB/c, and 129/J had intermediate multiplicities of 2-9 tumors, and C57BL/6J, DBA/2J, AKR, SJL, and C3H/HeJ were resistant to lung tumor induction (<1 tumor/mouse) (35). Similar patterns of susceptibility have been observed for spontaneous lung adenomas and tumors induced by other agents.

There have been extensive genetic studies of the sensitivity of strain A mice to lung tumor induction. In one of the earliest applications of quantitative genetic approaches to tumor induction, Heston (67) concluded that the high sensitivity of this strain relative to strain L mice was polygenic in origin. Analysis of segregating crosses between strain A mice and resistant mice carrying various mutant genes with visible phenotypes indicated linkage between susceptibility to lung tumor induction and several markers on chromosome 11 (68). However, the susceptibility gene(s) in this region accounted for a relatively small fraction of the difference in sensitivity between the parental stocks.

In subsequent studies, Bloom and Falconer (69) demonstrated that, in contrast to the intermediate susceptibility of most F_1 hybrids between A and resistant mice, the (A × C57BL)F_1 hybrid was nearly as sensitive as the parental strain A mice. Based on the analysis of tumor multiplicity in backcross and F_2 mice derived from A and C57BL strains, they suggested that a single locus accounted for 75% of the 20-fold difference in susceptibility between the two strains. This locus was designated *ptr* (*pulmonary tumor resistance*) based on the phenotype of the C57BL mice. Malkinson *et al.* (23) have also demonstrated the existence of a major locus conferring the high susceptibility phenotype in A/J mice by analysis of a set of 46 RI strains derived from A/J and C57BL/6J progenitors. The sensitivities of these RI strains to ethyl carbamate–induced lung carcinogenesis fell into four phenotypic classes ranging from the value observed for the resistant C57BL/6J parent to that for the susceptible A/J parent. These data were consistent with a three-locus model, with one locus, *Pas-1* (*Pulmonary adenoma sensitivity*), exerting a stronger effect than *Pas-2* or *Pas-3*. The *Pas-1* locus, which is equivalent to Falconer and Bloom's *ptr* gene, has not yet been identified or mapped to a specific chromosome. However, there is good evidence that the *Pas-2* gene is identical to the K-*ras*-2 proto-oncogene (see below).

The mechanisms governing strain variation in susceptibility to lung tumor induction are poorly understood. Early studies by Heston and Dunn (70) in which lung tissue from susceptible A and resistant L mice was explanted into F_1 animals indicated that the sensitivity to tumor induction was intrinsic to the target tissue. It is likely that the susceptibility genes predominantly influence post-initiation stages of carcinogenesis (*see* Chapter 5 for further discussion of multistage carcinogenesis). In addition to their high risk for the development of spontaneous lung tumors, A mice are highly susceptible to pulmonary carcinogenesis by a wide variety of chemicals (71). Although some studies have demonstrated strain-dependent differences in the level or persistence of DNA damage induced by some specific carcinogens (72), in general these effects are small and not correlated with variation in susceptibility to tumor induction. In two studies, the induction of lung cell proliferation by carcinogen treatment was correlated with the susceptibilities of several strains to tumor induction. Thaete *et al.* (73) observed that the ^{3}H-thymidine labeling index in type 2 pulmonary cells was significantly greater in ethyl carbamate–treated A mice than in similarly treated, resistant BALB/c or C57BL/6 mice. The proliferative response in alveolar cells following *N,N*-dimethylnitrosamine treatment was also significantly greater in susceptible GRS mice than in resistant C3H mice (74).

The histogenesis of lung tumors is also apparently under genetic control. While most tumors induced in A/J mice arise from alveolar type 2 cells, a high proportion of BALB/c lung tumors exhibit properties of Clara cells (41). The moderately susceptible BALB/c mouse is also significantly more sensitive to promotion of lung tumor induction by butylated hydroxytoluene (BHT). After treatment with ethyl carbamate, weekly treatment of BALB/c mice with BHT resulted in a two- to-four-fold increase in the yield of lung tumors relative to mice receiving only ethyl carbamate. In contrast, BHT was inactive as a tumor promoter in C57BL/6, 129, and C3H mice and weakly active in A, SWR, and RIIIS mice (35). Analysis of CXB recombinant inbred lines derived from BALB/c and C57BL/6 strains revealed that susceptibility to lung tumor induction by ethyl carbamate and its enhancement by BHT were determined by independent loci (75).

B. Liver Tumor Induction in Mice

Although Strong established the closely related C3H and CBA mouse strains to study the inheritance of susceptibility to mammary carcinogenesis, it was soon recognized that these two inbred strains developed an unusually high incidence of spontaneous liver tumors (76). Depending on the subline, the lifetime risk for spontaneous hepatocellular adenomas and carcinomas ranged from 20-100% for males and 17-60% for females. Subsequent studies demonstrated that these two inbred strains are the most susceptible to chemically-induced hepatocarcinogenesis among tested strains. We have compared directly ten inbred mouse strains for hepatocarcinogenesis by treatment of preweanling male mice with a single injection of *N*-ethyl-*N*-nitrosourea (ENU) (45) or diethylnitrosamine (DEN) (Table 2) (M. Bennett, T. Poole, M. Winkler, and N. Drinkwater, unpublished results). C3H/HeJ, CBA/J, and DBA/2J mice were the most susceptible with a mean tumor multiplicity in DBA/2J mice that was approximately 70% that for the two former strains. A moderate tumor yield (10-30% that for C3H mice) was obtained for AKR/J, BALB/cByJ, SM/J, and C57BR/cdJ mice, while A/J, C57BL/6J, and SWR/J mice were highly resistant to hepatocarcinogenesis. With the exception of the DBA/2 mouse, the relative susceptibilities of the above strains to ENU- or DEN-induced liver tumors was similar to that reported for other carcinogen treatment protocols and for the spontaneous incidence of liver tumors in male mice. Although DBA/2 mice are nearly as susceptible as C3H mice when treated perinatally with carcinogen, this strain has a low spontaneous incidence of liver tumors (33) and is relatively resistant to the induction of liver tumors by carcinogen treatment of adult animals (44).

The genetics and biology of hepatocarcinogenesis in the susceptible C3H mouse have been studied extensively by several laboratories. We have studied the genetic basis for the high susceptibility of C3H/HeJ male mice relative to C57BL/6J male mice by segregation analysis and by comparing RI strains derived from these two inbred strains (20). The simplest genetic model that could account for the observed distributions of tumor multiplicity included two independent loci, one of which accounted for approximately 85% of the 50-fold difference in susceptibility between the two inbred parental strains. This major locus, designated as *Hcs* (*Hepatocarcinogen sensitivity*), is autosomal and the C3H/HeJ and C57BL/6J alleles are semidominant, such that the heterozygous B6C3F$_1$ mouse is intermediate in sensitivity to the two parental strains. Comparison of the strain distribution patterns for chemically-induced and spontaneous hepatocarcinogenesis in male BXH RI mice (N. Drinkwater and M. Winkler, unpublished results) demonstrated a nearly perfect concordance between these two phenotypes, indicating that the same locus influences both traits.

The *Hcs* locus apparently controls susceptibility to hepatocarcinogenesis by regulating the growth rate of preneoplastic hepatic lesions. Dragani *et al.* (77, 78) observed that nodules induced by DEN or ethyl carbamate treatment were significantly larger at 30 weeks of age in susceptible C3H or B6C3F$_1$ mice than in resistant A, BALB/c, or (C57BL/6J × BALB/c)F$_1$ mice. We (79) have compared the kinetics for the development of preneoplastic, glucose-6-phosphatase–deficient, hepatic foci in C3H/HeJ and C57BL/6J male mice treated at 12 days of age with ENU. The most striking difference between the two strains was in the rate of growth of the preneoplastic lesions between 12 and 32 weeks of age. The 1.7-fold greater growth rate of the lesions in C3H/HeJ mice relative to C57BL/6J mice would have an exponential effect on the appearance of the large lesions presumed to be precursors of hepatocellular adenomas and carcinomas and would account for the differences in tumor multiplicities between the strains observed at later ages. Kakizoe *et al.* (80) and Pugh and Goldfarb (81) have also shown that the rate of growth of preneoplastic lesions in resistant C57BL/6 male mice was lower than that for susceptible C3H or B6C3F$_1$ male mice. However, in these studies the reduced growth rate of lesions in C57BL/6 mice was not observed until 18 weeks of age, and by 30 weeks of age the apparent growth rate of the lesions in these animals was only 20% that for C3H mice. The onset of the reduced growth rate was correlated with the development of inclusions of secretory proteins in the endoplasmic reticulum of hepatoctyes in C57BL/6 mice, but not in C3H mice. The incidence and severity of the protein inclusions in the hepatic lesions was inversely correlated with ^{3}H-thymidine labeling index.

The *Hcs* locus may also play an important role in the growth regulation of normal hepatocytes. The ^{3}H-thymidine labeling index for normal hepatocytes in untreated male C57BL/6J mice was approximately one half that observed for C3H/HeJ mice (79). Similarly, the response of C3H/HeJ mice to the proliferative stimulus of partial hepatectomy was significantly greater than that for C57BL/6J mice as measured by incorporation of ^{3}H-thymidine into hepatic DNA and labeling index during the first 48 hours following surgery (82).

The mechanisms by which the *Hcs* gene influences the proliferation of normal and preneoplastic hepatocytes are unknown. Studies of spontaneous (83) and chemically-induced (84) hepatocarcinogenesis in chimeric mice, derived by fusion of C3H and C57BL/6 embryos, demonstrated that the susceptibility phenotype was cell autonomous, *i.e.*, it was expressed at the level of the target hepatocyte. In studies by Lee *et al.* (84), in which C3H-C57BL/6 chimeric mice were treated as preweanlings with DEN, the preneoplastic hepatic lesions of C3H origin were five-fold larger than the lesions in the same livers derived from C57BL/6 cells. The *Hcs* locus may preferentially influence the growth of hepatic lesions containing mutations in the c-Ha-*ras* (c-Harvey-*ras*) gene. A high proportion of liver tumors induced in B6C3F$_1$ or C3H mice carried mutant Ha-*ras* genes, while these mutations were observed infrequently in liver tumors induced in C57BL/6, BALB/c, or (C57BL/6 × BALB/c)F$_1$ mice (85, 86).

Inbred mouse strains also vary in their responsiveness to hepatic tumor promoters (see also Chapter 5 on promotion). Several laboratories have demonstrated that C3H, DBA/2, and BALB/c mice are susceptible to the promoting effects of phenobarbital treatment, while the C57BL/6 mouse is resistant (44, 46, 87). Lee *et al.* (46) have also shown that clofibrate efficiently promotes hepatic carcinogenesis in C3H mice, but is ineffective in BALB/c and C57BL/6 mice. In contrast, hepatic tumor promotion by halogenated aromatic hydrocarbons is apparently independent of genetic background, when the genotype of the strain at the *Ah* locus (*see below*) is taken into account (10, 88).

Although genetic regulation of the development of liver tumors other than hepato-cellular adenomas and carcinomas has not been studied extensively, Diwan and coworkers (89) have described a potentially novel genetic mechanism for the control of susceptibility to hepatoblastoma development in reciprocal F$_1$ hybrids of C57BL/6N and DBA/2N mice. Treatment of D2B6F$_1$ male mice with a single injection of DEN, followed by chronic exposure to phenobarbital, resulted in a high incidence of hepatoblastomas by 47 weeks of age. In contrast, this type of tumor was observed rarely in similarly treated parental inbred or B6D2F$_1$ male mice. Although the basis for the difference between the F$_1$ hybrids in susceptibility to hepatoblastomas is unclear, this result is consistent with a role for genome imprinting (90), or epigenetic loss of heterozygosity, in the pathogenesis of the tumors.

C. Skin Tumor Induction in Mice

Boutwell (91) was the first to demonstrate the strong influence of genetic factors on the induction of skin tumors in mice by selective breeding of outbred mice for increased or decreased susceptibility. In these experiments, Rockland outbred mice were treated following a two-stage carcinogenesis protocol involving initiation by a single dose of 7,12-dimethylbenz[*a*]anthracene (DMBA) and promotion by repetitive treatment with croton oil. At each generation, the mice with the greatest (or lowest) tumor response were selected for breeding. Following eight generations of selection for increased tumor response, these animals were approximately 25-fold more sensitive to tumor induction than those animals selected for a reduced tumor response. Subsequent outcrossing of the sensitive stock with CD-1 outbred mice and further generations of selective breeding for a high tumor response has given rise to the Sencar outbred stock currently used for studies of skin carcinogenesis (92). The inbred strain designated SSIN has been derived from this stock (93).

Cope *et al.* (94) have similarly selected susceptible (PESTI) and resistant (PERTI) lines derived from CD-1 mice on the basis of responsiveness to tumor promotion by phorbol esters. Rather than using an outbred stock of mice as the starting point, Bangrazi *et al.* (95) constructed a foundation stock with high genetic variability by mating eight genetically diverse inbred strains, including A, DBA/2, P, SWR, SJL, CBA, BALB/c, and C57BL/6. This population was subjected to bidirectional selection by topical treatment with DMBA and 12-*O*-tetradecanoylphorbol-13-acetate (TPA) and using those animals that fell within the upper (or lower) 30% in tumor multiplicity as the parents for the next generation. Response to this selection protocol was rapid; in the fifth generation, the susceptible (Car-S) and resistant (Car-R) lines differed by 30-fold in tumor multiplicity after treatment according to the above initiation–promotion protocol.

While each of these selected lines exhibits a reproducible response to two-stage carcinogenesis in the skin, the genetic basis for the susceptibility phenotype is unknown. However, it is likely that multiple loci play a role in this response. First, even after several generations of selective breeding, further selection was effective in increasing the sensitivity of the animals to tumor induction. Given the strength of the selection in these studies, susceptible alleles would be fixed in a homozygous state within a few generations if only one or two loci regulated sensitivity to skin carcinogenesis. Second, the inbred SSIN strain and its outbred progenitor, Sencar, differed in their responses to skin carcinogenesis. Treatment of SSIN mice with initiating does DMBA or *N*-methyl-*N'*-nitro-*N*-nitrosoguanidine (MNNG) followed by promotion with TPA or benzoyl peroxide resulted in a three- to fivefold greater number of papillomas than similar treatment of Sencar mice (96). However, papillomas induced in Sencar mice were up to 20-fold more likely to progress to squamous cell carcinomas than papillomas in SSIN mice (97).

Unselected inbred strains of mice also show significant variation in skin tumor induction. The DBA/2 strain is highly susceptible to skin tumor induction by treatment with DMBA and TPA (98). C57BL/6 mice are less than 1% as responsive as DBA/2 mice to two-stage skin carcinogenesis while C3H/He and BALB/c mice are moderately susceptible (48, 99, 100). DiGiovanni and coworkers (99) have studied the inheritance of susceptibility to skin tumor induction in crosses between DBA/2N and C57BL/6N mice and demonstrated that sensitivity was semidominant. A high yield of tumors in B6D2F$_1$ × C57BL/6 backcross animals indicated that two or more loci were responsible for the high susceptibility of the DBA/2 mouse. Studies of skin tumor induction in 22 BXD recombinant inbred lines provided results consistent with this genetic model (25). The responses of these RI lines fell into four distinct phenotypic groups, ranging in susceptibility from that equivalent to the C57BL/6 parent to a value that exceeded the sensitivity of the DBA/2 parent. Approximately one half of the BXD lines were indistinguishable in phenotype from the C57BL/6 strain, indicating the existence of a major susceptibility locus that is epistatic to the other genes influencing skin tumor induction.

The high sensitivities of Sencar and DBA/2 mice apparently result from genetic effects on the promotion stage of skin carcinogenesis. Thus, the metabolic activation of polycyclic hydrocarbons and the DNA damage induced by these metabolites are similar in susceptible and resistant strains of mice (101). In addition, responsiveness to treatment with other initiating agents, such as MNNG, paralleled the sensitivity to DMBA treatment (98). Sencar mice have also been shown to be highly susceptible to the induction of skin tumors by ultraviolet light (50).

Studies in several laboratories have demonstrated that the best biological correlate of susceptibility to skin carcinogenesis is the observation of a sustained hyperplastic response in the epidermis following repetitive treatment with tumor promoters [(98, 102); for a detailed discussion, see Chapter 5]. In BXD recombinant inbred lines, the magnitude of the hyperplastic response following repetitive treatment with TPA was well correlated with the susceptibilities of the strains to tumor induction (25). The biochemical basis for these differences in cell proliferation is unknown. The promoting agent, TPA, used in most of the studies cited above exerts its effects by activation of protein kinase C. However, the differences in susceptibility to skin tumor induction appear to be unrelated to the early steps in this signal transduction pathway. Comparison of C57BL/6 and SSIN mice revealed no strain-dependent differences in the levels of protein kinase C isozymes in epidermis, activation of the enzyme by TPA, or in the early induction of ornithine decarboxylase (ODC) activity (102). In addition, the magnitude of ODC induction by TPA treatment in susceptible DBA/2 mice was lower than that for C57BL/6 mice and the SDPs for this response and skin tumor induction in BXD lines were highly discordant (25). Although there are quantitative differences in the relative susceptibilities of mouse strains to carcinogenic regimens involving other promoting agents, Sencar or DBA/2 mice are also highly responsive to promotion by benzoyl peroxide or anthralin derivatives (51). Transplantation studies have demonstrated that the high susceptibility of the Sencar mouse is intrinsic to the target tissue (103).

D. Colon Carcinogenesis in Mice

Although spontaneous tumors of the intestinal epithelium occur rarely in inbred mice, adenomas and adenocarcinomas of the colon are induced efficiently by repetitive treatment of adult animals with DMH (104). Several laboratories have demonstrated that there is substantial variation among inbred mouse strains in their susceptibilities to colon carcinogenesis (52–56). Treatment of SWR/J, ICR/Ha, A/J, and STS/A mice with DMH resulted in a yield of colon tumors that was 10- to 20-fold higher than that for moderately resistant C57BL/6 or BALB/c mice. Several strains, including AKR/J, C57BL/Ha, and DBA/2 mice, were extremely resistant to colon carcinogenesis by DMH and almost never developed colon tumors. Sublines of C57BL/6 mice also differed in their susceptibilities to colon tumor induction. Diwan and Blackman (55) observed that C57BL/6N mice were up to 40-fold more sensitive to DMH-induced colon carcinogenesis relative to C57BL/6Ha mice and that C57BL/6J mice had an intermediate phenotype.

Genetic studies of susceptibility to DMH-induced colon carcinogenesis revealed a complex pattern of inheritance for this trait, consistent with the involvement of multiple loci. Evans *et al.* (105) reported that the high susceptibility of ICR/Ha mice relative to C57BL/Ha mice was controlled by a single, autosomal dominant locus based on the analysis of tumor incidence in F_1, F_2, and backcross generations derived from this pair of strains. The incidence of colon tumors in ICR/Ha and F_1 mice was 100%, in C57BL/Ha mice it was O, and in the F_2 and male F_1 × C57BL/Ha mice it was 78 and 47%, respectively. However, a lower than expected incidence (32% *versus* 50% expected) of tumors was observed in female backcross mice, and semiquantitative scoring of the tumor burden in ICR/Ha, F_1, and F_2 animals indicated that susceptibility was semidominant rather than dominant. An analogous study by Deschner *et al.* (106), using susceptible SWR/J and resistant AKR/J parental mice, yielded somewhat different results. In that study, the incidence of colon tumors in F_1 and F_2 mice were 44 and 52%, respectively, while in F_1 × AKR/J backcross mice the incidence was only 7% — reflecting an important contribution of the resistant background to tumor yield. It was also observed that male mice from reciprocal F_1 hybrids of these strains differed by approximately twofold in sensitivity to colon tumor induction (107).

Recent studies by Fleiszer *et al.* (24) on the comparative susceptibilities of RI strains derived from C57BL/6J and A/J mice and from BALB/cHeA and STS/A mice strongly implicated the existence of multiple loci with significant effects on colon carcinogenesis. A smooth gradation of mean tumor multiplicities was observed among 23 strains derived from C57BL/6J and A/J mice, with some of the strains significantly more resistant to tumor induction than C57BL/6J mice and others more sensitive than A/J mice. Qualitatively similar results were obtained with a smaller set of BALB/c × STS RI strains. The complexity of the genetics of the susceptibility of STS mice to colon carcinogenesis was also demonstrated by studies of recombinant congenic (RC) strains derived from BALB/c and STS mice (28). As described above, the RC strains contain, on average, 12.5% of their genomes derived from the susceptible STS donor strain and are homozygous for the BALB/c alleles over the remainder of the genome. None of the RC strains were as susceptible as the donor STS strain, which developed a high tumor multiplicity by 27 weeks of treatment. By 32 weeks, approximately one half of the RC strains developed colon tumors with the moderate multiplicity characteristic of the BALB/c parent, whereas the remaining RC strains displayed a three- to tenfold higher yield of tumors. Tumor multiplicity and tumor size were found to vary independently among the RC strains. These results are consistent with the existence of two to four loci contributing to the susceptibility phenotype of the STS strain. The most susceptible RC strain (CcS-19) was studied further in backcrosses with BALB/c mice (29). Backcross animals heterozygous for the *CD44* locus on chromosome 2 had a twofold higher tumor multiplicity than animals homozygous for the BALB/c allele at that locus. Two other RC strains that carried the STS allele for *CD44* were also highly susceptible to colon tumor induction. Thus, the authors proposed that one susceptibility determinant, denoted as *Scc-1* (*Susceptibility to colon cancer*), is linked to *CD44*.

The mechanisms by which these genes modify susceptibility to colon carcinogenesis remain unknown. Several studies indicate that differences in the metabolism of DMH may account for some of the observed strain variation. Treatment of C57BL/6J mice with methylazoxymethanol (as the acetate), which is a proximate carcinogenic metabolite of DMH, resulted in a yield of colon tumors that was 50% of that observed for SWR/J mice, while these two strains differed by a factor of 10 in their responses to the parent compound, DMH (52). Analysis of DMH-induced DNA damage in the colon by alkaline elution or quantitation of methylated bases demonstrated a good correlation between these parameters and the sensitivities of DBA/2, C57BL/Ha, AKR/J, SWR/J, and ICR/Ha mice to colon carcinogenesis (108, 109). The level of DNA damage was only twofold greater in susceptible strains than in resistant strains, indicating that differences in the metabolism of the carcinogen does not play a predominant role in controlling sensitivity to colon tumor induction.

Mechanisms unrelated to carcinogen metabolism are also implicated by studies of tumor development in *Apc^{Min}* (see below) mutant mice. On a C57BL/6J genetic background, mice heterozygous for this mutation developed tumors throughout the intestinal tract, including the colon, with a mean multiplicity of approximately 30 by 120 days of age (7). However, on F_1 genetic backgrounds such as MA × C57BL/6 or AKR × C57BL/6, tumor development in heterozygous mutant mice was delayed by up to 200 days and the mean tumor multiplicity was only 25% that observed on the C57BL/6 background (110).

Comparative studies of the proliferative characteristics of normal colonic epithelial cells provide an alternative explanation for the high susceptibility of some mouse strains to colon carcinogenesis. Colonic crypts in susceptible CF1 (outbred) and A/J mice demonstrated a higher labeling index and wider proliferative compartment than those for moderately resistant C57BL/6J mice, while these parameters were lowest for resistant AKR/J mice (111, 112). The larger proliferative compartment in the colons of susceptible animals may result in a larger target cell population for initiation of carcinogenesis by

DMH than for resistant animals. These differences in the proliferative potential of normal cells may also apply to preneoplastic and neoplastic cells in the colon. The observation that tumors arising in the moderately resistant strains were significantly smaller than those in susceptible strains is consistent with this hypothesis (113).

E. Rat Mammary Carcinogenesis

Although less extensively studied than the mouse, variation among inbred strains of rats in susceptibility to carcinogenesis has been observed for a variety of sites, including the peripheral nervous system (63), liver (43), and mammary gland (57–60). The rat has provided an exceptionally fruitful model for genetic studies of mammary carcinogenesis.

Isaacs (60) compared ten inbred strains of rats for their sensitivities to mammary tumor induction by treatment of 50-day old females with a single dose of DMBA. Several strains, including OM, WF, NSD, LEW, and BUFF, were highly susceptible and developed >2 mammary tumors per rat, while the mean tumor multiplicities for F344, AUG, ACI, and WN rats ranged from 0.3 to 1.2 tumors/animal. One strain, COP, proved to be extremely resistant to mammary carcinogenesis. Gould (57) has examined the inheritance of suceptibility to mammary tumor induction in crosses between WF and F344 rats. These studies indicated that several autosomal dominant loci contributed to the greater sensitivity of the WF rat.

As noted above, the COP rat is extremely resistant to mammary carcinogenesis. This resistance is dominant in F_1 hybrids between COP and several strains of varying degrees of sensitivity (60). A single autosomal, dominant locus, designated *mcs* (*mammary carcinoma suppressor*), could account for the segregation of the resistant phenotype in segregating crosses between COP and susceptible rat strains (58, 114). Recent studies have demonstrated that the resistant phenotype can be overcome by neonatal treatment with *N*-methyl-*N*-nitrosourea (115) or by infection *in situ* of mammary epithelial cells by retroviral vectors containing a transforming *v*-Ha-*ras* gene (116).

Although the mechanism of action of the *mcs* gene is unknown, it is likely to influence mammary carcinogenesis through effects on the rate of malignant progression of preneoplastic lesions or the rate of growth of malignant lesions. COP and susceptible rats did not differ in the metabolic activation of chemical carcinogens or in the induction or repair of DNA lesions (59, 117). These animals were also similar in their relative levels of hormones, including estrogens, progesterone, and prolactin, that regulate mammary cell proliferation (60). Transplantation studies have demonstrated that the resistance of COP rats to carcinogenesis is intrinsic to the mammary epithelium (60, 118).

IV. EFFECTS OF SPECIFIC LOCI ON CARCINOGENESIS

The last decade has provided an explosive increase in our knowledge of the roles of specific gene products in carcinogenesis. A large number of cellular proto-oncogenes and tumor suppressor genes have been identified through molecular genetic studies of highly oncogenic retroviruses or human and animal tumors and by genetic analysis of inherited human cancer syndromes. Although this wealth of information is the foundation for modern studies of carcinogenesis, this section will focus more narrowly on specific loci that have been tested directly for their abilities to modulate spontaneous or chemically-induced carcinogenesis in mice through studies of variant alleles, and for which the chromosomal location and, in some cases, the biochemical function are known.

A. *A* (Agouti)

The *agouti* locus (chromosome 2) was identified through its effects on coat color by influencing the microenvironment of the hair follicle to regulate the distribution of phaeo-melanin and eumelanin pigments (119). However, this locus has pleiotropic effects on a variety of tissues. Several alleles are recessive, prenatal lethals (6, 120) and one of these, A^y, causes an increase in susceptibility to spontaneous or chemically-induced tumors of the liver, skin, mammary gland, and bladder in heterozygous animals (120, 121). Similar effects on susceptibility to carcinogenesis were observed for another allele, A^{vy}, which gives rise to viable homozygotes. On a susceptible C3H genetic background (see Section III.B above), the yield of spontaneous or phenobarbital-induced liver tumors in A^y or A^{vy} heterozygotes was two- to fourfold greater than that for A/a or A/A animals (121–124). The presence of the A^{vy} allele was also found to increase the rate of malignant progression in liver tumors induced by treatment of young C57BL/6 mice with a single dose of DEN (125). Although the mechanisms by which the A^y or A^{vy} alleles increase susceptibility to tumor development in the liver and other sites are unknown, the increased cancer risk is associated with a variety of alterations in energy metabolism and growth, including increased somatic growth, obesity, and elevated levels of circulating insulin (120).

B. *Ah* (Aromatic Hydrocarbon Responsiveness)

The *Ah* locus [chromosome 12 (126)] was first defined by differences between inbred strains in their responses to treatment with polycyclic aromatic hydrocarbons such as 3-methylcholanthrene. In most inbred strains (*e.g.*, C57BL/6), such treatment results in a large induction in hepatic cytochrome P_1-450 activity, while this response is not observed in DBA/2 mice and a few other strains (127). Poland and Glover (128) demonstrated that responsive strains, which carried the Ah^b allele, expressed a specific, high-affinity receptor for agonists such as 2,3,7,8-tetrachlorodibenzo-*p*-dioxin (TCDD) that induced hepatic monooxygenase activity, while DBA/2 and other nonresponsive strains expressed a low-affinity variant (Ah^d) of the receptor. Recent studies from several laboratories have demonstrated that the *Ah* locus encodes the ligand-binding subunit of a heterodimeric transcription factor that binds to specific DNA sequences (129, 130).

The *Ah* locus regulates susceptibility to carcinogenesis by distinct effects on both the initiation and promotion phases. The induction of xenobiotic metabolism mediated by the *Ah* receptor is observed in a variety of tissues and cell types and is an important determinant of the metabolic activation of polycyclic hydrocarbons (131). Inbred strains with an Ah^b genotype were significantly more susceptible to the induction of fibrosar-comas by subcutaneous injection of 3-methylcholanthrene or dibenz[*a,h*]anthracene than strains with an Ah^d genotype (65, 131) and susceptibility cosegregated with the *Ah* locus in crosses between responsive C57BL/6 mice and non-responsive DBA/2 mice (131). In addition to its effects on enzyme induction, the *Ah* locus also regulates the tissue-specific toxicity of TCDD and related compounds caused by alterations in the proliferation or differentiation of epithelial cells (132). Thus, promotion of liver tumor induction by 3,4,5,3′,4′,5′-hexabromobiphenyl (10) is dependent on the presence of the high-affinity Ah^b allele.

C. *Apc*^{Min} (Adenomatous Polyposis Coli)

The *Apc*^{Min} mutation (chromosome 18) was identified by Moser *et al.* (7) in a pedigree established by mating a C57BL/6J male mouse treated with ENU with an AKR/J female.

Some of the progeny in this pedigree developed an anemia as young adults that further investigation revealed to be the result of the presence of a large number of adenomas throughout the intestine. The phenotype of *multiple intestinal neoplasia (Min)* was a highly penetrant, autosomal dominant trait caused by a nonsense mutation in the murine homolog of the *Apc* locus, a candidate tumor suppressor gene which is responsible for familial adenomatous polyposis in humans (3, 133). Although all carriers of the Apc^{Min} mutation developed spontaneous intestinal tumors, the latency and severity of disease depended on the genetic background of the host (110) (see Section III.D, above).

D. *bg* (Beige)

Mice homozygous for the *bg* mutation (chromosome 13) exhibit a variety of defects in platelets, granulocytes, and melanocytes that have been attributed to alterations in lysosome function (6). These mice also suffer from a significant depression in natural killer (NK) cell activity similar to that for the analogous, human genetic disease, Chediak–Higashi syndrome (134). Presumably as a result of the defect in NK cell activity, *bg/bg* mutant mice were significantly more susceptible to the induction of experimental metastases by innoculation with B16 melanoma cells than phenotypically normal *bg/+* littermates (135). Argov *et al.* (136) have compared tumor induction in *bg/bg* and *bg/+* mice by oral administration of DMBA in order to test the hypothesis that NK cell function may also limit the induction of primary neoplasms. However, they observed only slight increases in the incidences or decreased latencies for skin tumors and nonthymic lymphomas in mutant mice relative to wild-type animals and no difference in the development of thymic lymphomas or hepatic neoplasms. Similarly, Malkinson and Beer (35) observed that *beige* mutant and wild-type mice were equally susceptible to lung tumor induction.

E. *bm* (Brachymorphic)

Homozygous *bm/bm* (chromosome 19) mutant mice suffer from a disproportionate dwarfing and a reduction in the development of the long bones (6). Sugahara and Schwartz (137) demonstrated that the reduced levels of sulfated glycosaminoglycans in cartilage observed in these mice was caused by a defect in the enzyme, adenylylsulfate kinase, that converts adenosine-5'-phosphosulfate to PAPS. In addition to its role as a sulfate donor for proteoglycans, PAPS is the cofactor for sulfotransferases involved in xenobiotic metabolism. The decreased tissue levels of PAPS in mutant mice can result in a reduction in the synthesis of electrophilic sulfuric acid esters for several proximate carcinogens. The Millers and their coworkers (9, 138, 139) have shown that treatment of *bm/bm* mutant mice with 1'-hydroxysafrole, 4-aminoazobenzene, or *N*-hydroxy-2-acetylaminofluorene resulted in levels of hepatic DNA adducts and yields of liver tumors that were 10–20% those observed in *bm/+* or *+/+* littermates.

F. *H-2* (Histocompatibility Complex-2)

The major histocompatibility complex (chromosome 17) is a highly polymorphic cluster of three classes of genes that play a role in the presentation of peptide antigens, encode complement components, or determine cytolytic immune responses, such as graft rejection (6). The availability of a large number of congenic strains that carry different *H-2* haplotypes has allowed the direct analysis of the role of this chromosomal region in determining susceptibility to tumor induction (31, 40, 140, 141). On a C57BL/10 genetic background, the lifetime incidence of spontaneous lung tumors was 26% for mice with the *H-2ᵃ* haplotype, but only 5% for animals carrying the *H-2ᵇ* haplotype (140). Oomen *et al.* (141) also observed that the yields of lung and intestinal tumors induced by perinatal treatment with ENU was two- to fourfold greater for *H-2ᵃ* than for *H-2ᵇ* mice on the C57BL/10 background. Comparison of strains with recombinant *H-2* haplotypes did not allow assignment of the susceptibility phenotype to a particular region of the complex, indicating that multiple loci within the region may play a role in tumor induction (140, 141). Although the roles of the *H-2* locus in various aspects of the immune response would appear to point toward an immunological basis for the effects of this locus on tumor induction, there is little direct evidence to support this hypothesis. For example, the observation that athymic, *nude (nu/nu)* mutant mice do not show increased susceptibility to spontaneous or induced carcinogenesis (142, 143) indicates that a T cell-mediated immune response does not play an important role in tumor induction. Oomen *et al.* (144) have recently shown that the modulation of lung and intestinal tumor induction by glucocorticoids depended on the *H-2* haplotype of the animals; these authors have argued that the *H-2* complex influences susceptibility to tumor induction through effects on the hormonal regulation of epithelial cell differentiation.

G. K-*ras*-2

A large proportion of lung tumors induced in mice carry somatically induced mutations in the K-*ras*-2 (Kirsten *ras*) proto-oncogene (chromosome 6) that presumably represent initiating events for carcinogenesis (145). Allelic variants of this gene may also contribute to susceptibility to tumor induction when inherited through the germ line. Ryan *et al.* (146) have identified a restriction fragment length polymorphism (RFLP) for this locus which gives rise to DNA fragments of 0.55 or 0.7 kb in inbred mouse strains. Among 13 strains typed for this RFLP and for susceptibility to spontaneous or ethyl carbamate–induced lung tumors, all five of the strains with a moderate or high susceptibility carried the 0.55-kb allele, while the resistant strains were homozygous for the 0.7-kb allele. Among the RI strains studied by Malkinson *et al.* (23), those homozygous for the 0.55-kb allele had a mean tumor multiplicity that was approximately threefold higher than that for the lines carrying the 0.7-kb allele. Similarly, Ryan *et al.* (146) observed a threefold difference in tumor yield for (C57BL/6J × A/J)F$_2$ mice, depending on the K-*ras*-2 genotype. You *et al.* (147) have analyzed a series of mutationally activated K-*ras*-2 genes in spontaneous lung tumors obtained from (A/J × C3H)F$_1$ mice. In 17 of 19 tumors, the allele in which the somatic mutation occurred was derived from the A/J parent. One hypothesis that could account for this result is that the two alleles are differentially expressed in the F$_1$ hybrid. This difference in the level of expression of the two alleles could also be responsible for their effects on susceptibility to lung tumor induction.

H. *Tfm* (Testicular Feminization)

Male mice are significantly more susceptible to liver tumor induction than female mice as a result of the contrasting effects on hepatocarcinogenesis of promotion by testosterone and inhibition by estrogen (45, 148). The promoting effects of testosterone are regulated by the *Tfm* locus (X-chromosome). Male mice hemizygous for the *Tfm* mutation do not express androgen receptor mRNA or functional receptor protein at detectable levels (149, 150). A greatly reduced yield of liver tumors in DEN-treated mutant male mice relative to normal males was observed even after chronic treatment with supraphysiological doses of testosterone, indicating that a functional androgen receptor is required for promotion of hepatocarcinogenesis by this hormone (11). However, analysis of tumors induced in heterozygous female mice for androgen receptor activity demonstrated that testosterone promotes tumor development by an indirect mechanism. Equal numbers of tumors that were deficient or expressed androgen receptors were induced in these mosaic animals when they were treated with DEN, ovariectomized, and received repetitive treatments with testosterone (11). These results indicate that the required receptor–hormone interaction does not take place in the target preneoplastic hepatocyte and implicates a second messenger produced in the liver or another tissue as the direct stimulus for promotion by androgens.

V. CONCLUDING REMARKS

Although several specific loci have been studied for their effects on tumor induction, the existence of a much larger number of risk-modifier genes may be inferred from studies of tissue-specific differences between inbred mouse or rat strains in susceptibility to carcinogenesis. As described in this review, many of these genes are likely to act during the promotion phase of carcinogenesis through effects on cellular growth controls. To date, none of these genes has been characterized in molecular terms. However, the recent development of dense genetic maps of the mouse (151) and rat (152) based on markers suitable for linkage analysis of cancer susceptibility genes and the development of methods for the physical analysis of complex genomes (153) provide encouragement that we will soon begin to understand the mechanisms by which the murine susceptibility genes influence carcinogenesis.

ACKNOWLEDGMENTS

Work in the author's laboratory was supported by Public Health Service Grants CA22484, CA07175, and CA09135.

REFERENCES

1. Friend, S. H., Bernards, R., Rogelj, S., Weinberg, R. A., Rapaport, J. M., Albert, D. M., and Dryja, T. P.: *Nature* **323**, 643 (1986).
2. Rose, E. A., Glaser, T., Jones, C., Smith, C. L., Lewis, W. H., Call, K. M., Minden, M., Champagne, E., Bonetta, L., Yeger, H., and Housman, D. E.: *Cell* **60**, 495 (1990).
3. Kinzler, K. W., Nilbert, M. C., Su, L., Vogelstein, B., Bryan, T. M., Levy, D. B., Smith, K. J., Preisinger, A. C., Hedge, P., McKechnie, D., Finniear, R., Markham, A., Groffen, J., Boguski, M. S., Altschul, S. F., Horii, A., Ando, H., Miyoshi, Y., Miki, Y., Nishisho, I., and Nakamura, Y.: *Science* **253**, 661 (1991).
4. Newman, B., Austin, M. A., Lee, M., and King, M.-C.: *Proc. Natl. Acad. Sci. U.S.A.* **85**, 3044 (1988).
5. Hall, J. M., Lee, M. K., Newman, B., Morrow, J. E., Anderson, L. A., Huey, B., and King, M.-C.: *Science* **250**, 1684 (1990).
6. Green, M. C: Catalog of Mutant Genes and Polymorphic Loci. *In* "Genetic Variants and Strains of the Laboratory Mouse" (M. F. Lyon and A. G. Searle, eds.). Oxford University Press, New York, 1989, p. 12.
7. Moser, A. R., Pitot, H. C., and Dove, W. F.: *Science* **247**, 322 (1990).
8. Levy, G. N., and Weber, W. W.: *Carcinogenesis* **10**, 705 (1989).
9. Lai, C.-C., Miller, J. A., Miller, E. C., and Liem, A.: *Carcinogenesis* **6**, 1037 (1985).
10. Drinkwater, N. R., Hanigan, M. H., and Kemp, C. J.: *Toxicol. Lett.* **49**, 255 (1989).

11. Kemp, C. J., Leary, C. N., and Drinkwater, N. R.: *Proc. Natl. Acad. Sci. U.S.A.* **86**, 7505 (1989).
12. Holland, J. M., Mitchell, T. J., Gipson, L. C., and Whitaker, M. S.: *J. Natl. Cancer Inst.* **61**, 1357 (1978).
13. Capecchi, M. R.: *Science* **244**, 1288 (1989).
14. Soriano, P., Montgomery, C., Geske, R., and Bradley, A.: *Cell* **64**, 693 (1991).
15. Schwartzenberg, P. L., Stall, A. M., Hardin, J. D., Bowdish, K. S., Humaran, T., Boast, S., Harbison, M. L., Robertson, E. J., and Goff, S. P.: *Cell* **65**, 1165 (1991).
16. Donehower, L. A., Harvey, M., Slagle, B. L., McArthur, M. J., Montgomery, C. A., Butel, J. S., and Bradley, A.: *Nature* **356**, 215 (1992).
17. Festing, M. F. W.: "Inbred Strains in Biomedical Research". Oxford University Press, New York, 1979, 483 pp.
18. Fitch, W. M., and Atchley, W. R.: *Science* **228**, 1169 (1985).
19. Morse, H. C.: The Laboratory Mouse — A Historical Perspective. *In* "The Mouse in Biomedical Research" (H. L. Foster, D. J. Small, and J. G. Fox, eds.). Academic Press, New York, 1981, Vol. 1, p. 1.
20. Drinkwater, N. R., and Ginsler, J. J.: *Carcinogenesis* **7**, 1701 (1986).
21. Bailey, D. W.: *Transplantation* **11**, 325 (1971).
22. Taylor, B. A.: Recombinant Inbred Strains. *In* "Genetic Variants and Strains of the Laboratory Mouse" (M. F. Lyon and A. G. Searle, eds.). Oxford University Press, New York, 1989, p. 773.
23. Malkinson, A. M., Nesbitt, M. N., and Skamene, E.: *J. Natl. Cancer Inst.* **75**, 971 (1985).
24. Fleiszer, D., Hilgers, J., and Skamene, E.: *Curr. Topics Microbiol. Immunol.* **137**, 243 (1988).
25. DiGiovanni, J., Imamoto, A., Naito, M., Walker, S. E., Beltran, L., Chenicek, K. J., and Skow, L.: *Carcinogenesis* **13**, 525 (1992).
26. Silver, J., and Buckler, C. E.: *Proc. Natl. Acad. Sci. U.S.A.* **83**, 1423 (1986).
27. Demant, P., and Hart, A. A. M.: *Immunogenetics* **24**, 416 (1986).
28. Moen, C. J. A., van der Valk, M. A., Snoek, M., van Zutphen, B. F. M., von Deimling, O., Hart, A. A. M., and Demant, P.: *Mammalian Genome* **1**, 217 (1991).
29. Moen, C. J. A., Snoek, M., Hart, A. A. M., and Demant, P.: *Oncogene* **7**, 563 (1992).
30. Lynch, C. J.: *J. Exp. Med.* **43**, 339 (1926).
31. Smith, G. S., and Walford, R. L.: Influence of the H-2 and H-1 Histocompatibility Systems upon Life Span and Spontaneous Cancer Incidences in Congenic Mice. *In* "Genetic Effects on Aging" (D. Bertsma and D. E. Harrison, eds.). Liss, New York, 1976, Vol. 14, p. 281.
32. Zurcher, C., van Zwieten, M. J., Solleveld, H. A., and Hollander, C. F.: Aging Research. *In* "The Mouse in Biomedical Research" (H. L. Foster, D. J. Small, and J. G. Fox, eds.). Academic Press, New York, 1982, Vol. 4, p. 11.
33. Smith, G. S., Walford, R. L., and Mickey, M. R.: *J. Natl. Cancer Inst.* **50**, 1195 (1973).
34. Rabstein, L. S., Peters, R. L., and Spahn, G. J.: *J. Natl. Cancer Inst.* **50**, 751 (1973).
35. Malkinson, A. M., and Beer, D. S.: *J. Natl. Cancer Inst.* **70**, 931 (1983).
36. Falconer, D. S., and Bloom, J. L.: *Br. J. Cancer* **16**, 665 (1962).
37. Trainin, N., Precerutti, A., and Law, L. L.: *Nature* **202**, 305 (1964).
38. Matsuyama, M., and Suzuki, H.: *Br. J. Cancer* **22**, 527 (1968).
39. Gorelik, E., and Herberman, R. B.: *J. Natl. Cancer Inst.* **67**, 1317 (1981).
40. Den Engelse, L., Oomen, L. C. J. M., Van derValk, M. A., Hart, A. A. M., Dux, A., and Emmelot, P.: *Int. J. Cancer* **28**, 199 (1981).
41. Beer, D. G., and Malkinson, A. M.: *J. Natl. Cancer Inst.* **75**, 963 (1985).
42. Anderson, L. M., Jones, A. B., and Kovatch, R. M.: *Cancer Lett.* **52**, 91 (1990).
43. Reuber, M. D.: *Toxicol. Appl. Pharm.* **37**, 525 (1976).
44. Diwan, B. A., Rice, J. M., Ohshima, M., and Ward, J. M.: *Carcinogenesis* **7**, 215 (1986).
45. Kemp, C. J., and Drinkwater, N. R.: *Cancer Res.* **49**, 5044 (1989).
46. Lee, G. H., Nomura, K., and Kitagawa, T.: *Carcinogenesis* **10**, 2227 (1989).
47. Andervont, H. B., and Edgcomb, J. H.: *J. Natl. Cancer Inst.* **17**, 481 (1956).
48. Wheldrake, J. F., Marshall, J., Ramli, J., and Murray, A. W.: *Carcinogenesis* **3**, 805 (1982).
49. Abbott, P. J.: *Cancer Res.* **43**, 2261 (1983).
50. Strickland, P. T., and Swartz, R. P.: *Cancer Res.* **47**, 6294 (1987).
51. DiGiovanni, J., Walker, S. C., Beltran, L., Naito, M., and Eastin, W. C.: *Cancer Res.* **51**, 1398 (1991).
52. Diwan, B. A., Dempster, A. M., and Blackman, K. E.: *Proc. Soc. Exp. Biol. Med.* **161**, 347 (1979).
53. Evans, J. T., Hauschka, T. S., and Mittelman, A.: *J. Natl. Cancer Inst.* **52**, 999 (1974).
54. Diwan, B. A., Meier, H., and Blackman, K. E.: *J. Natl. Cancer Inst.* **59**, 455 (1977).
55. Diwan, B. A., and Blackman, K. E.: *Cancer Lett.* **9**, 111 (1980).
56. Turusov, V. S., Lanko, N. S., Krutovskikh, V. A., and Parfenov, Y. D.: *Carcinogenesis* **3**, 603 (1982).
57. Gould, M. N.: *Cancer Res.* **46**, 1199 (1986).
58. Isaacs, J. T.: *Cancer Res.* **46**, 3958 (1986).
59. Moore, C. J., Tricomi, W. A., and Gould, M. N.: *Carcinogenesis* **9**, 2099 (1988).

60. Isaacs, J. T.: *Cancer Res.* **48,** 2204 (1988).
61. Beamer, W. G., Tennent, B. J., Shultz, K. L., Nadeau, J. H., Shultz, L. D., and Skow, L. C.: *Cancer Res.* **48,** 5092 (1988).
62. Shirai, T., Nakamura, A., Fukushima, S., Yamamoto, A., Tada, M., and Ito, N.: *Carcinogenesis* **11,** 793 (1990).
63. Naito, M., Naito, Y., and Ito A.: *Gann* **73,** 323 (1982).
64. Prehn, L. M., and Lawler, E. M.: *Science* **204,** 309 (1979).
65. Lubet, R. A., Connolly, G. M., Nebert, D. W., and Kouri, R. E.: *Carcinogenesis* **4,** 513 (1983).
66. Malkinson, A. M.: *Toxicology* **54,** 241 (1989).
67. Heston, W. E.: *J. Natl. Cancer Inst.* **3,** 69 (1942).
68. Heston, W. E., Deringer, M. K., Hughes, I. R., and Cornfield, J.: *J. Natl. Cancer Inst.* **12,** 1141 (1952).
69. Bloom, J. L., and Falconer, D. S.: *J. Natl. Cancer Inst.* **33,** 607 (1964).
70. Heston, W. E., and Dunn, T. B.: *J. Natl. Cancer Inst.* **11,** 1057 (1951).
71. Shimkin, M. B., and Stoner, G. D.: *Adv. Cancer Res.* **21,** 1 (1975).
72. Eastman, A., and Bresnick, E.: *Cancer Res.* **39,** 2400 (1979).
73. Thaete, L. G., Beer, D. G., and Malkinson, A. M.: *Cancer Res.* **46,** 5335 (1986).
74. DeMunter, H. K., Den Engelse, L., and Emmelot, P.: *Chem.-Biol. Interact.* **24,** 299 (1979).
75. Malkinson, A. M., and Beer, D. S.: *J. Natl Cancer Inst.* **73,** 925 (1984).
76. Andervont, H. B.: *J. Natl. Cancer Inst.* **11,** 581 (1950).
77. Dragani, T. A., Manenti, G., and Della Porta, G.: *J. Cancer Res. Clin. Oncol.* **113,** 223 (1987).
78. Dragani, T. A., Manenti, G., and Della Porta, G.: *Cancer Res.* **51,** 6299 (1991).
79. Hanigan, M. H., Kemp, C. J., Ginsler, J. J., and Drinkwater, N. R.: *Carcinogenesis* **9,** 885 (1988).
80. Kakizoe, S., Goldfarb, S., and Pugh, T. D.: *Cancer Res.* **49,** 3985 (1989).
81. Pugh, T. D., and Goldfarb, S.: *Cancer Res.* **52,** 280 (1992).
82. Bennett, L. M., Hanigan, M. H., Winkler, M. H., and Drinkwater, N. R.: *Proc. Am. Assoc. Cancer Res.* **31,** 152 (1990).
83. Condamine, H., Custer, R. P., and Mintz, B.: *Proc. Natl. Acad. Sci. U.S.A.* **68,** 2032 (1971).
84. Lee, G.-H., Nomura, K., Kanda, H., Kusakabe, M., Yoshiki, A., Sakakura, T., and Kitagawa, T.: *Cancer Res.* **51,** 3257 (1991).
85. Buchmann, A., Bauer-Hofmann, R., Mahr, J., Drinkwater, N. R., Luz, A., and Schwarz, M.: *Proc. Natl. Acad. Sci. U.S.A.* **88,** 911 (1991).
86. Dragani, T. A., Manenti, G., Colombo, B. M., Falvella, F. S., Gariboldi, M., Pierotti, M. A., and Della Porta, G.: *Oncogene* **6,** 333 (1991).
87. Weghorst, C. M., Pereira, M. A., Klaunig, J. E.: *Carcinogenesis* **10,** 1409 (1989).
88. Della Porta, G., Dragani, T. A., and Sozzi, G.: *Tumori* **73,** 99 (1987).
89. Diwan, B. A., Ward, J. M., and Rice, J. M.: *Carcinogenesis* **10,** 1345 (1989).
90. Sapienza, C.: *Mol. Carcinogenesis* **3,** 118 (1990).
91. Boutwell, R. K.: *Prog. Exptl. Tumor Res.* **4,** 207 (1964).
92. DiGiovanni, J., Slaga, T. J., and Boutwell, R. K.: *Carcinogenesis* **1,** 381 (1980).
93. Fischer, S. M., O'Connell, J. F., Conti, C. J., Tacker, K. C., Fries, J. W., Patrick, K. E., Adams, L. M., and Slaga, T. J.: *Carcinogenesis* **8,** 421 (1987).
94. Cope, F. O., Wagner, F. J., Conway, T., Burns, P. D., Johnston, D., Murphy, P., Triggs, G., and Wille, J.: *Mol. Carcinogenesis* **1,** 116 (1988).
95. Bangrazi, C., Mouton, D., Neveu, T., Saran, A., Covelli, V., Doria, G., and Biozzi, G.: *Carcinogenesis* **11,** 1711 (1990).
96. DiGiovanni, J., Walker, S. C., Beltran, L., Naito, M., and Eastin, W. C.: *Cancer Res.* **51,** 1398 (1991).
97. Gimenez-Conti, I. B., Bianchi, A. B., Fischer, S. M., Reiners, J. J., Conti C. J., and Slaga, T. J.: *Cancer Res.* **52,** 3432 (1992).
98. DiGiovanni, J., Prichett, W. P., Decina, P. C., and Diamond, L.: *Carcinogenesis* **5,** 1493 (1984).
99. Naito, M., Chenicek, K. J., Naito, Y., and DiGiovanni, J.: *Carcinogenesis* **9,** 639 (1988).
100. Ashman, L. K., Murray, A. W., Cook, M. G., and Kotlarski, I.: *Carcinogenesis* **3,** 99 (1982).
101. Ashurst, S. W., and Cohen, G. M.: *Int. J. Cancer* **27,** 357 (1981).
102. Fischer, S. M., Jasheway, D. W., Klann, R. C., Butler, A. P., Patrick, K. E., Baldwin, J. K., and Cameron, G. S.: *Cancer Res.* **49,** 6693 (1989).
103. Yuspa, S. H., Spangler, E. F., Donahoe, R., Geusz, S., Ferguson, E., Wenk, M., and Hennings, H.: *Cancer Res.* **42,** 437 (1982).
104. Thurnherr, N., Deschner, E. E., Stonehill, E. H., and Lipkin, M.: *Cancer Res.* **33,** 940 (1973).
105. Evans, J. T., Shows, T. B., Sproul, E. E., Paolini, N. S., Mittelman, A., and Hauschka, T. S.: *Cancer Res.* **37,** 134 (1977).
106. Deschner, E. E., Long, F. C., and Hakissian, M.: *Cancer* **61,** 478 (1988).
107. Deschner, E. E., Hakissian, M., and Long, F. C.: *J. Cancer Res. Clin. Oncol.* **115,** 335 (1989).

108. Cooper, H. K., Buecheler, J., and Kleuhues, P.: *Cancer Res.* **38**, 3063 (1978).
109. Bolognesi, C., Mariani, M. R., and Boffa, L. C.: *Carcinogenesis* **9**, 1347 (1988).
110. Moser, A. R., Dove, W. F., Roth, K. A., and Gordon, J. I.: *J. Cell Biol.* **116**, 1517 (1992).
111. Deschner, E. E., Long, F. C., Hakissian, M., and Herrmann, S. L.: *J. Natl. Cancer Inst.* **70**, 279 (1983).
112. Glickman, L. T., Suissa, S., and Fleiszer, D. M.: *Cancer Res.* **47**, 4766 (1987).
113. James, J. T., Shamsuddin, A. M., and Trump, B. F.: *J. Natl. Cancer Inst.* **71**, 955 (1983).
114. Gould, M. N., Wang, B., and Moore, C. J.: Modulation of Mammary Carcinogenesis by Enhancer and Suppressor Genes. *In* "Genes and Signal Transduction in Multistage Carcinogenesis" (N. H. Colburn, ed.). Marcel Dekker, New York, 1989, p. 19.
115. Lu, S.-J., Laroye, G., and Archer, M. C.: *Cancer Res.* **52**, 5037 (1992).
116. Wang, B., Kennan, W. S., Yasukawa-Barnes, J., Lindstrom, M. J., and Gould, M. N.: *Cancer Res.* **51**, 5298 (1991).
117. Lu, S.-J., Chaulk, E. J., and Archer, M. C.: *Carcinogenesis* **13**, 857 (1992).
118. Zhang, R., Haag, J. D., and Gould, M. N.: *Carcinogenesis* **11**, 1765 (1989).
119. Silvers, W. K.: The Agouti and Extension Series of Alleles—Umbrous and Sable. *In* "The Coat Colors of Mice" (W. K. Silvers, ed.). Springer-Verlag, New York, 1979, p. 6.
120. Wolff, G. L., Roberts, D. W., and Galbraith, D. B.: *J. Heredity* **77**, 151 (1986).
121. Heston, W. E., and Vlahakis, G.: *J. Natl. Cancer Inst.* **26**, 969 (1961).
122. Heston, W. E., and Vlahakis, G.: *J. Natl. Cancer Inst.* **40**, 1161 (1968).
123. Wolff, G. L.: *Cancer Res.* **30**, 1722 (1970).
124. Wolff, G. L., Morrissey, R. L., and Chen, J. J.: *Carcinogenesis* **7**, 1895 (1986).
125. Becker, F. F.: *Cancer Res.* **46**, 2241 (1986).
126. Poland, A., Glover, E., and Taylor, B. A.: *Mol. Pharmacol.* **32**, 471 (1987).
127. Nebert, D. W., Jensen, N. M., Shinozuka, H., Kunz, H. W., and Gill, T. J.: *Genetics* **100**, 79 (1982).
128. Poland, A., and Glover, E.: *Mol. Pharmacol.* **11**, 389 (1975).
129. Burbach, K. M., Poland, A., and Bradfield, C. A.: *Proc. Natl. Acad. Sci. U.S.A.* **89**, 8185 (1992).
130. Whitlock, J. P.: *Annu. Rev. Pharmacol. Toxicol.* **30**, 251 (1990).
131. Kouri, R. E., Ratrie, H., and Whitmire, C. E.: *J. Natl. Cancer Inst.* **51**, 197 (1973).
132. Poland, A., Knutson, J. C., and Glover, E.: *J. Invest. Dermatol.* **83**, 454 (1984).
133. Su, L.-K., Kinzler, K. W., Vogelstein, B., Preisinger, A. C., Moser, A. R., Luonog, C., Gould, K. A., and Dove, W. F.: *Science* **256**, 668 (1992).
134. Roder, J., and Duwe, A. K.: *Nature* **278**, 451 (1979).
135. Talmadge, J. E., Meyers, K. M., Prieur, D. J., and Starkey, J. R..: *J. Natl. Cancer Inst.* **65**, 929 (1980).
136. Argov, S., Cochran, A. J., Karre, K., Klein, G. O., and Klein, G.: *Int. J. Cancer* **28**, 739 (1981).
137. Sugahara, K., and Schwartz, N. B.: *Proc. Natl. Acad. Sci. U.S.A.* **76**, 6615 (1979).
138. Boberg, E. W., Miller, E. C., Miller, J. A., Poland, A., and Liem, A.: *Cancer Res.* **43**, 5163 (1983).
139. Delclos, K. B., Miller, E. C., Miller, J. A., and Liem, A.: *Carcinogenesis* **7**, 277 (1986).
140. Faraldo, M. J., Dux, A., Muhlbock, O., and Hart, G.: *Immunogenetics* **9**, 383 (1979).
141. Oomen, L. C. J. M., van der Valk, M. A., Hart, A. A. M., Demant, P., and Emmelot, P.: *Cancer Res.* **48**, 6634 (1988).
142. Stutman, O.: *Science* **183**, 534 (1974).
143. Stutman, O.: *Expl. Cell Biol.* **47**, 129 (1979).
144. Oomen, L. C. J. M., van der Valk, M. A., Hart, A. A. M., and Demant, P.: *J. Natl. Cancer Inst.* **81**, 512 (1989).
145. You, M., Canadrian U., Maronpot, R. R., Stoner, G. D., and Anderson, M. W.: *Proc. Natl. Acad. Sci. USA* **86**, 3070 (1989).
146. Ryan, J., Barker, P. E., Nesbitt, M. N., and Ruddle, F. H.: *J. Natl. Cancer Inst.* **79**, 1351 (1987).
147. You, M., Wang, Y., Stoner, G., You, L., Maronpot, R., Reynolds, S. H., and Anderson, M.: *Proc. Natl. Acad. Sci. U.S.A.* **89**, 5804 (1992).
148. Vesselinovitch, S. D., Itze, L., Mihailovich, N., and Rao, K. V. N.: *Cancer Res.* **40**, 1538 (1980).
149. Attardi, B., and Ohno, S.: *Cell* **2**, 205 (1974).
150. Gaspar, M.-L., Meo, T., Bourgarel, P., Guenet, J.-L., and Tosi, M.: *Proc. Natl. Acad. Sci. U.S.A.* **88**, 8606 (1991).
151. Dietrich, W., Katz, H., Lincoln, S. E., Shin, H.-S., Friedman, J., Dracopoli, N. C., and Lander, E. S.: *Genetics* **131**, 423 (1992).
152. Serikawa, T., Kuramoto, T., Hilbert, P., Mori, M., Yamada, J., Dubay, C. J., Lindpainter, K., Ganten, D., Guenet, J.-L., Lathrop, G. M., and Beckmann, J. S.: *Genetics* **131**, 701 (1992).
153. Schlessinger, D.: *TIG* **6**, 248 (1990).

NOTE ADDED IN PROOF

Since this chapter was written, the mouse genetic map based on simple sequence length polymorphisms has grown to include more than 4,000 marker loci [Dietrich, W. F., Miller, J. C., Steen, R. G., Merchant, M., Damron, D., Nahf, R., Gross, A., Joyce, D. C., Wessel, M., Dredge, R. D., Marquis, A., Stein, L. D., Goodman, N., Page, D. C., Lander, E. S.: *Nature Genetics* **7**, 220 (1994)]. The number of such markers, their high degree of polymorphism, and their ease of analysis by polymerase chain reaction have greatly facilitated the mapping of genes that influence the susceptibility of inbred strains to carcinogenesis. Several recent reports of the chromosomal localization of susceptibility genes are summarized below.

Pas-1: The major locus responsible for the high susceptibility of A/J mice to lung tumor induction (Sect. III.A) has been localized to mouse chromosome 6. This gene maps near, and may be identical to the K-*ras*-2 locus [Gariboldi, M., Manenti, G., Canzlan, F., Falvella, F. S., Radice, M. T., Pierotti, M. A., Della Porta, G., Binelli, G., Dragani, T. A.: *Nature Genetics* **3**, 131 (1993)].

Hcs: Several loci that contribute to the high susceptibility of C3H mice to liver tumor induction (Sect. III.B) have been mapped. Analysis of the segregation of susceptibility in C3AF$_2$ mice led to the identification of three loci, designated *Hcs-1, Hcs-2,* and *Hcs-3,* located near markers *D7Nds-1* (chromosome 7), *D8Mit-14* (chromosome 8), and *Odc-8* (chromosome 12), respectively [Gariboldi, M., Manenti, G., Canzian, F., Falvella, F. S., Pierotti, M. A., Della Porta, G., Binelli, G., Dragani, T. A.: *Cancer Res.* **53**, 209 (1993)]. The *Hcs* locus originally defined in segregating crosses between C3H/HeJ and C57BL/6J mice, now designated *Hcs-4,* has been localized to chromosome 1, near *D1Mit-15* [Bennett, L. M., Winkler, M. L., Drinkwater, N. R.: *Proc. Am. Assoc. Cancer Res.* **34**, 144 (1993)].

Mom-1: As noted above (Sect. III.D), the intestinal tumor phenotype induced by the *Apc^Min* mutation in mice is partially suppressed on AKR and MA genetic backgrounds. The locus responsible for this inhibition, *Mom-1 (modifier of Min)* has been mapped to a region of mouse chromosome 4, near the locus *D4Mit-13* [Dietrich, W. F., Lander, E. S., Smith, J. S., Moser, A. R., Gould, K. A., Luongo, C., Borenstein, N., Dove, W. F.: *Cell* **75**, 631 (1993)].

Mcs-1: The dominant suppressor of mammary carcinogenesis present in COP rats (Sect. III.E) has been mapped in crosses with WF rats to rat chromosome 2, near the marker *Mit-R1025* [Hsu, L., Kennan, W. S., Shepel, L. A., Jacob, H. J., Szpirer, C., Szpirer, J., Lander, E. S., Gould, M. N.: *Cancer Res.* **54**, 2765 (1994)].

CHAPTER **13**

Radiation Injury and Radiation Carcinogenesis with Special Reference to Combination Effects with Chemical Agents

Jeffrey L. Schwartz

I. INTRODUCTION

Radiation is a ubiquitous component of the environment. We are exposed to ultraviolet radiation from the sun; gamma rays from cosmic radiation; the decay of isotopes in building materials, air, water, and food; alpha particles from radon and radon-daughters that seep into our basements; and X-rays, gamma rays, and other radiation from man-made sources (such as those used in medical procedures or produced as a byproduct of nuclear power generation). All these radiations represent biological hazards and are associated with tumor induction. However, the mechanism of action of ultraviolet radiation (a nonionizing radiation) is different from those of X-rays, gamma rays, and other (particulate types of) ionizing radiations. This chapter focuses on radiation injury by ionizing radiations that leads to the emergence of tumors, and on the modulating effects of various biological factors and physical and chemical agents on this carcinogenic process.

The generation of radiation injury begins with physical interaction between the radiation and the biological medium resulting in an ionization event. This is followed by chemical processes that lead to alterations in biologically relevant molecules in the cell, which in turn lead to the biological effects, first at the genetic and cellular levels, and then ultimately at the level of a tissue or individual. It is important to bear in mind that all biological effects of ionizing radiation, be they mutation, cancer, cataracto-genesis, or acute lethality, begin with the ionization of some molecule in some cell that falls in the path of an X-ray or gamma ray beam or in the path of some energetic particle.

II. MECHANISM OF RADIATION INJURY

A. Radiation Interactions with Matter[1]

1. Subatomic Nature of the Interactions

Ionizing radiation refers to those types of radiation that produce the ejection of an orbital electron from atoms or molecules. This results in the breaking of chemical bonds and the formation of ion pairs, leading ultimately to biological effects. The ionization potential of most molecules in biological materials is 10–15 electron volts (eV), so in order to be ionizing, the radiation must be able to impart at least as much energy. Ionizing radiation can be either electromagnetic (X-rays and gamma rays) or particulate (neutrons and alpha particles). Some produce ionizations directly through interactions with orbital electrons, but most produce ionizations indirectly through the production of secondary electrons, recoil protons, and nuclei.

For radiation having an energy of 1–10 eV (nonionizing radiation), the major mode of energy transfer is by electron excitation at an atomic/molecular target. Excitation refers to the elevation of the energy level of an electron to an excited state. When the electron returns to the ground state, the excess energy is released in the form of visible light (fluorescence, phosphorescence) or it brings about chemical change (*e.g.*, pyrimidine dimer formation). Ultraviolet radiation is the major nonionizing radiation hazard, although excitation can be brought about with ionizing radiation as well. Whether excitation or ionization is produced depends on both the energy of the incident radiation and the type of interaction that occurs with the orbital electron.

For electromagnetic radiations, most ionizations occur primarily through indirect means. The incident radiation sets in motion an electron which then loses energy through excitation and ionization events. The initial interaction between the photon and atom is designated by the term "kerma" (kinetic energy released in the material). The term "dose" describes the energy absorbed within a defined volume.

There are three basic modes for energy transfer from electromagnetic radiation. In the low-energy range (10–100 keV), energy transfer is primarily via photoelectric effect, in which all the energy of the photon is transferred to the target electron, usually an inner shell electron. The electron is ejected at an energy equal to the energy of the incident photon less the binding energy of the electron. The probability of photoelectric processes occurring depends on the atomic number of the target as well as the photon energy.

At higher energies (0.1–3 MeV), only a fraction of the incident photon energy is transferred to the target electron, the outer orbital electron (Compton scattering). The incident photon is scattered with a lower energy and it continues to interact with other electrons until the energy is low enough for the photoelectric effect to predominate. The probability of Compton scattering is independent of atomic number and has only a modest dependence on photon energy.

When the incident photon energy is greater than 1.02 MeV, the photon may interact with the nucleus of the target atom and is converted into an electron and positron pair (pair production). This process is dependent on atomic number, and its probability of occurrence increases exponentially with higher (greater than 1.02 MeV) energies.

Once the electrons are set in motion through one of the three interactions mentioned above, they in turn interact with and eject other orbitally-localized electrons through coulombic interactions. Most of the energy of these secondary electrons (delta rays) is lost

---

[1] Two source books (1, 2) are recommended as general background to this section.

through the direct production of ionizations and excitations. In some instances photons are emitted as a result of electron deceleration (bremsstrahlung radiation).

Charged particles (alpha particles, protons, high Z particles) also lose energy primarily through coulombic interactions with electrons and nuclei and through the generation of bremsstrahlung radiation. The rate of energy loss is directly related to the charge of the particle and inversely related to its velocity. Energy loss is also dependent on the electron density of the target.

Since, with uncharged particles (such as neutrons) there can be no coulombic interaction, particle energy is lost through interactions with nuclei producing scattering events (elastic, inelastic, or nonelastic), capture reactions, or spallation events. In biological tissues, low-energy neutrons (< 10 MeV) interact primarily with hydrogen nuclei through an elastic scattering to produce recoil protons. (In elastic scattering there is no net loss of energy.) At higher energies (> 10 MeV), inelastic scattering, in which the neutron is reemitted from the nucleus along with a gamma ray, is more prevalent. At even higher energies (> 15 MeV), the neutrons interact with the nucleus, and a new particle (*e.g.*, alpha, proton) is emitted along with a gamma ray (nonelastic scatter). At very low neutron (thermal) energies, capture reactions predominate, while at very high energies spallation (nuclear fragmentation) may occur.

2. Linear Energy Transfer

Energy loss varies with the energy of the incoming photon or particle, the charge of the particle, and the character (atomic number, electron density) of the absorbing medium. The density of energy deposition along a track length has a profound influence on the subsequent biological effect. The spatial rate of energy loss along a track length is described by the term "linear energy transfer" (LET). LET is defined as the energy lost (in keV) per unit track length (in μm). For charged particles, it can be expressed as an average of LET distributions along a track, $t(L)$, or as an average of LET distributions in absorbed dose, $D(L)$. X-Rays and gamma rays are considered sparsely ionizing, low-LET radiations with ionizations or ionization clusters being spaced relatively far apart. The LET for ^{60}Co gamma rays (1.25 MeV) is 0.25 keV/μm, while that for 250 kVp X-rays is about 3.0 keV/μm.

Energetic particles tend to be more densely ionizing and have a higher LET than X-rays and gamma rays, although this is very dependent on the energy of the particle. The LET for a 2-MeV alpha particle is about 250 keV/μm. For energetic particles, the LET varies over the track length as the particle interacts and the energy spectrum changes. For high-energy particles, the density of ionizations at the beginning of the track is fairly sparse and the LET is correspondingly low. As the particle loses energy, the density of ionizations and the LET increases. At the end of the track, one may see a peak of ionization density (Bragg peak).

Knowledge of the LET is important in considering radiation effects, and it is commonly used to describe radiation quality. One weakness of the concept of LET is that it is an average measure and does not describe well what occurs in a more localized area. Two particles of the same type with the same energy may release very different amounts of energy in a small volume, just due to chance alone. Microdosimetry attempts to take into consideration small volumes as well as the probability of interaction. In microdosimetry, one uses the specific energy (z) rather than dose. Specific energy is defined as ϵ/m, where ϵ is the energy released from a single particle in a small volume (m). The mean z for large volumes is equivalent to the absorbed dose. The microdosimetric equivalent of LET is linear energy, defined as ϵ/d, where d is the mean cord length of the volume occupied by the mass m.

Depending on the type of radiation, the amount of energy released per ionization event can vary dramatically. One tends to see smaller energy events predominating with low-LET radiations and larger energy deposition events predominating with high-LET radiations, but both types will overlap (3, 4). Thus, with high-LET radiations, there will be energy losses that look to the cell as low-LET; and with low-LET radiations, there will be some events that appear high-LET in character. "Spurs" is the term used to describe low-energy (6-100-eV) events, "blobs" describes events in the 100-500-eV range, and "short tracks" describes 500-5000-eV energy deposition events.

3. Units of Dose and Activity

Radiation exposure is usually expressed as the amount of energy released per gram of tissue. The gray (Gy = 1 J/kg) is the Systéme Internationale (SI) unit of dose that is most often used. An older term still in use is the rad, which is equal to 0.01 Gy.

Because radiation effects are very dependent on the LET of the radiation, a dose equivalent is used to distinguish biologically effective radiation doses for radiations of different LET. The dose equivalent is calculated by multiplying the absorbed dose by a quality factor which takes into account the LET of the radiation. The quality factor for ^{60}Co gamma rays is 1. For high-LET radiations, the quality factor can be as high as 100. The original term used to compare radiations of different qualities was the rem (roentgen equivalent in man), which was equal to the dose in rads times a quality factor. The present SI term is the sievert (Sv), which is equal to the dose in Gy times a quality factor.

Radioactive isotopes decay, producing ionizing radiation at a rate specific for the type and concentration of the isotope. The intensity of the source (activity) is determined by the rate of nuclear transformations per unit time. The SI term used to describe activity is the becquerel (Bq), which is equal to 1 disintegration per second. The older term sometimes used is the curie (Ci), which was originally defined as the activity associated with 1 g of ^{222}Ra and later was defined as 3.7×10^{10} disintegrations per second. One Ci is equal to 3.7×10^{4} MBq.

B. Chemical Nature of Interactions[2]

1. Direct and Indirect Effects

The initial ionization event results in the formation of an ion pair. The ionization of water, for example, usually yields the ion pair $H_2O^+ + e^-$. This is an oxidation event and occurs very rapidly (on the order of 10^{-18} to 10^{-14} sec). For X-rays and gamma rays, it has been estimated that an average of 60-100 eV of energy is deposited for each event, and since only 34 eV is required to produce one H_2O ion pair, this means that each primary ionizing event results in a cluster of 2-3 ion pairs.

Where these ion pairs interact with each other or with other molecules, chemical reactions occur. For example, an electron may be trapped in a cluster of H_2O molecules, yielding a hydrated electron. An H_2O^+ ion can interact with an unchanged H_2O molecule to form a hydroxyl free radical ($HO^\bullet$) and a hydronium ion, H_3O^+. A water molecule in an excited form (H_2O^*) can yield hydrogen ($H^\bullet$) and hydroxyl ($HO^\bullet$) free radicals directly through dissociation. Other common species formed through the radiolysis of H_2O include H_2O_2 and molecular hydrogen. In general, the radiolysis of water yields hydrated electrons 45% of the time, $HO^\bullet$ 45% of the time, and $H^\bullet$ 10% of the time.

---

[2] For general reviews, *see* refs. 5, 6.

Chemical damage in the cell can result directly, as a result of ionization within an important biological molecule (direct effect) or through the interactions of free radicals such as those formed from H_2O (indirect effect). In the direct effect, absorption of energy by a DNA macromolecule leads to loss of an electron and then loss of a proton to yield a DNA radical:

$$DNAH \rightarrow DNAH^+ + e^-$$

$$DNAH^+ \rightarrow DNA^{\bullet} + H^+$$

This radical can then go on to produce strand breaks or base damage (*see below*).

In the indirect effect, free radicals react with DNA to produce DNA radicals either by abstraction or addition:

$$DNAH + R^{\bullet} \rightarrow DNA^{\bullet} + RH$$

$$DNAH + R^{\bullet} \rightarrow DNA(R)^{\bullet} + H^+$$

The $HO^{\bullet}$ radical is a very efficient oxidizing agent, which can extract an $H^{\bullet}$ from DNA:

$$DNAH + HO^{\bullet} \rightarrow DNA^{\bullet} + H_2O$$

The $HO^{\bullet}$ reacts rapidly with DNA and is thought to be a major cause of damage. It reacts mostly with bases, not sugar residues or phosphate moieties. However, radicals formed initially at a base may migrate to a sugar by $H^{\bullet}$ abstraction. Energy transfers are common and can be seen as far as 170 base-pairs away from the initial event.

In oxygenated solutions, $H^{\bullet}$ and aqueous electrons, both reducing agents, react rapidly with oxygen to form relatively unreactive superoxide radical anions (O_2^-), and therefore react little with DNA. In anoxic solutions, however, the reactions of $H^{\bullet}$ and aqueous electrons with DNA are more important.

Free radical formation is important in radiobiology because free radicals are very reactive. In addition, their life span in cells is much longer than the life span of ion pairs. The life span of water radicals is 100 times that of ion pairs, and the radicals may interact with other molecules to produce even longer-lived radicals such as organic peroxyl radicals. A longer life span means that radicals can diffuse and affect a much larger area than ion pairs. Free radicals can diffuse up to 30 nm in aqueous solutions. Free radical species have, therefore, the potential to interact with more sites within the cell. Damage produced by free radicals (indirect effect) will magnify the effects of low-LET ionizing radiation. With X-rays and gamma rays, about two-thirds of the effects of radiation are due to free radical–mediated (indirect) effects. With high-LET radiation, the yield of free radicals is lower, but still significant. However, while free radicals are produced, their contribution to the overall biological effect is much reduced because the density of ionizations is so high.

2. Interaction with Biological Targets

Since X-rays and gamma rays deposit energy randomly within the cell, there is no preferential molecular site of energy absorption; all components within a cell are potential targets. They are not, however, all of equal importance. Some molecules are ionized more often, simply because they make up a greater portion of the cell. For example, living organisms are mostly made up of water. Therefore, most of the radiation energy absorbed by the cell results in ionized water. This makes the radiolysis of water (see above) an important issue in radiation biology.

The frequency of ionization of some molecular species does not account for all its radiation effects. A very important factor is the biological function of the irradiated molecule and the essentiality of its function to cell life. Cells have many different components, including proteins, carbohydrates, lipids, and nucleic acids. Although each particular molecule is a potential target, most exist in multiple copies. Thus, if one particular protein molecule is damaged, it is likely that another molecule of that same protein exists in the cell in a functionally equivalent position, or may be resynthesized. Thus, ionization of most cellular components has no long-term effect. The important exception, of course, is DNA. Most of the genetic material is unique (*i.e.*, there are no multiple copies). Therefore, any permanent alteration in DNA may lead to mutation (defined as a permanent change in nucleotide sequence in DNA) or cell death.

The importance of maintaining the integrity of the DNA has been shown experimentally in a number of studies (7). A good example comes from studies with ^{80m}Br. This radioisotope decays with the production of a cascade of very low-energy electrons. All ionizations are limited to a very small radius around the atom. ^{80m}Br is toxic to a cell only when it is incorporated into the DNA as [^{80m}Br]5-bromo-2'-deoxyuridine. [^{80m}Br]Antipyrine, which uniformly distributes throughout the cell, is without effect on cell viability (8). Thus, the single critical site for cell killing, mutation, transformation, and most other radiation-induced changes is the DNA.

C. Radiation Effects on DNA

1. Induction of DNA Damage and Its Repair

There are three major effects of ionizing radiation on DNA structure: DNA–protein crosslink formation, base and sugar changes, and DNA strand breakage.

DNA–protein crosslinks are covalent bonds formed between DNA and the proteins of the nuclear matrix (9). DNA–protein crosslinks are induced linearly with dose at a frequency of about 150/Gy gamma rays (10). At high doses (>100 Gy), the number of crosslinks approaches a plateau value corresponding to the number of DNA attachment sites to the nuclear matrix. HO$^{\bullet}$ radicals are believed to be the primary agent responsible for crosslink production. Evidence suggests that these crosslinks do not play a major role in radiation-induced killing of cells (9, 10).

Radiation can cause many different changes in base structure (5, 11). Upon radiation exposure, for example, thymine (and cytosine) can undergo OH addition to the 5,6 double bond to form thymine glycol. Guanine may be modified to 8-hydroxyguanine; ring-opened pyrimidines and sugars are also found (5). The amount and type of damage is dependent on a number of factors, including chromatin structure (12–17). The radiation-induced changes in base and sugar structure are similar to those produced by oxidative stress (16–18), although there appear to be some important differences (19, 20).

Some of these base and sugar alterations appear to be benign, having no discernible biological effect. Some changes (coding lesions) lead to mutation through direct mispairing; that is, the polymerase reads the altered base and places "the wrong" complementary base in the new strand being synthesized. Thus, a permanent change in the DNA (mutation) results. One type of change that leads to mispair mutation is the deamination of cytosine, which yields uracil; this is read as thymidine and results in a C-to-T transition.

Adenine deamination yields hypoxanthine which is read as guanine, and produces therefore an A-to-G transition. The ionization of thymine causes it to be read as cytosine and to pair with guanine instead of adenine, resulting in a T-to-C transition. Transition mutations make up a large portion of radiation-induced mutations (20).

Radiation can also produce noncoding lesions such as thymine glycol or abasic sites. Abasic sites are formed when the bond between the base and sugar–phosphate backbone is broken (21). They can occur spontaneously, such as when the sugar on cytosine is ionized, or they can occur enzymatically as a result of repair. Noncoding lesions, such as abasic sites, may result in the loss of a base or the addition of a random base by polymerase action. With noncoding lesions such as thymine glycol or abasic sites, the polymerase could insert the wrong base 75% of the time. Actually, polymerases tend to add adenine opposite a noncoding lesion (22), so alterations at sites of thymine do not generally lead to mutation. Other examples of noncoding lesions include pyrimidine dimers and the 6,4-pyrimidine-pyrimidone product, both seen following ultraviolet or ionizing radiation exposure.

While the variety of base changes produced by ionizing radiation is large, the frequency with which these changes occur is relatively low as compared with DNA strand breakage. A single ionization in or near the DNA molecule has a very high probability of producing a DNA strand break. Most of these breaks are single-strand breaks, and evidence suggests that they are probably rejoined quite easily by most cells (23, 24). However, the repair process is complex and is not simply a single-step rejoining of the broken ends (ligation). Studies on the biochemistry of radiation-induced DNA strand breaks suggest that, in the process of producing a break, a base is often lost from the sugar–phosphate backbone (25). Thus, simple ligation would still result in at least one abasic site. In addition, the ends produced by ionizing radiation are not suitable for action by DNA ligase. The ends must be processed before repair can take place, and this usually results in the removal of additional bases.

The major DNA repair pathway in mammalian cells, which is involved in the repair of both base damage and strand breaks, is excision repair. The general outline of excision repair has been known for over 20 years (26). There are three basic steps. The first is recognition and removal of the damage by a specific endonuclease or exonuclease. Excision repair involves a number of very specific enzymes which recognize specific alterations in the DNA. Exonuclease III, for example, is believed to be identical to the bacterial enzyme involved in the recognition and repair of DNA strand breaks (27). Once identified, the damaged site is removed by nuclease action, along with some of the neighboring bases. In the second step, the undamaged complementary DNA strand is used as a template for the repair polymerase to fill in the nuclease-created gap. In the final step, the newly synthesized DNA is rejoined to the rest of the DNA molecule by DNA ligase.

Excision repair is a very important process in mammalian cells. It is responsible for the repair of most of the environmentally and endogenously produced DNA damage. It is also an error-free process. Mutations that affect excision repair can have dire consequences. Xeroderma pigmentosum (XP) is an autosomal recessive disease in which the initial recognition and excision of ultraviolet light–induced DNA damage is defective (28). Individuals with XP are very photosensitive and are prone to sunlight-induced skin cancer.

Normally, base damage and single-strand breaks are handled very well by most cells (18). Thus, they probably account for only a minor amount of the mutation and cell death seen after radiation exposure. They would probably be important only under conditions where the ability to repair damage has been altered or when they are found close to a replication fork and are not repaired prior to replication.

For X-rays, about 1 in 10 to 20 breaks span both strands of the DNA molecule. These double-strand breaks are believed to be the primary lethal and mutagenic lesions induced by ionizing radiation. There is much evidence to support the role of double-strand breaks in cell death and mutation. In yeast mutants that cannot repair DNA double-strand breaks, a single double-strand break is lethal (29). Similarly, in mammalian systems, cells that are not able to repair DNA double-strand breaks are very sensitive to ionizing radiation, while those defective in just single-strand break repair have only a slight sensitivity (24, 30). Although evidence supports the importance of DNA double-strand breaks in radiation-induced cell killing and mutation, this does not exclude base changes or single-strand breaks from also playing a role.

One reason for the lethality of DNA double-strand breaks is that, if left unrepaired, the effect of these breaks could be the loss of a whole group of bases that are distal to the centromere on the chromosome (see below) and therefore the loss of one or more genes. If these genes are crucial for the maintenance or reproduction of the cell, the result will be the death of the cell. DNA double-strand breaks are also more difficult to repair than DNA single-strand breaks or base alterations. Having no secondary structure to hold them together, the ends tend to come apart, making repair more difficult. As with single-strand breaks and base changes, double-strand break repair must involve some sort of excision repair process. But when damage is excised from both strands, overlapping gaps in the DNA will be generated; there will be, therefore, no complete intact complementary strand to use as a template.

To deal with this problem, cells use a recombinational repair pathway (26, 31). In recombinational repair, a homologous DNA strand, usually found on a separate chromosome, is used to supply missing information. This is a more complex system than excision repair and requires an intact DNA strand with homology to the damaged region. Recombinational repair is the major DNA double-strand break repair pathway in bacteria and in some yeast strains. It has been shown to occur in mammalian cells, but its relative importance is so far unknown.

Evidence for a second DNA double-strand break rejoining pathway has recently been presented. In this process, the broken ends are processed and then simply ligated (*e.g.*, 32). This must be an error-prone process, as some information will be lost. If the deletion is in a coding region, the result will be a gene mutation. If the gene is crucial for cell survival, the deletion will manifest itself as cytotoxicity. Many of the deletions occur in noncoding regions, however, and are therefore only of limited consequence. These small deletions will be balanced by the advantage of joining the broken ends and thus preventing loss of a much larger region of genetic material.

2. Effect on DNA Function

a. DNA Replication.   It has been known since 1942 that radiation will inhibit DNA synthesis (33). A semilog plot of the inhibitory effect of ionizing radiation on the incorporation of radionuclides into the DNA yields a two-component curve. At relatively low doses, there is a steep component to the curve, and at higher doses, the slope becomes more shallow. This two-component curve has been shown to reflect the effects of ionizing radiation on two components of DNA synthesis, initiation and chain elongation.

The organization of DNA replication in mammalian cells involves a large number of small replicating units (replicons). DNA synthesis initiates at specific sites in these replicons and then the DNA polymerase proceeds along the DNA molecule, extending the replication unit (chain elongation). When the replicon has been replicated, adjacent replicons are ligated. Adjacent replicons are grouped together in units of about 10 to 20 (replicon clusters). Replicons within a cluster initiate DNA synthesis synchronously.

Effects on chain elongation and initiation can be distinguished by analyzing the incorporation of radioactive label into newly replicated DNA of large (chain elongation) or small (initiation) size.

Breaks in the DNA molecule are blocks to DNA replication. When the DNA polymerase reaches these breaks, it stalls. This leads to an inhibition primarily in the chain elongation process. The effect on chain elongation is relatively small and is seen mostly at very high doses of radiation. This is a reflection of the large number of replicon units in the cell and the requirement to affect a significant proportion of the units in order to see an effect on overall replication. Low doses of radiation produce an inhibition of replication initiation. It was originally suggested that a single DNA break within a replicon cluster was sufficient to inhibit replicon initiation. This was based on the dose–response curve for DNA synthesis inhibition, which in turn suggested a target size of about 1000 kilobase (kb) for the effect on initiation. The target size for the inhibition of chain elongation was suggested to be about 50 kb, about the size of an individual replicon. The larger target size for initiation effects was thought to reflect the size of a replicon cluster. More recent studies (34, 35) suggest the existence of some intermediary transmediating factor involved in the inhibition of replicon initiation, so that breaks within replicon clusters may not be the signal for this effect. One excellent candidate for this factor is the p53 protein (36).

b. DNA Transcription. Information flow in protein synthesis is from DNA to RNA to protein. In transcription, the nucleotide sequences of RNA are determined by complementary base pairing between the polymerizing nucleotides and the sense strand of a duplex DNA template. Disruption of the DNA by DNA strand breaks or base changes will in turn disrupt transcription. However, because the target size of the genes involved are small, one needs rather large doses of radiation to inhibit overall transcription.

Until recently, the major effect of ionizing radiation on gene transcription was thought to be inhibition. There are an increasing number of reports, however, suggesting that radiation will turn on (up-regulate) the transcription of specific genes (37–39). Many of the genes identified as radiation-inducible turn out also to be induced by phorbol esters. The target for these effects may be protein kinase C (38, 40). The activation of protein kinase C will initiate a cascade of events, including the induction of a number of transcription factors such as c-*jun*, c-*fos*, *jun*-B, c-*myc*, and *egr*-1. These in turn will activate the transcription of a number of gene products. While radiation-induced activation of protein kinase C may be a major mechanism of gene induction by ionizing radiation, it is not the only mechanism; there is evidence for other pathways as well.

The role these activated genes play in cellular responses to ionizing radiation is not known. Inhibition of protein kinase C activity will sensitize cells slightly to ionizing radiation (41), but no known repair genes are activated by ionizing radiation. Many of the activated genes remain to be identified. A number of the genes induced by ionizing radiation appear to be involved in cell proliferation.

D. Induction of Chromosome Damage and Its Repair

Chromosome mutation, usually referred to as an aberration, is by definition a large change involving blocks of genes; it is, therefore, a more drastic change than a gene mutation. Chromosome aberrations are common, occurring in about 1% of human cells, and they can be seen under the light microscope. One or more chromosome aberrations are associated with about 35% of all spontaneous abortions (50% of all conceptions end in spontaneous abortions).

There are essentially three types of chromosome changes induced by ionizing radiation. Radiation can cause a change in the number of whole sets of chromosomes, as from diploid to triploid or tetraploid or haploid. These conditions are rare because they are not viable except under *in vitro* conditions or when they occur in tumor cells. Radiation can also cause a change in the number of one or more particular chromosomes of the basic set. This condition is called aneuploidy, and the change can be to a lesser (hypodiploid) or a greater (hyperdiploid) number. Aneuploidy is a much more common occurrence *in vivo*. There are many examples, such as Down's syndrome, which is usually a trisomy of chromosome 21. Aneuploidy is commonly seen in tumor cells.

Most often, radiation induces gross structural changes in the chromosomes. Radiation breaks DNA, which in turn results in chromosome breakage. Chromosome breaks evolve from DNA double-strand breaks. As chromosomes are uninemic, a single DNA double-strand break has the potential to form a chromosome break.

Broken chromosome ends can either (a) rejoin (restitute), (b) remain open, or (c) rearrange by joining to another broken end (misrepair). Aberrations are most often studied in mitotic cells, in which chromosomes have condensed sufficiently to be visible. Aberrations are classified as either chromosome-type, involving both sister chromatids, or chromatid-type, involving just one of the sister chromatids. The type of aberration reflects the stage of the cell cycle when the cell was irradiated. In G2 the break will affect only a single chromatid. Therefore, irradiation of cells in G2, after the S phase, results in almost entirely chromatid-type aberrations. Any breaks remaining in the genome by the onset of replication will be replicated, yielding breaks at identical sites in both sister chromatids. Irradiation before DNA replication, results therefore in chromosome-type aberrations.

Chromosome aberrations represent for the most part lethal mutations, and are often called dominant lethal mutations. As the cell divides, chromosomes or pieces of chromosomes without centromeres tend to be lost from the cell. Because the loss of a portion of a chromosome usually means the loss of one or more genes, the cell usually does not survive. Chromosome changes are thought to represent what occurs at the molecular level and have therefore been used to try to probe the mechanism of radiation-induced effects.

Much of our understanding of the genetic effects of radiation exposure comes from cytogenetic studies. For example, from the study of chromosome aberrations, we know that the number of aberrations increases with increasing dose and that there is no evidence for a threshold for the induction of aberration. The kinetics of induction at low doses follows a linear relationship (thought to reflect a single-hit event) while that at high doses follows a dose-squared relationship (thought to reflect a two-hit event). This relationship is:

$$F = A + \alpha D + \beta D^2$$

where F is the endpoint, A the background frequency, and D the dose; it is often seen in radiation-induced effects.

Almost all chromosome breaks are rejoined (42). Most aberrations seen reflect misrepair events where two broken ends have interacted. Only broken ends can interact. Telomeres prevent broken ends from joining with the end of an intact chromosome. Interestingly, telomerase, the enzyme responsible for telomere production, is able to act on certain broken chromosome ends (43, 44). Telomerase may influence chromosome aberration yield following radiation exposure. Many other literature sources (*e.g.*, 45–47) address DNA damage and repair.

E. Cell Response to Ionizing Radiation

There are four major cellular consequences to radiation exposure: delay of cell cycle progression, cell toxicity, mutation, and cell transformation.

1. Cell Cycle Effects

The mammalian cell division cycle is divided into four phases: G1 or presynthetic, S or DNA synthetic, G2 or postsynthetic, and M or mitosis. Ionizing radiation will slow cell growth, inducing transient delays in S phase (especially at the G1/S border) and in G2 (48, 49). The phenomenon of radiation-induced inhibition of DNA replication was mentioned earlier and accounts for the delay in S phase. A much more important source of radiation-induced cell cycle delay is the G2 block. Following radiation exposure, there is usually a buildup of cells transiently blocked in G2. The signal for this G2 delay is thought to be a double-strand break. In certain strains of yeast, a single DNA double-strand break is sufficient to block cells in G2, and cells will remain blocked until the break is repaired (50). Mammalian cells deficient in their ability to repair DNA double-strand breaks will delay for longer times in G2 (51).

Delays in cell cycle progression are probably beneficial to the cell because they allow the cell more time to repair damage before entering a critical phase of the cell cycle. S phase, for example, is critical because if unrepaired DNA damage is replicated the net result could be a permanent change in the DNA (mutation). For ionizing radiation damage mitosis is an even more critical phase, because any loose pieces of DNA, which would be expected with unrejoined DNA double-strand breaks, tend to be lost from the cell as it divides. Treatment of cells with agents which push G2 cells prematurely into mitosis, following radiation exposure, leads to increased cell toxicity (52). Cells with genetically altered shorter G2 delays following radiation are usually more radiosensitive (53). Conversely, delaying replication or mitosis will improve cell survival following radiation exposure. This is thought to be the basis for potentially lethal damage repair (PLDR) (see below).

2. Cell Toxicity

a. Interphase and Mitotic Death. Ionizing radiation is a potent cytotoxic agent. This is primarily because ionizing radiation is a potent inducer of DNA double-strand breaks, and DNA double-strand breaks are highly lethal lesions. There are two forms of lethality. For most cells and with moderate doses of radiation, cell death is not instantaneous. Cells will continue to grow and divide for 1-5 division cycles before dying (7). This is referred to as mitotic death. As cells go through successive mitoses, genetic material is lost through chromosome aberration. In addition, many lethal mutations are not immediately expressed. The expression of any mutation is dependent on cell division and on the resultant reduction in gene product with decay and dilution. Ultimately, as the lethal mutations are expressed, the cell finally succumbs and dies.

At very high doses of radiation, usually greater than 100 Gy, cells die almost immediately after irradiation or without any intervening mitotic division. This is termed interphase death (7), as it requires no cell division. The cause of interphase death is often damage to the cell membrane, leading to the cell being unable to maintain its integrity. For some cell lines, especially where interphase death is seen at relatively low doses (as in circulating lymphocytes, type A spermatogonia, and oocytes), ionizing radiation is thought to turn on a cell program which leads to DNA degradation and cell lysis. This programmed cell death is called apoptosis (54). It is believed to be an important process in development and may play a role in the response to radiation therapy.

> **b. Quantitation of Cell Toxicity.** Quantitation of cell toxicity is an extremely important topic in radiation biology and radiation oncology. Quantitation allows a more accurate description of effects and therefore better prediction of effects; prediction is important for both radiation protection and radiation therapy. Quantitation and the development of models to explain radiation toxicity also allows for a better understanding of radiation interactions with mammalian cells.

The quantitation of cell killing by radiation is usually expressed in the form of survival curves (7, 55). Survival curves are the plots of the fraction of cells surviving (N/N_0) or percent surviving, on the ordinate, *versus* dose (D) on the abscissa; N_0 is the initial number of cells and N the number surviving after a dose D. A typical survival curve for mammalian cells exposed to X-rays or gamma rays has a shoulder region at low doses where the rate of cell killing increases with dose, followed by an exponential portion at higher doses.

There are a variety of mathematical expressions that have been used to describe these curves. Early workers in radiation biology developed the target theory to describe survival or cell inactivation curves. The theory assumes that the production of an ionization (hit) in or near some molecular structure (target) is responsible for the effect noted (cell killing). The initial model assumed that only a single hit in a single target was required to inactivate the cell; however, the resulting mathematical relationship[3]

$$S(\%) = \exp(-kD)$$

yielded an exponential survival [$S(\%)$] curve. This was not seen with mammalian cells. Later the model was expanded to consider multiple targets. The resulting mathematical relationship

$$S(\%) = 1 - [1 - \exp(-kD)]^n$$

gives a better fit to the survival data, but still does not sufficiently describe survival at low doses. A linear–quadratic model

$$S(\%) = \exp[-(\alpha D + \beta D^2)]$$

better describes low-dose effects and is more often used.

Other models have also been proposed, but all have limitations. There are probably many reasons for the failure to accurately model radiation effects. The induction of damage, for example, is not only dependent on the biophysical nature of the radiation, but also on such variables as DNA conformation, intracellular oxygen tension, and the intracellular level of free radical scavengers. Repair or misrepair depends on many different enzymatic processes as well as chromosome conformation, which can modify damage and thereby change the shape of the survival curve.

Given the limitations of survival curve models, their importance lies in providing terms to describe a survival curve. The radiation sensitivity of a cell line is often quantified by D_0, the reciprocal of the slope of the exponential portion of the survival curve. D_0 is the dose that reduces survival by a factor of 0.37, as measured on the exponential portion.

---

[3] The mathematical notation exp(x) used for e^x is an alternative formalism to express exponential function.

If this curve had no shoulder, the D_0 would equal the D_{37}, the dose which results in 37% of the cells surviving. With a shoulder, the D_{37} is larger than the D_0. For mammalian cells in culture (mostly fibroblasts), D_0 values range from about 1.0 Gy to about 2.0 Gy (56). Fibroblasts from individuals with ataxia telangiectasia, a radiation-sensitive disorder, have D_0 values of about 0.5 Gy.

The shoulder of the survival curve is described in two ways. Extrapolation back to the ordinate yields the extrapolation number, n. The width of the shoulder is called the quasithreshold dose, or D_q. These terms are related to each other by the equation:

$$D_q = D_0 \ln(n)$$

Where one is interested in survival at relatively low doses, the α and β terms from the linear–quadratic model are used to describe the survival curve.

3. Induction of Mutation

One very important cellular consequence of radiation exposure is the induction of mutation. Ionizing radiation has been known to be a mutagen since 1928 (57). It is important to stress that the result of a misrepaired or unrepaired radiation-induced DNA lesion is a mutation. It may be as small as a single base change (as is found in sickle cell anemia) or it may involve thousands of genes (as when chromosomes are lost or duplicated).

Initial studies of radiation-induced genetic changes focused on cytogenetic changes (58), altered electrophoretic patterns of specific proteins (59), and studies with the specific locus systems in mice (60) and other species (61). Subsequently, *in vitro* cell systems were developed in which gene mutations could be detected at certain loci based on the resistance of the mutated cells to specific toxic drugs (62, 63). More recently, molecular techniques have been developed which allow for the examination of the types of molecular events that underlie the gene mutation in endogenous genes and in shuttle vector-based systems (64–66).

Based on cellular, cytogenetic, and molecular studies, it became possible to draw a number of general conclusions about the nature of ionizing radiation mutagenesis (64–66). Firstly, there appears to be no threshold for the induction of mutations. Mutations have been reported for X-ray doses as low as 0.01 Gy.

Secondly, the mutation rates following radiation exposure are very dependent on the genetic locus under study. Some loci, such as the *tk* locus, are very sensitive to mutation. Others are relatively insensitive, such as the *aprt* locus and the Na/K ATPase locus. Part of the difference in sensitivity has to do with genomic location and the molecular nature of mutations induced by ionizing radiation. Most radiation-induced mutations are deletions, no doubt a consequence of DNA double-strand breaks. The size of a deletion can vary from the loss of a single base (20) to loss of a whole chromosome (67). A major limitation on deletion size is the presence of nearby essential genes whose loss would result in cell death. Nearby essential genes probably account for the very different spectrum of radiation-induced mutations seen at the *aprt* locus (mostly point mutations) as compared to the *hprt* locus (50–90% deletions) and the *tk* locus (60–80% deletions). At the *tk* locus in mouse cells, one can find deletions that span multiple genetic loci. As most of the mutations are deletions, many of the induced mutations are recessive lethals, *in vivo*, and some have deleterious effects in the heterozygote (68).

DNA sequence and chromosome structure can also play a role in the types of mutations seen following radiation exposure. Runs of thymidine bases appear to be specially sensitive spots ("hotspots") for radiation-induced frameshifts (20). There is a suggestion for an ionizing radiation mutational hotspot at the DNA–nuclear matrix attachment site as well in the *hprt* locus (69).

The rates of radiation-induced mutation also seem to vary from cell type to cell type and between different species. There are differences in sensitivity between spermatogonia, postmeiotic male germ cells, and mature and immature oocytes as measured in murine systems (68). There also appear to be differences in mutation sensitivity between murine and human lymphoid cells (70, 71). Rodent cells appear to be more sensitive to the induction of mutations. This may reflect either the inbred nature of murine systems and the presence of more recessive lethals in human cells, or it may reflect differences in the repair of radiation-induced DNA damage in rodent *versus* human cells. Measurements of *in vivo*-induced mutations in murine systems also show greater radiation-induced frequencies than do similar measurements in human systems (72).

4. Cell Transformation

There are two basic types of cell transformation assays presently in use. One uses a short-term culture of rodent embryo cells in a clonal assay, where transformed colonies are identified by morphology. An example of this type of assay is the hamster embryo cell assay (73). A second assay uses established, immortal rodent cell lines such as the C3H 10T½ (74) or BALB/c 3T3 (75), where focus formation is the marker of transformation. Additional assays of transformation are being studied. Some tissues such as trachea, thyroid, cheek pouch, or breast can be irradiated *in vivo* and assayed for transformation either in a foot pad or soft agar assay (76, 77). There are also assays that use either human–rodent hybrids (78) or partially transformed human cells (79). While human primary cells have been transformed *in vitro* (80, 81), these systems are not sufficiently quantitative for use as a routine transformation assay.

The dose response for the transformation of cells by ionizing radiation is complex, reflecting a balance between the induction of radiogenic transformation and cell toxicity. With low-LET radiation, when transformation is plotted as a function of *cells surviving*, there is usually a linear or curvilinear increase in transformed clones which reaches a plateau at higher doses. If *cells at risk* are plotted, then the transformation frequency increases, plateaus, and then decreases at higher doses. Transformation frequency can be detected with doses as low as 0.01 Gy (X-ray). There are, however, some uncertainties concerning the dose response for cell transformation by ionizing radiation at low doses. Linear, linear–quadratic, and quadratic responses have all been reported for low-dose exposures. The basis for these different observations is not understood.

There has also been considerable effort using transformation systems to study the mechanism of radiation carcinogenesis. Studies by Kennedy *et al.* (82), and later Terzaghi *et al.* (76) and Clifton *et al.* (77), suggest that the initial event is a high-frequency one, affecting a large proportion of the irradiated population. It likely involves a generalized cellular response to radiation (*e.g.*, DNA damage) rather than a specific gene mutation. That the initial event is unlikely to be a single gene mutation is also inferred from a comparison of target sizes for radiation transformation and mutation. The target size for radiation-induced transformation is 30-100 times the size of an average gene (83). The second event that follows is probably a mutation, as it is much rarer, occurring with a frequency (10^{-6}) similar to that of spontaneous mutation.

Much work has gone into trying to identify the specific genes altered by ionizing radiation in transformed cells (84–86). Radiation-transformed cells have been shown to contain dominantly-transforming DNA sequences, but, with one exception (87), none appear to be any of the more than 14 known oncogenes for which these cells have been screened. Thus the role of specific oncogene activation in cell transformation remains unknown.

F. Radiation Carcinogenesis

1. General Considerations

Shortly after X-rays were discovered in 1895, reports appeared on the hazards of exposure (88). Dermatitis and alopecia associated with X-ray exposure were reported in 1896. Skin cancer was reported in 1902 and 1903. Cancer is the most important consequence of low to moderate exposure to ionizing radiation. It is the major limiting consideration for most *in vivo* exposures.

Information on the induction of cancer in human populations comes from epidemiological studies. The largest single group of exposed individuals are those Japanese who were exposed to the atomic bombs at Hiroshima and Nagasaki. About 280,000 individuals survived the immediate effects and about 80,000 have been followed for long-term effects (89, 90).

Many different types of cancer have been seen in the atomic bomb–exposed individuals. Initially, acute leukemia and chronic granulocytic leukemia were increased, presumably because of their short latency period. Chronic lymphocytic leukemia rates were not increased. Excesses in solid tumors showed up 5-10 years after the appearance of leukemias. By 1974, the cumulative excesses in solid tumors exceeded those of the leukemias. Absolute risk of solid tumors has been steadily increasing since 1950. For leukemias, risks have returned to normal levels. The major solid tumors found in excess in the atomic bomb survivors include thyroid, female breast, and lung. To a lesser extent, cancers of the esophagus, stomach, urinary tract, and lymphomas have been observed.

The weapons used on the two cities were very different. The one used on Nagasaki emitted mostly gamma rays and few neutrons. The one dropped on Hiroshima emitted a mixture of neutrons and gamma rays. There has recently been a reevaluation of the dosimetry (96), which has had a profound effect on risk estimates.

Other exposed populations include early radiation workers exposed occupationally, where increases in skin cancer, leukemias, and aplastic anemia were seen (91). The "radium dial painters" were a group (mostly women) whose work, around 1920, consisted in painting watch dials with radioactive solution of a radium salt, to create "luminescent dials". In the course of their work they ingested radium as a result of licking the tip of the brush to make it more pointed. The radium deposited in bone and resulted in very substantially increased incidences of bone cancers (92). An excess incidence of breast cancer was also seen in these individuals.

It has recently been recognized that a large portion of the average yearly exposure to ionizing radiation comes from exposure to radon and radon daughters. Much of the understanding of the carcinogenic effects of this exposure comes from studies on uranium mine workers. The alpha radiation exposure resulted in a higher incidence of lung cancer (93).

There are also a number of reports on individuals who were exposed to particulate radiation for diagnostic purposes. Thorotrast, a colloidal preparation of ^{232}Th-dioxide, was used as an X-ray contrast agent in the late 20s and early 1930s. Thorium is an alpha emitter which is permanently deposited in body tissues. Excess liver cancers and leukemias were seen in these individuals (89).

Other medically exposed populations include British ankylosing spondylitis patients. During the late 1930s, patients in Britain with ankylosing spondylitis were treated with radiation to reduce pain. An excess of leukemias has been reported in these individuals (89).

In the past, radiation has been used to reduce thymus size in children and also for the treatment of tinea capitis. These exposed children later showed excesses in the incidence of thyroid cancers (94, 95).

These and other smaller groups of exposed individuals serve as the human database for estimating risk for developing cancer following radiation exposure. They show a relatively wide range of neoplasms, latency periods, and dose exposure levels. It should be borne in mind, however, that most human exposures to radiation occur at doses substantially below 50 cGy, while most of the study populations received doses far in excess of that. In addition, most exposures are fractionated or chronic rather than acute, as was seen in the largest group of exposed individuals, the atomic bomb survivors. This has necessitated, therefore, an extrapolation of risk from high-dose exposures and from animal studies.

Studies on radiation carcinogenesis focused on the dose–response relationships and on the mechanisms of radiocarcinogenic action. Based on these studies, a number of conclusions have been drawn:

(i) The types of tumors seen following ionizing radiation exposure are usually the same as those seen spontaneously. Induction of cancer *by radiation* is inferred from the increase in frequency over background.

(ii) Radiation-induced tumors can appear in almost any tissue of the body, but sensitivity to induction varies greatly for specific tissues and organs. In general, tumors of the thyroid, the female breast, and certain leukemias are considered to be the most likely to be induced by ionizing radiation in humans, while induction of kidney, bone, skin, brain, and salivary gland tumors are considered to be the least likely. Lymphomas and lung, colon, liver, and pancreatic tumors are among those with moderate likelihood for induction (96). The differential sensitivity probably reflects a complex number of factors; it is not simply a reflection of spontaneous frequencies.

(iii) Sensitivity to tumor induction varies for different species and strains of animals and is also different for males and females. This variability suggests that the initial damage, which is presumed to be the same for a given dose and type of radiation, is subject to a number of host-related factors which modify response. Presumably these include repair capability, the presence of endogenous viruses, cell proliferation status (cell cycle stage), endocrine levels, immune competence, and factors related to genetic susceptibility (97).

(iv) The latent period of cancer induction by radiation varies with tumor type, radiation type, dose, and dose rate. Leukemias have the shortest latent periods (mean, 5-10 years), which no doubt accounts for their being the most frequently seen tumorigenic response following radiation exposures. Solid tumors show latencies of between 20 and 30 years.

(v) In general, the dose response for the induction of tumors by radiation follows a sigmoid response. At low doses there in little induction. This is followed by a steep increase, then a saturation plateau (and occasionally even a decrease in tumor frequency at high doses). The dose response will vary depending on tissue type, dose rate, and tumor latency time. As mentioned above, most of the available data on human carcinogenesis come from individuals exposed to relatively high doses of radiation. No human data exist for proven carcinogenic effects of radiation below 0.1 Gy. The dose response at low levels of exposure remains unknown; response in this region is predicted by extrapolation. Animal studies have suggested that the shape of this crucial portion of the curve may vary greatly from tissue to tissue and animal to animal. Depending on the model used to extrapolate from high-dose effects, one may underestimate or overestimate risk. This could result in extra costs for radiation protection or unnecessary risks to exposed populations. At present, linear extrapolation from high-dose effects is used to estimate risk for low doses of radiation. In addition, this extrapolation is made from acute exposures, while most human exposures are chronic or spread out over time.

(vi) Radiation risk is defined as the increase in the number of cancer deaths over that expected for an unirradiated population. It is expressed in units per person exposed per Gy of radiation. Estimates based on linear extrapolation of the atomic bomb data and on other more limited data from pooled results of various partial-body exposures give the total cancer mortality risks, for a general population exposed to whole-body radiation, as 1 to 4 $\times$ 10^{-2} per person-Gy (98).

2. Initiation, Promotion, and Progression

Ionizing radiation has been shown to be a complete carcinogen following either single or fractionated exposures. Thus, most of the studies with ionizing radiation have been designed on the premise that radiation is a complete carcinogen, and very few experiments have been designed to study, separately, the initiating and promoting effects of radiation. However, a few animal studies have provided clear evidence indicating that ionizing radiation initiates events which are retained in viable cells for long periods of time. In addition, experiments suggest that these lesions do not undergo further change or expression until a subsequent event is induced. Early work carried out by Berenblum and Shubik (99) established that ionizing radiation is an effective initiator. Later, Berenblum and Trainin (100) found that doses of X-rays, which alone were nonleukemogenic, resulted in an incidence of leukemia if followed by treatment with urethan. They interpreted these results to indicate that ionizing radiation at dose levels insufficient for complete carcinogenesis was an effective initiator.

Initiation probably involves the induction of a stable genetic alteration, presumably a gene mutation, that predisposes cells to neoplastic conversion. This could be through activation of a proto-oncogene or inactivation of a suppressor gene. While radiation has been shown to be an initiator, it appears to be a relatively weak one (100–106). The manifest effectiveness of radiation *as an initiator* may be dependent on the type of promoting agent used subsequently.

Since promoters are defined as agents that are (in principle) not carcinogenic by themselves, ionizing radiation is not a pure promoter, as it can act as a complete carcinogen. Radiation will induce protein kinase C activity (38, 40) and ornithine decarboxylase (107), which are also induced by classical tumor promoters such as phorbol ester and phenobarbital. When used in a tumor-promoting protocol, one can sometimes see evidence for radiation-induced promotion, although the evidence for this is mixed (108, 109). These may reflect cocarcinogenic processes rather than tumor promotion (see below).

Neoplastic progression is defined as changes seen from premalignant to malignant and aggressive type tumors. These are associated with activation or inactivation of specific genes. Jaffe *et al.* (108) have reported that ionizing radiation will enhance malignant progression in a mouse skin tumor model, while Mori *et al.* (110) reported evidence for radiation-induced progression in a rat liver model.

3. Molecular Aspects

Point mutation, chromosomal translocation, and deletion may all play a role in the initiation and progression of tumors following radiation exposure. Molecular analysis of radiation-induced gene mutations suggest that ionizing radiation can induce all these types of changes, although, depending on the genetic locus, deletions are usually the most frequent. Unlike with many chemical mutagens as well as ultraviolet light, there are no specific alterations associated with radiation exposure. This makes the detection of radiation-specific changes difficult. Activation of c-K-*ras* and c-*myc* oncogenes is frequently observed in carcinomas induced by ionizing radiation (111–114). Activation of *ras* is through point mutation and c-*myc* through gene rearrangement. The presence of non-*ras* dominant oncogenes has also been reported (113, 115), as have alterations in growth factors and growth factor receptors (116, 117). Mutations in the *p53* and *Rb* tumor-suppressors have also been reported in radiation-induced tumors (118). These mutations have included both point mutations, small deletions, and total gene deletions. Given the variety of changes seen and the lack of any radiation-specific alteration ("signature"), it is not clear whether these gene alterations occur subsequent to the radiation-initiating event or were directly induced by radiation.

III. MODIFICATION OF RESPONSE

There are many different agents and conditions that will modify response to ionizing radiation. Some act at very early stages, affecting energy transfer or the nature of the initial physical interactions. Some act at much later stages, modifying enzymatic repair of damage or host responses to cellular changes. These modifiers can be grouped into physical, biological, and chemical categories.

A. Physical Modifiers

1. LET Effects and Relative Biological Effectiveness[4]

Different qualities of ionizing radiation, distinguished by their LET, produce very different biological effects. In general, as the LET of the radiation increases, the biological effects seen also increase in severity. Relative biological effectiveness (RBE) is the term used to describe the relative efficiencies of different radiation types. It was originally defined as the ratio of doses that produce some defined endpoint with a standard radiation (usually either 250 kVp X-rays or ^{60}Co gamma rays) to the dose producing the same effect for the test radiation. For radiation protection considerations, ^{60}Co gamma rays are the standard. As the dose required to produce an effect increases, the RBE also increases. A more useful term now used is an RBE based on the ratio of initial slopes from the dose–response curves of radiations of different quality.

RBE increases with LET up to about 100 keV/μm. As LET increases beyond this point, RBE usually declines. This reflects "overkill", where individual ionization events are not less effective, but the increasing amounts of the energy released per ionization event are wasted. RBE is also very dependent on the endpoint studied: for fission–spectrum neutrons the RBE for toxicity is about 3-4; for the induction of mutations it is about 5-10; for the induction of tumors it can be between 20-50.

The basis for the increased efficiency with which high-LET induces biological effects is not fully understood. The effect of high-LET radiations probably does not reflect the production of increased numbers of lesions per unit dose. High-LET radiation produces similar numbers of DNA double-strand breaks as low-LET radiations and actually induces fewer DNA single-strand breaks and base alterations (119). Many have suggested that the quality of the lesion induced by high-LET radiation is different. Some investigators suggested that there is a lesser capability to repair this lesion than the lesion produced by low-LET radiations (119–122). Evidence that these lesions are indeed less

---

[4] For a general textbook to this section *see* ref. 55.

well repaired also comes from studies of repair-deficient cell lines (123, 124). Although these cell lines are much more sensitive to low-LET radiations than their repair-proficient parents, there is little difference in high-LET responses.

2. Oxygen Effects and the Oxygen Enhancement Ratio[5]

Molecular oxygen is a potent modifier of radiation sensitivity. Reducing oxygen tension in cells reduces the sensitivity of these cells to radiation effects. The effect of oxygen is described by the oxygen enhancement ratio (OER). The OER is the ratio of D_0 values for cells irradiated under oxygenated conditions, as compared to the same cells irradiated under hypoxic conditions. For X-rays and gamma rays, the OER ranges between 2.5 and 3.0. As the LET of the radiation increases, the OER decreases, reaching a minimum at 1.0. The OER for neutrons is about 1.6.

For the oxygen effect to be seen, oxygen must be present at the time of irradiation (or at least within 5 msec of irradiation). Very little oxygen is required to see the effect. An increase of oxygen tension from 0 to 3 mmHg at 37°C will result in a radiosensitivity halfway between anoxia and full oxygenation. The oxygen tension of most normal tissues ranges from 20 to 40 mmHg.

Oxygen sensitization is believed to be due to the interaction of oxygen with free radical species. In the absence of oxygen, free radicals can be annihilated by their reaction with hydrogen atom or by electron donation. However, in the presence of oxygen, free radicals interact with the oxygen to form peroxy radicals, which are highly reactive, but cannot be annihilated by reaction with hydrogen atom or by electron donation.

3. Dose Rate

Many of the effects seen from low-LET radiation suggest that they are due to the interaction of two lesions. Fractionating the dose or reducing the dose rate will in general lead to a reduction in the effectiveness of the radiation by allowing time for repair of these sublethal lesions (125, 126). Dose rate sparing is seen for all effects, including cell toxicity, induction of mutation, transformation, and carcinogenesis. The sparing is generally larger for rodent cells than for human cells.

The effectiveness of fractionated or low–dose-rate irradiation for inducing tumors is quite different for low-LET and high-LET radiation. Most studies on fractionated low-LET radiations have resulted in a reduction of tumor incidence for a given total dose. Presumably, fractionation of the dose allows for time to repair sublethal and subcarcinogenic damage. In contrast, fractionation of high-LET radiation or low-dose exposure usually has little effect on radiation-induced cellular or genotoxicity (127–130). The lack of sparing at low dose rates is presumed to be due to the inability of cells to repair damage induced by high-LET radiations. That is, the damage produced by high-LET radiations is thought to be qualitatively different than that from low-LET radiations and less well repaired (as discussed above).

For some types of radiation, such as fission–spectrum neutrons, reduction of the dose rate actually leads to increased transformation and more tumors. This is known as the inverse dose-rate effect. Much of the evidence for an inverse dose-rate effect comes from *in vitro* studies of oncogenic transformation, although there is also evidence for an inverse dose-rate effect for the induction of mutation (131–133). Elkind and associates were the first to report an inverse dose-rate effect for fission–spectrum neutrons in the induction of transformation in C3H 10T½ cells (129). They found that for a given low dose of

---

neutrons (5 to 30 cGy), the transformation incidence was much higher if the radiation was delivered at low dose rate or in a series of fractions over 5, as compared to a single acute dose. Similar results were seen for hamster embryo cells (134).

Evidence for inverse dose-rate effect for neutrons and other high-LET radiations also comes from *in vivo* studies of life-shortening tumor induction and cataract induction in laboratory animals (135–139). There are also some epidemiological studies that support the animal studies (140–142).

The largest inverse dose-rate effects are seen for fission–spectrum neutrons, with monoenergetic neutrons yielding less enhancement (129, 143, 144). Charged particles having LETs above 120 kev/μm produce little or no enhancement (145–147). The inverse dose-rate effect is most prominent at low doses (<20 cGy) and low dose rates (<0.5 cGy/min).

The basis for the inverse dose-rate effect is not known, although a number of suggestions have been made (143, 148–152). Some suggested that the enhancement is related to cell cycle–specific sensitivity. Others have postulated that DNA repair/misrepair processes or radiation-mediated tumor promotion might underlie the phenomenon.

B. Biological Modifiers

1. Tissue Origin

There are many different biological factors that play a role in the cellular responses to ionizing radiation. For example, the origin of the tissue defines to some extent radiation responses. Different tissues show different sensitivities to cancer induction following radiation exposure. This can also be seen in *in vitro* cell cultures. Tumor cell lines derived from different tissues show a characteristic distribution of radiosensitivities (153, 154). These differences may reflect alterations in DNA repair ability, chromosome structure, cell cycle, or some other difference in radiation response.

2. Ploidy

Differences in DNA or chromosome content may play some modifying role in radiation response. There have been reports that more aneuploid tumors tend not to respond as well as more diploid tumors to cytotoxic therapies (including radiation). *In vitro* studies in general suggest no clear relationship between DNA content and radiation sensitivity; however, larger nuclear size is associated with increased radiation sensitivity (155–159).

3. DNA Repair[6]

The inherent ability of cells to repair DNA damage has a profound effect on the responses to radiation. Cells deficient in their ability to rejoin DNA single- or double-strand breaks are very sensitive to the cytotoxic effects of ionizing radiation (125, 126). The extent of DNA repair ability will affect both the frequency and type of gene or chromosome mutation induced by ionizing radiation (70, 125, 126, 160). Individuals with the autosomal recessive genetic disease, xeroderma pigmentosum, are prone to sunlight-induced skin cancer (28). Cells from such individuals are unable to excise ultraviolet light–induced pyrimidine dimers. Individuals with the autosomal recessive

---

[6] For a general textbook on the repair of radiation-induced cell damage, *see* ref. 55.

disorder, ataxia telangiectasia, are similarly hypersensitive to ionizing radiation (28). This is also associated with a defect in the repair of radiation-induced DNA damage.

a. Sublethal Damage Recovery.[7] The shoulder on the survival curve is thought to represent the ability of a cell to accumulate and repair sublethal damage. This can be demonstrated by dose fractionating experiments. For example, if a 10-Gy dose of X-rays is split into two 5-Gy doses separated by a 6-hour time interval, the survival level seen will be higher than if the 10-Gy dose is given all at once. As one continues to divide the dose into smaller and smaller fractions, survival continues to increase up to a maximum related to the initial slope of the survival curve. This is equivalent to reducing the dose rate. In general, as dose rate decreases, the effects of ionizing radiation also decrease. There are some exceptions to this general rule (such as the inverse dose rate effect seen with high-LET radiations).

Split-dose recovery or sublethal damage recovery (SLDR) has been seen in almost all cell systems where it has been studied. The amount of SLDR seen is related to the size of the shoulder on the survival curve. High-LET radiations, which produce little or no shoulder, also produce little or no SLDR. The length of interval between doses suggests that the repair of damage underlying SLDR takes about 3 to 4 hours. This can vary from cell line to cell line (162). SLDR is cell cycle dependent, being greatest in G1.

b. Potentially Lethal Damage Repair.[8] Delaying cell cycle progression following radiation damage will also improve cell survival (164, 165). This phenomenon has been termed potentially lethal damage repair (PLDR). Potentially lethal damage is operationally defined as damage which, if left unrepaired, is lethal. It is measured many different ways. Usually, cells are irradiated in a noncycling condition, then the cycling block is released at various times following irradiation, and survival is subsequently measured. Delaying the cell cycle (cycling block) can be achieved by different means: by the addition of cycloheximide (a protein synthesis inhibitor), by reducing temperature, by serum depletion in the medium, or by maintaining cells in a confluent state. DNA synthesis inhibitors and nonisotonic solutions of certain salts inhibit PLDR and convert potentially lethal lesions to lethal lesions. The ratio: the number of surviving cells determined following some length of duration of cycling block, divided by the number of surviving cells immediately released from cycling block following irradiation, is the PLDR ratio. PLDR is observed for the three endpoints: survival, mutation, and cell transformation, following radiation exposure. The PLDR ratio is also dose dependent.

Potentially lethal lesions are repaired with a half-time of between 1 and 2 hours. Most lesions are repaired within 4 to 6 hours (166, 167). Repair takes place throughout the cell cycle, but is greatest in G1.

Most studies suggest that DNA double-strand breaks are likely to be the molecular lesions involved in both SLDR and PLDR (24, 168, 169). Some of the evidence for this comes from cell lines deficient in DNA double-strand break repair. These lines are deficient in SLDR and PLDR and are, therefore, less affected by alterations in the dose rate. The exact nature of the molecular event(s) involved in PLDR and SLDR remains unclear.

4. Cell Cycle[9]

Almost all mammalian cells show variations in radiation sensitivity across the cell cycle. Mitosis and the G2 phase are usually the most sensitive phases toward radiation

---

[7] For further discussion, *see* refs. 55, 161.
[8] For further discussion, *see* refs. 55, 163.
[9] For a general textbook to this section *see* ref. 55.

toxicity. The most resistant phase is the late S phase, followed by G1 and early S phase. These changes in sensitivity are associated with both effects on D_0 and the shoulder, although effects on the shoulder predominate. There are probably a number of different molecular events underlying the different radiation sensitivities. DNA repair is one factor. Cell lines defective in DNA double-strand break repair show less differences in cell cycle phase radiosensitivity (170). There is also evidence for cell cycle–specific repair processes (171). Recombination, for example, might be favored in late S/G2. There is generally an inverse relationship between survival and the induction of mutation, with S phase being the most sensitive to mutation (172).

5. Chromosome Structure

The multiple levels of organization of DNA in chromosomes are important not only for efficient packing of the genetic material, but are also important for DNA function (173). For example, the process of DNA replication is initiated at specific sites located at the base of supercoiled loops of DNA attached to the nuclear matrix, and these sites are also involved in the control of transcription. Chromosome structure also exerts a profound effect on the induction and repair of DNA damage. For example, chromatin proteins may act as free radical scavengers. Moreover, the organization of the DNA affects the access of free radicals to DNA bases or sugar–phosphate bonds (12, 13). Chromosome structure could also affect the repair of DNA damage (162, 174).

Associations between alterations in chromosome structure and radiation sensitivity have been reported for human tumor cell lines (162, 174), monolayer (*versus* spheroid) V79 cells (175, 176), the mouse cell line Ly5178Y-S (177), radiosensitive Chinese hamster ovary cell lines (178), and cell lines from patients with ataxia telangiectasia (179).

C. Chemical Modifiers

The biological effects of many chemical agents interact with the effects of ionizing radiation in the induction of tumors. Some of these agents act at very early stages in carcinogenesis and have to be present before or during irradiation. Other agents can interact with radiation effects at much later stages, long after the initial radiation exposure. Many of the agents that are protective against radiation-induced injury are also protective against the toxic effects of a variety of chemical agents. There is an overlap of the time periods when, relative to radiation exposure, these agents can affect radiation-induced cancer incidence. It is likely that the most effective agents act by multiple mechanisms.

The effect of a particular agent on radiation carcinogenesis will also vary depending on dose, time of addition, type of tumor induced, and the animal strain studied. Some agents can act as cocarcinogens in one experimental protocol and as anticarcinogens in another protocol. This reflects the complex and multiple mechanisms by which these agents act. The action of these agents can best be understood in the context of how radiation injury develops.

1. Mechanisms of Action[10]

a. Free Radical Scavenging. A major source of damage produced by ionizing radiation, and also by many chemical carcinogens, are free radicals. Thus, agents that

---

[10] For general references, *see* refs. 180–182.

interfere with free radical levels affect tumor frequency following radiation exposure. Free radicals are also normal byproducts of cell respiration. Not surprisingly, cells have evolved systems to protect and repair free radical damage. Endogenous thiols such as glutathione are thought to be major cellular radioprotectors. They act by scavenging free radicals before they can damage important cellular targets.

$$2R^\bullet + 2RSH \rightarrow 2RH + RSSR$$

The importance of endogenous thiols in protecting cells from radiation damage by free radical scavenging is underscored by the observations that chemical agents that deplete cells of thiols, such as D,L-buthione-S,R-sulfoxime (BSO) or diazenedicarboxylic acid bis(N,N-dimethylamine) diamide, sensitize cells to radiation-induced effects. BSO interferes with glutathione biosynthesis and the diamide oxidizes reduced glutathione to its disulfide. Other agents which are sulfhydryl-binding or oxidizing agents also sensitize cells to ionizing radiation; these agents usually act by stabilizing the radicals or enhancing their ability to damage macromolecules.

Most of the protective agents that act by influencing free radical levels must be present during or prior to irradiation to affect induction of DNA damage.

b. Chemical Repair. The initial attack on DNA can lead to the formation of a DNA radical (DNA$^\bullet$). At this stage, the damage can be repaired through a chemical process in which protons or electrons are added back to the DNA radical, so that the reactivity of the DNA site bearing the unpaired electron is abolished.

For example, with thiols,

$$2DNA^\bullet + 2RSH \rightarrow 2DNAH + RSSR$$

or

$$2DNA^\bullet + 2RS^- \rightarrow 2DNA^- + RSSR$$

followed by

$$DNA^- + H^+ \rightarrow DNAH$$

This reaction occurs because, in general, SH bonds are weaker than CH bonds so that transfer of H$^\bullet$ from RSH is energetically favored. This probably accounts for the greater protection seen with thiols as compared with alcohols.

Oxygen affects this chemical repair process and sensitizes cells to DNA damage presumably because of its ability to form peroxy radicals which are highly reactive, but cannot be rendered nonreactive by the addition of hydrogen atom or by electron donation. Agents that reduce oxygen tension and produce hypoxia provide protection to cells against radiation effects. In contrast, chemical agents, that mimic the ability of oxygen to form peroxy radicals, sensitize cells to radiation effects. Agents that influence this chemical repair process must be present within milliseconds of radiation exposure.

c. Enzymatic Repair Processes. Once DNA damage has occurred, the next stage at which chemical agents can interfere with the carcinogenic process is at the level of DNA repair. Thus, defective repair leads to increased sensitivity to ionizing radiation. Eukaryotic DNA repair processes involve many enzymes and cofactors, and there is a multitude of agents that can disrupt repair. Agents that inhibit DNA strand-break rejoining are particularly effective with ionizing radiations, as are also a number of agents (primarily DNA intercalating agents) which affect chromosome structure and thereby the fidelity of DNA repair.

In contrast, there are just a handful of agents that seem to enhance repair processes. These provide some protection against radiation effects. There are also agents which provide protection through their ability to inhibit DNA synthesis or prolong G2 delay, allowing more time to repair DNA damage.

As repair processes are usually rapid, taking minutes to hours to complete, agents that affect repair have to be present shortly after radiation exposure so as to affect the outcome.

d. Effects on Tumor Promotion and Progression.   Cancer is a multistage process. Once it has been initiated, presumably through gene mutation, it evolves through stages of promotion and progression. These later events are associated with changes in gene expression and clonal expansion. Thus, agents that affect cell growth and gene expression, such as various cytokines and hormones, will affect tumor frequency. The effect of these agents is very cell-type–specific, but they can act on carcinogenesis caused by many different agents, not just by ionizing radiations. As free radicals are believed to play an important role in tumor promotion and progression, agents that affect free radical levels should also affect promotion and progression.

Agents that affect carcinogenesis at the level of promotion or progression must be present at these later stages of tumor development.

e. Microvasculature Changes.   Ionizing radiation will produce physiologic changes in vascular function and architecture. Large doses will damage the vasculature, yielding perivascular fibrosis and restricting blood flow; this will result in cell toxicity and may be in part responsible for the antagonistic effects sometimes seen in cancer induction by combinations of radiation and chemical carcinogens. In contrast, low doses of radiation cause more subtle changes in microvasculature, which appear to enhance chemical and physical carcinogenesis rather than inhibit it (183). Microvasculature changes might also be induced by various chemical agents, especially cytokines.

f. Immune Effects.   A major target of radiation action is the hematopoietic system. Ionizing radiation depresses immune function primarily through bone marrow depletion. Depression of the immune system can contribute to tumor induction. It is well established that immunosuppression, whether spontaneous, chemically induced, or radiation induced, is associated with higher frequencies of tumors (184–187). Depending on the dose and tumor system, radiation can sometimes lead to tumor suppression, due to the fact that suppressor T cells and their precursors are radiosensitive (188). Alterations in immune response will also affect viral oncogenesis.

2. Examples of Radioprotectors and Anticarcinogens

a. Thiols.   In 1949, Patt and coworkers (189) reported that cysteine protects mice against the lethal effects of gamma radiation. At about the same time, Bacq *et al.* (190) reported that the decarboxylated form of cysteine, 2-mercaptoethylamine, was even more radioprotective. Thiols and their disulfides, including endogenous thiols such as glutathione and exogenous thiols such as synthetic derivatives of cysteine, are perhaps the largest and most studied group of radioprotectors. The endogenous thiols, cysteine, glutathione, and γ-glutamylcysteine, are present in all mammalian cells and are responsible for a variety of metabolic functions. The levels of these agents are specific for cell type and can be modulated by various metabolic inhibitors such as BSO (191). In general, a lowering of endogenous thiol levels will sensitize cells to ionizing radiation effects, although radioprotection usually requires very low levels of thiols (192). Conversely, more substantial increase in thiol levels will provide modest increases in protection.

Free radical scavenging has long been thought to be a major mechanism underlying the radioprotective effects of thiols and related agents. Thiols will compete efficiently with DNA for free radicals because they react with most radicals at similar diffusion-controlled rates as DNA. One apparent contradiction with free radical scavenging, as a major mechanism of radioprotection by thiols, is that in solution high concentrations of thiols are required to effectively reduce free radical concentrations. *In vivo*, radioprotection is achieved at much lower concentrations. For example, Ward (193) has estimated from chemical data that protection with the aminothiol WR-1065 (see below) should be seen at intracellular concentrations of 73 mM, whereas in fact protection is seen at intracellular concentrations as low as 2-3 mM. One explanation for this discrepancy is that thiols and related radioprotectors may compartmentalize near DNA. There is indeed evidence for compartmentalization of glutathione and related enzymes (181) and for the binding of WR-1065 to DNA (194). However, even with this caveat, free radical scavenging probably cannot explain all instances of radioprotection, as some efficient non-SH hydroxyl radical scavengers are poor radioprotectors.

Eldjarn and Pihl (195) have proposed that the thiol groups of certain enzymes are radiosensitive sites and that endogenous thiols could form transient mixed disulfides at these sites. Free radical attack would then lead to the reduction of one of the sulfur atoms while the other is oxidized (sulfhydryl shielding). The net result would be that only half of the molecules are damaged. The major flaw of this hypothesis is that it fails to explain protection of the major target molecule, DNA, which does not contain sulfhydryl groups.

The capability to donate electrons and protons to radical species is also unable to fully explain the radioprotective effects of thiols, because of the variations in the radioprotective ability of agents unrelated to their electron-donating ability. Thiols may also act in part by producing hypoxia. Oxygen can be depleted by thiol addition itself. Thiols added to growth medium will deplete oxygen in 10-30 minutes (196). Thus, thiols and related compounds act most likely through a combination of mechanisms. *See also* Chapter 4.

b. Aminothiols. In the late 1950s, the U.S. Army began the development of chemical radioprotective agents. Many of the compounds developed were thiophosphate derivatives of cysteamine; the role of the phosphate group was to reduce toxicity. These WR (Walter Reed series) compounds have been extensively studied. The aminothiols (WR-2721 and related compounds) protect against acute and late-arising radiation injuries both *in vitro* and *in vivo*. For example, when added to cells in culture prior to irradiation, aminothiols reduce the cytotoxic (197), clastogenic (198), mutagenic (199), and transforming (200, 201) effects of ionizing radiation. They have similar effects on lethality, induction of mutation, and of tumorigenesis in *in vivo*-exposed animals (202–208). The effects of aminothiols have been shown mostly for low-LET radiation such as X-rays and gamma rays, but they also provide protection against high-LET radiation such as fission–spectrum neutrons (208).

The aminothiols are thought to act similarly to thiols, affecting primarily the induction of DNA damage. The fact that most radioprotectors usually have to be present at the time of irradiation to affect survival argues against any postirradiation mechanism as the basis of action of these agents. However, there is evidence for aminothiols affecting later stages of radiation injury, such as repair. Grdina *et al.* (199) reported a post-irradiation effect of aminothiols on the induction of mutation. The mechanism underlying this postirradiation effect may be related to the ability of aminothiols to prolong G2 delay (209) or may be related to the reported effects of thiols on DNA repair enzymes (210).

Aminothiols might also act on chromosome structure. Brown (182) has suggested that aminothiols act to stabilize the DNA helix and inhibit DNA synthesis by binding to non-histone-containing regions. This would reduce both primary damage by localized free radical scavenging and secondary damage by maintaining structure and preventing shortening or chemical alteration of single-strand breaks. Also, by inhibiting DNA replication, more time would be available for repair.

c. Antioxidants. Given the importance of free radicals in radiation-induced transformation and tumor promotion, it is not surprising that antioxidants such as *p*-aminoacetophenone have radioprotective effect. There are also naturally occurring agents that either act as antioxidants themselves, or act to increase antioxidant levels in cells. These include ascorbic acid (vitamin C), retinoids (such as vitamin A), selenium, and α-tocopherol (vitamin E). All these agents have been shown to be potent inhibitors of radiation-induced transformation *in vitro* and carcinogenesis *in vivo*. They appear to act both at early stages, preventing tumor initiation, and can act after carcinogen exposure, affecting promotional and tumor progression stages.

The activity of the above agents is very carcinogen-specific and appears to involve overlapping, but distinct mechanisms. For example, retinoids act as inducers of electrophile detoxification enzymes such as glutathione transferase, UDP-glucuronyl transferase, and NADPH-quinone reductase. Vitamin E is a free-radical scavenger. Organic selenium is an essential constituent of glutathione peroxidase. Glutathione peroxidase uses reducing equivalents from glutathione to detoxify hydrogen peroxide and organic hydroperoxides. Selenium also plays a role in the transport and storage of vitamin E. Nontoxic levels of selenium are associated with enhanced levels of cellular peroxidase and catalase activities, which are unaffected by vitamin E treatment.

The role of antioxidants has been extensively studied in the last 15 years (*e.g.*, 211–216); *see also* Chapters 4 and 9/Sects. III and IV.

d. Protease Inhibitors. Protease inhibitors are agents that have been extensively studied for their anticarcinogenic effects (*e.g.*, 217–219). These agents reduce radiation-induced transformation both *in vivo* and *in vitro*. The protease inhibitors that show anticarcinogenic effect include leupeptin, antipain, and soybean trypsin inhibitor. These are low–molecular-weight compounds that are trypsin or trypsin chymotrypsin inhibitors.

The mechanism of anticarcinogenic action of protease inhibitors is not known. Protease inhibitors will inhibit both tumor initiation and promotion. Identifying the specific target of the inhibitors is difficult, because measured protease activity is frequently the sum of a cascade of protease activities involving a number of different proteases. One effect of protease inhibitors is to inhibit the "respiratory burst" response of polymorphonuclear leukocytes, which is seen in inflammatory responses. The respiratory burst involves the release of O_2^- and H_2O_2, which may promote tumor induction. Other effects that have been reported for protease inhibitors include effects on gene amplification and oncogene expression.

e. Immunologic and Cell Growth Modifiers. Agents that enhance immune function such as glucan (β-1,3-polyglucose) will reduce tumor incidence following irradiation. These agents inhibit tumorigenesis by enhancing host resistance to post-irradiation infections and enhancing hematopoietic regeneration. Cytokines and glucocorticoids, which influence tumor cell growth, will also reduce tumor incidence following radiation exposure. As with many of the agents so far described, the effects appear to be on both the initiation and promotion levels. What is observed depends on the particular agents studied, the tumor system, and the time period when treatment is applied (*e.g.*, 220, 221).

3. Examples of Radiosensitizers and Cocarcinogens

a. Hypoxic Cell Sensitizers[11]. Electrophilic agents mimic oxygen and act as radiosensitizers. The sensitizing effects are related to the redox potential of the agent. The agents are usually most effective in hypoxic cells. *p*-Nitroacetophenone was one of the first hypoxic cell sensitizers studied. Over the years, there has been much study of the ability of derivatives of 5-nitroimidazoles and 2-nitroimidazoles to act as hypoxic cell sensitizers *in vivo*. Metronidazole (5-nitroimidazole) and misonidazole (2-nitroimidazole) are two drugs that have been studied for their clinical efficacy in potentiating tumor cell killing, in combination with ionizing radiation therapy.

b. Halogenated Pyrimidines. Halogenated pyrimidines such as 5-bromo-deoxyuridine, chlorodeoxyuridine, and iododeoxyuridine are structural analogs of thy-midine. They are incorporated into DNA during replication and, once incorporated, they act as radiosensitizers. The degree of sensitization is in general related to the relative amount of halogenated pyrimidine that is incorporated into DNA. Iododeoxyuridine produces the greatest sensitization to the effects of X-rays, followed by bromodeoxyuri-dine and then chlorodeoxyuridine.

The exact mechanism of sensitization by these thymidine analogs is not known. These agents affect a variety of cellular activities, including chromosome structure and protein binding to DNA. More breaks are seen in irradiated cells that contain incorporated halogens, suggesting that the effect of incorporation is to increase DNA sensitivity to strand breakage. The halogens may be interacting with radiation-induced free radicals (*e.g.*, aqueous electrons) or the halogen may be making the phosphate links more labile due to electrostatic interactions to cause increased frequency of strand breaks.

For further discussion of halogenated pyrimidines and their role in sensitization, *see* refs. (222–225).

c. DNA Synthesis Inhibitors. Some of the agents that inhibit DNA synthesis act by affecting DNA strand-break rejoining and will thus sensitize cells to radiation effects. Aphidicolin is an inhibitor of α-polymerase, an enzyme involved in DNA repair as well as in replicative DNA synthesis. Aphidicolin will sensitize cells to the cytotoxic and mutagenic effects of ionizing radiation. These effects are dependent on nucleotide pool sizes and may be cell-cycle-specific.

9-β-D-Arabinofuranosyladenine (ara A) and 1-β-D-arabinofuranosylcytosine (ara C) are two other inhibitors of DNA synthesis that have been shown to act on both polymerase α and polymerase β. Polymerase β is believed to be involved in repair synthesis. It is not entirely clear how these analogs inhibit DNA synthesis; however, most evidence points to their acting as chain terminators. These agents are incorporated into DNA. Like aphidicolin, ara A and ara C will sensitize cells to the cytotoxic and mutagenic effects of ionizing radiation. The increased toxicity seen with combinations of radiation and these analogs might be due to (a) inhibition of DNA repair, (b) interactions between radiation-induced DNA damage and the damage produced by ara A or ara C, or (c) combined effects of radiation and ara A/ara C on apoptosis.

Hydroxyurea is an inhibitor of ribonucleotide reductase and acts to inhibit DNA

---

[11] For source books on this subject *see* refs. 55, 222.

synthesis by lowering deoxyribonucleotide pools. Hydroxyurea has indeed been reported to affect repair of radiation damage; both increases and decreases in repair endpoints have been reported. The effect is believed to be on the polymerase step of excision repair.

DNA synthesis inhibitors have been studied extensively during the last quarter century (*e.g.*, 226–247).

d. Poly(ADP-ribose) Inhibitors

d. Poly(ADP-ribose) Inhibitors Poly(ADP-ribose) polymerase is a chromatin-associated enzyme of 116 kDa that acts in response to DNA strand breakage and synthesizes long polymers of ADP-ribose, using NAD^+ as a substrate. In the process, cellular NAD^+ levels are depleted. These polymers are covalently attached to a number of protein targets including poly(ADP-ribose) polymerase itself, DNA ligase, topoisomerase II, various histone proteins, and certain other nuclear proteins. The ADP-ribose modifications in general alter protein structure, reducing the activity of the affected enzymes, and altering chromatin protein binding to DNA. The polymers are short-lived (in the order of minutes), being rapidly degraded by a specific glycohydrolase. The physiological role of the polymerization/degradation cycle is unclear.

There are a number of agents that inhibit this ADP ribosylation. Many of these inhibitors act as competitive inhibitors of the enzyme, being structurally similar to NAD^+. Inhibition of this enzyme sensitizes cells to the cytotoxic and clastogenic effects of ionizing radiation. Increases in mutagenicity and transformation have also been reported, but the results are conflicting as there are other reports of a lack of effect on these endpoints. Part of this conflict may be explained by the observation that the effects of poly(ADP-ribose) inhibitors are oncogene-specific (248). Alternatively, the effects of the inhibitors may be on later promotional stages (249).

The effect of poly(ADP-ribose) polymerase inhibition on radiation-induced cellular and cytogenetic effects may be due to the action of poly(ADP-ribose) polymerase on chromatin structure (250). It is interesting to note that most ribosylations are associated with the DNA nuclear matrix (251), which has been suggested to play an important role in radiation response (162). Alterations in chromatin structure may affect the rate and accuracy of DNA strand-break rejoining (162). Strand-break rejoining is slower and less accurate in the presence of poly(ADP-ribose) polymerase inhibitors.

Several other references (252–254) discuss poly(ADP-ribose) inhibitors.

e. Methylxanthines.

e. Methylxanthines. Methylxanthines, such as the purine analog caffeine, have been extensively studied as potential modifiers of radiation response (255–260). The mechanism of action of the methylxanthines is not clear. They may act by inhibiting postreplication repair synthesis of DNA, by their ability to inhibit poly(ADP-ribose) polymerase, through effects on DNA synthesis; or they may act through cell cycle effects, such as reducing G2 delay following radiation exposure.

f. Hormones.

f. Hormones. Certain hormones will act in concert with radiation to increase the incidence and shorten the latency of tumors. Usually, these are hormone-responsive tumors such as mammary tumors. Shellabarger and coworkers (261, 263), Segaloff and Maxfield (262), and Yokoro and Furth (264) have published extensively on diethylstilbestrol, estradiol, and prolactin effects on radiation-induced murine mammary tumors. The enhanced tumor induction is seen when hormone treatment is combined with either high- or low-LET radiations. They are thought to reflect hormonal influences on promotion and progression of radiation-initiated transformed foci. The effects are strain specific and variable in expression.

g. Cocarcinogens.

g. Cocarcinogens. Several chemical agents act as cocarcinogens in combination with ionizing radiation acting as the carcinogen. Pyrene is one example of such a cocarcinogen. It is nonmutagenic and noncarcinogenic, but in combination with ionizing radiation it enhances the transforming effects of a single gamma ray exposure without influencing, however, the cytotoxicity (265–271). The mechanism of action of pyrene and related compounds is not known. Atcheson *et al.* (270) suggested that they may interfere with DNA repair. Many tumor promoters can also act as cocarcinogens, which suggests that the mechanism underlying tumor promotion might be similar to that underlying cocarcinogenesis.

h. Chemical Carcinogens. The interactions of ionizing radiation and various chemical carcinogens (complete carcinogens) have been studied for many decades. In some cases, synergism has been reported. In other cases, additivity or even antagonistic effects have been seen. The results and conclusions of such studies stress the importance of dose, time and sequence of treatments, strain of animal studied, and target tissue. Synergism is observed most often, and the combination of effects is the greatest, when the chemical treatment *follows* radiation. Thus, in these cases the chemical agent appears to act as a tumor promoter. Reversing the order sometimes results in simple additivity or sometimes results in reduced tumor frequencies. When tumor yields are less than additive, it is usually assumed to be due to the toxicity of the combined treatments, but other mechanisms have also been suggested. Similarly, there is no clear understanding of the mechanism of synergism. All the mechanisms mentioned above probably play a role in different instances.

Among the polycyclic hydrocarbons studied in this context, synergism with ionizing radiation has been reported for 7,12-dimethylbenz[*a*]anthracene, benzo[*a*]pyrene, and 3-methylcholanthrene (272–274). Synergism is seen for both low- and high-LET radiations. Benzo[*a*]pyrene is one agent that has been extensively studied. Benzo[*a*]pyrene is a component of cigarette smoke, and smoking has a multiplicative effect on tumor induction by ionizing radiation. Enhancement of tumorigenesis (synergism) has been reported for benzo[*a*]pyrene combined with gamma rays and alpha particles.

Synergism has also been reported for combinations of ionizing radiations and a variety of alkylating agents. Synergistic induction of tumors is seen when mice, irradiated *in utero*, are treated with *N*-ethyl-*N*-nitrosourea (275). The effect is dose dependent. Higher doses of radiation resulted in a suppression of *N*-ethyl-*N*-nitrosourea-induced tumors. Synergism has also been reported for 4-nitroquinoline *N*-oxide, the effect being greatest when the chemical carcinogen *followed* radiation treatment (276). Other agents showing synergistic interactions with radiation include *N*-2-fluorenylacetamide, 4-ethyl-sulfonyl-naphthalene-1-sulfonamide, and procarbazine (277–279).

Ethyl carbamate (urethan), which is moderately carcinogenic, synergistically increases leukemogenesis in X-irradiated mice when exposure to the chemical *follows* radiation exposure. However, when urethan exposure precedes radiation exposure, an antagonistic effect in tumor induction is sometimes seen (280).

i. Miscellaneous Agents. There are a number of other agents which potentiate radiation effects. They include agents that affect chromatin structure, like bisbenzimidazole (281) and actinomycin D, and agents that inhibit protein phosphorylation (41). Given the pleiotropic influences of chromosome structure and protein phosphorylation on cell metabolism, these agents probably produce effects via several pathways.

ACKNOWLEDGMENTS

The writing of this chapter was supported by the U.S. Department of Energy under contract W-31-109-ENG-38 (JLS) and grant No. DE-FG02-88ER60661, and by a Faculty Research Award from the American Cancer Society.

U.S. GOVERNMENT COPYRIGHT LICENSE

REFERENCES

1. Johns, H. E., and Cunningham, J. R.: "The Physics of Radiology". Charles C Thomas, Springfield, Illinois, 1969.
2. Goodwin, P. N., Quimby, E. H., and Morgan, R. H.: "Physical Foundations of Radiology". Harper & Row, New York, 1970.
3. Goodhead, D. T.: *Int. J. Radiat. Biol.* **56**, 623 (1989).
4. Goodhead, D. T., and Nikjoo, H.: *Int. J. Radiat. Biol.* **55**, 513 (1989).
5. Sonntag, C. von: "The Chemical Basis of Radiation Biology". Taylor & Francis, London, 1987.
6. Michaels, H. B., and Hunt, J. W.: *Radiat. Res.* **74**, 23 (1978).
7. Lea, D. E.: "Actions of Radiations on Living Cells". 2nd ed. Cambridge Univ. Press, Cambridge, 1956.
8. DeSombre, E. R., Harper, P. V., Hughes, A., Mease, R. C., Gatley, S. J., DeJesus, O. T., and Schwartz, J. L.: *Cancer Res.* **48**, 585 (1988).
9. Oleinick, N. L., Chiu, S., Friedman, L. R., Xue, L., and Ramakrishnan, N.: "Mechanism of DNA Damage and Repair". Plenum Press, New York, 1986, p. 181.
10. Ramakrishnan, N., Chiu, S., and Oleinick, N. L.: *Cancer Res.* **47**, 2032 (1987).
11. Hutchinson, F.: *Prog. Nucleic Acid Res. Mol. Biol.* **32**, 115 (1985).
12. Ward, J. F., and Kuo, I.: *Radiat. Res.* **75**, 278 (1978).
13. Ward, J. F.: *Radiat. Res.* **104**, S-103 (1985).
14. Waters, R. L., and Childers, T. J.: *Radiat. Res.* **90**, 584 (1982).
15. Patil, M. S., Locher, S. E., and Hariharan, P. V.: *Int. J. Radiat Biol.* **48**, 691 (1985).
16. Frenkel, K., Chrzan, K., Troll, W., Teebor, G., and Steinberg, J.: *Cancer Res.* **46**, 5533 (1986).
17. Ames, B. N.: *Free Radical Res. Commun.* **7**, 121 (1989).
18. Frankenberg-Schwager, M.: *Radiat. Environ. Biophys.* **29**, 273 (1990).
19. McBride, T., Preston, B., and Loeb, L.: *Biochemistry* **30**, 207 (1991).
20. Turkington, E., and Strauss, B. G.: *Mutat. Res.* **251**, 187 (1991)
21. Kunkel, T. A.: *Proc. Natl. Acad. Sci. U.S.A.* **81**, 1494 (1984).
22. Strauss, B. S.: *Bio Essays* **13**, 79 (1991).
23. Dikomey, E., and Franzke, J.: *Radiat. Environ. Biophys.* **25**, 189 (1986).
24. Schwartz, J. L., Giovanazzi, S. M., and Weichselbaum, R. R.: *Radiat. Res.* **111**, 58 (1987).
25. Henner, W. D., Rodriguez, L. O., Hecht, S. M., and Haseltine, W. A.: *J. Biol. Chem.* **258**, 711 (1983).
26. Hanawalt, P., Cooper, P., Ganeson, A., and Smith, C.: *Annu. Rev. Biochem.* **48**, 783 (1979).
27. Jorgensen, T. J., Kow, Y. W., Wallace, S. S., and Henner, W. D.: *Biochemistry* **26**, 6436 (1987).
28. Cleaver, J. E., and Bootsma, D.: *Annu. Rev. Genet.* **9**, 19 (1975).
29. Frankenberg, D., Frankenberg-Schwager, M., Blöcher, D., and Harbich, R.: *Radiat. Res.* **88**, 524 (1981).
30. Jeggo, P. A., and Kemp, L. M.: *Mutat. Res.* **112**, 313 (1983).
31. Hutchinson, F.: DNA Strand Break Repair in Eukaryotes: A Workshop Summary. *In* "DNA Repair Mechanisms" (P. C. Hanawalt, E. C. Friedberg, and C. F. Fox, eds.). Academic Press, New York, 1978, p. 457.
32. Ozenberger, B. A., and Roeder, G. S.: *Mol. Cell Biol.* **11**, 1222 (1991).
33. Painter, R. B.: *Int. J. Radiat. Biol.* **49**, 771 (1986).
34. Lamb, J. R., Petit-Frere, C., Broughton, B. C., Lehmann, A. R., and Green, M. H.: *Int. J. Radiat. Biol.* **56**, 125 (1989).
35. Cleaver, J. E., Rose, R., and Mitchell, D. L.: *Radiat. Res.* **124**, 294 (1990).
36. Kaston, M. B., Onyetueve, O., Sidransky, D., Vogelstein, B., and Craig, R. W.: *Cancer Res.* **51**, 6304 (1991).
37. Hallahan, D. E., Spriggs, D. R., Beckett, M. A., Kufe, D. W., and Weichselbaum, R. R.: *Proc. Natl. Acad. Sci. U.S.A.* **86**, 10104 (1989).
38. Woloschak, G. E., Chang-Liu, C-M., and Shearin-Jones, P.: *Cancer Res.* **50**, 3963 (1990).
39. Boothman, D. A., and Lee, S. W.: *Proc. Am. Assoc. Cancer Res.* **32**, 74 (1991).

40. Hallahan, D. E., Sukhatme, V. P., Sherman, M. L., Virudachalam, S., Kufe, D. W., and Weichselbaum, R. R.: *Proc. Natl. Acad. Sci. U.S.A.* **88**, 2156 (1991).
41. Hallahan, D. E., Virudachalam, S., Schwartz, J. L., Panje, N., Mustafi, R., and Weichselbaum, R. R.: *Radiat Res.* **129**, 345 (1992).
42. Cornforth, M. N., and Bedford, J. S.: *Science* **222**, 1141 (1983).
43. Harrington, L. A., and Greider, C. W.: *Nature* **353**, 451 (1991).
44. Morin, G. B.: *Nature* **353**, 454 (1991).
45. Evans, H. J.: *Int. Rev. Cytol.* **13**, 221 (1962).
46. Bender, M.: *Am. J. Pathol.* **43**, 26a (1963).
47. Edwards, A. A., Lloyd, D. C., and Prosser, J. S.: Chromosome Aberrations in Human Lymphocytes — A Radiobiological Review. *In* "Low Dose Radiation: Biological Bases of Risk Assessment" (K. F. Baverstock and J. W. Stather, eds.). Taylor & Francis, London, 1989, p. 423.
48. Terasima, T., and Tolmach, L. J.: *Biophys. J.* **3**, 11 (1963).
49. Sinclair, W. K., and Morton, R. A.: *Radiat. Res.* **29**, 450 (1966).
50. Weinert, T. A., and Hartwell, L. H.: *Science* **241**, 317 (1988).
51. Weibezahn, K. F., Lohrer, H., and Herrlich, P.: *Mutat. Res.* **145**, 177 (1985).
52. Grinfeld, S., and Jacquet, P.: *Int. J. Radiat. Biol.* **54**, 257 (1988).
53. McKenna, W. G., Iliakis, G., Weiss, M. C., Bernhard, E. J., and Muschel, R. J.: *Radiat. Res.* **125**, 283 (1991).
54. Arends, M. J., Morris, R. G., and Wyllie, A. H.: *Am. J. Pathol.* **136**, 593 (1990).
55. Hall, E. J.: "Radiobiology for the Radiologist", 3rd ed. Lippincott, Philadelphia, 1988.
56. Little, J. B., Nove, J., Strong, L. C., and Nichols, W. W.: *Int. J. Radiat. Biol.* **54**, 899 (1988).
57. Muller, H. J.: *Science* **67**, 82 (1928).
58. Searle, A. G.: Evidence from Mammalian Studies on Genetic Effects of Low Level Irradiation. *In* "Low Dose Radiation: Biological Bases of Risk Assessment" (K. F. Baverstock and J. W. Stather, eds.). Taylor and Francis, London, 1989, p. 123.
59. Valcovic, L. R., and Malling, H. U.: *Environ. Health Perspect.* **6**, 301 (1973).
60. Russell, W. L.: *Cold Spring Harbor Symp. Quant. Biol.* **16**, 327 (1951).
61. de Serres, F. J.: Specific-Locus Studies with Two-Component Heterokaryons of *Neuorospora crassa* Predict Differential Recovery of Mutants in Mammalian Cells. *In* "Mammalian Cell Mutagenesis", Banbury Rep. 28 (M. M. Moore, D. M. DeMarini, F. J. de Serres, and K. R. Tindall, eds.). Cold Spring Harbor Laboratory, Cold Spring Harbor, New York, 1987, p. 55.
62. Hsie, A. W., O'Neill, J. P., and McElheny, V. K., eds.: "Mammalian Cell Mutagenesis," Banbury Report 2. Cold Spring Harbor Laboratory, Cold Spring Harbor, New York, 1979.
63. Liber, H. L., and Thilly, W. G.: *Mutat. Res.* **94**, 467 (1982).
64. Breimer, L. H.: *Br. J. Cancer* **57**, 6 (1988).
65. DeMarini, D. M., Brockman, H. E., de Serres, F. J., Evans, H. H., Stankowski, L. F., Jr., and Hsie, A. W.: *Mutat. Res.* **220**, 11 (1989).
66. Sankaranarayanan, K.: *Mutat. Res.* **258**, 75 (1991).
67. Waldren, C., Corell, L., Soginer, M. A., and Puck, T. T.: *Proc. Natl. Acad. Sci. U.S.A.* **83**, 4839 (1986).
68. Searle, A. G.: *Adv. Radiat. Biol.* **4**, 131 (1974).
69. Morgan, T. L., Fleck, E. W., Poston, K. A., Denovan, B. A., Neuman, C. N., Rossiter, B. J. F., and Miller, J. H.: *Mutat. Res.* **232**, 171 (1990).
70. Evans, H. H., Mencl, J., Harng, M-F., Ricanati, M., Sanchez, C., and Hozier, J.: *Proc. Natl. Acad. Sci. U.S.A.* **83**, 4379 (1986).
71. Liber, H. L., Yandell, D. W., and Little, J. B.: *Mutat. Res.* **216**, 9 (1989).
72. Neel, J. V.: *Environ. Mol. Mutagen.* **14**, 55 (1989).
73. Borek, C., and Sachs, L.: *Nature* **210**, 276 (1966).
74. Reznikoff, C. A., Bertram, J. S., Brankow, D. W., and Heidelberger, C.: *Cancer Res.* **33**, 3239 (1973).
75. Kakunaga, T.: *Int. J. Cancer* **12**, 463 (1973).
76. Terzaghi, M., Klein-Szanto, A., and Nettesheim, P.: *Cancer Res.* **43**, 1461 (1983).
77. Clifton, K. H., Tanner, M. A., and Gould, M. N.: *Cancer Res.* **46**, 2390 (1986).
78. Redpath, J. L., and Sun, C.: *Radiat. Res.* **121**, 206 (1990).
79. Thraves, P., Salehi, Z., Dritschilo, A., and Rhim, J. S.: *Proc. Natl. Acad. Sci. U.S.A.* **87**, 1174 (1990).
80. Borek, C.: *Nature* **283**, 776 (1980).
81. Milo, G. E., and Casto, B. C.: *Cancer Lett.* **31**, 1 (1986).
82. Kennedy, A. R., Cairns, J., and Little, J. B.: *Nature* **276**, 825 (1978).
83. Goodhead, D. T.: Deductions from Cellular Studies of Inactivation, Mutagenesis, and Transformation. *In* "Radiation Carcinogenesis: Epidemiology and, Biological Significance" (J. D. Boice, Jr. and J. F. Fraumeni, Jr., eds.) Progr. Cancer Res. Therap., Vol. 26 Raven Press, New York, 1984, p. 369.
84. Borek, C., Ong, A., and Mason, H.: *Proc. Natl. Acad. Sci. U.S.A.* **84**, 794 (1987).

85. Krolewski, B., and Little, J. B.: *Mol. Carcinogenesis* **2**, 27 (1989).
86. Little, J. B.: The Relevance of Cell Transformation to Carcinogenesis *in vivo*. *In* "Low Dose Radiation: Biological Bases of Risk Assessment" (K. F. Baverstock and J. W. Stather, eds.). Taylor & Francis, London, 1989, p. 396.
87. Sawey, M. J., and Kennedy, A. R.: Activation of Oncogenes in Radiation-Induced Malignant Transformation. *In* "Low Dose Radiation: Biological Bases of Risk Assessment" (K. F. Baverstock and J. W. Stather, eds.). Taylor & Francis, London, 1989, p. 433.
88. Furth, J., and Lorenz, E.: Carcinogenesis by Ionizing Radiations". *In* "Radiation Biology" (A. Hollaender, ed.), Vol. I, Part II. McGraw-Hill, New York, 1954, p. 1145.
89. Boice, J. D., and Land, C. E.: Ionizing Radiation. *In* "Cancer Epidemiology and Prevention" (D. Schottenfeld and J. F. Fraumeni, eds.). Saunders, Philadelphia, 1982 p. 231.
90. Beebe, G. W., Kata, H., and Land, C. E.: *Radiat. Res.* **75**, 138 (1978).
91. Matanoski, G. M., Seltser, R., Sartwell, P. E.: *Am. J. Epidemiol.* **101**, 199 (1975).
92. Stebbings, J. H., Lucas, H. F., and Stehney, A. F.: *Am. J. Ind. Med.* **5**, 435 (1984).
93. Archer, V. E., Gillam, J. D., and Wagoner, J. K.: *Ann. N.Y. Acad. Sci.* **271**, 280 (1976).
94. Ron, E., and Modan, B.: *J. Natl. Cancer Inst.* **65**, 7 (1980).
95. Shore, R. E., Albert, R. E., and Pasternack, B. S.: *Arch. Environ. Health* **31**, 21 (1976).
96. Committee on the Biological Effects of Ionizing Radiations: "Health Effects of Exposure to Low Levels of Ionizing Radiation" (BEIR V). National Academy Press, Washington, D. C., 1990.
97. Weissman, I. L.: *Int. J. Radiat. Oncol. Biol. Phys.* **11**, 57 (1985).
98. Kohn, H. I., and Fry, R. J. M.: *N. Engl. J. Med.* **310**, 504 (1984).
99. Berenblum, I., and Shubik, P.: *Br. J. Cancer* **3**, 384 (1949).
100. Berenblum, I., and Trainin, N.: *Science* **132**, 40 (1960).
101. McGregor, J. F.: *J. Natl. Cancer Inst.* **56**, 429 (1976).
102. Hoshino, H., and Tanooka, H.: *Cancer Res.* **35**, 663 (1975).
103. Kitagawa, T., Nomura, K., and Sasaki, S.: *Cancer Res.* **45**, 6078 (1985).
104. Kaufmann, W. K., MacKenzie, S. A., and Kaufman, D. G.: *Teratogen. Carcinogen. Mutagen.* **7**, 551 (1987).
105. Jaffe, D. R., and Bowden, G. T.: *Radiat. Res.* **106**, 156 (1986).
106. Jaffe, D. R., and Bowden, G. T.: *Cancer Res.* **47**, 6692 (1987).
107. Fujiki, H., Mori, M., and Tanooka, H.: *Cancer Lett.* **12**, 15 (1982).
108. Jaffe, D. R., Williamson, J. F., and Bowden, G. T.: *Carcinogenesis* **8**, 1753 (1987).
109. Ootsugama, A., and Tanooka, H.: *Jpn. J. Cancer Res.* **78**, 1203 (1987).
110. Mori, H., Iwata, H., Morishita, Y., Mori, Y., Ohno, T., Tanaka, T., and Sasaki, S.: *Jpn. J. Cancer Res.* **81**, 975 (1990).
111. Sawey, M. J., Hood, A. T., and Burns, F. J.: *Mol. Cell. Biol.* **7**, 932 (1987).
112. Diamond, L. E., Guerrero, I., and Pellicer, A.: *Mol. Cell Biol.* **8**, 2233 (1988).
113. Newcomb, E. W., Steinberg, J. J., and Pellicer, A.: *Cancer Res.* **48**, 5514 (1988).
114. Sturm, S. A., Strauss, P. G., Adolph, S., Hameister, H., and Erfle, V.: *Cancer Res.* **50**, 4146 (1990).
115. Jaffe, D. R., and Bowden, G. T.: *Carcinogenesis* **10**, 2243 (1989).
116. Leung, F. C.: *Radiat. Environ. Biophys.* **30**, 191 (1991).
117. Leung, F. C., Bohn, L. R., and Dagle, G. E.: *Proc. Soc. Exp. Biol. Med.* **196**, 385 (1991).
118. Brachman, D. G., Hallahan, D. E., Beckett, M. A., Yandell, D. W., and Weichselbaum, R. R.: *Cancer Res.* **51**, 6393 (1991).
119. Furuno, I., Yada, T., Matsudaira, H., and Maruyama, T.: *Int. J. Radiat. Biol.* **36**, 639 (1979).
120. Ritter, M. A., Cleaver, J. E., and Tobias, C. A.: *Nature* **266**, 653 (1977).
121. Roots, R., Yang, T. C., Craise, L., Blakely, E. A., and Tobias, C. A.: *Radiat. Res.* **78**, 38 (1979).
122. Hendry, J. H.: *Radiat. Res.* **128**, S-111 (1991).
123. Shadley, J. D., Whitlock, J. L., Rotmensch, J., Atcher, R. W., Tang, J., and Schwartz, J. L.: *Mutat. Res.* **248**, 73 (1991).
124. Schwartz, J. L., Shadley, J. D., Atcher, R. W., Tang, J., Whitlock, J. L., and Rotmensch, J.: *Environ. Mol. Mutagen.* **16**, 178 (1990).
125. Elkind, M. M., and Sutton, H.: *Nature* **184**, 1293 (1959).
126. Elkind, M. M.: *Radiat. Res.* **100**, 425 (1984).
127. Ngo, F. Q. H., Han, A., and Elkind, M. M.: *Int. J. Radiat. Biol.* **32**, 507 (1977).
128. Han, A., and Elkind, M. M.: *Cancer Res.* **39**, 123 (1979).
129. Hill, C. K., Carnes, B. A., Han, A., and Elkind, M. M.: *Radiat. Res.* **102**, 404 (1982).
130. Han, A., Hill, C. K., and Elkind, M. M.: *Radiat. Res.* **99**, 249 (1984).
131. Grahn, D., Carnes, B. A., and Farrington, B. H.: *Mutat. Res.* **162**, 81 (1986).
132. Kubota, N., Jones, C. A., and Hill, C. K.: The Influence of Low Dose Rate Irradiations with Neutrons on Mutation Induction in Chinese Hamster Cells and Human Diploid Fibroblasts. *In* "Proc. 8th Int.

Congr. Radiat. Res.", July 1987, Edinburgh (E. M. Fielden, J. F. Fowler, J. H. Hendry, and D. Scott, eds.), Vol. I. Taylor & Francis, Philadelphia, 1989, p. 132.

133. Kronenberg, A., and Little, J. B.: Enhancement of Neutron-Induced Mutation Frequency in Human B-Lymphoblastoid Cells by Continuous Low Dose-Rate Exposure. *In* "Proc. 8th Int. Congr. Radiat. Res.", July 1987, Edinburgh (E. M. Fielden, J. F. Fowler, J. H. Hendry, and D. Scott, eds.), Vol. I. Taylor & Francis, Philadelphia, 1989, p. 135.

134. Jones, C. A., Sedita, B. A., Hill, C. K., and Elkind, M. M.: Influence of Dose Rate on the Transformation of Syrian Hamster Embryo Cells by Fission-Spectrum Neutrons. *In* "Low Dose Radiation: Biological Bases of Risk Assessment" (K. F. Baverstock and J. W. Stather, eds.). Taylor & Francis, London, 1989, p. 539.

135. Ullrich, R. L.: *Radiat. Res.* **86,** 587 (1984).

136. Upton, A. C., Randolph, M. L., and Conklin, J. W.: *Radiat. Res.* **41,** 467 (1970).

137. Cross, F. T., Evidence of Lung Cancer from Animal Studies. *In* "Radon and Its Decay Products in Indoor Air" (W. W. Nazaroff and A. V. Nero, Jr., eds.). Wiley, New York, 1988, p. 373.

138. Little, J. B., Kennedy, A. R., and McGandy, R. B.: *Radiat. Res.* **103,** 293 (1985).

139. Worgul, B. V., Merriam, G. R., Jr., Medvedovsky, C., and Brenner, D. J.: *Radiat. Res.* **118,** 93 (1989).

140. Hornung, R. W., and Meinhardt, T. J.: *Health Phys.* **52,** 417 (1987).

141. Darby, S. C., and Doll, R.: *Nature* **344,** 824 (1990).

142. Chemlevsky, D., Kellerer, A. M., Land, C. E., Mays, C. W., and Spiess, H.: *Radiat. Environ. Biophys.* **27,** 91 (1988).

143. Hill, C. K., Han, A., and Elkind, M. M.: *Int. J. Radiat. Biol.* **46,** 11 (1984).

144. Miller, R. C., Brenner, D. J., Geard, C. R., Komatsu, K., Marino, S. A., and Hall, E. J.: *Radiat. Res.* **114,** 589 (1988).

145. Miller, R. C., Brenner, D. J., Randers-Pherson, G., Marino, S. A., and Hall, E. J.: *Radiat. Res.* **124,** 562 (1989).

146. Hieber, L., Ponsel, G., Roos, H., Fenn, S., Fromke, E., and Kellerer, A. M.: *Int. J. Radiat. Biol.* **52,** 859 (1987).

147. Yang, T. C., Craise, L. M., Mei, M. T., and Tobias, C. A.: *Adv. Space Res.* **6,** 137 (1987).

148. Barendson, G. W.: *Int. J. Radiat. Biol.* **47,** 731 (1985).

149. Burch, P. R. J., and Chesters, M. S.: *Int. J. Radiat. Biol.* **49,** 495 (1986).

150. Elkind, M. M.: *Radiat. Res.* **128,** 547 (1991).

151. Rossi, H. H., and Kellerer, A. M.: *Int. J. Radiat. Biol.* **50,** 353 (1986).

152. Sykes, C. E., and Watt, D. E.: *Int. J. Radiat. Biol.* **55,** 925 (1989).

153. Weichselbaum, R. R., Rotmensch, J., Ahmed-Swann, S., and Beckett, M. A.: *Int. J. Radiat. Biol.* **56,** 553 (1989).

154. Schwartz, J. L., Beckett, M. A., Mustafi, R., Vaughan, A. T. M., and Weichselbaum, R. R.: Radiation Research: A Twentieth-Century Perspective. *In* "Proc. 9th Int. Congr. Radiat. Res." (W. C. Dewey, M. Edington, R. J. M. Fry, E. J. Hall, and G. F. Whitmore, eds.). Vol. II. Academic Press, San Diego, 1992, p. 716.

155. Bedford, J. S., and Hall, E. J.: *Radiat. Res.* **31,** 679 (1967).

156. Burki, H. J., and Carrano, A. V.: *Mutat. Res.* **17,** 277 (1973).

157. Radford, I. R., and Hodgson, G. S.: *Int. J. Radiat. Biol.* **51,** 765 (1987).

158. Szumiel, I.: *Adv. Radiat. Biol.* **9,** 281 (1981).

159. Schwartz, J. L.: *Radiat. Res.* **129,** 96 (1992).

160. Darroudi, F., and Natarajan, A. T.: *Mutat. Res.* **212,** 123 (1989).

161. Elkind, M. M.: *Radiat. Res.* **100,** 425 (1984).

162. Schwartz, J. L., and Vaughan, A. T. M.: *Cancer Res.* **49,** 5054 (1989).

163. Phillips, R. A., and Tolmach, L. J.: *Radiat. Res.* **29,** 413 (1966).

164. Hahn, G. M., and Little, J. B.: *Top. Radiat. Res. Quart.* **8,** 39 (1972).

165. Weiss, B. G., and Tolmach, L. J.: *Biophys. J.* **7,** 779 (1967).

166. Little, J. B.: *Nature* **224,** 804 (1969).

167. Hahn, G. M., and Little, J. B.: *Int. J. Radiat. Biol.* **23,** 401 (1973).

168. Thacker, J., and Stretch, A.: *Mutat. Res.* **146,** 99 (1985).

169. Frankenberg, D., Frankenberg-Schwager, M., and Jarbich, R.: *Int. J. Radiat. Biol.* **46,** 541 (1984).

170. Iliakis, G. E., and Okayasu, R.: *Int. J. Radiat. Biol.* **57,** 1195 (1990).

171. Giaccia, A., Weinstein, R., Hu, J., and Stamato, T. D.: *Somatic Cell. Mol. Genet.* **11,** 485 (1985).

172. Jostes, R. F., Bushnell, K. M., and Dewey, W. C.: *Radiat. Res.* **83,** 146 (1980).

173. van Holde, K. E.: "Chromatin". Springer-Verlag, New York, 1990.

174. Vaughan, A. T. M., Milner, A. M., Gordon, D. G., and Schwartz, J. L.: *Cancer Res.* **51,** 3857 (1991).

175. Olive, P. L., Hilton, J., and Durand, R. E.: *Radiat. Res.* **107,** 115 (1986).

176. Gordon, D. J., Milner, A. E., Beaney, R. P., Grdina, D. J., and Vaughan, A. T. M.: *Radiat. Res.* **121,** 174 (1990).

177. Kapiszewska, M., Wright, W. D., Lange, C. S., and Roti, J. L.: *Radiat. Res.* **119**, 569 (1989).
178. Schwartz, J. L., Shadley, J. D., Jaffe, D. R., Whitlock, J., Rotmensch, J., Cowan, J. M., Gordon, D. J., and Vaughan, A. T. M.: Association between Radiation Sensitivity, DNA Repair, and Chromosome Organization in the Chinese Hamster Ovary Cell Line xrs-5. *In* "Mutation and the Environment", Part A: Basic Mechanisms. (M. L. Mendelsohn and R. J. Albertini, eds.). Wiley-Liss, New York, 1990, p. 255.
179. Taylor, Y. C., Duncan, P. G., Zhang, X., and Wright, W. D.: *Mutat. Res.* **146**, 99 (1991).
180. Copeland, E. S.: *Photochem. Photobiol.* **28**, 839 (1978).
181. Livesey, J. C., and Reed, D. J.: *Adv. Radiat. Biol.* **13**, 285 (1987).
182. Brown, P. E.: *Nature* **213**, 363 (1967).
183. Lurie, A., Coghill, J., and Rippey, R. M.: *Radiat. Res.* **103**, 46 (1985).
184. Gatti, R. A. and Good, R. A.: *Cancer* **28**, 89 (1971).
185. McKhann, C. F.: *Transplantation* **8**, 209 (1969).
186. Borella, L. and Webster, R. G.: *Cancer Res.* **31**, 420 (1971).
187. Stewart, A. M., and Kneale, G. W.: *Cancer Immunol. Immunother.* **14**, 110 (1982).
188. North, R. J.: *J. Exp. Med.* **164**, 1652 (1986).
189. Patt, H. M., Tyree, E. B., Straube, R. L., and Smith, D. E.: *Science* **110**, 213 (1949).
190. Bacq, Z. M., Herve, A., Lecomte, J., Fischer, P., Blavier, J., Dechamps, G., LeBihan, H., and Rayet, P.: *Arch. Int. Physiol.* **59**, 442 (1951).
191. Meister, A.: *Science* **220**, 472 (1983).
192. Mitchell, J. B., and Russo, A.: *Cancer* (Suppl. VIII) **55**, 96 (1987).
193. Ward, J. F.: Chemical Aspects of Radioprotection. *In* "Radioprotectors and Anticarcinogens" (O. F. Nygaard and M. G. Simic, eds.). Academic Press, New York, 1983, p. 73.
194. Meechan, P. J., Vaughan, A. T. M., Giometti, C. S., and Grdina, D. J.: *Radiat. Res.* **125**, 152 (1991).
195. Eldjarn, L., and Pihl, A.: *J. Biol. Chem.* **223**, 341 (1956).
196. Purdie, J. W., Inhaber, E. R., Schneider, H., and Labelle, J. L.: *Int. J. Radiat. Biol.* **43**, 517 (1983).
197. Purdie, J. W.: *Radiat. Res.* **77**, 303 (1979).
198. Schwartz, J. L., Giovanazzi, S. M., Karrison, T., Jones, C., and Grdina, D. J.: *Radiat. Res.* **113**, 145 (1988).
199. Grdina, D. J., Nagy, B., Hill, C. K., Wells, R. L., and Peraino, C.: *Carcinogenesis* **6**, 929 (1985).
200. Grdina, D. J., Peraino, C., Carnes, B. A., and Hill, C. K.: *Cancer Res.* **45**, 5379 (1985).
201. Hill, C. K., Nagy, B., Peraino, C., and Grdina, D. J.: *Carcinogenesis* **7**, 665 (1988).
202. Milas, L., Hunter, N., Stephens, C. L., and Peters, L. J.: *Cancer Res.* **44**, 5567 (1984).
203. Sigdestad, C. P., Grdina, D. J., Connor, A. M., and Hanson, W. R.: *Radiat. Res.* **106**, 224 (1986).
204. Gupta, R., and Devi, P. U.: *Br. J. Cancer* **59**, 625 (1986).
205. Benova, D.: *Int. J. Radiat. Oncol. Biol. Phys.* **13**, 117 (1987).
206. Afzal, S. M. J., and Ainsworth, E. J.: *Radiat. Res.* **109**, 118 (1987).
207. Grdina, D. J., Carnes, B. A., Grahn, D., and Sigdestad, C. P.: *Cancer Res.* **51**, 4125 (1991).
208. Kataoka, Y., Basic, I., Perrin, J., and Grdina, D. J.: *Int. J. Radiat. Biol.* **61**, 387 (1992).
209. Sigdestad, C. P., Guilford, W., Perrin, J., and Grdina, D. J.: *Cell Tissue Kinet.* **21**, 193 (1988).
210. Holwitt, E. A., Koda, E., and Swenberg, C. E.: *Radiat. Res.* **124**, 107 (1990).
211. Scott, D. L., Kelleher, J., and Lobowsky, M. S.: *Biochim. Biophys. Acta* **497**, 218 (1977).
212. Borek, C., Ong, A., Mason, H., Donahue, L., and Biaglow, J. E.: *Proc. Natl. Acad. Sci. U.S.A.* **83**, 1490 (1986).
213. Orfanos, C. E., Ehlert, R., and Gollnick, H.: *Drugs* **34**, 459 (1987).
214. Harisidiadis, L., Miller, R. C., Hall, E. J., and Borek, C.: *Nature* **274**, 486 (1978).
215. Gensler, H., and Bowden, G. T.: *Cancer Lett.* **22**, 71 (1984).
216. Rutz, H. P., and Little, J. B.: *Carcinogenesis* **10**, 2183 (1989).
217. Troll, W., Frenkel, K., and Wiesner, R.: *J. Natl. Cancer Inst.* **6**, 1245 (1984).
218. Kennedy, A. R.: Prevention of Radiation - Induced Transformation *in Vitro*. *In* "Vitamins, Nutrition and Cancer" (H. Prasad, ed.). Karger, Basel, 1984, p. 166.
219. Kennedy, A. R., and Billings, P. C.: Anticarcinogenic Actions of Protease Inhibitors. *In* "Proc. 2nd Int. Conf. Anticarcinogens and Radiation Protection" (P. Cerutti, O. F. Nygaard, and M. Simic, eds.). Plenum Press, New York, 1987, p. 285.
220. DiPaolo, J. A., Evans, C. H., DeMarinis, A. J., and Doniger, J.: *Cancer Res.* **44**, 1465 (1984).
221. Patchen, M. L.: *Surv. Immunol. Res.* **2**, 237 (1983).
222. Alpen, E. L.: "Radiation Biophysics". Prentice-Hall, New Jersey, 1990.
223. Nori, D., Kim, J. H., Hilaris, B. S., and Chu, F.: *Cancer Invest.* **2**, 321 (1984).
224. Sawada, S., and Okada, S.: *Radiat Res.* **41**, 145 (1970).
225. Ragni, G., and Szybalski, W.: *J. Mol. Biol.* **4**, 338 (1962).
226. Ikegami, S., Taguchi, T., Ohashi, M., Oguro, M., Nagano, H., and Mano, Y.: *Nature* **275**, 458 (1978).

227. Snyder, R. D., van Houlen, B., and Regan, J. G.: "DNA Repair and Its Inhibition". IRL Press, Oxford, 1984, p. 13.

228. Berger, N. A., Kurohara, K. K., Petzold, S. J., and Sikorski, G. W.: *Biochem. Biophys. Res. Commun.* **89**, 218 (1979).

229. Moore, R. C., and Bender, M. A.: *Radiat. Res.* **110**, 385 (1987).

230. Iliakis, G., Pantelias, G., Okayasu, R., and Seaner, R.: *Int. J. Radiat. Oncol. Biol. Phys.* **16**, 1261 (1989).

231. Yoshida, S., Yamada, M., and Masaki, S.: *Biochim. Biophys. Acta* **477**, 144 (1977).

232. Ohno, Y., Spriggs, D., Ohno, A., and Kufe, D. W.: *Cancer Res.* **48**, 1494 (1988).

233. Moore, R. C., and Randall, C.: *Mutat. Res.* **178**, 73 (1987).

234. Virsik-Peuckert, R. P., and Harder, D.: *Int. J. Radiat. Biol.* **49**, 103 (1986).

235. Preston, R. J.: *Teratogen. Carcinogen. Mutagen.* **1**, 147 (1980).

236. Obe, G., and Natarajan, A. T.: *Mutat. Res.* **152**, 205 (1985).

237. Pantelias, G. E., and Wolff, S.: *Mutat. Res.* **151**, 65 (1985).

238. Gunji, H., Kharbanda, S., and Kufe, D.: *Cancer Res.* **51**, 741 (1991).

239. Ben-Hur, E., and Ben-Ishai, R.: *Photochem. Photobiol.* **13**, 337 (1971).

240. Cleaver, J. E.: *Radiat. Res.* **37**, 334 (1969).

241. Collins, A. R. S., Schor, S. L., and Johnson, R. T.: *Mutat. Res.* **42**, 413 (1977).

242. Djordjevic, B., and Tolmach, L. J.: *Radiat. Res.* **32**, 327 (1967).

243. Horikawa, M., Fukuhara, M., Suzuku, F., Nikaido, O., and Sugahara, T.: *Exp. Cell Res.* **70**, 349 (1972).

244. Prempree, T., and Merz, T.: *Nature* **244**, 603 (1969).

245. Wolff, S.: *Mutat. Res.* **15**, 435 (1972).

246. Clarkson, J. M.: *Mutat. Res.* **52**, 273 (1978).

247. Hunting, D. J., and Dresler, S. L.: *Carcinogenesis* **10**, 1525 (1985).

248. Diamond, A. M., Der, C. J., and Schwartz, J. L.: *Carcinogenesis* **10**, 383 (1989).

249. Borek, C., and Cleaver, J. E.: *Biochem. Biophys. Res. Commun.* **134**, 1334 (1986).

250. de Murcia, G., Huletsky, A., and Poirier, G. G.: *Biochem. Cell Biol.* **66**, 626 (1988).

251. Cardenas-Corona, M. E., Jacobson, E. J., and Jacobson, M. K.: *J. Biol. Chem.* **262**, 14863 (1987).

252. Shall, S.: *Adv. Radiat. Biol.* **11**, 1 (1983).

253. Boulikas, T.: *Toxicol. Lett.* **67**, 129 (1993).

254. Cleaver, J. E., and Morgan, W. F.: *Mutat. Res.* **257**, 1 (1991).

255. Roberts, J. J.: Mechanism of Potentiation by Caffeine of Genotoxic Damage Induced by Physical and Chemical Agents. *In* "DNA Repair and its Inhibition" (A. Collins, C. S. Downes, and R. Johnson, eds.). IRL Press, Oxford, 1984, p. 193.

256. Zwelling, L. A., and Kohn, K. W.: Platinum complexes. *In* "Pharmacological Principles in Cancer Treatment" (B. Chabner, ed.). Saunders, Philadelphia, 1982, p. 309.

257. Levi, V., Jacobson, E. L., and Jacobson, M. K.: *FEBS Lett.* **88**, 144 (1978).

258. Murnane, J. P., Byfield, J. E., Ward, J. F., and Calabro-Jones, P.: *Nature* **285**, 326 (1980).

259. Painter, R.: *J. Mol. Biol.* **143**, 289 (1980).

260. Lau, C. C., and Pardee, A. B.: *Proc. Natl. Acad. Sci. U.S.A.* **79**, 2942 (1982).

261. Stone, J. P., Holtzman, S., and Shellabarger, C. J.: *Cancer Res.* **40**, 3966 (1980).

262. Segaloff, S., and Maxfield, W. S.: *Cancer Res.* **31**, 166 (1971).

263. Shellabarger, C. J., Stone, J. P., and Holtzman, S.: *Cancer Res.* **36**, 1019 (1976).

264. Yokoro, K., and Furth, J.: *Proc. Soc. Exp. Biol. Med.* **107**, 921 (1961).

265. Weinstein, I. B.: *J. Environ. Pathol. Toxicol.* **3**, 89 (1980).

266. Williams, G. M.: *Fund. Appl. Tox.* **4**, 325 (1984).

267. Chen, F. U.: *Nucleic Acids Res.* **11**, 7231 (1983).

268. Van Duren, B. L., Wita, G., and Goldschmidt, B. M.: Structure-Activity Relationships of Tumor Promoters and Cocarcinogens and Interaction of Phorbol Myristate Acetate and Related Esters with Plasma Membranes. *In* "Mechanisms of Tumor Promotion and Cocarcinogenesis" (T. Slaga, A. Sivak, and R. K. Boutwell, eds.), Carcinogenesis – A Comprehensive Survey, Vol. 2. Raven Press, New York, 1978, p. 491.

269. Baturay, N., and Kennedy, A. R.: *Cell Biol. Toxicol.* **2**, 21 (1986).

270. Atcheson, M., Chu, C., Kakunaga, T., and Van Duuren, B. L.: *J. Natl. Cancer Inst.* **69**, 503 (1982).

271. Kennedy, A. R.: Promotion and Other Interactions Between Agents in the Induction of Transformation in vitro in Fibroblasts. *In* "Mechanisms of Tumor Promotion" Vol. III: Tumor Promotion and Carcinogenesis In Vitro (T. J. Slaga, ed.) CRC Press, Boca Raton, Florida, 1984, p. 13.

272. Metivier, H., Wahrendorf, J., and Masse, R.: *Br. J. Cancer* **50**, 215 (1984).

273. Farber, E.: *Am. J. Pathol.* **106**, 271 (1982).

274. Temple, L. A., Marks, S., and Blair, W. J.: *Int. J. Radiat. Biol.* **2**, 143 (1977).

275. Schmahl, W.: *Carcinogenesis* **9**, 1493 (1988).

276. Hoshino, H., Tanooka, H., and Fukuoka, F.: *Jpn. J. Cancer Res.* **59**, 43 (1968).

277. Nagano, T., Ho, M., and Yamada, S.: *Jpn. J. Cancer Res.* **63**, 143 (1972).
278. Flaks, A., Hamilton, J. M., Clayson, D. B., and Burch, P. R. J.: *Br. J. Cancer* **28**, 227 (1973).
279. Arseneau, J. C., Fowler, E., and Bakemeier, R. F.: *J. Natl. Cancer Inst.* **59**, 423 (1977).
280. Burkard, W., and Fritz-Niggli, H.: *Int. J. Radiat. Biol.* **51**, 1031 (1987).
281. Smith, P. J., and Anderson, C. O.: *Int. J. Radiat. Biol.* **46**, 331 (1984).

EDITORS' NOTE ADDED IN PROOF

For overviews on the topic, not covered in this chapter, of tumor induction by *ultraviolet radiation* and its combination effects with chemical carcinogens the reader is referred to the following sources:

1. IARC: "Solar and Ultraviolet Radiation". Monograph Vol. 55. Internat. Agency for Res. on Cancer (WHO), Lyon, France, 1992.
2. Urbach, F.: Cutaneous Photocarcinogenesis. *Environ. Carcino. Rev.* **C5**, 211–234 (1987).
3. Kripke, M. L., Pitcher, H., and Longstreth, J. D.: Potential Carcinogenic Impacts of Stratospheric Ozone Depletion. *Environ. Carcino. Rev.* **C7**, 53–74 (1989).
4. Passchier, W. F., and Bosnjakovic, B. F. M., eds.: "Human Exposure to Ultraviolet Radiation". Excerpta Medica, Amsterdam, 1987.
5. Parrish, J. A., Kripke, M. L., and Morison, W. L.: "Photoimmunology". Plenum Press, New York, 1983.
6. Kripke, M. L., and Sass, E. R., eds.: "Ultraviolet Carcinogenesis". DHEW Publication (NIH) 78-1532. National Cancer Institute, Bethesda, Maryland, 1978.
7. Fitzpatrick, T. B.: "Ultraviolet Carcinogenesis: Experimental, Global and Genetic Aspects". Univ. Tokyo Press, Tokyo, 1974.
8. Urbach, F., ed.: "The Biologic Effects of Ultraviolet Radiation". Pergamon, Oxford, 1969.
9. Blum, H. F.: "Carcinogenesis by Ultraviolet Light". Princeton Univ. Press, Princeton, New Jersey, 1959.

CHAPTER 14

Mechanisms of Viral Tumorigenesis and the Combination Effects of Viruses and Chemical Carcinogens*

Contents: **Introduction.** **Section I:** General Characteristics of Tumor Viruses. Viral and Cellular Oncogenes. Nonviral Oncogene Activators. **Section II:** Molecular Biology of Virally-Induced Cell Transformation and Tumorigenesis. **Section III:** Viral-Chemical Combination Effects in Tumorigenesis. **Speculative Closing Note.**

Introduction

Joseph C. Arcos

Cancer is a large group of diseases representing the outcome of highly diverse patterns of dysfunction of cellular homeostasis, as was discussed in some detail in Chapter 7 and the Prefatory Chapter. Crucial advances in the last three decades, that led to an explosively growing understanding of the induction of cancer in animals and humans, came from studies on tumor viruses. This is because through the discovery of oncogenes these studies opened an ever-expanding vista on the functioning of the genome and of the network of normal cellular regulatory pathways (including more recently the tumor-suppressor genes) which maintain normal cellular homeostasis. Hence, the significance of these studies far supersedes the scope of viral tumorigenesis proper as they will probably lead to the elucidation of the mechanisms of action of all types of carcinogenic agents.

Normal cellular genes—that code for the components of the regulatory pathways (receptors, signal transducer proteins, transcription and translation regulator proteins,

---

*Cellular genes and retroviral oncogenes are, in general, designated here in lowercase italics, whereas the terms for proteins named for their coding genes *begin* with a capital letter and are not italicized. However, terms for tumor-suppressor genes and transforming genes (in italics) of DNA tumor viruses and the respective proteins coded for (not italics) are, in general, all in capital letters. Growth factor terminology used here follows the recent convention that designates variants by capital letters and the respective receptors by Greek letters, *e.g.*, PDGF **A**, PDGF **B**, and PDGF α, PDGF β.

tumor-suppressor gene products) — as well as the regulatory proteins themselves that are expressed by these genes, may be targets of oncogenic effectors. Certain RNA tumor viruses may alter such cellular genes directly via *cis-* or *trans*-activation. These altered cellular genes (cellular oncogenes), in turn, produce inappropriately expressed or altered proteins that interfere with, subvert the functioning of components of the regulatory network. Alternatively, RNA tumor viruses may transduce certain normal cellular genes (proto-oncogenes) which, in their altered forms, become viral oncogenes. Once integrated into the infected cell's genome a retroviral oncogene will code for a mutated or overexpressed or inappropriately expressed analog of the protein product of the original normal cellular gene and, hence, will subvert its regulatory function. The genomes of most DNA tumor viruses, on the other hand, express genuine viral proteins which — while having no cellular sequence origin — may block, amplify, or bypass the functioning of the normal regulatory proteins of the infected cell. Again, alternatively, many nonviral tumorigenic agents (chemical carcinogens, radiations, etc.) may alter the above-mentioned normal cellular genes by mutation of either their protein-coding or gene-regulatory segments or both, or by bringing about dysregulation through the induction of gene translocation(s) to elsewhere in the chromosomes.

To lay the background for a perspective on syncarcinogenic interactions in combinations of viral and chemical agents (*in* Section III), the Chapter begins (*in* Sections I and II) with overviews on viral and nonviral oncogene activation, on some representative retroviral oncogenes and DNA tumor viruses, and on cellular targets of viral and nonviral effectors of oncogenic transformation (signal transduction cascades, transcription-regulatory proteins, and tumor-suppressor genes and their protein products).

General Characteristics of Tumor Viruses.
Viral and Cellular Oncogenes.
Nonviral Oncogene Activators[1]

Joseph C. Arcos, Lawrence R. Boone, and William C. Phelps *

The first evidence for the existence of a transmissible animal tumor virus is due to the discovery in 1911 by Peyton Rous, that a filterable agent from "Chicken Tumor No. 1" induced sarcomas in chickens. The original spontaneous tumor, a spindle cell sarcoma, was successively transplanted in Plymouth Rock chickens, the breed of the original host, and after many passages became transplantable to other breeds. Rous found that tumors with histological properties of the original tumor were rapidly induced at the site of inoculation by filtrates that passed through Berkefeld filter candles, which excludes tumor cells and bacteria. This finding prompted Rous to go on to study tumorigenesis by this new nonbacterial agent and isolate others (*rev. 1*).

Rous's original discovery clearly marks the birth of Tumor Virology, and provided considerable stimulus for the development of all other areas of virology. The tumor viruses recognized at present are a large and biologically diverse group belonging to seven distinct taxonomic families[2] (*rev. 2*). Tumor viruses include both RNA viruses and DNA viruses. The classification of tumor viruses is summarized in Table 1.

I. RNA TUMOR VIRUSES

RNA tumor viruses belong to the family of retroviruses (*Retroviridae*), characterized by the presence in the virus of RNA-dependent DNA-polymerase (reverse transcriptase).

---

*The three authors contributed equally to this section.
[1]The Abbreviations Used in this Section are given on p. 536.
[2]The International Committee on the Taxonomy of Viruses (ICTV) established in 1966 a universal system of virus taxonomy. The ICTV recognizes three hierarchical levels: *family* (in some cases *subfamily*), *genus,* and *species.* For example, the species Epstein-Barr virus is a member of the *Herpesviridae,* subfamily *Gammaherpesviridae,* genus *Lymphocryptovirus.* Taxonomic classification is based on: (a) the geometric properties of the virion, (b) properties of the genome, (c) properties of the viral proteins, (d) characteristics of the viral life cycle, (e) physicochemical properties, and (f) infectivity and other biological properties (3).

TABLE 1.   Currently Recognized Tumor Viruses[a]

Genome	Virus group	Representative viral species	Common host species	Type of tumors induced in *susceptible* host species
RNA	*Oncovirus*			
	Avian leukosis-sarcoma (ALSV) (resembles mammalian C-type)	Rous sarcoma virus (RSV) Avian myeloblastosis virus (AMV) Avian erythroblastosis virus (AEV) Rous-associated virus (RAV)	Chickens, pheasant	Leukemia-lymphoma-sarcoma diseases
	Mammalian C-type	Harvey murine sarcoma virus (HaMSV) Murine leukemia viruses •Moloney (Mo-MLV) •Abelson (A-MuLV) Feline leukemia virus (FeLV) Simian sarcoma virus (SSV) *Numerous* mammalian-type leukemia-sarcoma-inducing viruses	Rodents, reptiles, fish, birds, ox, cat, dog, primates	Leukemia-lymphoma-sarcoma diseases
	B-type	Mouse mammary tumor viruses (MMTV)	Mouse	Mammary adenocarcinoma
	D-type	Human T-cell leukemia viruses (HTLV I and II) Bovine leukemia virus (BLV)	Human, ox	T-cell lymphoma, B-cell lymphoma,
DNA	*Hepadnavirus*	Human hepatitis B virus (HBV) Woodchuck hepatitis virus (WHV) Duck hepatitis B virus (DHBV) Ground squirrel hepatitis virus (GSHV)	Human, woodchuck, duck, heron, squirrel	Hepatocellular carcinoma
	Papillomavirus (Papova A)	Bovine papillomaviruses (BVP) Shope papillomavirus (SV) [also known as cottontail rabbit papillomavirus (CRPV)] Canine papillomaviruses Equine papillomaviruses Human papillomaviruses (HPV)	Ox, rabbit, dog, horse, sheep, elk, deer, primates, human	Benign papilloma, squamous cell carcinoma
	Polyomavirus (Papova B)	Polyomavirus Hamster papovavirus (HapV) Simian vacuolating virus 40 (SV40) Lymphotropic papovavirus (LPV) BKV JCV	Rodents, birds, hamster, primates, human	Unknown[b] (but highly transforming in cultures)
	Adenovirus	Human adenovirus (Ad) (at least 37 types) Ovine adenovirus	Human, sheep	Adenoma/unknown

TABLE 1. *(Continued)*

Genome	Virus group	Representative viral species	Common host species	Type of tumors induced in *susceptible* host species
DNA (cont.)	Herpesvirus (about 100 species, classified into three subfamilies: alpha, beta, and gamma)	Baboon herpesvirus Chimpanzee herpesvirus Squirrel monkey virus Marek's disease (avian) Turkey herpesvirus Human herpesvirus 6 (HHV-6) Epstein-Barr virus (EBV) Herpes simplex virus (HSV) (?)[c] Cytomegalovirus (?)[c]	Chicken, turkey, squirrel monkey, primates, human	Lymphosarcoma, leukemia, lymphoma, Burkitt's lymphoma, nasopharyngeal carcinoma
	Poxvirus	Shope fibromavirus (rabbit) Yaba virus Molluscum contagiosum	Rabbit, squirrel, primates, human	Fibroma, benign histiocytoma, benign molluscum bodies

[a]Compilation based primarily on data abstracted from B.N. Fields, D.M. Knipe, R.M. Chanock, M.S. Hirsch, J.L. Melnick, T.P. Monath, and B. Roizman, eds.: ["Virology", 2nd ed. Raven Press, New York, 1990].

[b]Induced in *newborn* mice a wide range of tumors including osteosarcomas [S.E. Stewart, B.E. Eddy, M. Irwin, and S. Lee: *Nature* **186,** 615 (1960)] and in *3-week-old* Syrian hamsters lymphocytic leukemia, lymphosarcomas, reticulum cell sarcomas, and osteosarcomas [G.T. Diamandopoulos: *J. Natl. Cancer Inst.* **50,** 1347 (1973)].

[b]Causal association with tumor induction has not been firmly established.

The life cycle of retroviruses is simple. Once the virus core has entered the cell, the reverse transcriptase transcribes the single-stranded RNA viral genome into double-stranded DNA copies. The original viral RNA becomes degraded and the viral DNA copy becomes integrated into the host genome (provirus). The virus then may proceed to the subsequent two stages of its life cycle: (i) transcription of the provirus to yield viral mRNA (some of which is spliced) for coding of the viral proteins [the Gag/Pro proteins (matrix, capsid, nucleocapsid, and protease), the Pol proteins (reverse transcriptase and integrase), and the envelope proteins] and genomic RNA used in assembling the daughter virions; (ii) viral protein synthesis coded by the mRNA portion and assembly of the daughter virions; assembly includes the establishment of the diploid RNA core (two genomic RNA copies, linked by noncovalent bonds, primarily hydrogen bonds near the 5' end, for each virion) (4, 5). Figure 1 shows a highly schematized representation of the internal organization of a retroviral virion.

Now, at some point during their life cycles some retroviruses have accidentally acquired (*transduced*) from their host's genome an *initially* normal sequence (which may have been adjacent to the site of integration of the viral DNA). The *original* normal cellular function of such a host gene sequence (proto-oncogene or c-*onc*) detected in these viruses is to code for a protein with some key regulatory, structural, or differentiation function (such as a receptor, protein kinase, GTP-binding GTPase, nuclear gene regulatory protein, growth factor, membrane protein) (*e.g.,* 4, 6–11a). However, in the process of transduction most original proto-oncogenes become altered (by point mutations, insertions, deletions, or by becoming truncated) and their expression is now initiated

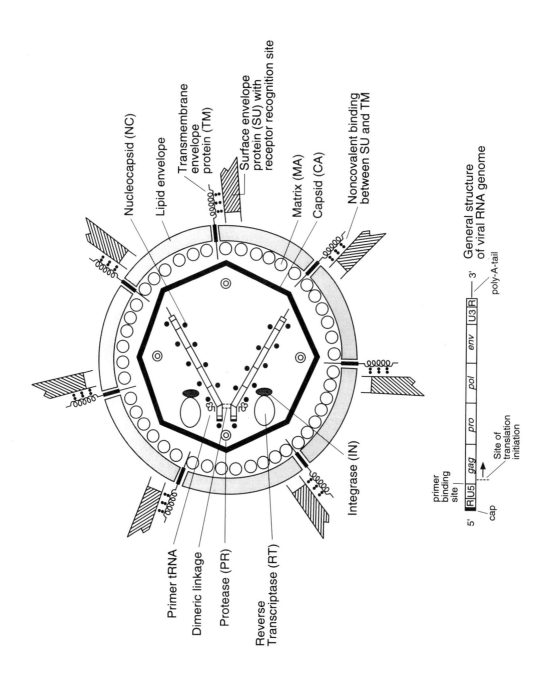

Nucleocapsid (NC)

Lipid envelope

Transmembrane
envelope
protein (TM)

Surface envelope
protein (SU) with
receptor recognition site

Matrix (MA)

Capsid (CA)

Noncovalent binding
between SU and TM

Integrase (IN)

Primer tRNA

Dimeric linkage

Protease (PR)

Reverse
Transcriptase (RT)

General structure
of viral RNA genome

poly-A-tail

Site of
translation
initiation

primer
binding
site

5'   R U5   gag   pro   pol   env   U3 R   3'

cap

514

FIGURE 1. General scheme of the structural organization of a retroviral virion. The two units of the RNA genome are linked together by secondary valence forces, primarily hydrogen bonds, near the 5′ end. The size of the RNA genome unit varies between 3.5 and 9.0 kb in different retroviruses. Each unit of the dimeric RNA core carries with it a tRNA primer which is specific for a retrovirus group. Also packaged within the capsid are: the reverse transcriptase (RT); the integrase (IN), which has the function of integrating the proviral DNA into the host genome; nucleocapsid (NC), which is/are nucleic-acid-binding protein(s) providing structural stability to the genomic core within the capsid; and a protease (PR), which has the functional role of proteolytically cleaving the Gag and Gag-Pro-Pol precursor polyproteins. The matrix serves as a packaging intermediary between the capsid and the lipid envelope and envelope proteins. The surface envelope protein (SU) knobs and the transmembrane protein (TM) helixes schematize the key functional roles of the two envelope glycoproteins (*see* below) in viral infectivity. The solid cylinder within the backbone of TM represents the membrane-spanning helix. Under the structural scheme is shown the distribution of the typical retroviral genomic sequences. At the 5′ end a small polynucleotide segment known as the "capping group" has the sequence of $m7G5′ppp5′G_mp$; at the 3′ end there is a chain of about 200 adenylate residues, sometimes referred to as the "poly-A tail". Most cellular mRNAs contain a cap structure and a poly-A tail. Adjacent to the capping group and the poly-A tail there are important regulatory signal sequences, RU5 and U3R, respectively. These sequences are usually noncoding for protein synthesis but provide different regulatory signals for RNA and DNA synthesis and processing. The long terminal repeat (LTR) at each end of the DNA provirus is composed of a duplication and rearrangement of the U5 and U3 sequences through a complex process mediated by template strand-switching during reverse transcription. Through this mechanism the transcription promoter element, which lies upstream of the RNA start site and thus not copied into RNA, is regenerated from a downstream copy (U3) and returned to its functional position outside of the transcriptional unit. Usually, but not in all types of viruses, the internal regions of the genome have exclusively protein coding functions. The *gag* gene expresses a polyprotein that is cleaved to a matrix protein (MA), a capsid protein (CA), and the NC protein(s). Thus, *gag* determines the group-specific antigenicity of the virus. The *pro* gene codes for the PR enzyme, the proteolytic processing function of which was mentioned above. The *pol* gene codes for a polyprotein yielding two proteins, the RT and the IN. The *env* gene codes for the two glycoprotein components of the viral envelope: the larger SU protein which includes a recognition site for cell surface receptors and the TM protein; thus, by coding for SU, the *env* gene determines the host range of a virus. The TM protein is responsible for fusing the viral envelope to the cell surface once recognition has been made. This fusion is accomplished at one or two viral sites through the TM's hydrophobic amino acid sequence (fusogenic moiety) on the viral surface. In the free, unattached virus the fusogenic moiety of TM (represented by the helical motifs) is masked by its binding to SU. The nature of binding between TM and SU is different for various viruses; noncovalent bonds and disulfide linkage (*e.g.,* in Rous sarcoma virus) may be involved. Upon cell surface recognition SU undergoes an allosteric transition and unmasks the reactive fusogenic moiety of TM. Beyond the extracellularly fixed fate of the viral envelope proteins, little is known about the stepwise details of retroviral uncoating and penetration into the cell. It is not unreasonable to suppose that fusion to the cell membrane initiates a transenvelope signal propagated by allosteric changes through the TM protein, actuating extravasation of the capsid into the cytoplasm. The RT, IN, PR, and NC proteins (and possibly capsid components) remain together with the genome during penetration.

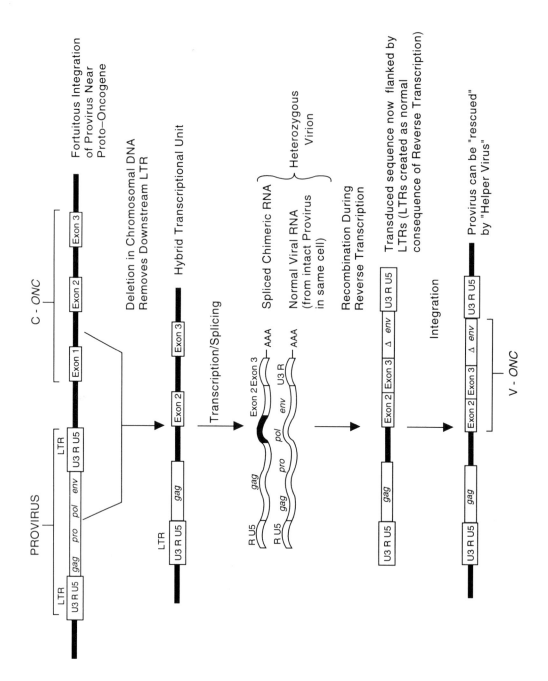

FIGURE 2.   Schematic representation of the transduction of a host proto-oncogene (c-*onc*) into the viral genome. Integration of viral DNA (produced by reverse transcription of virion RNA early after infection) into the host chromosome to form a provirus is a required step in the replication of all retroviruses. The chance integration near a c-*onc* gene is likely to be the first step in the transduction process. Although other mechanisms can be envisioned, a deletion removing the downstream LTR and possibly some portion of the c-*onc* gene allows for RNA transcription initiated in the viral LTR to proceed into the cellular gene before termination. Polyadenylation and splicing create a functional mRNA and also an RNA capable of being packaged into a virion, if the *cis*-acting packaging signals near the 5' end of *gag* are included. Incorporation into a virion also depends on the presence of a normal, undeleted provirus elsewhere in the cell, or on reinfection at a later time to produce a functional provirus. The normal provirus provides the virion proteins required for packaging, in *trans* to the chimeric RNA. Furthermore, heterozygous virions can be produced that contain the normal viral RNA and the viral/cellular chimeric RNA. The chimeric RNA , at this point in the scheme, cannot serve, *singly,* as a template for reverse transcription into an integration-competent viral DNA. However, the chimeric RNA can serve as a co-template for DNA synthesis by reverse transcriptase, by participating in a template-strand-switching mechanism of recombination (not shown) involving normal viral RNA transcribed from intact provirus in the same cell. Thus, it can become incorporated into an integration-competent structure with two LTRs. In the vast majority of cases some viral sequences of the normal viral RNA will be lost; thus, the integrated provirus will be defective for replication but not defective for expression. Expression of the transduced c-*onc* gene leads to transformation of the target cell. A helper virus is required for replication of the transforming gene (now termed v-*onc*)-containing retrovirus. The convention Δ (as in Δ*env*) indicates an incomplete sequence.

from the retroviral LTR[3] (10, 11a). Such an acquired but mutated gene, which originated from a host, is a retroviral oncogene or v-*onc*. The v-*onc* genes contain no noncoding intron spacer sequences, so they resemble more the processed RNA form rather than the genomic form of the respective original c-*onc* genes. Oncogene-carrying retroviruses are known as *transducing retroviruses*. A large number of transducing retroviruses carrying a variety of oncogenes have been identified (*rev.* 2, 4, 10, 11a). Illustrative examples of retroviral oncogenes are given in Table 2.

There is probably more than one mechanism operative in the transduction of a proto-oncogene sequence (*rev.* 2, 4, 10, 11a). A model based on the one of Swanstrom *et al.* (11b), that is consistent with most of the features of transduced oncogenes, involves an RNA intermediate and recombination during the reverse transcription process. This model is schematically illustrated in Figure 2. Integration of a provirus near a c-*onc* locus and a subsequent deletion including the downstream LTR can bring the c-*onc* gene, or a portion of it, under the control of the strong retroviral promoter sequence. Such an arrangement as a *cis*-acting mechanism could lead to transformation, as discussed elsewhere in this chapter. However, if the cell was producing virions expressed from a normal provirus integrated elsewhere in the same cell or later became infected with another normal retrovirus, then the scene would be set for creating a recombinant virus in which the oncogene becomes stably transduced. Since retroviruses package two copies

---

[3]The *l*ong *t*erminal *r*epeat (LTR) present at each end of the DNA proviral form provides noncoding regulatory signals for the viral life cycle. LTR is composed of U3, R, and U5 sequences. U3 contains about 170 to 1260 nucleotides, R (for "redundant") 20 to 80 nucleotides, and U5 about 70 to 100 nucleotides. In the RNA viral form the U3 sequence is present only at the 3' end (*i.e.,* as a *U*nique 3' sequence) and the U5 sequence is present only at the 5' end (*i.e.,* as a *U*nique 5' sequence) (Fig. 1). The binding site for the tRNA primer is adjacent to U5; it is from this site that reverse transcription of DNA is initiated. A small sequence of about 9 to 15 purine moieties (polypurine tract, PPT) between U3 and *env* provides initiation for the synthesis of the complementary DNA strand.

TABLE 2.   Some Examples of Known Retroviral Oncogenes

Oncogene	Typical viral vector	Host species of origin	Biochemical function displayed by oncoprotein	Tumor induced
abl	Abelson leukemia virus (Ab-MLV)	Mouse	Protein tyrosine kinase	Lymphoid leukemia
erb-A	Avian erythroblastosis virus (AEV)	Chicken	Thyroid hormone receptor	Erythroleukemia
erb-B	Avian erythroblastosis virus (AEV)	Chicken	EGF receptor tyrosine kinase	Sarcoma
ets	E26 avian erythroblastosis virus	Chicken	Gene regulatory protein	Myeloid leukemia
fes	Snyder-Theilen feline sarcoma virus (St-FeSV)	Cat	Protein tyrosine kinase	Sarcoma
fps (homol. to *fes*)	Fujinami sarcoma virus	Chicken	Protein tyrosine kinase	Sarcoma
fgr	Gardner-Rasheed feline sarcoma virus	Cat	Protein tyrosine kinase	Sarcoma
fms	Susan McDonough feline sarcoma virus	Cat	Macrophage CSF receptor tyrosine kinase	Sarcoma
fos	FBJ osteosarcoma virus	Mouse	Component of AP-1 gene regulatory protein (together with *jun* prod.)	Osteosarcoma
jun	Avian sarcoma virus 17	Chicken	Component of AP-1 gene regulatory protein (together with *fos* prod.)	Fibrosarcoma
kit	Hardy-Zuckerman-4 feline sarcoma virus (Hz-fsv)	Cat	Steel factor receptor protein tyrosine kinase	Sarcoma
mos	Moloney sarcoma virus (Mo-MSV)	Mouse	Protein serine/threonine kinase	Sarcoma
myb	E26 avian myeloblastosis virus	Avian	Gene regulatory protein	Myeloid leukemia
myc	Myleocytomatosis virus 29 (MC29)	Chicken	Gene regulatory protein of the HLH type	Sarcoma/leukemia
raf	3611 Murine sarcoma virus (MSV-3611)	Mouse	Protein serine/threonine kinase	Sarcoma
raf	Mill-Hill 2 virus (MH2 virus)	Chicken	Protein serine/threonine kinase	Sarcoma
H-*ras*	Harvey murine sarcoma virus (Ha-MSV)	Mouse/rat	GTP-binding GTPase	Sarcoma
K-*ras*	Kirsten murine sarcoma virus (Ki-MSV)	Mouse/rat	GTP-binding GTPase	Sarcoma

TABLE 2. *(Continued)*

Oncogene	Typical viral vector	Host species of origin	Biochemical function displayed by oncoprotein	Tumor induced
rel	Reticuloendothelial virus, strain T	Turkey	Regulatory protein to the NFkB binding site on DNA	Reticuloendotheliosis
sis	Simian sarcoma virus (SSV)	Woolly monkey	PDGF B-chain	Sarcoma
sis	Parodi-Irgens feline sarcoma virus (Pi-FeSV)	Cat	PDGF B-chain	Sarcoma
ski	SKV 770 virus	Chicken	Gene regulatory protein	Sarcoma
src	Rous sarcoma virus (RSV)	Chicken	Protein tyrosine kinase	Sarcoma

of the RNA genome per virion (Figure 1), the chimeric RNA transcript that contains viral sequences together with cellular sequences can be copackaged along with a normal viral RNA transcript to yield a heterozygous virion. According to the model (11b), the two units of the diploid RNA core participate in serving *jointly* as template for reverse transcription into a single viral DNA. This is because the reverse transcriptase can switch back and forth between the two templates (which is known to occur at high frequency) and synthesize a viral DNA that contains sequences from each RNA genome. Thus, when a provirus is formed from a heterozygous virion it can be a recombinant in which the cellular sequences are now embedded within the viral DNA genome. This is usually at the expense of some genuine viral genes and the provirus is thus replication defective. The transformed cell — in which the transduced mutated cellular sequences, now part of the host's genome, are continually expressed — is, therefore, a "nonproducer" with respect to viral replication unless and until it becomes coinfected with a replication competent "helper virus". Although the replication- defective transforming virus does not replicate as a virus in the absence of a "helper", it is nevertheless perpetuated as part of the genome of the transformed cell. More dramatic, however, is the amplification and virus spread that occurs with the rescue of the transforming genome by "helper virus". In a manner similar to the above description of the original transduction event, when the nonproducer cells become infected with a replication-competent helper virus, they become "producers" of virions that contain the transforming virus genome (either heterozygous or homozygous) along with more helper virus. Virions containing replication-defective v-*onc* genomes are infectious and efficiently transform cells, but always require co-infection with helper virus to produce more infectious virus particles. Transforming retroviruses isolated from tumors are thus usually a mixture of replication-competent helper and replication-defective transforming virus. For this reason cell transformation represents a selective advantage for an oncogene embedded in a replication-defective virus, because the provirus can be rescued and amplified by a helper virus. Although the integration of an oncogene into a retrovirus is a rare event, it has been occasionally observed experimentally (12). Presumably cellular genes other than oncogenes can be transduced by retroviruses, but, without this selective advantage the virus containing them will be lost. [It is noteworthy that the utility of retroviruses as vectors for gene therapy is based precisely on this feature, that any gene inserted into the viral genome and replacing some viral sequence will be integrated and expressed as part of a provirus in the absence of further replication.]

The gene loss in a chimeric RNA transcript is probably consistent with the space limitation when this transcript and the normal viral RNA transcript are co-packaged into the capsid during viral assembly. The gene loss in a chimeric RNA can entail most of the viral genome, since the normal viral RNA transcript can provide the *gag, pro, pol,* and *env* functions for synthesis of the recombinant viral DNA. Ultimately, all that is required for a replication-defective virus to be "viable" is that the totality of viral sequences and the acquired host gene—which are co-packaged into the capsid as a unit—have enough functional features to yield a provirus which, although replication defective, can be rescued by a "helper virus". Thus, a "minimal" chimeric RNA must have the 5′ and 3′ end sequences to provide essential replication regulatory signals (*see* Legend to Figure 1), including sequences at the 5′ end to provide initiation (primer binding) site for proviral DNA synthesis, as well as a packaging signal (Psi) for viral assembly (*cf.* 2, 4). In fact, a retrovirus may accommodate two independent oncogenes; examples for this are the AEV strain ES4 which carries an *erb*-A and an *erb*-B oncogene and the Mill-Hill 2 (MH2) avian sarcoma virus which carries a *raf* and a *myc* oncogene. Consistent with their highly flexible functional features are the generally high mutation rates of the retroviruses.

When a viral oncogene is expressed it is generally transcribed together with a segment of the viral *gag* gene (coding for the polyprotein precursor of the capsid) or with a segment of the *env* gene (coding for viral envelope glycoprotein) to yield a "fusion protein"[4]. This depends on where the oncogene was incorporated, more toward the 5′ end or more toward the 3′ end. For example, the Susan McDonough feline sarcoma virus' (SM-FeSV) provirus will express a Gag-v-Fms fusion protein, whereas the Moloney murine sarcoma provirus will express an Env-v-Mos fusion protein. These genuine viral protein/v-Onc viral fusion proteins are *transforming oncoproteins*. Transforming, because the v-Onc moieties of the fusion proteins—owing to their close similarity to but nonidentity with various cellular regulatory proteins, receptors, growth factors, etc., to which they bear some degree of sequence homology—represent abnormal stimuli or can create abnormal bypass channels. Thus, they bring about drastic perturbations in the pathways of intracellular signal transduction and intercellular communication that govern the control of growth and of normal phenotypic behavior. For example, such cells are no longer able to regulate exit from the cell cycle and undergo differentiation. Hence, these fusion proteins induce cell transformation *in vitro* or tumorigenesis *in vivo*. Transducing retroviruses are the most rapidly acting carcinogens known. The surprisingly short latency period (days) with which transducing retroviruses can bring about cell transformation (2) is probably related to the fact that among the different types of tumor viruses they are the only ones to introduce into the cell machinery "ready-made" altered templates which originated from and have a high sequence homology to normal host genes. These altered templates have, therefore, a very high specificity for reorienting the network of normal cellular homeostasis; they represent "subversion of growth regulatory pathways" (13). Also, consistent with the molecular similarity of the virally-encoded oncoproteins with some components of the cellular regulatory network is the generally very low cytotoxicity of transducing retroviruses.

It is precisely the homology of the sequences of the acquired, but now viral genes with genes in normal cellular genomes that led to the realization of the cellular origin of the former. This was first noted with the *src* gene of the Rous sarcoma virus. Other examples are the Sis oncoprotein of the simian sarcoma virus (SSV), which has an about 88%

---

[4]A common convention is to include all components of the fusion protein produced by a given virus in its designation (*e.g.,* Gag-Myc, Gag-Pol-Myc). In most cases, the segment expressed by genuine viral gene(s) is incomplete. Often a capital delta (Δ) adjacent to the incomplete protein is used to denote incompleteness. (*e.g.,* ΔGAG-Myc, GAG-ΔPol-Myc). This convention is not used in this chapter. The completeness and functionality of gene products of any remaining viral genes in replication-defective transforming retroviruses is highly variable. Selective pressure is on the expression of the transforming gene and not the genuine viral genes, since all gene products required for replication can be provided by helper virus.

sequence identity with the B-chain of the human platelet-derived growth factor (PDGF), the Erb-A protein which is homologous with the thyroid hormone receptor, and the Erb-B protein which is homologous with the epidermal growth factor receptor (2, 4, 10, 11a).

There are several retroviruses which do not carry a v-*onc,* and yet are capable of inducing tumors in animals (although not *in vitro* cell transformation). The mechanism of tumorigenesis by these retroviruses involves the alteration of cellular proto-oncogenes into activated cellular oncogenes by the insertion of viral sequences in the immediate vicinity or even within proto-oncogene sequences (*insertional mutagenesis*). These viruses are known as *cis*-activating retroviruses (2, 4, 11a). Examples for *cis*-activating retroviruses are the two Rous-associated virus strains (RAV-1 and RAV-2) which are avian viruses, the mouse mammary tumor virus (MMTV), and the spleen focus-forming virus (SSFV) which is one of the two components of Friend murine leukemia infective virus stock.

Regarding the nature of *cis*-activation, it should be noted that actual sequence alteration(s), mutation, of the gene region coding for protein sequence is not essential for a proto-oncogene to bring about cell transformation. Because of the finely-tuned structural interlinkages between various signal transduction pathways, between receptors and signal transduction pathways, and between signal transduction pathways and gene regulatory proteins, any excess or ill-timed production of a protein with some regulatory function—such as receptor, cytoplasmic signal transduction intermediary, or growth factor—can bring about cell transformation (*cf.* 13). Insertion of the provirus close to a host gene (or insertion adjacent to the host gene and fusing it to the viral sequences) brings the host gene under the control of the viral enhancer and this leads to excess production (or hyperactivity). This is the basis for cell transformation by overexpression[5] of a proto-oncogene (15). In some cases viral insertion can lead to secondary mutations in the proto-oncogene (4).

The third type of mechanism whereby retroviruses can induce cell transformation is *trans*-activation. *Trans*-activating retroviruses do not carry a v-*onc* either. However, *trans*-activating retroviruses contain sequences that express nonstructural regulatory protein(s) which enhance transcription by the viral LTR. These viral proteins also bring about overexpression[5] of certain cellular genes and induce thereby cell transformation. This mechanism of *trans*-activation by certain retroviruses is similar to the mechanism of action of those DNA viruses that transform via genuine viral oncoproteins (papillomaviruses, polyomaviruses, adenoviruses, and herpesviruses); *see* below in "II. DNA Tumor Viruses." An example of *trans*-activating retroviruses is the human T-cell leukemia virus I (HTLV-I). The latency period for malignant transformation is much longer for *cis*-activating retroviruses (weeks/months) and *trans*-activating retroviruses (months/years) than for the very rapidly acting transducing retroviruses (days), as we have seen above.

Taxonomically, retroviruses are subdivided into three subfamilies: oncoviruses, lentiviruses, and spumaviruses. Only the oncoviruses (also known as oncornaviruses)— the largest subfamily—are tumor viruses. Following a classification, initiated by Bernhard in 1960 (16), retroviruses are further described as type ALSV (avian leukosis–sarcoma virus), and types B, C, and D. Classification is based on: virion shape and morphology, endogenous or exogenous transmission, host range, presence or absence of an oncogene, and aspects of pathogenicity. The mammalian type-C virus group includes the largest number of exogenous and endogenous RNA tumor viruses that have been identified.

---

[5]That overexpression alone of a proto-oncogene can lead to cell transformation is well established for *myc* and holds probably for all nuclear oncogenes. However, expression of the Src protein (a plasma membrane localized oncoprotein) was reported not to induce transformation in NIH 3T3 cells (14).

TABLE 3.   Brief Synopsis of DNA Tumor Virus Transforming Oncoproteins

Virus group (typical representative)	
Hepadnaviruses (HBV)	There are no experimental data on the existence of any dominant viral oncogene, although the X-gene has been suspected to play a role in some instances. X-transformed NIH 3T3 cells are tumorigenic in nude mice. Hepatitis B virus, the typical representative of this group, may act by insertional activation of *myc* genes, by chromosomal aberrations produced at viral integration sites, by an indirect mechanism involving chronic inflammation of the liver, fibrosis, and consequent mitogenic stimulation of hepatocyte regeneration, or by a combination of these mechanisms.
Papillomaviruses (BPV, HPV)	Genes encoding "early" proteins (*i.e.,* proteins expressed in the early part of the viral life cycle) are designated *E1* to *E8*. These proteins have the capability to immortalize and transform different cell lines. Some of them can complement the transforming capability of adeno- and polyomaviruses. The most extensively studied were the BPV-1 E5 protein (44 amino acids, 6–7 kDa; the smallest transforming protein known), BPV-1 E6 (127 amino acids, 15.5 kDa), and HPV E7 (98 amino acids).
Polyomaviruses (Polyomavirus, SV40)	Oncogenes and oncoproteins of polyomaviruses have been characterized probably in the greatest detail among the transforming genes and their products of all DNA viruses. The transforming proteins encoded by their oncogenes are designated as T (for tumor) antigens. Polyomavirus encodes three T antigens: large-T (100 kDa), middle-T (55 kDa), and small-T (22 kDa). The SV40 encodes a large-T (94 kDa) and a small-T (17 kDa). The 421 amino acid middle-T antigen is an effective agent which can transform, alone, established cell lines. It is a multifunctional protein which interacts with two key enzymes of the signal transduction network: the Src tyrosine protein kinase and PI 3-kinase.
Adenoviruses (Human, many types; and types specific to various animal species)	Proteins coded by two regions of the adenovirus genome, *E1A* and *E1B*, were shown to be involved in Ad-induced cell transformation. Protein expressed by the *E1A* region can bring about, alone, the transformation of established but not primary cell lines (in the absence of *E1B*). *E1B* can also bring about transformation, but its expression is under the control of the product of the *E1A* gene. The *E1A* region encodes two closely related proteins, of 243 (26 kDa) and 289 (32 kDa) amino acid size; the two proteins differ only in a segment of 46 amino acids, specific to the 289 amino acid protein. The *E1B* region encodes a 179 amino acid protein (19 kDa) and a 495 amino acid protein (55 kDa). Of these, only the 19 kDa protein is essential for cell transformation.
Herpesviruses (EBV)	Various proteins expressed by EBV may play different roles in cell transformation. These are latent infection proteins: EBNA-1 and EBNA-2, EBNA-3A, -3B, and -3C, and EBNA-LP, the lipoprotein membrane (LMP) proteins, and EBER proteins. EBNA-1 is a 641 amino acid (76 kDa) protein, whereas EBNA-2 consists of 443 amino acids. The *EBNA-3* genes encode three closely related 900 to 1,000 amino acid proteins. EBNA-3 proteins, which are highly hydrophilic, as well as EBNA-LP accumulate in the nucleus of the infected cells.
Poxviruses (SFV)	There is no evidence of integration of viral DNA into the infected cell's genome. Many poxviruses produce hyperplastic responses. A 19 kDa gene product of vaccinia virus has a region analogous to a site in EGF and TGFα, which possibly provides a mechanism for the hyperplastic response. An expressed protein, VGF (vaccinia growth factor), binds to the EGF receptor and induces its autophosphorlation as well as brings about anchorage-independent growth.

II. DNA TUMOR VIRUSES

Unlike the oncogenes of retroviruses which are accidental acquisitions from and show sequence homology with host genomes, the sequences of DNA viral genomes have no cellular counterpart in any host genomes. As we have seen, retroviral oncogenes, consistent with their accidental presence in a virus, play no role in the viral life cycle. On the other hand, the recognized oncogenes of DNA viruses are genuine viral genes and perform essential functions in the viral life cycle.

The interaction of a DNA tumor virus with its target cell can result in a "productive" infection, in which the virus completes its life cycle, produces progeny virus, and often kills the cell; retroviruses, in contrast, have usually no cytocidal effect as mentioned above. Infection with a DNA virus can also be "nonproductive", in which case the virus produces no progeny but transforms the cell, becomes integrated into the host genome, and continues to express gene function thereby maintaining the transformed state. Once inserted, a tumor virus can become latent, and for RNA viruses this is the basis of the transgenerational genetic permanence of the viral genome, if established in germ cells (2, 15).

With the apparent exception of the hepadnaviruses and poxviruses, the transformation of target cells by the other DNA tumor viruses is mediated by various transforming proteins coded for by viral genes; these will be discussed in some detail in Section II of this chapter. The role of these proteins in cell transformation and their respective intracellular molecular targets vary from virus to virus and from host species to host species. But, as already mentioned, the transforming proteins of DNA tumor viruses play a necessary functional role in the early part of the respective viral life cycles (as well as in cell transformation). No gene coding for any transforming protein has been identified in hepadnaviruses and poxviruses, and the exact molecular mediator or mechanism of their tumorigenic action is not known.

DNA tumor virus oncoproteins are generally multifunctional and this underlies their ability to act pleiotropically and bring about the multiplicity of changes that accompany cell transformation (2, 11a, *cf.* 13). This multifunctionality, multivalent specificity resides in the fact that they contain several structural domains which can act independently as well as cooperatively, depending on the cell compartment and the cellular proteins with which they form complexes (2). Two types of interactions are relevant to cell transformation, those that activate proto-oncogene products and those that inactivate tumor-suppressor gene products. A brief synopsis of transforming oncoproteins of DNA tumor viruses is given in Table 3.

The formal taxonomic terms for the six major families of DNA tumor viruses derive from the vernacular names: hepadnaviruses, polyomaviruses, papillomaviruses, adenoviruses, herpesviruses, and poxviruses, by affixing the suffix *-viridae,* such as *Hepadnaviridae* and *Polyomaviridae*. The sequence of the above listing parallels the sequence of the magnitude of the viral genomes: 2, 3, 5, 20, 90, and 120 in 10^6 dalton units of molecular weight, respectively (17, 18). The hepadnaviruses are among the smallest and the poxviruses are the largest of all animal viruses. The polyomaviruses and papillomaviruses have been grouped together, historically, to form the *Papovaviridae* family (from the contraction of rabbit *pa*pillomavirus, mouse *po*lyomavirus, and simian *va*cuolating virus); papillomaviruses are A-type and polyomaviruses are B-type papovaviruses. Some viral species representative of the DNA tumor virus families, their hosts, and the tumors induced are shown in Table 1.

III. VARIETIES OF NONVIRAL ONCOGENE ACTIVATORS

Under "I. RNA Tumor Viruses" and "II. DNA Tumor Viruses" it was briefly discussed that cell transformation and tumorigenesis by transducing retroviruses and by most DNA tumor viruses are mediated by various oncoproteins. Transducing retrovirus oncoproteins are coded by initially-nonviral acquired host genes alien to the virus, whereas DNA tumor virus oncoproteins are coded by genuine viral genes which have essential functions in the viral life cycle and have no counterpart in the host genome. It is important to bear in mind at this point that these two categories of oncogenes are *exogenous* to a cell being infected and are imported by the virus. Oncogenes may also be generated, however, from proto-oncogenes in the cell, *in situ*. The transforming capability of such *cellular oncogenes* (mutated, overexpressed, or amplified) is ascertained by the transfection assay (usually in NIH 3T3 cells) and by tumorigenicity tested most often in thymus-deficient "nude" mice (BALB/c *nu/nu*).

In "I. RNA Tumor Viruses" above we have already mentioned the *in situ* activation of proto-oncogenes by the insertion in its vicinity of *cis*-activating retroviruses, which are not oncogene carriers. However, beyond insertion mutagenesis a proto-oncogene may also be altered/enhanced by other mutagenic events caused by chemical carcinogens, radiations, as well as by spontaneous chromosome translocations, excess chromosomes acquired in faulty meiosis, and by some special circumstances of cellular stress discussed under D. below. Agent-induced mutagenic events may be: point-mutation and/or deletion(s) in the protein coding sequence of the gene, induced chromosome transloca- tions, or they may result in overexpression or gene amplification[6] (*ref.* 19, Sect. 5.7.2). Also, a substantial number of transforming *cellular* oncogenes have been described that have no counterpart in transducing retroviruses (4, 10, 20). The above depicted perspective underlies the realization that the discovery of viral and cellular oncogenes and of their relationship to the proto-oncogenes created a heuristic conceptual framework for the elucidation of the mechanism of action of most (if not all) types of carcinogenic agents.

A. Chemical Carcinogens

Chemical carcinogens may be genotoxic by the criteria of inducing gene mutations (point-mutation, frameshift mutation) and/or chromosome mutations (chromosomal aberrations, aneuploidy). Genotoxic agents that induce gene mutations are electrophilic reactants as such (direct acting carcinogens) or may become electrophiles by metabolic activation (*e.g.*, 21–23). These electron-deficient species can attack many types of nucleophilic sites in the cell, most importantly sites in nucleic acids with which they form covalent adducts [*e.g.*, 21 and 19 (Appendix V)]. It is well established that virtually all carcinogens, which covalently bind to DNA, are mutagens (*e.g.*, 24).

Regarding the mechanism of this mutagenicity, the formation of carcinogen covalent adducts at hydrogen-bonding sites of base-pairs can result in miscoding. But miscoding may also be caused by the presence of carcinogen moieties linked to other DNA sites close by, through electron charge displacements influencing hydrogen bonding. Some forms of DNA damage can undergo errorless repair (25). However, if the cell replicates before DNA repair can take place, the molecular alteration in DNA will become permanent as mutation(s). Hence, DNA repair is a limiting factor in the process of carcinogenesis. This is illustrated by several inheritable human diseases, *e.g.*, xeroderma pigmentosum,

---

[6]In overexpression a gene is transcribed to mRNA at an elevated rate. In amplification gene transcription yields a high copy number because of an abnormal multiplication of the coding sequence, owing to a cascading error of chromosome replication (provided this error remains unchecked due to a lack of or mutated/inactive p53 tumor-suppressor gene product). Independent double minute chromosomes and homogeneously staining regions, if seen, are cytogenetic abnormalities indicative of gene amplification (15).

ataxia-telangiectasia, and Fanconi's anemia, which are characterized by deficient DNA repair as well as by increased incidence of cancer.

Covalent binding of an electrophile, if it occurs in or in close vicinity of a proto-oncogene DNA sequence, can bring about its activation. It was known since about 1980 that activated oncogenes are present in cultured cells transformed by chemical carcinogens (*e.g.*, 26, rev. 27). At the time of this writing most of the information available on the activation of specific oncogenes by chemical carcinogens is on the *ras* and *myc* family. There are four mammalian *ras* genes (H-, K-, N-, and R-*ras*); they encode closely related p21 proteins, cytoplasmic G-protein-like GPT-binding GTPases, which are elements of signal transduction pathways and, thus, have critical roles in the normal control of cell proliferation and differentiation. There are four *myc* genes (c-, N-, L-, and R-*myc*); they encode nucleus-localized helix-loop-helix (HLH) type, leucine zipper (LZ) domain-containing gene regulatory proteins, which have key roles as transcriptional regulators in controlling the cell response to stimulation by growth factors and the rate of cell proliferation through the cell cycle (4, 15). Activation of *ras* usually involves a single point-mutation at a specific codon. These amino acid substitutions are at positions 12, 13, 59, 61 or 63; they are located at the loop region representing the GDP-binding domain or at the effector domain of the Ras protein (2). In contrast to *ras, myc* genes are activated most often not by mutation within the protein coding region of the gene, but in gene regulatory control regions; thus, transforming *myc* genes are usually overexpressed or amplified (4, 10, 11a, 15, 28).

1. Activation of ras

Activated *ras* oncogene was detected in tumors induced by various chemical carcinogens (*e.g., revs.* 20, 29, 30) and is also present in many human tumors (*e.g.,* 4, 11a, and 19, Sect. 5.7.2). The ubiquitousness of activated *ras* oncogenes spans virtually all the types of carcinogens and tumors that have been studied; this is consistent with the key role of the normal *ras* encoded p21 proteins which function as an allosteric switch device in the phosphatidylinositol second messenger cascade (15). For example, activated *ras* oncogenes have been found in mouse skin tumors induced by polycyclic aromatic hydrocarbons (31), in neurogenic tumors induced by ethylnitrosourea (32), in mouse liver and rat liver, mammary and renal tumors induced by various nitroso compounds other than ethylnitrosourea (33, rev. 34), and in mouse skin tumors initiated by ethylcarbamate (35a).

In some instances the specific activating mutation of *ras* was identified. For example, Barbacid and coworkers traced the activation of H-*ras* in tumors induced by *N*-methyl-*N*-nitrosourea to a single point-mutation (from G to A) at the 12th codon (35b). Balmain *et al.* (36) observed the activation as well as overexpression of H-*ras* in papillomas and squamous cell carcinomas initiated by 7,12-dimethylbenz[*a*]anthracene (DMBA) and promoted by 12-*O*-tetradecanoylphorbol-13-acetate (TPA) in mice. The point-mutation produced by DMBA is an A to T mutation at the 61st codon; about 90% of the skin tumors bore this mutation (37, 38). Activation of H-*ras* in transformed cells, in skin tumors initiated by and in lung tumors (in A/J mice) induced by ethylcarbamate, as well as in mouse hepatomas induced by vinyl carbamate (a putative proximate carcinogen of ethylcarbamate) was also shown to be an A to T mutation at the 61st codon (39).

2. Augmentation of ras

Besides mutational activation of *ras,* the overproduction of Ras protein through the amplification of *ras* has been reported. In NIH 3T3 cells this leads to increased responsiveness to bombesin (a normal autocrine growth factor produced in excess by small-cell lung carcinoma cells), measured by the turnover rate of the phosphatidylinositol pathway (40) as one facet of cell transformation in culture through *ras* amplification (41). Elevated levels of the Ras protein, p21, have been found in human bladder, colon, and prostate tumors, and in some instances the degree of *ras* expression could be correlated with the histopathological tumor grade (4).

3. Augmentation and Activation of myc

Like *ras*, *myc* is also a ubiquitously found oncogene. It has most often been detected in tumors in an augmented form. In general, expression of *myc* rises sharply in cells that are stimulated to proliferate. Enhanced expression of *myc* is associated with experimentally induced tumors as well as in spontaneously occurring tumors in humans (4). For example, in the studies of Balmain, Barbacid, and their coworkers (36–38), *myc* genes were noted to be overexpressed or amplified (besides the activation of *ras* genes discussed above). Also, amplification of N-*myc* was reported in *N*-acetoxy-*N*-acetylaminofluorene-induced tumors (42).

Investigation reported in 1993–1994 established important mutation(s) in a functional domain of the *myc* encoded regulatory protein. The transcriptional activation function of Myc resides in its amino-terminal domain. The regulation of this function is carried out through heterodimeric complexing with a related protein, Max, via an HLH-LZ domain present in both proteins. Myc-Max complexes stimulate transcription and cell proliferation, whereas Max-Max homodimers and heterodimers of Max and Mad (another HLH-LZ protein) act as transcriptional repressors (*rev.* 43). The activity of the Myc-Max complexes requires the transcriptional activation domain which is present only in the Myc moiety of the complex. The activity of this domain appears to be regulated by protein-protein interaction with the p107 protein which—although it is highly related structurally to the retinoblastoma (Rb) suppressor protein—regulates different targets during the cell cycle (*rev.* 43). The p107 protein complexes with Myc *in vivo* and suppresses the functioning of its transcriptional activation domain; on the other hand, the Rb protein is completely inactive in suppressing transcriptional activation by Myc (43). Mutant varieties of *myc* from Burkitt lymphoma cell lines—which contain mutations in the sequences coding for the Myc transcriptional activation domain—are resistant to the functional suppression of the domain (43). Multiple point-mutations in the Myc transcriptional activation domain have also been reported in human lymphomas and plasmacytomas (44, 45).

4. Collaboration between ras and myc

It has been known for some time that transfected *ras* oncogenes do not transform or transform only poorly nonestablished normal primary cells in culture (46, 47). There are a number of oncogenes that collaborate with *ras* oncogenes to enable them to transform cultured primary cells; *myc* oncogenes are among the ones that can cooperate in this cell transformation (47). Cells transformed by a pair of collaborating oncogenes express high levels of each oncogene product and there appears to be no evidence for sequence modification of p21 from these transformed cells. In fact, *ras* has been shown to inhibit cell proliferation upon removal of the collaborating activity from the culture (48).

An interesting sequence-dependent phenomenon in the *ras-myc* collaboration was observed when c-H-*ras* and c-*myc* oncogenes were transfected into rat embryo primary cell line. When *ras* and *myc* were transfected *one at a time,* the cells treated with *ras* at first were not converted to a tumorigenic phenotype by subsequent transfection with *myc,* but cells transfected and immortalized with *myc* first readily underwent transformation by subsequent transfection with *ras* (49). Thus, *myc*-immortalized cells appear more permissive to transformation via a secondary treatment. In these sequentially transfected cultures *myc* expression was high irrespective of whether it preceded or succeeded *ras* in the transfections, whereas the expression of *ras* was the highest when it was transfected into the cells subsequent to *myc* (precisely the transfection sequence which was transforming) (49).

The capability of oncogene collaboration extends to oncogenes other than *ras* and *myc* proper but loosely related to them in terms of function and subcellular localization. The products of "*ras*-like" oncogenes are localized in the membrane/cytoplasm and include members of the Ras family, also Ral, Mel, as well as Src and related protein kinases (*e.g.,* Yes, Ros, Fms, Fps/Fes, Mil/Raf, Abl, Neu, Erb-B). The products of "*myc*-like" oncogenes are localized in the nucleus and include members of the Myc family as well as Myb, Fos, Ski, p53, SV40 large T antigen, polyoma large T antigen, and adenovirus E1A protein (*ref.* 19, Sect. 5.7.2.4; 20).

5. Activation/Enhancement of Other Oncogenes

Less is known at the time of this writing about the activation or augmentation of oncogenes other than *ras* and *myc*. For example, transforming *neu* oncogene, active in NIH 3T3 cells, was found in neurogenic tumors induced transplacentally by ethylnitrosourea in BDIX (50) and F344 (32) strain rats. Interestingly, exposure of rat embryo central nervous system cells in culture to ethylnitrosourea *depresses* the expression of the *src* proto-oncogene (51); there was a significant decrease in the level of Src pp60 protein product (as well as in the level of the 200 kDa neurofilament protein). Since there is a marked increase in the levels of these proteins and in Src tyrosine kinase activity at the time of neuronal differentiation, these decreases appear to represent markers of the developmental toxic effect of ethylnitrosourea, which is both carcinogenic and teratogenic (52).

In squamous cell carcinomas, initiated by DMBA or *N*-methyl-*N*-nitroso-*N'*-nitroguanidine and promoted by TPA in the mouse skin, all tumors exhibited very high levels of the RNA transcripts of stromelysin, which is an extracellular matrix degrading metalloproteinase encoded by the transin gene (39). Papillomas exhibited very little expression of the transin gene (39). It was also observed that TPA treatment of normal mouse epidermis induces a temporary expression of the transin gene (53). Stromelysin, when activated, can degrade a variety of protein components of the basement membrane, a facet of the malignant invasive phenotype. Conversion to a malignant phenotype is usually accompanied by acquisition of the constitutive expression of stromelysin (39). Induction of the expression of stromelysin by TPA represent, hence, the epigenetic equivalent of a collaborating oncogene (47). Indeed, TPA has been shown to promote the transformation by *ras* alone of nonestablished embryo fibroblasts (54), as well as two-stage carcinogenesis in the mouse skin with v-*ras* gene from Harvey or BALB murine sarcoma viruses, as initiators (55). It appears then that oncogene activation by chemical carcinogens possibly represents the first stage of the carcinogenic process currently known as "initiation" (38, 56, 57).

Conclusion. The complex network of cell regulation involves a multiplicity of dimeric and trimeric interactions between elements of signal transduction pathways as well as yet unspecified interactions between these pathways and gene regulation through nuclear receptors. Hence signal channeling in the network is in a constant flux depending on autocrine, paracrine, and endocrine factors, as well as xenobiotics, that will specify or emphasize different paths by way of action on receptors and in some instances possibly through direct action on allosteric signal transduction components (*cf.* 13, 15; *see also* under D. below).

Depending on the proto-oncogene or groups of proto-oncogenes that are activated or enhanced by a particular carcinogenic agent — chemical, viral, or other — the regulatory network, in constant interchange with the genome, will respond accordingly with a modification of the phenotype. This underlies the morphological and functional differences between cells transformed by various agents. It follows that if tumor induction is in different tissue types (or transformation in different cell lines) even with a given etiological agent, cell transformation will involve activation of different groups of multiple proto-oncogene pathways (*e.g.*, 58, *cf.* 39, 47, 59). Consistent with this is that certain viruses can induce more than one tumor type, depending on the type of cell infected and the experimental conditions (4). It was predicted in 1985 (60) that:

> the field of carcinogenesis is being increasingly recognized as a vast area of molecular biology concerned with the cellular regulatory mechanisms. Through interaction with different areas of the genome, involving activation of oncogenes or otherwise affecting gene expression, and/or interaction with other macromolecular systems (as in various epigenetic mechanisms), chemical carcinogens induce tumor cells which display an almost limitless variety of enzymatic and morphological patterns. The types of cellular interactions of and the target tissues affected by carcinogens are determined by their reactivity, molecular geometry, and physicochemical characteristics. Chemical carcinogens represent, hence, specific molecular tools affecting different structural areas underlying the feedback network of cellular homeostasis.

B. Radiations

The large genetic lesions produced by ionizing radiation (chromosomal aberrations, DNA strand breaks, DNA-protein crosslinks, large deletions, gene rearrangements) and their biochemical functional correlates have been discussed in Chapter 13 in some detail. Although point-mutations (base substitutions, frameshifts, and small deletions) have been observed to occur as a consequence of radiation exposure (*e.g.*, 61), ionizing radiation is a relatively weak point mutagen (39).

Proto-oncogenes are important target genes for chemical carcinogens and for certain types of viruses (*cis*-activating), and some degree of structural specificity probably plays a role in gene targeting by such agents. While specificity in the structural sense cannot play a role in the targeting of proto-oncogenes by radiations, these cellular genes are *as a category* key macromolecular targets in radiation carcinogenesis. In the spectrum of the presently known proto-oncogenes (over 100), some have been detected with much greater frequency than others in the mutated or augmented oncogene form in various tumor cells. These genes belong mostly to the *ras* and the *myc* families and they are also the ones most commonly detected in mutated or augmented form in radiation-induced malignancies.

1. Ionizing Radiations

a. Activation of ras *Genes.* Activated K-*ras* was found in ionizing radiation-induced thymomas in (AKR × RF/J)F$_1$ mice (30), in skin carcinomas (62) and thyroid tumors (63) in rats. Activation of solely K-*ras* appears to be more prevalent with ionizing radiation, whereas thyroid tumors induced by *N*-methyl-*N*-nitrosourea displayed activated H-*ras* but not K-*ras* (63). Activated H-*ras* was also detected in a strontium-90 induced mouse osteosarcoma cell line (64). Surprisingly, in other experiments (65), transforming DNAs from various mouse skin tumors (papillomas, and squamous and basal cell carcinomas) initiated with X-irradiation and promoted with TPA were reported to carry dominant transforming genes — detectable through transfection into NIH 3T3 cells — but which were concluded to be other than H-*ras*, K-*ras*, N-*ras*, erb-B, B-*lym*, *met*, *neu*, or *raf*. Based on Southern blot analysis the oncogene sequences of the primary NIH 3T3 transformant DNAs were considered by the authors (65) to be distinctly non-*ras* transforming genes.

As expected (*cf.* 58, 60), even within one oncogene family, genetic factors (species and strain) will determine which gene will be activated. Thus, in radiation-induced thymomas both K-*ras* and N-*ras* were found activated in RF/J strain mice, whereas in thymomas induced in C57BL/6J mice mainly activated N-*ras* was detected (66, 67). Activated c-N-*ras* was also found in nonlymphocytic leukemia induced in the dog by a cobalt-source gamma radiation (68); this mutation involved the 12th codon aspartic acid.

The most common positions of activation of *ras* appear to be mutations at the 12th and 61st codons. While gamma radiation follows this typical activation pattern in inducing mutations in *ras*, neutron radiation was found to activate K-*ras* via an unusual position, at codon 146 (69).

In *established* Chinese hamster embryo cell culture incorporation of iodine-125 selectively amplified c-K-*ras* and c-H-*ras*, as well as the integrated SV40 sequences (70). However, in embryo cell culture lines from Syrian golden hamster (regarded to be a taxonomically different species) X-irradiation produced neither amplification (detectable by Southern blot analysis) or overexpression of any culture tested for v-*myc*, v-H-*ras* or N-*ras* related oncogenes, nor the activation of any oncogene that would be detectable in the NIH 3T3 transfection assay (71). Yet, all irradiated cell lines did show tumorigenesis when injected s.c. into nude mice (BALB/c *nu/nu*). Karyotypic analysis showed trisomy of chromosome 9 in 8 of 10 cell lines, which may have an important role in the X-ray-induced neoplastic transformation (71).

b. Augmentation of *myc* Genes.

In a number of ionizing radiation-induced mouse tumors overexpression and amplification of the c-*myc* gene were observed (72); also in ionizing radiation-induced rat skin tumors c-*myc* overexpression and amplification (in addition to c-K-*ras* activation) were seen (62). Overexpression of c-*myc* was also noted in some radiation-induced osteosarcomas (73, 74) and in thymomas (75) in the mouse. Different lines of evidence support the view that the amplification of c-*myc* confers a significant selective advantage on a cell subpopulation in these tumors. First, there is a correlation between c-*myc* copy number and tumor growth (76) and a molecular heterogeneity among the c-*myc* copies within individual cells (77). Second, in experiments on the cooperative effect of oncogene (*myc* or *ras*) transfection and cesium-137 gamma irradiation, specifically c-*myc* but not c-*ras* was found to create a permissive state to enable the subsequently applied radiation to transform rat embryo cells (49). In these experiments gamma irradiation did not increase expression of *myc* beyond the level in the *myc*-immortalized cells. It is noteworthy, however, that cobalt-60 gamma radiation did bring about a further increase in the expression of c-*myc* — beyond the spontaneous overexpression of this oncogene — in SV40-transformed fibroblasts from ataxia-telangiectasia patients (78).

2. Nonionizing Radiations

Activated *ras* oncogenes have been identified in human skin cancers. The presence of *ras* oncogenes in benign and self-regressing keratoacanthomas suggest that they play a role in the early stages of carcinogenesis; therefore, *ras* oncogenes must remain latent for a long period of time (*rev.* 79). It is well known that defective DNA repair in xeroderma pigmentosum (XP) patients renders them particularly susceptible to skin carcinogenesis by ultraviolet light; altered *ras* and *myc* genes have indeed been detected in skin tumors of XP patients (*rev.* 80). Demonstration was given that ultraviolet radiation can activate a *ras* gene *in vitro*. Proto-N-*ras,* as part of a plasmid, was directly exposed to UV light and thereby became capable of transforming cells in a Rat-2 cell line; this activated N-*ras* gene showed mutations at the typical codon positions 12 or 61 (81). Ultraviolet radiation was also found to modify the expression of the c-*fos* gene; UV light exposure induces c-*fos* expression in Chinese hamster ovary cells (82), but decreases the level of c-*fos* expression together with enhanced c-*myc* expression in C3H 10T1/2 cells (83).

C. Chromosome Translocations: Spontaneous and Induced; Intrinsically Fragile Sites. Excess Chromosomes Acquired in Meiosis

It has been an early observation in cytogenetics that specific chromosomal translocations correlate with many different leukemias and lymphomas. Klein (84) came to the insight in 1981 that chromosome breaks and translocations may lead to the activation of proto-oncogenes located at or near the breakpoints. This insight has since been fully confirmed. The activation of proto-oncogenes (as well as the inactivation of tumor-suppressor genes) results from the structural alteration(s), mutations, in these genes as the consequence of the breaks. Moreover, the chromosomal translocation that follows a breakage brings the genes at or near the breakpoints under the influence of transcriptional control regions of other genes and, thus, brings about the dysregulation of gene expression as distinct from mutational alteration of the gene(s). In some typical instances this leads to the overexpression/amplification of proto-oncogenes.

Chromosome breakage and translocation can result from a "spontaneous" (*i.e.,* genetically determined) karyotypic instability or may represent a chromosome mutation induced by a viral or chemical agent, radiation, or by special circumstances of cellular stress (*see* under D. below). Only the former are reviewed here. Genetically determined karyotypic instability is displayed in the group of "chromosome instability syndromes" (CIS): the better known syndromes, Fanconi's anemia, Bloom's syndrome, ataxia-telangiectasia, xeroderma pigmentosum (15, 85–89) and the less well known glutathione reductase deficiency syndrome (*cited in* 90). These autosomal recessive disorders are characterized by greatly increased rate of chromosome breakage and high incidence of leukemia, carcinoma, and lymphoreticular neoplasia (85–90). With the possible exception of the glutathione deficiency syndrome, probably none of neoplasias arising in the CIS is of single-gene origin.

Other cancer-prone chromosomal aberrations, which bring genes under the transcriptional control regions of different genes, are seen in the syndromes with excess chromosomes: Down syndrome and Klinefelter's syndrome. In Down syndrome the chromosomal aberration is an extra chromosome 21 (trisomy 21) attached to chromosome 14 [translocation t(14;21)] (87); the incidence of live birth with Down syndrome increases considerably with maternal age—the median is approximately 1/700. In Klinefelter's syndrome, occurring with about the same incidence in *male* births, there is an extra chromosome X attached to the Y chromosome, represented as 47,XXY (87). Patients with Down syndrome develop leukemia at a rate that is about 15 times higher than that of the normal population (87). Males with Klinefelter's syndrome are at greatly increased risk for breast cancer, approaching the risk of normal women (about 66 times the risk of normal men) (85).

The chromosome translocation–initiated disorder in which the molecular biology of neoplastic transformation is the best understood is chronic myelogenous leukemia (CML); this is characterized by a great increase of mature granulocytes primarily in the bone marrow, but also at extramedullary sites (*e.g.,* spleen, liver). Because of this infiltration of malignant cells, the liver and especially the spleen are enlarged; splenomegaly may become extreme with the progression of the disease. The translocation-induced oncogene activation which underlies this syndrome will be discussed below in some detail. Why chromosome breakage and translocation/transposition (except for Klinefelter's syndrome involving sex chromosomes) lead predominantly to leukemias and tumors of the lymphatic tissue is not understood. The karyotypic instability in CIS and CML is the consequence of the existence of *fragile sites* in the chromosomes. Such sites are less stable than other sites and these specific loci of genetic instability are inherited in Mendelian fashion. One may speculate that the structural integrity of all large complex macromolecular structures requires that they be able to withstand the molecular stress of the dynamics of cell life upon the chemical bonds. Hence, sites that are of higher than "normal" (excess) fragility are comparatively prone to breakage, and the resulting chemically reactive fragments may reattach at (translocate to) other macromolecular areas as determined by the topographic position of the particular break.

1. Summary Clinical Picture of Chromosome Instability Syndromes

Various faults in DNA repair and replication underlie or are key components in all CIS. For some the defective steps have been determined. For example, in Bloom's syndrome there is a defect in DNA ligation, whereas in xeroderma pigmentosum the defect is in the nucleotide excision repair process; there is suggestive evidence that in Fanconi's anemia there is a deficiency in an exonuclease that removes DNA cross- links before normal repair of DNA begins. Manifestations of these syndromes begin very early in life and the patients generally show stunted growth. To briefly characterize the severe manifestations of these diseases: (a) In *Fanconi's anemia* (a form of aplastic anemia) there is early onset of pancytopenia and the principal symptom is thrombocytopenia, causing bleeding. There is brown pigmentation of the skin, fibrosis of the pancreas with bronchiectasis, often malformation of the kidneys and renal dysfunction. The associated neoplasms are acute myelomonocytic leukemia, carcinoma of the mucocutaneous junction, and hepatic adenoma or carcinoma (85, 86, 91, 92). (b) In *Bloom's syndrome* a readily evident manifestation is photophobia/severe sun sensitivity of the skin leading to lesions. However, the associated neoplasms are leukemia and intestinal cancer. Among the various chromosomal aberrations seen, there is a characteristic quadriradial chromosome configuration specifically associated with Bloom's syndrome. In most cases there are severe immunoglobulin deficiencies (85, 86, 93). (c) *Ataxia-telangiectasia* is a multisystem syndrome, which is primarily neurologic but with endocrine and vascular abnormalities and deficiencies. There is muscle weakness and atrophy leading to severe disability. Most patients show progressive mental retardation linked to the cerebellar ataxia and immune defects (lack of serum and secretory IgA, occasionally antibodies to IgA, deficiency of IgE, and very low T-cell immunity). A very typical symptom is the telangiectatic veins in the skin and the cornea. The associated neoplasms are leukemia, carcinoma of the stomach, brain tumors, and various lymphoreticular malignancies (85, 86, 94). (d) *Xeroderma pigmentosum* is a disfiguring disease, characterized by disseminated pigmented spots, telangiectasis, atrophy and contraction of the skin, particularly in areas exposed to sunlight. The skin lesions are wart-like and soon turn into carcinomas. There is photophobia, generally familial. Progressive neurological disorders and enzyme defects are associated also with this syndrome (85–87).

2. Excess Chromosome Syndromes

Unlike in the CIS in which the chromosome translocations/aberrations develop progressively following birth, the chromosomal aberrations in Down syndrome and in Klinefelter's syndrome are of very early developmental origin. If during meiosis the homologues (male and female version) of a particular chromosome fail to separate (known as nondisjunction), some haploid cells will have more than one copy of that chromosome, whereas in others that chromosome will be absent. In Down syndrome an extra chromosome 21 becomes attached to chromosome 14 as the result of nondisjunction; similarly, in Klinefelter's syndrome, the extra X chromosome is acquired through meiotic nondisjunction (mainly maternal) (87). This brings about dysregulation of gene expression in the affected chromosomes, just as in genetically determined or agent-induced chromosome translocations.

The clinical picture of patients with Down syndrome is that of stunted growth, normal to increased head size, prominent jaw, and protruding small ears. The bridge of the nose is flattened, the tongue is large and protruding from the mouth, most often held open; the hands are short and broad. The mean IQ is about 50. Congenital heart disease (in about 35% of the patients: structural defects in the atrioventricular canal and ventricular septum) and predisposition to acute leukemia limits the maximum life span to 45–55 years.

Individuals affected by Klinefelter's syndrome are tall, eunuchoid, with small firm fibrotis testes, and display gynecomastia. Facial hair is light. Some patients with Klinefelter's syndrome may have more than two X chromosomes (up to five) together with the Y chromosome. The mental deficits (mainly verbal) and constitutional malfunctions increase with the number of X chromosomes (87).

3. Chromosome Translocation in Chronic Myelogenous Leukemia

Chromosome translocation and the resulting activation/enhancement of oncogenes has been the most extensively studied in CML and in Burkitt's lymphoma; the latter is discussed in some detail in Section II of this chapter.

The characteristic translocation in CML (present in 90–95% of the patients) is a t(9;22) reciprocal translocation between chromosomes 9 and 22, yielding an abnormal chromosome, known as the Philadelphia chromosome (Ph[1]), in the leukocytes. On chromosome 9 the breakpoint is at q34 and on chromosome 22 at q11.[7] So the concise cytogenetic description of the *translocation* is t(9;22)(q34;q11).

The translocation moves the *abl* proto-oncogene (normally present in chromosome 9) to chromosome 22 close to the breakpoint and moves the *sis* proto-oncogene (normally present on chromosome 22) to chromosome 9. The translocated *abl* gene is expressed as a 210 kDa Bcr-Abl fusion protein, where Bcr is the product of the "breakpoint cluster region" (*bcr*) sequence at q11. The Bcr-Abl protein shows increased tyrosine kinase activity compared to the normal (120 kDa) Abl protein. Yet, despite the similarity of

---

[7]The cytogenetic designation "q" is for the long arm of a chromosome and "p" for the short arm of a chromosome. The number that follows designates the chromosome band that can be visualized by staining procedure. The concise designation of the position of these *bands* is 9(q34) and 22(q11).

bcr-abl with the v-*abl* oncogene of the Abelson murine leukemia virus (which also shows increased tyrosine kinase activity), *bcr-abl,* unlike v-*abl,* is inactive in the NIH 3T3 cell transformation assay. This appears to be due to the nature of the N-terminus of the fusion protein since insertion of a viral *gag* sequence into the 5′ region of *bcr-abl* enables the fusion protein to transform NIH 3T3 fibroblasts (*rev.* 4, 20).

Besides CML and Burkitt's lymphoma, which are the best studied examples of oncogene activation/enhancement by chromosome translocation, recurring translocations have been detected in various leukemias (*e.g.,* human chronic B-cell leukemia, promyelocytic leukemia) and lymphoid tumors (*e.g.,* B-cell lymphomas). Translocations between chromosome 14 and regions of chromosome 11 or 18 are the ones seen in these malignancies. In various mouse lymphomas the *myc* proto-oncogene is translocated from its normal site on chromosome 15 to the IgH-chain locus on chromosome 12. This translocation has also been detected in mouse plasmacytomas.

D. Conditions of Sustained Cellular Stress

Beyond the induction of hepatic tumors by the administration of a lipotrope (specifically choline)-deficient diet, discussed in Chapter 9 (Section III) and in the Prefactory Chapter, there are three intriguing modalities of tumor induction (or cell transformation) which proceed in the absence of any carcinogenic agent, promoter, or other modifying agent. These modalities are: the subcutaneous implantation of films or platelets of plastics (or any other chemically inert solid material), the spontaneous transformation of cells in culture maintained for an extended period of time, and the subcutaneous injection of *hypertonic* solutions of glucose, sodium chloride, or other normal physiological substance. These represent sustained conditions of cellular stress. In the first two, stress is due to the deprivation of the cells from chemical signals of intercellular and systemic communication by mechanical confinement or by cytological isolation; in the third, stress is due to osmolarity crisis. Studies in these areas have been reviewed in some detail in the previous volume of this series (*see ref.* 19, Sections 5.5.3, 5.6.2, and 5.6.3), consequently only working summaries on these phenomena are given here:

- *Solid-state carcinogenesis* (SSC) is the term for the induction of local sarcomas by the (usually subcutaneous) implantation of films or platelets made of any type of inert, solid, insoluble material (various plastics, glass, ivory, parchment paper, various metals, etc.). Independently from the chemical nature of the material, implanted foreign bodies produce histopathologically very similar tumors. Local sarcomas have been induced with a high incidence in rats and mice and with a low incidence in hamsters and dogs, by means of SSC. Even in susceptible species the incidence depends on the size, shape, porosity, and surface properties of the implant; the implantation of powders or threads of the same material does not produce sarcomas. A given amount of material fashioned into a platelet may be highly effective in inducing local sarcomas, whereas implantation of the same amount of material fashioned in the shape of a small ball may be totally ineffective. Platelets (disk or square) of at least 0.5 cm in diameter or length are sarcomatogenic; tumor incidence decreases and latent period increases with the decrease of the diameter or length. Fragmented implants or implants made porous are less effective or ineffective in inducing sarcomas; if the implants are made porous, tumor incidence varies inversely with the number and size of the pores (implants with pore diameters greater than 0.22 μm do not yield tumors). Tumors have been induced by the subcutaneous implantation of Millipore filters into rats and tumor incidence was found to vary inversely with the pore diameter.

- *Spontaneous malignant transformation (SMT)* in vitro. The first observation by Gey dates back to 1941. He observed that normal rat mesenchymal cells undergo spontaneous transformation in culture if maintained for a prolonged period of time. Two years later Earle observed the spontaneous transformation of mouse embryo fibroblasts in culture. These early observations have been fully confirmed in a number of studies using various normal cell types from rats, mice, hamsters, and humans. The new properties of the cells, indicative of transformation, may appear several weeks or months after the establishment of the culture line. The time required for spontaneous transformation depends on the serum used to support cell growth; "transformed" properties appear less rapidly in media containing *fetal* calf serum than in those containing calf or horse serum.

- *Osmolarity-crisis-induced sarcomatogenesis (OSIC)* was first reported in 1935 by Japanese workers and was confirmed repeatedly. Subcutaneous injections of concentrated *hypertonic* solutions of glucose, sodium chloride and of a variety of normal physiological substances, if performed repeatedly for a long term, induce local sarcomas in rats and less effectively in mice. In cell cultures, high osmolarity has been shown to induce gene mutations in Chinese hamster ovary cells and in L5178Y mouse lymphoma cells, and to significantly increase the number of transformed foci in BALB/c 3T3 cells. High osmolarity due to monovalent salts (NaCl, KCl, NaF, and KF) is more effective than sucrose in bringing about the clastogenic effects. It has often been observed that cultures of different tissues show bridge formation and clumping in chromosomes when maintained in high salt media.

1. Deprivation from Extracellular Signals

As already mentioned earlier in this section, the common feature of SSC and SMT is the partial or total loss of chemical signals of intercellular and systemic communication to some cells: due to mechanical shielding/confinement in the former case and produced by cytological isolation in the latter.

The existence of tumors or transformed cell cultures that are devoid of activated/enhanced oncogenes has not been reported (or confirmed) so far. It does remain that tumors induced in solid-state carcinogenesis or cell cultures that have undergone spontaneous transformation have not been investigated for the presence of oncogenes. For this reason, the key role of allostery in receptor function and signal transduction prompts an examination of the question: Does the deprivation/limitation of extracellular chemical signals alter the dynamics of some allosteric transitions in the cell—alterations that may become "locked-in" at the gene level if sustained long enough? This would lead eventually to the activation/enhancement of proto-oncogenes to cellular oncogenes in the absence of any viral or chemical agent or radiation.

Consider that cells of complex organisms function in concert in a sea of regulatory chemical signals which modulate myriad interlocking negative and positive feedback loops that underlie the functioning of a multicellular organization. The signals—which may originate from adjacent identical or different cell types (autocrine or paracrine signals), from distant organs (endocrine hormonal signals), or may derive from the external environment of the organism (xenobiotics)—activate different areas of the signal transduction network and/or act on nuclear receptors (*e.g., revs.* 13, 95, 96; *see also in* 15). This enables the cell to adapt to change occurring in the tissue, organismic or external environment.

As briefly alluded to above, a critically important feature of the signal transduction network is the allosteric nature of many or most of its control elements (*e.g., revs.* 96–98; *see also in* 15). Since the definition of allosteric effects in 1963 by Monod et al. (99, *rev.* 100, 101), an enormous literature has developed on the allosteric regulation of various control elements of signal transduction, gene expression, and cell metabolism (illustrative of recent literature, *see* 96–98, 102–115). In eukaryotic cells 10 up to 30% of total proteins may undergo phosphorylation often at multiple sites (*e.g.*, 116, 117)—the reaction that drives and is indicative of allosteric transitions—in response to a variety of extracellular signals.

Allosteric effects are defined as indirect interactions between topographically distinct binding sites mediated by the protein molecule through conformational changes (100). Although most allosteric effects have been observed in oligomeric enzymes, monomeric enzymes may also be subject to allosteric regulation. As described by Monod *et al.* (99), allosteric interaction between two identical molecules, a homotropic interaction, can lead to cooperativity or anticooperativity in binding; an allosteric interaction between two different molecules (*e.g.*, substrate and an inhibitor or activator) is a heterotropic interaction. Normally, the kinetics of binding of a substrate to an enzyme follows a hyperbolic function, but in oligomeric allosteric enzymes the kinetics of binding follows a sigmoidal curve. Allosteric enzymes exist in at least two conformational states; these are in an equilibrium and differ in their affinities for the ligands. To illustrate the ligand-induced conformational shift, consider the case when the excess one of the ligands, *e.g.*, an activator, would shift the kinetics toward a steeper response, then an excess of an inhibitor would shift the kinetics toward a response less steep than the sigmoidal binding isotherm (100). In the absence of one of the ligands the conformational equilibrium shifts back toward the sigmoidal isotherm and this conformational shift brings about preferential binding of the other ligand (99–101); this binding, in turn, stabilizes the respective conformational state (*cf.* 118).

In the actual functioning of the signal transduction network in normal cells, the extensive protein phosphorylations (and associated with it the conformational states of allosteric intermediaries) are only transient. Beneath the high level of total phosphorylation of cell proteins there is a perpetually ongoing rapid changeover of phosphorylation sites (and conformational states) that are phosphorylated by a very large number of distinct protein kinases, then reversed by phosphatases, and so on. The disappearance or chronic dearth of extracellular regulatory signals, normally acting upon the conformational states of certain membrane-localized receptors and nuclear receptors, will "lock-in" these receptors as well as other allosteric regulatory elements (*e.g.*, G proteins and MAP kinases in the signal transduction cascades) in a fixed conformational mode. If sustained, this dysregulation will eventually be reflected in alterations of DNA structure and gene expression. Hence, expectably activated/enhanced cellular oncogenes will be found in SSC- and SMT-induced malignancies.

Genetically locked-in structural alterations in allosteric membrane-localized receptors, signal transduction intermediates, and nuclear receptors, brought about by the sustained absence of extracellular regulatory signals, may be regarded as a "functional disuse atrophy" at the molecular level that precedes cell transformation/tumorigenesis. It is noteworthy that there is an analogy at higher organizational level: tissue atrophy is regarded to be a precancerous condition (*e.g.*, 119–121, *see also* 19, Sect. 5.7.4).

2. Osmolarity Crisis

Deviation of the extracellular milieu from isotonicity generates intercellular biochemical signals through cell volume change that force adjustments in the topography of the cytoskeleton and conformational shifts in some allosteric elements of signal transduction. Exposure of cultured mammalian cells to nonisotonic media has been reported to cause an increase in protein tyrosine phosphorylation (122), suggesting that one or more protein kinases are activated by the osmotic shock (123).

The existence of an osmosensing signal transduction pathway in mammalian cells (123) and in yeast (123, 124) has been reported. Similarly to osmotic shock, mechanical stimulus that forces cell deformation/shape change generates biochemical signals; the second messengers generated in response to cell deformation have been reviewed (125).

Several components of the signal transduction network have been implicated in osmosensing. The Jnk signal transduction pathway (126, 127) is activated in Chinese hamster ovary cells by exposure to hyperosmolar media, and phosphorylation is required to activate Jnk-1 (123). The actual osmotic sensor in the Jnk protein kinase cascade is, however, not known. Jnk kinases have been implicated in the regulation of the function of intercellular transporter proteins which have a role in increased gene expression in osmotically shocked cells (128, 129). Jnk may also more directly regulate gene expression. In this context Jnk was found to bind to the transcription factor protein Jun, resulting in increased transcriptional activity. Osmotic shock induces the expression of Jun and in some tissues of Fos, components of the AP-1 gene regulatory protein (*rev.* 123).

Hyperosmolarity was also found to activate a different signalling cascade involving p38 tyrosine kinase (130); this pathway is also activated by lipopolysaccharides that is regarded as a cellular stress signal (130). The p38 kinase is a member of the family of MAP kinases which are involved in the regulation and coordination of various signalling cascades (131–133).

The existence of osmosensing and osmoregulatory pathways, which are being actively explored at the time of this writing, underlies the capability of many eukaryotic cells to increase their internal osmolarity in response to the increase of external osmolarity (134). It remains that the p38 kinase and possibly all other osmosensing members of the signalling cascades are the products of a group of genes that are termed stress genes (*cited in* ref. 130).

In conclusion, it should be borne in mind that while the osmoregulatory capability enables the cells to compensate to an extent so as to avoid imminent cell death, hyperosmolarity results in the loss of the optimum ionic environment, which is necessary for the functional and structural integrity of the genome (135). This is consistent with the observed effects of ion type and salt concentration on supercoiled DNA properties, which may be important for strand recombination and transcription requiring favorable conformational states (*e.g.,* 136–138). Moreover, salt concentration may influence recognition interactions with DNA-binding protein possibly through the regulatory role of salt on the functions of looped DNA segments (137, 138). These phenomena may account for the clastogenic, mutagenic, and transforming effects of hyperosmolarity in cell cultures (*ref.* 19, Sect. 5.6.2) and are indicators of the virtual presence in these cultures of activated/enhanced oncogenes, but not studied in this context so far. Investigations are needed to formally explore the presence of oncogenes in all three categories of cellular stress-induced malignant transformation reviewed above.

Abbreviations Used: ALSV, avian leukosis-sarcoma virus; B-cell, leukocyte (maturing in bone marrow); *bcr,* breakpoint cluster region; CA, capsid protein; CIS, chromosome instability syndromes; CML, chronic myelogenous leukemia; CSF, colony stimulating factor; c-*onc*, proto-oncogene; c-*onc* (activated), cellular oncogene; DMBA, 7,12-dimethylbenz[*a*]anthracene; *env,* retroviral gene sequence coding for the cell-recognition-site-bearing and the transmembrane envelope proteins; *gag,* retroviral gene sequence coding for the matrix, capsid, and nucleocapsid proteins; HLH, helix-loop-helix (type protein); HTLV, human T-cell leukemia virus(es); G protein, guanine-nucleotide-binding protein; ICTV, International Committee on the Taxonomy of Viruses; Ig, immunoglobulin; IN, integrase; IQ, intelligence quotient; LZ, leucine zipper; LTR, long terminal repeat; MA, matrix protein; MH2, Mill-Hill 2 avian sarcoma virus; MMTV, mouse mammary tumor virus; NC, nucleocapsid (nucleic-acid-binding protein);

OCIS, osmolarity-crisis-induced sarcomatogenesis; PDGF, platelet-derived growth factor; Ph^1, Philadelphia chromosome; *pol,* retroviral gene sequence coding for the reverse transcriptase and integrase; poly-A tail, 3′ terminal polyadenylate sequence; PPT, polypurine tract; PR, protease; *pro,* retroviral gene sequence coding for the protease; Psi, (viral) packaging signal; R, "redundant" (sequence); RAV, Rous-associated virus; RSV, Rous sarcoma virus; RT, reverse transcriptase; SFFV, spleen focus-forming virus; SM-FeSV, Susan McDonough feline sarcoma virus; SMT, spontaneous malignant transformation; SSC, solid-state carcinogenesis; SSV, simian sarcoma virus; SU, viral envelope protein, larger (cell-recognition-site-bearing); SV40, simian vacuolating virus, type 40; T-cell, leukocyte (maturing in the thymus); TM, viral envelope protein, smaller (transmembrane); TPA, 12-*O*-tetradecanoylphorbol-13-acetate; U, "Unique" (sequences at 5′ and 3′ termini); v-*onc,* viral oncogene; XP, xeroderma pigmentosum.

REFERENCES

1. Gross, L.: "Oncogene Viruses", 3rd ed., Vol. I. Pergamon, New York, 1983. *See* Chap. 7, The Rous Chicken Sarcoma, p. 123.
2. Benjamin, T., and Vogt, P. K.: Cell-Transformation by Viruses. *In* "Fundamental Virology" (B. N. Fields and D. M. Knipe, chief eds.). Raven Press, New York, 1991, p. 291.
3. Murphy, F. A., and Kingsbury, D. W.: Virus Taxonomy. *In* "Fundamental Virology" (B. N. Fields and D. M. Knipe, chief eds.). Raven Press, New York, 1991, p. 9.
4. Burck, K. B., Liu, E. T., and Larrick, J. W.: "Oncogenes — An Introduction to the Concept of Cancer Genes". Springer-Verlag, New York, 1988.
5. Coffin, J. M.: Retroviridae and Their Replication. *In* "Fundamental Virology" (B. N. Fields and D. M. Knipe, chief eds.). Raven Press, New York, 1991, p. 645.
6. Muller, R.: *Trends Biochem. Sci.* **11,** 129 (1986).
7. Nishimura, S., and Sekiya, T.: *Biochem. J.* **243,** 313 (1987).
8. Brickell, P.: *Int. J. Exp. Pathol.* **72,** 97 (1991).
9. Corcoran, G. B., Fix, L., Jones, D. P., Treinen Moslen, M., Nicotera, P., Oberhammer, F. A., and Buttyan, R.: *Toxicol. Appl. Pharmacol.* **128,** 169 (1994).
10. Reddy, E. P., Skalka, A. M., and Curran, T., eds.: "The Oncogene Handbook". Elsevier, New York, 1988.
11a. Weinberg, R. A., ed.: "Oncogenes and the Molecular Origin of Cancer", Monograph 18. Cold Spring Harbor Laboratory Press, Cold Spring Harbor, New York, 1990.
11b. Swanstrom, R., Parker, R. C., Varmus, H. E., and Bishop, J. M.: *Proc. Natl. Acad. Sci. U.S.A.* **80,** 2519 (1983).
12. Rapp, U. R., Reynolds, F. H., and Stephenson, J. R.: *J. Virol.* **45,** 914 (1983).
13. Heldin, C.-H., Betsholtz, C., Claesson-Welsh, L., and Westermark, B.: *Biochim. Biophys. Acta* **907,** 219 (1987).
14. Shalloway, D., Coussens, P. M., and Yaciuk, P.: *Proc. Natl. Acad. Sci. U.S.A.* **81,** 7071 (1984).
15. Alberts, B., Bray, D., Lewis, J., Raff, M., Roberts, K., and Watson, J. D.: "Molecular Biology of the Cell", 3rd ed. Garland, New York, 1994, Chap. 24, p. 1255.
16. Bernhard, W.: *Cancer Res.* **20,** 712 (1960).
17. Fields, B. N., and Knipe, D. M., chief eds.: "Fundamental Virology". Raven Press, New York, 1991.
18. Sheinin, R., Mak, T. W., and Clark, S. P.: Viruses and Cancer. *In* "The Basic Science of Oncology" (I. F. Tannock and R. P. Hills, eds.). Pergamon, New York, 1987, p. 52.
19. Woo, Y.-t., Lai, D. Y., Arcos, J. C., and Argus, M. F.: "Chemical Induction of Cancer — Structural Bases and Biological Mechanisms", Vol. IIIC: Natural, Metal, Fiber and Macrmolecular Carcinogens. Academic Press, San Diego, 1988.
20. Minden, M. A.: Oncogenes. *In* "The Basic Science of Oncology" (I. F. Tannock and R. P. Hill, eds.). Pergamon, New York, 1987, p. 72.
21. Miller, E. C., and Miller, J. A.: *Cancer* **47,** 2327 (1981).
22. Zedeck, M. S.: *J. Environ. Pathol. Toxicol.* **3,** 537 (1980).
23. Arcos, J. C., Woo, Y.-t., Argus, M. F., and Lai, D. Y.: "Chemical Induction of Cancer — Structural Bases and Biological Mechanisms", Vol. IIIA: Aliphatic Carcinogens. Academic Press, New York, 1982.
24. Ames, B. N.: *Science* **204,** 587 (1979).
25. Maher, V. M., and McCormick, J. J.: DNA Repair and Carcinogenesis. *In* "Chemical Carcinogens and DNA" (P. L. Grover, ed.), Vol. II. CRC Press, Boca Raton, Florida, 1979, p. 133.

26. Sukumar, S., Pulciani, S., Doniger, J., Di Paolo, J. A., Evans, C. H., Zbar, B., and Barbacid, M.: *Science* **223**, 1197 (1984).

27. Weinberg, R. A.: *Adv. Cancer Res.* **36**, 149 (1982).

28. Cole, M.: *Annu. Rev. Genet.* **20**, 361 (1987).

29. Archer, M. C.: Chemical Carcinogenesis. *In* "The Basic Science of Oncology" (I. F. Tannock and R. P. Hill, eds.). Pergamon, New York, 1987, p. 89.

30. Belinsky, S. A., and Anderson, M. W.: Activation of the *ras* Proto-oncogene in Rodent Model Systems: Implications for Understanding Mechanisms of Carcinogenicity. *In* "New Horizons in Molecular Toxicology" (G. S. Probst, M. J. Vodicnik, and M. A. Dorato, eds.). Eli Lilly, Indianapolis, Indiana, 1991, p. 9.

31. Bizub, D., Wood, A. W., and Skalka, A. M.: *Proc. Natl. Acad. Sci. U.S.A.* **83**, 6048 (1986).

32. Perantoni, A. O., Rice, J. M., Reed, C. D., Watatami, M., and Wenk, M. I.: *Proc. Natl. Acad. Sci. U.S.A.* **84**, 6317 (1987).

33. Stower, S. J., Maronpot, R. R., Reynolds, S. H., and Anderson, M. W.: *Environ. Health Perspect.* **75**, 81 (1987).

34. Balmain, A., and Brown, K.: *Adv. Cancer Res.* **51**, 147 (1988).

35a. Bonham, K., Embry, T., Gibson, D., Jaffe, D. R., Roberts, R. A., Cress, A. E., and Bowden, G. T.: *Molec. Carcinogenesis* **2**, 34 (1989).

35b. Sukumar, S., Notario, V., Martin-Zanca, V., and Barbacid, M.: *Nature* **306**, 658 (1983).

36. Balmain, A., Ramsden, M., Bowden, G. T., and Smith, J.: *Nature* **307**, 658 (1984).

37. Quintanilla, M., Brown, K., Ramsden, M., and Balmain, A.: *Nature* **322**, 78 (1986).

38. Zarbl, H., Sukumar, S., Arthur, A. V., Martin-Zanca, D., and Barbacid, M.: *Nature* **315**, 382 (1985).

39. Bowden, G. T., and Krieg, P.: *Environ. Health Perspect.* **93**, 51 (1991).

40. Wakelam, M. J. O., Davies, S. A., Houslay, M. D., McKay, I., Marshall, C. J., and Hall, A.: *Nature* **323**, 173 (1986).

41. Chang, E. H., Furth, M. E., Scolnick, E. M., and Lowry, D. R.: *Nature* **297**, 479 (1982).

42. Schimke, R. T.: *Cancer Res.* **44**, 1735 (1984).

43. Gu, W., Bhatia, K., Magrath, I. T., Dang, C. V., and Dalla-Favera, R.: *Science* **264**, 251 (1994).

44. Bhatia, K., Huppi, K., Spangler, G., Siwarski, D., Iyer, R., and Magrath, I.: *Nature Genet.* **5**, 56 (1993).

45. Yano, T., Sander, C. A., Clark, H. M., Dolezal, M. V., Jaffe, E. S., and Raffield, M.: *Oncogene* **8**, 2741 (1993).

46. Land, H., Parada, I. F., and Weinberg, R. A.: *Nature* **304**, 596 (1983).

47. Ruley, H. E.: *Cancer Cells* **2**, 258 (1990).

48. Hirakawa, T., and Ruley, H. E.: *Proc. Natl. Acad. Sci. U.S.A.* **85**, 1519 (1988).

49. Endlich, B., Salarati, R., Sullivan, T., and Ling, C. C.: *Radiat. Res.* **132**, 301 (1992).

50. Bergman, C. I., Hung, M.-C., and Weinberg, R. A.: *Nature* **319**, 226 (1986).

51. Faustman, E. M., and Sweeney, C.: *Toxicol. Appl. Pharmacol.* **128**, 182 (1994).

52. Wechsler, M.: Carcinogenic and Teratogenic Effects of Ethylnitrosourea and Methylnitrosourea During Pregnancy in Experimental Rats. *In* "Transplacental Carcinogenesis" (L. Tomatis and U. Mohr, eds.). IARC, Lyon, France, 1973, p. 127.

53. Krieg, P., Finch, J., Fürstenberger, G., Melber, K., Matrisian, L., and Bowden, G. T.: *Carcinogenesis* **9**, 95 (1988).

54. Dotta, G. P., Parada, L. F., and Weinberg, R. A.: *Nature* **318**, 472 (1985).

55. Brown, K., Quintanilla, M., Ramsden, M., Kerr, I. B., Young, S., and Balmain, A.: *Cell* **46**, 447 (1986).

56. Barbacid, M.: Involvement of *ras* Oncogenes in the Initiation of Carcinogen-Induced Tumors. *In* "Oncogenes and Cancer" (S. A. Aaronson, J. M. Bishop, T. Sugimura, M. Terada, K. Toyoshima, and P. K. Vogt, eds.). Japan Sci. Soc. Press, Tokyo, 1987, p. 43.

57. Sukumar, S.: *Curr. Top. Microbiol. Immunol.* **148**, 93 (1989).

58. Garte, S. J.: *J. Theoret. Biol.* **129**, 177 (1987).

59. Egan, S. E., Wright, J. A., and Greenberg, A. H.: *Environ. Health Perspect.* **93**, 91 (1991).

60. Woo, Y.-t., Lai, D. Y., Arcos, J. C., and Argus, M. F.: "Chemical Induction of Cancer—Structural Bases and Biological Mechanisms", Vol. IIIB: Aliphatic and Polyhalogenated Carcinogens. Academic Press, Orlando, 1985, *in* "Preface".

61. Grosovsky, A. J., de Boer, J. G., de Jong, P. J., Drobetsky, E. A., and Glickman, B. W.: *Proc. Natl. Acad. Sci. U.S.A.* **85**, 185 (1988).

62. Sawey, M. J., Hood, A. T., Burns, F. J., and Garte, S. J.: *Molec. Cell Biol.* **7**, 932 (1987).

63. Lemoine, N. R., Mayall, E. S., Williams, E. D., Thurston, V., and Wyford-Thomas, D.: *Oncogene* **3**, 541 (1988).

64. Merregaert, J., Michiels, L., van der Rauwelaert, E., Lommel, M., Gel-Winkler, R., and Janowski, M.: *Leukemia Res.* **10**, 915 (1986).

65. Jaffe, D. R,. and Bowden, G. T.: *Carcinogenesis* **10**, 2243 (1989).

66. Newcomb, E. W., Diamond, L. E., Sloan, S. R., Carominas, M., Guerrero, I., and Pellicer, A.: *Environ.*

Health Perspect. **81,** 33 (1989).

67. Newcomb, E. W., Steinberg, J. J., and Pellicer, A.: *Cancer Res.* **48,** 5514 (1988).
68. Gumerlock, P. H., Meyers, F. J., Foster, B. A., Kawakami, T. G., and deVere White, R. W.: *Radiat. Res.* **117,** 198 (1989).
69. Sloan, S. R., Newcomb, E. W., and Pellicer, A.: *Molec. Cell. Biol.* **10,** 405 (1990).
70. Ehrfeld, A., Planes-Bohne, F., and Lucke-Huhle, C.: *Radiat. Res.* **108,** 43 (1986).
71. Suzuki, K., Yasuda, N., Suzuki, F., Nikaido, O., and Watanabe, M.: *Int. J. Cancer* **44,** 1057 (1989).
72. Niwa, O., Enoki, Y., and Yokoro, K.: *Jpn. J. Cancer Res.* **80,** 212 (1989).
73. Schon, A., Michiels, L., Janowski, M., Merregaert, J., and Erfle, V.: *Int. J. Cancer* **38,** 67 (1986).
74. van der Rauwelaert, E., Maisin, J. R., and Merregaert, J.: *Oncogene* **2,** 215 (1988).
75. Bandyopadhyay, S. K., D'Andrea, E., and Fleissner, E.: *Oncogene Res.* **4,** 311 (1989).
76. Garte, S. J., Burns, F. J., Ashkenazi-Kimmel, T., Felber, M., and Sawey, M. J.: *Cancer Res.* **50,** 3073 (1990).
77. Garte, S. J., and Burns, F. J.: *Environ. Health Perspect.* **93,** 45 (1991).
78. Lucke-Huhle, C.: *Int. Radiat. Biol.* **65,** 665 (1994).
79. Ananthaswamy, H. N., and Pierceall, W. E.: *Photochem. Photobiol.* **52,** 1119 (1990).
80. Suarez, H. G.: *Anticancer Res.* **9,** 1331 (1989).
81. van der Lubbe, J. L., Rosdorf, H. J., Bos, J. L., and van der Ebb, A. J.: *Oncogene Res.* **3,** 9 (1988).
82. Hollander, M. C., and Fornace, A. J.: *Cancer Res.* **49,** 1687 (1989).
83. Shuin, T., Billings, P. C., Lillehaug, J. R., Patierno, S. R., Roy-Burman, P., and Landolph, J. R.: *Cancer Res.* **46,** 5302 (1986).
84. Klein, G.: *Nature* **294,** 313 (1981).
85. Mulvihill, J. J.: Congenital and Genetic Diseases. *In* "Persons at High Risk of Cancer — An Approach to Cancer Etiology and Control" (J. F. Fraumeni, ed.). Academic Press, New York, 1975, p. 3.
86. Schroeder, T. M.: Chromosome Instability and Malignancy. *In* ' "Chemical and Viral Oncogenesis", Vol. 2 (P. Bucalossi, U. Veronesi, and N. Cascinelli, eds.). Proc. 9th Int. Cancer Congr. Excerpta Medica, Amsterdam, 1975, p. 62.
87. Davidson, R. G.: General Principles of Medical Genetics. *In* "The Merck Manual", 16th ed. (R. Berkow, editor-in-chief). Merck Res. Labs., Rahway, New Jersey, 1992, p. 2285, *see* "Genetics of Malignant Disease" and "Population Genetics".
88. Paterson, M. C.: Heritable Cancer-Prone Disorders Featuring Carcinogen Hypersensitivity and DNA Repair Deficiency. *In* "Host Factors in Carcinogenesis" (H. Bartsch and B. Armstrong, eds.). IARC Sci. Publ. No. 39. IARC, Lyon, France, 1992, p. 57.
89. Taylor, A. M. R., and Edwards, M. J.: Malignancy, DNA Damage, and Chromosomal Aberrations in Ataxia Telangiectasia. *In* "Host Factors in Carcinogenesis" (H. Bartsch and B. Armstrong, eds.), IARC Sci. Publ. No. 39. IARC, Lyon, France, 1982, p. 119.
90. Schroeder, T. M., and Kurth, R.: *Blood* **37,** 96 (1971).
91. Gmyrek, D., and Syllm-Rappaport, A.: *Kinderheilkunde* **91,** 297 (1964).
92. "The Merck Manual", 16th ed. (R. Berkow, editor-in-chief). Merck Res. Lab., Rahway, New Jersey, 1992: "Hematology and Oncology", *see* "Hypoplastic (Aplastic) Anemias", p. 1153.
93. German, J.: *Am. J. Human Genet.* **22,** 196 (1969).
94. "The Merck Manual", 16th ed. (R. Berkow, editor-in-chief). Merck Res. Lab., Rahway, New Jersey, 1992: "Immunology–Allergic Disorders", *see* "Specific Immunodeficiencies", p. 313.
95. Schüller, H.: *Biochem. Pharmacol.* **42,** 1511 (1991).
96. Simon, M. I., Strathman, M. P., and Gautam, N.: *Science* **252,** 802 (1991).
97. Oliveira, L., Paiva, A. C. M., Sander, C., and Vriend, G.: *Trends Pharmacol. Sci.* **15,** 170 (1994).
98. Adhya, S., and Garges, S.: *J. Biol. Chem.* **265,** 1079 (1990).
99. Monod, J., Changeux, J. F., and Jacob, F.: *J. Molec. Biol.* **6,** 306 (1963).
100. Hammes, G. G., and Wu, C.-W.: *Science* **172,** 1205 (1971).
101. Perutz, M. F.: "Mechanisms of Cooperativity and Allosteric Regulation in Proteins". Cambridge Univ. Press, New York, 1990.
102. Wroblewski, J. T., Fadde, E., Mazzetta, J., Lazarewicz, J. W., and Costa, E.: *Neuropharmacology* **28,** 447 (1989).
103. Jasmin, C., Allouche, M., Le Bousse-Kerdiles, C., Smadja-Joffe, F., Krief, P., Georgoulias, V., and Boucheix, C.: *Leukemia Res.* **14,** 695 (1990).
104. Birnbaumer, L., Abramowitz, J., and Brown, A. M.: *Biochim. Biophys. Acta* **1031,** 163 (1990).
105. Farrar, W. L., Brini, A. T., Harel-Bellan, A., Korner, M., and Ferris, D. K.: *Immunol. Ser.* **49,** 379 (1990).
106. Irvine, R. F.: *FEBS Lett.* **263,** 5 (1990).
107. MacDonald, M. J.: *Diabetes* **39,** 19461 (1990).
108. Theroux, S. J., Stanley, K., Campbell, D. A., and Davis, R. J.: *Molec. Endocrinol.* **6,** 1849 (1992).
109. Johnson, L. N.: *FASEB J.* **6,** 2274 (1992).

110. Shoelson, S. E., Sivaraja, M., Williams, P., Hu, P., and Schlessinger, J.: *EMBO J.* **12,** 795 (1993).
111. Du, X., Gu, M., Weisel, J. W., Nagaswami, C., Bennett, C. S., Bowditch, R., and Ginsberg, M. H.: *J. Biol. Chem.* **268,** 23087 (1993).
112. Herskovits, J. S., Shpetner, H. S., Burgess, C. C., and Vallee, R. B.: *Proc. Natl. Acad. Sci. U.S.A.* **90,** 11468 (1993).
113. Samama, P., Pei, G., Costa, T., Cotecchia, S., and Lefkowitz, R. J.: *Molec. Pharmacol.* **45,** 390 (1994).
114. Lee, J., and Pilch, P. F.: *Am. J. Physiol.* **266** (2, Pt.1), C319 (1994).
115. Smith, J. L., Zaluzec, E. J., Wey, J.-P., Niu, L., Switzer, R. L., Zalkin, H., and Satow, Y.: *Science* **264,** 1427 (1994).
116. Hunter, T.: *Cell* **50,** 823 (1987).
117. Pelech, S. L., Sanghera, J. S., and Daya-Makin, M.: *Biochem. Cell. Biol.* **68,** 1297 (1990).
118. Pace, C. N.: Conformational Stability of Globular Proteins. *In* "Proteins: Form and Function" (R. A. Bradshaw and M. Burton, eds.). Elsevier Trends Journals publ., Cambridge, UK, 1990, p. 117.
119. Crile, G., Jr.: *J. Natl. Cancer Inst.* **20,** 229 (1958).
120. Snell, K. C., Stewart, H. L., and Morris, H. P.: *Gann Monogr. No.* **8,** 125 (1969).
121. Stewart, H. L.: Comparison of Sites of Multiple Neoplastic and Atrophic Lesions Induced by Carcinogenic Hydrocarbons and Fluorenylamine Compounds. *In* "Multiple Primary Malignant Tumours" (L. Severi, ed.), 5th Perugia Quadrennial Int. Conf. Cancer. Perugia Univ. Med. Sch., Div. Cancer Res. publ., Perugia, Italy, 1973, p. 947.
122. Tilly, B. C., van den Berghe, N., Tertoolen, L. G. J., Edixhoven, M. J., and de Jonge, H. R.: *J. Biol. Chem.* **268,** 19919 (1993).
123. Galcheva-Gargova, Z., Dérijard, B., Wu, I.-H., and Davis, R. J.: *Science* **265,** 806 (1994).
124. Brewster, J. L., de Valoir, T., Dwyer, N. D., Winter, E., and Gustin, M. C.: *Science* **259,** 1760 (1993).
125. Watson, P. A.: *FASEB J.* **5,** 2013 (1991).
126. Dérijard, B., Hibi, M., Wu, I. H., Barrett, T., Su, B., Deng, T., Karin, M., and Davis, R. J.: *Cell* **76,** 1025 (1994).
127. Hibi, M., Liu, A., Smeal, T., Minden, A., and Karin, M.: *Genes Dev.* **7,** 2135 (1993).
128. Dall'Asta, V., Rossi, P. A., Bussolati, O., and Garzola, G. C.: *J. Biol. Chem.* **269,** 10485 (1994).
129. Paredes, A., McManus, M., Kwon, H. M., and Stronge, K.: *Am. J. Physiol.* **263,** C1282 (1992).
130. Han, J., Lee, J.-D., Bibbs, L., and Ulevitch, R. J.: *Science* **265,** 808 (1994).
131. Davis, J. R.: *J. Biol. Chem.* **268,** 14553 (1993).
132. Lange-Carter, C. A., Pleiman, C. M., Gardner, A. M., Blumer, K. J., and Johnson, G. L.: *Science* **260,** 315 (1993).
133. Nishida, E., and Gotoh, Y.: *Trends Biochem. Sci.* **18,** 128 (1993).
134. Chamberlin, M. E., and Strange, K.: *Am. J. Physiol.* **257,** 159 (1989).
135. Arcos, J. C., and Argus, M. F.: "Chemical Induction of Cancer", Vol. I. Academic Press, New York, 1968, *in* Sect. 3.4.4.
136. Anderson, C. F., and Bauer, W.: *Biochemistry* **17,** 594 (1978).
137. Bednar, J., Furrer, P., Stasiak, A., Dubochet, J., Engelman, E. H., and Bates, A. D.: *J. Molec. Biol.* **235,** 825 (1994).
138. Schlick, T., Li, B., and Olson, W. K.: *Biophys. J.* **67,** 2146 (1994).

Molecular Biology of Virally-Induced Cell Transformation and Tumorigenesis[1]

Lawrence R. Boone, K. Gregory Moore, William C. Phelps, and Yin-tak Woo*

Following the introductory discussion in Section I of the general characteristics of tumor viruses, this section endeavors to provide a systematic overview of the molecular biology of viral carcinogenesis. However, before coming to specific examples of RNA or DNA tumor viruses we will review some of the important methodological and conceptual tools to provide a framework for understanding many of the aspects discussed in the subsections on the tumor viruses. Thus, the section begins with a discussion of the assay systems for cell transformation and oncogenesis and of the properties of transformed cells (in subsection I). This is followed (in subsection II) by an illustrative, systematic review of the vast area of the signal transduction network which functions principally in the cytoplasm in eukaryotic cells. Although in many cases the oncogenic property of a virally-transduced gene may have provided the first insight into, and experimental handle on, the functions of various components of this highly complex network, we have chosen to outline normal function first. In subsection III we discuss and exemplify the tumor-suppressor genes, a number of which play key roles in the control of normal cell cycling and the regulation of cell proliferation.

After these brief reviews of experimental approaches toward and concepts of the intricate biochemical systems that control normal cell proliferation and differentiation, we discuss specific examples of oncogenic RNA and DNA viruses in animals and humans. Perhaps the most important lesson that can be learned from the examples is that viruses can subvert the normal control of cell proliferation in about as many different ways as there are different components and connections in the signal transducing network and in other cellular regulatory pathways. The study of transformation by viruses has clearly been of great value in the larger effort of trying to understand the mechanisms responsible for both neoplasia and normal cell proliferation. From early studies with oncogenic viruses—primarily with the Rous sarcoma virus and the polyomavirus—the important concept emerged that one or a small number of genes could be responsible for the neoplastic transformation. Thus, it was principally through the study of RNA and DNA viruses that theories on the mechanisms of carcinogenesis evolved ultimately to the gene level.

One of the striking differences between RNA and DNA tumor viruses lies in their

---

[1]For the Abbreviations Used see p. 594.
*The four authors have contributed equally to this section.

oncogene-mediated mechanisms for bringing about cell transformation/oncogenesis. The RNA tumor viruses induce cell transformation most frequently through dominant transforming genes carried by the virus. In contrast, many of the DNA tumor viruses rely on interference with tumor-suppressor genes. Although there are several exceptions, the mechanisms of transformation by these two virus groups can be roughly divided on this basis. Another important difference (as we have seen in Section I) is that DNA viral oncogenes are genuine viral genes which express proteins with essential roles in the viral life cycle but which are also transforming toward the host cell. In contrast, the oncogenes of transducing retroviruses are alien to the virus and express proteins that are transforming but play no role in viral replication. The examples described in subsections IV and V will provide a sense of the interesting and important virological aspects and put in focus the critical connections with the mechanisms of the induction of cancer by nonviral oncogene activators reviewed in some detail in Section I.

I. ASSAYS FOR CELL TRANSFORMATION AND ONCOGENESIS; PROPERTIES OF THE TRANSFORMED CELL

To supplement the conventional two-year bioassays for carcinogenesis, a number of *in vitro* assays for cell transformation and specialized *in vivo* assays for oncogenesis have been developed for rapid screening as well as for mechanistic studies with chemical carcinogens. These assays have also played and continue to maintain a pivotal role in the discovery of and studies on viral oncogenes and cellular proto-oncogenes.

A. *In vitro* Assays for Cell Transformation

In vitro assays use cultured primary organ cells or established cell lines (*see* definition below) to detect cell transformation which results from treatment with chemicals or from introduction of oncogenic DNA into cells. These assays are inexpensive and can be done within a short period of time. The cell transformation assay is the only *in vitro* assay that directly scores for malignant transformation, rather than for mutagenesis. The assay has been used as a model for studying multistage carcinogenesis; under appropriate conditions, it can be used to detect genotoxic as well as epigenetic carcinogens.

1. *Properties of Cultured Cells: Cell Strains, Established Cell Lines, and Transformed Cells*

There are two main types of cultured cells used in *in vitro* cell transformation assays: *cell strains* and established *cell lines* (1–3). Their respective properties are summarized below along with a description of the properties of transformed cells.

Cell strains are cultured cells with a finite life span. They are usually obtained directly from animals and cultured for a few cell divisions or generations (primary cultures). Typically, they can only live, grow, and divide for several generations (up to about 50 doublings for fetal fibroblasts, but considerably fewer for adult cells) and then die even if provided with fresh nutrients, growth factors, or serum (this is the phenomenon known as *cell senescence*). Phenotypically, these cells appear "normal" and resemble the cells of their origin anatomically and functionally. They normally grow to a particular density and then stop; growth may be resumed following proper dilution. Cultured fibroblasts grow in a monolayer and stop growing when the cells are in contact (the phenomenon known as *contact inhibition*). Cytogenetically, the cells tend to maintain normal diploid chromosome complement and remain homogeneous until they die or undergo transformation. The main disadvantages of primary cultures are the difficulties of growing cell cultures, high variability, and low sensitivity.

Cell lines are cultured cells that escape cell senescence and become *immortalized;* this means that they do not die and can be maintained indefinitely in culture. The most commonly used cell lines include BALB/c 3T3, C3H 10T½, and mouse prostate cells (1). Although not totally "normal" [because immortalization involves some mutational event(s)], they still retain most of the normal cell characteristics, such a contact inhibition and inability to induce tumor when injected into syngeneic animals. Cell lines, such as BALB/c 3T3, can be easily transformed by chemicals, viral infection, or introduction of tumor DNA.

The properties of transformed cells may change progressively with time. This is consistent with the multistage nature of the process leading to malignancy. They are usually phenotypically abnormal, do not resemble the cells from which they originate, and may be heterogeneous among themselves (*pleomorphism*). They grow in a nonordered way, tend to have lost their ability to respond to contact inhibition, and, therefore, may pile up and can be seen as foci/colonies. Transformed cells also display significantly reduced requirements for serum and reduced anchorage-dependence for growth. They undergo a variety of structural and morphologial changes affecting the cytoskeleton (as indicated by a loss of stress fibers, and rearrangement of actin bundles and microfilaments), the cell surface (as indicated by the acquired ability to be agglutinated by plant lectins) and their extracellular matrix (*cf.* 4). Cytogenetically, they tend to be aneuploid often with rearranged or altered chromosomes. Single transformed cells can be cloned in soft agar, where they can grow and divide to form a discrete colony. Transformed cells, when injected into syngeneic or immunosuppressed nonsyngeneic animals, are capable of inducing tumors.

2. Basic Methodology of in vitro *Cell Transformation Assays*

In vitro cell transformation assays may use cells with a finite life span [*e.g.,* Syrian hamster embryo (SHE) cells], some established cell lines (e.g., BALB/c 3T3 cells), or cells containing latent tumor virus (1). In a typical procedure (*see* ref. 5) using BALB/c 3T3 cells, a series of 25 cm^2 flasks seeded with 10^4 cells per flask are incubated for 24 hours and then treated with the test substance, the positive control (usually 3-methylcholanthrene), or the negative control (solvent) and then incubated for a 3-day exposure period. Cells are then washed and further incubated for 4 weeks with refeeding twice a week. The assay should be terminated by fixing the cell monolayers with methanol and staining with Giemsa. When examined by eye or low power microscope, normal cells yield a uniformly stained monolayer of round, closely-packed cells, whereas transformed cells form a dense mass (focus or colony) that stains deeply and is superimposed on the surrounding monolayer of normal cells. Although not routinely done, most transformed clones when collected from unstained transformation plate and injected into syngeneic host animals will produce malignant tumors.

3. Study of Tumor Viruses Using Cell Transformation Assays

In vitro cell transformation assays have played a pivotal role in detecting many tumor viruses, in particular in the hepadna, papilloma, papova B, adeno, herpes, and retrovirus families (6). In most of these studies, normal cells (usually fibroblasts) are infected with a tumor virus under conditions which do not result in lysis of all the cells. Some of the surviving cells may undergo viral transformation giving rise to transformed cells which proliferate and pile up to form identifiable foci/colonies. Transformed cells can then be harvested from these foci. Injection of such transformed cells into adult animals of the appropriate syngeneic background can lead to formation of transplantable tumors. The ability of transformed cells to grow to transplantable tumor (to "take") is the confirmation that the foci contain malignant cells. *In vitro* cell transformation is also a crucial assay for the study of human tumor viruses, which cannot ethically be evaluated by *in vivo* tests. Instead, transformed human cells can be tested for tumor induction in susceptible experimental animals, such as the immune-deficient athymic "nude mice" (*see* below).

4. Cell Transformation in DNA Transfection Assays

Besides detecting tumor viruses by viral infection, *in vitro* cell transformation assays are also crucial for the discovery of new viral and cellular oncogenes through transfection experiments. Transfection is the technique of introducing naked DNA into intact cells. When DNA is mixed in a buffer containing calcium phosphate/chloride and applied to cultured cells in precipitated form, by some as yet unknown mechanism cells become receptive to uptake of the foreign DNA. The technique has wide applicability for both prokaryotic and eukaryotic cells. If the DNA contains viral or cellular oncogenes, cell transformation may ensue. When the transfection technique was used, it was possible to transform BALB/c 3T3 cells to a malignant phenotype with DNA from a variety of histological types of human tumors. However, the transfection assay is often quite variable and sometimes inconsistently reproducible (7). With the advancement in gene splicing and cloning techniques, however, more effective transformation is now possible by transfecting with cloned viral or cellular oncogenic DNA. Like *in vivo* assays, *in vitro* cell transformation assay is also useful for demonstrating "oncogene collaboration"—the synergistic action of two or more specific oncogenes to transform cells (*see* Sect. I). If normal rat embryo fibroblasts are transfected with a *ras* oncogene or *myc* oncogene alone, complete transformation does not occur. Transfection with both oncogenes, together, is needed in most instances in order to successfully transform primary or secondary cultured cells (3).

5. Use of the Cell Transformation Assay for Screening Potentially Carcinogenic Chemical Agents

In vitro cell transformation assays have been extensively used in screening for potential carcinogens and tumorigenesis promoters. The cell systems used include: (i) primary and secondary cultures of Syrian hamster embryo (SHE) cells; (ii) established BALB/c 3T3, C3H 10T½, and mouse prostate cell lines; and (iii) cultured cells with latent tumor virus (*e.g.,* rat embryo cells with RLV leukemia retrovirus, SHE cells with simian adenovirus SA7, mouse embryo cells with AKR leukemia virus) that can be activated by chemical agents to induce viral transformation. The detailed protocols, advantages/disadvantages, and test performance of each of these systems have been reviewed and evaluated under the Gene-Tox Program of the U.S. Environmental Protection Agency. In general, there is a reasonably good correlation between the results of the cell transformation assay and *in vivo* carcinogenesis bioassay (3).

B. Specialized *in vivo* Assays for Oncogenesis

For studying the multifactorial nature of oncogenesis, conventional long-term bioassays and *in vitro* assays are of limited usefulness. During the past decade, two specialized *in vivo* assays — the "nude mice" and "transgenic mice" — have emerged as powerful research tools for mechanistic and *in vivo* multifactorial interaction studies as well as for developing predictive assays and therapeutic/preventive strategies.

1. The "Nude Mice" Assay

The "nude mice" are a special (hairless) strain of mice which lack thymus and therefore do not have mature T lymphocytes and functional cellular immunity (*see* ref. 2). The immune deficiency impairs the ability of the mice to reject xenografts, making them ideal subjects for transplantation studies. When nude mice are used, tumor cells from human or other animal species, chemically- or virally-transformed cells can all be tested for their ability to produce tumors *in vivo* (without the complication of foreign-body rejection by the animal). The impaired immune system also makes the nude mice more susceptible to chemical carcinogenesis, because of the lack of immune surveillance. In addition, the lack of animal hair in nude mice offers an advantage for dermal bioassays, because their dermal absorption characteristics better approximate the human skin.

2. The Transgenic Mice Assay

Transgenic mice are genetically manipulated mice which carry engineered genes permanently inserted into their germ line or stem cells. By inserting activated oncogene(s) or "knocking out" tumor-suppressor gene(s), specialized cancer-prone transgenic mice have been developed. These mice have provided invaluable means for studying the role of specific genetic alterations as predisposing factors for chemical carcinogenesis (the multistage process) and for developing improved methods for risk assessment.

a. *Basic Principles/Methodology in Making Transgenic Mice*   The methodology for constructing transgenic mice has been described in many publications (3, 8–10). Essentially, there are two main techniques: zygote injection and gene targeting. Zygote injection involves microinjection or transfection of DNA into a pronucleus of zygotes. The subsequent homologous or nonhomologous recombination incorporates the foreign DNA into the host genome as an inheritable trait. The DNA introduced into a germ line usually consists of the intended gene(s) together with promoter sequence(s) which can regulate the expression of the inserted gene(s). For example, by constructing a DNA fragment containing the intended oncogene together with a promoter sequence for immunoglobulin heavy chain ($E\mu$) gene, the oncogene will be expressed only in lymphoid cells of transgenic mice.

For construction of transgenic mice with specific alterations of certain endogeneous genes (*e.g.,* knocking out a tumor-suppressor gene), gene targeting is the preferred technique. Gene targeting involves the insertion of a DNA fragment that contains an intended mutant gene (*e.g.,* mutated *p53* gene) into a retroviral vector, and introducing therewith the retrovirus-carried DNA into a special line of embryo-derived mouse stem cells (ES cells). After a period of cell proliferation, the rare colonies of ES cells, in which a homologous recombination with gene replacement did take place, are isolated by selection techniques and injected into an early mouse embryo to produce transgenic mice with specifically altered endogenous genes. Through crossbreeding, transgenic mice with multiple altered genes can be constructed to study the role of oncogene synergy.

   b.   Transgenic Models of Tumor Development   Transgenic mice allow definitive tests of the role of a candidate oncogene or tumor-suppressor gene in the induction of specific type of tumors and in contributing to a specific a step in the multistage carcinogenesis process. With the use of transgenic mice, over two dozen tumor types (*e.g.,* mammary tumors using *myc, ras, erb*-B2, or *int* transgene and liver tumors using *HBV* or *myc* transgene) have been modeled (11). The approximately 30 transgenes thus far used encode representatives from each major class of proteins implicated in neoplasia including: growth factors (TGF-α, Wnt-1, Int-2), cytokine receptors (Erb-B2, Ret), signal-transducer proteins (Ras, Pim-1, Abl, Fps, Lck), a cytoplasmic protein for cell survival (Bcl-2), and nuclear proteins that serve as transcription factors or regulators of cell replication (Myc, Fos, Jun, p53). These studies made significant contributions to the understanding of the mechanisms of oncogenesis.

   Transgenic mice have also been used to test for synergism/cooperativity between/ among oncogenes and for the interaction(s) of oncogene(s) with other exogenous/ endogenous factors, in order to widen our understanding of the multifactorial, multistage nature of carcinogenesis. With the use of transgenic cross-breeding to construct transgenic mice with two or more activated oncogenes, or by retroviral delivery of a second oncogene to transgenic mice already carrying one activated oncogene, *in vivo* oncogene cooperativity has been demonstrated (11). The Myc nuclear oncoprotein has been shown to collaborate with cytoplasmic oncoproteins (H-Ras, N-Ras, K-Ras, v-Abl, v-Raf, Bcl-2, and Pim-1) as well as with nuclear T antigen and Bmi-1. The mechanism of collaboration remains to be elucidated. Based on complementary functions, perhaps related to distinctly separate signal transduction pathways, at least three different complementary groups — represented by the protein products of *myc* for cell self-renewal, of *bcl-2* for prevention of cell death, and of *ras/raf* for relieving growth factor requirement — have been identified.

   The effect of genetic background on the expression of cancer-prone gene in transgenic mice has been studied using the Eμ-*myc* construct. The transgene favored the induction of B lymphomas in C57BL/6 mice, but T lymphomas in C3H/HeJ mice (11). The synergistic interaction between aflatoxins and the *HBV* gene carried by transgenic mice is discussed in Section III of this Chapter. Studies on possible interaction between other chemical carcinogens and oncogenes in transgenic mice have also been reported (9).

   c.   Transgenic Mice in Tests of Potential Carcinogens, for Exploring Therapeutic Strategies, and Risk Assessment   Transgenic mice with activated oncogene and/or mutated tumor-suppressor gene are highly predisposed to carcinogenesis, rendering them potentially useful as a sensitive test system for potential carcinogens. Several transgenic strains have demonstrated heightened sensitivity to specific classes of carcinogens: *pim-1* mice to lymphoma induction by nitrosourea, *HBV* mice to liver carcinogens, and H2K-*fos* mice to skin carcinogens (11). However, their utility for general carcinogen identification remains to be evaluated. As pointed out by Tennant *et al.* (12), because constitutively expressed transgenic oncogenes often result in elevated levels of spontaneous tumorigenesis, only highly potent carcinogens can possibly produce demonstrable increases of the incidence or acceleration of the onset of tumors. Transgenic mice with gene(s) commonly involved in human tumors (*e.g., p53, myc, ras*) but with relatively low spontaneous incidence should be selected for carcinogen screening.

   Cancer-prone transgenic mice should prove to be highly useful for exploring therapeutic strategies. For example, retinoic acid has been shown to inhibit the induction of skin papilloma in transgenic H-*ras* mice (13). Chemopreventive agents can be tested to counter the anticipated action of activated oncogene(s) or mutated/deleted tumor-suppressor gene(s). Such studies should provide invaluable insights toward the design of therapeutic or preventive measures for individuals carrying genes predisposing to cancer.

Two specialized strains (Big Blue™, Muta™Mouse) of transgenic mice have recently been commercially developed for measuring *in vivo* mutations as a result of exposure to chemicals (10). These animal models involve insertion of the *Escherichia coli lac I* (lac repressor) and *lac Z* (β-galactosidase) genes into the mouse genome, in the germ line or in embryonic stem cells. These bacterial genes are then present in the mouse genomic DNA in all tissues and serve as targets for *in vivo* mutation. Following *in vivo* exposure to genotoxic chemicals, the bacterial target genes can be isolated from various tissues and evaluated for mutation. These animal models should render accessible an improved accuracy of measurements of the internal dosage of carcinogens, which is useful for more realistic risk assessment. Transgenic animals can also be used to study the role of indirect/secondary mutations in response to exposure to nongenotoxic chemicals and would, thus, provide mechanistic insights.

II. SIGNAL TRANSDUCTION CASCADES: NON-DNA TARGETS OF VIRAL EFFECTORS

Many extracellular ligands are unable to effectively enter the cell and they act through high affinity binding to their specific transmembrane receptors. These receptors—which comprise an extracellular ligand-binding domain, a transmembrane segment, and a cytoplasmic effector domain—are initiating components of signal transduction pathways (revs. 14–18, *see also* Chap. 11, Section I). Other ligands, such as steroids and retinoids, can easily pass through the plasma membrane and bind to receptors in the cytoplasm and nucleus, respectively. Such ligands, which bind to intracellular receptors, tend to act upon the cellular signalling pathways at later points. The signal transduction pathways of both types of receptors may follow branched routes that either cross over into other signalling cascades, feed back into earlier points in the same pathway, or directly funnel to the nucleus. This subsection focuses predominantly on pathways of signal transduction in mammalian cells initiated at transmembrane receptors, pathways that are non-DNA targets of viral effectors in cell transformation/oncogenesis. In view of the enormous complexity of the signal transduction network, the intent of the subsection is merely to *illustrate* the complexity and to provide a perspective by exemplifying some of its more extensively studied transducer protein components and their interactions. The subsection does not specifically cover proto-oncogenes, that are gene targets of certain viral effectors by *cis*-activation; this topic is touched upon in Section I above as well as here in this Section under "IV. Retroviral Oncogenes . . ." in G. Neither does this subsection aim to cover genes or transcription factors which may be targets of gene products of *trans*-activating retroviruses.

The two major categories of extracellular ligands that bind to transmembrane receptors are growth factors [*e.g.,* epidermal growth factor (EGF) and platelet-derived growth factor (PDGF)] and cytokines [*e.g.,* the various interferons and interleukins (ILs)]. Many mammalian cellular signalling pathways are shared by different receptors; it is currently unknown how precise specificity is achieved leading to the transcription of specific sets of genes (*rev.* 14–19). An early event appears to be the rapid stimulation of tyrosine kinase activity, which is associated with the activation of transmembrane receptors, followed by phospholipid hydrolysis, and linked to a common signalling pathway resulting in the activation of Ras. Activated Ras induces sequential cascading activation of several tiers of serine/threonine kinases belonging to the mitogen-activated protein kinase (MAPK) family (*rev.* 20, 21).

Signalling pathways diverge in the nucleus with the stimulation of specific transcription factors such as c-Myc and c-Jun (*rev.* 20–22). The transcription of a few general response genes (*i.e., c-fos*) is stimulated by the binding of diverse ligands to their receptors, but the transcription of numerous genes is stimulated only by the binding of a specific ligand to its receptor. Some of the genes the transcription of which is initiated by the binding of ligands to transmembrane receptors are proto-oncogenes (*rev.* 23). As was discussed briefly in Section I in this chapter, proto-oncogenes are normal cellular genes often involved in growth and development. Proto-oncogenes were probably evolutionarily acquired from primordial genes. This ontogeny possibly accounts for the fact that the transcription of proto-oncogenes and control of their corresponding products are tightly regulated in mammalian cells.

A. Transmembrane Receptors and Protein Tyrosine Kinase Activity

Transmembrane receptors tend to fall into two basic groups: (i) receptors that contain an intracellular protein tyrosine kinase (PTK) domain that becomes activated after binding of its ligand, and (ii) receptors which do not contain an intracellular PTK domain but which must interact with and activate cytoplasmic tyrosine kinases after binding of its ligand (*rev.* 14–19). Many growth factor receptors contain a PTK domain while many cytokine receptors do not contain a PTK domain and require cytoplasmic tyrosine kinases (*e.g.,* the JAK or Src family kinases) for their intracellular signalling. The key role that tyrosine kinase activity plays in cellular signalling pathways has been demonstrated by the use of tyrosine kinase-deficient mutant cells; the transmembrane receptors of these are able to bind ligands but are unable to signal to the nucleus. Phosphorylation of tyrosine residues on proteins is a highly-regulated short-lived process. Specific cellular tyrosine phosphatases exist that can rapidly remove the phosphate group from tyrosine residues in activated receptors and in signalling proteins, reverting them in most cases to an inactive form.

The activation of transmembrane receptors brought about by ligand binding frequently involves receptor dimerization (*rev.* 14–17). Such dimerization may involve identical receptors or, in some cases, different related receptors. Receptor dimerization usually brings into close proximity two PTK domains which transphosphorylate specific intracellular tyrosine residues on each receptor. These short-lived phosphorylated tyrosine residues serve as the recognition sites of an activated receptor and are bound by cytoplasmic signalling proteins containing Src-homology 2 (SH2) domains (24, 25). An example is shown in Fig. 1 with the activated PDGF receptor. Signalling proteins that contain SH2 domains are often phosphorylated after binding to the activated receptor. Alternatively, activated receptors containing PTK domains may directly phosphorylate specific intracellular proteins that do not contain SH2 domains. For example, the EGF receptor can directly phosphorylate cytoplasmic proteins such as annexin I (*rev.* 14). Some activated receptors do not bind to multiple signalling proteins, however. For example, the phosphorylated insulin receptor binds the insulin receptor substrate 1 (IRS1), but other signalling proteins do not appear to bind to the activated insulin receptor (*rev.* 26). Phosphorylated IRS1 serves as the major agent of insulin receptor-mediated signal transduction by becoming bound to numerous cytoplasmic signalling proteins containing SH2 domains. Receptors that do not possess intrinsic PTK domains also often dimerize and indirectly promote phosphorylation of the tyrosine kinases needed by them to transduce their signal to the nucleus (*rev.* 18, 19).

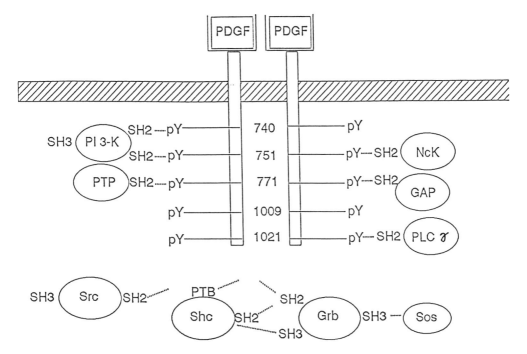

FIGURE 1. Interaction of cellular signalling proteins with the activated PDGF receptor. Occupied PDGF receptors dimerize and become phosphorylated on tyrosine residues 740, 751, 771, 1009, and 1021. The phosphorylated PDGF receptors are specifically bound at the phosphotyrosine residues by signalling proteins possessing SH2 domains and PTB domains. Another means of interaction between cellular signalling proteins is mediated by the SH3 domains of the proteins. The interaction between phosphotyrosine residues and SH2 domains as well as the interaction between SH3 domains and proline-rich sequences in signalling proteins is shown by dotted lines. Most of the information contained in this figure is derived from M. Joly, A. Kazlauskas, F. S. Fay, and S. Corvera [*Science* **263**, 684 (1994)] and W. M. Kavanaugh and L. T. Williams [*Science* **266**, 1862 (1994)].

B. "Signalling Motifs": The Functional Domains in Proteins That Enact Signal Transduction

Three signalling motifs have been identified that allow proteins involved in signal transduction to interact: the SH2 domain (24, 25) and the phosphotyrosine-binding (PTB) domain (27), both of which specifically bind phosphotyrosine and adjacent residues in signalling proteins, and the SH3 domain which specifically binds proline-rich sequences in signalling proteins (*rev.* 28–30). The SH2 domains and the SH3 domains, which are found in many cytoplasmic signalling proteins, are non-catalytic regions of roughly 100 and 70 amino acids, respectively, that share strong homology with similar domains in v-Src, the product of the *src* gene of Rous sarcoma virus. Numerous proteins involved in signal transduction use SH2 domains to interact with other signalling proteins containing phosphorylated tyrosine residues, such as the Src family of tyrosine kinases, phosphatidylinositol (PI) 3-kinase, growth-factor-receptor-bound protein 2 (Grb 2), IRS1, and Shc proteins (24, 25, *rev.* 15–19).

Another motif, used by signalling proteins to bind phosphotyrosine residues associated with activated transmembrane receptors, has recently been described (14). The PTB domain, containing roughly 186 amino acid residues, has thus far been identified in Shc and Sck. The latter, Sck, is a protein of unknown function. The Shc proteins have been implicated in signalling through Ras by interaction with Grb2 and with Son of Sevenless protein (Sos). By alternate splicing, the *shc* gene encodes 46 kDa, 52 kDa, and 62 kDa proteins which are tyrosine phosphorylated in response to the binding of several growth factors to their receptors. Some of the Src family tyrosine kinases have been shown to phosphorylate Shc proteins. The SH2 domain is at the carboxy terminal region in the Shc proteins; this domain binds to activated receptors. The middle region of the Shc proteins contains a binding site for the Grb2 transporter protein. The amino terminal region of Shc contains the phosphotyrosine phosphatase (PTP) domain which, after stimulation of cells with growth factors, binds to certain tyrosine phosphorylated proteins collectively known as pp145 (a group of proteins of unknown function but which are also phosphorylated after growth factor treatment). The pp145 proteins can not be effectively dephosphorylated when complexed to Shc proteins, suggesting that pp145 binding to the PTB domain of Shc proteins protects their phosphotyrosine residues from tyrosine phosphatase action.

The SH3 domain of proteins mediate protein-protein interactions through binding to proline-rich sequences, interactions that are important in signal transduction (*rev. 28–30*). Two types of consensus sequences that bind to SH3 regions have been identified: (i) one type that binds to the consensus sequence

Arg-X-Leu-Pro-Pro-Z-Pro

(where Z = Leu for Src SH3; Z = Arg for PI 3-kinase SH3; and X = any amino acid), and (ii) another type that binds to the consensus sequence

X-Pro-Pro-Leu-Pro-X-Arg.

The stabilization of the complex between a protein containing an SH3 domain and a protein containing a specific proline-rich sequence is mainly achieved by hydrophobic interactions and involves the formation of a polyproline helix in the latter protein.

Numerous proteins involved in signal transduction use SH3 domains for protein-protein interactions such as the Src family of tyrosine kinases, PI 3-kinase, Grb2, Sos, Csk, phospholipase C (PLC) gamma, and Nck. The SH2 domain and the SH3 domain in a protein may act synergistically to transduce cellular signals. For example, the SH2 domains and SH3 domains of Grb2 and PLC gamma work in concert to link the activated receptor and its associated protein tyrosine kinase activity to the Ras signal transduction pathway and phosphatidylinositol hydrolysis, respectively (*rev. 28, 30, 31*).

C. Phosphatidylinositol-Associated Intracellular Signalling Pathways

Phosphatidylinositol (PI) metabolism has been associated with the intracellular signalling of many different transmembrane receptors and may play an important role in mitogenesis induced by growth factors (32–35, *rev.* 31, 36–40). Two enzymes, well characterized by driving PI signalling pathways, are PI 3-kinase (32–34, *rev.* 36, 37, 40) and PI-specific PLC (*rev.* 38, 39). After treatment of cells with growth factors (such as EGF or PDGF), PI 3-kinase phosphorylates PI and phosphorylated forms of PI (at the D3 position of its inositol ring), and there is rapid accumulation of PI 3-phosphate, PI 3,4-diphosphate, and PI 3,4,5-triphosphate. The function of the phosphorylated forms of PI in signal transduction is still unclear and may be involved in an as yet uncharacterized signal transduction pathway.

PI 3-kinase is a dimer composed of an 85 kDa subunit and a 110 kDa subunit. At least three genes (alpha, beta, and gamma) are known to encode the 85 kDa subunit which has no catalytic activity and is thought to regulate the kinase activity of the 110 kDa catalytic subunit. Two SH2 domains, located at the carboxy terminus of the 85 kDa subunit, have been shown to bind to tyrosine-phosphorylated receptors and intracellular proteins. The amino terminal region of the 85 kDa subunit contains an SH3 domain. Five closely related forms of the 110 kDa protein may exist and their PI 3-kinase activity appears to reside in the carboxy terminal region (34).

Either phosphotyrosine-containing proteins or peptides can cause activation of PI 3-kinase activity. Treatment of PI 3-kinase *in vitro* with either tyrosine-phosphorylated PDGF receptor or a phosphopeptide, an analog containing the phosphorylated tyrosine moiety at 751 in the PDGF receptor, activates PI 3-kinase's catalytic activity. Similarly, treatment of PI 3-kinase *in vitro* with either phosphorylated IRS1 or an analog phosphopeptide containing its putative phosphorylation sites likewise activates PI 3-kinase activity.

PI 3-kinase may be involved in directing activated receptor trafficking (35). A Hep G2 cell line mutant, containing a PDGF receptor lacking only the PI 3-kinase binding site, failed to be internalized after binding of PDGF. Restoration of the PI 3-kinase binding site on the mutant PDGF receptor enabled the activated PDGF receptor to be internalized, suggesting that PI 3-kinase is necessary for endocytic trafficking of the activated PDGF receptor.

A rapid increase in PI-specific PLC activity has been found after treatment of cells with growth factors, such as EGF and PDGF (*rev.* 38, 39). PLC catalyzes the hydrolysis of PI 4,5-diphosphate to generate 1,2-diacylglycerol (DAG) and inositol 1,4,5-triphosphate, which act as intracellular second messengers by activating the serine/threonine kinase and protein kinase C (PKC), and by increasing the level of intracellular calcium levels, respectively. Increased intracellular calcium levels can activate the calcium-dependent phospholipase A2 (PLA2) enzyme which can hydrolyze membrane phospholipids to form arachidonic acid, that can then be metabolized to form potent second messengers such as the eicosanoids. The PLC family of isozymes contains SH2 and SH3 domains to interact with other signalling proteins. Growth factor treatment of cells can cause PLC to become rapidly associated with the growth factor's activated receptor and to become phosphorylated on tyrosine and serine residues.

D. Grb2 and Sos: The Link Between the Activated Receptor and Ras

Grb2 is a widely expressed non-catalytic protein important in linking the activated receptor to Ras signalling (41, 42). With its one SH2 domain and two SH3 domains, Grb2 is believed to function as a ubiquitous mediating protein, by binding to one or more signalling proteins and promoting their interaction. Grb2 binds to tyrosine-phosphorylated receptors, such as the EGF receptor and the PDGF receptor, via its SH2 domain. The SH3 domain of Grb2 has been shown to bind to the Sos protein (*rev.* 15, 43). The Sos protein is a guanidine nucleotide exchange molecule which can facilitate the conversion of Ras-GDP to Ras-GTP. Microinjection experiments have shown that injection of either Grb2 or H-Ras protein singly into quiescent rat fibroblasts has little effect on DNA synthesis, whereas microinjection of the two proteins together into rat fibroblasts stimulates DNA synthesis. The discovery of the interaction between Grb2 and Sos directly links activated receptors and their associated tyrosine kinase activity to Ras activation.

E. Ras: The Molecular Switch of Cellular Signalling

Three closely related genes (H-*ras,* K-*ras,* and N-*ras*) encode 21 kDa Ras proteins that act as molecular switches for the signalling cascades that control cellular growth and differentiation (*rev.* 43–46). Ras is located at the inner side of the plasma membrane and is activated by binding GTP. Microinjection studies have demonstrated that the Ras-GTP complex is biologically active, whereas the Ras-GDP complex is inactive. The dissociation of Ras from GDP is mediated by specific proteins termed guanine-nucleotide-releasing factors (GRFs). Two types of GRF proteins have been identified: (i) a 140 kDa protein which is chiefly expressed in brain tissue, and (ii) the two 175 kDa Sos proteins which are widely expressed. GRF-induced binding of GTP to Ras causes a conformational change in Ras which allows an effector protein (*i.e.,* Raf) to bind to it. After transient cell signalling, the GTP on Ras is hydrolyzed by Ras itself which has an intrinsically weak GTPase activity, but which is greatly enhanced by interaction with specific GTPase-activating proteins (GAPs), such as p120^{GAP}. These proteins recognize Ras in the GTP-bound state and accelerate GTP hydrolysis.

F. Raf and the 14-3-3 Family Proteins

Raf was first described as a product of the murine transforming retrovirus 3611-MSV and as a product of the avian transforming sarcoma virus MH2 (*rev.* 44, 46, 47). The viral forms of Raf are constitutively active because they are truncated at the amino terminus and lack a putative regulatory region found in the cellular proto-oncogene product, Raf1. In normal mammalian cells, many growth factors can trigger the phosphorylation of cytoplasmic Raf1 and activate its serine/threonine kinase activity. One of the major roles associated with Raf is its ability to phosphorylate mitogen-activated protein kinase kinase (MEK) which in turn phosphorylates MAPK, leading to stimulation of the transcription of previously quiescent genes.

Ras plays a critical role in targeting Raf to the plasma membrane. Ras contains a CAAX box (a signal for farnesylation) at the carboxy terminus and an adjacent polybasic domain of six lysine residues, which serves as a targeting signal for Raf (48, *rev.* 46). A fusion protein, that is composed of Raf plus the targeting motif only of Ras, localizes exclusively at the plasma membrane and shows constitutive kinase activity completely independent of Ras expression. These results indicate that the only role the Ras-GTP complex plays in Raf activation and in the MAPK cascade is to promote the localization of Raf to the plasma membrane where other proteins activate its kinase activity.

Recent evidence suggests that the "14-3-3" proteins play a role in Raf activation after its localization to the plasma membrane (49, 50). The 14-3-3 proteins are a family of ubiquitous, highly-conserved proteins found in plants, invertebrates, and mammals. In mammals, these proteins have been associated with inhibition of PKC activity and activation of tyrosine and tryptophan hydroxylases. Two isoforms of 14-3-3 (14-3-3-beta and 14-3-3 zeta) interact with the amino terminal regulatory region and the carboxy terminal kinase region of Raf. An additional undescribed Factor X must be involved, however, in Raf activation because the interaction between Raf and 14-3-3 proteins is insufficient for full activation of the kinase activity of Raf.

G. The MAP Kinase Cascade

An important convergence point involved in the signal transduction pathways of many different growth factors, hormones, and cytokines is the MAPK cascade (*rev.* 20, 21, 51). Two tiers of upstream kinases have been identified that lead to the activation of MAPK. The first tier of the MAPK cascade contains Raf, Mos, and MEKK (MAPK kinase kinase) which phosphorylate MEK1 (MAPK kinase 1) and MEK2. The second tier of the MAPK cascade contains MEK1 and MEK2 which phosphorylate the two forms of MAPK (ERK1 for extracellular-regulated kinase 1; and ERK2). The MEKs are dual specific kinases which sequentially phosphorylate the tyrosine 185 and threonine 183 of MAPK. MAPK is only active after both the threonine and tyrosine residues are phosphorylated by MEK.

Activated MAPK phosphorylates and regulates numerous cellular signalling proteins. These proteins include receptors, phospholipases, cytoplasmic kinases, and transcription factors. Phosphorylation of PLA2 by MAPK greatly increases its lipase activity and production of second messengers. The p90Rsk and MAPKAP (MAPK-activated protein kinase) are activated by MAPK phosphorylation. Phosphorylated MAPK and p90Rsk migrate to the nucleus and are thought to play a key role in promoting the transcription of cellular genes by phosphorylation of transcription factors such as c-Myc, c-Fos, c-Jun, and ATF2 (*rev.* 20, 21, 51, 52). Such phosphorylation has been shown to stimulate transcription factor activity and induce the transcription of numerous genes involved in cellular growth. A full diagram of cellular signalling cascades is shown in Figure 2.

Phosphatases and feedback loops probably regulate the MAPK cascade (*rev.* 20, 21, 51). Protein phosphatase (PP) 2A and a specific MAPK phosphatase (MAPKP) (53) can directly regulate MAPK activity. MAPK has been shown to phosphorylate activated receptors, such as the EGF receptor, and may decrease the affinity of a receptor for its ligand. Upstream kinases, such as Raf1 and MEK1, can be phosphorylated by MAPK. The MAPK serine/threonine phosphorylation sites on these signalling proteins are unique sites used for activation; phosphorylation of these sites may regulate their activity and decrease MAPK activation.

H. The Src Family Tyrosine Kinases

Many members of the Src family of tyrosine kinases, each with an SH2 and SH3 functional interaction domain, have been described in mammalian cells as being essential to early intracellular signalling by transmembrane receptors (*rev.* 16). Some Src family kinases, such as c-Src, Fyn, and Yes, are ubiquitously expressed, but some Src family kinases show restricted tissue distribution, such as Lck, Blk, and Lyn in lymphocytes, and Hck and Fes in granulocytes and monocytic/macrophage series cells.

One example of the importance of an Src family kinase is the critical role of Lck in T lymphocyte activation (*rev.* 54). Cross-linking of either the CD4 or CD8 transmembrane molecules of T lymphocyte activates Lck kinase activity, which is essential for intracellular signalling. Src, Fyn, and Yes are activated during intracellular signalling initiated by both receptors that contain a PTK domain (such as the PDGF receptor) and receptors that do not contain a PTK domain (such as the colony stimulating factor-1 receptor, the IL-2 receptor, and the IL-3 receptor). Src potentiates the response of cells to EGF and is a critical component of signalling by occupied PDGF receptor. Mutant cells that do contain Src cannot enter S phase of the cell cycle after treatment with PDGF.

The cellular proto-oncogene-coded Src family proteins have tyrosine kinase activity that is highly regulated through phosphorylation of a carboxy terminal tyrosine residue by specific tyrosine kinases, such as Csk. After an Src family kinase is phosphorylated at this carboxy terminal tyrosine moiety, its SH2 domain can bind to the phosphotyrosine tail. This causes a conformational change in the kinase which change is believed to inactivate its tyrosine kinase activity. Binding of an Src family kinase to an activated receptor is believed to suppress the ability of the carboxy terminal tyrosine residue to be phosphorylated, and its tyrosine kinase activity remains, therefore, activated. After the transmembrane receptor is returned to an inactive stage—often by conformational changes induced by enzymatic phosphorylation on serine/threonine residues of the receptor's cytoplasmic portion or by the action of tyrosine phosphatases—the Src family kinase usually dissociates from the receptor and becomes inactivated.

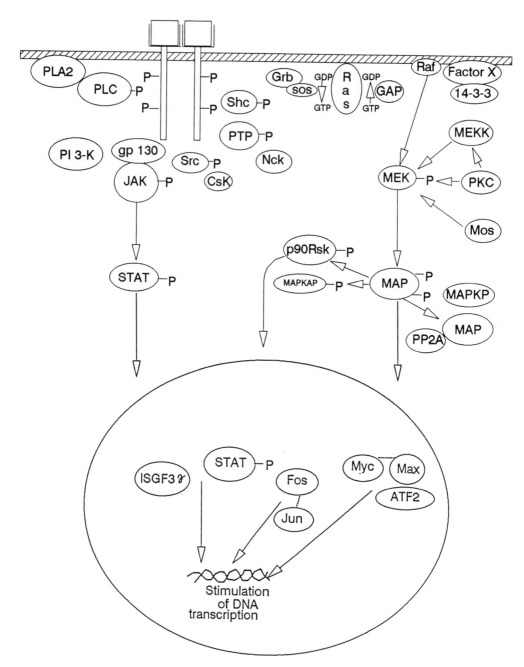

FIGURE 2. Signal transduction cascades in mammalian cells. Multiple routes lead from the activated cellular receptor to the nucleus. Two major signalling pathways are exemplified: (i) the Ras-dependent pathway where phosphorylated MAPK and phosphorylated p90Rsk enter the nucleus and activate DNA transcription factors such as Myc-Max and Fos-Jun; (ii) the Ras-independent pathway where phosphorylated STAT enters the nucleus and directly binds to specific DNA sequences. Also shown are some of the feedback loops used to regulate cellular signalling such as the inactivation of Ras by GAP and the inactivation of MAPK by the phosphatase action of PP2A and MAPKP.

I. JAKs and the STAT Family: Ras-Independent Signalling

The Janus or "just another" kinase (JAK) family of cytoplasmic tyrosine kinases have been implicated in signal transduction induced by cytokines and growth factors (*rev.* 18, 19). Family members such as JAK1, JAK2, and TYK2 are ubiquitous, whereas JAK3 is predominantly expressed in T lymphocytes (55, 56). Studies with mutant cells that do not express JAK1, JAK2, or TYK2 show that their activation is essential for the signal transduction pathways of the interferon alpha receptor, interferon beta receptor, and interferon gamma receptor, which do not contain intrinsic PTK domains. Specific ligand binding to the erythropoietin, IL-2, IL-3, and growth hormone receptors also induce tyrosine kinase activation of JAK family members and their association with the occupied receptors. JAK family kinases may either phosphorylate each other or be phosphorylated by an as yet undescribed tyrosine kinase. Different cytokines can activate cells via phosphorylation of distinct JAK family members (57). In some cells, the membrane-associated gp130 protein has been implicated in induction of JAK family phosphorylation, although gp130 itself has no known kinase activity (58).

Some of the specificity of ligand signalling to the cell nucleus is thought to be accomplished by the STAT (signal transducer and activators of transcription) proteins which can be selectively phosphorylated on tyrosine residues by JAK family kinases and by some receptors containing PTK activity (*rev.* 18, 19, 59). The STAT proteins are highly similar in their amino terminal region, but each protein contains a unique carboxy terminal region thought to be essential for its selective activity. Currently six STAT proteins have been described ranging in molecular weight from 84–94 kDa (STAT1-alpha, STAT1-beta, STAT3, STAT4, STAT5, STAT6) to 113 kDa (STAT2). STAT1-alpha, STAT1-beta, and STAT2 are phosphorylated after treatment of cells with interferon alpha. Interferon alpha seems to promote phosphorylated STAT1 and STAT2 to form heterodimers that can interact with a 48 kDa DNA-binding protein called ISGF3-gamma (interferon-stimulated growth factor 3). This complex then moves to the nucleus and binds to specific sites, called "interferon-stimulated response elements", on cellular DNA to enhance the transcription of cellular genes. After treatment of cells with interferon gamma, however, STAT1-alpha and -beta are phosphorylated, but STAT2 is not phosphorylated. Interferon gamma treatment of cells induces STAT1 (alpha or beta) to form a DNA-binding homodimer by interaction of its tyrosine-phosphorylated residues with the SH2 domain of the other STAT1 molecule. STAT3 becomes activated by phosphorylation on a tyrosine residue, as a DNA-binding protein, after treatment of cells with EGF and IL-6, but not after treatment with interferon gamma. STAT1 and STAT3 may form heterodimers that bind to specific cellular DNA sequences. Similarly, STAT6 and STAT5 become phosphorylated and acquire DNA-binding capability following treatment of cells with IL-4 and prolactin, respectively (59–61). Taken together, differential activation and association of the various STAT proteins, as either homo-complexes or hetero-complexes in response to ligand binding to its receptor, may contribute to the specificity of cellular signalling to the nucleus (*rev.* 19, 62).

J. Transcription Factors Associated with Signal Transduction

Transcription factors are proteins that bind to specific cellular DNA sequences and enhance their transcription. There are Ras-dependent pathways and Ras-independent pathways that stimulate DNA transcription. Ras-dependent pathways are embodied by MAPK and p90Rsk entering the nucleus and activating transcription factor partners such as c-Myc/Max and c-Fos/c-Jun (*rev.* 22, 63–67). Ras-independent pathways are represented by STAT proteins moving into the nucleus and directly activating DNA transcription (*rev.* 19, 62). The short-lived Myc phosphoproteins can bind to DNA and activate the transcription of specific cellular genes. Given their nuclear localization and contiguous regions containing the basic region/helix-loop-helix/leucine zipper motifs, Myc phosphoproteins are thought to be the key transcription-activating factors of growth-related genes that mediate the action of many growth factors. Several different forms of Myc have been described: (i) c-Myc, the product of the cellular proto-oncogene, c-*myc;* (ii) v-Myc, the analog derived from retrovirus-infected chicken cells; (iii) 1-Myc, an isoform described in small-lung-cell carcinoma; and (iv) N-Myc, which is expressed in neuroblastoma cells. Each Myc can form a heterodimer with the protein Max through its carboxy terminal leucine-zipper region and bind to specific cellular DNA sequences containing the motif CAC(G/A)TG. The c-Myc/Max heterodimer is thought to positively regulate the transcription of growth-related genes. In contrast, the Max homodimer negatively regulates the transcription of the same genes. Max can also form inhibitor heterodimers with two other proteins, Mad and Mxi-1.

Treatment of cells with many growth factors induces high levels of c-Myc expression, whereas the level of Max does not increase (*rev.* 22, 63–65). Experimental evidence suggests that in quiescent cells, where low levels of c-Myc are present, either Max homodimers or Max/Mad or Max/Mxi-1 heterodimers predominate, which inhibits the transcription of growth-related genes. Treatment of cells with growth factors induces rapid expression of high levels of c-Myc, which form a complex with Max that induces the transcription of growth-related genes. MAPK can phosphorylate c-Myc and increase its transcriptional activity. Overexpression of c-Myc in cells can cause profound effects. For example, in some breast cancers the c-Myc levels are highly elevated; this changes the PTK activity associated with the EGF receptor and the fibroblast growth factor receptor from being simply mitogenic to being capable of inducing cellular transformation (amplification and overexpression of c-*myc* is discussed in greater detail in Section I, as well as here in this Section in "IV. Retroviral Oncogenes . . ." under F. and in "V. DNA Tumor Viruses . . ." under E). In other cell models, increased expression of c-*myc* was found to be associated with programmed cell death (apoptosis).

The transcriptional complex AP-1 (activator protein-1), the role of which is intimately associated with cell proliferation and transformation, is composed of members of the Fos and Jun family of bZIP proteins (*rev.* 66, 67). These dimeric complexes bind to cellular genes containing either an AP-1 site or phorbol ester response element and induce their transcription. The levels of c-Jun and c-Fos increase after treatment of cells with many growth factors, cytokines, and tumor promoters. c-Jun expression is increased by a two-step mechanism: (i) preexisting c-Jun is posttranslationally modified into an activated form, and (ii) modified c-Jun activates its own transcription and the expression of AP-1 dependent genes. Both c-Jun and c-Fos can be regulated by phosphorylation. Phosphorylation of c-Jun near its DNA-binding site by an uncharacterized protein kinase inhibits DNA binding activity, while dephosphorylation stimulates DNA binding. In contrast, phosphorylation of c-Fos by p90Rsk and MAPK stimulates DNA transcription. The transcriptional activity of c-Jun is regulated by other transcriptional factors, such as nuclear hormone receptors and the Myo D family of regulatory factors.

K. Closing Note: A Perspective on the Requirement for Complexity in the Signal Transduction Network

The focus of this subsection was on the major pathways of intracellular signalling; of necessity it omitted the associated branching pathways. The obvious teleological question is why have such a complex network of proteins that selectively phosphorylate/ dephosphorylate each other, move GTP around, and hydrolyze phospholipids? Why not have simply on/off proteins that recognize an activated receptor, travel to the nucleus, and activate the transcription of specific genes? The mechanistic rationale lies in the operational need for amplification, regulation, and specificity. The advantage of a kinase cascade is the potential increase in the number of activated target proteins that can greatly amplify an intracellular signal to the nucleus. These targets can undergo negative cross-regulation by other signalling pathways. The GTP-regulated Ras protein has been suggested to be a more effective sensor of cellular activation than kinases, essentially functioning as a rheostat (*rev.* 46).

Tightly-regulated multiple signalling proteins and pathways can provide the specificity needed for the transcription of the plethora of different genes and the performance of different cellular effects. In PC12 cells, for example, activation of Ras and MAPK by nerve growth factor induces differentiation, but activation of Ras and MAPK by EGF induces proliferation (*rev.* 20). Furthermore, some cellular processes require the sequential expression of proteins. For example, the cell cycle is driven by the sequential expression of specific cyclins that activate cyclin-dependent kinases at precise moments, or else a "mitotic catastrophe" can occur (68, *rev.* 69). Thus, only a highly complex, interwoven network of signal transduction pathways can provide the precision needed to fine-tune cellular responses.

III. TUMOR-SUPPRESSOR GENES: TARGETS OF VIRAL EFFECTORS

Tumor-suppressor genes, also known as antioncogenes, are negative regulators of cell division. The first evidence that tumor-suppressor genes existed arose from experiments involving the somatic hybridization of normal and tumor cells (*rev.* 70, 71). These experiments demonstrated that the normal genome contains genes that are able to restore the responsiveness of a tumor cell to growth factor control. Subsequent experiments have shown that even cells which have undergone malignant transformation through multiple changes in several genes can be restored to normal responsiveness by the introduction of a certain normal-cell-derived single gene. These observations illustrate the far-reaching power of tumor-suppressor genes to be able to overcome the effects of multiple genes involved in tumor progression. The accumulation of multiple genetic alterations that occur during carcinogenesis has been suggested to involve the sequential alterations of multiple tumor-suppressor genes; this may be the dominant feature of the malignant transformation, rather than the acquisition of oncogenes, in some tumors (*rev.* 70–73).

The proteins encoded by tumor-suppressor genes are generally thought to act as DNA transcription factors. However, some tumor-suppressor gene products also bind to and regulate the function of non-nuclear cellular proteins involved in growth and differentiation; for example, MTS1 is a cyclin Cdk4 inhibitor, NF1 is an activator of Ras GTPase activity, and DCC is a cell adhesion protein (*rev.* 70–72, 74). Some transforming oncoproteins bind to tumor-suppressor gene products which may inhibit/block their regulatory functions in various cellular processes.

At least 17 tumor-suppressor genes have so far been identified and 10 of these (*Rbl, WT1, p53, MTS1, NF1, NF2, VHL, FAP, DCC,* and *RET*) have been cloned (3, 4). The three that have been probably the most extensively studied so far are: (i) the *p53* gene (*rev.* 70–74); (ii) the retinoblastoma gene (*Rb*) (*rev.* 70, 72, 75, 76); and (iii) the Wilms'-tumor-suppressor gene (*WT1*) (*rev.* 70, 72, 77). Some features and the biological actions exerted by these suppressor-genes are briefly described below.

A. The *p53* Tumor-Suppressor Gene

The *p53* gene [at chromosome location 17(p13)], also known as the *TP53* gene, encodes a 53 kDa nuclear phosphoprotein which is involved in gene transcription, DNA synthesis and repair, and programmed cell death (*rev.* 70–74). The *p53* gene was originally described as an oncogene because its overexpression could immortalize rodent cells. Subsequent studies established that the *p53* genes that had been previously characterized and reported were mutated forms of the *p53* gene, and that the normal "wild-type" form of the *p53* gene does suppress tumor growth. Since that time, loss of normal *p53* gene function has been correlated with the transformation of numerous cell lines *in vitro* and with the emergence of various tumors *in vivo*. Mutations in the *p53* tumor-suppressor gene is associated with the appearance of many types of cancer. The *p53* gene is constitutionally mutant in most patients with Li-Fraumeni syndrome, which is dominantly inherited and predisposes to several types of cancer (although never to all forms in any one individual) (*rev.* 72).

The amino terminus of the p53 protein contains an acidic domain similar to those found in other transcription factors. The middle hydrophobic region of p53 (amino acids 100–295) is essential for growth suppression, because this region determines the specific binding to DNA consensus regions and sequence-specific transcriptional activity. The carboxy region of p53 contains a basic nuclear localization sequence (amino acids 316–325) and an oligomerization domain (amino acids 319–360). The formation of p53 dimers or tetramers greatly enhances DNA binding and stimulation of DNA transcription. Binding of the polyomavirus middle-T or large-T antigen, the SV40 large-T antigen, the adenovirus E1B protein, or the papillomavirus E6 protein to certain regions of p53 is thought to inhibit its tumor-suppressor action.

B. The Retinoblastoma Tumor-Suppressor Gene

The *Rb* gene [at chromosome location 13(q14)], also known as *RB1* gene, encodes a 110 kDa nuclear protein that acts as a regulator of the cell cycle at the G1 phase (*rev.* 70, 75, 76). Germline mutations in the gene product of *Rb* has been directly correlated with the occurrence of retinoblastoma and osteosarcoma but does not predispose to other forms of cancer. Somatic mutation of the *Rb* gene, however, has been associated with many forms of cancer including carcinomas of the lung, breast, and bladder (78, 79). Introduction of the *Rb* gene into various tumor cells which lack the gene product of *Rb* suppresses growth of the tumor cells *in vitro* and tumorigenicity *in vivo*.

The gene product, Rb, is a regulator of the cell cycle depending on its state of phosphorylation. Unphosphorylated Rb blocks the cycle through G_1 to S, probably by complexing with a transcription factor, such as E2F, which would activate cell cycle genes. Phosphorylated Rb does not combine with E2F and does not inhibit this cell cycle passage (72). The gene product Rb also plays a key role in differentiation and programmed cell death. Loss of *Rb* gene function during early stages of cell differentiation leads to uncontrolled cellular proliferation, whereas loss of *Rb* gene function during later stages of differentiation leads to programmed cell death. Like the p53 tumor-suppressor protein, the gene product Rb is also targeted by the transforming proteins of the polyomaviruses, adenoviruses, and papillomaviruses.

C. The Wilms'-Tumor-Suppressor Gene

The *WT1* gene [at chromosome location 11(p13)] encodes a 52–54 kDa (or 45kDa) nuclear protein which acts as a transcription factor (*rev.* 70, 72, 77). Germline mutation(s) in the *WT1* gene has been linked to the formation of Wilms' tumor, one of the most frequent solid tumors seen in children. Somatic mutation of *WT1* is associated with nephroblastoma (*rev.* 73). Unlike the products of the *Rb* and *p53* tumor-suppressor genes, WT1 is a highly tissue-specific and developmentally-regulated transcription factor. The gene product of *WT1* contains a DNA binding domain composed of four zinc finger motifs and a proline-glutamine rich region which are involved in the regulation of DNA transcription. Like the *Rb* and *p53* tumor-suppressor genes, *WT1* is believed to block the transcription of growth-promoting genes and stimulate the transcription of differentiation inducing genes.

IV. RETROVIRAL ONCOGENES – AN ILLUSTRATIVE SAMPLING: EFFECTORS OF ONCOGENIC TRANSFORMATION

Retroviral transduction converts proto-oncogenes into retroviral oncogenes which play dominant roles in virally-induced cell transformation and oncogenesis. Accordingly, retroviral oncogenes may be classified following the biochemical functions and cellular locations of the gene products of the proto-oncogenes from which they have originated and conserve a homology to. Thus, a retroviral oncogene may represent a mutant form of a gene coding for: a growth factor (*e.g.,* PDGF **B**); a growth-factor-receptor acting via tyrosine protein kinase activity (*e.g.,* CSF-1 receptor); a GTP-binding GTPase (Ras); a membrane-bound nonreceptor tyrosine protein kinase (Src); a cytoplasmic tyrosine protein kinase (*e.g.,* Fes); a cytoplasmic serine/threonine-specific protein kinase (*e.g.,* Mos); a steroid-type growth factor receptor (*e.g.,* thyroid hormone receptor); or a nuclear regulatory protein (*e.g.,* Myc). Moreover, certain retroviruses that do not carry oncogenes may be tumorigenic via *cis*-activation of c-*onc* gene(s) (*e.g.,* MMTV) or via *trans*-activation (*e.g.,* HTLV-I). As an illustration of the varieties of oncogenic transformation by retroviruses, the nature and molecular mechanisms of action of several of these viral oncogenes and of nontransducing retroviruses are discussed below.

A. *sis*: Homology to Human PDGF B, a Mutated Growth Factor Analog

The simian sarcoma virus (SSV) was isolated from a naturally occurring multicentric fibrosarcoma of a pet woolly monkey in 1971 (80). Multiple tumor foci were present but without the histologic pattern indicative of a primary tumor with metastasis. This appearance was similar to known virally-induced fibrosarcomas of chickens, mice, and cats. Electron microscopy revealed C-type and immature virus particles and subsequent studies established the viral etiology of the tumor. SSV is able to induce fibrosarcomas and glioblastomas *in vivo* (81) and transform cells in culture (82). A non-transforming replication-competent virus, simian sarcoma-associated virus (SSAV), was found in association with SSV (82, 83). Probably SSAV was the evolutionary predecessor of SSV; SSAV serves as helper virus in an infectious viral stock.

Hybridization studies using probes from a 1 kbp segment in the *env* region of SSV, not homologous with SSAV, demonstrated the cellular origin of this sequence, the v-*sis* oncogene (84–87). The proto-oncogene c-*sis* was shown to be highly conserved among various species, a common theme for proto-oncogenes. The c-*sis* proto-oncogene was also transduced by another retrovirus, the Parodi-Irgens feline sarcoma virus (88, 89).

The human c-*sis* gene contains 7 exons with rather long 5' and 3' non-coding regions (90, *rev.* 91). The first exon is predominantly non-coding and is missing from v-*sis*. All of the remaining coding sequences are included in v-*sis*. The seventh exon is entirely non-coding and is largely missing in the viral version. The product of the SSV v-*sis* is a 28 kDa Env-Sis fusion glycoprotein (92). Translation from a spliced message begins at the normal SSAV *env* initiation codon and continues for 51 amino acids before reaching the recombination junction and the Sis-specific amino acids beginning with exon 2. In addition to serving as the site for the initiation of translation, the viral Env segment serves as a signal peptide for translocation across the endoplasmic reticulum and has a site for N-linked glycosylation (93). The Env segment is essential for transformation and serves in place of similar signals from the missing c-*sis* exon 1 coded region. The v-*sis* product is proteolytically processed at the carboxy and amino terminal ends and rapidly forms dimers in the Golgi apparatus (94).

A most exciting finding was the discovery of the close amino acid sequence similarity between the human platelet-derived growth factor (PDGF) **B** chain and the v-Sis oncoprotein (95–97). PDGF is stored in platelet alpha-granules and is the major protein growth factor in serum for cells of mesenchymal origin (98, *rev.* 99). PDGF is a disulfide-linked dimer of two closely related peptides, PDGF A and PDGF **B** (100–102). These proteins share approximately 60% homology. Homodimers of each, as well as heterodimers, are known to exist in nature and to bind PDGF α and β receptors (103–105). Ligand binding results in receptor dimerization and activation of an intracellular tyrosine kinase domain (106, *rev.* 107).

The c-*sis* gene was demonstrated to be the gene for PDGF **B** (108–110). This defined for the first time a function for a proto-oncogene and linked the structural alteration of a growth factor to a pathway to neoplastic transformation. The v-Sis oncoprotein, derived from the PDGF **B** gene, functions therefore as a **BB** homodimer and activates the PDGF receptor. A mechanism of transformation that was immediately obvious was the constitutive activation of a proliferation signal via an autocrine loop. That such a mechanism is valid was strongly supported by the observation that only cells expressing the PDGF receptor were transformed by v-Sis (111). This specificity also explains the novel ability of SSV to induce gliomas at high frequency, since glial cells, as well as other connective tissue cells, express PDGF receptors (112).

An intracellular autocrine loop, in which newly synthesized Sis interacts with the PDGF receptor, is thought to be the mechanism of transformation. A small portion of v-Sis reaches the cell surface and remains tightly associated with the membrane. Very little of the v-Sis produced is secreted (94, 113). Various membrane-anchored forms of v-Sis have been experimentally constructed and shown to be transforming (114).

As expected from the above-summarized mechanism of transformation by v-*sis,* the experimental expression of normal c-*sis* gene, if linked to viral long terminal repeat (LTR), for example, is also transforming for cells with PDGF receptors (115, 116). Many human fibrosarcomas and glioblastoma cell lines express c-Sis (PDGF **B**) (117, 118). A PDGF autocrine loop-driven proliferation is a possible mechanism involved in the early stages of tumor progression (*rev.* 119). It has recently been shown, using an inducible v-*sis* gene expression system, that a reversible stage of transformation proceeds the irreversible stage of transformation involving presumably additional genetic changes (120).

The crystal structure of human PDGF **BB** homodimer has been determined to a 3Å resolution (121). The polypeptide chain is folded into two highly twisted anti-parallel β-strand pairs. Three intramolecular disulfide bonds are identified in an unusual knotted arrangement. Three surface loops at each end of the dimer are presumably involved in receptor recognition. Transforming growth factor B (TGF-B) and nerve growth factor (NGF) also have a similar cystine-knot plus beta-strand topology (122).

It has been assumed that disulfide-linked dimer formation was essential for biological activity. Reduction of disulfide bonds was correlated with loss of dimerization and loss of activity. However, recent evidence has demonstrated that intrachain disulfide bond(s) may be more important features of a functional structure. Mutant proteins were constructed that retained the intrachain disulfide(s) but were unable to establish interchain disulfide bonds (123). Sis proteins constructed in this way were shown to be active as mitogens. The monomeric protein was able to fold properly and associate into noncovalent dimers and retain activity. Interchain disulfide bonds increase stability, but appear not to be essential for dimerization and activity.

B. *fms*: Mutated Analog of CSF-1 Receptor

The relationship between the v-*fms* onocogene of feline sarcoma virus (FeSV) and the proto-oncogene c-*fms* has been well described and illustrates several important aspects of viral oncogenes (*rev.* 124). The Susan McDonough strain (SM) and the Hardy-Zuckerman-5 strain (HZ 5) of FeSV are independent isolates, both of which contain the v-*fms* oncogene. These viruses are acutely transforming and replication defective. The transduced cellular gene that v-*fms* is derived from, designated c-*fms,* is the gene for the colony stimulating factor-1 (CSF-1) receptor (CSF-1R) (125). Other strains of FeSV have transduced other cellular genes (c-*kit* by HZ4 FeSv, c-*fes* by HZ1-, ST-, and GA-FeSV). SM-FeSV and HZ5-FeSV were isolated from fibrosarcomas in domestic cats, and cause fibrosarcomas when injected into kittens (126, 127). CSF-1, also known as macrophage colony stimulating factor (M-CSF), is an important hematopoietic and inflammatory cytokine that stimulates the growth and differentiation of macrophages, monocytes, and committed bone marrow progenitors cells (128, *rev.* 129). It is interesting that although its oncogene is derived from a cell lineage-specific growth factor receptor gene, SM-FeSV can transform a wide variety of mammalian fibroblast and epithelial cell lines in culture as well as macrophage and myeloid cell lines. SM-FeSV can infect bone marrow cells and cause or contribute to a wide variety of hematopoietic neoplasias and proliferative disorders under certain experimental conditions (130).

The products of the v-*fms* and c-*fms* genes are membrane bound glycoproteins with an extracellular ligand-binding domain, single transmembrane segment and a cytoplasmic domain with tyrosine kinase activity. CSF-1R shares sequence homology with PDGF-R (131), c-Kit (132), and the receptor for basic fibroblast growth factor (FGF-R) (133). CSF-1R is adjacent to PDGF-R on human chromosome 5 and these genes are thought to arise from duplication of a common ancestor (134).

CSF-1 binding to the external domain of the CSF-1R activates the tyrosine kinase activity of the cytoplasmic domain, resulting in autophosphorylation and the phosphorylation of other cytoplasmic components. PI 3-kinase is involved in the pathway (135) that leads to expression of c-*fos, jun-B,* and c-*myc* (136–138). Ligand binding results in a rapid down-regulation of CSF-1R. Exposure of cells to the phorbol ester, 12-*O*-tetradecanoylphorbol-13-acetate (TPA), causes a transmodulation of CSF-1R that is mediated by proteolytic cleavage of the extracellular domain (139). In contrast to CSF-1, the tyrosine kinase activity of v-Fms is constitutively activated. CSF-1R and v-Fms are also biochemically distinguished by the inability of v-Fms to be transmodulated by TPA and by a relatively slow maturation and transit of v-Fms through the Golgi complex (140).

The recombination event that captured sequences of c-*fms* into feline leukemia virus (FeLV) resulted in a *gag*-v-*onc* fusion as is common with acutely transforming replication-defective retroviruses. Some of the FeLV *gag* and virtually all of the *pol* gene were deleted in the process. The fusion protein includes 5′ sequences normally untranslated in c-Fms. The Gag portion of Gag-v-Fms peptide is cleaved at the Gag-v-Fms junction by a signal peptidase, so it is not a component of the mature oncoprotein and has no effect on the transformation potential of this oncoprotein. There are important differences throughout the v-Fms oncoprotein compared to c-Fms that are responsible for the transforming activity. Most studies have compared v-Fms to the human c-Fms and are thus complicated by species differences between feline and human c-Fms. There are point mutations that distinguish the extracellular domains of v-Fms and feline c-Fms. Also, 50 amino acids of the 3′ end of c-Fms are missing from v-Fms (SM strain) and are replaced by 11 unrelated acids. A different transduction event occurred in the creation of HZ5-FeSV that also makes the carboxy terminus different from that of the c-Fms protein. In both cases the region deleted contains a tyrosine residue that is thought to be an important negative regulatory element in CSF-1R. Certain mutations in the extracellular domain (*e.g.* residue 301) of CSF-1R confer constitutive protein tyrosine kinase activity and consequently transforming activity (141, 142). This transforming activity is enhanced by mutations in the carboxy terminal tail. In particular, tyrosine 969 is an important negative regulator. This mutation alone is not transforming, but contributes to a proliferative advantage and factor-independence in certain hematopoietic progenitors (143, 144). Activation of the feline c-Fms requires mutations at 301 and 374 (141). Mutations at amino acid residues 301 and 969 have been detected in myelodysplasia and myeloid leukemia patients (145, 146).

Chimeric receptors containing the extracellular domain of CSF-1R and the cytoplasmic kinase domain of v-Fms respond to ligand binding by autophosphorylation and down-modulation. This chimeric receptor is not transforming. The chimera is still unresponsive to TPA-induced down-regulation. The cytoplasmic kinase domain is likely to be the site for protein kinase C (PKC)-mediated phosphorylation and down-regulation in c-Fms.

An autocrine mechanism of transformation has been suggested in some human myeloid leukemias and can be experimentally created by transducing genes expressing CSF-1 and c-Fms in NIH 3T3 cells (147). Although the gene for CSF-1 can make a murine macrophage cell line factor-independent, it does not make it tumorigenic. Expression of v-*fms* in this cell line does both. Evidence from a variety of sources indicates that v-Fms is not simply the equivalent of ligand activated c-Fms (*rev.* 129).

Much like FeSV/v-*fms,* the gene for the epidermal growth factor (EGF) receptor has been captured in an avian retrovirus to create avian erythroblastosis virus (AEV) (*rev.* 148). The transduced oncogene is v-*erb*-B. In the ES4 strain of AEV a second transduced gene, v-*erb*-A, contributes to the oncogenicity of the virus, but is not essential. The v-*erb* A oncogene is derived from thyroid hormone receptor gene. Another strain of AEV, the H-strain, contains only v-*erb*-B. The EGF receptor has a structure similar to that described above for CSF-1. Furthermore, like v-Fms, the membrane localization of v-Erb-B is essential for its transforming activity. Unlike v-Fms, the ligand-binding domain is deleted in v-Erb-B. The ES4 strain contains a deletion in the carboxy terminal regulatory domain.

C. *ras:* Mutated Analog of GTP-Binding GTPase

The first mammalian sarcoma virus was isolated by Jennifer Harvey in 1964 during animal passage experiments with Moloney murine leukemia virus (Mo-MuLV) (149). Plasma from a rat with leukemia induced by Mo-MuLV was inoculated into newborn BALB/c mice. Approximately one month later anaplastic sarcomas arose unexpectedly at the site of inoculation in 5 of 15 animals and the animals had splenomegaly. Typically, Mo-MuLV does not induce symptoms of leukemia before 8 weeks following infection and was not known to cause solid tumors. Rats and hamsters were also found to be susceptible to rapid tumor induction with this new agent, the Harvey murine sarcoma virus (Ha-MSV). A very similar sequence of events involving rat passage of a murine leukemia virus resulted in the isolation of the Kirsten strain of MSV (Ki-MSV) (150, *rev.* 151).

It was later shown that the transforming gene sequences of both Ha-MSV and Ki-MSV were indeed transduced by the leukemia virus during passage in the rat host and are actually rat-drived oncogenes. Although it was realized early on that these viruses contained rat genetic information, the complex arrangement of the transduced sequences was not clearly understood until molecular cloning and DNA sequence analysis. In both viruses, a major portion of the MuLV was replaced by recombination with a rat endogenous 30 S virus-like RNA (VL30). The transduced H-*ras* and K-*ras* genes are located within these VL30 sequences (152, 153).

The H-*ras* gene of mouse origin has been transduced by murine leukemia viruses (BALB-MSV and AF1) and an independent isolate of rat H-*ras* has also been reported (154–156). The BALB-MSV genome has a large deletion in the *pol* region and H-*ras* is substituted for the *env* gene, a structure more typical of transforming retroviruses (157). As rat VL30 sequences are not part of the BALB-MSV genome, they are not considered essential for the transforming activity of Ha-MSV or Ki-MSV. A 21 kDa phosphoprotein, p21, is the only translation product of MSV and has been shown to be essential for the initiation and maintenance of transformation (*rev.* 158).

The v-H-*ras* and v-K-*ras* genes are related members of a gene family, but ironically it was the rat VL30 sequences that first led to the belief that the transduced sequences of these viruses were related. The third known mammalian *ras* gene is N-*ras,* isolated as a transforming gene by transfection of DNA from a neuroblastoma cell line (159). No instance is known of N-*ras* transduction by a retrovirus. A so-called superfamily of Ras proteins has been defined based on the structural homology of its members to the Ras proteins. The Ras superfamily includes R-Ras, K- Rev-1/Rap, TC21, Rho, and Rac. Ras proteins have been found to be key regulators of a variety of cell growth and differentiation pathways in all eukaryotic cells. In addition to transforming assays in cell culture, the biological activity of various wild type and mutant *ras* genes is often assayed in yeast and *Xenopus* oocyte systems among others.

All three mammalian c-*ras* genes code for a 189 amino acid 21 kDa protein. The gene structure is similar for all three with one non-coding and four coding exons (*rev.* 158). The proteins are highly homologous in the first 164 amino acid segment, but diverge in the last 25 amino acid segment. c-K-*ras* has alternate fourth coding exons A and B, making two protein products that also differ in the carboxy terminal end. The three c-*ras* genes differ greatly in size due to large differences in intron size. They also differ with respect to distribution of tissue expression. H-*ras* expression is highest in the skin and skeletal muscle, whereas K-*ras* is lowest in the skin and muscle and highest in the testis and thymus (160).

It was realized early on that Ras proteins are similar to G- proteins in binding guanine nucleotides and in having an intrinsic GTPase activity. The normal cellular role of Ras is involved in signal transduction and in the control of cell proliferation. In particular, it was found that the binding of GTP or GDP determines turning on or off the intrinsic GTPase activity of Ras; thus, Ras is active when GTP is bound and becomes inactive when GTP has been hydrolyzed to GDP. The transforming ability of c-Ras is activated by various mutations that shift the balance to favor the activated GTP-bound form. The v-H-Ras and v-K-Ras proteins carry an activating mutation at residue 12 and a threonine at 59, not present in c-Ras. The threonine-59 is autophosphorylated, but the importance of this for transformation is doubtful.

Clearly, a major reason for the explosion of research on Ras is due to the finding that a mutated *ras* gene is responsible for the transforming activity of DNA from a human bladder cancer cell line (161–164). The *ras* oncogene was the first and is the most frequent example of an activated human transforming gene present in tumor cell DNA as detected in the NIH 3T3 transformation assay (165). The lure of establishing a mechanistic connection between the oncogenes of transforming retroviruses and activation of the normal counterpart in human cancer created an intense search for additional human oncogenes.

The most common mutation in c-*ras* genes isolated from tumor cell DNA are substitutions at codon 12, 13, or 61 (*rev.* 158). Activating mutations at codons 12 and 61 cause the protein to have impaired GTPase activity and, perhaps more importantly, decreased sensitivity to GTPase activating proteins (GAP) and neurofibromin which stimulate inactivation. GAP are of major importance in the regulation of Ras. Other, often mutated residues detected in transforming *ras* gene products are at sites 63, 116, 119, or 146. These mutations cause an increase in the normally slow dissociation of bound nucleotide. The consequence is that dissociation of GDP will result in the rebinding of GTP, since GTP is more abundant in the cell, and Ras will remain activated. NIH 3T3 transformation can also occur by transfection of overexpressed normal c-*ras,* indicating that there must be more than one single mechanism of transformation by *ras.*

Ras is a key component in a wide variety of signal transduction pathways in all eukaryotes. Raf and some other serine/threonine kinases involved in mitogenic pathways are Ras-dependent. A kinase that activates the mitosis-activated protein (MAP) kinase, referred to as MAP kinase kinase, is included in this group. In yeast, adenyl cyclase is a major Ras target. This is not the case in higher eukaryotes where GAP may be targets for Ras in the signal transduction network in addition to their role in negative regulation of Ras (*rev.* 158, *see* Signal Transduction, this Section).

A critical determinant of the transforming ability of Ras is its association with the inner surface of the plasma membrane. Ras associates with the plasma membrane as a result of several posttranslational modifications leading to the addition of a farnesyl group to a cysteine near the carboxy terminus (*rev.* 166). The membrane bindng of Ras is also greatly enhanced by a basic domain or a palmitylated cysteine (167, *rev.* 168). Farnesylation is essential for oncogenic transformation by Ras; thus, the enzyme responsible, protein farnesyltransferase, has become an important target for the development of compounds that inhibit transformation by Ras (166, 169, 170). Specific inhibitors of farnesyltransferase have been recenty described that block the growth of Ras-dependent tumors in nude mice (171).

D. *src:* Membrane-Bound Mutated Nonreceptor Tyrosine Protein Kinase

The Rous sarcoma virus (RSV) is the first oncogenic virus to be isolated (172) and the first retrovirus that was shown to have transduced a cellular gene (173). But, the Rous sarcoma virus is also associated with many other scientific "firsts". The first quantitative cell culture transformation system was developed by Temin and Rubin in 1958 using this virus (174). Reverse transcriptase was discovered by Temin and Mizutani using RSV (175) at the same time that Baltimore discovered the same enzymatic activity with murine leukemia virus (176). Furthermore, pp60[Src] was the first retroviral oncoprotein and tyrosine protein kinase to be identified (177–180).

All RSV strains are thought to derive from "Chicken Tumor No. 1" of Rous's original investigations. The extensively studied genetics of RSV provided many important insights into retroviral replication and oncogenic transformation decades before site-directed mutagenesis and other modern molecular biology techniques were introduced to dissect the activities of viral genes and of oncogene products. The observation, that viral oncogenes were necessary for the initiation and maintenance of the transformed phenotype, came from studies of temperature-sensitive RSV mutants (181–183). The partial transformation phenotype induced by some RSV mutants led to the realization that transforming proteins can have multiple targets, some of which were quantitatively or qualitative altered by the mutation (184, 185).

The c-*src* gene in chickens (and humans) has 12 exons and all are included in v-*src*. The first exon is non-coding but nevertheless is intact in the transduced version. An abbreviated model for the process of transduction is shown in Figure 2 of Section I in this chapter. Most models include two recombination steps. The first is at the chromosomal DNA level between an integrated provirus and an adjacent cellular oncogene. The observation, that recombination between the transducing virus and the cellular gene is often within an intron of the cellular gene, argues that the first step is at the chromosomal DNA level (186). The second proposed recombination step, during reverse transcription, is known to occur with high frequency during retrovirus replication.

It is ironic that RSV, the prototype for most features of the acutely transforming retroviruses, is not at all typical in its ability to replicate in the absence of helper virus. The Schmidt-Ruppin subgroup A and Prague subgroup C strains of RSV are both replication competent. The v-*src* gene is inserted at the 3′ end of the genome, between the *env* gene and the LTR, and is expected as the only product of a spliced message. The other viral genes are undisturbed by the insertion. The Bryan high-titer (BH) strain of RSV is, however, replication-defective (187) by virtue of an *env* deletion (188–190). The requirement of a helper virus for a defective transforming virus to replicate was first described with the BH strain. When diluted beyond the endpoint for transformation, a non-transforming virus, designated as the Rous-associated virus (RAV), was discovered in BH-RSV stocks by RAV's ability to interfere in the transformation by RSV. This interference phenomenon, termed "homologous interference", is common with retroviruses and is due to the saturation of available virus receptors by the Env glycoprotein of the virus being produced. Thus, new infection by viruses using the same receptor are blocked. This interference phenomenon is the basis of a system used to classify retroviruses into various subgroups.

RAV is a prototype "helper virus" complementing the replication functions absent in the defective transforming virus, analogous to helper phage in bacteriophage systems. RAV is non-transforming in cell culture, but does cause leukemia after a long latent period.

Replication-defectiveness of acutely transforming retroviruses has turned out to be the rule, and the Schmidt-Ruppin A and Prague C strains are the exception. It is not clear, however, whether the original virus was replication-competent or -defective. The BH strain may have arisen by deletion of the *env* gene of a replication-competent transforming virus or the replication- competent viruses could have arisen from recombination of helper virus with a more typical replication-defective virus. There is some evidence to suggest that BH-RSV arose by recombination between c-*src* and RAV-2 rather than by deletion of *env* (188). Furthermore, early isolates of RSV are thought to be defective (*cited in ref*. 188). It may not be possible, nor is it a critical point, to know the order of these events. The important lesson is that replication-defectiveness is not an absolute property of acutely transforming retroviruses, but is the predominant characteristic.

The chicken c-Src protein is 533 amino acids in length, whereas the v-Src protein is 526 amino acids in length. Although there are scattered mutations throughout the gene (10 for Schmidt-Ruppin A and 19 for Prague C), a 39 bp segment at the 3′ end of v-*src* not present in c-*src* accounts for the largest difference in the two genes (*rev*. 191). The two products are thus distinctly different at their carboxy terminal ends. In RSV infected cells v-*src* is expressed at higher levels than c-*src,* but the product has a shorter half-life: approximately 6 hours for v-Src and approximately 24 hours for c-Src.

The pp60^{Src} protein is a protein kinase that phosphorylates tyrosine and autophosphorylates itself on tyrosine-416 (180). The tyrosine protein kinase activity was shown to be essential for transformation by RSV (192); however, the phosphorylation of Src on tyrosine-416 is not necessary (193). Phosphorylation of tyrosine-527 in c-Src serves as a negative regulatory element. This residue is absent in v-Src. Tyrosine protein kinase activity was shown to be an important property of other transforming proteins (194).

One of the apparent targets observed early was vinculin, a component of "adhesion plaques" (*rev.* 195). The major phosphotyrosine-containing protein in RSV-transformed cells has a molecular weight of 36 kDa (196). Other identified targets for pp60^{Src} are enolase, phosphoglycerate mutase, and lactate dehydrogenase (*rev.* 195). Many of the proteins phosphorylated following infection and transformation by RSV are likely to be irrelevant targets for the induction of neoplasia.

A wide variety of cytoplasmic proteins have been found to share homology with regions of Src. These have been defined as "Src homology" (SH) domains. The SH1 domain is the tyrosine kinase domain. Other oncogenes and tyrosine protein kinases share extensive homology with Src and are considered to be members of the Src family. The Src family includes Yes, Lyn, Fyn, Lck, Blk, Fgr, Hck, and Yrk. Some homology, primarily in the ATP-binding domain, exists between Src and serine/threonine kinases.

SH2 domains are of fundamental importance in signal transduction networks initiated by tyrosine kinase growth factor receptors. As there are many SH2-containing proteins and they bind differentially to other components of pathways, the specificity for binding is determined by structural elements beyond the phosphotyrosine itself. The SH2 domain (approximately 100 amino acids) is responsible for binding to phosphotyrosine-containing proteins, most likely by recognition of a small 3–4 amino acid consensus motif on the carboxy-terminal side of a phosphotyrosine residue (*rev.* 197). The functional roles of the SH domains in signal transduction were discussed in additional detail under "II. Non-DNA Targets of Viral Effectors: Signal Transduction Cascades."

The amino terminal region of Src targets the protein to localize at the inner surface of the plasma membrane. The membrane association of Src is not due to a hydrophobic transmembrane domain, but rather to a co-translational addition of myristate to the amino terminal glycine after the initiator methionine is removed. Myristate alone is not enough to anchor a protein to the membrane. Actually, two signals are required for membrane binding (*rev.* 168). It has been recently reported that for Src family proteins three alternating lysine residues or a palmitylated cysteine near the amino terminus contribute to membrane binding (198, 199).

The crystal structure of Src has been determined (200) and additional details of structure and function continue to emerge in the literature.

E. *mos*: Unscheduled Expression of Cytoplasmic Serine/Threonine Protein Kinase

The *mos* oncogene is the transforming component of the Moloney murine sarcoma virus (Mo-MSV), a replication-defective virus that has been isolated from a BALB/c mouse sarcoma (201, 202). Mo-MSV transforms fibroblasts in culture and causes fibrosarcomas *in vivo* (203). The *mos* gene was among the earliest retroviral oncogenes to be molecularly cloned and studied; it is a particularly interesting oncogene because mutations are not required to activate the transforming potential of the respective proto-oncogene. Indeed, normal mouse c-*mos* gene linked to a viral LTR transforms mouse fibroblasts as efficiently as v-*mos* (204); in this respect there is a similarity to normal c-*sis* which — when linked to a viral LTR — becomes transforming (toward cells containing PDGF receptors) (*see* "A. *sis* . . ." above). It has been shown that the c-*mos* proto-oncogene can also be activated via a promoter insertion mechanism by intracisternal A-particles (IAP) (which are retrotranposon elements) (205–207), by a process similar to the activation of *myc* by avian leukosis virus (ALV).

The v-*mos* oncogene is transduced into the *env* gene region of the parental Mo-MuLV and the product is an Env-Mos fusion protein (208). The first 5 codons are contributed by the *env* gene followed by an additional 26 in-frame codons upstream of the normal c-*mos* ATG initiation codon, and finally the normal c-*mos* coding exon. The c-*mos* gene is unusual in having a single coding exon. The carboxy termini of v-*mos* and c-*mos* are identical, as termination occurs within the transduced sequence. The *pol* region of Mo-MSV contains large deletions and *env* is virtually absent. Although the *gag* coding region is not disrupted by the inserted cellular sequence, *gag* is unexpressed in some strains (209). v-Mos and c-Mos are 39 kDa cytoplasmic proteins with serine/threonine kinase activity (210, 211). A variant strain of MSV124, termed ts110, produces an 85 kDa Gag-Mos fusion protein (212). The v-*mos* mutants lacking kinase activity fail to transform cells (213, 214).

With the exception of the additional amino terminus amino acids mentioned previously, the sequence of v-Mos protein of the HT-1 strain of Mo-MSV is identical to mouse c-Mos (215). The HT-1 strain was isolated from a hamster tumor induced by an early passage of the original MSV stock (216). Some well-studied Mo-MSV strains, such as 124 and m1 obtained from later passages, do contain mutations, however. Since transforming activity is a property of the normal cellular gene product when expressed in an inappropriate context, it is clear that these mutations are not critical for transformation. The v-Mos and c-Mos proteins are distinguishable by their half-lives: the c-Mos protein has a short half-life (0.5–2.0 hours), whereas v-Mos has a half-life of greater than 10 hours (217, 218). Cells acutely infected with Mo-MSV have 30–100 times more v-Mos protein than stably transformed cells (217). The high levels of v-Mos expressed during acute Mo-MSV infection are toxic and result in a selection for lower levels in stably transformed cells. Very low levels of Mos protein are sufficient for transformation (219).

The murine c-*mos* gene is a potent transforming gene when experimentally expressed in an inappropriate context. Differences in transformation efficiency of up to 100-fold have been reported for the c-*mos* genes of various species (220–223). Much higher levels of protein are required for transformation with the human c-*mos* gene as compared to the mouse gene, for example. Lower transformation efficiencies of the c-*mos* of certain species correlate with lower ability to induce *Xenopus* oocyte maturation, arrest cell cleavage in developing embryos, and *in vitro* autophosphorylation (224) (see discussion below concerning the role of *mos* in oogenesis).

The c-*mos* RNA is expressed at low or undetectable levels in most adult tissues, but is highly expressed in germ cells suggesting a role in gametogenesis (225). The first evidence for a role in oogenesis came from studies with the *Xenopus* oocyte *in vitro* system (226). The c-*mos* RNA in *Xenopus* oocytes is translationally-regulated maternal RNA, and c-Mos protein is not synthesized until maturation is induced with progesterone. Micro-injection of *mos* antisense oligonucleotides into progesterone-stimulated oocytes inhibits pp39[Mos] expression and germinal vesicle breakdown (GVBD), a step in meiotic maturation. Work in the *Xenopus* oocyte system has demonstrated that c-*mos* expression is required for the 1st and 2nd meiotic divisions and is involved in the arrest of unfertilized eggs in metaphase II (227, 228). The *mos* gene product has also been shown to be necessary for normal meiotic maturation in mouse oocytes (229–231). Mos is required for the activation of the maturation promoting factor (MPF), a cytoplasmic factor that induces oocyte maturation and controls entry into mitosis (226). MPF, consisting of the p34^{Cdc2} homolog and cyclin, promotes transition from G2 into meiosis and mitosis in eukaryotic cells. Cytostatic factor (CyF) is an activity responsible for stabilization of MPF at metaphase II that can be experimentally measured by the induction of cleavage arrest in one blastomere of a 2-cell embryo. Mos was shown to be identical to CyF, or is the catalytic component of CyF (227), and v-Mos can substitute for c-Mos^{Xe} protein as a component of CyF (228). Mos has been shown to activate MEK *in vitro;* MAP kinases function at G1/S and G2/M points of the cell cycle of somatic and germ cells.

The mechanism of transformation by *mos* is thought to be related to the normal function of the Mos serine/threonine protein kinase in triggering the cell cycle during meiosis. Insights into the manner in which v-Mos perturbs the cell cycle in transformed NIH 3T3 cells have recently been gained (232). NIH 3T3 cells transformed by *mos* are growth arrested in the absence of serum; however, these cells do not enter a quiescent state as do serum-starved normal NIH 3T3 cells. The *mos* transformed cells reenter S phase more rapidly than untransformed NIH 3T3 cells and the growth-arrest-specific product of the *gas*-1 gene is not expressed. Thus, v-*mos* appears to prevent NIH 3T3 cells from exiting the cell cycle.

F. *myc:* Codes for Mutated and/or Excessive Nuclear Regulatory Protein

An acutely transforming replication-defective virus, designated MC29, was isolated in 1964 from spontaneous myelocytomatosis in a Rhode Island Red chicken (233). MC29 is the prototype of v-*myc* containing retroviruses. MC29 and other *myc* containing viruses rapidly induce fatal neoplastic diseases including myelocytomas, endotheliomas, sarcomas, and carcinomas of the liver and kidney (234–236). These viruses have the capacity to transform macrophage-like cells as well as fibroblasts and epithelial cells *in vitro* (237–239).

The independently isolated avian retroviruses CMII, OK10, and MH2 have also transduced *myc* (240, 241, *rev.* 242). MH2 is one of a few examples where two oncogenes have been transduced in the same virus. In MH2 the second gene has been designated *mht* or *mil* (243–246), and is now known to be the same as *raf* (247, 248). More recently the feline leukemia virus (FeLV) has also been shown to transduce *myc* in naturally occurring leukemia (249–251).

In MC29 a portion of *gag,* all of *pol,* and a portion of *env* is replaced by approximately 1600 bp of the transduced oncogene v-*myc* (252, 253). The original source of v-*myc,* the c-*myc* gene of chickens, as well as of rodents and humans, contains 3 exons. The first exon is not translated and is deleted in all 4 v-*myc* containing avian retroviruses (*rev.* 242). Two transcription start sites are utilized to produce a 439 amino acid protein and a 453 amino acid protein at low levels in a wide variety of tissues. The different virus isolates vary with respect to the length of upstream and downstream non-coding regions retained and also where precisely in the viral genome the v-*myc* resides, but they all include exon 2 and the coding portion of exon 3, largely unchanged. There are a few mutations in the various v-*myc* genes relative to chicken c-*myc* (only 8 base changes in MC29). In addition to the deregulated expression attributed to viral LTR, an important mutation that contributes to transformation is the loss of a key phosphorylation site at threonine-58 (254–256).

In MC29, the transforming protein is expressed as a 110 kDa Gag-Myc fusion protein translated from an unspliced genomic-length transcript (257, 258). In a similar fashion, a 90 kDa Gag-Myc fusion protein is expressed from CMII (259). Like c-Myc, these products are phosphorylated and located predominantly in the nucleus (260). The OK10 strain differs in that two *myc* transcripts are produced. One is a complete genomic transcript translated into a 200 kDa Gag-Pol-Myc fusion protein, whereas the other is spliced from a splice donor in *gag* and produces a p57 Gag-Myc fusion protein (261, *rev.* 242). Whereas c-Myc and the Gag-Myc proteins are nuclear, the p200 Gag-Pol-Myc protein is located in the cytoplasm, a property most likely determined by the large viral polyprotein portion (262). The transforming activity is attributable probably to the nuclear p57 Gag-Myc protein. The MH2 strain also produces v-Myc as a spliced gene product, but an unspliced genomic message is also produced and is responsible for the expression of the cytoplasmic Gag-Mht (Raf) protein.

Transduction is not the only way that retroviruses activate *myc*. Replication-competent leukemogenic retroviruses are unable to transform cells *in vitro* and cause neoplastic disease in animals only after a long latent period. A finding of major importance, which led to the understanding of the mechanism by which such viruses cause neoplasia, came from studies on ALV- induced bursal lymphoma (263–266). The sites of retrovirus integration into the host cell chromosome are considered to be predominantly random. Chronically infected animals are subjected to a great many retrovirus integration events and occasionally one will be in the vicinity of a gene that is important for some aspect of cell proliferation. Host genes at the site of integration may be inactivated by insertional mutagenesis or their oncogenic expression may be activated by several different mechanisms that basically rely on the transcriptional regulatory activity of the viral LTR. In ALV-induced bursal lymphomas, integrations in the non-coding exon 1 or, more frequently, in intron 1 near the start of exon 2 of c-*myc* leads to neoplasia. Often the upstream LTR has been deleted and the downstream LTR serves to drive the expression of the c-*myc* coding exons (267). Less often, integrations in lymphomas have been observed in the opposite orientation to the c-*myc* gene or even downstream of the c- *myc* gene. It is thought that in these cases the expression of c-*myc* is deregulated by the presence of the enhancer sequences in the viral LTRs. Leukemias induced by murine leukemia viruses have also involved promoter insertion activation of c-*myc* (268, 269).

Beyond virally-induced insertional mutagenesis, c-*myc* can also be activated by virally- or nonvirally-triggered chromosomal translocations and gene amplifications (*rev.* 242, *see also* Section I in this chapter). Gene amplification appears to be a late event in tumor progression. In Burkitt's lymphoma, c-*myc* on chromosome 8(q24) is translocated to chromosome 14(q22), 2(p12), or 22(q11) in a head-to-head arrangement (*see* role of EBV in Burkitt's lymphoma later in this Section). In mouse plasmacytomas the *myc* locus on chromosome 15 is translocated to the immunoglobulin locus on the distal arm of chromsome 12 or 6 by a reciprocal exchange. Typically, this involves a break point in exon 1 or intron 1, similar to the mechanism by which provirus integration disrupts the normal regulation of c-*myc*.

The *myc* oncogene is considered to play a cell immortalization role in the transformation of primary cells in culture (270). Cooperation with *ras* in the transformation of primary rat embryo fibroblasts (REF cells) and other experimental systems is briefly described in Section I.

Other genes related to c-myc have been discovered by virtue of their amplification in tumors and hybridization (at reduced stringency to detect distantly-related sequences) to *myc* probes: N-*myc* from human neuroblastoma (271–273) and L-*myc* from human lung small-cell carcinoma (274).

The c-*myc* gene is expressed in a wide variety of cell types. Expression is elevated following mitogenic signals and is thus higher in proliferating tissues such as regenerating liver (*see also* in Section I).

It has been known since the early studies on Myc that these proteins are phosphorylated, are located predominantly in the cell nucleus, and have DNA binding activity (*rev.* 233). The c-Myc protein contains a basic helix-loop-helix (bH-L-H) domain, a leucine-zipper in the carboxy terminal region, and transactivating activity in the amino terminal region (*rev.* 233). The structural similarity of Myc to known transcription factors has been realized for quite some time. A satisfactory understanding of Myc function, however, has lagged behind some of the other nuclear oncoproteins such as Fos and Jun. The finding of heterodimerization with another nuclear protein, designated as Max, was an important step in focusing on the role(s) of Myc in the regulation of transcription (275). Max forms homodimers and heterodimers with Myc and other proteins including Mad and Mxi-1 (276, 277). c-Myc/Max heterodimers bind to a specific DNA sequence (designated as an E box) and transactivate adjacent genes (278–282). Max homodimers and Max/Mad heterodimers, on the other hand, repress genes that include this binding site because of the lack of a transactivating domain.

Phosphorylation plays a key role in regulating the activity of many transcription factors (*see* Section I and in this Section above) and c-Onc proteins. Alterations in Myc phosphorylation sites have been shown to be related to transforming activity. Mutations of threonine-58 are common in Burkitt's lymphoma, mouse plasmacytomas (283), and v-Myc (254). The transforming activity of c-*myc* is increased by mutation corresponding to threonine-58 (255) and that of v-*myc* decreased by restoring threonine-58 in the oncoprotein (284). Recent characterization of phosphorylation sites, their regulation, and the kinases involved have suggested an interdependence and a hierarchical order of phosphorylation of key sites in the transactivating amino terminal domain (178). Evidence has been presented that the phosphorylation of threonine-58 and serine-62 residues is carried out in the cytoplasm, whereas the phosphorylation of serine-71 appears to occur in the nucleus. Phosphorylation sites serine-2 and serine-11 in the Max protein have been identified as important regulators of the formation of homodimers versus Max/Myc heterodimers (285). The role that c-Myc plays in the transcription of genes involved in cell proliferation and differentiation will continue to be unraveled as the specificities of the various dimer partners become better understood.

G. *Cis*-Activation of c-*onc* Genes: MuLV and MMTV

Many replication-competent retroviruses are associated with leukemias, lymphomas, and carcinomas. These viruses, some of which are carried in the germline of animal species, are unable to transform cells in culture and they cause neoplastic disease *in vivo* typically after long latent periods. For neoplasia to result, certain additional independent genetic events may be required, or the viruses may only rarely trigger an event that eventually leads to neoplasia.

The first glimpse at a potential mechanism by which leukemogenic viruses are oncogenic came from the observations that ALV integrations into or near the c-*myc* gene were causally related to the development of avian bursal lymphoma (*see* F., this subsection). This phenomenon, variably termed insertional mutagenesis, downstream promotion, promoter insertion, or enhancer insertion, among others, is involved in neoplasia induced by many retroviruses that do not contain an oncogene. Proviruses can be inserted upstream or downstream of the target gene, in the same transcriptional orientation as the target gene, or the opposite orientation. For "promoter insertion" to be functional, as often observed in the avian bursal lymphomas, the provirus must be upstream and in the same transcriptional orientation as the target gene. However, a target gene does not have to be transcribed by read-thru from the viral LTR for expression to be activated by presence of the provirus. The enhancer sequence in the LTR functions in an orientation-independent manner and can be upstream or downstream. Usually, the proviral transcription is in the opposite direction to the target gene for enhancer activation, but not always (286). The term *cis*-activation of oncogenes conveys the importance of the proximity of the integrated provirus to the proto-oncogene, but without the mechanistic implication of "promotion insertion" or "enhancer insertion" (*rev.* 4).

A hallmark of tumors induced by proviral insertion rather than by oncogenes carried by the virus is the clonality of the tumors. This is particularly obvious when most of the cells in a tumor have in common one or a small set of proviral integrations. Such integration events could be shared by the majority of the cells in the tumor only if they occurred early in the clonal proliferation of that tumor. Common integrations within a single tumor do not provide evidence for causality, however. Hybridization probes made from DNA sequences adjacent to a particular integrated provirus common in one tumor made it possible to detect proviral integrations in the same region in independent tumors. These findings were strongly suggestive that the common integration regions contained genes that contributed to neoplasia. Oncogenes familiar to us in other contexts have been found to be activated by the *cis*-activation mechanism and, more significantly, new oncogenes have been revealed for the first time. Indeed, many putative oncogenes have been identified in this way in the past decade, some of which have also turned out to be very important developmental genes.

Two examples in virally-induced mouse tumor models illustrate the discovery of new oncogenes. Friend, Moloney, and Rauscher leukemia viruses make up a related group that induces a variety of neoplasias, such as T-cell, B-cell, and myeloid leukemias in certain mouse strains. A common integration site for MuLV in T-cell tumors induced by these viruses has been observed and designated *pim*-1 (for proviral integration MuLV) (*rev.* 287). Insertion of MuLV near *pim*-1 enhances transcription of the *pim*-1 gene. That *pim*-1 expression can play a role in neoplasia has been directly demonstrated by transgenic experiments (288). Pim-1 has serine/threonine protein kinase activity (289), an activity shared by the known oncoproteins Mos and Raf. The *pim*-1 gene has been shown to actually code for two serine/threonine protein kinases using alternative translation initiations (290).

Another integration site activated by proviral insertion in the late stages of Friend virus-induced erythroleukemia is designated *spi*-1 (*rev.* 291). The *spi*-1 gene encodes the PU-1 oncoprotein, a transcription factor related to the Ets oncoprotein family.

Friend erythroleukemia is a complex multistage disease and at least two additional very interesting aspects are virally mediated. The early proliferative phase is caused by the spleen focus-forming virus (SSFV) component of the Friend virus complex. SFFV is a replication-defective virus, but its "oncogene" its not a cell-derived gene. SFFV differs from the replication-competent helper virus component in having a truncated *env* gene that expresses a gp55 protein rather than the full length gp70. The gp55 functions as an oncoprotein by activating the erythropoietin receptor (EPO-R) and thus—possibly by mimicking an erythropoiesis-independent mitogen (4)—it stimulates erythroblast proliferation (*rev.* 292a,b). Indeed, the gp55 protein is not structurally similar to erythropoietin (EPO) and the basis of the interaction—that appears to occur in the endoplasmic reticulum—is not fully understood. This seemingly unique mechanism of retroviral Env glycoprotein activation of cell receptors may be more widespread than currently realized. The other virally-mediated event in Friend erythroleukemia is proviral insertional inactivation of the *p53* tumor-suppressor gene (*rev.* 291). Thus, *cis*-activation and *cis*-inactivation may play a role in this viral disease.

Another well-studied viral neoplasia and example of *cis*-activation is mammary carcinoma induced by the mouse mammary tumor virus (MMTV). MMTV has, of course, been known since the 1930's from the pioneering work of J. J. Bittner (*rev.* 293). MMTV does not carry an oncogene, and the mechanism of transformation was poorly understood until proviral insertions allowed investigators to identify some of the important genes. Although the way *cis*-activated genes lead to malignancy is not precisely understood, at least five genes are now known to be involved in the induction of mammary carcinomas through their activation by MMTV integrations. They all appear to be involved in or interfere with extracellular signalling, *i.e.,* intercellular communication (*rev.* 294). The first of these, *int*-1, was actually the first new oncogene identified by proviral insertions (295). It is now known that this gene is a homolog of the developmentally important *wingless* gene of *Drosophila*. In light of this relationship *int*-1 has been renamed *wnt*-1 (*rev.* 294). The second gene that was identified by MMTV insertion, *int*-2 (296), is now known to be a homolog of *fgf*-3. Often, both of these genes are *cis*- activated in the same tumor, suggesting a possible cooperation. Another member of the fibroblast growth factor gene family, *fgf*-4, is also activated by MMTV insertion and is otherwise known as *hst*-1/k-FGF (297). Another common MMTV insertion site has implicated yet another member of the *wnt* gene family, *wnt*-3, in tumorigenesis (298). These four genes express secretory glycoproteins which are thought to act as growth factors. Interestingly, *int*-3, another locus identified by MMTV integrations in mammary carcinomas, does not code for a secreted product but for a protein likely to be a transmembrane receptor (299, 300). Deregulation of any of these genes may lead to hyperproliferation in the mammary gland, allowing subsequent genetic events to accumulate and, thus, resulting in full malignancy.

H. *Trans*-Activation of c-*onc* Genes: HTLV-I

Human T-cell leukemia virus type I (HTLV-I) was the first human retrovirus isolated (301). HTLV-I is distinct from the other retroviruses discussed in this chapter in having a more complex genome that includes a gene regulation mechanism. This complex genome structure is also shared by bovine leukemia virus (BLV) which causes B-cell lymphoma in cattle and sheep, simian T-cell leukemia virus (STLV), and another human virus (designated HTLV-II) with approximately 60% sequence homology to HTLV-I. These viruses make up a separate subgroup of the oncoviruses. Sequences in addition to those coding for familiar viral enzymes and structural proteins are present near the 3' end of the genome and code for the Tax and Rex regulatory proteins. Both products are essential for virus replication and Tax is responsible for the transactivating oncogenic property of HTLV- I (*revs.* 302, 303).

HTLV-I is the etiologic agent of an adult T-cell leukemia (ATL) (304) and a neurological disorder known as tropical spastic paraparesis (TSP) or HTLV-I associated myelopathy (HAM) (305, 306). ATL is an aggressive, fatal $CD4^+$, $IL-2R\alpha^+$ T-cell malignancy first recognized in 1977 in Japan (307). The virus is endemic in certain regions of the world, primarily in the southwest of Japan, central Africa, the Caribbean basin, New Guinea, South America, and the southeastern United States. In some areas 10% or more of the adults are carriers of the virus. HTLV-I is highly infectious only as cell-associated virus. Blood transfusion and sexual transmission, predominantly male to female, are well-documented routes of transmission. The major route of HTLV-I transmission that leads to a lifelong carrier state and risk of ATL is from mother to infant, predominantly by breastfeeding. Fortunately, most individuals will remain asymptomatic for life. The cumulative risk for developing ATL is approximately 2.5% over a normal 70-year life span (*revs.* 308, 309). The typical age of onset is in the 40s and 50s, although the range is broad, beginning in the 20s. Four subtypes of the disease have been defined: acute, chronic, smoldering, and lymphoma. The acute and lymphoma subtypes have a poor prognosis, with survival times from weeks to months. The events that push a chronic/smoldering disease into acute phase are unknown. This very long latent period makes it difficult to clearly understand the mechanism, but the epidemiology and molecular biology studies make a strong case for HTLV-I to be a key component in this disease. ATL cells are clonal or oligoclonal, and always have an integrated HTLV-I provirus. Viral gene expression is virtually undetectable in ATL cells, although the provirus is usually intact. In cases where the provirus is defective, the *tax* gene region is intact, strongly suggesting a role for this gene product in the malignancy. No common integration sites that would implicate oncogene activation have been observed, ruling out the *cis*-activation mechanism that was discussed previously (*see* above in G.). Although chromosomal aberrations are frequent, there are none that are characteristic of ATL.

HTLV-I may cause the chronic demyelinating disease TSP/HAM via the chronic activation of T-cells. There appears to be a strong chronic inflammation/immunological component to the pathology, and HTLV-I levels are much higher in TSP/HAM patients than in ATL patients or asymptomatic individuals. TSP has a much more rapid onset than ATL − 2 years rather than 20 years or more for ATL − and is more likely to be the consequence of transmission by blood transfusion rather than by sexual transmission or the mother to child route.

The p40 Tax product is a transcription transactivating protein that stimulates viral gene expression, while the Rex protein modulates RNA splicing and therefore controls the shift in expression from early (multiply spliced) to late (single and unspliced) mRNAs. Tax is not a DNA binding protein, but activates transcription from the viral LTR by virtue of interacting with cellular factors that recognize the 21 bp repeat elements. One of the characterized group of factors involved in regulating viral RNA expression are the cAMP response element binding proteins (CREB). Also, the Tax product is capable of stimulating cellular genes that have nuclear factor *k*B (NF-*k*B)/Rel family binding sites. The Tax product can, thus, transactivate a variety of genes that are involved in T-cell proliferation, primarily the genes coding for IL-2, the IL-2 receptor α chain and GM-CSF, as well as the c-*fos,* and c-*jun* genes, among others. The oncogenic activity of this virus is likely to involve a gene transactivating mechanism − thus the *tax* gene may be regarded as the "oncogene" of HTLV-I. The *tax* gene is essential for virus replication and has no homology to cellular proto-oncogenes. In this regard HTLV-I resembles DNA tumor viruses rather than the other oncogenic retroviruses.

HTLV-I is able to transform or immortalize human T-cells *in vitro.* Because the virus is not very infective as cell-free virus, transformation of human T-cells is usually done by co-culture of irradiated producer cells with peripheral blood mononuclear cells. Early polyclonal proliferation of IL-2 and IL-2R expressing cells precedes the emergence of immortalized T-cell clones. *In vitro* transformed T-cells typically express HTLV-I, whereas ATL cells do not. The mechanism by which the HTLV-I genome is repressed *in vivo* is not understood. Recent studies suggest that the NF-*k*B2 p100 gene product forms a noncovalent complex with Tax and this leads to the inhibition of Tax transactivation activity (310).

Tax exhibits transforming activity in transgenic animals (311, 312) and in fibroblast cell line transfection assays (313, 314), and has been shown to cooperate with Ras in transforming primary rat embryo fibroblasts (315).

HTLV-I particles are mitogenic for resting T-cells, possibly by interaction of the Env gp46 with a cellular receptor (316, *rev.* 303). Both activities, mitogenic stimulation by a virion component and Tax-mediated transactivation (*e.g.,* IL-2/IL-2R autocrine loop) may play roles in the early proliferative phase which, together with other events, lead to ATL.

Tax has been shown to repress certain cellular genes. Of particular interest in this regard is DNA polymerase β involved in DNA repair (*rev.* 303). The DNA polymerase β

gene, and perhaps others, are repressed by Tax through its interaction with bH-L-H proteins (317). It is reasonable to assume that DNA damage accumulates as a result of the repression of repair functions and this contributes to progression to full neoplasia.

V. DNA TUMOR VIRUSES: EFFECTORS OF ONCOGENIC TRANSFORMATION

This subsection on DNA tumor viruses begins with a review on interrelated experimental studies of adenoviruses, polyomaviruses, and papillomaviruses. The first evidence that viral oncoproteins could transform cells through interaction with cell cycle regulatory factors grew out of parallel studies with the adenoviruses (*Adenoviridae*) and polyomaviruses (*Papovaviridae*). The relevance to human disease was then established through the conceptual extension to another related member of the papovaviruses, the human papillomaviruses. The latter half of the subsection discusses individual examples from other virus families the mechanisms of oncogenic actions of which are not as yet clearly established. These examples from the *Hepadnaviridae, Herpesviridae,* and *Poxviridae* families are present in order of increasing genomic complexity.

A. Adenoviridae Family

In humans, adenoviruses (Ad) are highly infectious agents that may be transmitted through direct contact or via aerosols, and most commonly cause acute, febrile respiratory illnesses or ocular keratoconjunctivitis. Some 42 distinct human serotypes have been described, and, although infection in human populations is quite widespread, there has been no association to date with any form of human malignancy. However, these viruses are of substantial interest to experimental and molecular oncology, and have been for a number of years one of the premier systems used in mechanistic studies on eukaryotic transcription and replication.

1. General Features

The Ad viruses have non-enveloped, icosahedral capsids enclosing a linear, double-stranded DNA genome about 36,000 bp in length. Expression of Ad is relatively complicated in that 6 different transcriptional units are expressed early after infection, and 3 late regions are transcribed after the initiation of viral DNA synthesis (318). Early viral proteins are, parallel with other DNA viruses, those proteins whose functions within the viral life cycle are required prior to viral DNA replication. Late proteins, which normally include capsid proteins, are not required until after viral DNA replication has begun. For the adenoviruses, the polyomaviruses, and the papillomaviruses, it is a subset of the early proteins that perturbs normal cell growth, and which by virtue of certain biological and biochemical properties are designated as transforming proteins.

2. Cell Transformation

In the early 1960s, infection of rodents with the Ad 12 serotype was found to cause tumors (319). These studies represented the first example of the use of a human pathogenic virus for the direct induction of malignant tumors in an animal model system. In subsequent studies, it became clear that the oncogenic potential of the different human Ad viruses was variable, and could be used to classify the serotypes according to the degree of their tumorigenic activity in animals (320). A different classification scheme based on the degree of DNA sequence homology (A–E) fits neatly into that derived from consideration of the relative oncogenicity. Group A members (*e.g.,* Ad 12) are "highly oncogenic" in rodents, and group B members (*e.g.,* Ad 3, Ad 7) are considered to be "weakly oncogenic," requiring many months for the appearance of tumors. Ad groups C, D, and E are considered to represent the "non-oncogenic" Ad because they do not cause tumors in rodents.

It is important to note, however, that all of the Ad will induce morphological transformation of rodent fibroblasts in tissue culture. *In vitro* Ad-transformed cells possess many of the prototypic growth characteristics discussed above in "I. Assays for Cell Transformation and Oncogenesis; Properties of the Transformed Cell", including anchorage-independent growth, loss of contact inhibition, and a reduced requirement for growth factors. Through genetic studies of the induction of transformation of rodent cells *in vitro,* it was shown that only two Ad genes, *E1A* and *E1B,* are required for transformation.

3. Transforming Proteins

a. E1A. Transformation of primary cells in culture by Ad has been shown to be accompanied by the expression of the *E1A* and *E1B* regions, and to indeed require both early viral gene products (321, 322). The *E1A* gene is a complex transcriptional unit encoding numerous mRNA species derived through alternative splicing (323). Two major gene products are translated, a 289 amino acid protein and an internally spliced 243 amino acid product in Ad2 with slight differences among different serotypes. Through analysis of host range mutants, bearing alterations in the *E1A* region, the transactivating transcriptional modulatory function of E1A was defined (324). In the absence of an intact *E1A* gene, virus infection can not proceed due to a broad defect in the expression of early viral genes. A direct, independent role for the products of the *E1A* gene in the transformation of primary cells grew out of studies of the "immortalizing" function of E1A. It was observed that expression of Ad5 *E1A* alone, in primary rodent cells, would allow the cells to be passaged indefinitely in culture without senescence (325).

An important experimental technique developed in the 1980s was used to examine the cooperativity of viral and cellular oncogenes in primary cell cultures. The introduction of multiple oncogenes into primary rodent cells mimics the natural progression of genetic changes associated with the development of cancer in animals and humans. Transfection of polyomavirus (Py) middle-T antigen or an activated *ras* oncogene, which efficiently transforms established rodent cells, has no effect on primary cells. However, co-transfection with pairs of viral and cellular oncogenes – Py middle plus large-T antigen coding regions, or *ras* plus *myc*, or *ras* plus *E1A*, or *E1A* plus *E1B* – was found to efficiently transform primary rodent cells (270, 326, 327). These and subsequent studies led to the classification of cellular and viral oncogenes into two groups, the cytoplasmic and nuclear oncogenes (328). The co-transformation assay became an important tool for dissection of the genetic determinants of *E1A*-induced transformation (329).

b. E1B. The *E1B* region is also a complex transcriptional unit encoding at least 5 different mRNA species, and plays an important role in both virus replication and cell transformation. Past analyses of Ad mutants with alterations in the *E1B* region suggested a role in the shutoff of host mRNA synthesis, with concomitant stabilization of late viral mRNAs (330). The *E1B* region encodes two major proteins from overlapping reading frames, a 19 kDa and a 55 kDa protein. More recent mutation analysis of the two proteins has revealed a complex, somewhat pleiotropic series of phenotypes. For example, specific mutations in the 19 kDa protein resulted in increased cytopathic effects, a large plaque phenotype, and cell-dependent host DNA degradation suggestive of a negative regulatory role in the virus life cycle (331–333). However, at least some mutations in the 19 kDa protein inhibit transforming functions (334, 335). Surprisingly, both the 19 kDa and 55 kDa protein can independently and additively cooperate with Ad E1A for the transformation of primary rodent cells (336, 337).

4. A Dual Link to Tumor-Suppressor Genes

Examination of the amino acid sequences of the E1A gene products of a series of different Ad serotypes reveals that three regions are highly conserved: CR1, CR2, and CR3 (CR for conserved region) (338). Genetic studies subsequently showed that CR1 and CR2 are critical to the cellular transforming functions of *E1A*. In contrast, the transcriptional activating functions were genetically mapped to the CR3 domain (329). Immunoprecipitation analysis of *E1A*-transformed cells showed that E1A is specifically associated with a series of host cellular proteins (339, 340). It was hypothesized that the transformation functions of E1A might be mediated through interaction with these cellular proteins. It was further shown that the domains of E1A required for cellular transformation are critical for interaction with the host factors (341).

The seminal link between the transforming functions of viral oncoproteins and tumor-suppressor genes was established when it was discovered that one of the cellular proteins which interacted with the E1A protein is the product of the retinoblastoma gene (*Rb*) (342). In subsequent studies, it was shown that this is a common pathway of cellular transformation since oncoproteins of other DNA tumor viruses, namely SV40 T antigen (343), the other polyomavirus T antigens (344), as well as the human papillomavirus (HPV) E7 protein (345) interact with the Rb protein. This conserved association between viral oncoproteins and cellular tumor-suppressor proteins immediately suggested a biochemical mechanism for viral transformation involving interaction of normal cell growth regulators through direct protein-protein interaction. This interaction is only the beginning of a complex cascade of events which culminate in the induction of the cell cycle. More recent studies have revealed that the Rb protein is a member of a family of proteins which also includes p107 and a p130 protein (346–348). It is thought that the mechanism whereby viral oncoproteins, such as E1A, drive resting cells into the S phase of the cell cycle is through displacement of other cellular proteins that normally complex with the Rb protein (349). One important set of cellular proteins that binds specifically to the Rb protein is the E2F family of transcription factors (350, 351). Displacement of the transcription factor from the Rb complex is thought to activate E2F resulting in the induction of E2F-responsive cellular genes. Cellular genes that encode an E2F DNA binding-site in their promoters include a number of genes important for cellular (and viral) DNA synthesis such as those coding for dehydrofolate reductase (DHFR), thymidine kinase, ribonucleotide reductase, thymidylate synthetase, DNA polymerase α, CDC-2, c-*myc*, N-*myc*, c-*myb* (352–354).

The second link between the viral oncogenes and the tumor-suppressor genes features the p53 cellular protein. In cells transformed by DNA tumor viruses, p53 was found to be in complex with the SV40 large-T antigen (355, 356), or with the 55 kDa Ad E1B protein (357), or with the HPV E6 protein (358). Missense mutations in the *p53* gene are one of the most common genetic alterations found in human malignancies (359). The wild-type form of *p53* is experimentally defined as a tumor-suppressor gene because its expression can suppress the growth of transformed murine (360) and human (361) cells in culture. Interaction with viral transforming proteins, such as the E1B 55 kDa, results in the inactivation of the growth-suppressive functions of p53 (362).

More recently, studies of the role of p53 in programmed cell death (apoptosis) provide an additional perspective on the role of the viral oncoproteins in the stimulation of host cell growth. Apoptosis is a normal and important part of eukaryotic tissues and organismic development. In addition, it is thought to be a defensive mechanism for the elimination of genetically damaged cells from a normal population. The presence in an infected cell of an inappropriate (*i.e.,* viral) nucleic acid may stimulate the host cell's apoptotic response. Adenoviruses encode the E1B 19 kDa protein which can inhibit p53-mediated apoptosis (363), and, furthermore, this protein activity is required for co-transformation of primary rodent cells with Ad E1A (364). Interestingly, the E1B 19 kDa protein has functional and partial structural similarity to the cellular *bcl*-2 gene, which gene can complement an *E1B*-mutant Ad and inhibit apoptosis (365).

B. *Papovaviridae* Family

1. *Polyomaviruses*

The mouse polyomavirus (Py) was discovered by Ludwik Gross in the 1950s as the etiological agent causing unexpected salivary gland tumors induced by passage from leukemic mice. Subsequent studies revealed that Py induces a wide variety of tumors by inoculation to rodents (*rev.* 366). The simian vacuolating virus (SV40) was discovered in 1960 through examination of monkey cell lines used for the production of poliovirus vaccine stocks. The first association of polyomaviruses with a human disease was progressive multifocal leukoencephalopathy (PML), caused by the human JC virus (367).

As with the Ad, the most important contributions that the study of polyomaviruses made to the field of oncology are not related to their association with human disease, but rather to their use as experimental model systems both *in vitro* and *in vivo*. Primarily through studies more than a quarter century ago with Py and SV40 as well as Rous sarcoma virus, cancer came to be perceived not as a disease of the whole organism, but, instead, as the alteration of single cells in a population. Characteristics of transformation could be induced with relatively small amounts of genetic information delivered through viral infection (368).

a. General Features. Py and SV40 have naked, icosahedral capsids, and contain a covalently closed circular DNA genome about 5000 bp in length. The genomes are bisected into an early and late region according to the roles of the encoded viral proteins. The early region of Py encodes three proteins, originally called tumor antigens (T antigens), which are expressed from overlapping reading frames. The early viral proteins of mouse Py are named according to their relative sizes: small T-antigen (sT), middle-T antigen (mT), and large-T antigen (LT). In contrast, SV40 encodes only two T antigens, small and large.

Py and SV40 are generally species-specific and replicate in the nucleus of infected cells. The natural host for Py is the mouse and the predominant site of virus replication *in vivo* is the kidney. Experimental inoculation of newborn mice can lead to the induction of tumors in more than a dozen different tissues. The natural host for SV40 is the Asian macaque monkey in which the virus causes an inapparent infection of the kidney.

In the late 1950s and early 1960s, millions of Americans, who were immunized against poliovirus, were inadvertently inoculated with SV40 virus, a then unknown contaminant of the monkey cell lines used for vaccine production (369). Fortunately, no disease resulted from this accidental exposure.

Infections with the human papovaviruses JC and BK usually occur in young children. Following primary infection, the virus persists as a clinically inapparent, latent infection. Reactivation of latent BK and JC is associated with immunological suppression in bone marrow transplant recipients (370) and in AIDS patients. JC virus-associated PML has become a significant problem in HIV-infected patients as a cause of AIDS-related dementia (371). Thus far, the association with human malignancy is uncertain, although BK virus has been isolated from pancreatic islet cell tumors and some brain tumors (372). Both the BK and JC viruses will induce tumors in newborn hamsters when inoculated subcutaneously or intracranially.

b. Cell Transformation. Py and SV40 cause lytic infections in mouse and monkey fibroblasts in cell culture. In other cells, such as rat or hamster, Py and SV40 will undergo abortive replication and induce morphological transformation of the infected cells. Alternatively, in permissive mouse or monkey cells, transformation can be induced without lytic replication by transfection of the early viral oncogenes in the absence of the late viral genes. In cells thus transformed the viral genes are normally found to be integrated into the host chromosome, and viral transcription is restricted to the early region. Both the BK and JC viruses will transform a wide variety of cells in culture including those of mouse, hamster, rat, rabbit, and monkey. As with Py and SV40, transformed cells contain integrated BK and JC viral DNA. Transgenic mice harboring the JC and BK virus early regions develop tumors that are reflective of their different cell tropisms. BK transgenic mice develop adrenal neuroblastomas, whereas JC transgenic mice develop renal and hepatic tumors (373).

c. Transforming Proteins: T Antigens. As already mentioned above, the mouse Py expresses three distinct T antigens from the early region of the genome. All three proteins share a common 79 amino acid amino terminus and, in addition, sT and mT share 112 amino acids not found in LT. Translation of these overlapping open reading frames (ORF) is facilitated through alternative splicing from a common primary transcript. The analysis of cDNA clones, which only express the individual T antigens, has been important for the definition of the independent functions of these early viral proteins.

Large T antigen is the major replicative protein in both SV40 and Py, and is the major transforming protein of SV40. The Py LT, like the SV40 LT, is a site-specific DNA binding protein which recognizes a pentanucleotide sequence (374, 375). In addition, Py LT has ATPase and helicase activities (376) important for unwinding viral DNA at the origin of replication. Unlike the SV40 LT, the Py LT does not complex with the p53 tumor-suppressor protein (377); however — like the SV40 LT, the Ad E1A, and the HPV E7 proteins — the Py LT does complex with the Rb tumor-suppressor protein (344). Induction of cellular DNA synthesis following Py infection, which was noted many years ago (378), is dependent upon the interaction of Py LT with the Rb protein (379). Through this interaction it may be possible to coordinate the replicative cycle of the virus with the progression of the virus-induced host cell cycle. The SV40 LT and Py LT antigens are functionally similar, and differ primarily in their capacity to directly associate with the p53 tumor-suppressor protein.

The role of sT in the viral life cycle or in cell transformation is not yet clear. The sT from both SV40 and Py potentiate the transformation of cells in culture, and may be involved in transcriptional regulation (380). The sT of the SV40, Py, and BK viruses, as well as the mT of Py, can form specific complexes with serine/threonine protein phosphatase 2A (PP2A) (381). Association with sT inhibits the phosphatase activity of PP2A preventing dephosphorylation of a variety of protein targets, such as myelin basic protein, myosin light chain, p53, and LT (382, 383).

Stable transformation of nonpermissive cells in culture by mouse Py is primarily due to the expression of mT (384, 385). To mediate its transforming effects, Py mT utilizes a unique pathway relative to other DNA tumor viruses. Immunoprecipitation studies of Py mT from transformed cells revealed that a tyrosine kinase activity remained stably associated with mT during purification (386). This kinase activity was subsequently shown to be due to the presence of $pp60^{c-Src}$, the cellular homolog of $pp60^{v-Src}$ from Rous sarcoma virus. Mutational studies of mT found a good correlation between the transforming potential of mT and the ability to associate with $pp60^{c-Src}$ (387). In addition, mT has been shown to interact with other related tyrosine kinases including c-*yes* and c-*fyn* (388–391). The association with mT results in a 10- to 100-fold enhancement of the kinase activity of $pp60^{c-Src}$ (392). In addition, mT has an associated phophatidylinositol (PI) kinase activity through interaction with the p85 subunit of PI 3-kinase (135, 393, 394). Biochemical and transforming functions homologous to those of mT antigen are not found in other members of the *Papovaviridae* family. It is perhaps the unique transforming function of the mouse Py which is responsible for the broad range of tissues which can be malignantly transformed through Py infection of mice.

2. Papillomaviruses

Benign warts or papillomas have been recognized in animals and in humans for centuries (395). As early as the 9th century A.D., a stablemaster of the Caliph of Baghdad described warts in horses. The infectious nature of papillomas was first investigated around the beginning of this century by experimental transmission of canine (396), equine (397), and human (398) warts. In the 1930s, Richard Shope (399) and Peyton Rous (400) described the cottontail rabbit papillomavirus (CRPV) and its oncogenic potential. Although the first observations of the progression of benign papillomas to carcinomas were made more than 50 years ago, the precise role of the virus in malignant progression is still not completely understood.

a. General Features. The papillomaviruses (PVs) are members of the *Papovaviridae* family of DNA tumor viruses. The nonenveloped, icosahedral capsid encloses a single copy of a double-stranded DNA genome approximately 8000 bp in length. Viral DNA is found complexed to cellular histones within the nucleus of infected cells. PVs infect most higher vertebrates with a characteristically stringent host and tissue specificity.

PV infection of cutaneous or mucosal epidermis induces a distinctive hyperplasia of the suprabasal cells. Benign neoplastic warts may arise through the combined effects of accelerated cell division and delay of normal keratinocyte maturation, leading to an increase in the transit time of cells prior to being sloughed from the surface (401). The PV life cycle is highly dependent upon the progressive vertical differentiation that occurs during normal keratinocyte maturation.

b. Animal Papillomaviruses. As mentioned above, infection of cottontail and domestic rabbits with CRPV has been studied for many years. This model system has been used to study viral epidemiology and transmission, host immune response to viral infection, and the extrinsic and intrinsic factors which play a role in the malignant progression of benign tumors. CRPV infection of rabbits induces papillomas which can either regress, persist, or, over the course of several years, undergo malignant transformation to invasive, metastatic, squamous carcinomas. Spontaneous enzootic disease in wild cottontail rabbits is primarily restricted to the upper midwestern United States. Experimental laboratory infection of domestic rabbits is readily accomplished using extracts of papillomas from wild rabbits. Interestingly, although rapidly growing benign warts are induced in domestic rabbits, the infection can not be transmitted using extracts of domestic rabbit warts (402) because little or no infectious virus is produced (403, 404). However, benign warts of domestic rabbits progress to carcinoma at a much higher frequency than similar lesions of wild rabbits (400, 405). These early observations with CRPV illustrate the importance of as yet undefined genetic factors which can influnce both productive viral infection and malignant progression.

A second major concept which is illustrated by the early work with CRPV is related to the multistep nature of cancer. The rate of malignant progression of CRPV-induced benign warts can be substantially enhanced by the repeated application of a complete carcinogen acting as a tumor-promoting agent, such as coal tar or 3-methylcholanthrene (406, 407). In this model, the carcinogen acts in concert with CRPV in the malignant progression.

Bovine papillomavirus types 1 and 2 (BPV-1, BPV-2) induce strictly benign fibropapillomas in cattle at cutaneous and perigenital sites (408). In contrast, alimentary papillomas in cattle induced by BPV-4 have been associated with a geographically restricted, but high incidence of malignant conversion (409). BPV-4 induced alimentary tract papillomas were observed to become malignant only in areas of Scotland where cattle consumed bracken fern. It has subsequently been shown that bracken fern contains radiomimetic and immunosuppressive plant metabolites when grown in certain geographic areas (410). Under these circumstances, the bracken fern substances synergise/promote BPV-4 in the malignant conversion of benign lesions.

    c. Human Papillomaviruses. The most commonly recognized manifestations of infection by human papillomaviruses (HPV) are palmar or plantar warts on the hands and feet. These benign lesions, caused by HPV types 1–4, are virtually ubiquitous, although they are somewhat more common in children than in adults. To date, more than 70 different HPV types have been isolated from a wide variety of cutaneous and mucosal epithelial lesions (411, 412). HPVs can be broadly divided into two groups: mucosal-associated and cutaneous-associated. Although infection of the epidermis with HPV normally results in a benign hyperplastic epithelial tumor, certain HPV types are associated with an increased risk for malignant conversion to invasive carcinoma. Among the two dozen HPV types routinely detected in lesions of the genital and oral mucosa, two distinct groups, low and high risk, are recognized according to their relative associations with the development of invasive cancer (413).

Infection by HPV types 6 and 11 is the etiological cause of sexually transmitted genital warts or condyloma acuminatum (414–416). These are generally benign, exophytic lesions on external or internal genital mucosal surfaces. Although genital warts can be persistent, infectious, and resistant to therapy, they are associated with a relatively low rate of malignant progression. During pregnancy, condyloma are often observed to increase in both size and number, possibly due to direct hormonal effects on HPV transcription or host immunity (417, 418).

Numerous epidemiological studies suggested that human cervical cancer has an infectious etiology. This led to the consideration of many sexually transmitted viral and bacterial agents including herpes simplex virus type 2 (419). In the late 1970s, it became clear that the cytological abnormalities which are the diagnostic basis for the Pap (Papanicolaou) screen are, in fact, cytopathic effects resulting from HPV infection (420, 421). With the advent of molecular cloning and technical improvements in nucleic acid hybridization in the 1980s, an etiological relationship between HPV infection and cervical cancer was established. More than 85% of cervical carcinoma tissues examined have been found to maintain and express HPV sequences (413). In general, it is a subgroup of HPVs referred to as the "high-risk" types which are found in premalignant and malignant lesions of the genital and oral mucosa. This group of "high-risk" HPVs is represented by types 16 and 18 which together are found in almost two thirds of the biopsies from cervical carcinomas. Epidemiological confirmation of a causal role for HPV infection is currently being established through prospective case-control studies of large cohorts of HPV-infected women (422).

    d. *Transformation of Cells in Culture by Papillomaviruses.* Although PVs cannot be routinely propagated in tissue culture, morphological transformation of cells in culture has been studied since the 1960s (423). A quantitative focal assay for BPV-1 transformation of mouse cells was developed in the late 1970s (424), which permitted the genetic analysis of the transformation and replication functions of BPV (425, 426). BPV-transformed mouse cells possess many of the typical characteristics of transformed cells, such as morphological changes (cuboidal to spindle-shaped), loss of contact inhibition and anchorage-dependence, and tumorigenicity in athymic nude mice. An unusual characteristic of BPV-1 transformed mouse cells is that the viral DNA is maintained as a multicopy extrachromosomal episome (427). This is analogous to PV-induced benign papillomas of animals and humans where the viral DNA is normally found as a physically distinct, episomal replicon.

    Similar assays systems for the study of the transforming functions of the HPVs have also been developed (428, 429), although the efficiency of transformation by the HPVs is substantially lower. Transfection of HPV-16 or -18 DNA will induce morphological transformation or immortalization of primary rodent and human fibroblasts and keratinocytes (430–437). These systems have been used for the identification of the transforming genes of the animal and human PVs.

    e. *Transforming Proteins of Papillomavirus.* E5 Protein. Principally by the study of BPV-1 transformation of C127 mouse cells, the E5 protein has been identified as the smallest transforming protein yet described. The E5 ORF encodes a 44 amino acid polypeptide with a strongly hydrophobic amino terminus for localization to cellular membranes, and a hydrophilic carboxy terminus (438, 439). The E5 protein has been shown to complex with (440–442) and disrupt normal processing and turnover of the cellular platelet-drived growth factor receptor (PDGFR) resulting in constitutive activation of the receptor (443). Activation of PDGFR may be mediated through interaction with other cellular proteins such as the 16 kDa subunit of the vacuolar H^+ ATPase which can complex with the BPV-1 E5 protein (444, 445). Mutational analyses have revealed that only 8 specific amino acids together with the overall hydrophobic nature of BPV-1 E5 are absolutely required for transformation of rodent fibroblasts (446–449). The relatively small number of amino acids required for cell transformation makes it unlikely that the E5 protein possesses any intrinsic enzymatic activity. The E5 protein physically associates with the endogenous β subunit of PDGFR, resulting in constitutive stimulation of the tyrosine kinase activity of the growth factor receptor.

    The relatively poorly conserved HPV *E5* gene also encodes a small, hydrophobic protein, albeit with a weaker transforming capacity. Expression of HPV-6 *E5* in NIH 3T3 cells leads to morphological transformation and tumorigenicity in nude mice (450). Other studies have suggested that expression of HPV-16 *E5* will perturb normal cycling of the epidermal growth factor receptor (EGFR) (451–453) leading to enhancement of EGF-mediated mitogenic stimulation of cell growth. This is a potentially intriguing mechanism, as EGF is an important growth factor for keratinocytes (454) and EGFR has been found to be overexpressed in many cervical dysplasias (455). In contrast, deletion of the *E5* ORF in the rabbit CRPV model system resulted in only a modest effect on the development of cutaneous warts, suggesting that expression of *E5* may not be absolutely required for induction of *benign* tumors (456).

E6 and E7 Proteins. In HPV-associated carcinomas, viral DNA is frequently integrated into one or more apparently random locations in the host chromosome (457–459). However, with regard to the viral genome, integration preferentially occurs within the *E1* and/or *E2* ORFs leading to disruption of functions involved in viral DNA replication and transcriptional regulation. The *E6* and *E7* genes are invariably spared of disruption and found to be constitutively expressed in virtually all HPV-associated carcinomas (460–463). Genetic analysis of cellular immortalizing or transforming functions of the HPVs has indicated that, in contrast to BPV where *E5* encodes the predominant viral transforming function, the major transforming genes of the HPVs are the *E6* and *E7* proteins.

The HPV E6 protein encoded by the "high-risk" HPVs (*e.g.*, types 16 and 18), cooperates with the HPV E7 protein in the immortalization of primary human keratinocytes (459, 464–467). The E6 protein from the "high-risk" associates with a key cell cycle regulatory protein, p53, and promotes the rapid proteolytic degradation of the protein (358, 468, 469). Mutational inactivation of the *p53* gene is one of the most common genetic alterations found in human cancers (359). This suggests that inactivation of its tumor-suppressor function is a critical step in malignant conversion of human cells. The HPV E6 protein, in association with another cellular protein, E6-AP (E6-associated protein), binds specifically to p53 and accelerates ubiquitin-dependent proteolytic digestion of p53 (470–472). In support of this mechanism, the levels of p53 in HPV-immortalized cells or HPV-positive cervical carcinoma lines are consistently lower than those in primary keratinocytes (473, 474). In human keratinocytes that express the HPV-16 E6 protein the intracellular half-life of the endogenous p53 is reduced from 3 hours to approximately 20 minutes (475). Therefore, inactivation of the cell-cycle regulatory functions of p53 is thought to result from the ability of HPV E6 to target cellular p53 for degradation. Several lines of evidence indicate that the reduced levels of p53 in HPV-E6-expressing cells are accompanied by functional inactivation, including interference with p53 transcriptional repression (476), and abrogation of the p53-mediated cellular response to DNA damage (477).

The HPV E7 protein also associates with a cell-cycle regulatory factor, the retinoblastoma tumor-suppressor protein (Rb) (345, 478). Insight into the activity of the E7 protein followed recognition of the functional and structural similarity to the Ad E1A protein (433). HPV E7, like Ad E1A and SV40 T antigen, can transactivate the Ad E2 promoter and cooperate with an activated *ras* gene for the transformation of primary rodent cells in culture (432, 433). In addition to the functional homology, the E7 protein shares regions of significant amino acid sequence similarity with Ad E1A and SV40 T antigen (433). These conserved regions were found to be involved in binding to the Rb protein (342–345). As with HPV E6 association with p53, binding of E7 to the Rb protein is thought to functionally inactivate its cell-cycle-regulatory functions so as to permit progression of cells into S phase. An apparent consequence of the interaction between HPV E7 and the Rb family of proteins (p105, p107, and p130) (479, 480) is the displacement of a cellular transcription factor, E2F (350, 481, 482). The E2F family of transcription factors is thought to modulate the expression of a number of cellular genes important to cell-cycle progression and cellular DNA synthesis, as discussed above (in A.4).

The PVs do not encode their own DNA polymerase, primase, or any enzymes necessary for nucleotide synthesis. Thus, to accomplish viral DNA replication, infection of basal cells in the epithelium is accompanied by a delay in normal terminal differentiation of keratinocytes, and stimulation of unscheduled G_1/S transition for the induction of the host DNA synthetic machinery. Therefore, in the context of the virus life cycle, expression of E7, association with Rb, and dissociation of E2F may provide the means for induction of S-phase-specific catalytic enzymes required for viral DNA replication (483).

Infection with virtually all papillomaviruses induces epithelial hyperproliferation; however, only a relatively small proportion of the lesions will progress to carcinoma. Although expression of the "high-risk" HPV E6 and E7 proteins are required for malignant progression, clearly other cellular events may be necessary in the progression toward invasive cancer. Thus, elucidation of the biochemical differences between the transforming proteins of the "high"- and "low"-risk HPVs may significantly contribute to our understanding of the role that viral infection can play in human and animal cancer.

C. Hepatitis Viruses

Acute inflammation of the liver can be observed in association with many infectious agents. Hepatitis is often recognized by the pathognomic jaundice or yellow discoloration of the skin and conjunctiva, due to deposition of bile pigments normally removed by a healthy liver. "Viral hepatitis" is generally used to refer to infections due to one of at least five different virus types designated as hepatitis A–E (HAV, HBV, HCV, etc.) viruses. HAV is a single-stranded RNA virus, a picornavirus; it causes an acute "infectious hepatitis" which is primarily spread through fecal contamination of water or food sources. Although HAV infection can in some cases be fulminant and fatal, complete recovery is the most common outcome. In contrast, infection with the other human hepatitis viruses, *e.g.,* HBV and HCV, are associated with both acute and chronic phases of infection, and with a substantially elevated, long-term risk for the development of hepatocellular carcinoma (HCC). It has been estimated that more than 500,000 deaths per year can be attributed to liver cancer, making it one of the most common human malignancies in the world (484).

1. Hepatitis B Virus

a. Internal Organization and Replication Features. Proof for the viral etiology of "serum hepatitis" grew out of immunogenetic studies of Blumberg and others in the 1960s (485–487) who made the connection between the Australian antigen and its specific relationship to clinical hepatitis. In 1970 Dane *et al.* (488) were first to observe by electron microscopy the complete 42 nm size spherical HBV virions in the serum of hepatitis patients. HBV is characterized by three antigens. The viral surface antigen, HBsAg, which is the target of neutralizing antibody, is located on the phospholipid-containing envelope. The 22–25 nm size electron-dense inner core displays the core (HBcAg) and the "e" (HBeAg) antigens.[2] The core encloses the viral DNA genome. The

---

[2]The surface (envelope) antigen specificity (HBsAg) is contained in three HBV envelope polypeptides, ranging from 24 to 33 kDa in the nonglycosylated form and encoded by the pre-S2

packaged DNA genome is a 3–3.3 kb, partially double-stranded circle consisting of a full-length strand of negative polarity, base-paired to a complementary positive strand, comprising 15–60% of the full circle (1,700–2,800 bases) (489). The HBV genomic organization is highly compact and efficient. Every nucleotide is contained within a translated ORF, and approximately 50% of the viral DNA is translated in more than one ORF. The viral genome contains 4 long ORFs: the *C* gene (core and "e" antigens), the *S* gene (surface antigens), the *P* gene (polymerase or reverse transcriptase), and the *X* gene (X protein) (490).

The mode of viral DNA replication in the *Hepadnaviridae* family is unique. Early studies of Summers and Mason, who analyzed the replication of duck hepatitis B virus (DHBV) *in vivo* from infected livers, revealed that HBV replication utilizes an RNA intermediate synthesized by a virally-encoded reverse transcriptase (RT) (491). Following infection of liver cells, the partially double-stranded viral genome is converted to a closed circular (cc-DNA) form by completion of the positive strand of HBV DNA. Viral cc-DNA is used as a template for the synthesis of HBV mRNA and a 3.4 kb full-length transcript. Viral mRNA is synthesized in the nucleus by the host cellular RNA polymerase II. The full-length RNA serves as a template for reverse transcription into a DNA minus-strand with concomitant degradation of the RNA template by RNase H activity of the RT. The nascent minus-strand of DNA, in turn, serves as a template for synthesis of the complementary plus-strand. Replication of the viral DNA occurs within immature nucleocapsids in the cytoplasm of infected hepatocytes. Once genome replication is complete, the mature nucleocapsids can exit through the cellular membrane by budding, retaining a portion of the host membrane as the viral glycoprotein envelope.

b. Epidemiological Linkage to HCC. HBV infection can be acquired either perinatally or postnatally, with the former being most common in highly endemic areas of the world such as Asia and Africa. In Europe and North America, the most common route of transmission is postnatal. The clinical course of disease following HBV exposure is highly variable and, at least in part, is dependent upon the immunological response of the host. Many HBV infected patients (>60%) will develop subclinical infections and about 90% of infected adults will recover completely. Rarely, infection can result in acute, fulminant hepatitis, which is often fatal. Approximately 2–10% of HBV infected adults will become chronic carriers following the acute phase of the disease. Perinatal infection of the immunologically immature newborn often results in the establishment of a chronic infection (492), although this can vary according to the serological status of the mother. A high proportion (70–90%) of HBeAg-positive mothers will transmit virus to their newborns; in contrast, among HBsAg-positive women the frequency of transmission is much lower (493, 494).

It has been estimated that there are over 250 million chronic carriers of HBV in the world. Chronic HBV carriers have a 100- to 200-fold increased lifetime risk for the development of hepatocellular cancer. The epidemiological linkage between chronic HBV infection and HCC is compelling evidence that HBV infection can play a significant role

---

and the S region of the S ORF. Both nucleocapsid (core protein) specificities (HBcAg and HBeAg) reside in a 22 kDa *C*-gene encoded polypeptide. The HBcAg specificity in undisrupted core particles appears to be due to the intact conformation of the 22 kDa polypeptide, which conformation masks the HBeAg specificity. The soluble HBeAg is a truncated 16 kDa segment of the 22 kDa polypeptide in which residual determinants of HBcAg specificity are masked in the serum by avid and specific binding to serum albumin, immunoglobulin, and α-antitrypsin. HBeAg may be extracted from intact virion core by strong detergent. In the serum of infected individuals the HBeAg found is possibly generated by proteolytic self-cleavage of the 22 kDa polypeptide (*rev.* 489).

in the development of liver cancer. Examination of HCC tissues from HBV infected patients has revealed that 75–85% of the tumors retain viral DNA (495–497). In the majority of the cases where HBV DNA is retained, multiple copies of the viral DNA are found to have integrated into the host genome. HCC tumors are typically of clonal origin with respect to the locus of HBV DNA integration. This suggests that integration precedes malignant progression in the infected hepatocytes and, furthermore, that integration of viral sequences may play a direct role in the development of HBV-associated liver cancer.

Additional evidence of a role for hepadnaviruses in liver cancer comes from animal model studies, in particular those with the woodchuck hepatitis virus (WHV). As noted above, there is a close epidemiological association between HBV infection in humans and HCC. The linkage between WHV infection of woodchucks and HCC is even more compelling. Virtually 100% of naturally or experimentally infected animals will develop HCC within 2 to 4 years after infection (498, 499). Ground squirrels naturally infected with their species-specific hepatitis virus (GSHV) were observed in captivity, and no HCC was seen prior to 4.5 years; however, by 7 years, two thirds of the infected squirrels had died of HCC (500).

c. Viral Mechanisms of Neoplastic Conversion. Oncogenes or Insertional Activation.

The molecular mechanisms potentially responsible for the progression of HBV-infected hepatocytes can be broadly divided into two catgories: direct and indirect. Persuasive evidence for HBV playing either (or both) a direct or an indirect role in malignant progression has recently become available.

If HBV plays a direct role in the development of HCC, the virus must either encode a dominant-acting oncogene, directly induce a cellular oncogene, or inactivate a tumor-suppressor gene. Most proto-oncogenes, as discussed previously, have been detected through transduction by rodent, feline, and avian retroviruses. Although hepadnaviruses and retroviruses utilize similar modes of genomic replication, there is no experimental data to suggest that the hepadnaviruses encode a dominant viral oncogene such as *ras, myc, fos, src,* or *myb*. Furthermore, there is a relatively long delay after infection, prior to the development of HCC: 20–30 years in humans, 2–4 years in woodchucks, and 5–9 years in ground squirrels. Such a long latency period is more consistent with a less direct mechanism of tumor induction.

Consideration of the mode of cell transformation by *cis*-activating retroviruses may be helpful at this point. Regarding the length of the latency period in retroviral transformation of cells in culture, two distinct groups are recognized: acutely transforming viruses which induce cell transformation within weeks or even days, and those which remain latent for 6 months or more prior to transformation. The leukemia or leukosis viruses such as MuLV (murine leukemia virus) and ALV (avian leukosis virus) do not carry a dominant oncogene; instead, these tumors induce transformation by insertional activation of cellular oncogenes (*see* IV.G above). For example, inoculation of young chickens with ALV will induce a B-cell lymphoma after a latency period of 6 months or greater. Examination of the tumor cell DNA shows that the majority of the cellular genomes have a proviral insert adjacent to the c-*myc* proto-oncogene so that the expression of c-*myc* is under control of the viral LTR. The consequence of this insertional event is that the levels of c-*myc* mRNA are substantially elevated due to the "promoter insertion" (263).

Does evidence exist to suggest that the hepadnaviruses induce transformation through insertional activation? Efforts to routinely identify cellular oncogenes in the vicinity of integrated HBV genomes in human HCC have been essentially unsuccessful. Several individual examples, however, have been reported, including integration adjacent to the genes coding for the retinoic acid receptor (501, 502), cyclin A (503), and the erb-β/EGF receptor (504). More extensive analysis of human HCC has failed to identify common integration sites associated with HBV integration (505). In contrast, recent studies in the woodchuck animal model system reveal a somewhat different story, and suggest that insertional activation may play a role in malignant progression of WHV infected animals. In 30 to 40% of the woodchuck HCC tumors examined, WHV DNA is found to have integrated in the vicinity of the c-*myc*, N-*myc*, or N-*myc* 2 cellular genes (506–508). These studies suggest that induction of the *myc* gene through insertional activation may play an important role in malignant progression of hepadnavirus-associated HCC.

Chromosome Mutations. Gross chromosomal alterations, including duplications, deletions, and translocations, have been observed in HBV-associated HCC at the site of HBV integration (509). Such chromosomal rearrangements might contribute to loss of growth control during malignant progression through inactivation of tumor-suppressor genes. Restriction fragment length polymorphism (RFLP)[3] studies of HCC tumor DNA have revealed loss of heterozygosity (LOH) on several chromosomes, including 11p, 13q, 16q (510–512), and on 17p including the *p53* locus (513). Indeed, analysis of HCC samples from high-risk areas of China for alterations of the often mutated *p53* revealed a strikingly narrow spectrum of mutations. A high proportion of the biopsies contained guanine to thymine transversions at codon 249 of the *p53* gene (514, 515). The selective occurrence of this mutation in HCC from endemic areas is particularly intriguing as aflatoxin B, which is a potent mutagen in cell culture, is preferentially associated with transversions at codon 249 of the *p53* gene (516). It has been noted that dietary exposure to fungal aflatoxin B is also high in these areas and may therefore be a synergistic risk factor for the development of HCC (517); *see* Section III of this chapter for further discussion of this topic.

Transcriptional Regulation. An alternative mechanism for HBV activation of cellular oncogenes has focused on the viral *X*-gene product. The role of the X-protein is somewhat enigmatic. It is a promiscuous transcriptional transactivator (518–520) and encodes a serine/threonine protein kinase activity (521). Expression of the *X*-gene is not required for virus replication in cell culture (522), although it may be important for replication *in vivo* (523). The HBV X-protein does not bind directly to DNA, but instead mediates its transcriptional effects through interaction with host cellular transcription factors including CREB, ATF-2, and AP-2 (524, 525). Disruption of normal transcriptional control in infected hepatocytes may contribute to malignant progression in HCC through deregulation of cellular proto-oncogenes such as N-*myc*. In support of this model, transgenic mice which express the X-protein have been reported to develop liver

---

[3]Restriction enzymes cut DNA at specific sequences and this yields "restriction fragments" of different lengths. RFLP analysis is based on the characteristic pattern of band lengths, due to polymorphism, yielded by these fragments in a Southern blot after hybridization with a specific DNA probe. Only complementary DNA will hybridize and can be made visible by autoradiography following ^{32}P labeling of the DNA preparation. When a combination of different restriction enzymes is used, the various regions of DNA yield "restriction maps" that are specific to each particular genetic region; thus, restriction maps may be useful markers for comparing the same region in different individuals or different species, without the determination of the respective nucleotide sequences. Moreover, the number and size of the DNA fragments and the amount of radioactivity associated with them may serve as indicators of relative gene abundance; conversely, RFLP analysis can also indicate the absence of certain fragments, the loss of key suppressor-genes.

cancer (526), although Lee *et al.* (527) found that HBV *X* was not tumorigenic in transgenic mice.

Indirect Mechanism. Alternatively, the link between HBV infection and HCC may be less direct. It has been known for many years that a high risk for the development of HCC is also independently associated with alcoholic cirrosis. Chronic liver damage by HBV infection or alcohol abuse is characterized by inflammation, fibrosis, and hepatocyte regeneration. Continuous tissue destruction and mitogenic stimulation of cell division over a period of years may permit the selection of additional somatic mutations and chromosomal rearrangements, which promote the development of the malignant phenotype in HCC (528). In an elegant series of experiments, Chisari *et al.* (529) created transgenic mice which expressed different amounts of HBV capsid proteins in the liver. The disproportionate expression of the capsid proteins led to the accumulation of "subviral filamentous particles" in the endoplasmic reticulum of the mouse hepatocytes. Agglomeration of the capsid glycoproteins in the endoplasmic reticulum was toxic to the hepatocytes and led to necrosis, inflammation, and hepatocellular regeneration. In two independent transgenic lines with high levels of HBV capsid protein retention, a high proportion of the mice developed HCC (530). Thus, in this model system, accumulation of HBV capsid proteins is sufficient to induce chronic hepatocellular injury which is likely to lead to the development of liver cancer (531).

2. Hepatitis C Virus

HCV, the major etiological cause of "non-A,non-B hepatitis" (NANB), is an RNA virus. HCV is discussed here because — as with HBV — infection with this agent represents a long-term elevated risk for the development of HCC. HCV is an enveloped virus with a positive polarity, single-stranded RNA genome of approximately 9.4 kb. Due to its genomic organization, HCV is classified with the flaviviruses and pestiviruses, which includes the yellow fever virus. HCV is associated with the majority of blood-transfusion-associated cases of hepatitis, and with a substantial proportion of the sporadic cases of NANB (532). A cDNA clone of HCV, isolated in 1989 (533), provided the molecular reagents for the rapid development of diagnosic assays to screen blood products for transfusion (534). HCV infection results in disease which can range from an asymptomatic course to severe, chronic active hepatitis with cirrhosis. Although acute HCV infections are often clinically less severe than those caused by HBV or HAV, patients are much more likely to become chronic carriers with attendant cirrhosis of the liver and an elevated risk for the development of HCC (535–537). Some 60–70% of the HBV-negative HCC patients have circulating antibodies to HCV, strongly suggesting that chronic HCV infection, like HBV, can play a dominant role in the development of hepatic cancer (538, 539).

HCV infection is primarily localized in the liver, and is associated with characteristic alterations in the ultrastructure of the infected hepatocytes (540). Liver damage may result from either the cytotoxic effects, which can accompany virus replication, or from the host inflammatory response. Like HBV, HCV does not encode any known oncogenic proteins and, furthermore, it does not replicate through any DNA intermediate which might permit integration into the host genome. A specific mechanism for the role of HCV in the development of HCC has, thus, not been defined. However, it seems likely that, as with HBV infection, chronic liver damage and regenerative hyperplasia due to HCV replication may drive the selection of somatic chromosomal alterations which lead to malignant progression.

D. *Herpesviridae* Family

1. *The Epstein-Barr Virus*

The Epstein-Barr virus (EBV) is a human herpesvirus which infects both B lymphocytes and epithelial cells, and is the etiological cause of infectious mononucleosis. EBV is also associated with human malignancies: Burkitt's lymphoma (BL), nasopharyngeal carcinoma, and B-cell lymphomas in immunocompromised patients. Although EBV is ubiquitous in human populations and is one of the most efficient transforming viruses known in any species, it is most often nonpathogenic and only rarely causes malignant disease (541), except in a particular region in Africa where BL is the most prevalent tumor affecting children and young adults, especially males. BL is rare in the United States.

EBV virions were first observed by Epstein in 1964 (542) by electron microscopy of a cell line derived from one of the clinical BL tissue samples of Denis Burkitt, the English surgeon who first described (543, 544) this lymphoma occurring in children living in the so-called "lymphoma belt" region of Africa. That EBV was also the cause of infectious mononucleosis was demonstrated by serological studies based upon viral antigens produced by BL cells (545).

a.   General Features.   EBV has a linear, double-stranded genome approximately 170 kb in length, and was the first herpesvirus to be completely sequenced (546). The genome has 0.5 kb tandemly reiterated terminal repeats and a sequential series of 3 kb internal direct repeats which divide the genome into the short and long unique regions (547). Individual EBV isolates tend to maintain a constant number of tandemly-arranged terminal repeats through sequential passage *in vivo* and *in vitro* (548, 549). Two EBV types have been defined, EBV-1 and EBV-2 (also called types A and B), which are highly related but differ in the sequence and arrangement of viral genes associated with latency (550).

EBV is commonly transmitted through oral secretions due to permissive replication in the epithelial cells of the nasopharynx. At some point in the course of the primary infection, EBV will infect B-lymphocytes and establish a latent infection. EBV infection of B-cells is mediated through direct association between the outer envelope glycoprotein, gp350/220 (551) and the CD21 type 2 complement receptor (552–555).

One of the hallmarks of the EBV life cycle is the highly adapted mode of virus latency. Bone marrow transplantation can result in replacement with the donor's EBV serotype, suggesting that latent virus is maintained in the hematopoietic compartment (556). Although the small B-cell is thought to be the primary reservoir of latent virus, other hematopoietic stem cells may be involved since EBV has been found associated with Hodgkin's lymphomas and some T-cell lymphomas (541).

In vitro infection of primate B-lymphocytes with EBV will lead, with high efficiency, to the establishment of a latently and persistently infected population of immortalized cells. Furthermore, the immortalized lymphocytes are tumorigenic in athymic or SCID mice (557). Immortalized, latently infected lymphocytes can be stimulated to productive infection either spontaneously (558) or by various exogenous agents, such as phorbol esters or 5-azacytidine (559). In contrast, lymphocytes infected *in vivo,* such as BL cells or B-lymphocytes from patients with mononucleosis, can be induced from latency to productive replication simply through continued growth in laboratory culture.

The clinical association of EBV with various lymphoproliferative diseases is thought to be due to the ability of the virus to efficiently induce indefinite proliferation of lymphocytes in cell culture. Nearly 100% of the well-differentiated B-lymphocytes in culture can be immortalized through EBV infection (560, 561). The EBV genome is normally found in immortalized cells as a circular extrachromosomal replicon, although integration can occur (562). Immortalized B-lymphocytes normally maintain and replicate a large fraction of the EBV genome, and up to 10 different viral gene products are expressed. EBV gene products expressed in immortalized lymphocytes include 6 EBV nuclear antigens (EBNAs), two latent infection membrane proteins (LMP-1 and LMP-2), and two small RNAs (EBER-1 and EBER-2) which have extensive sequence similarity to adenovirus VA and VA2 RNAs (547).

b. Burkitt's Lymphoma. The characterization of BL as a disease entity and the detection of EBV a few years later represents a classic example of epidemiological investigation. Following his initial finding of this unusual lymphatic tumor (543), Burkitt recognized that in areas representing the "lymphoma belt" in tropical East Africa, the tumor incidence fluctuated with environmental parameters, such as elevation, rainfall, and temperature. This suggested that a biological agent was the etiology of the disease, prior to linking this epidemiology to the electronmicroscopic observation of Epstein (542, *cf.* 544).

It has been noted that the African regions endemic for BL are also highly endemic for malaria. Infection with EBV or with malaria parasites induces massive B lymphocyte proliferation. Simultaneous and constant exposure of lymphocytes to these mitogenic stimuli is believed to represent a synergistic combination that predisposes to the chromosome translocation characteristic of BL (*see below; see also* Chap. 5, Sect. IIIA.).

The specific and requisite role of EBV infection in the development of BL is not entirely clear. In endemic areas of Africa, more than 90% of BL contains EBV DNA, while in other areas of the world where the incidence of BL is sporadic only 15–20% is associated with EBV infection. BL predominantly occurs in children 4–8 years old, and is initially recognized as a tumor of the jaw often with associated abdominal disease of the kidney, liver, or gut (563). Histopathologically, the tumor is characterized as a poorly differentiated, high-grade lymphoma interspersed with a high density of macrophages commonly thought to have a "starry sky" appearance (564). Cytogenetic analysis of BL tumors indicates that they are monoclonal in origin, expressing only kappa or lambda immunoglobulin light chain and one isozyme of glucose-6-phosphate dehydrogenase (565). Although Burkitt's lymphoma is one of the most rapidly growing types of tumors in children, the tumors are highly responsive to therapeutic intervention with appropriate chemotherapy, and are curable in more than 80% of the patients (563).

Although not used for routine clinical diagnosis, the best marker of BL is the characteristic cytogenetic abnormality of an 8;14 (less frequently 8;2 or 8;22) chromosomal translocation invariably found in BL tumor cells (566, 567). The chromosomal rearrangement occurs in both endemic and sporadic cases of BL, and in *both* EBV-positive and -negative tumors. Interestingly, the 8;14 translocation is not observed in peripheral lympocytes or hematopoietic stem cells from BL patients, but appears to be restricted to the tumor cells. The translocation is reciprocal, involving the c-*myc* oncogene on the long arm of chromosome 8(q24) and the immunoglobulin locus on the long arm of chromosome 14(q32). This chromosomal rearrangement results in the juxtaposition of the c-*myc* coding sequences to the strong transcriptional enhancer of immunoglobulin genes leading to deregulation of expression of the c-*myc* gene (568) (*see also* Section I).

In normal cells, c-*myc* expression is tightly regulated through both transcriptional and post-transcriptional mechanisms. The c-*myc* oncogene, which has been discussed in greater detail elsewhere in this chapter, plays a critical regulatory role in normal cell proliferation. It is one of the immediate early response genes which are rapidly induced when quiescent cells are mitogenically stimulated. Conversely, induction of quiescence or growth arrest by removal of growth factors leads to down regulation of c-*myc* expression (569). As a consequence of the chromosomal translocation associated with BL, the c-*myc* gene is brought under the control of the immunoglobulin locus and can no longer be down-regulated in B-lymphocytes. Constitutive expression of c-*myc* is thought to result in the continued replication of the affected lymphocytes and disruption of their customary ability to enter a resting state after transient stimulation. Indeed, elevation or deregulation of expression of the *myc* gene is associated with a wide range of tumors suggesting that *myc* activation plays a pivotal role in neoplastic growth and malignant progression (570). Studies in transgenic mice revealed that targeted overexpression of c-*myc* in B-cells, using the immunoglobulin promoter, leads to a high incidence of B-cell lymphomas (571). The tumors that arise in the transgenic mice are monoclonal, suggesting that additional somatic mutations are still required for malignant conversion. The secondary genetic alteration(s) that are required for BL tumor formation have not been specifically identified, although mutations in the *p53* tumor-suppressor gene may play an important role (572–574).

c. Nasopharyngeal Carcinoma. Nasopharyngeal carcinoma (NPC) is an epithelial malignancy that occurs most often in adults 20–50 years of age, and less frequently in children and adolescents (575). EBV DNA is found in virtually all cases of NPC regardless of geographic location (576, 577). Episomal EBV DNA can vary in size due to the inclusion of propagation of a variable number of terminal repeats. Utilizing this molecular barcode, it has been shown that a single clone of EBV DNA is associated with each NPC tumor (578). Karyotypic analysis of clonal tumors has, thus far, not identified a consistent, diagnostically indicative chromosomal abnormality, nor any evidence for the alteration of expression of a cellular proto-oncogene. Furthermore, in contrast to BL, mutations in the *p53* tumor-suppressor gene are not associated with NPC tumors (579).

Several genetic and environmental cofactors have been suggested to underlie the emergence of NPC. Individuals of southern Chinese heritage have a roughly 10-fold higher incidence of NPC irrespective of where they live; furthermore, the ratio of males to females who develop NPC is about 2 to 1. These two observations are consistent with the existence of a genetic prediposing component (575). Certain environmental or dietary cofactors have also been suggested as contributing to NPC, most notably nitrosamines in salted fish.

The expression of EBV DNA associated with NPC has been characterized as "abortive replication". Only a subset of the latent infection proteins, EBNA-1 and LMP, is expressed in the majority of NPC tumors (580, 581). Passage of NPC tumors in nude mice can induce EBV replication and virion production (578), although *p53* mutations may also be selected during *in vivo* passage (579).

d. Immunodeficiency-Associated Lymphomas. Individuals with broad immunodeficiencies including patients with AIDS, ataxia-telangiectasia, severe combined immunodeficiency, or organ transplant recipients are at increased risk for the development of EBV-associated polyclonal lymphomas (582–584) or fatal mononucleosis. The EBV-associated lymphomas are highly dependent on the immune status of the patient. For example, in organ transplant recipients undergoing immunosuppressive therapy with cyclosporin A, immunoproliferative disorders normally regress after cessation of drug treatment. These results emphasize the importance of continuously ongoing immune surveillance in the elimination of EBV-transformed B-cells (585). Although EBV-associated tumors are initially polyclonal, over the course of the disease the tumors may become oligoclonal or monoclonal (586, 587). Together, these findings suggest that multiple EBV-associated immortalizing events are initiated and followed by growth selection *in vivo* which is only permitted in the context of systemic immunodeficiency. The nature of the *in vivo* selection is unclear, although tumor progression does not appear to involve alterations in the *p53* tumor-suppressor gene (588). B-cells of the polyclonal lymphomas of immunosuppressed patients resemble those immortalized *in vitro* through EBV infection (541), in that they express 6 EBNA proteins and the latent membrane proteins LMP-1 and -2 (589).

     e. Transforming Proteins. In EBV-associated malignancy, the viral genome is maintained in a latent state and expresses a small number of viral genes. The latent state of EBV can be reestablished *in vitro* through the infection of resting B-cells. The immortalized cell lines that result are the lymphoblastoid cell lines (LCLs), used to study lymphocyte immortalization and EBV latency. As mentioned above, 10 distinct EBV gene products are expressed in latently infected B-lymphocytes (547): 6 nuclear and 3 membrane proteins. Thus far, only LMP-1 was shown to display a dominant and independent cellular transforming activity. The small RNAs, the EBERs, as well as EBNA-3B and LMP-2 are not required for the establishment of latent infection or immortalization of B-lymphocytes (590–593). The EBV gene products required for lymphocyte immortalization or latent infection include EBNA-1, -2, -3A, -3C, LMP-1, and EBNA-LP.

     The EBNA-1 protein is a sequence-specific DNA binding protein (594) which binds at the origin of replication (oriP), and is used for episomal or plasmid-like viral DNA replication. Binding of EBNA-1 to oriP is required for extrachromosomal replication of the EBV genome (595, 596). EBNA-1 is also a transcriptional activator (597) and may promote association of the EBV episome with metaphase chromosomes (598, 599).

     EBNA-2 is a nuclear phosphoprotein that associates with the chromatin and nuclear matrix, and is a transcriptional activator. Expression of *EBNA-2* induces, in turn, the expression of *LMP-1* and *LMP-2* (600–602), as well as the expression of several cellular genes (603–605). A proline-rich domain of EBNA-2 mediates binding to a cellular protein, J kappa, which enhances sequence-specific DNA binding to EBNA-2 responsive elements (606, 607). Variants of EBV with deletions in the *EBNA-2* gene (608) are commonly seen in oral hairy leukoplakia, an epithelial lesion of the tongue commonly seen in HIV-infected patients (609). Although *EBNA-2* is required for the immortalization of B-lymphocytes by EBV, its role in productively or latently infected epithelial cells is not clear.

     EBNA-3 is composed of EBNA-3A and EBNA-3B (also called EBNA-3 and -4), and 3-C (also called EBNA-6), which are partially related hydrophilic structures encoded by 3 tandem genes. EBNA-3B is not required for lymphocyte transformation, but both -3A and -3C are required. EBNA-3C is thought to play a regulatory role in EBV expression. It is a nuclear phosphoprotein with a leucine-zipper motif adjacent to a putative DNA-binding domain (610). Expression of *EBNA-3C* leads to the induction of the EBV *LMP-1* gene in late G_1 of the cell cycle (611).

     Although the explicit function of the *LMP-1* gene has not been fully clarified, its product is the only EBV protein yet shown to induce transformation of established rodent cells in culture, an often cited benchmark of a dominant oncogene. LMP-1 induces morphological transformation of Rat-1 (612) and BALB/c 3T3 (613) fibroblasts in culture. In EBV-infected cells, LMP-1 is anchored in the plasma membrane through 6 hydrophobic transmembrane domains (614). Deletion analysis has shown that the amino terminus domain and the transmembrane domain are absolute requirements for the transforming activity of LMP-1, whereas the role of the carboxy terminal cytoplasmic domain is less well understood (615–617). Although LMP-1 displays little sequence homology with known viral and cellular proteins, the overall structure is reminiscent of cell membrane receptors. Furthermore, LMP-1 has been observed to associate with components of the cytoskeleton (618), suggestive of a role in signal transduction.

EBNA-LP (also called EBNA-5) is largely associated with the nuclear matrix in infected cells and localizes to discrete intranuclear particles. The *EBNA-LP* coding sequence is created through splicing of the leaders of the other EBNA mRNAs. The protein expressed contains an internal domain with a highly repetitive internal amino acid sequence. Although the expression of other EBV transformation associated proteins are unaffected by mutation of *EBNA-LP,* the growth of the infected lymphocytes is altered. These observations suggest that EBNA-LP may regulate a growth factor or a receptor important to the immortalized B-cell (619).

2. Marek's Disease Virus

Marek's disease virus (MDV) is an oncogenic avian herpesvirus which causes T-cell lymphomas we well as peripheral nerve demyelination and paralysis in chickens (620). It was named for a Hungarian pathologist, Joseph Marek, who first described the disease in 1907. Experimental transmission was demonstrated in 1967 (621) through co-cultivation of cells from infected birds with naive chicken or duck fibroblasts. Attenuation of MDV in tissue culture led to the rapid development of an effective vaccine to prevent infection of commercial poultry stocks (622). Although MDV has received considerable attention in veterinary and poultry sciences, it is often overlooked in the consideration of DNA tumor viruses. In fact, the early success of the vaccination program in the 1970s was a disincentive to more detailed studies of the pathobiology of the virus. However, MDV remains an attractive model system for the study of the induction of lymphoma by a herpesvirus and the effective prevention through vaccination.

a. General Features. MDV was originally classified as a gamma herpesvirus, although the overall genomic structure is similar to that of the alpha herpesviruses which include varicella zoster and herpes simplex (623). Although the virus infects T lymphocytes, infectious particles are primarily found associated with the follicular epithelium of the feathers. Latently-infected T-cells can be readily established in culture as immortalized lymphoblastoid cell lines. As with EBV, latently-infected MDV cell lines express a small subset of viral antigens and will undergo reactivation and lytic replication to varying degrees in response to agents such as iododeoxyuridine (624).

b. Transforming Genes. Relatively little is known about the MDV gene functions that lead to transformation of cells in culture or T-cell lymphomas *in vivo*. It has been noted that serial passage of virulent MDV in primary cell culture will attenuate MDV tumorigenicity (625, 626). Analysis of the attenuated viral genome revealed that a 132 bp repeat sequence had been amplified, leading to the alterations in the expression of individual viral RNA transcripts (627, 628). cDNA analysis of this altered region revealed two spliced transcripts, 1.5 and 1.9 kb, although protein products have not been specifically assigned (629). Recently, a homolog of the cellular *fos/jun* proto-oncogene called *meq* has been mapped to an adjacent region of the inverted repeat segment. The *meq* gene encodes a 40 kDa basic leucine-zipper protein found only in MDV-transformed lymphocytes (630). Two additional viral proteins have been identified in MDV-transformed cells, a 38 kDa (631) and a 14 kDa (632) protein. Much work remains both in the identification and functional characterization of the viral genes involved in MDV-induced cellular transformation, and in the elucidation of their role in virus-associated lymphomas.

E. *Poxviridae* Family

The poxvirus family is a large, heterogeneous group of DNA viruses with a very wide host range which includes both vertebrate and invertebrate species. The most familiar member of the family is variola, the etiological agent of smallpox. Infection with many of the poxviruses induces an epithelial hyperplastic response resulting in the formation of benign skin tumors. Induction of benign lesions is most common with fowlpox, Yaba, Shope fibroma, and molluscum contagiosum viruses. Of primary interest for the study of the tumor biology of poxviruses is the observation that many of them encode a viral analog of the cellular epidermal growth factor (EGF), which is thought to be involved in the characteristic, virally-induced epithelial proliferation (633).

1. General Features

The poxviruses are the largest animal viruses yet described with a virion diameter of 200–400 nm. The enveloped virion contains a linear double-stranded DNA genome that ranges from 130,000 to 300,000 bp. The poxviruses are extraordinarily complex viruses. For example, they encode an independent transcriptional system which can express functional mRNA that is capped and methylated at the 5' end and polyadenylated at the 3' end (634, 635). Indeed, the poxviruses are the only eukaryotic DNA viruses that encode their own DNA-dependent RNA polymerase. Numerous other enzymatic activities have been associated with pox virions including topoisomerase, ligase, ATPase, protein kinase, polynucleotide kinase, ribonuclease, and alkaline protease (633). By virtue of their extensive synthetic capacity, poxviruses are able to express and replicate somewhat autonomously in the cytoplasm of the host cell, even being able to replicate in enucleated cells (636).

Shope fibroma virus (SFV) was first described in the 1930s as a naturally occurring infection of wild rabbits in the United States (637). Laboratory infection with SFV causes benign fibromas at the site of inoculation in both wild and domestic rabbits. Yaba monkey tumor virus was first isolated from transient subcutaneous histiocytomas on the hands and limbs of African rhesus monkeys (638). Molluscum contagiosum was identified as a serologically distinct poxvirus in 1931 (639). The benign lesions induced by these groups of viruses can persist for many months as hyperplastic foci; however, under most circumstances, they will eventually regress.

2. Virally-Encoded Growth Factors

Although the relationship between virus infection and tumor induction is not well understood, it has been suggested that poxvirus-infected cells excrete a growth-promoting factor that is responsible for the characteristic regional hyperplasia (640). Indeed, most members of the poxvirus family encode specific growth factors that are structurally or evolutionarily related to the epidermal growth factor (EGF) family of mitogenic proteins (641, 642). These viral genes, which appear not to be essential for virus replication, significantly contribute, however, to the pathogenesis of the resulting disease (643, 644). For example, replacement of the gene coding for the myxoma growth factor (MGF) in myxoma virus recombinants with related genes—such as the growth factor genes from Shope fibroma (SFGF) or from vaccinia viruses (VGF), or with the gene of rat TFGα—resulted in the reconstitution of the gross pathological features of rabbit myxomatosis (645). These results suggest that, at least in the context of myxomavirus infection, different EGF-like growth factors have similar biological activities. Amino acid sequence homology among the viral and cellular members of the EGF family is as high as 40–50%. Binding studies indicated that, like TGFα, the poxvirus growth factors can bind and activate the EGF receptor (646–649). Comparison of the sequences of SFGF and MGF revealed that these growth factors lack the characteristic membrane-spanning domain, which is normally located in the carboxy terminus of EGF-related polypeptides. Consequently, these growth factors may differ somewhat in their subcellular localization, as well as in their biological activities (645). Further studies of the subtle biochemical and pathobiological features of these viral growth factors will yield additional insights into the role of EGF in epithelial cancers.

Abbreviations Used: Ad, adenovirus; AEV, avian erythroblastosis virus; ALV, avian leukosis virus; AP-1, activator protein-1; ATL, adult T-cell leukemia; bH-L-H, basic helix-loop-helix; BH-RSV, Bryan high-titer strain RSV; BL, Burkitt's lymphoma; BLV, bovine leukemia virus; bp, base pairs; BPV, bovine papillomavirus; cc-DNA, covalently-closed, circular DNA; CR, conserved region; CREB, cAMP response element binding (proteins); CRPV, cottontail rabbit papillomavirus; CSF-1, colony stimulating factor-1; CSF-1R, colony stimulating factor-1 receptor; CyF, cytostatic factor; DAG, 1,2-diacylglycerol; DHBV, duck hepatitis B virus; DHFR, dihydrofolate reductase; E6-AP, E6-associated protein; EBV, Epstein-Barr virus; EGF, epidermal growth factor; EGF-R, epidermal growth factor receptor; EPO, erythropoietin; EPO-R, erythropoietin receptor; ERK, extracellular-regulated kinase; ES cells, embryonic stem cells; FeLV, feline leukemia virus; FeSV, feline sarcoma virus; FGF-R, basic fibroblast growth factor receptor; GAP, GTPase-activating proteins; Grb2, growth-factor-receptor-bound protein 2; GRF, guanine-nucleotide-releasing factor; GSHV, ground squirrel hepatitis virus; GVBD, germinal vesicle breakdown; HAM, HTLV-I associated myelopathy; Ha-MSV, Harvey murine sarcoma virus; HAV, hepatitis A virus; HBcAg, hepatitis B virus core antigen; HBeAg, hepatitis B "e" antigen; HBsAg, hepatitis B viral surface antigen; HBV, hepatitis B virus; HCC, hepatocellular carcinoma; HCV, hepatitis C virus; HPV, human papillomavirus; HTLV-I, human T-cell leukemia virus type I; HZ, Hardy-Zuckerman (strains of feline sarcoma virus); IAP, intracisternal A-particles; IFN, interferon; IL, interleukin; IL-2R, interleukin-2 receptor; IRS1, insulin receptor substrate 1; ISGF, interferon-stimulated growth factor; JAK, Janus or "just another" kinase; Ki-MSV, Kirsten murine sarcoma virus; LCL, lymphoblastoid cell line; LOH, loss of heterozygosity; LT, large-T antigen; LTR, long terminal repeat; MAP, mitogen-activated proteins; MAPK, mitogen-activated protein kinase; MAPKAP, MAPK-activated protein kinase; MAPKP, mitogen- activated protein kinase phosphatase; M-CSF, macrophage colony stimulating factor; MDV, Marek's disease virus; MEK, mitogen- activated protein kinase kinase; MEKK, MAPK kinase kinase; MGF, myxoma growth factor; MMTV, mouse mammary tumor virus; Mo-MSV, Moloney murine sarcoma virus; Mo-MuLV, Moloney murine leukemia virus; MPF, maturation promoting factor; MSV, murine sarcoma virus; mT, middle-T antigen, MuLV, murine leukemia virus; NANB, non-A,non-B hepatitis; NF-kB, nuclear factor kB; NGF, nerve growth factor; NPC, nasopharyngeal carcinoma; ORF, open reading frame; oriP, origin of replication; PDGF, platelet-derived growth factor; PDGF-R, platelet-derived growth factor receptor; PI, phosphatidylinositol; PKC, protein kinase C; PL, phospholipase; PLA2, phospholipase A2; PLC, phospholipase C; PML, progressive multifocal leukoencephalopathy; PP, protein phosphatase; PTB, phosphotyrosine-binding; PTK, protein tyrosine kinase; PTP, phosphotyrosine phosphatase; PV, papillomavirus; Py, polyomavirus; RAV, Rous-associated virus; *Rb,* retinoblastoma gene (gene term in italics); Rb, retinoblastoma protein (protein term not italics); REF cells, primary rat embryo fibroblasts; RFLP, restriction fragment length polymorphism; RSV, Rous sarcoma virus; RT, reverse transcriptase; SFFV, spleen focus-forming virus; SFGF, Shope fibroma growth factor; SFV, Shope fibroma virus; SH, Src homology; SH2, Src-homology 2; SH3, Src-homology 3; SHE, Syrian hamster embryo; SM, Susan McDonough (strain of feline sarcoma virus); Sos, Son of Sevenless protein; SSAV, simian sarcoma-associated virus; SSV, simian sarcoma virus; sT, small-T antigen; STAT, signal transducers and activators of transcription; STLV, simian T-cell leukemia virus; SV40, simian vacuolating virus, type 40; T antigen, tumor antigen (transforming oncoproteins expressed by polyomaviruses); TGF, transforming growth factor; TPA, 12-*O*-tetradecanoylphorbol-13-acetate; TSP, tropical spastic paraparesis; VGF, vaccinia growth factor; VL30, virus-like 30S RNA; WHV, woodchuck hepatitis virus; *WT1,* Wilms' tumor gene.

REFERENCES

1. Heidelberger, C., Freeman, A. E., Pienta, R. J., Sivak, A., Bertram, J. S., Casto, B. C., Dunkel, V. C., Francis, M. W., Kakunaga, T., Little, J. B., and Schechtman, L. M.: *Mutat. Res.* **114**, 283 (1983).
2. Burck, K. B., Liu, E. T., and Larrick, J. W.: "Oncogenes—An Introduction to the Concept of Cancer Genes". Springer-Verlag, New York, 1988.
3. Albert, B., Bray, D., Lewis, J., Raff, M., Robert, K., and Watson, J. D.: "Molecular Biology of the Cell", 3rd ed. Garland, New York, 1994, p. 1280.
4. Benjamin, T., and Vogt, P. K.: Cell Transformation by Viruses. *In* "Fundamental Virology" (B. N. Fields and D. M. Knipe, chief eds.). Raven Press, New York, 1991, p. 291.
5. Brusick, D.: Genetic Toxicology. *In* "Principles and Methods of Toxicology" (A. Wallace Hayes, ed.). Raven Press, New York, 1982, p. 223.
6. Sheinin, R., Mark, T. W., and Clark, S. P.: Viruses and Cancer. *In* "The Basic Science of Oncology" (I. F. Tanock and R. P. Hill, eds.). Pergamon, New York, 1987, p. 51.
7. Minden, M. A.: Oncogenes. *In* "The Basic Science of Oncology" (I. F. Tannock and R. P. Hill, eds.). Pergamon, New York, 1987, p. 72.
8. Merlino, G. T.: *FASEB J.* **5**, 2996 (1991).
9. Goldsworthy, T. L., Recio, L., Brown, K., Donehower, L. A., Marsalis, J. C., Tennant, R. W., and Purchase, I. F.: *Fund. Appl. Toxicol.* **22**, 8 (1994).
10. Mirsalis, J. C., Monforte, J. A., and Winegar, R. A.: *CRC Crit. Rev. Toxicol.* **24**, 255 (1994).
11. Adams, J. M., and Cory, S.: *Science* **254**, 1161 (1991).
12. Tennant, R. W., Rao, G. N., Russfield, A., Seilkop, S., and Braum, A. G.: *Carcinogenesis* **14**, 29 (1993).
13. Leder, A., Kuo, A., Cardiff, R. D., Sinn, E., and Leder, P.: *Proc. Natl. Acad. Sci. U.S.A.* **87**, 9178 (1990).
14. Carpenter, G.: *Annu. Rev. Biochem.* **56**, 881 (1987).
15. Pawson, T.: *Dev. Genet.* **14**, 333 (1993).
16. Courtneidge, S. A.: *Semin. Cancer Biol.* **5**, 239 (1994).
17. Claesson-Welsh, L.: *Prog. Growth Factor Res.* **5**, 37 (1994).
18. Wilks, A. F., and Harpur, A. G.: *Bioessays* **16**, 313 (1994).
19. Ihle, J. N., Witthuhn, B. A., Quelle, F. W., Yamamoto, K., Thierfelder, W. E., Kreider, B., and Silvennoinen, O.: *Trends Biochem. Sci.* **19**, 222 (1994).
20. Guan, K.-L.: *Cell. Signalling* **6**, 581 (1994).
21. Nishida, E., and Gotoh, Y.: *Trends Biochem. Sci.* **18**, 128 (1993).
22. Kato, G. J., Wechsler, D. S., and Dang, C. V.: *Cancer Treat. Res.* **63**, 313 (1992).
23. Turcanu, V.: *Rev. Med. Chir. Soc. Med. Nat. Iasi.* **96**, 13 (1992).
24. Songyang, Z., Shoelson, S. E., Chaudhurl, M., Gish, G., Pawson, T., Haser, W. G., King, F., Roberts, T., Ratnofaky, S., Lechiedider, R. J., Neel, B. G., Birge, R. B., Fajardo, J. E., Chou, M. M., Hanafusa, H., Schaffhausen, B., and Cantley, L. C.: *Cell* **72**, 767 (1993).
25. Moran, M. F., Koch, C. A., Anderson, D., Ellis, C., England, L., Martin, G. S., and Pawson, T.: *Proc. Natl. Acad. Sci. U.S.A.* **87**, 8622 (1990).
26. Myers, M. G., Jr., Sun, X. J., and White, M. F.: *Trends Biochem. Sci.* **19**, 289 (1994).

27. Kavanaugh, W. M., and Williams, L. T.: *Science* **266**, 1862 (1994).
28. Pawson, T., and Gish, G. D.: *Cell* **71**, 359 (1992).
29. Feng, S., Chen, J. K., Yu, H., Simon, J. A., and Schreiber, S. L.: *Science* **266**, 1241 (1994).
30. Pawson, T., Olivier, P., Rozakis-Adcock, M., McGlade, J., and Henkemeyer, M.: *Phil. Trans. R. Soc. Lond. B. Biol. Sci.* **340**, 279 (1993).
31. Schlessinger, J.: *Curr. Opin. Genet. Dev.* **4**, 25 (1994).
32. Skolnik, E. Y., Margolis, B., Mohammadi, M., Lowenstein, E., Fischer, R., Drepps, A., Ullrich, A., and Schlessinger, J.: *Cell* **65**, 83 (1991).
33. Cohen, B., Liu, Y., Druker, B., Roberts, T. M., and Schaffhausen, B. L.: *Molec. Cell. Biol.* **10**, 2909 (1990).
34. Dhand, R., Hara, K., Hiles, I., Bax, B., Gout, I., Panayotou, G., Fry, M. J., Yonezawa, K., Kasuga, M., and Waterfield, M. D.: *EMBO J.* **13**, 511 (1994).
35. Joly, M., Kazlauskas, A., Fay, F. S., and Corvera, S.: *Science* **263**, 684 (1994).
36. Kapeller, R., and Cantley, L. C.: *Bioessays* **16**, 565 (1994).
37. Nishibe, S., and Carpenter, G.: *Semin. Cancer Biol.* **1**, 285 (1990).
38. Cockcroft, S., and Thomas, G. M.: *Biochem. J.* **288**, 1 (1992).
39. Jones, G., and Carpenter, G.: *Prog. Growth Factor. Res.* **4**, 97 (1992).
40. Liscovitch, M., and Cantley, L. C.: *Cell* **77**, 329 (1994).
41. Lowenstein, E. J,. Daly, R. J., Li, W., Batzer, A. G., Margolis, B., Lammers, R., Ullrich, A., Skolnik, E., Bar-Sagi, D., and Schlessinger, J.: *Cell* **70**, 431 (1992).
42. Batzer, A. G., Rotin, D., Urena, J. M., Skolnik, E. Y., and Schlessinger, J.: *Molec. Cell. Biol.* **14**, 5192 (1994).
43. Schlessinger, J.: *Trends Biochem. Sci.* **18**, 273 (1993).
44. Avruch, J., Zhang, X., and Kyriakis, J. M.: *Trends Biochem. Sci.* **19**, 279 (1994).
45. Satoh, T., Nakafuku, M., and Kaziro, Y.: *J. Biol. Chem.* **267**, 24149 (1992).
46. Hall, A.: *Science* **264**, 1413 (1994).
47. Magnuson, N. S., Beck, T., Vahidi, H., Hahn, H., Smola, U., and Rapp, U. R.: *Semin. Cancer Biol.* **5**, 247 (1994).
48. Stokoe, D., Macdonald, S. G., Cadwallader, K., Symons, M., and Hancock, J. F.: *Science* **264**, 1463 (1994).
49. Irie, K., Gotoh, Y., Yashar, B. M., Errede, B., Nishida, E., and Matsumoto, K.: *Science* **265**, 1716 (1994).
50. Freed, E., Symons, M., Macdonald, S. G., McCormick, F., and Ruggieri, R.: *Science* **265**, 1713 (1994).
51. Cobb, M. H., Hepler, J. E., Cheng, M., and Robbins, D.: *Semin. Cancer Biol.* **5**, 261 (1994).
52. Chen, R.-H., Tung, R., Abate, C., and Blenis, J.: *Biochem. Soc. Trans.* **21**, 895 (1993).
53. Sun, H., Tonks, N. K., and Bar-Sagi, D.: *Science* **266**, 285 (1994).
54. Mustelin, T., and Burn, P.: *Trends Biochem. Sci.* **18**, 215 (1993).
55. Kamamuru, M., McVicar, D. W., Johnston, J. A., Blake, T. B., Chen, Y., Lal, B. K., Lloyd, A. R., Kelvin, D. J., Staples, E., Ortaldo, J. R., and O'Shea, J. J.: *Proc. Natl. Acad. Sci. U.S.A.* **91**, 6374 (1994).
56. Silvennoinen, O., Schindler, C., Schlessinger, J., and Levy, D. E.: *Science* **261**, 1736 (1993).
57. Barber, D. L., and D'Andrea, A. D.: *Molec. Cell. Biol.* **14**, 6506 (1994).
58. Lutticken, C., Wegenka, U. M., Yuan, J., Buschmann, J., Schindler, C., Ziemiecki, A., Harpur, A. G., Wilks, A. F., Yasukawa, K., Taga, T., Kishimoto, T., Barbieri, G., Pellegrini, S., Sendtner, M., Heinrich, P. C., and Horn, F.: *Science* **263**, 89 (1994).
59. Darnell, J. E., Jr., Kerr, I. M., and Stark, G. R.: *Science* **264**, 1415 (1994).
60. Yamamoto, K., Quelle, F. W., Thierfelder, W. E., Kreider, B. L., Gilbert, D. J., Jenkins, N. A., Copeland, N. G., Silvennoinen, O., and Ihle, J. N.: *Molec. Cell. Biol.* **14**, 4342 (1994).
61. David, M., Petricoin III, E. F., Igarashi, K., Feldman, G. M., Finbloom, D. S., and Larner, A. C.: *Proc. Natl. Acad. Sci. U.S.A.* **91**, 7174 (1994).
62. Zhong, Z., Wen, Z., and Darnell, J. E., Jr.: *Science* **264**, 95 (1994).
63. Amati, B., and Land, H.: *Curr. Opin. Genet. Dev.* **4**, 102 (1994).
64. Koskinen, P. J., and Alitalo, K.: *Semin. Cancer Biol.* **4**, 3 (1993).
65. Kato, G. J., and Dang, C. V.: *FASEB J.* **6**, 3065 (1992).
66. Castellazzi, M., and Sergeant, A.: *Bull. Cancer (Paris)* **80**, 757 (1993).
67. Karin, M., Yang-Yen, H. F., Chambard, J. C., Deng, T., and Saatcioglu, F.: *Eur. J. Clin. Pharmacol.* **45** (Suppl. 1), S9 (1993).
68. Shi, L., Nishioka, W. K., Th'ng, J., Bradbury, E. M., Litchfield, D. W., and Greenberg, A. H.: *Science* **263**, 1143 (1994).
69. Pines, J.: *Trends Biochem. Sci.* **18**, 195 (1993).
70. Klein, G.: *FASEB J.* **7**, 821 (1993).
71. Yokota, J., and Sugimura, T.: *FASEB J.* **7**, 920 (1993).

72. Knudson, A. G. *Proc. Natl. Acad. Sci. U.S.A.* **90**, 10914 (1993).
73. Ahmed, F. E.: *Environ. Carcinog. Ecotoxicol. Revs.* **C13**, 1 (1995).
74. Greenblatt, M. S., Bennett, W. P., Hollstein, M., and Harris, C. C.: *Cancer Res.* **54**, 4855 (1994).
75. Wiman, K. G.: *FASEB J.* **7**, 841 (1993).
76. Hael, P. A., Phillips, R. A., Muncaster, M., and Gallie, B. L.: *FASEB J.* **7**, 846 (1993).
77. Rauscher, F. J.: *FASEB J.* **7**, 896 (1993).
78. Hansen, M. F., and Cavenee, W. K.: *Trends Genet.* **4**, 125 (1988).
79. Weinberg, R. A.: *Trends Biochem. Sci.* **15**, 199 (1990).
80. Theilen, G. H., Gould, D., Fowler, M., and Dungworth, D. L.: *J. Natl. Cancer Inst.* **47**, 881 (1971).
81. Wolfe, L. G., Deinhardt, F., Theilen, G. J., Rabin, H., Kawakami, T., and Bustad, L. K.: *J. Natl. Cancer Inst.* **47**, 1115 (1971).
82. Wolfe, L. G., Smith, R. K., and Dienhardt, R.: *J. Natl. Cancer Inst.* **48**, 1905 (1972).
83. Aaronson, S. A.: *Virology* **52**, 562 (1973).
84. Aaronson, S. A., Stephenson, J. R., Hino, S., and Tronick, S. R.: *Proc. Natl. Acad. Sci. U.S.A.* **80**, 731 (1975).
85. Wong-Staal, F., Dalla-Favera, R., Gelmann, E. P., Manzari, V., Szala, S., Josephs, S. F., and Gallo, R. C.: *Nature* **294**, 273 (1981).
86. Robbins, K. C., Hill, R. L., and Aaronson, S. A.: *J. Virol.* **41**, 721 (1982).
87. Devare, S. G., Reddy, E. P., Law, J. D., Robbins, K. C., and Aaronson, S. A.: *Proc. Natl. Acad. Sci. U.S.A.* **80**, 731 (1983).
88. Irgens, K., Wyers, M., Moraillon, A., and Fortuny, V.: *C.R. Acad. Sci.* **26**, 1783 (1973).
89. Besmer, P., Snyder, H. W., Jr., Murphy, J. E., Hardy, W. D., Jr., and Parodi, A.: *J. Virol.* **46**, 606 (1983).
90. Rao, C. D., Igarashi, H., Chiu, I.-M., and Aaronson, S. A.: *Proc. Natl. Acad. Sci. U.S.A.* **83**, 2392 (1986).
91. Robbins, K. C., and Aaronson, S. A.: The *sis* Oncogene. *In* "The Oncogene Handbook" (E. P. Reddy, A. M. Skalka, and T. Curran, eds.). Elsevier, New York, 1988, p. 427.
92. Robbins, K. C., Devare, S. G., Reddy, E. P., and Aaronson, S. A.: *Science* **218**, 1131 (1982).
93. Hannick, M., and Donoghue, D. J.: *Science* **226**, 1197 (1984).
94. Robbins, K. C., Leal, F., Pierce, J. H., and Aaronson, S. A.: *EMBO J.* **4**, 1783 (1985).
95. Doolittle, R. F.: *Science* **214**, 149 (1981).
96. Doolittle, R. F., Hunkapiller, M. W., Hood, L. E., Devare, S. G., Robbins, K. C., Aaronson, S. A., and Antoniades, H. N.: *Science* **221**, 275 (1983).
97. Waterfield, M. D,. Scrace, G. T., Whittle, N., Stroobant, P., Johnsson, A., Wasteson, A., Westermark, B., Heldin, C. H., Huang, H. S., and Deuel, T. F.: *Nature* **304**, 35 (1983).
98. Ross, R., Glomset, J., Kariya, B., and Harker, L.: *Proc. Natl. Acad. Sci. U.S.A.* **71**, 1207 (1974).
99. Scher, C. D., Shepard, R. C., Antoniades, H. N., and Stiles, C. D.: *Biochim. Biophys. Acta* **560**, 217 (1979).
100. Antoniades, H. N., Scher, C. D., and Stiles, C. D.: *Proc. Natl. Acad. Sci. U.S.A.* **76**, 1809 (1979).
101. Deuel, T. F., Huang, J. S., Proffitt, R. T., Baensiger, J. U., Chang, D., and Kennedy, B. B.: *J. Biol. Chem.* **256**, 8896 (1981).
102. Antoniades, H. N., and Hunkapiller, M. W.: *Science* **220**, 693 (1983).
103. Johnsson, A., Heldin, C.-H., Westmark, B., and Wasteson, A.: *Biochem. Biophys. Res. Commun.* **104**, 66 (1982).
104. Yarden, Y., Escobedo, J. A., Kung, W.-J., Yang-Feng, T. L., Daniel, T. O., Tremble, P. M., Chen, E. Y., Ando, M. E., Harkin, R. N., Francke, U., Fried, U. A., Ullrich, A., and Williams, L. T.: *Nature* **323**, 226 (1986).
105. Matsui, T., Heidaran, M., Miki, T., Popescu, N., LaRochelle, W., Kraus, M., Pierce, J., and Aaronson, S.: *Science* **243**, 800 (1989).
106. Ek, B., Westermark, B., Wasteson, A., and Heldin, C.-H.: *Nature* **295**, 419 (1982).
107. Cross, M., and Dexter, T. M.: *Cell* **64**, 271 (1991).
108. Chui, I.-M., Reddy, E. P., Givol, D., Robbins, K. C., Tronick, S. R., and Aaronson, S. A.: *Cell* **37**, 123 (1984).
109. Johnsson, A., Heldin, C.-H., Wasteson, A., Westermark, B., Deuel, T. F., Huang, J. S., Seeburg, H., Gray, A., Ullrich, A., Scrace, G., Stroobant, P., and Waterfield, M. D.: *EMBO J.* **3**, 921 (1984).
110. Josephs, S. F., Guo, C., Ratner, L., and Wong-Staal, F.: *Science* **223**, 487 (1984).
111. Leal, F., William, L. T., Robbins, K. C., and Aaronson, S. A.: *Science* **230**, 327 (1985).
112. Heldin, C.-H., Westermark, B., and Wasteson, A.: *Proc. Natl. Acad. Sci. U.S.A.* **78**, 3664 (1981).
113. Lokeshwar, V. B., Huang, S. S., and Huang, J. S.: *J. Biol. Chem.* **265**, 1665 (1990).
114. Xu, Y. F., Myer, A. N., Webster, M. K., Lee, B. A., and Donoghue, D. J.: *J. Cell Biol.* **123**, 549 (1993).
115. Gazit, A., Igarashi, H., Chiu, I.-M., Srinivasan, A., Yaniv, A., Tronick, S. R., Robbins, K. C., and Aaronson, S. A.: *Cell* **39**, 89 (1984).
116. Josephs, S. F., Ratner, L., Clarke, M. F., Westin, E. H., Reitz, M. S., and Wong-Staal, F.: *Science* **225**,

636 (1984).

117. Eva, A., Robbins, K. C., Andersen, P. R., Srinivasan, A., Tronick, S. R., Reddy, E. P., Ellmore, N. W., Galen, A. T., Lautenberger, J. A., Papas, T. S., Westin, E. H., Wong-Staal, F., Gallo, R. C., and Aaronson, S. A.: *Nature* **295**, 116 (1982).

118. Westin, E. H., Wong-Staal, F., Gelmann, E. P., Dalla-Favera, R., Papas, T. S., Lautenberger, J. A., Eva, A., Reddy, E. P., Tronick, S. R., Aaronson, S. A., and Gallo, R. C.: *Proc. Natl. Acad. Sci. U.S.A.* **79**, 2490 (1982).

119. Heldin, C.-H., and Westermark, B.: Role of PDGF-like Growth Factors in Cell Transformation. *In* "Theories of Carcinogenesis" (O. H. Iversen, ed.). Hemisphere Publ., New York, 1988, p. 81.

120. Mercola, D., Carpenter, P. M., Grover-Bardwick, A., and Mercola, M.: *Oncogene* **7**, 1793 (1992).

121. Oefner, C., D'Arcy, A., Winkler, F. K., Eggimann, B., and Hosang, M.: *EMBO J.* **11**, 3921 (1992).

122. Murray-Rust, J., McDonald, N. Q., Blundell, T. L., Hosang, M., Oefner, C., Winkler, F., and Bradshaw, R. A.: *Structure* **1**, 153 (1993).

123. Kenney, W. C., Haniu, M., Herman, A. C., Arakawa, T., Costigan, V. J., Lary, L., Yphantis, D. A., and Thomason, A. R.: *J. Biol. Chem.* **269**, 12351 (1994).

124. Sherr, C. J., Downing, J. R., and Roussel, M. F.: Colony- Stimulating Factor 1 Receptor (fms): Signal Transduction and Hematopoietic Cell Transformation. *In* "Origins of Human Cancer: A Comprehensive Review". Cold Spring Harbor Laboratory Press, Cold Spring Harbor, New York, 1991, p. 473.

125. Sherr, C. J., Rettenmeir, C. W., Sacca, R., Roussel, M. F., Look, A. T., and Stanley, E. R.: *Cell* **41**, 665 (1985).

126. McDonough, S. K., Larsen, S., Brodey, R. S., Stock, N. D., and Hardy, W. D., Jr.: *Cancer Res.* **31**, 953 (1971).

127. Sarma, P. S., Sharar, A. L., and McDonough, S.: *Proc. Soc. Exp. Biol. Med.* **140**, 1365 (1972).

128. Stanley, E. R., Guilbert, L. J., Tushinski, R. J., and Bartelmez, S. H.: *J. Cell Biochem.* **21**, 151 (1983).

129. Sherr, C. J.: *Blood* **75**, 1 (1990).

130. Heard, J. M., Roussel, M. F., Rettenmeier, C. W., and Sherr, C. J.: *Cell* **51**, 663 (1987).

131. Das, S. K., and Stanley, E. R.: *J. Biol. Chem.* **257**, 1367 (1982).

132. Kawasaki, E. S., Ladner, M. B., Wang, A. M., Van Arsdell, J., Warren, M. K., Coyne, M. Y., Schweickart, V. L., Lee, M. T., Wilson, K. J., Boorman, A., Stanley, E. R., Ralph, P., and Mark, D. F.: *Science* **230**, 291 (1985).

133. Guilbert, L. J., and Stanley, E. R.: *J. Cell Biol.* **85**, 153 (1980).

134. Roberts, W. M., Look, A. T., Roussel, M. F., and Sherr, C. J.: *Cell* **55**, 655 (1988).

135. Kaplan, D. R., Whitman, M., Schaffhausen, B., Palles, D. C., White, M., Cantley, L., and Roberts, T. M.: *Cell* **50**, 1021 (1987).

136. Bravo, R., Neuberg, M., Burckhardt, J., Almendral, J., Wallich, R., and Muller, R.: *Cell* **48**, 251 (1987).

137. Orlofsky, A., and Stanley, E. R.: *EMBO J.* **6**, 2947 (1987).

138. Roussel, M. F., Shurtleff, S. A., Downing, J. R., and Sherr, C. J.: *Proc. Natl. Acad. Sci. U.S.A.* **87**, 6738 (1990).

139. Downing, J. R., Roussel, M. F., and Sherr, C. J.: *Molec. Cell. Biol.* **9**, 2890 (1989).

140. Sherr, C. J.: *Biochim. Biophys. Acta* **948**, 225 (1988).

141. Woolfold, J., McAuliffe, A., and Rohrschneider, L. R.: *Cell* **55**, 965 (1988).

142. Roussel, M. F., Downing, J. R., Rettenmier, C. W., and Sherr, C. J.: *Cell* **55**, 979 (1988).

143. Kato, J.-Y., Roussel, M. F., Ashmun, R. A., and Sherr, C. J.: *Molec. Cell. Biol.* **9**, 4069 (1989).

144. Borzillo, G. V., Ashmun, R. A., and Sherr, C. J.: *Molec. Cell. Biol.* **10**, 2703 (1990).

145. Ridge, S. A., Worwood, M., Oscier, D., Jacobs, A., and Padua, R. A.: *Proc. Natl. Acad. Sci. U.S.A.* **87**, 1377 (1990).

146. Tobal, K., Pagliuca, A., Bhatt, B., Bailey, N., Layton, D. M., and Mufti, C. J.: *Leukemia* **4**, 486 (1990).

147. Roussel, M. F., Dull, T. J., Rettenmier, C. W., Ralph, P., Ullrich, A., and Sherr, C. J.: *Nature* **325**, 549 (1987).

148. Vennstrom, B., and Damm, K.: The *erbA* and *erbB* Oncogenes. *In* "The Oncogene Handbook" (E. P. Reddy, A. M. Skalka, and T. Curan, eds.). Elsevier, New York, 1988, p. 39.

149. Harvey, J. J.: *Nature* **204**, 1104 (1964).

150. Kirsten, W. H. and Mayer, L. A.: *J. Natl. Cancer. Inst.* **39**, 311 (1967).

151. Lacal, J. C., and Tronick, S. R.: The *ras* Oncogene. *In* "The Oncogene Handbook" (E. P. Reddy, A. M. Skalka, and T. Curran, eds.). Elsevier, New York, 1988, p. 257.

152. Ellis, R. W., DeFeo, D., Maryak, J. M., Young, H. A., Shih, T. Y., Chang, E. H., Lowy, D. R., and Scolnick, E. M.: *J. Virol.* **36**, 408 (1980).

153. Tsuchida, N., and Uesugi, S.: *J. Virol.* **38**, 720 (1981).

154. Peters, R. L., Rabstein, L. S., Louise, S., Van Vleck, R., Kelloff, G. J., and Huebner, R. J.: *J. Natl. Cancer Inst.* **53**, 1725 (1974).

155. Rasheed, S., Gardner, M. B., and Huebner, R. J. (1978). *Proc. Natl. Acad. Sci. U.S.A.* **75**, 2972 (1978).

156. Franz, T., Lohler, J., Fusco, A., Pragnell, I., Nobis, P., Pauda, R., and Ostertag, W.: *Nature* **315**, 149

(1985).

157. Reddy, E. P., Lipman, D., Andersen, P. R., Tronick, S. R., and Aaronson, S. A.: *J. Virol.* **53**, 984 (1985).
158. Lowy, D. R., and Willumsen, B. M.: *Annu. Rev. Biochem.* **62**, 851 (1993).
159. Shimizu, K., Goldfarb, M., Suard, Y., Perucho, M., Li, Y., Kamata, T., Feramisco, J., Stavnezer, E., Fogh, J., and Wigler, M. H.: *Proc. Natl. Acad. Sci. U.S.A.* **80**, 2112 (1983).
160. Leon, J., Guerrero, I., and Pellicer, A.: *Molec. Cell. Biol.* **7**, 1535 (1987).
161. Goldfarb, M. P., Shimizu, K., Perucho, M., and Wigler, M.: *Nature* **296**, 404 (1982).
162. Santos, E., Tronick, S. R., Aaronson, S. A., Pulciani, S., and Barbacid, M.: *Nature* **298**, 343 (1982).
163. Parada, L. F., Tabin, C. J., Shih, C., and Weinberg, R. A.: *Nature* **297**, 474 (1982).
164. Der, C. J., Krontiris, T. G., and Cooper, G. M.: *Proc. Natl. Acad. Sci. U.S.A.* **79**, 3637 (1982).
165. Bos, J. L.: *Cancer Res.* **49**, 4682 (1982).
166. Gibbs, J. B.: *Cell* **65**, 1 (1991).
167. Hancock, J. F., Paterson, H., and Marshall, C. J.: *Cell* **63**, 133 (1990).
168. Resh, M.: *Cell* **76**, 411 (1994).
169. Kohl, N. E., Mosser, S. D., deSolms, S. J., Giuliani, E. A., Pompliano, D. L., Graham, S. L., Smith, R. L., Scolnick, E. M., Oliff, A., and Gibbs, J. B.: *Science* **260**, 1934 (1993).
170. James, G. L., Goldstein, J. L., Brown, M. S., Rawson, T. E., Somers, T. C., McDowell, R. S., Crowley, C. W., Lucas, B. K., Levinson, A. D., and Marsters, J. C., Jr.: *Science* **260**, 1937 (1993).
171. Kohl, N. E., Wilson, F. R., Mosser, S. D., Giuliani, E., DeSolms, S. J., Conners, M. W., Anthony, N. J., Holtz, W. J., Gomez, R. P., Lee, T.-J., Smith, R. L., Graham, S. L., Hartman, G. D., Gibbs, J. B., and Oliff, A.: *Proc. Natl. Acad. Sci. U.S.A.* **91**, 9141 (1994).
172. Rous, P.: *J. Exp. Med.* **13**, 397 (1911).
173. Stehelin, D., Varmus, H. E., Bishop, J. M., and Vogt, P. K.: *Nature* **268**, 170 (1976).
174. Temin, H., and Rubin, H.: *Virology* **6**, 669 (1958).
175. Temin, H. M., and Mizutani, S.: *Nature* **226**, 1211 (1970).
176. Baltimore, D.: *Nature* **226**, 1209 (1970).
177. Brugge, J. S., and Erickson, R. L.: *Nature* **269**, 346 (1977).
178. Collett, M. S., and Erikson, R. L.: *Proc. Natl. Acad. Sci. U.S.A.* **75**, 2021 (1978).
179. Levinson, A. D., Opperman, H., Levintow, L., Varmus, H. E., and Bishop, J. M.: *Cell* **15**, 561 (1978).
180. Hunter, T., and Sefton, B.: *Proc. Natl. Acad. Sci. U.S.A.* **77**, 1311 (1980).
181. Bader, J. P.: *J. Virol.* **10**, 267 (1972).
182. Kawai, S., and Hanafusa, H.: *Virology* **46**, 470 (1971).
183. Martin, G. S.: *Nature* **227**, 1021 (1970).
184. Becker, D., Kurth, R., Critchley, D., Friis, R., and Bauer, H.: *J. Virol.* **21**, 1042 (1977).
185. Friis, R. R., Schwarz, R. T., and Schmidt, M. F. G.: *Med. Microbiol. Immunol.* **164**, 155 (1977).
186. Swanstrom, R., Parker, R. C., Varmus, H. E., and Bishop, J. M.: *Proc. Natl. Acad. Sci. U.S.A.* **80**, 2519 (1983).
187. Hanafusa, H., Hanafusa, T., and Rubin, H.: *Proc. Natl. Acad. Sci. U.S.A.* **49**, 572 (1963).
188. Lerner, T. L., and Hanafusa, H.: *J. Virol.* **49**, 549 (1984).
189. Scheele, C. M., and Hanafusa, H.: *Virology* **45**, 401 (1971).
190. Duesberg, P. H., Kawai, S., Wang, L.-H., Vogt, P. K., Murphy, H. M., and Hanafusa, H.: *Proc. Natl. Acad. Sci. U.S.A.* **72**, 1569 (1975).
191. Golden, A., and Brugge, J. S.: The *src* Oncogene. *In* "The Oncogene Handbook" (E. P. Reddy, A. M. Skalka, and T. Curran, eds.). Elsevier, New York, 1988, p. 149.
192. Sefton, B. M., Hunter, T., Beemon, K., and Eckhart, W.: *Cell* **20**, 807 (1980).
193. Snyder, M. A., Bishop, J. M., Colby, W. W., and Levinson, A. D.: *Cell* **32**, 891 (1983).
194. Hunter, T., Sefton, B. M., and Beemon, K.: Phosphorylation of Tyrosine: A Mechanism of Transformation Shared by a Number of Otherwise Unrelated RNA Tumor Viruses. *In* "ICN-UCLA Symposium on Animal Tumor Virus Genetics" (B. M. Fields and R. Jaenisch, eds.). Academic Press, New York, 1980, p. 499.
195. Weber, M. J.: Malignant Transformation by Rous Sarcoma Virus: From Phosphorylation to Phenotype. *In* "Advances in Viral Oncology" (G. Klein ed.). Raven Press, New York, 1984, p. 249.
196. Martinez, R., Nakamura, K. D., and Weber, M. J.: *Molec. Cell. Biol.* **2**, 653 (1982).
197. Birge, R. B., and Hanafusa, H.: *Science* **262**, 1522 (1993).
198. Silverman, L., and Resh, M.: *J. Cell. Biol.* **119**, 415 (1992).
199. Silverman, L., Sudol, M., and Resh, M. D.: *Cell Growth Differ.* **4**, 475 (1993).
200. Waksman, G., Shoelson, S. E., Pant, N., Cowburn, D., and Kuriyan, J.: *Cell* **72**, 779 (1993).
201. Blumenschein, G. R., and Moloney, J. B.: *J. Natl. Cancer Inst.* **42**, 123 (1969).
202. Perk, K., and Moloney, J. B.: *J. Natl. Cancer Inst.* **37**, 581 (1966).
203. Levy, J. P., and Leclerc, J. C.: *Adv. Cancer Res.* **24**, 1 (1977).
204. Blair, D. G., Oskarsson, M., Wood, T. G., McClements, W. L., Fischinger, P. J., and Vande Woude,

G. G.: *Science* **212**, 941 (1981).

205. Canaani, E., Dreazen, O., Klar, A., Rechavi, G., Ram, D., Cohen, J. B., and Givol, D.: *Proc. Natl. Acad. Sci. U.S.A.* **80**, 7118 (1979).
206. Gattoni-Celli, S., Hsiao, W.-L. W., and Weinstein, I. B.: *Nature* **306**, 795 (1983).
207. Cohen, J. B., Unger, T., Rechavi, G., Canaani, E., and Givol, D.: *Nature* **306**, 797 (1983).
208. Van Breven, C., van Straaten, F., Galleshaw, J. A., and Verma, I.: *Cell* **27**, 97 (1981).
209. Seth, A., and Vande Woude, G. F.: The *mos* Oncogene. *In* "The Oncogene Handbook" (E. P. Reddy, A. M. Skalka, and T. Curran, eds.). Elsevier, New York, 1988, p. 195.
210. Maxwell, S. A., and Arlinghaus, R. B.: *Virology* **143**, 321 (1985).
211. Papkoff, J., Nigg, E. A., and Hunter, T.: *Cell* **33**, 161 (1983).
212. Arlinghaus, R. B.: *J. Gen. Virol.* **66**, 1845 (1985).
213. Singh, B., Hannink, M., Donoghue, D. J., and Arlinghaus, R. J.: *J. Virol.* **60**, 1148 (1986).
214. Singh, B., Wittenberg, C., Hannink, M., Reed, S. I., Donoghue, D. J., and Arlinghaus, R. B.: *Virology* **164**, 114 (1988).
215. Seth, A., and Vande Woude, G. F.: *J. Virol.* **56**, 144 (1985).
216. Huebner, R. J., Hartley, J. W., Rowe, W. P., Lane, W. T., and Capps, W. I.: *Proc. Natl. Acad. Sci. U.S.A.* **56**, 1164 (1966).
217. Papkoff, J., Verma, I. M., and Hunter, T.: *Cell* **29**, 417 (1982).
218. Paules, R. S., Resnick, J., Kasenally, A. B., Ernst, M. K., Donovan, P., and Vande Woude, G. F.: *Oncogene* **7**, 2489 (1992).
219. Papkoff, J., Lai, M. H., Hunter, T., and Verma, I. M.: *Cell* **27**, 109 (1981).
220. Blair, D. G., Oskarsson, M. K., Seth, A., Dunn, K. J., Dean, M., Zweig, M., Tainsky, M. A., and Vande Woude, G. F.: *Cell* **46**, 785 (1986).
221. Paules, R. S., Propst, F., Dunn, K. J., Blair, D. G., Kaul, K., Palmer, A. E., and Vande Woude, G. F.: *Oncogene* **3**, 59 (1988).
222. Schmidt, M., Oskarsson, M. K., Dunn, J. K., Blair, D. G., Hughes, S., Propst, F., and Vande Woude, G. F.: *Molec. Cell. Biol.* **8**, 923 (1988).
223. Freeman, R. S., Pickham, K. M., Kanki, J. P., Lee, B. A., Pena, S. V., and Donoghue, D. J.: *Proc. Natl. Acad. Sci. U.S.A.* **86**, 5805 (1989).
224. Yew, N., Oskarsson, M., Daar, I., Blair, D. G., and Vande Woude, G.: *Molec. Cell. Biol.* **11**, 640 (1991).
225. Propst, F., and Vande Woude, G. F.: *Nature* **315**, 516 (1985).
226. Sagata, N., Oskarsson, M., Copeland, T., Brumbaugh, J., and Vande Woude, G. F.: *Nature* **335**, 519 (1988).
227. Sagata, N., Watanabe, N., Vande Woude, G. F., and Ikawa, Y.: *Nature* **342**, 512 (1989).
228. Freeman, R. S., Kanki, J. P., Ballantyne, S. M., Pickham, K. M., and Donoghue, D. J.: *J. Cell Biol.* **111**, 533 (1990).
229. Paules, R. S., Buccione, R., Moschel, R. C., Vande Woude, G. F., and Eppig, J. J.: *Proc. Natl. Acad. Sci. U.S.A.* **86**, 5395 (1989).
230. O'Keefe, S. J., Wolfes, H., Kiwssling, A. A., and Cooper, G. M.: *Proc. Natl. Acad. Sci. U.S.A.* **86**, 7038 (1989).
231. Zhao, X., Batten, B., Singh, B., and Arlinghaus, R. B.: *Oncogene* **5**, 1727 (1990).
232. Rhodes, N., Hicks, R., Kasenally, A. B., Innes, C. L., Paules, R. S., and Propst, F.: *Exp. Cell Res.* **213**, 210 (1994).
233. Kato, G. J., Wechsler, D. S., and Dang, C. V.: DNA Binding by the Myc Oncoproteins. *In* "Oncogenes and Tumor Suppressor Genes" (C. C. Benz and E. T. Liu, eds.). Kluwer, Boston, 1993, p. 313.
234. Mladenov, T., Heine, U., Beard, D., and Beard, J. W.: *J. Natl. Cancer Inst.* **38**, 251 (1967).
235. Beard, J. W., Hillman, E. A., Beard, D., Lapis, K., and Heine, U.: *Cancer Res.* **35**, 1603 (1975).
236. Beard, J. W., Chabot, J. F., Beard, D., Hein, U., and Houts, G. E.: *Cancer Res.* **36**, 339 (1976).
237. Langlois, A. J., Fritz, R. B., Heine, U., Beard, U., Bolognesi, D. P., and Beard, J. W.: *Cancer Res.* **29**, 2056 (1969).
238. Graf, T.: *Virology* **54**, 398 (1973).
239. Moscovici, C., Gazzolo, L., and Moscovici, M. G.: *Virology* **68**, 173 (1975).
240. Sheiness, D., Fanshier, L., and Bishop, J. M.: *J. Virol.* **28**, 600 (1978).
241. Roussel, M., Saule, S., Lagron, C., Rommens, C., Beug, H., Graf, T., and Stehelin, D.: *Nature* **281**, 452 (1979).
242. Erisman, M. D., and Astrin, S. M.: The *myc* Oncogene. *In* "The Oncogene Handbook" (E. P. Reddy, A. M. Skalka, and T. Curran, eds.). Elsevier, New York, 1988, p. 341.
243. Duesberg, P. H., and Vogt, P. K.: *Proc. Natl. Acad. Sci. U.S.A.* **76**, 1633 (1979).
244. Coll, J., Righi, M., De Taisne, C., Dissous, C., Gegonne, A., and Stehelin, D.: *EMBO J.* **2**, 2189 (1983).
245. Kan, N. C., Flordellis, C. S., Garon, C. F., Duesberg, P. H., and Papas, T. S.: *Proc. Natl. Acad. Sci. U.S.A.* **80**, 6566 (1983).
246. Jansen, H. W., Ruckert, B., Lurz, R., and Bister, K.: *EMBO J.* **2**, 1969 (1983).

247. Kan, N. C., Flordellis, C. S., Mark, G. E., Duesberg, P. H., and Papas, T. S.: *Science* **223**, 813 (1984).
248. Sutrave, P., Bonner, T. I., Rapp, U. R., Janse, H. W., Patschinsky, T., and Bister, K.: *Nature* **309**, 85 (1984).
249. Levy, L. S., Gardner, M. B., and Casey, J. W.: *Nature* **308**, 853 (1984).
250. Mullins, J. I., Brody, D. S., Binari, R. C., Jr., and Cotter, S. M.: *Nature* **308**, 856 (1984).
251. Neil, J. C., Hughes, D., McFarlane, R., Wilkie, N. M., Onions, D. E., Lees, G., and Jarret, O.: *Nature* **308**, 814 (1984).
252. Alitalo, K., Bishop, J. M., Smith, D. H., Chen, E. Y., Colby, W. W., and Levinson, A. D.: *Proc. Natl. Acad. Sci. U.S.A.* **80**, 100 (1983).
253. Reddy, E. P., Reynolds, R. K., Watson, D. K., Schulz, R. A., Lautenberger, J., and Papas, T. S.: *Proc. Natl. Acad. Sci. U.S.A.* **80**, 2500 (1983).
254. Papas, T. S., and Lautenberger, J. A.: *Nature* **318**, 237 (1985).
255. Frykberg, L., Graft, T., and Vennstrom, B.: *Oncogene* **1**, 415 (1990).
256. Lutterbach, B., and Hann, S. R.: *Molec. Cell. Biol.* **14**, 5510 (1994).
257. Bister, K., Hayman, M. J., and Vogt, P. K.: *Virology* **82**, 431 (1977).
258. Sheiness, D., Vennstrom, B., and Bishop, J. M.: *Cell* **23**, 291 (1981).
259. Hayman, M. J., Kitchener, G., and Graf, T.: *Virology* **98**, 191 (1979).
260. Hann, S. R., Abrams, H. D., Rohrschneider, L. R., and Eisenman, R. N.: *Cell* **34**, 789 (1983).
261. Hayflick, J., Seeburg, P. H., Ohlsson, R., Pfeifer, S. E., Ohlsson, S., Watson, D., Papas, T., and Duesberg, P. H.: *Proc. Natl. Acad. Sci. U.S.A.* **82**, 2718 (1985).
262. Bunte, T., Greiser-Wilke, I., and Moelling, K.: *EMBO J.* **2**, 1087 (1983).
263. Hayward, W. S., Neel, B. G., and Astrin, S. M.: *Nature* **290**, 475 (1981).
264. Neel, B. G., Hayward, W. S., Robinson, H. L., Fang, J., and Astrin, S.: *Cell* **23**, 323 (1981).
265. Payne, G. S., Courtneidge, S. A., Crittenden, L. B., Fadly, A. M., Bishop, J. M., and Varmus, H. E.: *Cell* **23**, 311 (1981).
266. Payne, G. S., Bishop, J. M., and Varmus, H. E.: *Nature* **295**, 209 (1982).
267. Westaway, D., Payne, G., and Varmus, H. E.: *Proc. Natl. Acad. Sci. U.S.A.* **81**, 843 (1984).
268. Steffen, D.: *Proc. Natl. Acad. Sci. U.S.A.* **81**, 2097 (1984).
269. Li, Y., Holland, C. A., Hartley, J. W., and Hopkins, N.: *Proc. Natl. Acad. Sci. U.S.A.* **81**, 6801 (1984).
270. Land, H., Parada, L. F., and Weinberg, R. A.: *Nature* **304**, 596 (1983).
271. Schwab, M., Alitalo, K., Klempnauer, K. H., Varmus, H. E., Bishop, J. M., Gilbert, F., Brodeur, G., Goldstein, M., and Trent, J.: *Nature* **305**, 245 (1983).
272. Schwab, M., Varmus, H. E., Bishop, J. M., Grzeschik, K. H., Naylor, S., Sakaguchi, A., Brodeur, G., and Trent, J. H.: *Nature* **308**, 288 (1984).
273. Kohl, N. E., Kanda, N., Schreck, R. R., Burns, G., Latt, S. A., Gilbert, F., and Alt, F.: *Cell* **135**, 359 (1986).
274. Nau, M. M., Brooks, B. J., Battey, J., Sausville, E., Gazdar, A., Kirsch, I., McBride, O. W., Bertness, V., Hollis, G. F,. and Minna, J. D.: *Nature* **318**, 69 (1985).
275. Blackwood, E. M., and Eisenman, R. N.: *Science* **251**, 1211 (1991).
276. Ayer, D. E., Kretzner, L., and Eisenman, R. N.: *Cell* **72**, 211 (1993).
277. Zervos, A. S., Gyuris, J., and Brent, R.: *Cell* **72**, 223 (1993).
278. Blackwood, E. M., Kretzner, L., and Eisenman, R. N.: *Curr. Op. Genet. Dev.* **2**, 227 (1992).
279. Kato, G. J., Lee, W. M. F., Chen, L., and Dang, C. V.: *Genes Dev.* **6**, 81 (1992).
280. Littlewood, T. D., Amati, B., Land, H., and Evan, G. I.: *Oncogene* **7**, 1783 (1992).
281. Amati, B., Dalton, S., Brooks, M. W., Littlewood, T. D,. Evan, G. I., and Land, H.: *Nature* **359**, 423 (1992).
282. Amati, B., Brooks, M. W., Levy, N., Littlewood, T. D., Evan, G. I., and Land, H.: *Cell* **72**, 235 (1993).
283. Bhatia, K., Huppi, K., Spangler, G., Siwarski, D., Iyer, I., and Magrath, I.: *Nature Genet.* **5**, 56 (1993).
284. Symonds, G., Hartshorn, A., Kennewell, A., O'Mara, M.-A., Bruskin, A., and Bishop, J. M.: *Oncogene* **4**, 285 (1989).
285. Bousset, K., Henriksson, M., Luscher-Firzlaff, J. M., Litchfield, D. W., and Luscher, B.: *Oncogene* **8**, 3210 (1993).
286. Clausse, N., Baines, D., Moore, R., Brookes, S., Dickson, C., and Peters, G.: *Virology* **194**, 157 (1993).
287. Berns, A., Selten, G., Cuypers, H. T., and Domen, J.: The *pim*-1 Oncogene. *In* "The Oncogene Handbook" (E. P. Reddy, A. M. Skalka, and T. Curran, eds.). Elsevier, New York, 1988, p. 121.
288. Van Lohuizen, M., Verbeek, S., Krimpenfort, P., Domen, J. L., Saris, C., Radaszkiewicz, T., and Berns, A.: *Cell* **56**, 673 (1989).
289. Padma, R., and Nagarajan, L.: *Cancer Res.* **51**, 2486 (1991).
290. Saris, C. J. M., Domen, J., and Berns, A.: *EMBO J.* **10**, 655 (1991).
291. Ben-David, Y., and Bernstein, A.: *Cell* **66**, 831 (1991).
292a. D'Andrea, A. D.: *Cancer Surveys* **15**, 19 (1992).
292b. Yew, N., Mellini, M. L., and Vande Woude, G. F.: *Nature* **355**, 649 (1992).

293. Gross, L.: "Oncogenic Viruses", 3rd ed., Vol. I. Pergamon, New York, 1983, *see* Chap. 10, Mouse Mammary Carcinoma, p. 262.

294. Nusse, R., and Varmus, H. E.: *Cell* **69**, 1073 (1992).

295. Nusse, R., and Varmus, H. E.: *Cell* **31**, 99 (1982).

296. Dickson, C., Smith, R., Brookes, S., and Peters, G.: *Cell* **37**, 529 (1984).

297. Peters, G., Brookes, S., Smith, R., Placzek, M., and Dickson, C.: *Proc. Natl. Acad. Sci. U.S.A.* **86**, 5678 (1989).

298. Roelink, H., Wagenaar, E., Lopes da Silva, S., and Nusse, R.: *Proc. Natl. Acad. Sci. U.S.A.* **87**, 4519 (1990).

299. Gallahan, D., and Callahan, R.: *J. Virol.* **61**, 66 (1987).

300. Robbins, J., Blondel, B. J., Gallahan, D., and Callahan, R.: *J. Virol.* **66**, 2594 (1992).

301. Poiesz, B. J., Ruscetti, F. W., Gazdar, A. F., Bunn, P. A., Minna, J. D., and Gallo, R. C.: *Proc. Natl. Acad. Sci. U.S.A.* **77**, 7415 (1980).

302. Yoshida, M., and Fujisawa, J.: Positive and Negative Regulation of HTLV-I gene Expression and Their Roles in Leukemogenesis in ATL. *In* "Advances in Adult T-Cell Leukemia and HTLV-I Research," Gann Monogr. Vol. 39. Japan. Sci. Soc. Press, Tokyo, 1992, p. 217.

303. Feuer, G., and Chen, I. S. Y.: *Biochim. Biophys. Acta* **1114**, 223 (1993).

304. Yoshida, M., Miyoshi, I., and Hinuma, Y.: *Proc. Natl. Acad. Sci. U.S.A.* **79**, 1031 (1982).

305. Osame, M., Usuku, K., Izumo, S., Ijichi, N., Amitani, H., Igata, A., Matsumoto, M., and Tara, M.: *Lancet* **i**, 1031 (1986).

306. Bhagarati, S., Ehrlich, G., Kula, R. W., Kwok, S., Sninsky, J., Udani, V., and Poiesz, B. J.: *New Engl. J. Med.* **318**, 1141 (1988).

307. Uchiyama, T., Yodoi, J., Sagawa, K., Takatsuki, K., and Uchino, H.: *Blood* **50**, 481 (1977).

308. Yamaguchi, K.: *Lancet* **343**, 213 (1994).

309. Kaplan, M. H.: *Clin. Infect. Dis.* **17** (Suppl. 2), S400 (1993).

310. Beraud, C., Sun, S.-H., Ganchi, P., Ballard, D. W., and Greene, W. C.: *Molec. Cell. Biol.* **14**, 1374 (1994).

311. Hinrichs, S. H., Nerenberg, M., Reynolds, K., Khoury, G., and Jay, G.: *Science* **237**, 1340 (1987).

312. Nerenberg, M., Hinrichs, S. H., Reynolds, R. K., Khoury, G., and Jay, G.: *Science* **237**, 1324 (1987).

313. Smith, M. R., and Greene, W. C.: *J. Clin. Invest.* **88**, 1038 (1991).

314. Tanaka, A., Takahashi, C., Yamaoka, S., Nosaka, T., Maki, M., and Hatanaka, M.: *Proc. Natl. Acad. Sci. U.S.A.* **87**, 1071 (1990).

315. Pozzatti, R., Vogel, J., and Jay, G.: *Mol. Cell. Biol.* **10**, 413 (1990).

316. Casse, H., Girerd, Y., Gazzzolo, L., and Duc-Dodon, M.: *J. Gen. Virol.* **75**, 1909 (1994).

317. Uittenbogaard, M. N., Armstrong, A. P., Chiaramello, A., and Nyborg, J. K.: *J. Biol. Chem.* **269**, 22466 (1994).

318. Shenk, T.: Oncogenesis by DNA Viruses: Adenovirus. *In* "Oncogenes and the Molecular Origins of Cancer" (R. A. Weinberg, ed.). Cold Spring Harbor Laboratory Press, Cold Spring Harbor, New York, 1989, p. 239.

319. Trentin, J. J., Yabe, Y., and Taylor, G.: *Science* **137**, 835 (1962).

320. Huebner, R. J., Casey, M. J., Chanock, R. M., and Schell, K.: *Proc. Natl. Acad. Sci. U.S.A.* **54**, 381 (1965).

321. Graham, F. L., van der Eb, A. J., and Heijneker, H. L.: *Nature* **251**, 687 (1974).

322. van den Elsen, P., Houweling, A., and van der Eb, A. J.: *Virology* **128**, 377 (1983).

323. Stephens, C., and Harlow, E.: *EMBO J.* **6**, 2027 (1987).

324. Jones, N., and Shenk, T.: *Proc. Natl. Acad. Sci. U.S.A.* **76**, 3665 (1979).

325. Houweling, A., van den Elsen, P. J., and van der Eb, A. J.: *Virology* **105**, 537 (1980).

326. Rassoulzadegan, M., Nagashfar, Z., Cowie, A., Carr, A., Grisoni, M., Kamen, R., and Cuzin, F.: *Proc. Natl. Acad. Sci. U.S.A.* **80**, 4354 (1983).

327. Ruley, H. E.: *Nature* **304**, 602 (1983).

328. Weinberg, R. A.: Oncogenes and Multistep Carcinogenesis. *In* "Oncogenes and the Molecular Origins of Cancer" (R. A. Weinberg, ed.), Cold Spring Harbor Laboratory Press, Cold Spring Harbor, New York, 1989, p. 307.

329. Moran, E., and Mathews, M. B.: *Cell* **48**, 177 (1987).

330. Babiss, L. E., Ginsberg, H. S., and Darnell, J. E.: *Molec. Cell. Biol.* **5**, 2552 (1985).

331. Barker, D. D., and Berk, A. J.: *Virology* **156**, 107 (1987).

332. Pilder, S., Logan, J., and Shenk, T.: *J. Virol.* **52**, 664 (1984).

333. White, E., and Stillman, B.: *J. Virol.* **61**, 426 (1987).

334. Bernards, R., de Leeuw, G. W., Houweling, A., and van der Eb, A. J.: *Virology* **150**, 126 (1986).

335. Chinnadurai, G.: *Cell* **33**, 759 (1983).

336. White, E., and Cipriani, R.: *Molec. Cell. Biol.* **10**, 120 (1990).

337. McLorie, W., McGlade, C. J., Takayesu, D., and Branton, P. E.: *J. Gen. Virol.* **72**, 1467 (1991).

338. Kimelman, D., Miller, J. S., Porter, D., and Roberts, B. E.: *J. Virol.* **53**, 399 (1985).
339. Yee, S., and Branton, P. E.: *Virology* **147**, 142 (1985).
340. Harlow, E., Whyte, P., Franza, B. R., and Schley, C.: *Molec. Cell. Biol.* **6**, 1579 (1986).
341. Whyte, P., Ruley, H. E., and Harlow, E.: *J. Virol.* **62**, 257 (1988).
342. Whyte, P., Buchkovich, K. J., Horowitz, J. M., Friend, S. H., Raybuck, M., Weinberg, R. A., and Harlow, E.: *Nature* **334**, 124 (1988).
343. DeCaprio, J. A., Ludlow, J. W., Figge, J., Shew, J.-Y., Huang, C.- M., Lee, W.-H., Marsilio, E., Pancha, E., and Livingston, D. M.: *Cell* **54**, 275 (1988).
344. Dyson, N., Bernards, R., Friend, S. H., Gooding, L. R., Hassell, J. A., Major, E. O., Pipas, J. M., Vandyke, T., and Harlow, E.: *J. Virol.* **64**, 1353 (1990).
345. Dyson, N,. Howley, P. M., Münger, K., and Harlow, E.: *Science* **243**, 934 (1989).
346. Ewen, M., Xing, Y., Lawrence, J. B., and Livingston, D. M.: *Cell* **66**, 1155 (1991).
347. Zhu, L., Vandeheuvel, S., Helin, K., Fattaey, A., Ewen, M., Livingston, D., Dyson, N., and Harlow, E.: *Genes Develop.* **7**, 1111 (1993).
348. Hannon, G. J., Demetrick, D., and Beach, D.: *Genes Develop.* **7**, 2378 (1993).
349. Nevins, J. R.: *Science* **258**, 424 (1992).
350. Chellappan, S., Hiebert, S., Mudryj, M., Horowitz, J. M., and Nevins, J. R.: *Cell* **65**, 1053 (1991).
351. Bandara, L. R., and LaThangue, N. B.: *Nature* **351**, 494 (1991).
352. Hiebert, S. W., Chellappan, S. P., Horowitz, J. M., and Nevins, J. R.: *Genes Develop.* **6**, 177 (1992).
353. Blake, M. C., and Azizkhan, J. C.: *Molec. Cell. Biol.* **9**, 4994 (1989).
354. Kim, S.-J., Lee, H.-Y., Robbins, P. D., Busam, K., and Sporn, M. B.: *Proc. Natl. Acad. Sci. U.S.A.* **88**, 3052 (1991).
355. Lane, D. P., and Crawford, L. V.: *Nature* **278**, 261 (1979).
356. Linzer, D. I. H., and Levine, A. J.: *Cell* **17**, 43 (1979).
357. Sarnow, P., Ho, Y. S., Williams, J., and Levine, A. J.: *Cell* **28**, 387 (1982).
358. Werness, B. A., Levine, A. J., and Howley, P. M.: *Science* **248**, 76 (1990).
359. Vogelstein, B., and Kinzler, K. W.: *Cell* **70**, 523 (1992).
360. Finlay, C. A., Hinds, P. W., and Levine, A. J.: *Cell* **57**, 1083 (1989).
361. Baker, S. J., Markowitz, S., Fearon, E. R., Willson, J. K. V,. and Vogelstein, B.: *Science* **249**, 912 (1990).
362. Yew, P. R., and Berk, A. J.: *Nature* **357**, 82 (1992).
363. White, E., Sabbatini, P., Debbas, M., Wold, W. S. M., Kusher, K. I., and Gooding, L.: *Molec. Cell. Biol.* **12**, 2570 (1992).
364. Rao, L., Debbas, M., Sabbatini, P., Hockenbery, D., Korsmayer, S., and White, E.: *Proc. Natl. Acad. Sci. U.S.A.* **89**, 7742 (1992).
365. Chiou, S., Tseng, C., Rao, L., and White, E.: *J. Virol.* **68**, 6553 (1994).
366. Miller, J. F. A. P.: *Adv. Cancer Res.* **6**, 291 (1961).
367. Padgett, B. L., Walker, D. L., Zu Rhein, G. M., Eckroade, R. J., and Dessel, B. H.: *Lancet* **1**, 1257 (1971).
368. Weinberg, R. A.: Oncogenes, Tumor-Suppressor Genes, and Cell Transformation: Trying to Put It All Together. *In* "Origins of Human Cancer" (J. Brugge, T. Curran, E. Harlow, and F. McCormick, eds.). Cold Spring Harbor Laboratory Press, Cold Spring Harbor, New York, 1991, p. 1.
369. Shah, K., and Nathanson, N.: *Am. J. Epidemiol.* **103**, 1 (1976).
370. Arthur, R. R., Shah, K. V., Charache, P., and Saral, R.: *J. Infect. Dis.* **158**, 563 (1988).
371. Berger, J. R., Kaszovita, B., Donovan Post, J., and Dickinson, G.: *Ann. Intern. Med.* **107**, 78 (1987).
372. Shah, K. V.: Polyomaviruses. *In* "Virology" (B. N. Fields and D. M. Knipe, chief eds.). Raven Press, New York, 1990, p. 1609.
373. Small, J. A., Khoury, G., Jay, G., Howley, P. M., and Scangos, G. A.: *Proc. Natl. Acad. Sci. U.S.A.* **83**, 8288 (1986).
374. Cowie, A., and Kamen, R.: *J. Virol.* **52**, 750 (1984).
375. Scheller, A., and Prives, C.: *J. Virol.* **54**, 532 (1985).
376. Seki, M., Enomoto, T., Eki, T., Miyajima, A., Murakami, Y., Hanaoka, F., and Ui, M.: *Biochemistry* **29**, 1003 (1990).
377. Wang, E. H., Friedman, P. N., and Prives, C.: *Cell* **57**, 379 (1989).
378. Dulbecco, R., Hartwell, L. H., and Vogt, M.: *Proc. Natl. Acad. Sci. U.S.A.* **53**, 403 (1965).
379. Freund, R., Bauer, P. H., Crissman, H. A., Bradbury, E. M., and Benjamin, T. L.: *J. Virol.* **68**, 7227 (1994).
380. Loeken, M. R., and Brady, J.: *J. Biol. Chem.* **264**, 6572 (1989).
381. Pallas, D. C., Shahrik, L. K., Martin, B. L., Japsers, S., Miller, T. B., Brautigan, D. L., and Roberts, T. M.: *Cell* **60**, 167 (1990).
382. Scheidtmann, K. H., Mumby, M. C., Rundell, K., and Walter, G.: *Molec. Cell. Biol.* **11**, 1996 (1991).
383. Yang, S., Lickteig, L., Estes, R., Rundell, K., Walter, G., and Mumby, M. C.: *Molec. Cell. Biol.* **11**, 1988 (1991).

384. Treisman, R., Novak, U., Favaloro, J., and Kamen, R.: *Nature* **292**, 595 (1981).
385. Kaplan, P. L., Simon, S., and Eckhart, W.: *J. Virol.* **56**, 1023 (1985).
386. Courtneidge, S. A., and Smith, A. E.: *Nature* **303**, 435 (1983).
387. Markland, W., and Smith, A. E.: *Biochim. Biophys. Acta* **907**, 299 (1987).
388. Cheng, S. H., Harvey, R., Espino, P., Semba, K., Yamamoto, T., Toyoshima, K., and Smith, A. E.: *EMBO J.* **7**, 3845 (1988).
389. Horak, I. D., Kawakami, T., Gregory, F., Robbins, K. C., and Bolen, J. B.: *J. Virol.* **63**, 2343 (1989).
390. Kornbluth, S., Sudol, M., and Hanafusa, H.: *Nature* **325**, 171 (1987).
391. Kypta, R. M., Hemming, A., and Courtneidge, S. A.: *EMBO J.* **7**, 3837 (1988).
392. Bolen, J. B., Thiele, C. J., Israel, M. A., Yonemoto, W., Lipsich, L. A., and Brugge, J. S.: *Cell* **38**, 767 (1984).
393. Whitman, M., Kaplan, D. R., Schaffhausen, B., Cantley, L., and Roberts, T. M.: *Nature* **315**, 239 (1985).
394. Courtneidge, S. A., and Heber, A.: *Cell* **50**, 1031 (1987).
395. Lancaster, W. D., and Olson, C.: *Microbiol. Rev.* **46**, 191 (1982).
396. McFadyean, J., and Hodbay, F.: *J. Comp. Pathol. Ther.* **11**, 341 (1898).
397. Cadeac, M.: *Bull. Soc. Sci. vet. Med. Comp. (Lyon)* **4**, 280 (1901).
398. Ciuffo, G.: *Giorn. Ital. Mal. Venereol.* **48**, 12 (1907).
399. Shope, R. E.: *J. Exp. Med.* **58**, 607 (1933).
400. Rous, P., and Beard, J. W.: *J. Exp. Med.* **62**, 523 (1935).
401. Broker, T. R., and Botchan, M.: Papillomaviruses: Retrospectives and Prospectives. *In* "DNA Tumor Viruses: Control of Gene Expression and Replication" (M. Botchan, T. Grodzicker, and P. Sharp, eds.). Cold Spring Harbor Laboratory Press, Cold Spring Harbor, New York, 1986, p. 17.
402. Shope, R. E.: *Proc. Soc. Exp. Biol. Med.* **32**, 830 (1935).
403. Osato, T., and Ito, Y.: *J. Exp. Med.* **126**, 881 (1967).
404. Noyes, W. F., and Mellors, R. C.: *J. Exp. Med.* **106**, 555 (1957).
405. Syverton, J. T.: *Ann. N.Y. Acad. Sci.* **54**, 1126 (1952).
406. Rous, P., and Kidd, J. G.: *J. Exp. Med.* **67**, 399 (1938).
407. Rous, P., and Friedewald, W. F.: *J. Exp. Med.* **79**, 511 (1944).
408. Lancaster, W. D., and Olson, C.: *Virology* **89**, 371 (1978).
409. Jarrett, W. F. H., McNeil, P. E., Grimshaw, W. T. R., Selman, I. E., and McIntyre, W. I. M.: *Nature* **274**, 215 (1978).
410. Woo, Y.-t., Lai, D. Y., Arcos, J. C., and Argus, M. F.: "Chemical Induction of Cancer – Structural Bases and Biological Mechanisms", Vol. IIIC: Natural, Metal, Fiber and Macromolecular Carcinogens. Academic Press, San Diego, 1988, p. 159.
411. De Villiers, E. M.: *J. Virol.* **63**, 4898 (1989).
412. De Villiers, E.: Human Pathogenic Papillomavirus Types: An Update. *In* "Human Pathogenic Papillomaviruses" (H. zur Hausen, ed.). Springer-Verlag, Berlin, 1994, p. 1.
413. zur Hausen, H., and Schneider, A.: The Role of Papillomaviruses in Human Anogenital Cancers. *In* "The Papovaviridae", Vol. 2 (N. Salzman and P. M. Howley, eds.). Plenum Press, New York, 1987, p. 245.
414. De Villiers, E., Gissmann, L., and zur Hausen, H.: *J. Virol.* **40**, 932 (1981).
415. Gissmann, L., and zur Hausen, H.: *Int. J. Cancer* **25**, 605 (1980).
416. Gissman, L., Wolnik, L., Ikenberg, H., Koldovsky, U., Schnurch, H. G., and zur Hausen, H.: *Proc. Natl. Acad. Sci. U.S.A.* **80**, 560 (1983).
417. Chan, W.-K., Klock, G., and Bernard, H.-U.: *J. Virol.* **63**, 3261 (1989).
418. Pater, M., Hughes, G., Hyslop, D., Nakshatri, H., and Pater, A.: *Nature* **335**, 832 (1988).
419. Rawls, W. E., Tompkins, W. A. F., Figueroa, M. E., and Melnick, J. L.: *Science* **161**, 1255 (1968).
420. Meisels, A., and Fortin, R.: *Acta Cytol.* **20**, 505 (1976).
421. Purola, E., and Savia, E.: *Acta Cytol.* **21**, 26 (1977).
422. Schiffman, M. H.: *J. Natl. Cancer Inst.* **84**, 394 (1992).
423. Black, P. H., Hartley, J. W., Rowe, W. P., and Huebner, R. J.: *Nature* **199**, 1016 (1963).
424. Dvoretzky, I., Shober, R., Chattopadhyay, S. K., and Lowy, D. R.: *Virology* **103**, 369 (1980).
425. Lowy, D. R. Dvortzky, I., Shober, R., Law, M.-F., Engel, L., and Howley, P. M.: *Nature* **287**, 72 (1980).
426. Lambert, P. F., Baker, C. C., and Howley, P. M.: *Annu. Rev. Genet.* **22**, 235 (1989).
427. Law, M., Lowy, D. R., Dvoretzky, I., and Howley, P. M.: *Proc. Natl. Acad. Sci. U.S.A.* **78**, 2727 (1981).
428. Watts, S. L., Phelps, W. C., Ostrow, R. S., Zachow, K. R., and Faras, A. J.: *Science* **225**, 634 (1984).
429. Yasumoto, S., Burkhardt, A. L., Doninger, J., and DiPaolo, J.: *J. Virol.* **57**, 572 (1986).
430. Dürst, M., Dzarlieva-Petrusevska, R. T., Boukamp, P., Fusenig, N. E., and Gissmann, L.: *Oncogene* **1**, 251 (1987).
431. Kanda, T., Watanabe, S., and Yoshiike, K.: *Virology* **165**, 321 (1988).
432. Matlashewski, G., Schneider, J., Banks, L., Jones, N., Murray, A., and Crawford, L.: *EMBO J.* **6**, 1741 (1987).
433. Phelps, W. C., Yee, C. L., Münger, K., and Howley, P. M.: *Cell* **53**, 539 (1988).

434. Pirisi, L., Yasumoto, S., Fellerey, M., Doninger, J. K., and DiPaolo, J. A.: *J. Virol.* **61**, 1061 (1987).
435. Schlegel, R., Phelps, W. C., Zhang, Y.-L., and Barbosa, M.: *EMBO J.* **7**, 3181 (1988).
436. Watanabe, S., and Yoshiike, K.: *Int. J. Cancer* **41**, 896 (1988).
437. Bedell, M. A., Jones, K. H., Grossman, S. R., and Laimins, L. A.: *J. Virol.* **63**, 1247 (1989).
438. Schlegel, R., Wade-Glass, M., Rabson, M., and Yang, Y. C.: *Science* **233**, 464 (1986).
439. DiMaio, D.: *Adv. Cancer Res.* **56**, 133 (1991).
440. Petti, L., and DiMaio, D.: *Proc. Natl. Acad. Sci. U.S.A.* **89**, 6736 (1992).
441. Goldstein, D. J., Li, W., Wang, L., Heidaran, M. A., Aaronson, S., Shinn, R., Schlegel, R., and Pierce, J. H.: *J. Virol.* **68**, 4432 (1994).
442. Petti, L., and DiMaio, D.: *J. Virol.* **68**, 3582 (1994).
443. Petti, L., Nilson, L. A., and DiMaio, D.: *EMBO J.* **10**, 845 (1991).
444. Goldstein, D. J., Andresson, T., Sparkowski, J. J., and Schlegel, R.: *EMBO J.* **11**, 4851 (1992).
445. Goldstein, D. J., Finbow, M. E., Andresson, T., McClean, P., Smith, K., Bubb, V., and Schlegel, R.: *Nature* **352**, 347 (1991).
446. Horwitz, B. J., Weinstat, D. L., and DiMaio, D.: *J. Virol.* **63**, 4515 (1989).
447. Horwitz, B. J., Burkhardt, A. L., Schlegel, R., and DiMaio, D.: *Molec. Cell. Biol.* **8**, 4071 (1988).
448. Kulke, R., Horwitz, B., Zibello, T., and DiMaio, D.: *J. Virol.* **66**, 505 (1992).
449. Sparkowski, J., Anders, J., and Schlegel, R.: *J. Virol.* **68**, 6120 (1994).
450. Chen, S., and Mounts, P.: *J. Virol.* **64**, 3226 (1990).
451. Leechanachai, P., Banks, L., Moreau, F., and Matlashewski, G.: *Oncogene* **7**, 17 (1992).
452. Pim, D., Collins, M., and Banks, L.: *Oncogene* **7**, 27 (1992).
453. Straight, S. W., Hinkle, P. M., Jewers, R. J., and McCance, D. J.: *J. Virol.* **67**, 4521 (1993).
454. Rheinwald, J. G., and Green, H.: *Nature* **265**, 421 (1977).
455. Kohler, M., Janz, I., Wintzer, H. O., Wagner, E., and Bauknecht, T.: *Anticancer Res.* **9**, 1537 (1989).
456. Brandsma, J. L., Yang, Z., DiMaio, D., Barthold, S. W., and Xiao, W.: *J. Virol.* **66**, 6204 (1992).
457. Boshart, M., Gissmann, L., Ikenberg, H., Kleinheinz, A., Scheurlen, W., and zur Hausen, H.: *EMBO J.* **3**, 1151 (1984).
458. Dürst, M., Kleinheinz, A., Hotz, M., and Gissmann, L.: *J. Gen. Virol.* **66**, 1515 (1985).
459. Dürst, M., Croce, C. M., Gissmann, L., Schwarz, E., and Huebner, K.: *Proc. Natl. Acad. Sci. U.S.A.* **80**, 3812 (1987).
460. Schwarz, E., Freese, U. K., Gissmann, L., Mayer, W., Roggenbuck, B., Stremlau, A., and zur Hausen, H.: *Nature* **314**, 111 (1985).
461. Schneider-Gädicke, A., and Schwarz, E.: *EMBO J.* **5**, 2285 (1986).
462. Matsukura, T., Koi, S., and Sugase, M.: *Virology* **172**, 63 (1989).
463. Baker, C. C., Phelps, W. C., Lindgren, V., Braun, M. J., Gonda, M. A., and Howley, P. M.: *J. Virol.* **61**, 962 (1987).
464. Hawley-Nelson, P., Vousden, K. H., Hubbert, N. L., Lowy, D. R., and Schiller, J. T.: *EMBO J.* **8**, 3905 (1989).
465. Hudson, J. B., Bedell, M. A., McCance, D. J., and Laimins, L. A.: *J. Virol.* **64**, 519 (1990).
466. Barbosa, M. S., Vass, W. C., Lowy, D. R., and Schiller, J. T.: *J. Virol.* **65**, 292 (1991).
467. Münger, K., Phelps, W. C., Bubb, V., Howley, P. M., and Schlegel, R.: *J. Virol.* **63**, 4417 (1989).
468. Scheffner, M., Werness, B. A., Hulbregtse, J. M., Levine, A. J., and Howley, P. M.: *Cell* **63**, 1129 (1990).
469. Scheffner, M., Münger, K., Huibregtse, J. M., and Howley, P. M.: *EMBO J.* **11**, 2425 (1992).
470. Huibregtse, J. M., Scheffner, M., and Howley, P. M.: *EMBO J.* **10**, 4129 (1991).
471. Huibregtse, J. M., Scheffner, M., and Howley, P. M.: *Molec. Cell. Biol.* **13**, 775 (1993).
472. Scheffner, M., Huibregtse, J. M., Vierstra, R. D., and Howley, P. M.: *Cell* **75**, 495 (1993).
473. Band, V., DeCaprio, J. A., Delmolino, L., Kulesa, V., and Sager, R.: *J. Virol.* **65**, 6671 (1991).
474. Scheffner, M., Münger, K., Byrne, J. C., and Howley, P. M.: *Proc. Natl. Acad. Sci. U.S.A.* **88**, 5523 (1991).
475. Hubbert, N. L., Sedman, S. A., and Schiller, J. T.: *J. Virol.* **66**, 6237 (1992).
476. Lechner, M. S., Mack, D. H., Finicle, A. B., Crook, T., Vousden, K. H., and Laimins, L. A.: *EMBO J.* **11**, 3045 (1992).
477. Kessis, T. D., Slebos, R. J., Nelson, W. G., Kastan, M. B., Plunkett, B. S., Han, S. M., Lorincz, A. T., Hedrick, L., and Cho, K. R.: *Proc. Natl. Acad. Sci. U.S.A.* **90**, 3988 (1993).
478. Münger, K., Werness, B. A., Dyson, N., Phelps, W. C., Harlow, E., and Howley, P. M.: *EMBO J.* **8**, 4099 (1989).
479. Dyson, N., Guida, P., Münger, K., and Harlow, E.: *J. Virol.* **66**, 6893 (1992).
480. Dyson, N., Dembski, M., Fattaey, A., Ngwu, C., Ewen, M., and Helin, K.: *J. Virol.* **67**, 7641 (1993).
481. Phelps, W. C., Bagchi, S., Barnes, J. A., Raychaudhuri, P., Kraus, V., Münger, K., Howley, P. M., and Nevins, J. R.: *J. Virol.* **65**, 6922 (1991).
482. Chellappan, S., Kraus, V. B., Kroger, B., Münger, K., Howley, P. M., Phelps, W. C., and Nevins, J. R.: *Proc. Natl. Acad. Sci. U.S.A.* **89**, 4549 (1992).

483. Münger, K., and Phelps, W. C.: *Biochim. Biophys. Acta* **1155**, 111 (1993).
484. Flehmig, B., Mauler, R. F., Noll, G., Weinmann, E., and Gregersen, J. P.: Progress in the Development of an Attenuated, Live Hepatitis A Vaccine. *In* "Viral Hepatitis and Liver Disease" (A. J. Zuckerman, ed.). Alan R. Liss, New York, 1988, p. 87.
485. Blumberg, B. S., Gerstley, B. J. S., Hungerford, D. A., London, W. T., and Sutnick, A. I.: *Ann. Intern. Med.* **66**, 924 (1967).
486. Blumberg, B. S., Alter, H. J., and Visnich, S.: *JAMA* **191**, 541 (1965).
487. Prince, A. M.: *Proc. Natl. Acad. Sci. U.S.A.* **60**, 814 (1968).
488. Dane, D. S., Cameron, C. H., and Briggs, M.: *Lancet* **1**, 695 (1970).
489. Robinson, W. S.: Hepadnaviridae and Their Replication. *In* "Fundamental Virology" (B. N. Fields and D. M. Knipe, chief eds.). Raven Press, New York, 1991, p. 989.
490. Ganem, D.: Replication Cycle of Hepatitis B Viruses: Implications for Viral Persistence and Oncogenesis. *In* "Origins of Human Cancer" (J. Brugge, T. Curran, E. Harlow, and F. McCormick, eds.). Cold Spring Harbor Laboratory Press, Cold Spring Harbor, New York, 1991, p. 715.
491. Summers, J., and Mason, W. S.: *Cell* **29**, 403 (1982).
492. Mazzur, S., Blumberg, B. S., and Friedlaender, J.: *Nature* **274**, 41 (1974).
493. Beasley, R. P., Trepo, C., Stevens, C. E., and Szmuness, W.: *Am. J. Epidemiol.* **105**, 94 (1977).
494. Okada, K., Kamiyama, I., Inomata, M., Imai, M., Miyakawa, Y., and Mayumi, M.: *N. Engl. J. Med.* **294**, 746 (1976).
495. Brechot, C., Hadchouel, M., Scotto, J., Fonck, M., Potet, F., Vyas, G. N., and Tiollais, P.: *Proc. Natl. Acad. Sci. U.S.A.* **78**, 3906 (1981).
496. Miller, R. H., Lee, S. C., Liaw, Y. F., and Robinson, W. S.: *J. Infect. Dis.* **151**, 1081 (1985).
497. Shafritz, D. A., Shouval, D., Sherman, H., Hadziyannis, S., and Kew, M.: *N. Engl. J. Med.* **305**, 1067 (1981).
498. Popper, H., Roth, L., Purcell, R. H., Tennant, B. C., and Gerin, J. L.: *Proc. Natl. Acad. Sci. U.S.A.* **84**, 866 (1987).
499. Gerin, J. L., Cote, P. J., Korba, B. E., Miller, R. H., Purcell, R. H., and Tennant, B. C.: Hepatitis B Virus and Liver Cancer: The Woodchuck as an Experimental Model of Hepadnavirus-Induced Liver Cancer. *In* "Viral Hepatitis and Liver Disease" (F. B. Hollinger, S. M. Lemon, and H. Margolis, eds.). Williams & Wilkins, Baltimore, 1991, p. 556.
500. Marion, P. L., Van Davelaar, M. J., Knight, S. S., Salazer, F. H., Garcia, G., Popper, H., and Robinson, W. S.: *Proc. Natl. Acad. Sci. U.S.A.* **83**, 4543 (1986).
501. Dejean, A., Bougeleret, L., Grzeschik, K., and Tiollais, P.: *Nature* **322**, 70 (1986).
502. de Thé, H., Marchio, A., Tiollais, P., and Dejean, A.: *Nature* **330**, 667 (1987).
503. Wang, J., Chenivesse, X., Henglein, B., and Brechot, C.: *Nature* **343**, 555 (1990).
504. Zhang, X. K., Egan, J. O., Huang, D., Cun, Z. L., Chien, V. K., and Chiu, J. F.: *Biochem. Biophys. Res. Commun.* **188**, 344 (1992).
505. Tokino, T., and Matsubara, K.: *J. Virol.* **65**, 6761 (1991).
506. Fourel, G., Trepo, C., Bougueleret, L., Hengelein, B., Ponzetto, A., Tiollais, P., and Buendia, M. A.: *Nature* **347**, 294 (1990).
507. Hsu, T. Y., Moroy, T., Etiemble, J., Louise, A., Trepo, C., Tiollais, P., and Buendia, M. A.: *Cell* **55**, 627 (1988).
508. Wei, Y., Fourel, G., Ponzetto, A., Silvestro, M., Tiollais, P., and Buendia, M. A.: *J. Virol.* **66**, 5265 (1992).
509. Hino, O., Shows, T. B., and Rogler, C. E.: *Proc. Natl. Acad. Sci. U.S.A.* **83**, 8338 (1986).
510. Wang, H. P., and Rogler, C. E.: *Cytogenet. Cell Genet.* **48**, 72 (1988).
511. Beutow, K. H., Murray, J. C., Israel, J. L., London, W. T., Smith, M., Kew, M., Blanquet, V., Brechot, C., Redeker, A., and Govindarajah, S.: *Proc. Natl. Acad. Sci. U.S.A.* **86**, 8852 (1989).
512. Zhang, W., Hirohashi, S., Tsuda, H., Shimosato, Y., Yokota, J., Terada, M., and Sugimura, T.: *Jpn. J. Cancer Res.* **81**, 108 (1990).
513. Slagle, B. L., Zhou, Y., and Butel, J. S.: *Cancer Res.* **51**, 49 (1991).
514. Bressac, B., Kew, M., Wands, J., and Ozturk, M.: *Nature* **350**, 429 (1991).
515. Hsu, I. C., Metcalf, R. A., Sun, T., Welsch, J. A., Wang, N. J., and Harris, C. C.: *Nature* **350**, 427 (1991).
516. Aguilar, F., Hussain, S. P., and Cerutti, P.: *Proc. Natl. Acad. Sci. U.S.A.* **90**, 8586 (1993).
517. Harris, C. C., and Hollstein, M.: *N. Engl. J. Med.* **329**, 1318 (1993).
518. Aufiero, B., and Schneider, R. J.: *EMBO J.* **9**, 497 (1990).
519. Colgrove, R., Simon, G., and Ganem, D.: *J. Virol.* **63**, 4019 (1989).
520. Rossner, M. T.: *J. Med. Virol.* **36**, 101 (1992).
521. Wu, J. Y., Zhou, Z., Judd, A., Cartwright, C. A., and Robinson, W. S.: *Cell* **63**, 687 (1990).
522. Blum, H. E., Zhang, Z., Galun, E., von Weizsacker, F., Garner, B., Liang, T. J., and Wands, J. R.: *J. Virol.* **66**, 1223 (1992).

523. Chen, H., Kaneko, S., Girones, R., Anderson, R. W., Hornbuckle, W. E., Tennant, B. C., Cote, P. J., Gerin, J. L., Purcell, R. H., and Miller, R. H.: *J. Virol.* **67**, 1218 (1993).
524. Maguire, H. F., Hoeffler, J. P., and Siddiqui, A.: *Science* **252**, 842 (1991).
525. Unger, T., and Shaul, Y.: *EMBO J.* **9**, 1889 (1990).
526. Kim, C., Koike, K., Saito, I., Miyamura, T., and Jay, G.: *Nature* **351**, 317 (1991).
527. Lee, T., Finegold, M. J., Shen, R., DeMayo, J. L., Woo, S. L. C., and Butel, J. S.: *J. Virol.* **64**, 5939 (1990).
528. Ganem, D.: *Nature* **347**, 230 (1990).
529. Chisari, F. V., Filippi, P., Buras, J., McLachlan, A., Popper, H., Pinkert, C. A., Palmiter, R. D., and Brinster, R. L.: *Proc. Natl. Acad. Sci. U.S.A.* **84**, 6909 (1987).
530. Chisari, F. V., Klopchin, K., Moriyama, T., Pasquinelli, C., Dunsford, H. A., Sell, S., Pinkert, C. A., Brinster, R. L., and Palmiter, R. D.: *Cell* **59**, 1145 (1989).
531. Chisari, F. V.: Multistage Hepatocarcinogenesis in Hepatitis B Virus Transgenic Mice. *In* "Origins of Human Cancer" (J. Brugge, T. Curran, E. Harlow, and F. McCormick, eds.). Cold Spring Harbor Laboratory Press, Cold Spring Harbor, New York, 1991, p. 727.
532. Alter, H. J., Purcell, R. H., Shih, J. W., Melpolder, J. C., Houghton, M., Choo, Q., and Kuo, G.: *N. Engl. J. Med.* **321**, 1494 (1989).
533. Cho, Q., Kuo, G., Weiner, A., Overby, L. R., Bradley, D. W., and Houghton, M.: *Science* **244**, 359 (1989).
534. Kuo, G., Choo, Q., Alter, H. J., Gitnick, G. L., Redeker, A. G., Purcell, R. H., Miyamura, T., Dienstag, J. L., Alter, M. J., Stevens, C. E., Tegtmeier, G. E., Bonino, F., Colombo, M., Lee, W., Kuo, C., Berger, K., Shusher, J. R., Overby, L. R., Bradley, D. W., and Houghton, M.: *Science* **244**, 362 (1989).
535. Alter, H. J.: Chronic Consequences of Non-A Non-B. *In* "Current Prespectives in Hepatology" (L. B. Seef and J. H. Lewis, eds.). Plenum Press, New York, 1989, p. 83.
536. Choo, Q., Weiner, A. J., Overby, L. R., Kuo, G., Houghton, M., and Bradley, D. W.: *Br. Med. Bull.* **46**, 423 (1990).
537. Saito, I., Miyamura, T., Ohbayashi, A., Harada, H., Katayama, T., Kiluchi, S., Watanabe, T. Y., Koi, S., Onji, M., Ohta, Y., and Choo, Q.: *Proc. Natl. Acad. Sci. U.S.A.* **87**, 6547 (1990).
538. Colombo, M., Kuo, G., Choo, Q., Donato, M. F., Del Ninno, E., Tommasini, M. A., Dioguardi, N., and Houghton, M.: *Lancet* **ii**, 1006 (1989).
539. Bruix, J., Calvet, X., Costa, J., Ventura, M., Bruguera, M., Castillo, R., Barrera, J. M., Ercilla, G., Sanchez-Tapias, J. M., Vall, M., Bru, C., and Rodes, J.: *Lancet* **ii**, 1004 (1989).
540. Plagemann, P. G. W.: *Arch. Virol.* **120**, 165 (1991).
541. Klein, G.: *Cell* **77**, 791 (1994).
542. Epstein, M. A., Achong, B. G., and Barr, Y. M.: *Lancet* **i**, 702 (1964).
543. Burkitt, D. P.: *Br. J. Surg.* **46**, 218 (1958).
544. Burkitt, D. P.: *Lancet* **ii**, 1229 (1969).
545. Henle, G., Henle, W., and Diehl, V.: *Proc. Natl. Acad. Sci. U.S.A.* **59**, 94 (1968).
546. Baer, R., Bankier, A. T., Biggin, M. D., Deininger, P. L., Farrell, P. J., Gibson, T. J., Hatfull, G., Hudson, G. S., Satchwell, S. C., Sequin, C., Tuffnell, P. S., and Barrell, B. G.: *Nature* **310**, 207 (1984).
547. Kieff, E., and Liebowitz, D.: Epstein-Barr Virus and Its Replication. *In* "Fundamental Virology" (B. N. Fields and D. M. Knipe, chief eds.). Raven Press, New York, 1991, p. 897.
548. Heller, M., Dambaugh, T., and Kieff, E.: *J. Virol.* **38**, 632 (1981).
549. Katz, B. Z., Niederman, J. C., Olson, B. A., and Miller, G.: *J. Infect. Dis.* **157**, 299 (1988).
550. Rowe, M., Young, L. S., Cadwallader, K., Petti, L., Kieff, E., and Rickinson, A. B.: *J. Virol.* **63**, 1031 (1989).
551. Tanner, J., Weis, J., Fearon, D., Whang, Y., and Kieff, E.: *Cell* **50**, 203 (1987).
552. Fingeroth, J. D., Weis, J. J., Tedder, T. F., Strominger, J. L., Biro, P. A., and Fearson, D. T.: *Proc. Natl. Acad. Sci. U.S.A.* **81**, 4510 (1984).
553. Frade, R., Barel, M., Ehlin-Henriksson, B., and Klein, G.: *Proc. Natl. Acad. Sci. U.S.A.* **82**, 1490 (1985).
554. Nemerow, G., Wolfert, R., McNaughton, M., and Cooper, N.: *J. Virol.* **55**, 347 (1985).
555. Weis, J. J., Tedder, T. F., and Fearon, D. T.: *Proc. Natl. Acad. Sci. U.S.A.* **81**, 881 (1984).
556. Gratama, J. W., Oosterveer, M. A. P., Zwaan, F. E., Lepoutre, J., Klein, G., and Ernberg, I.: *Proc. Natl. Acad. Sci. U.S.A.* **85**, 8693 (1988).
557. Rowe, M., Young, L., Crocker, J., Stokes, H., Henderson, S., and Rickinson, A.: *J. Exp. Med.* **173**, 147 (1991).
558. Gerber, P., Nkrumah, F., Pritchett, R., and Kieff, E. D.: *Int. J. Cancer* **17**, 71 (1976).
559. Ben-Sasson, S. A., and Klein, G.: *Int. J. Cancer* **28**, 131 (1981).
560. Henderson, E., Miller, G., Robinson, J., and Heston, L.: *Virology* **76**, 152 (1977).
561. Sugden, B., and Mark, W.: *J. Virol.* **23**, 503 (1977).
562. Henderson, A., Ripley, S., Heller, M., and Kief, E.: *Proc. Natl. Acad. Sci. U.S.A.* **80**, 1987 (1983).

563. Bouffet, E., Frappaz, D., Pinkerton, R., Favrot, M., and Philip, T.: *Eur. J. Cancer* **27**, 504 (1991).
564. O'Connor, G. T., Rappaport, H., and Smith, E. B.: *Cancer* **18**, 330 (1965).
565. Fialkow, P. J., Klein, E., Klein, G., Clifford, P., and Singh, S.: *J. Exp. Med.* **138**, 89 (1973).
566. Manolov, Y., and Manolova, Y.: *Nature* **237**, 33 (1972).
567. Croce, C. M., and Nowell, P. C.: *Blood* **65**, 1 (1985).
568. Dalla-Favera, R., Brejni, M., Erikson, J., Patterson, D., Gallo, R. C., and Croce, C. M.: *Proc. Natl. Acad. Sci. U.S.A.* **79**, 7824 (1982).
569. Dean, M., Levine, R. A., Ran, W., Kindy, M. S., Sonenshein, G. E., and Campisi, J.: *J. Biol. Chem.* **261**, 9161 (1986).
570. Field, J. K., and Spandidos, D. A.: *Anticancer Res.* **10**, 1 (1990).
571. Adams, J. M., Harris, A. W., Pinkert, C. A., Concoran, L. M., Alexander, W. S., Cory, S., Palmiter, R. D., and Brinster, R. L.: *Nature* **318**, 533 (1985).
572. Bhata, K. G., Gutierrez, M. I., Huppi, K., and Magrath, I.: *Cancer Res.* **52**, 4273 (1992).
573. Farrell, P. J., Allan, G. J., Shanahan, F., Vousden, K. H., and Crook, T.: *EMBO J.* **10**, 2879 (1991).
574. Giadano, G., Ballerini, P., Gong, J. Z., Inghirami, G., Neri, A., Newcomb, E. W., Magrath, I., Knowles, D., and Dalla-Favera, R.: *Proc. Natl. Acad. Sci. U.S.A.* **88**, 5413 (1991).
575. Miller, G.: Epstein-Barr Virus. *In* "Virology" Vol. 2 (B. N. Fields and D. M. Knipe, eds.). Raven Press, New York, 1990, p. 1921.
576. zur Hausen, H., Schulte-Holthausen, H., Klein, G., Henle, W., Henle, G., Clifford, P., and Sanesson, L.: *Nature* **228**, 1056 (1970).
577. Raab-Traub, N., Flynn, K., Pearson, G., Huang, A., Levine, P., Lanier, A., and Pagano, J.: *Int. J. Cancer* **39**, 25 (1987).
578. Raab-Traub, N., and Flynn, K.: *Cell* **22**, 257 (1986).
579. Effert, P., McCoy, R., Abdel-Hamid, M., Flynn, K., Zhang, Q., Busson, P., Tursz, T., Lui, E., and Raab-Traub, N.: *J. Virol.* **66**, 3768 (1992).
580. Fåhraeus, R., Hu, L., Ernberg, I., Finke, J., Rowe, M., Klein, G., Falk, K., Nilsson, E., Yadav, M., Busson, P., Tursz, T., and Kallin, B.: *Int. J. Cancer* **42**, 329 (1988).
581. Raab-Traub, N., Hood, R., Yang, C,. Henry, B., and Pagano, J. S.: *J. Virol.* **48**, 580 (1983).
582. Chappuis, B. B., Muller, H., Stutte, J., Hey, M. M., Hubner, K., and Muller-Hermelink, M. K.: *Pathology* **58**, 199 (1990).
583. Hanto, D. W., Frizzera, G., Gajl-Peczalska, K. J., Sakamoto, K., Purtillo, D. T., Balfour, H. H., Simmons, R. L., and Najarian, J. S.: *N. Engl. J. Med.* **306**, 913 (1982).
584. Katz, B. Z., Raab-Traub, N., and Miller, G.: *J. Infect. Dis.* **160**, 589 (1989).
585. Starzl, T. E., Nalesnik, M. A., Porter, K. A., Ho, M., Iwatsuki, G., Griffith, B. P., Rosenthal, J. T., Hakala, T. R., Shaw, Jr., B. W., Hardesty, R. L., Atchison, R. W., Jaffe, R., and Bahnson, H. T.:*Lancet* **17**, 583 (1984).
586. Brown, N. A., Liu, C., Wang, Y., and Garcia, C. R.: *J. Virol.* **62**, 962 (1988).
587. Cleary, M. L., Nalesnik, M. A., Shearer, W. T., and Sklar, J.: *Blood* **72**, 349 (1988).
588. Edwards, R. H., and Raab-Traub, N.: *J. Virol.* **68**, 1309 (1994).
589. Gratama, J. W., Zutter, M. M., Minarovits, J., Oosterveer, M. A., Thomas, E. D., Klein, G., and Ernberg, I.: *Int. J. Cancer* **47**, 188 (1991).
590. Swaminathan, S., Tomkinson, B., and Kieff, E.: *Proc. Natl. Acad. Sci. U.S.A.* **88**, 1546 (1991).
591. Tomkinson, B., and Kieff, E.: *J. Virol.* **66**, 2893 (1992).
592. Longnecker, R., Miller, C. L., Miao, X. Q., Tomkinson, B., and Kieff, E.: *J. Virol.* **67**, 2006 (1993).
593. Longnecker, R. C., Miller, C. L., Tomkinson, B., Miao, X. Q., and Kieff, E.: *J. Virol.* **67**, 5068 (1993).
594. Jones, C. H., Hayward, S. D., and Rawlins, D. R.: *J. Virol.* **63**, 101 (1989).
595. Reisman, D., Yates, J., and Sugden, B.: *Molec. Cell. Biol.* **5**, 1822 (1985).
596. Ytes, J. L., Warren, N., and Sugden, B.: *Nature* **313**, 812 (1985).
597. Middleton, T., and Sugden, B.: *J. Virol.* **66**, 1795 (1992).
598. Lafemina, R. L., Pizzorno, M. C., Mosca, J. D., and Hayward, G. S.: *Virology* **172**, 584 (1989).
599. Harris, A., Young, B. D., and Griffin, B. E.: *J. Virol.* **56**, 328 (1985).
600. Abbot, S. D., Rowe, M., Cadwallader, K., Ricksten, A., Gordon, J., Wang, F., Rymo, L., and Rickinson, A. B.: *J. Virol.* **64**, 2126 (1990).
601. Wang, F., Tsang, S. F., Kurilla, M. G., Cohen, J. I., and Kieff, E.: *J. Virol.* **64**, 3407 (1990).
602. Zimber-Strobl, U., Suentzenich, K. O., Laux, G., Eick, D., Cordier, M., Calender, A., Billaud, M., Lenoir, G. M., and Bornkamm, G. W.: *J. Virol.* **65**, 415 (1991).
603. Cordier, M., Calender, A., Billaud, M., Zimber, U., Rousselet, G., Pavlish, O., Banchereau, J., Tursz, T., Bornkamm, G., and Lenoir, G. M.: *J. Virol.* **64**, 1002 (1990).
604. Wang, F., Kikutani, H., Tsang, S. F., Kishimoto, T., and Kieff, E.: *J. Virol.* **65**, 4101 (1991).
605. Knutson, J. C.: *J. Virol.* **64**, 2530 (1990).
606. Grossman, S. R., Johannsen, E., Tong, X., Yalamanchili, R., and Kieff, E.: *Proc. Natl. Acad. Sci. U.S.A.* **91**, 7568 (1994).

607. Ling, P. D., Rawlins, D. R., and Hayward, S. D.: *Proc. Natl. Acad. Sci. U.S.A.* **90**, 9237 (1993).
608. Walling, D. M., Perkins, A. G., Webster-Cyriaque, J., Resnick, L., and Raab-Traub, N.: *J. Virol.* **68**, 7918 (1994).
609. Greenspan, J. S., Greenspan, D., Lennette, E., Abrams, K. I., Conant, M. A., Petersen, V., and Freese, U. K.: *N. Engl. J. Med.* **313**, 1564 (1985).
610. Allday, M. J., Crawford, D. H., and Thomas, J. A.: *J. Gen. Virol.* **74**, 361 (1993).
611. Allday, M. J., and Farrell, P. J.: *J. Virol.* **68**, 3491 (1994).
612. Wang, D., Liebowitz, D., and Kieff, E.: *Cell* **43**, 831 (1985).
613. Baichwal, V. R., and Sugden, B.: *Oncogene* **2**, 461 (1988).
614. Liebowitz, D., Wang, D., and Kieff, E.: *J. Virol.* **58**, 233 (1986).
615. Baichwal, V. R., and Sugden, B.: *Oncogene* **4**, 67 (1989).
616. Wang, D., Liebowitz, D., and Kieff, E.: *J. Virol.* **62**, 2337 (1988).
617. Moorthy, R., and Thorley-Lawson, D. A.: *J. Virol.* **67**, 1638 (1993).
618. Liebowitz, D., Kopan, R., Fuchs, E., Sample, J., and Kieff, E.: *Molec. Cell. Biol.* **7**, 2299 (1987).
619. Kieff, E., Wang, F., Birkenbach, M. J. C., Sampl, J., Tomkinson, B., Swaminathan, S., Longnecker, R., Marchini, A., Mannick, J., Tsang, S., Sample, C., and Kurilla, M.: Molecular Biology of Lymphocyte Transformation by Epstein-Barr Virus. *In* "Origins of Human Cancer: A Comprehensive Review" (J. Brugge, T. Curran, E. Harlow, and F. McCormick, eds.). Cold Spring Harbor Laboratory Press, Cold Spring Harbor, New York, 1991, p. 563.
620. Calnek, B. K.: *Crit. Rev. Microbiol.* **12**, 293 (1985).
621. Churchill, A. E., and Biggs, P. M.: *Nature* **215**, 528 (1967).
622. Churchill, A. E., Payne, L. N., and Chubb, R. C.: *Nature* **221**, 744 (1969).
623. Fukuchi, K., Sudo, M., Lee, Y. S., Tanaka, A., and Nonoyama, M.: *J. Virol.* **51**, 102 (1984).
624. Calnek, B. W., Aldinger, H. K., and Kahn, D. E.: *Infection Immunity* **34**, 483 (1981).
625. Fukuchi, K., Tanaka, A., Shierman, L. W., Witter, R. L., and Nonoyama, M.: *Proc. Natl. Acad. Sci. U.S.A.* **82**, 751 (1985).
626. Silva, R. F., and Witter, R. L.: *J. Virol.* **54**, 690 (1985).
627. Bradley, G., Hayashi, M., Lancz, G., Tanaka, A., and Nonoyama, M.: *J. Virol.* **63**, 2534 (1989).
628. Bradley, G., Lancz, G., Tanaka, A., and Nonoyama, M.: *J. Virol.* **63**, 4129 (1989).
629. Peng, F., Bradley, G., Tanaka, A., Lancz, G., and Nonoyama, M.: *J. Virol.* **66**, 7389 (1992).
630. Jones, D., Lee, L., Liu, J., Kung, H., and Tillotson, J. K.: *Biochemistry* **89**, 4042 (1992).
631. Chen, X., Sondermeijer, P. J. A., and Velicer, L. F.: *J. Virol.* **66**, 85 (1992).
632. Hong, Y., and Coussens, P. M.: *J. Virol.* **68**, 3593 (1994).
633. Moss, B.: Poxviridae and Their Replication. *In* "Fundamental Virology" (B. N. Fields and D. M. Knipe, chief eds.). Raven Press, New York, 1991, p. 953.
634. Kates, J., and Beeson, J.: *J. Molec. Biol.* **50**, 19 (1970).
635. Wei, C. M., and Moss, B.: *Proc. Natl. Acad. Sci. U.S.A.* **72**, 318 (1975).
636. Pennington, T. H., and Follett, E. A.: *J. Virol.* **13**, 488 (1974).
637. Shope, R. E.: *J. Exp. Med.* **56**, 803 (1932).
638. Niven, J. S. F., Armstrong, J. A., Andrewes, C. H., Pereira, H. G., and Valentine, R. C.: *J. Pathol. Bacteriol.* **81**, 1 (1961).
639. Goodpasture, E. W., and Woodruff, C. E.: *Am. J. Pathol.* **7**, 1 (1931).
640. Chang, W., Macaulay, C., Hu, S., Tam, J. P., and McFadden, G.: *Virology* **179**, 926 (1990).
641. Brown, J. P., Twardzik, K. R., Marquardt, H., and Todaro, G. J.: *Nature* **313**, 491 (1985).
642. Twardzik, D. R., Brown, J. B., Ranchalis, J. E., Todaro, G. J., and Moss, B.: *Proc. Natl. Acad. Sci. U.S.A.* **82**, 5300 (1985).
643. Buller, R. M., Chakrabarti, S., Cooper, J. A., Twardzik, D. R., and Moss, B.: *J. Virol.* **62**, 866 (1988).
644. Opgenorth, A., Strayer, D., Upton, C., and McFadden, G.: *Virology* **186**, 175 (1992).
645. Opgenorth, A., Nation, N., Graham, K., and McFadden, G.: *Virology* **192**, 701 (1993).
646. Stroobant, P., Rice, A. P., Gullick, W. J., Cheng, D. J., Kerr, I. M., and Waterfield, M. D.: *Cell* **42**, 383 (1985).
647. King, C. S., Cooper, J. A., Moss, B., and Twardzik, D. R.: *Molec. Cell. Biol.* **6**, 332 (1986).
648. Ye, Y. K., Lin, Y. Z., and Tam, J. P.: *Biochem. Biophy. Res. Commun.* **154**, 497 (1988).
649. Lin, Y. Z., Caproaso, G., Chang, P. Y., Ke, X., and Tam, J. P.: *Biochemistry* **27**, 5640 (1988).

Viral–Chemical Combination Effects in Tumorigenesis[1]

Yin-tak Woo

Shortly after the discovery of the first tumor virus by Rous (1) in 1911 and the first experimental demonstration of chemical induction of cancer in rabbit skin by painting coal tar by Yamagiwa and Ichikawa (2) in 1915, Rous and Kidd (3, 4) reported that tar enhanced the carcinogenic activity of the Shope papillomavirus for the rabbit skin. Since then, numerous reports of interaction between viruses and chemical carcinogens have been published (*revs.* 5–15) with the majority of these showing synergism. These findings have attracted increasing attention as evidence is mounting that human populations are often exposed to both viruses and chemical carcinogens and that the high incidence of human cancer in certain geographic areas can be attributed to viral–chemical synergistic action. The focus of this section is to review studies indicative of viral–chemical interaction in tumorigenesis in humans, experimental animals, and cell culture systems.

I. EPIDEMIOLOGIC EVIDENCE OF POSSIBLE SYNERGISTIC INTERACTIONS BETWEEN TUMOR VIRUSES AND CHEMICAL CARCINOGENS/PROMOTERS IN HUMAN

Epidemiologic studies indicative of synergistic interactions between tumor viruses and chemical carcinogens/promoters in humans are summarized in Table 1. The viruses known to involve synergistic interactions include: (a) hepatitis B virus (HBV), (b) Epstein-Barr virus (EBV), (c) human papillomavirus (HPV), and (d) human T-cell leukemia viruses (HTLV).

Viral hepatitis has long been suspected to act synergistically with aflatoxin (and possibly other hepatocarcinogens) in the development of hepatocellular carcinoma (HCC) in humans (26, 27). Epidemiologic studies listed in Table 1 have shown clear association between aflatoxin exposure and liver cancer in many tropical or subtropical countries such as Thailand, Senegal, Kenya, Mozambique, and Swaziland (*see also* Section 5.3.1.1.1.5.1 of ref. 28); moreover, it is estimated that 75–90% of HCC cases are attributable to HBV

---

[1]For the Abbreviations Used *see* p. 619.

TABLE 1.   Evidence Indicative of Synergistic Interactions Between Viruses and Chemical
Carcinogens/Promoters in Humans

Virus[a]	Carcinogen	Geographic area	Cancer type	Reference
Hepadnavirus				
HBV	Aflatoxin	Southern Africa and Southeast China	Hepatocellular carcinoma	16–20
Herpesvirus				
EBV	*Euphorbia* plants	Kenya, Tanzania	Burkitt's lymphoma	21
	Aflatoxin	Kenya, Uganda	Burkitt's lymphoma	12
	Aleurites plants, tung oil	Southern China	Nasopharyngeal carcinoma	22
	N-Nitrosamines	Southern China	Nasopharyngeal carcinoma	23
Papillomavirus				
HPV-16	Betel quid	Taiwan	Oral cancer	24
Retrovirus				
HTLV-I	Diterpene esters	Southwestern Japan	Adult T-cell leukemia	25

[a]Abbreviations used: HBV, hepatitis B virus; EBV, Epstein-Barr virus; HPV, human papillomavirus; HTLV, human T-cell leukemia virus.

(29). The DNA of HBV is found integrated into the genome of HCC cells; the HBV *X* gene codes for the HBV X-protein that causes mutation and inactivates the gene product of the *p53* tumor suppressor gene (*rev.* 30). Transgenic mice containing the HBV *X* gene in their germline have an increased frequency of HCC (31). Numerous investigators have found concomitant HBV infection and *p53* mutations in the same tumors. Their results indicate that HBV alone does not influence the rate of *p53* mutation but that the combination of aflatoxin exposure and HBV infection is highly effective in causing mutation in *p53* (*rev.* 30). A recent prospective cohort study of 18,244 people in China has provided convincing evidence that aflatoxin B_1 (AFB_1) has an etiological role in HCC and indicates a synergy between AFB_1 and HBV. This case-control analysis shows statistical association between the presence of AFB_1 and its metabolites in urine specimens, serum HBV surface antigen positivity, on one hand, and the risk of HCC, on the other (19, 20). There is suggestive evidence that AFB_1 selectively causes mutation at codon 249 in the *p53* gene and that the hepatocyte clone carrying this specific mutant has a selective growth advantage in HBV-infected patients (*see* 30). These studies lend support to international efforts to develop methods for the biomonitoring of individual aflatoxin exposure (*rev.* 32) and to establish vaccination programs against HBV for the prevention of HCC in high-risk areas (33).

The epidemiologic evidence indicative of synergism between EBV and chemical carcinogens and/or tumorigenesis promoters has been reviewed by Henderson (12) and Osato *et al.* (21). It is estimated that EBV is associated with 95% of endemic Burkitt's lymphoma (BL) in Africa and with 10–20% of sporadic form of BL outside Africa. In a classic prospective seroepidemiological study, de Thé *et al.* (34) demonstrated that African children with high antibody titers to EBV antigens are at high risk of developing BL. However, despite the high incidence of EBV infection, less than one child in a thousand develop BL, suggesting that other cofactors may be involved. One such cofactor may be the plant *Euphorbia tirucalli,* which grows densely in the villages around Lake Victoria where most BL cases in Kenya and Tanzania are encountered. The plant is used as herbal medicine in the treatment of headache, sore throat, diarrhea, and stick wounds. A number of Euphorbiaceae species are known to contain the potent tumor promoter 12-*O*-tetradecanoylphorbol-13-acetate (TPA). Osato and coworkers (21) have shown that extracts of *E. tirucalli* stalks, leaves, and roots contain TPA-like substance(s) capable of enhancing EBV-induced cell transformation by activating latent EBV genes. Even the soil, vegetables, and reservoir drinking water near areas where these plants grow contain the TPA-like substance(s). Extracts of these plants are also capable of causing immunosuppression. In addition to the *Euphorbia* plants, AFB_1 has also been implicated. The geographical distribution of AFB_1 contamination of foodstuffs parallels that of endemic BL (35). There is some evidence that AFB_1 interacts with and causes damage to DNA in human lymphocytes and lymphoblastoid cell lines (*rev.* 12).

In addition to BL, EBV has been implicated as an/the etiologic agent in nasopharyngeal carcinoma (NPC) in humans (36). As in the induction of BL, environmental cofactors together with EBV play a role. *N*-Nitrosamines in salted fish together with EBV are believed to contribute to the high incidence of NPC in southern China (23). Tumorigenesis promoters present in medicinal plants have also been suspected. Ito and coworkers (22) screened a variety of medicinal plants used in southern China and found substantial EBV-activating and/or tumor promoting activities in many of these plants. In particular, they isolated a potent tumor promoter (12-*O*-hexadecanoyl-16-hydroxyphorbol-13-acetate, HHPA) from *Aleurites fordii,* a plant commonly grown in southern China and used medicinally in the treatment of intestinal and respiratory disorders. This plant is also a well-known source of a major industrial product, tung oil, which has been used in oil paints, varnishes, waterproofing agents, anticorrosives, and printing inks. In the NPC endemic area of southern China, tung oil trees are abundantly planted and blossom in late April. Extracts of these flowers have been found to contain EBV-activating activity. Local residents may be exposed to the tumor promoters through inhalation of air contaminated with soil dusts mixed with fallen and decaying flowers. Several other Chinese herbal medicines have been identified as plants in the Euphorbiaceae and Thymeloeaceae families, known to contain TPA and TPA-like substances.

Although the cooperation between papillomaviruses and chemical carcinogens in the induction of tumors has been clearly demonstrated in cows and rabbits, there is only limited epidemiological evidence of such cooperative effects between HPV and chemical carcinogens. There are more than 60 types of HPVs, of which several have been implicated as causative agents of anogenital, oral, respiratory and skin tumors. The E6 and E7 oncoproteins of HPV (types 16 and 18) have been shown to bind to and promote degradation of the gene products of *p53* and retinoblastoma tumor-suppressor genes, respectively (*rev.* 15). An epidemiologic study of Taiwanese patients with oral epidermoid carcinoma showed a high prevalence of HPV-16 infection and high frequency of betel quid chewing, suggesting their cooperative action in the induction of oral cancer (24). A number of epidemiological studies have shown that cigarette smokers are at a higher risk for both cervical (*rev.* 37) and anal (38) cancers. A possible cooperation between HPV and smoking-related carcinogenic/cocarcinogenic/immunosuppressive activities has been suggested (15).

Human T-cell leukemia viruses (HTLV-I and HTLV-II) have been etiologically implicated with human adult T-cell leukemia (ATL) and T-cell variant hairy cell leukemia, respectively (14, 39). Ito and coworkers (25) reported unusually high incidence of clinical manifestation of ATL in HTLV-infected individuals in southwestern Japan, where the population is exposed to plant-derived diterpene esters. In these regions, trees containing the tumor-promoting substances are widely used as street and garden decorative plants or cultivated for industrial wax production. A synergistic action between HTLV and diterpene esters has been suggested.

II. COMBINATION EFFECTS BETWEEN TUMOR VIRUSES AND CHEMICAL CARCINOGENS/PROMOTERS IN ANIMALS

Combination effects between tumor viruses and chemical carcinogens/promoters in animals have been extensively investigated; some representative studies are summarized in Table 2. The viruses involved may be introduced by exogenous inoculation, are endogenously present and are activated, or are introduced by transfection in the use of transgenic mice. The variety of viruses used in these studies are summarized below.

Hepadnaviruses. The close association of endemic HBV infection with HCC has attracted an intense interest in the study of the role of the hepadnaviruses in the development of this neoplasm in animal models and their possible interaction with

TABLE 2.   Representative Studies Indicative of Synergistic/Potentiating Interactions Between Viruses and Chemical Carcinogens in Animals

Virus (source)[a]	Carcinogen[b]	Species/strain	Target organ	Reference
Hepadnavirus				
HBV (transgenic)	DAB, DEN	Mice (C3H/He)	Liver	40
	AFB$_1$, DEN	Mice (C57BL/6)	Liver	41
Papillomavirus				
SPV (exogenous)	Tar, 3-MC, B[a]P	Rabbit	Skin	3,4,42,43
BPV-2 (exogenous)	Bracken fern	Cow	Urinary bladder	15
BPV-4 (exogenous)	Bracken fern	Cow	G.I. tract	44–46
Polyomavirus				
Polyomavirus (exogenous)	DMBA, croton oil	Mice (Swiss)	Parotid gland	47,48
	B[a]P	Mice (Swiss)	Skin	47,48
Poxvirus				
SFV (exogenous)	3-MC, B[a]P or tar	Rabbit	Skin	49
Fowl pox (exogenous)	3-MC	Chicken	Skin	6
Retroviruses				
RSV (exogenous)	3-MC	Chicken	Local sarcoma	50
MuLV (endogenous)	1,3-Butadiene	Mice (B6C3F$_1$)	Thymic lymphoma	51
Viruses That Are Not Known to Be Oncogenic				
Herpes simplex virus (exogenous)	3-MC	Mice (Swiss)	Skin	52
West Nile virus (exogenous)	3-MC, B[a]P	Mice (Swiss)	Skin	52
Vaccinia virus (exogenous)	3-MC	Mice (Swiss)	Skin, lymphatic system	5–7
Influenza virus (exogenous)	Urethan	Mice (AxZb F$_1$)	Lung	53
	B[a]P and other PAHs	Mice (C57BL)	Lung	54,55
	DEN	Mice (XMRI)	Lung	56

[a]Source of viral infection may be: (a) by exogenous inoculation, (b) by induction of endogenous virus, or (c) by transfecting active viral gene into transgenic mice. Abbreviations: HBV, hepatitis B virus; SPV, Shope papillomavirus; HPV, human papillomavirus; SFV, Shope fibroma virus; MuLV, murine leukemia virus.

[b]Abbreviations of carcinogens: DAB, 4-dimethylaminoazobenzene; DEN, diethylnitrosamine; AFB$_1$, aflatoxin B$_1$; 3-MC, 3-methylcholanthrene; DMBA, 7,12-dimethylbenz[a]anthracene; B[a]P, benzo[a]pyrene; PAHs, polycyclic aromatic hydrocarbons.

chemical carcinogens. Woodchuck hepatitis virus (WHV) and ground squirrel hepatitis virus (GSHV) have been clearly shown to induce HCC in their respective host, whereas duck hepatitis B virus (DHBV) is only marginally hepatocarcinogenic (*rev.* 57) possibly because DHBV lacks the HBV *X* gene (58). Three studies using congenitally DHBV-infected ducks and ducks inoculated with DBHV after hatching showed no evidence of syncarcinogenesis with AFB_1 (*rev.* 32). However, the discovery of HCC in domestic congenitally DHBV-infected ducks in Qidong, China, has been suspected to be attributable to possible DHBV and AFB_1 synergism (59). Convincing syncarcinogenesis data have been obtained using transgenic mice carrying the integrated HBV DNA. Sell and coworkers (41) found 2 HCC and 10 hepatic adenomas in 10 HBV-activated transgenic mice given three i.p. doses of 2 mg/kg body weight AFB_1 and maintained under observation for 15 months. No such tumors were detected in untreated transgenic mice or AFB_1-treated nontransgenic mice. Similar synergism has also been observed using diethylnitrosamine or 4-dimethylaminoazobenzene as the hepatocarcinogen (40, 41), whereas phenobarbital was inactive (41).

Papillomaviruses. Shope papillomavirus (SPV) has been shown to induce squamous cell carcinomas in rabbits. In the wild, SPV-induced tumors occur as a spontaneous enzootic disease of cottontail rabbits living in certain areas in the United States (60, 61); hence, SPV is also known as CRPV, for cottontail rabbit papillomavirus. About 50% of the lesions in cottontail rabbits undergo spontaneous regression (62). However, in domestic rabbits, experimental SPV infection leads to characteristic squamous cell papillomas which persist in more than 90% of animals. About 75% of these papillomas become malignant within an average of 9 months, as compared with the cottontail rabbit in which only 25% of the papillomas do so (62). This different behavior of the SPV-induced tumors in the wild and domestic strain has been attributed to differences in the host reactivity.

The role of synergism, regarded to be of crucial importance in SPV-induced carcinogenesis, was studied by Rous and coworkers (3, 4, 42, 43). 3-Methylcholanthrene (3-MC) or tar, when applied repeatedly to SPV-induced papillomas of domestic rabbits, caused the tumors to undergo malignant transformation more rapidly and at multiple sites. The same effect was observed when tar and SPV were applied concurrently (43). Repeated tarring in itself rarely led to carcinomas, but subsequent intravenous inoculation with SPV yielded squamous cell carcinomas in a high percentage of animals (4). SPV was readily recoverable from papillomas that arose in skin treated with the virus followed by 3-MC. The likely explanation is that coal tar or 3-MC modified the development of neoplasms from cells previously transformed by the virus. Hyperplasia of cells transformed by 3-MC treatment is not likely to be a valid rationale, since turpentine–acetone mixture, which was inactive in synergizing SPV (42), has the same type of irritant effect. 3-MC and related polycyclic hydrocarbons are also known to interfere with the host's immunocompetence (*see* Chapter 8, *this volume*); however, to explain the effects in the above system it would have to be assumed that the locally applied doses were large enough for a systemic immunosuppressive effect. These early studies suggest that chemical carcinogens and SPV play a synergistic role in the genesis of squamous cell carcinomas in rabbits. The role of tarring was to apparently increase the susceptibility of the ear skin to the effect of SPV.

Another potential animal model of the human disease is the alimentary tract papilloma-to-carcinoma progression in cattle observed in the high-incidence areas of Scotland (44–46). However, this papilloma-to-carcinoma progression was demonstrated only in cattle fed a diet containing bracken fern. Evidence has been presented on the presence of bovine papillomavirus type 4 (BPV-4) DNA in squamous cell papillomas, but not in carcinomas developing from papillomas (44–46). The bracken fern from the highlands of Scotland contains a radiomimetic substance, which is thought possibly to act as a cofactor cooperating with the BPV-4 in the progression of the lesions to squamous cell carcinomas of the upper alimentary tract. The carcinomas of the upper alimentary tract are often accompanied by adenomas and adenocarcinomas of the lower gastrointestinal tract, as well as by carcinomas and hemangiosarcomas of the urinary bladder. Bracken ferm is also known to contain carcinogenic substances and powerful immunosuppressants (*rev.* Section 5.3.2.1 of ref. 28). In addition to BPV-4, there is also some evidence that bracken fern and BPV-2 can act synergistically in the induction of urinary bladder tumors in the cow (15).

Polyomaviruses.   In 1961, Rowson *et al.* (47) studied the effect of polyomavirus on 7,12-dimethylbenz[*a*]anthracene (DMBA)/croton oil-induced skin carcinogenesis. Newborn Swiss mice from polyomavirus-free parents were inoculated with the virus and then skin-painted with the following chemical agents at 7 weeks of age: (a) a single subcarcinogenic dose of DMBA, (b) DMBA followed after 3 weeks by 15 once-weekly applications of croton oil, and (c) 15 weekly applications of croton oil alone. A control group was inoculated with the virus but received no further treatment. In parallel with the 4 polyomavirus-treated groups, 4 groups of mice were injected with polyoma-free tissue culture material at birth. The results showed no evidence of viral enhancement of DMBA/croton oil-induced skin carcinogenesis. The incidence of the parotid gland tumors was, however, increased in all the three groups that received treatment with the chemical agents. Further experiments reported by Rowson *et al.* (48) focused on the combination effect of neonatal polyoma inoculation and subsequent twice-weekly applications of benzo[*a*]pyrene (BaP). In contrast to the 3-MC study, there was definite evidence that skin tumors of the type normally induced by the application of BaP arose earlier and in higher incidence of the polyoma-treated group.

Poxviruses.   Many poxviruses induce hyperplastic responses and tumors in the skin of infected animals. These effects are most pronounced with the three fowl poxviruses: Shope fibroma virus (63), Yaba virus (64, 65), and molluscum contagiosum virus (66, 67). Ahlström and Andrewes (49) studied the combination effects of polycyclic aromatic hydrocarbons and Shope fibroma virus (SFV). They injected rabbits with 3-MC, BaP, or coal tar and then inoculated the same animals with SFV by various routes. Massive tumors developed at the site of s.c. inoculation of the virus, and general fibromatosis followed its i.v. inoculation. SFV was recoverable from the tumors and fibromatosis lesions. Without the chemical agents, the systemic inoculation of SFV has no significant carcinogenic effect. Since the titer of circulating antibodies to the virus was unaffected by treatment with chemical agents in this study, it was postulated that the enhancement of viral tumorigenesis by chemical agents was not due to interference with immune mechanisms.

Retroviruses.   Retroviruses have been shown to act synergistically with a variety of chemical carcinogens in *in vitro* carcinogenesis in cell culture systems (*see* Section IV, below). There is some evidence that this synergism may also occur *in vivo*. Carr (50) reported that inoculation of Rous sarcoma virus together with 3-MC injection led to injection-site tumor induction in a strain of chickens not normally sensitive to the virus. Carcinogenesis studies with 1,3-butadiene indicated that $B6C3F_1$ mice are substantially more susceptible to the leukemogenic activity of the chemical than Sprague-Dawley rats (68). Irons (51) attributed this marked species difference to the endogenous ecotropic retroviral background of mice [a number of strains (including $B6C3F_1$) of mice contain proviral genes that code for murine leukemia virus (MuLV)]. He found that the leukemogenic activity of 1,3-butadiene in NIH Swiss mice (which has truncated proviral ecotropic sequence so that the virus cannot be expressed) is at least four times lower than in B6C3F$_1$ mice and suggested that the high susceptibility of B6C3F$_1$ mice may be due to the combined effect of the chemical and MuLV.

III. POTENTIATION OF CHEMICAL CARCINOGENS BY VIRUSES NOT KNOWN TO BE ONCOGENIC

In addition to reports of syncarcinogenesis between tumor viruses and chemical carcinogens, potentiation of chemical carcinogenesis by a number of viruses, not known to be overtly oncogenic, has also been observed. These viruses are: herpes simplex virus, West Nile virus, vaccinia virus, and influenza virus (*see* Table 2).

Herpes Simplex Virus. Tanaka and Southam (52) reported that the intradermal inoculation of herpes simplex virus into mice during a 5-day course of skin painting with 3-MC gave rise to an earlier appearance and a higher incidence of skin papillomas than 3-MC treatment alone. Most of the skin tumors tended to arise close to the site of virus inoculation. Inoculation with noninfective control preparations was without tumor-enhancing effect. The virus alone had no tumorigenic activity. The enhancing effect of the virus could not be observed if given 7 days prior to or 14 days after 3-MC treatment. It appears that 3-MC facilitates the proliferation of the virus and augments the severity of the inflammatory lesions which it produces. The resultant wound healing and hyperplasia promote the development of tumors in the 3-MC- treated skin.

West Nile Virus. Besides the herpes simplex virus, Tanaka and Southam (52) also studied the combined effect of West Nile virus (an RNA arborvirus) with 3-MC or BaP in mice. When given intraperitoneally during a 10-day course of skin painting with 3-MC or BaP, the virus increased the incidence of both benign and malignant skin tumors. The virus itself is not known to induce skin tumors in mice or in any other species of animals. Virus inoculation after the completion of 3-MC or BaP treatment was ineffective.

Vaccinia Virus. Duran-Reynals (5) developed an experimental protocol for studying the combined effects of a strain of vaccinia virus (VV) and of other agents in cortisone-treated mice. Non-inbred Swiss Carworth mice first received 10 skin paintings with 3-MC and, next, s.c. injections of cortisone followed by an intradermal inoculation of VV into the 3-MC-painted flank. Ulcers developed at the site of virus inoculation. These healed with the formation of hyperplastic keloid scars from which skin tumors developed in 66% of cases; 50% of the tumors were malignant. In mice pretreated with benzene instead of 3-MC, no skin tumors developed. Subsequent experiments of Duran-Reynals (6, 7) revealed that 3-MC applied shortly after VV inoculation was more effective than 3-MC applied before VV inoculation in the induction of skin tumors. Prior immunization of mice with VV abolished this enhancement of carcinogenesis by 3-MC. A further finding was that, after treatment with cortisone and VV followed by 3-MC, the incidence of malignant lymphoma was much higher than after treatment with any one or two of the agents alone. Again, prior immunization of mice with VV abolished the effect of the triple combination of lymphoma incidence.

The applications of 3-MC after VV and cortisone treatment increased the amount of VV recoverable from the skin on the 8th day, but on the 14th day no virus was recoverable from either 3-MC-treated mice or controls. The explanation of the first experiment could be that the application of 3-MC, before the inoculation of VV, facilitated the entry of VV into cells or enabled the rapid replication and lateral spread of the virus before the level of circulating antibodies was high enough to limit the process. It is possible that a noncarcinogenic irritant would have had the same effect, as was the case in the experiments of Pound and Withers (68). In any case, the result of the prior treatment with 3-MC was a considerable increase in the severity of the inflammatory response to the virus with resultant ulceration and scarring. The latter effects promoted the development of skin tumor formation initiated by 3-MC. The promoting effect of such a wound healing is well documented (*see* Chapter 5, *this volume*). Rous and Kidd (69) noted the phenomenon in rabbit ear skin previously treated with either coal tar or 3-MC, and others have reported a promoting effect of deep wounding in mouse skin (70, 71). But perhaps the most relevant examples of the phenomenon are those described by Salaman and Glendenning (72). These authors introduced three irritants—phenol, proflavine hemisulfate, or ethanolamine oleate—intradermally into mouse skin previously treated with a subcarcinogenic dose of DMBA. Tumors eventually arose at the edge of the scars that resulted from the intradermal injections. This is suggestive that the tumors arising in Duran-Reynals' experiment were induced by 3-MC, and that the virus and cortisone treatment only modified the development of these tumors. However, the experiments of Mazurenko (73) in a different strain of mice (inbred CC57Br) support the view that the lymphomas seen by Duran-Reynals (6, 7) were induced by a virus other than vaccinia. Nonetheless, they also suggest that VV may specifically activate a lymphoma virus. Mazurenko showed that the inoculation of newborn mice of this strain with VV-enhanced lymphoma development (before 6 months of age) from 1.1% in untreated controls to between 10% and 45%. Under similar conditions, influenza virus produced a less-marked enhancement, and Newcastle disease virus, BCG vaccine, and heat-inactivated VV were without effect. However, these early experiments, as suggestive as they were, could not provide conclusive evidence for true multifactorial carcinogenesis.

Influenza Virus. The synergistic/potentiating action of influenza virus (type A_2, A/PRS, B, Sendai) on various chemical carcinogens (urethan, BaP, cigarette smoke, ozonized gasoline, diethylnitrosamine) in the induction of lung tumors has been extensively studied (*rev.* 74). Influenza viral infection was suspected to have synergistic/potentiating potential after reports of histologic evidence of proliferative changes with characteristics of epithelial tumors were found in lungs of survivors of influenza pandemic in 1918 (75). Imagawa and coworkers (53) were the first to report in 1957 that $(A \times Zb)F_1$ hybrid mice, given influenza virus intranasally and urethan intraperitoneally, had high incidence of lung tumors. Kotin and Wiseley (54) reported that exposure of strain A or strain C57BL mice to aerosols of ozonized gasoline resulted in the development of adenocarcinomas and synergism between influenza viruses and ozonized gasoline. Harris and Negroni (55) reported similar results in experiments in which mice were exposed to a combination of influenza viruses and tobacco smoke. Schmidt-Ruppin and Papadopulu (56) administered influenza A_2-Bethesda or A/PRS/EKI virus to XMRI mice. After the subsidence of the stage of infection, the animals were given diethylnitrosamine (DEN) in the drinking water for 6 months. The lung tumor incidence were 78.2% for those given A_2 + DEN, 58% for those given A/PRS + DEN, and 10% for those given DEN alone.

IV. COMBINED EFFECT OF VIRUSES AND CHEMICAL CARCINOGENS/ PROMOTERS IN CELL CULTURES

The combination effects of viruses and chemical carcinogens/promoters have also been extensively studied in cell culture. Table 3 summarizes some representative studies

TABLE 3. Studies Illustrative of Synergistic Interactions Between Viruses and Carcinogens/Promoters in Cell Culture Systems

Virus[a]	Carcinogen/promoter[b]	Cell culture system	Reference
Papillomavirus			
BPV-1	TPA, mezerein, PRA	C3H/10T½ cells	76
BPV-4 + *ras*	Quercetin	Primary bovine cells	77
BPV-4	DMBA, TPA	Bovine palatine tissue	15
HPV-16	MNNG	NIH 3T3 cells	78
HPV-18	MNU + TPA	Human keratinocytes	79
Papova B (Polyoma) Virus			
Polyomavirus	TPA	Rat fibroblasts	80
SV40	4-NQO	Chinese hamster embryo cells	81
	3-MC	Human urinary tract epithelial cells	82
	TPA	Chinese hamster lung cells	83
Herpesvirus			
EBV	TPA	Primary human skin epithelial cells	84
	TPA	Human leukocytes	85
	Euphorbia plants	Primary human B lymphocytes	21
	MNNG	Human umbilical cord and adult peripheral blood lymphocytes	12
	DMN, DEN, MNU, AFB$_1$	Human adult peripheral blood lymphocytes	12
Adenovirus			
Simian adenovirus SA7	A wide variety of carcinogens[c]	Syrian hamster embryo cells	86–88
Human adenovirus 5	DMBA, B[a]P, TPA or DMBA + TPA	Rat embryo cells	89,90
Human adenovirus 12	MNNG	Rat embryo cells	89
Retroviruses			
MLV	DEN	Rat embryo cells	91
Moloney MLV	3-MC	NRK cell clone	14
	DMBA	NRK cell clone	14
Friend MLV + SFFV complex	TPA	BALB/c 3T3 cells	92
Rauscher leukemia virus	DMBA	Rat embryo cells	93
Mouse mammary tumor virus	DMBA	Mammary epithelial cell clone	94
HTLV-I	Diterpene esters	Lymphocytes	95
Nononcogenic viruses			
Influenza virus	Urethan	Human embryo lung cells	96

[a]Abbreviations of viruses: BPV, bovine papillomavirus; EBV, Epstein-Barr virus; HPV, human papillomavirus; HTLV, human T-cell leukemia virus; MLV, murine leukemia virus; SFFV, Friend spleen focus-forming virus; SV40, simian virus 40.

[b]Abbreviations of carcinogens: 2-AAF, 2-acetylaminofluorene; AFB$_1$, aflatoxin B$_1$; B[a]P, benzo[a]pyrene; DEN, diethylnitrosamine; DB[a,h]A, dibenz[a,h]anthracene; DMBA, 7,12-dimethylbenz[a]anthracene; DMN, dimethylnitrosamine; MAMAc, methylazoxymethanol acetate; 3-MC, 3-methylcholanthrene; MMS, methyl methanesulfonate; MNNG, N-methyl-N-nitroso-N'-nitroguanidine; MNU, N-methyl-N-nitrosourea; 4-NQO, 4-nitroquinoline-N-oxide. Abbreviations of promoters: RPA, phorbol-12-retinoate-13-acetate; TPA, 12-O-tetradecanoylphorbol-13-acetate.

[c]Chemical carcinogens that showed positive results include DB[a,h]A, MMS, MAMAc, MNNG, N-acetoxy-AAF, As, Cd, Cr, and Sb salts. However, Ni salt and a number of indirect acting carcinogens such as DMN, DEN, and 2-AAF were inactive.

illustrative of synergistic interactions between viruses and chemical carcinogens/ promoters. These studies involve a variety of tumor viruses and chemical carcinogens/ promoters in different cell culture systems ranging from primary cell cultures to established cell lines. Several potent promoters (*e.g.,* TPA, mezerein) and TPA-containing plant extracts (*e.g., Euphorbia* plant) appear to be as effective as complete carcinogens. In fact, induction of virus production and enhancement of virally-induced transformation have been used as assays for screening promoters (*revs.* 97, 98). Whereas a detailed discussion of these *in vitro* studies is beyond the scope of this section, they may provide mechanistic insights toward the understanding of the combination of effects and of the multifactorial nature of carcinogenesis as well as could serve as predictors of synergistic interactions in animals and humans.

V. CONCLUDING NOTE

Despite the extensive data on synergistic interactions between viruses and chemical carcinogens/promoters, their mechanism remains elusive. It is likely that a mechanism may be specific for a specific pair of interacting virus and chemical. This is further complicated by the sometimes identical consequence of viral oncoprotein expression and chemical treatment; for example, the chromosome abnormalities induced by the E7 oncoprotein of HPV-16 (99) are basically indistinguishable from those induced by the carcinogen/ promoter quercetin (100). For synergistic interaction between tumor viruses and chemical carcinogens/promoters, a variety of possible mechanisms have been suggested (6, 12–14, 32, 48). In general, chemicals may enhance viral carcinogenesis by: (a) enhancing viral replication, (b) activating latent viruses, (c) increasing the susceptibility of target cells to viral infection or transformation, and (d) impairing the immunologic response of the host to the virus. Viruses may enhance chemical carcinogenesis by: (a) changing the permeability of target cells to facilitate uptake of chemical carcinogens; (b) enhancing metabolic activation and/or inhibiting detoxification of chemical carcinogens; (c) increasing mitotic activity of target cells, thus providing a more favorable condition for fixation of errors resulting from DNA adduct formation; and (d) impairing immune surveillance of the host. For effective synergism in the host, it is most likely that the tumor virus and chemical carcinogen collaboration involve action on both nuclear and cytoplasmic/membrane-linked regulatory proteins and/or their coding proto-oncogenes. Alternatively, it is possible that the action of one of the agents creates a selective advantage to the cell vis-à-vis the second agent. For example, there is suggestive evidence that AFB_1 selectively causes mutation at codon 249 in the *p53* gene and that the hepatocyte clone carrying this specific mutant has a selective growth advantage in HBV-infected patients (*see* 30). Further mechanistic studies of AFB_1-HBV and other synergistically interacting pairs of virus and chemical carcinogen should provide insights into a better understanding of the basis of high tumor incidence in susceptible subpopulations and eventually lead to preventive measures.

Abbreviations Used: AFB_1, aflatoxin B_1; ATL, adult T-cell leukemia; BaP, benzo[*a*]pyrene; BL, Burkitt's lymphoma; BPV, bovine papillomavirus; CRPV, cottontail rabbit papillomavirus; DEN, diethylnitrosamine; DHBV, duck hepatitis B virus; DMBA, 7,12-dimethylbenz[*a*]anthracene; EBV, Epstein-Barr virus; GSHV, ground squirrel hepatitis virus; HBV, hepatitis B virus; HCC, hepatocellular carcinoma; HHPA, 12-*O*-hexadecanoyl-16-hydroxyphorbol-13-acetate; HPV, human papillomavirus; HTLV, human T-cell leukemia virus; 3-MC, 3-methylcholanthrene; MuLV, murine leukemia virus; NPC, nasopharyngeal carcinoma; SFV, Shope fibromavirus; SPV, Shope papillomavirus; TPA, 12-*O*-tetradecanoylphorbol-13-acetate; VV, vaccinia virus; WHV, woodchuck hepatitis virus.

REFERENCES

1. Rous, R.: *JAMA* **56,** 198 (1911).
2. Yamagiwa, K., and Ichikawa, K.: *Mitt. Med. Fakult. Kais. Jpn.* **15,** 295 (1915).
3. Rous, P., and Kidd, J. G.: *Science* 83, 468 (1936).
4. Rous, P., and Kidd, J. G.: *J. Exp. Med.* **67,** 399 (1938).
5. Duran-Reynals, F.: *Texas Repts. Biol. Med.* **15,** 306 (1957).
6. Duran-Reynals, M. L.: *Prog. Exp. Tumor Res.* **3,** 148 (1963).
7. Duran-Reynals, M. L.: *Acta Unio Intern. Contra Cancrum* **19,** 792 (1963).
8. Tennant, R. W., and Rascati, R. J.: Mechanisms of Cocarcinogenesis Involving Endogenous Retroviruses. *In* "Modifiers of Chemical Carcinogenesis" (T. J. Slaga, ed.). Raven Press, New York, 1980, p. 185.
9. Southam, C. M., Tanaka, S., Arata, T., Simkovic, D., Miura, M., and Petropulos, S. F.: *Prog. Exp. Tumor Res.* **11,** 194 (1969).
10. Yamamoto, N.: *Rev. Physiol. Biochem. Pharmacol.* **101,** 111 (1984).
11. Harris, C. C., and Sun, T.-T.: *Cancer Surveys* **5,** 765 (1986).
12. Henderson, E. E.: *J. Natl. Cancer Inst.* **80,** 476 (1988).
13. Weinstein, I. B.: *Cancer, Detection Prev.* **14,** 253 (1989).
14. Aboud, M., Rosner, M., Dombrovsky, A., Revazova, T., Feldman, G., Tolpolar, L., Strilitz-Hassan, Y., and Flugel, R. M.: *Leukemia Res.* **16,** 1061 (1992).
15. Jackson, M. E., Campo, M. S., and Gaukroger, J. M.: *Crit. Rev. Oncogenesis* **4,** 277 (1993).
16. Van Rensburg, S. J., Cook-Mozaffari, P., Van Schalkwyk, D. J., Van der Watt, J. J., Vincent, T. J., and Purchase, I. F.: *Br. J. Cancer* **51,** 713 (1985).
17. Peers, F., Bosch, X., Kaldor, J., Linsell, A., and Pluijmen, M.: *Int. J. Cancer* **39,** 545 (1987).
18. Yeh, F. S., Yu, M. C., Mo, C. C., Luo, S., Tong, M. J., and Henderson, B. E.: *Cancer Res* **49,** 2506 (1989).
19. Ross, R. K., Yuan, M. J., Yu, M. C., Wogan, G. N., Qian, G. S., Tu, J. T., Groopman, J. D., Gao, Y. T., and Henderson, B. E.: *Lancet* **339,** 943 (1992).
20. Qian, G. S., Ross, R. K., Yu, M. C., Yuan, J. M., Gao, Y. T., Henderson, B. E., Wogan, G. N., and Groopman, J. D.: *Cancer Epidemiol. Biomarkers Prev.* **3,** 3 (1994).
21. Osato, T., Imai, S., Kinoshita, T., Aya, T., Sugiura, M., Koizumi, S., and Mizuno, F.: Epstein-Barr Virus, Burkitt's Lymphoma, and an African Tumor Promoter. *In* "Immunobiology and Prophylaxis of Human Herpesvirus Infections" (C. Lopez, ed.). Plenum Press, New York, 1990, p. 147.
22. Ito, Y., Tokuka, H., Ohigashi, H., and Koshimizu, K.: Distribution and Characterization of Environmental Promoter Substances as Assayed by Synergistic Epstein-Barr Virus-Activating System. *In* "Cellular Interactions by Environmental Tumor Promoters" (H. Fujiki, ed.). Japan Sci. Soc. Press, Tokyo, 1984, p. 125.
23. Ho, J. H. C., Huang, D. P., and Fong, Y. Y.: *Lancet* **ii,** 626 (1978).
24. Chang, K. W., Chang, C. S., Lai, K. S., Chou, M. J., and Choo, K. B.: *J. Med. Virol.* **28,** 57 (1989).
25. Ito, Y., Matsuda, S., Tokuda, H., and Nakao, Y.: Tumor Promoting Diterpene Esters as Possible Environmental Co-factors of ATL. *In* "Human T-Cell Leukemia/Lymphoma Virus and Adult T-Cell Leukemia" (R. C. Gallo, M. Essex, and L. Gross, eds.). Cold Spring Harbor Laboratory Press, Cold Spring Harbor, New York, 1984, p. 69.
26. Lutwick, I. L.: *Lancet* **i,** 755 (1979).
27. Munoz, N. M., and Bosch, F. X.: Epidemiology of Hepatocellular Carcinoma. *In* "Neoplasms of the Liver" (K. Okuda and K. G. Ishak, eds.). Springer-Verlag, Tokyo, 1987, p. 3.
28. Woo, Y.-t., Lai, D. Y., Arcos, J. C., and Argus, M. F.: "Chemical Induction of Cancer—Structural Bases and Biological Mechanisms," Vol. IIIC: Natural, Metal, Fiber and Macromolecular Carcinogens. Academic Press, San Diego, 1988.
29. Beasley, R. P.: *Cancer* **61,** 1942 (1988).
30. Greenblatt, M. S., Bennett, W. P., Hollstein, M., and Harris, C. C.: *Cancer Res.* **54,** 4855 (1994).
31. Kim, C. M., Koike, K., Saito, I., Miyamura, T., and Jay, G.: *Nature* **351,** 317 (1991).
32. Wild, C., Jansen, L. A. M., Cova, L., and Montesano, R.: *Environ. Health Perspect.* **99,** 115 (1993).
33. The Gambia Hepatitis Study Group: *Lancet* **i,** 1057 (1989).
34. de Thé, G., Geser, A., and Day, N. E.: *Nature* **274,** 756 (1978).
35. Shank, R. C.: Epidemiology of Aflatoxin Carcinogenesis. *In* "Environmental Cancer" (H. F. Kraybill and M. A. Mehlman, eds.). Wiley, New York, 1977, p. 301.
36. Henle, W., Henle, G., and Ho, H. C.: *J. Natl. Cancer Inst.* **44,** 225 (1970).
37. Winkelstein, W.: *Am. J. Epidemiol.* **131,** 945 (1990).
38. Holly, E. A., Whittemore, A. S., Aston, D. A., Ahn, D. K., Nickoloff, B. J., and Kristiansen, J. L.: *J. Natl. Cancer Inst.* **81,** 1726 (1989).
39. Cann, A. J., and Chen, I. S. Y.: Human T-Cell Leukemia Virus Types I and II. *In* "Virology" (B. N.

Fields and D. M. Knipe, eds.), 2nd ed. Raven Press, New York, 1990, p. 1501.
40. Dragani, T. A., Manenti, G., Farza, H., Della Porta, G., Tiollais, P., and Pourcel, C.: *Carcinogenesis* **11**, 953 (1989).
41. Sell, S., Hunt, J. M., Dunsford, H. A., and Chisari, F. V.: *Cancer Res.* **51**, 1278 (1991).
42. Rous, P., and Friedewald, W. F.: *J. Exp. Med.* **79**, 511 (1944).
43. Rogers, S., and Rous, P.: *J. Exp. Med.* **93**, 459 (1951).
44. Jarrett, W. F. H.: *Bull. Cancer* **65**, 191 (1978).
45. Campo, M. S., Moar, M. H., Jarrett, W. F. H., and Laird, H. M.: *Nature* **286**, 180 (1980).
46. Campo, M. S.: *Cancer Surveys* **6**, 39 (1987).
47. Rowson, K. E. K., Roe, F. J. C., Ball, J. K., and Salaman, M. H.: *Nature* **191**, 893 (1961).
48. Roe, F. J. C., and Rowson, K. E. K.: *Int. Rev. Exp. Pathol.* **6**, 181 (1968).
49. Ahlström, C. G., and Andrewes, C. N.: *J. Pathol. Bacteriol.* **47**, 65 (1938).
50. Carr, J. G.: *Br. J. Exp. Pathol.* **23**, 221 (1942).
51. Irons, R. D.: *Environ. Health Perspect.* **86**, 49 (1990).
52. Tanaka, S., and Southam, C. M.: *J. Natl. Cancer Inst.* **34**, 441 (1965).
53. Imagawa, D. T., Yorhimori, M., and Adams, J. M.: *Proc. Am. Assoc. Cancer Res.* **2**, 217 (1957).
54. Kotin, P., and Wiseley, D. V.: *Prog. Exp. Tumor Res.* **3**, 186 (1963).
55. Harris, R. J., and Negroni, C.: *Br. Med. J.* **58**, 6337 (1967).
56. Schmidt-Ruppin, K. H., and Papadopulu, G.: *Z. Krebsforsch.* **77**, 150 (1972).
57. Sherker, A. H., and Marion, P.: *Annu. Rev. Microbiol.* **45**, 475 (1991).
58. Rogler, C. E.: *Curr. Top. Microbiol. Immunobiol.* **168**, 104 (1991).
59. Cova, L., Duflot, A., Prave, M., and Trepo, C.: *Arch. Virol. [Suppl.]* **8**, 81 (1993).
60. Shope, R. E., and Hurst, E. W.: *J. Exp. Med.* **58**, 607 (1933).
61. Lancaster, W. D., and Olson, C.: *Microbiol. Rev.* **46**, 191 (1982).
62. Syverton, J. T.: *Ann. NY Acad. Sci.* **54**, 1126 (1952).
63. Shope, R. E.: *J. Exp. Med.* **56**, 803 (1932).
64. Andrewes, C., Allison, A. C., Armstrong, J. A., Bearcroft, G., Niven, J. S. F., and Pereira, H. S.: *Acta Unio Int. Contra Cancrum* **15**, 760 (1959).
65. Bearcroft, W. G. C., and Jamieson, M. F.: *Nature* **182**, 195 (1958).
66. LaPlaca, M., Portolani, M., Mannini-Palenzona, A., Barbanti-Brodano, G., and Bernardini, A.: *J. Microbiol.* **15**, 205 (1967).
67. Vreeswijk, J., Leene, W., and Kalsbeek, G. L.: *J. Invest. Dermatol.* **69**, 249 (1977).
68. Pound, A. W., and Withers, H. R.: *Br. J. Cancer* **17**, 460 (1963).
69. Rous, P., and Kidd, J. G.: *J. Exp. Med.* **73**, 365 (1941).
70. Deelman, H. T.: *Z. Krebsforsch.* **18**, 261 (1923).
71. Pullinger, B. D.: *J. Pathol. Bacteriol.* **57**, 477 (1945).
72. Salaman, M. H., and Glendenning, O. M.: *Br. J. Cancer* **11**, 434 (1957).
73. Mazurenko, N. P.: *Probl. Oncol.* (USSR). (English Transl.) **6**, 873 (1960).
74. Šula, J.: *Neoplasma* **26**, 1 (1979).
75. Askanazy, M.: *Zentrabl. allg. Pathol. pathol. Anat.* **30**, 443 (1919).
76. Tsang, S. S., and Stich, H. F.: *Cancer Lett.* **43**, 93 (1988).
77. Pennie, W. D., and Campo, M. S.: *Virology* **190**, 861 (1992).
78. Mitrani-Rosenbaum, S., and Tsvieli, R.: *Intervirology* **33**, 76 (1992).
79. Garrett, L. R., Perez-Reyes, N., Smith, P. P., and McDougall, J. K.: *Carcinogenesis* **14**, 329 (1993).
80. Self, R.: *J. Virol.* **36**, 421 (1980).
81. Diamond, L., Knorr, R., and Shimizu, Y.: *Cancer Res.* **34**, 2599 (1974).
82. Reznikoff, C. A., Loretz, L. J., Christian, B. J., Wu, S.-Q., and Meisner, L. F.: *Carcinogenesis* **9**, 1427 (1988).
83. Martin, R. G., Stelow, V. P., and Edwards, C. A. F.: *J. Virol.* **31**, 596 (1979).
84. Tomei, L. D., Noyes, I., Blocker, D., Holliday, J., and Glaser, R.: *Nature* **329**, 73 (1987).
85. Yamamoto, N., and zur Hausen, H.: *Nature* **280**, 244 (1979).
86. Casto, B. C.: *Cancer Res.* **33**, 402 (1973).
87. Casto, B. C., Pieczynski, W. J., and DiPaolo, J. A.: *Cancer Res.* **34**, 72 (1974).
88. Casto, B. C., Meyer, J., and DiPaolo, J. A.: *Cancer Res.* **39**, 193 (1979).
89. Fisher, P. B., Weinstein, I. B., Eisenberg, D., and Ginsberg, H.: *Proc. Natl. Acad. Sci. U.S.A.* **75**, 2311 (1978).
90. Fisher, P. B., Mufson, R. A., Weinstein, I. B., and Little, J. B.: *Carcinogenesis* **2**, 183 (1981).
91. Freeman, A. E., Price, P. J., Igel, H. J., Young, J. C., Maryak, J. M., and Huebner, R. J.: *J. Natl. Cancer Inst.* **44**, 65 (1970).
92. Lipp, M., Scherer, B., Lips, G., Brandner, G., and Hunsmann, G.: *Carcinogenesis* **3**, 261 (1982).
93. Rhim, J. S., Vass, W., Cho, H. Y., and Huebner, R. J.: *Int. J. Cancer* **7**, 65 (1971).
94. Howard, D. K., Schlom, J. H., and Fisher, P. B.: *In Vitro* **19**, 58 (1983).

95. Matsuda, S., Nakao, Y., Ohigashi, H., Koshimizu, K., and Ito, Y.: *Int. J. Cancer* **38**, 859 (1986).
96. Frolov, A. F., Sherbinskaya, A. M., and Botsman, N. E.: *Folia Biol.* **17**, 521 (1971).
97. zur Hausen, H., Yamamoto, N., and Bauer, G.: Virus Induction by Tumor Promoters. *In* "Carcinogenesis", Vol. 7 (E. Hecker, ed.). Raven Press, New York, 1982, p. 617.
98. Yamamoto, N.: *Rev. Physiol. Biochem. Pharmacol.* **101**, 111 (1984).
99. Hashida, T., and Yamamoto, S.: *J. Gen. Virol.* **72**, 1569 (1991).
100. Ishidate, M.: "Data Book on Chromosome Aberration Tests *in vitro*". Elsevier, Amsterdam, 1988.

Speculative Closing Note

Joseph C. Arcos

Different mechanisms proposed previously by other authors to provide a rationale for the syncarcinogenic interactions between viruses and chemical carcinogens/promoters have been cited in Section III. This Note is an attempt to create an alternative viewpoint on this synergism.

Possible cellular and systemic effects that viruses and chemical carcinogens/promoters may display individually were considered in Section III. Different combinations of these effects may underlie a synergistic response depending on the particular pair of virus and chemical agent. However, beyond the individual gene-alteration-based effects, an *overall* genomic characteristic drives the progress of the nascent, preneoplastic clone through the selection process toward increasing autonomy, dedifferentiation, and ability to metastasize. This selective pressure favors such aspects as increasing freedom from external growth factor requirements (*i.e.,* the progressive development of autocrine features), the ability to bypass senescence and apoptosis, the abolishment of antiproliferative genes or inactivation of their products, the ability to escape immune surveillance, the ability to increasingly vascularize the growing tumor so as to ensure its independent blood supply, and derepression of genes coding for proteolytic enzymes so as to be able to invade surrounding tissue. The facilitating common denominator behind all these phenomena is the genomic instability of premalignant and tumor cells; this same characteristic enables tumor cells to rapidly evolve when subjected to some new selective pressure (such as chemotherapy or trauma). Figure 1 posits this instability as a component of a network of interrelationships between oncogene activators, proto-oncogenes/oncogenes, tumor-suppressor genes, and some of their devolving cellular consequences.

Indeed, most tumor cells—especially when totally free from restraining tissue signals, such as in culture—show often extraordinary instability of their karyotypes. The restrictive growth conditions of the nascent, preneoplastic clone may represent precisely the selective pressure that selects (or induces) cells which are genetically increasingly unstable. In the shuffling, chromosomes are translocated or may become duplicated or lost; genes adjacent to or near the breakpoint of translocation may undergo mutation. There are, however, tumors and leukemic cells without microscopically visible alteration of the karyotype. This is because individual genes may undergo mutation, amplification, or deletion—alterations that may be sufficient for the progression of particular clones to full malignancy. Chromosome translocation may also produce the overexpression or unscheduled expression of nonmutated genes by bringing them under the influence of transcriptional control regions (possibly near active promoters) of other genes at the point

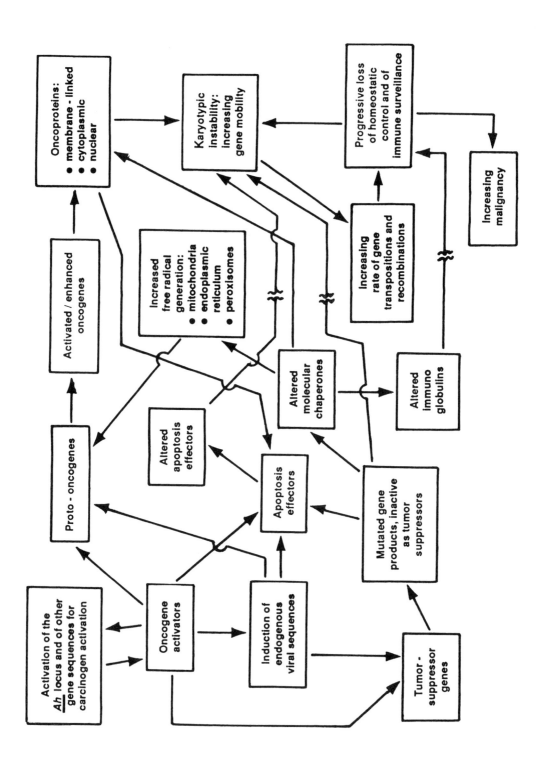

624

of reattachment. Thus, because of the continuously ongoing genetic shuffling during tumor progression each instance of full malignancy is characterized by its own array of genetic lesions.

The onset of destabilization of the karyotype may be due to mutations in various tumor-suppressor genes (or continuous inactivation of suppressor proteins), in particular of *p53*. For example, cells with damaged DNA, but lacking functional p53 protein will pass through the p53-dependent control point in the G_1 phase of the cell cycle despite the DNA damage. Through several cell divisions this will produce an accumulation of genetic/chromosomal alterations: gene amplifications, chromosome fragmentation and reattachment — leading eventually to a highly unstable karyotype.

The destabilization of the karyotype may also begin with the largely random, direct action of carcinogens on DNA, such as radiations or attachment of reactive electrophilic chemical moieties. If unrepaired or misrepaired these lesions will result in mutations and an increase in the relative fragility of the chromosome in the region. Viral integrations also represent regions of relatively increased chromosome fragility. Moreover, carcinogen/ promoter- or virally-induced chromosomal lesions may significantly accelerate the normally very slow traffic of some intrinsic transposable elements, in particular retro-transposons, in the mammalian genome. Such direct effects on DNA are likely to be mutually amplifying and this may represent the underlying basis of the synergistic nature of random genetic alterations known for some years. Once the alterations/ destabilization of the genome, due to random direct action on DNA, begins to affect the expression of suppressor-genes, it will accelerate the onset of tumorigenesis and maximize the degree of synergism (possibly by advancing it to multiplicative synergism).

Reviewing tumorigenesis by viral–chemical combinations, clear antagonism between these two categories of agents was found to be exceedingly rare, if nonexistent (*see* Section III above). This is consistent with the findings that antagonism between carcinogenic agents occurs when two agents are highly similar in their chemical structure and/or physical nature so that there is an overlap between the carcinogenesis rate-limiting steps (*see* Chapter 2, this volume). Overwhelmingly, viral–chemical combination tumorigenesis data reported show synergistic effects between the two categories of agents (*see* Section III above). This is in accordance with the findings that synergism occurs in instances when two agents differ greatly in chemical structure and in their physical nature, so that the rate-limiting steps of tumorigenesis are different (Chapters 2 and 3, this volume). Thus,

---

FIGURE 1.   A partial network of interrelationships between oncogene activators, proto-oncogenes, and tumor-suppressor genes in affecting genomic stability and the rate of progress of the malignant transformation: a speculative schematic. The "Oncogene activators" may be viral (exogenous), chemical, radiation, or cellular stress. The arrows symbolize the direction of the relationships. For example, the action of "Oncogene activators" upon "Tumor-suppressor genes" yields "Mutated gene products, inactive as tumor suppressors". The latter, in turn, affects the process of apoptosis ("Apoptosis effectors") as well as the molecular chaperone function of stress proteins ("Altered molecular chaperones"); this can lead to "Altered immunoglobulins" and, hence, to impaired immune surveillance (as indicated by a broken arrow). Tumor-suppressor gene products and apoptosis effectors, when mutated/altered cannot counteract the consequences of karyotypic instability, also denoted by breaks in the respective arrows. "Karyotypic instability: increasing gene mobility" drives the "Increasing rate of gene transpositions and recombinations". This, together with "Altered immunoglobulins", leads to the "Progressive loss of homeostatic control and of immune surveillance". In fact, "Karyotypic instability . . .", "Increasing rate of gene transpositions . . .", and "Progressive loss of homeostatic control . . ." represent a positive feedback loop; the spin-off of the loop is "Increasing malignancy".

tumor viruses and chemical carcinogens tend to activate/express oncogenes or inactivate/block tumor-suppressor genes which function in different compartments, in largely different areas of the cellular regulatory network. In this sense then carcinogenesis by viral–chemical combinations may be compared to malignant transformation brought about by oncogene collaboration.

CHAPTER **15**

Effect of Stress On Tumor Induction

Wolfgang H. Vogel

1. INTRODUCTION

It has become established over the past decades that a number of variables, for example, diet, pollutants, drugs, or the presence of certain diseases, can modulate the carcinogenic process (1-6). The foregoing chapters in the present volume reviewed and discussed different exogenous and endogenous variables which influence tumor induction and the progression of tumors. Another parameter, stress, has been recognized more recently to markedly modulate the induction and growth of tumors. However, although stress has been firmly established as a parameter in carcinogenesis, it usually receives very little attention. A computer survey with the key words "carcinogenesis" or "stress" over the last 3 years revealed hundreds of papers in each category, but only three which were cross-referenced. Stress is often intentionally neglected or even omitted in scientific investigations in order to reduce and minimize the number of confounding variables (7). While such studies then produce "exact" scientific data, it is difficult and is *in fact* inaccurate and improper to extrapolate such results to the human population in which individuals are often affected by periods of intense stress.

This chapter discusses the biochemical, physiological, and behavioral changes that occur during periods of stress, the evidence that stress does indeed modulate carcinogenesis, and the possible mechanisms of how stress might affect the action of carcinogens on their respective target tissues.

II. STRESSOR, STRESS, AND HEALTH CONSEQUENCES

In the past, it was generally assumed that certain stressful events, termed "stressors", cause a stress response in an individual. Stress can be defined as any change away from an existing homeostasis. These changes may be behavioral (*e.g.*, fear, tension, anxiety), physiological (*e.g.*, increased gastrointestinal tract activity, tachycardia, and increased blood pressure), and/or biochemical (*e.g.*, rise of plasma catecholamine or steroid levels). The stressors can be external (*e.g.*, job pressure, loss of a beloved one) or internal (*e.g.*, pain, illness) events. If stress is very intense or chronic, it can cause the well-known stress-related diseases (*e.g.*, depression, headache, hypertension, ulcer). However, while the original definitions are still valid, the understanding of the sequential emergence of these parameters has undergone a gradual change (7-10).

It is the *highly individualized nature* of the stress response that has changed the concept of the sequence; this is now conceived as follows: an event is being perceived by an individual and assessed as to its importance and personal consequences. If the event is deemed of no importance, then no stress occurs and the homeostasis remains unaffected: the event remains just "an event". However, if this event is felt to be important (*e.g.*, threatening), then it is properly evaluated and the individual now searches for the appropriate coping strategies which can involve active or passive actions. If properly evaluated and if proper coping mechanisms can be devised, then, again, homeostasis remains unchanged and no stress is experienced: the event remains, again, just "an event". In contrast, if the event is misinterpreted (out of proportion or wrongly) or if proper coping strategies are not available, then homeostasis changes and stress are experienced because the event is designated as a challenge or a stressor (11–14). Rats exposed to a foot shock, which they can control, show significantly less biochemical changes or stress than do rats which receive identical, but not controllable foot shocks (15, 16).

Exposure to chronic stress can sometimes lead to adaptation or a gradual reduction in stress response. In some instances chronic stress produces no change in stress response. Conversely, chronic stress may bring about sensitization with an increase in the stress response over time (17, 18). The high variation among individuals probably reflects the plasticity of the evaluation process as well as the availability of coping mechanisms.

Stress does not always lead to detrimental health consequences or to occurrence of stress-related diseases. Again, health consequences are highly individualized. While some individuals show no stress-related diseases even during periods of intense stress, others experience significant stress-related problems and pathology even under less stressful conditions. Not all individuals who experience stress and display stress-related pathology show stress-related diseases. Individuals usually express selectivity in their responses regarding the organs affected (*e.g.*, headache or hypertension or ulcer or depression, but not all simultaneously). This difference and selectivity have been explained on the basis of organ vulnerability (19); if a person has no organ vulnerability, stress will not cause stress-related problems, no matter how severe the stress reaction might be. If there is organ vulnerability, however, then the particular organ will respond pathologically to stress while the other organs will remain unaffected. This explains the selectivity and specificity of stress-related pathology.

The high variability of the stress response and organ vulnerability, their possible changes over time, and detrimental health consequences are caused by genetic and environmental/experiential factors. Certain strains of rats and mice will show more intense stress responses to the same type of environmental stimulus than will other strains (20, 21). Animals can actually be bred selectively for their stress responses; one half of the members of a particular strain of hamsters develops a cardiomyopathy later in life, while the other half remains free of this pathology. Stress has no detrimental effects on the healthy members of this strain, but markedly worsens the onset and outcome of the cardiomyopathy in the other members (19).

While many of these effects have been observed *during* stress, stress can also produce effects long after a particular stress response has ceased to exist. Moreover, stress response may be physiologically beneficial in some instances. Exposure to a 4-hour immobilization period (a stressor) provided long-lasting protection by unknown mechanisms against sudden death caused by tetracaine; tetracaine killed 6 of 12 nonstressed rats, but caused no death if these animals have been stressed by immobilization 28 days earlier (22). Stress aftereffects can originate already during fetal development and can last into later life. Prenatal stress exposure caused offspring to show altered drug responses during adulthood in that they were considerably more sensitive to caffeine exposure than were the offspring of nonstressed rats (23).

Thus, stress is a *highly selective experience* of an individual in response to outside or inside stimuli. This response is based on the perception, evaluation, and coping strategies of the individual. If stress is experienced, the stimulus becomes a stressor and pathology can ensue, but only if the individual has a stress-susceptible organ system. All these processes and pathological events are under the control of genetic and environmental factors. Thus, we create our own stress experiences, sometimes transform plain events into stressors, and, if vulnerable, cause our own stress-related diseases.

III. HOMEOSTATIC CHANGES DURING STRESS

During stress a wide variety of behavioral, physiological, and chemical changes occur in the brain and/or body of the stressed individual.

Most widely studied have been the stress-induced changes in the levels of "stress chemicals": epinephrine, norepinephrine, and corticosterone/cortisol (corticosterone is the major circulating adrenocortical hormone in animals, while cortisol is the dominant hormone in humans). In the plasma, the levels of the catecholamines rise immediately at the beginning of stress, increase up to 20 times their original levels, start to return toward normal at the end of the stressful experience, and reach baseline levels 30 to 60 min after the stressor has ceased to exist (24–26). In the brain, the turnover of the adrenergic system is increased and levels of norepinephrine start to decline, in particular in the hypothalamus (27, 28). Corticosterone levels increase in the plasma only after a delay of a few minutes, rise usually two- to fourfold, and then start to decline at the end of the stressful experience to reach baseline values at 30 to 60 minutes after cessation of the stressor (29–31). In addition to these changes, many other biochemicals such as lipids, amino acids, and electrolytes are affected in the stressed organism (32–34).

Among the physiological/organ systems, the cardiovascular and the gastrointestinal have been widely studied. Heart rate and blood pressure may increase often to pathological levels during stressful experience. While the blood pressure returns soon to normal, increase in heart rate might persist for long periods of time (35–37). Intestinal activity can also be affected, leading to change in the rate of passage of food, drugs, and/or toxins through the intestinal tract (38, 39). In addition, other systems, most importantly the immune system (*see below*), change drastically during stress.

Among the behavioral manifestations, feelings of fear, anxiety, tension, and apprehension might predominate and repeated stressful experiences might lead to depression (28, 40, 41). These changes will affect various bodily systems, including the immune system, which is now recognized to be influenced in many of its aspects by the emotional state of the brain (*see below*). These feelings may be so intense that the individual is completely dominated by them and might change his or her normal habits, including the abuse of drugs which will place him/her at additional risk (*see below*).

As it has been mentioned in Section II above, it has been shown in animal experiments that if the opportunity is allowed for the animal to control the aversive event or it is allowed to cope successfully with the situation, then these physiological/behavioral changes will occur at lower intensities or not at all. While animals which cannot control an electric shock show large decreases in hypothalamic norepinephrine levels, animals which can control the shock maintain normal levels of this neurotransmitter (16, 28).

IV. SPECIFIC HOMEOSTATIC CHANGES POSSIBLY AFFECTING CARCINOGENESIS

All the above-mentioned as well as other as yet unexplored changes during stress may have a direct bearing on the effects of carcinogens in tumor initiation, progression, and spread. Conceivably, they may affect the transport and metabolism of carcinogens in the body, modify DNA synthesis and repair, and alter the activity of the immune system. Some of these possibilities are outlined below:

(i) Changes in the activity of the gastrointestinal tract, of the liver, and the kidney can change blood flow, mixed-function oxidase and other enzyme activities, as well as renal excretion rates. This can directly affect the toxicokinetics of a chemical. Plasma levels of amphetamine and its major metabolite after oral administration of the drug were found to be significantly altered in rats during immobilization stress as compared to resting rats (42). Foot shock stress decreases the plasma and tissue levels of nicorandile, a vasodilator, but significantly increases the levels of its metabolite (43). Chronic stress increases the half-life of antipyrine and markedly reduces its clearance (43). The latter results were taken as an indication of stress-induced inhibition of hepatic oxidative metabolism. Triorthotolyl caused significant neurotoxicity in chickens, which was significantly delayed by stress, most probably resulting from a reduction in microsomal mixed-function oxidase activities and the formation of the toxic metabolites (44). It is a most interesting finding that the availability of coping strategies can change toxic effects. For example, the pesticide dieldrin was observed to cause significant escape deficits only in those animals that were exposed to inescapable foot shock, but not in animals which were exposed to the same foot shock, but given the chance to control or terminate the stressful stimulus (45). Thus, it is quite conceivable that a carcinogen could be differently absorbed, distributed, metabolized, and/or excreted during stress with the result that the levels of the actual carcinogenic chemical acting on the macromolecular target(s) in the cell are either increased or decreased, resulting in enhanced or reduced carcinogenesis.

(ii) The rise and/or occurrence of specific stress chemicals in the system could affect the promotion and progression of tumor cells and their spread. During stress many chemicals, including the biogenic amines, steroids, and endorphines, rise markedly in the blood. Biogenic amines have been shown to be involved not only in the homeostatic control of normal cells, but also in tumor cell proliferation; drugs which inhibit amine uptake into tumor cells have been shown to reduce the proliferation of these cells (46–48). It has been suggested that tumor cells must take up biogenic amines before the cells can be stimulated (46) and that these effects are caused *via* second messenger systems involving cAMP or cGMP (49–51). Steroids, such as corticosterone or cortisol, which are well known to suppress the immune system and tumor cell surveillance, interfere with intracellular receptors by binding to specific proteins in the cytosol and thereby inhibit the interaction of hormone receptor complexes with DNA; this can affect DNA synthesis and cell division (52, 53). Endorphins rise during stress and act at various receptors to affect functions of the central nervous system (54, 55), the immune system (56), and/or tumor cells where endorphin receptors have been shown to affect tumor growth and spread (57, 58). Thus, stress-induced changes in these and other stress hormones can affect carcinogenesis on many different levels.

(iii) Cellular receptors, including those directly affecting the function of DNA, can be changed during stress either directly or through an action of stress chemicals, leading to alteration in the number of and/or affinity to receptors, as well as to impaired repair mechanisms. This can lead to an increased or decreased chemical–receptor interaction or impaired or enhanced DNA synthesis or repair. All these effects can result in the modulation of carcinogenesis to different degrees. The high affinity of ethanol to the opioid receptor is markedly altered during stress (59). As expected, the monoamine oxidase (MAO) inhibitor phenelzine reduces markedly MAO activity in resting rats, but enzyme inhibition is considerably reduced in stressed rats (60). Neither stress nor carbon tetrachloride *alone* causes significant rise in glutamate transaminase activity in resting rats, but enzyme activity increases 12-fold in response to this chemical during and after stress (61). Animals housed under more or less stressful conditions change their serotonin receptor characteristics (62). Immobilization stress induced interleukin-1 beta mRNA selectively in the rat hypothalamus (63). Benzodiazepine receptor binding is changed in mice subjected to acute or chronic defeat stress (64).

Thus stress-induced changes in DNA-related enzyme systems affect the response of these systems to the effects of different toxins; analogously, it will increase or decrease their interactions with carcinogens and enhance or reduce carcinogenesis.

(iv) It is now well recognized that stress modulates the immune system in a variety of ways. There can be a direct effect, since the immune system and the brain form a feedback loop in which the immune system informs the brain about its status and in which the brain responds by affecting the immune system through nerve impulses or through chemical means (65–67). It has been shown that many neurotransmitter systems, such as the norepinephrine, dopamine, serotonin, and endorphine systems, change their activities during stress, resulting in modified mood states and altered messages to the immune system. In addition, the immune system can be affected indirectly through changes in peripheral stress chemicals, such as epinephrine or steroids. Brief exposure to electric shock or immobilization can initially increase and then decrease circulating leukocytes, in general, and lymphocytes, in particular (68, 69). A 1-hour foot shock to rats reduced T-lymphocyte proliferation by 74% and natural killer (NK) cell cytotoxicity by 59%; these effects were also seen in adrenalectomized animals, but were significantly blunted in animals pretreated with antibodies to the hypothalamic hormone, corticotropin-releasing factor (70); this hormone is the key mediator of the endocrine and probably the autonomic and visceral responses to stress. Immobilization decreased the number of T-lymphocytes and T-helper and T-suppressor cells in rats (71)). Immobilization and electric shock also decreased splenic NK cell activity (69, 72–74). Delayed-type hypersensitivity, phagocytosis, and NK cell activity were reduced in mice by foot shock (75). Macrophages obtained from stressed mice showed reduced phagocytic activity (76). Splenic mononuclear cells isolated from rats exposed to as little as 5 minutes of restraint or 2 minutes of foot shock showed significantly reduced responses (77). A pure social stress, such as separation of the infant from the mother, caused marked suppression of the mitogen-induced lymphocyte proliferation response in the offspring; the response was restored to normal after reunion with the mother (78). Using another pure psychological stressor, by placing the animal in an environment in which they had received aversive stimuli, markedly reduced mitogenic responsiveness (79). The response of the immune system seems to depend on the intensity of the stressor; mitogen response in the spleen showed a linear correlation with the duration of foot shock experienced (80), and rats exposed to a graded series of stressors showed effects on lymphocyte stimulation which were again proportional to the intensity of the stressor (81). Also, age will play a role in the response of the immune system to stress. Isolation stress reduced NK cell activity markedly in old, but only slightly in young rats (82). Response to a stressor also carries a significant genetic component. Mice of three different strains were exposed to the same stressor, but the strains responded quite differently in their decrease of NK cell cytotoxicity (83). Again, availability of coping responses can nullify the effects of an otherwise stressful situation; lymphocyte proliferation was suppressed in rats which were not allowed to cope, but remained normal in rats which were allowed to cope with an electric shock (84). Again, any change in the immune system, produced directly or indirectly during stress, could conceivably affect tumor cell surveillance and increase or decrease the emergence, growth, and spread of tumors.

(v) Stress can influence carcinogenesis by changing the lifestyle of a stressed individual. Stress has been implicated in the etiology of anxiety, depression, obesity, or drug abuse (85–87). Mice with high caloric intake had more spontaneous tumors than mice with low caloric intake, and 7,12-dimethylbenz[*a*]anthracene (DMBA)-induced tumors grew more rapidly in rats fed a diet high in fat as compared to animals on a low-fat diet (88–90). Depression in humans has been found to be associated with higher incidences of immune suppression and cancer (91–94). The abuse of tobacco or alcohol carries by itself a higher risk of cancer and can potentiate the action of carcinogenic chemicals as well (95, 96). Thus, stress can indirectly cause certain life changes which can enhance the formation, growth, and spread of tumor cells. In conclusion, stress can change many different aspects of the homeostasis of an organism and with it the response to carcinogens, drugs, and other xenobiotics.

V. STRESS AND CARCINOGENESIS IN ANIMALS

Whereas the carcinogenic effects of many chemicals in resting (nonstressed) animals have been widely investigated, the effects of stress on carcinogenesis have received comparatively very little attention. Nevertheless, the relatively few studies that have been carried out obtained results which definitively show that stress affects carcinogenesis significantly, although the exact nature of the interactions is still unknown. The data are often contradictory, but this is not surprising since different chemicals have been studied, different species and strains were employed, stress was induced by different means and to different degrees of intensity and duration, and the physical and environmental conditions in these experiments varied often markedly.

It is, moreover, abundantly established that different species and strains can show enormously different susceptibilities to the carcinogenic action of chemical agents. For example, Sprague–Dawley rats are much more susceptible than hooded Long–Evans rats to mammary tumor induction by DMBA (97–100). Chapter 12 in this volume discusses the nature of genetic susceptibility to carcinogenesis, which is the underlying basis of such differences. Thus, when comparing studies on the effect of stress on carcinogenesis in different species and strains, the stress effect must be regarded as being superimposed on the genetically determined effects.

It has been shown in various studies that stress promotes DMBA-induced tumor induction, progression, and spread. Female Fischer 344 rats receiving 15 mg DMBA by gastric intubation were kept at rest or were stressed by restraint 30 min a day for 18 weeks; stressed rats developed a higher incidence of mammary tumors (and earlier) than nonstressed rats (*e.g.*, 27% as compared to 12% at the 15th week). Tumor growth could be suppressed by the administration of naloxone, implicating a role of the stress-activated opioid system in accelerated tumor growth. From parallel experiments with naltrexone and measurement of hypothalamic endorphin levels, it was suggested that stress facilitates endorphin and prolactin release and that naltrexone antagonizes the effects of endorphin on mammary tumor induction (101). A single intubation of 15 mg DMBA to female F344 rats, stressed by restraint, developed tumors earlier (by about 12 weeks) and showed a 57% increase of tumor incidence compared to the rats which were not stressed; this increase of tumor incidence was related to the prolactin levels and the opioid system, since the latter could be blocked by naltrexone, which also reduced the tumor incidence by one half (102). In another investigation, rats receiving DMBA were housed under different social conditions: (a) in stable groups after weaning, (b) in isolation after weaning, and (c) in groups after weaning, but switched to isolation at the beginning of the experiment. Tumor mean weight at sacrifice in these groups of animals varied and was 4.7, 0.7, and 13.9 g, respectively (103). In studies with mice, implantation of DMBA pellets into the submandibular glands caused more rapid tumor growth and larger mammary tumors when the animals were stressed by a 3°C environment, as compared to room temperature; no difference in the time of onset of tumor development was noted, however (104).

Other studies indicate, in contrast, an enhancing effect of stress on resistance to carcinogenesis. DMBA was administered at five weekly doses to Sprague–Dawley rats and the animals were subjected to daily 3-hour sessions of restraint 5 days a week for 9 weeks beginning the day after the third dose; this stress regimen decreased mammary tumor incidence from 90 to 70% and tumor weight from an average of 6.0 to 2.7 g. One acute stress session has no effect (96). Measurement of striatal dopamine-stimulated adenylate cyclase in these animals showed that chronic stress increased enzyme activity, but no correlation was found between the activity of this enzyme and the tumor incidence (96). In another study, the inhibitory effects of stress on DMBA-induced mammary tumorigenesis was found to correlate with increased levels of estradiol and decreased levels of prolactin (97). DMBA was injected into caudal blood vessels of female Sprague–Dawley and Charles River CD rats three times and the animals were restrained for 5 or 10 hour daily; the stress delayed the time of emergence of the tumors and significantly reduced the final tumor incidence (105). Female Sprague–Dawley rats received 5 mg DMBA weekly for 5 weeks and were stressed by electroconvulsive shock, noise, immobilization, or foot shock; in all cases stress did not affect tumor incidence, but reduced significantly tumor weight (106). In the same investigation, chlorpromazine was found to inhibit the stress-induced reduction in tumor growth. Female Sprague–Dawley rats received three intubations of 5 mg DMBA and were stressed by electric shock for various durations; the tumor incidence was reduced in the animals stressed for 85 and 40 days but not in the animals stressed for only 25 days (107). Another study explored the effect of the timing of stress on its inhibition of DMBA-induced tumorigenesis; this study found that stress does not reduce the tumor incidence when applied either during the preinduction or in the induction periods, but reduces the tumor incidence only if applied after the induction period (108).

N-Methyl-N'-nitro-N-nitrosoguanidine induces gastric tumors, but susceptibility depends on the strain of rats used. After 52 weeks of exposure to the carcinogen in the drinking water, spontaneously hypertensive rats showed a significantly greater incidence and tumor multiplicity than Wistar Kyoto and Wistar rats. Hypertensive rats are supposed to be more stress sensitive and to show more autonomic hyperactivity. All tumors induced in the glandular stomach were adenocarcinomas and no differences were noted in the histopathology of these three strains (100).

N-Nitrosodiethylamine induces hyperplastic foci in liver and hepatocellular tumors (adenomas and carcinomas) when fed to mice, and simultaneous administration of a benzodiazepine tranquilizer promoted this tumorigenic process (109). Although different mechanisms could be involved in this facilitatory response, it can be argued that the tranquilizer reduced the stress in these animals and that the reduction of stress promoted tumor development.

3-Methylcholanthrene (3-MC) was given subcutaneously to female Simonsen rats at a single dose of 2 mg and the animals were housed in either a 2 or 25°C environment. Lower tumor incidence was seen in the cold-stressed animals, but latency period and survival rates were the same (110). A single injection of 0.25 mg MC was given to mice from different strains which were then exposed to crowded living conditions and electroshock; though both stressors affected body and adrenal weights, no difference was found between control and experimental groups in cancer incidence or time of tumor appearance (111).

Eugenol induces hepatic tumors, and the incidence of these tumors was found to be influenced by the mere positioning of the cages in a room; male mice housed in cages close to a source of "normal" noise had a greater number of tumor bearers than those housed in cages distant from the noise source (112). 2-Acetylaminofluorene induced neoplasms (reticulum cell sarcomas, lymphomas, adrenocortical adenomas, and lung alveolar cell tumors) in mice, beginning later in those animals that were housed higher in a cage rack as compared to those housed lower in the same rack (113). However, the induction of colorectal carcinomas in rats by dimethylhydrazine was not affected by the application of these mild stressors (114).

Thus, obvious stressors such as foot shock, immobilization, low ambient temperature—as well as less obvious stressors, such as different housing conditions—can indeed influence carcinogenesis. However, it is unknown why stress did sometimes enhance, but at other times attenuate, tumor induction. The reasons are probably the different, but highly individualized stress responses of the animals.

VI. EFFECT OF STRESS ON VIRALLY-INDUCED TUMORS AND ON TUMOR CELL GROWTH

Although not the focal point of this chapter, a substantial number of investigations explored the effects of stress on the "take" and growth of transplanted tumors and on the appearance of virally-induced tumors. These studies have the advantage that tumor development and growth can be controlled more precisely, and that tumor emergence is more reliable and occurs in a shorter span of time for most virally-induced tumors.

The stress of simple housing conditions was found to markedly enhance the growth of virally-induced mammary tumors in mice (115). Mice with transplanted Lewis lung carcinomas showed a higher incidence of spontaneous lung metastases if kept in a high-stress environment; transfer of mice from a low-stress environment to a higher stress environment enhanced lung metastasis (116). No difference in tumor growth was found after mammary tumor cell transplantation in male or female rats housed in a customary manner either individually or in groups; however, tumor growth was doubled in rats which had been initially housed in groups and then switched to isolation before the beginning of the experiment (117). Female mice carrying the Bittner oncogenic virus and housed under stressful conditions of isolation, crowding, and repeated handling showed an increased risk of developing mammary carcinomas (115). Isolation of mice led to a increase in survival of animals with tumor grafts (leukemia, melanoma), whereas the abrupt change in social conditions from group housing to isolation increased tumor weight (118). These findings were supported by other results showing that abrupt change in social conditions markedly reduces resistance to tumors (119). In contrast, mice reared in isolation and switched to social groups at the beginning of receiving implants of mammary-cell carcinoma cells showed reduced tumor growth (120). Mice receiving P815 mastocytoma cells *and* foot shock showed lower tumor rejection rates than did non-stressed controls (121). Fischer 344 rats injected with MADB-106 tumor cells and exposed to stress showed a substantial decrease in NK cell cytotoxicity and an increase in surface lung metastases (122). The antitumor action of *Corynebacterium parvum* against mastocytoma ascites cells was affected by housing and foot shock; the bacterium inhibited tumor growth in nonstressed and individually housed animals, but group housing and stress negated the antitumor action of this microorganism (123). In contrast, rats receiving implants of mammary adenocarcinoma cells and subjected to restraint stress showed increased tumor burden during the stress period, which was significantly reduced during the recovery period (124). Virus-induced tumors grew more slowly in animals receiving foot shock, but faster *after* the stress period (125). Rats inoculated with 256 Walker carcinoma cells, and stressed, showed enhanced tumor development, but significantly reduced metastasis (126). Chronic cold stress decreased L 1210 tumor count, but intermittent cold stress increased the magnitude of this variable (127).

The availability of coping strategies can affect these results. When rats were able to control or terminate an electric shock, they rejected the implanted tumors more readily than did the rats which received the same shocks, but could not terminate the stressor (119, 121).

VII. STRESS AND SPONTANEOUS TUMORS

The development of spontaneously occurring tumors is also influenced by stress. Mice living in isolation developed spontaneous mammary tumors earlier than did their littermates living in groups (128). The incidence of reticuloendothelial tumors was found to increase from 17 to 37% in animals housed from the bottom to the top of the same rack

(129). Mice housed in plastic cages showed more spontaneous tumors than those housed in stainless steel cages (130). Mild foot shock for 1 month followed by whole-body gamma irradiation lowered the cumulative prevalence of malignant tumors in male rats (testes and lungs), whereas the prevalence of malignant tumors in females was increased (mammaries, lungs, ovaries). Mild stress represented by light–dark shift changes had no significant effect on spontaneous tumor development in NB female rats, although a trend toward reduction was noted (131).

Since stress has an effect on spontaneous tumor development, it will affect not only the experimental, but also the control groups. Therefore, care must be exercised by housing all groups under very similar conditions.

VIII. TRAUMA

Trauma implies physical injury, but most probably consists of both the physical insult to bodily tissues and the physiological consequence of such damage. Thus, effects observed in carcinogenesis can be the result of either or of both.

Laparotomy, and fever induced by the prostaglandin (PGE2), were found to increase the levels of epinephrine and corticosterone, as well as that of interleukin 6 (132). Surgical stress and progressive tumor burden independently and codependently impaired NK cell activity (133). Partial hepatectomy enhanced liver carcinogenesis, perhaps due to increased cell proliferation (134, 135). However, partial hepatectomy performed 10 weeks prior to carcinogen administration still enhanced tumorigenesis following exposure to nitrosodiethylamine (136). The chemical SQ18506 was more hepatocarcinogenic in female mice with hepatic hyperplasia induced by deposition of schistosome eggs in the liver and enhanced by administration of hycanthone (137). Partial hepatectomy reduced the toxicity of benzene, probably by decreasing hepatic metabolism of benzene to toxic metabolites (138). Pancreatic tumorigenesis by azaserine was enhanced in rats which were submitted to partial pancreatectomy (139). Chickens injected with Rous sarcoma virus developed primary tumors, and wounding the animals gave rise to secondary tumors at the site of the injury (140). Rats with undamaged or damaged nasal mucosa were exposed to formaldehyde; after 28 weeks, nasal squamous cell carcinomas were found in rats with wounded, but not with intact nasal mucosa (141). In contrast, hamsters subjected to oral DMBA, followed by incisions and manipulations of the buccal carcinomas, showed no different tumor growth as compared to controls (142). Surgical stress in rats did not significantly affect the growth or rejection time of sarcomas (143). In humans, NK cell cytotoxicity was significantly decreased postoperatively, perhaps caused by a direct "toxic" effect on these cells (144). Patients undergoing total gastrectomy or esophageal resection showed significantly depressed T-helper and NK cell activity 1 day after surgery (145).

Again, these data point out that animals or humans subjected to trauma can be expected to be at special risk to carcinogenic substances or viruses during and after the period of injury.

IX. STRESS, IMMUNITY, AND CARCINOGENESIS IN HUMANS

Although no formal epidemiological or case studies have been carried out in humans, it is now generally accepted that a definitive relationship exists between certain mood states including stress, the functioning of the immune system, and the occurrence of cancer.

Individuals experiencing a major life crisis with signs of depression showed reduced lymphocyte numbers (146). Individuals who cared for terminally ill patients and were chronically stressed showed reduced numbers of T-lymphocytes, T-helper cells, and T-suppressor cells (147). Examination stress reduced interferon production and NK cell activity in medical students; the effect on NK cells was more pronounced in those individuals who reported higher levels of distress (148, 149). Healthy women were divided according to exposure to "life stresses" and challenged with an antigen; women with higher levels of distress had lower baselines and 3-week post-immunization immunoglobulin levels than did women with lower levels of stress (150). Immunosuppressive effects were most frequently found in individuals who felt overwhelmed by psychosocial events, were lonely and helpless, and lacked proper social support (151). The effects of stress on the immune system may be modified by age. Exposure of younger and older individuals to a brief psychological stressor showed that younger individuals increase their immune response; this was not observed in the older individuals (152). This would suggest that the redundancy and "reserve" of the immune system decreases with age. Like in animal studies, controllability of the stressor is extremely important. Subjects were exposed to a mild shock and noise which they could control or not control; subjects who could not control the challenge showed more deterioration of immune functions than did individuals who could cope with the situation (153).

Similarly, the impact of stress on the emergence, growth, and spread of cancer in humans is well established, although definite relationships have not been identified. Women with metastatic breast cancer were assigned to a social support group to buffer the stress of the illness or left to routine medical care only; patients in the support group had a mean survival time of 37 months, whereas the mean survival time of the other group was 19 months (154, 155). Patients with leukemia and lymphoma survived longer if assigned to home-based intervention and special educational programs (156). Workers chronically exposed to asbestos and high stress levels showed a higher incidence of smoking and an increased risk of developing lung cancer (157) (although the increased risk could also be ascribed to the synergism between asbestos and tobacco chemicals). This shows that stress can affect the immune system directly, but *also* indirectly, in that stress might cause the individual to smoke or use drugs and alcohol, which would then, in turn, affect cancer development (55, 94). However, the absence of effects between stress and cancer has also been reported (158, 159).

Thus, stress can affect individuals very differently, and this probably contributes to the wide variations seen in humans who are occupationally or environmentally exposed to chemical carcinogens.

X. CLOSING NOTE

Stress is a highly individualized reaction in response to exogenous or endogenous stimuli. We all experience stress, depending on our genetic and experiential backgrounds. It is *the response* which determines if a stimulus is a stressor. Stress causes a variety of significant biochemical and physiological changes in the brain and body, which could give rise to stress-related diseases, if the individual has certain organ vulnerabilities. The stress-related mood changes, most notably anxiety, tension, and fear, can drastically alter many biochemical and physiological aspects of the organism, including the response to and action of chemicals with carcinogenic potential. These changes can alter the toxicokinetics and toxicodynamics of these chemicals in that their toxic actions can be enhanced or attenuated, and evidence is available which demonstrates that, indeed, stress can markedly affect carcinogenesis.

If animal studies are conducted to assess the carcinogenic potential of chemical compounds, stress should not be neglected or omitted as a confounding variable. Stress is an important parameter that must be considered when designing studies for testing the carcinogenic potential of the compounds themselves, in view of extrapolation of the significance of animal data to humans. Consider that stress has an ever-increasing presence in the lives of human societies.

The inclusion of stress factors in the design of animal bioassay studies would not only contribute to the justification of extrapolation from animal data to humans, but such studies might also be useful in identifying certain personality types which are at higher risk to chemically induced carcinogenesis. Moreover, a better understanding of the basic mechanisms of the stress response and its interaction with the biological effect of carcinogens might provide important additional clues on the detailed mechanisms which underlie chemically induced carcinogenesis.

REFERENCES

1. Abelson, P. H.: *Science* **255**, 141 (1992)
2. Henderson, B. E.: *Science* **254**, 1131 (1991)
3. Ross, K., and Pike, M. C.: *Science* **254**, 141 (1991)
4. Rossi, J. S.: *Science* **254**, 501 (1991)
5. Fry, R. J. M., and Staffeldt, E., *J. Natl. Cancer Inst.* **51**, 1349 (1973)
6. Clough, G.: *Neurobiol. Aging* **12**, 653 (1991)
7. Vogel, W. H.: *Trends Pharmacol. Sci.* **8**, 35 (1987)
8. Cannon, W. B., and de la Paz, D.: *Am. J. Physiol.* **28**, 64 (1911)
9. Fortier, C., Yrarrazaval, S., and Selye, H.: *Am. J. Physiol.* **165**, 466 (1951)
10. Schuckil, M. A.: *J. Clin. Physiol.* **44**, 31 (1983)
11. Chrousos, G. P., and Gold, P. W.: *JAMA* **267**, 1244 (1992)
12. Lazarus, R. S., and DeLongis, A.: *Am. Psychol.*, March issue, p. 245, 1983.
13. Vogel, W. H.: *Neuropsychobiology* **13**, 129 (1985)
14. Rutter, M.: *Am. J. Psychiatry* **143**, 1077 (1986)
15. Weiss, J. M., Stone, E. A., and Harrel, N.: *J. Comp. Physiol.* **72**, 153 (1970)
16. Swenson, R. M., and Vogel, W. H.: *Biochem. Pharmacol. Behav.* **18**, 689 (1983)
17. Quirce, C. M., and Maickel, R. P.: *Psychoneuroendocrinology* **6**, 91 (1981)
18. Vogel, W. H., and Jensh, R.: *Neurosciences* **87**, 183 (1988)
19. Tapp, W. N., and Natelson, B. H.: *FASEB J.* **2**, 2268 (1988)
20. Taylor, J., Weyers, P., Harris, N., and Vogel, W. H.: *Physiol. Behav.* **46**, 853 (1989)
21. Vogel, W. H., Harris, N., and Taylor, J.: *NIDA Res. Monogr.* **20**, 103 (1990)
22. Antelman, S. M., DeGiovanni, L. A., and Kocan, D.: *Life Sci.* **44**, 210 (1989)
23. Pohorecky, L. A., Roberts, P., Colter, S., and Carbone, J. J.: *Pharmacol. Biochem. Behav.* **33**, 55 (1988)
24. Popper, L. W., Chiueh, C. C., and Kopin, I. J.: *J. Pharmacol. Exp. Therap.* **202**, 144 (1977)
25. DeTurck, K. H., and Vogel, W. H.: *Pharmacol. Biochem. Behav.* **13**, 129 (1980)
26. Pashko, S., DeTurck, K. H., and Vogel, W. H.: *Pharmacol. Biochem. Behav.* **13**, 471 (1980)
27. DeTurck, K. H., and Vogel, W. H.: *J. Pharmacol Exp. Therap.* **233**, 348 (1982)
28. Weiss, J. M.: *Brain Res. Rev.* **3**, 167 (1981)
29. Feurer, G.: *J. Physiol.* **169**, 43 (1963)
30. Natelson, B. H., Tapp, W. M., Mittler, J. E., and Levin, E. B.: *Physiol. Behav.* **29**, 1049 (1981)
31. Abel, E. L.: *Physiol. Behav.* **50**, 151 (1991)
32. Conahan, S. T., Narayan, S., and Vogel, W. H.: *Pharmacol. Biochem. Behav.* **23**, 147 (1985)
33. Milakofsky, L., Hare, T., Miller, J., and Vogel, W. H.: *Life Sci.* **36**, 753 (1984)
34. Hershock, D., and Vogel W. H.: *Life Sci.* **45**, 157 (1989)
35. Graffy-Sparrow, S. M., Roggendorf, H., and Vogel, W. H.: *Life Sci.* **50**, 2551 (1987)
36. Conahan, S. T., and Vogel, W. H.: *Res. Commun. Chem. Pathol. Pharmacol.* **53**, 301 (1986)
37. Taylor, J., Harris, N., Krieman, M., and Vogel, W. H.: *Biochem. Behav.* **34**, 349 (1989)
38. Brady, J. V.: *Sci. Am.* **199**, 95 (1958)
39. Selye, H.: "Stress". Acta Medica Publ., Montreal (Quebec), 1950.
40. Wise, R. A.: *Brain Res.* **152**, 215 (1978)

41. Wise, R. A., *Behav. Brain Res.* **8,** 178 (1985)
42. Pashko, S., and Vogel, W. H.: *Biochem. Pharmacol.* **29,** 22 (1980)
43. Motoo, Y., Yutaka, G., and Ryozo, O.: *Life Sci.* **48,** 2065 (1991)
44. Ehrich, M., and Gross, B.: *Toxicol. Appl. Pharmacol.* **70,** 249 (1983)
45. Carlson, J. N., and Rossellini, R. A.: *Psychopharmacology* **91,** 122 (1987)
46. Kristoffer, H., Svante, H., and Orjans, K: *J. Immunol.* **134,** 409 (1985)
47. Tutton, P. J. M. and Barkla, D. H.: *Anticancer Res.* **7,** 1 (1987)
48. Nieman, D. C., Berk, L. S., Simpson-Westerberg, M., Arabatzis, K., Youngberg, S., Tan, S. A. and Eby, W. C.: *Int. J. Sports Med.* **10,** 317 (1989)
49. Rebhun, L. I: *Int. J. Cytol.* **9,** 1 (1977)
50. Plotnikoff, N., Murgo, A., Faith, R., and Wybran, J., eds: "Stress and Immunity". CRC Press, Boca Raton, Florida, 1991.
51. Felten, D. L., Ackerman, K. D., Weigand, S. J., and Felten, S. Y.: *J. Neurosci. Res.* **18,** 28 (1987)
52. Felten, D. L. Felten, S. Y., Bellinger, D. L., Carlson, S. L., Ackerman, K. D., Madden, K. S., Olschowki, T. A., and Livnat, S.: *Immunol. Res.* **100,** 235 (1987)
53. Pratt, W. B.: *J. Cell Biochem.* **35,** 51 (1987)
54. Landman, M. A., Buergisser, E., Wesp, M., and Buehler, F. R.: *J. Recept. Res.* **4,** 47 (1984)
55. Koff, W. C., and Dunegan, M. A.: *J. Immunol.* **125,** 350 (1985)
56. Dinarello, C. A., and Mier, J. W.: *Annu. Rev. Med.* **37,** 137 (1986)
57. Godowski, P. J., Picard, D., and Yamamoto, K. R.: *Science* **241,** 812 (1988)
58. Plotnikoff, N. P., Faith, R. E., Murgo, A. J., and Good, R. A., eds: "Enkephalins and Endorphins". Plenum Press, New York, 1986.
59. Przewlocka, B., and Wladyslaw, L.: *Pol. J. Pharmacol.* **42,** 137 (1990)
60. Clow, A., Glover, V., Oxenkrug, G. F., and Sandler, M.: *Neurosci. Lett.* **107,** 331 (1989)
61. Iwai, M., Saheki, S., Ohta, Y., and Shimazu, T.; *Biomed. Res.* **7,** 145 (1986)
62. Essman, E. J., and Valzelli, P. G.: *Pharmacol. Res. Commun.* **16,** 401 (1984)
63. Kuraishi, Y., Yamaguchi, J., Nakai, S., Hirai, Y., and Sotoh, M.: *Neurosci. Lett.* **123,** 254 (1991)
64. Barnhill, J. G., Miller, J., Greenblat, D. J., Thompson, M. L., Ciraulo, D. A., and Shader, R. I.: *Pharmacology* **42,** 181 (1991)
65. Besedovski, H., and Sorkin, E.: *Clin. Exp. Immunol.* **26,** 1 (1977)
66. Dunn, A. J.: *J. Recept. Res.* **8,** 589 (1988)
67. Besedovski, H., DelReye, A., Sorkin, E., DaPrada, M., and Levin, T. A.: *Science* **221,** 564 (1983)
68. Vogel, W. H., and Bower, D.: *Abstr. Soc. Neurosci.* **12,** 171 (1986)
69. Steplewski, Z., Vogel, W. H., Ehya, H., Porvpatich, C., and McDonald-Smith, J.: *Cancer Rev.* **45,** 5128 (1985)
70. Jain, R., Zwickler, D., Hollander, C. S., Brand, H., Saperstein, A., Hutchinson, B., Brown, C., and Aduhya T.: *Endocrinology* **128,** 1329 (1991)
71. Keller, T., and Stromberg, G. T.: *Proc. Natl. Acad. Sci. U.S.A.* **46,** 17 (1988)
72. Morley, J. E., Key, N. E., Solomon, G. F., and Plotnikoff, N. P.: *Life Sci.* **41,** 5278 (1987)
73. Shavit, Y., Lewis, J. W., and Terman, G. W.: *Science* **223,** 188 (1984)
74. Odio, T., and Maickel, R.: *Immunol. Lett.* **13,** 25 (1986)
75. Esterling, B., and Rabin, B. S.: *Behav. Neurosci.* **101,** 115 (1987)
76. Schultz, R. M., Shirigos, M. A., Stoychkov, J. N., and Pavlidis, N. A.: *J. Reticuloendoth. Soc.* **26,** 83 (1987)
77. Halper, J. P., Miller, A. H., and Trestman, R. L.: *J. Neuroimmunol.* **32,** 241 (1991)
78. Laudenslager, M. L., Reite, M., and Harbeck, R. J.: *Behav. Neur. Biol.* **36,** 40 (1982)
79. Lysle, D. T., Cunnick, J. E., Fowler, H., and Rabin, B.: *Life Sci.* **42,** 2185 (1988)
80. Lysle, D. T., Lyte, M., Fowler, H., and Rabin, B.: *Life Sci.* **41,** 1805 (1987)
81. Keller, S. E.: *Science* **213,** 1397 (1981)
82. Ghonuem, M., Gill, G., Assanah, P., and Stevens, W.: *Immunology* **60,** 461 (1987)
83. Zalcman, S., Irwin, J., and Anisman, H.: *Pharmacol. Biochem. Behav.* **39,** 361 (1991)
84. Laudenslager, M. L., Ryan, S., Drugan, R. C., Hyson, R. I., and Maier, S. F.: *Science* **221,** 568 (1983)
85. Doll, R., and Peto, R.: *J. Natl. Cancer Inst.* **66,** 1191 (1981)
86. O'Doherty, F.: *Drug Alcohol. Dep.* **29,** 97 (1991)
87. Dohrenwend, B. P., Levav, I., Shrout, P. E., Schwartz, S., Neveh, G., Link, B. G., Skodol, A. E., and Stueve, A.: *Science* **225,** 946 (1992)
88. McCay, P. B., King, M., Rikous, L. E., and Pitha, J. V.: *J. Environ. Pathol. Toxicol.* **3,** 451 (1981)
89. National Research Council, Committee on Diet, Nutrition and Cancer. *In* "Diet, Nutrition, and Cancer": Lipids (Fat and Cholesterol). National Academy Press, Washington, D.C., 1982, p. 73.
90. Tannebaum, A.: *Cancer Res.* **5,** 609 (1945)
91. Whitlock, F. A., and Siskind, M.: *Psychol. Med.* **9,** 747 (1979)

92. Schmale, A. H. and Ker, H. P. J.: *Psychosom. Med.* **28,** 714 (1966)
93. Shekelle, R. B., Raynor, W. J., Ostfeld, A. M., Garron, D. C., Shuguey, C. L., Maliza, C., and Ogelsby, P.: *Psychosom. Med.* **43,** 117 (1981)
94. Rogers, M., Dubey, D., and Reich, P.: *Psychosom. Med.* **41,** 147 (1979)
95. Tuyns, A. J.: *Int. J. Cancer* **5,** 152 (1970)
96. Department of Health, Education and Welfare: "Smoking and Health". Washington, D.C., 1964, p. 57.
97. Goldman, P. R., and Vogel, W. H.: *Cancer Lett.* **25,** 227 (1985)
98. Boyland, E., and Sydnor, K. L.: *Br. J. Cancer* **16,** 731 (1962)
99. Masahura, T., Hiroyasu, I., Mityako, B., and Haruo, M.: *Cancer Res.* **49,** 794 (1989)
100. Pradhan, S. N., and Prabhati, R.: *J. Natl. Cancer Inst.* **53,** 1241 (1974)
101. Tejwani, G. A., Gudchithlu, K. P., Hanissian, S. H., Gienapp, L. E., Whitacre, C. C., and Malarkey, W. B.: *Carcinogenesis* **12,** 637 (1991)
102. Berger, W. C.: *Adv. Biosci.* **75,** 615 (1989)
103. Goldman, P. R., and Vogel, W. H.: *Carcinogenesis* **5,** 971 (1984)
104. Turbiner, S.: *Oral Surg. Oral Med. Oral Pathol.* **29,** 130 (1970)
105. Newberry, B. H., Gildow, J., Wogan, J., and Reese, R. L.: *Psychosom. Med.* **38,** 155 (1976)
106. Sydnov, K. L., Butenandt, O., Brillantes, F. P., and Huggins, C.: *J. Natl. Cancer Inst.* **29,** 805 (1962)
107. Newberry, B. H., Frankie, G., Beatty, P. A., Maloney, B. D. and Gildchrist, J. C.: *Psychosom. Med.* **37,** 295 (1972)
108. Newberry, B. H.: *J. Natl. Cancer Inst.* **61,** 725 (1978)
109. Bhalchandra, D., Rice, J. M., and Ward, J. M.: *Carcinogenesis* **7,** 789 (1986)
110. Baker, D. G.: *Cancer Res.* **37,** 3939 (1977)
111. Weber, R.: *J. Natl. Cancer Inst.* **41,** 967 (1968)
112. Young, S. S.: *Fundam. Appl. Toxicol.* **8,** 1 (1987)
113. Greenman, M., Kodell, R. L., and Sheldon, N. G.: *J. Natl. Cancer Inst.* **73,** 107 (1984)
114. Andrianopoulos, G. D., Nelson, R. L., Barch, D. H., Bombeck, C. T., and Nyhus, L. M.: *Cancer Detect. Prevent.* **15,** 557 (1990)
115. Riley, V.: *Science* **185,** 465 (1975)
116. Giraldi, T.: *Eur. J. Cancer Clin. Oncol.* **25,** 1583 (1989)
117. Steplewski, Z., Goldman, P. R., and Vogel, W. H.: *Cancer Lett.* **34,** 257 (1987)
118. Dechambre, R. P., and Gosse, C.: *Cancer Res.* **33,** 140 (1973)
119. Sklar, L. S., and Anisman, H.: *Science* **205,** 513 (1979)
120. Emmerman, J. T., and Weinberg, J.: "Molecular Biology of Stress". Liss, New York, 1989, p. 295.
121. Visintainer, M. A., Volpicelli, J. R., and Seligman, M. P.: *Science* **216,** 437 (1982)
122. Ben-Eliyahu, S., Yirmiya, R., Liebeskind, J. C., Taylor, A. N., and Gale, R. P.: *Brain Behav. Immun.* **5,** 193 (1991)
123. Turney, T. H., Harmsen, A. G., and Jarpe, M. A.: *Phys. Behav.* **37,** 555 (1986)
124. Vogel, W. H., and Steplewski, Z.: *Neurosci. Lett.* **62,** 277 (1985)
125. Amkraut, A., and Solomon, G. F.:*Cancer Res.* **32,** 1428 (1972)
126. Zimel, H.: *Neoplasma* **24,** 151 (1975)
127. Lahiri, T., and Dilip, R.: *Indian J. Exp. Biol.* **25,** 285 (1987)
128. Andervont, H. B.: *J. Natl. Cancer Inst.* **4,** 579 (1944)
129. Lagakos, S., and Mosteller, F.: *J. Natl. Cancer Inst.* **66,** 197 (1981)
130. Finkel, S., and Scribner, T.: *Br. J. Cancer* **9,** 464 (1955)
131. Kort, W. J.: *J. Natl. Cancer Inst.* **76,** 439 (1986)
132. vanGool, J., Van Vugt, H., Helle, M. and Aarden, L. A.: *Clin. Immunol. Immunopathol.* **57,** 200 (1990)
133. Pollack, E. R., Bobcock, G. F., Romsdahl, M. M., and Nishioka, K.: *Cancer Res.* **44,** 3888 (1984)
134. Hollander, C. F., and Bentvelzen, P.: *J. Natl. Cancer Inst.* **41,** 1303 (1968)
135. Brady, J.: *Cancer Res.* **20,** 1469 (1960)
136. Bartsch, H., Preat, V., Aito, A., Cabral, J. R. P., and Roberfroid, M.: *Carcinogenesis* **9,** 2315 (1988)
137. Haese, W. H., Smith, D. L., and Bueding, E.: *J. Pharmacol. Exp. Therap.* **186,** 430 (1973)
138. Lee, E. W., Kocsis, J. J., and Snyder, R.: *J. Toxicol. Environ. Health* **5,** 785 (1979)
139. Denda, A., Inui, S., Sunagawa, M., Takahasi, S., and Konishi, Y.: *Gann* **69,** 633 (1978)
140. Sieweke, M. H., Stoker, A. W., and Bissell, M. J.: *Cancer Res.* **49,** 6419 (1989)
141. Wourtersen, R. A., van Garderen-Hoetmer, T., Bruijntjes, J. P., Zwart, A., and Ferron, V. J.: *J. Appl. Toxicol.* **9,** 39 (1989)
142. Shklar, G.: *Cancer Res.* **28,** 2180 (1968)
143. Radosevic-Stasic, B.: *Anesth. Analg.* **69,** 570 (1989)
144. Pollock, R. E., Lotzovia, E., and Stanford, S. D.: *Arch. Surg.* **126,** 338 (1991)
145. Toge, T., Kegoya, Y., Yamaguchi, Y., Baba, N., Kunisnobu, H., Takayama, T., Yanagawa, E., and Hattori, T.: *Gan to Kaz Ryo* **16,** 115 (1989)

146. Willis, L., Thomas, P., and Garry, P. J.: *Gerontol. J.* **42**, 627 (1987)
147. Glaser, R., Shuttleworth, E. G., Dyer, C. S., Rocki, P., and Speiolo, L. E.: *Psychosom. Med.* **49**, 523 (1987)
148. Glaser, R., Rice, J., Speicher, C. E., Stout, J. C., and Kilcolt-Glaser, J. K.: *Behav. Neurosci.* **100**, 675 (1986)
149. Kilcolt-Glaser, J. K., Garner, W., Speicher, C., Penn, G. M., Holliday, J., and Glaser, R.: *Psychosom. Med.* **46**, 7 (1984)
150. Snyder, B. K., Roghmann, K. J., and Sigal, L. H.: *J. Adolesc. Health Care* **11**, 472 (1990)
151. Bergler, R., and Zipperling, C.: *Zentralbl. Hyg. Umweltmed.* **191**, 241 (1991)
152. Naliboff, B. D., Benton, D., Solomon, G. F., Morely, J. E., Fahey, J. L., and Coon, T. L.: *Psychosom. Med.* **53**, 121 (1991)
153. Weisse, C. S., Pato, C. N., McAllister, C. G., Littman, R., Breier, A., Paul, S. M., and Baum, A.: *Brain Behav. Immun.* **4**, 330 (1991)
154. Spiegel, D., and Bloom, J. R.: *Lancet* **II**, 1447 (1989)
155. Spiegel, D.: *J. Natl. Inst. Health* **3**, 61 (1991)
156. Shelton, D. R., Kailo, M., and Levine, A. M.: *J. Clin. Oncol.* **8**, 35 (1990)
157. Lebovits, A. H., Byrne, M., Bernstein, J., and Strain, J. J.: *J. Occup. Med.* **30**, 49 (1988)
158. Morgenstern, H., Gillert, G. A., Walter, S. D., Ostfeld, A. M., and Siegel, B. S.: *J. Chron. Dis.* **37**, 273 (1984)
159. Fox, B.: *J. Psychosoc. Oncol.* **1**, 17 (1983)

EDITORS' NOTE ADDED IN PROOF

Stress Proteins:
Heat-Shock Proteins/Molecular Chaperones

Investigations in the last few years led to the discovery of stress proteins and their catalytic roles in the folding of nascent proteins, as well as in the maintenance of/refolding native functional protein conformations in the face of stress-related insult. Insult to the cell environment activates a set of genes which express proteins that can repair stress-induced molecular damage to proteins and reestablish normal homeostasis. The standardized form of stress that has been used in studies with prokaryotic and eukaryotic cell cultures is exposure to unusually elevated temperatures (*e.g.,* 42°C). This evokes a heat-shock response by inducing the dramatically enhanced expression of *heat-shock-proteins* (Hsp) to stabilize and reestablish partially denatured protein conformations. Under normal conditions Hsp's are expressed at relatively low levels.

The Hsp's are key components of the system of *molecular chaperones,* which are a diverse group of proteins that mediate the folding of polypeptide chains, the assembly of protein modules, protein transport, and the establishment of the respective final tertiary structures of nascent proteins — but without becoming themselves components of these structures. Nascent protein backbones fold at first spontaneously into a conformation which already contains correctly folded secondary structure elements (α-helices and β-chains), but which is still flexible and can assume various tertiary structures. This flexible, "open" conformation is termed the *molten globule* intermediate [K. Kuwajima: *Proteins* **6**, 87 (1989)]. The role of molecular chaperones appears to start from this stage on to rapidly guide the folding process to the correct, native tertiary conformation [J. Martin *et al.*: *Nature* **352**, 36 (1991)]. This is thought to be accomplished by noncovalent (mainly hydrophobic bonding) interactions with transiently exposed surfaces of the protein molecule during nascent synthesis, folding, and oligomerization. The net effect of chaperone participation in these processes is a reduction of inappropriate protein-protein interactions that may produce a nonfunctional protein structure. Consistent with these compartmentalized roles, different chaperones may function along a protein maturation pathway (StressGen Biotechnologies, Victoria, BC, *1994 Product Specifications Newsletter*). The serial interactions of molecular chaperones with nascent proteins have been likened to a "protein massage". Since "protein massage" is an energy-requiring process, chaperones have ATPase activity that provides the energy support for the binding-release cycles (B. Alberts *et al.*: "Molecular Biology of the Cell," 3rd ed. Garland, New York, 1994, p.214). Considerable advances have been made in very recent years on major Hsp's as molecular chaperones [*e.g., revs.* C. Georgopoulos and W. J. Welch: *Annu. Rev. Cell Biol.* **9**, 601 (1993); R. J. Ellis, R. A. Laskey, and H. Lorimer: "Molecular Chaperones". Chapman & Hall, New York, 1994; R. I. Morimoto, A. Tissieres, and C. Georgopoulos: "The Biology of Heat-Shock Proteins and Molecular Chaperones", Monograph 26. Cold Spring Harbor Laboratory Press, Cold Spring Harbor, New York, 1994]. Originally identified as stress-inducible proteins, many chaperones are essential for cell viability.

Many stress proteins have been identified as being molecular chaperones and these include the major Hsp families: Hsp 60 (60 kDa),Hsp 70 (70 kDa), Hsp 90 (90 kDa), and the "small heat-shock protein" (sHsp) family (a diverse group of proteins ranging from 15 to 30 kDa, *e.g.,* sHsp 25, sHsp 27, sHsp 30). Eukaryotes as well as prokaryotes have their specific Hsp's; in fact, molecular chaperones were first identified in *E. coli*. Moreover, different Hsp's function in different compartments in the cell. A subset of molecular chaperones, refered to as "chaperonins" (cpn's), are present in all bacteria, in mitochondria, and in plastids; for example, GroEL (cpn 60) is the *E. coli* homolog of Hsp 60 and DnaK (cpn 70) is the homolog of Hsp 70 (StressGen., *loc. cit.*). Studies with DnaK mutants, such as delta DnaK 52, suggest that the most significant physiological function of DnaK in the metabolism of unstressed *E. coli* cells is their role in the regulation of Hsp genes [B. Bukau and G. C. Walker: *EMBO J.* **9**, 4027 (1990)]. The cytosolic chaperonins belong to the Hsp 70 family; Hsp 70 ensures the correct folding of cytosolic proteins, and Hsp 60 and Hsp 70 ensure the translocation of proteins through the membranes of mitochondria and the endoplasmic reticulum [Alberts *et al., loc. cit.* pp. 571, 572; W. T. Wickner: *Science* **266**, 1197, 1250 (1994)]. Many chaperones are highly immunogenic; some have been implicated as key antigens in microbial infection and in autoimmune diseases [StressGen, *loc.cit.*; S.J. Thompson *et al.*: *Autoimmunity* **11**, 35 (1991)].

The Hsp 70-type chaperones act early in the life span of a protein; they bind to a sequence of about seven amino acids (a critical hydrophobic set) before the nascent polypeptide leaves the ribosome (Alberts *et al., loc. cit.*, p. 214). Constitutively synthesized, moderately stress-inducible members of the Hsp 70 family include: Hsc 70 in the cytosol and the nucleus, BiP ('binding protein", also known as Grp 78) in the endoplasmic reticulum lumen, and Grp 75 in the mitochondrial matrix. The most strictly stress-inducible member of the family, Hsp 70 itself—present in the cytosol and the nucleus—is usually not detectable under normal conditions (except in primates) and is therefore regarded as a diagnostic marker of stress (StressGen, *loc. cit.*). Thus, even within the Hsp 70 family, different members are distinctly localized in various cell compartments. Hsp 70-type proteins are thought to perform the chaperone-like protein folding and assisting functions most typically by cyclic transient interactions with hydrophobic polypeptide surfaces (the "protein massage" referred to above).

Molecules of Hsp 60-type chaperones consist of two stacked "doughnut-like" rings, each composed of seven identical subunits. This large barrel-shaped structure acts on protein folding following the action of Hsp 70. The incompletely folded or misfolded protein is fed into the cavity of Hsp 60. While the mechanism of Hsp 60 action is not clearly understood, the ATP-driven high energy cavity is thought to provide the low entropy environment that can maximize the refolding of the protein. An alternate possibilty is that nascent and incompletely-folded proteins are vulnerable to ubiquitin-tagging-dependent proteolysis which competes with the folding process; enclosure of the nascent protein within the Hsp 60 provides temporary protection against being targeted for proteolysis.

Hsp 90 has been shown to fold inactive basic helix-loop-helix (bH-L-H) proteins (from *E. coli*) into their active conformations. A 48-amino-acid region of Hsp 90 confers the bH-L-H folding activity upon Hsp 90. This region is required for the activation of DNA binding of homodimers and heterodimers formed between two bH-L-H proteins, MyoD and E12 [G. Shue and D. S. Kohtz: *J. Biol. Chem.* **269**, 27707 (1994)].

The sHsp's are probably the most strongly stress-inducible among the chaperones. A key feature of sHsp's is their rapid and pronounced phosphorylation not only following stress but also following exposure to a variety of stimuli such as steroid hormones, tumor promoters, mitogens, calcium ionophores, and during cell differentiation and development. In lower eukaryotes multiple sHsp genes exist, but higher eukaryotes (mammals) generally contain only a single gene type. Following stress, the sHsp's, like other cytoplasmic stress proteins, display redistribution of intracellular localization, a portion localizing in the nucleus. The chaperone activities of the sHsp's have been implicated in the regulation of actin cytoskeleton organization (StressGen, *loc. cit.*).

An intriguing question concerns the mechanism by which the protein folding machinery is regulated. For example, it is known that the synthesis of BiP (Grp 78) is strongly induced by the level of unfolded/misfolded proteins in the endoplasmic reticulum. But how the levels of unfolded/misfolded molecules are monitored, and how this information is used to regulate the level BiP synthesis, is not known [R. W. Doms *et al.*: *Virology* **133**, 545 (1993)]. A partial answer may be provided by investigations showing that agents which mobilize sequestered intracellular Ca^{2+} disrupt early processing in the endoplasmic reticulum, inhibit translation initiation,, and trigger the induction of *Grp 78* (BiP). In the intact pituitary cell lines (GH3), used in these studies referenced below, this was accompanied by a 5-fold increase in the phosphorylation of elF-2α and a 50% reduction of elF-2B activity, two translation initiation factors. With continued exposure to the ionophore used, the rates of amino acid incorporation partially recovered, elF-2α became dephosphorylated and the inhibition of elF-2B activity was abolished. The observation may represent the manifestations of a signaling system of the endoplasmic reticulum through the alteration of elF-2 activity via regulation of the CA^{2+} level [Prostko *et al.*: *J. Biol. Chem.* **267**, 16751 (1992)].

By far, most investigations to date on heat-shock proteins/chaperones have been carried out in prokaryotic systems, often aiming at insights into the mechanism of microbial pathogenesis. Studies more directly relevant to the mechanism of carcinogenesis are scant.

The tumor promoters, 12-*O*-tetradecanoylphorbol-13-acetate (TPA) and okadaic acid, were found to strongly induce the phosphorylation of various Hsp's in BALB/3T3 and BALB/MK-2 cell lines; however, the human tumor necrosis factor alpha (TNF-α) is about 1000-fold more effective in BALB/3T3 cells than the promoters [A. Komori *et al.*: *Cancer Res.* **53**, 1982 (1993); A. Kasahara *et al.*: *Europ. J. Biochem.* **213**, 1101 (1993)]. The level of phosphorylation was promoter-dose dependent. The results suggest that chemical tumor promoters act via induction of the secretion of TNF-α which then acts as an endogenous tumor promoter (Komori *et al., loc. cit.*).

HeLa cells possess a cytosolic/nuclear tumor-promoter-specific binding protein (CN-TPBP), a 66–68 kDa protein which lacks protein kinase C activity. Following treatment with TPA, CN-TPBP translocates into the nucleus. CN-TPBP, which forms a complex with Hsp 90, has the characteristics of the nuclear receptors for glucocorticoids and 2,3,7,8-tetrachlorodibenzo-*p*-dioxin. The findings suggest that CN-TPBP acts as a nuclear receptor for tumor promoters which exert their biological effects through this receptor [J. Hashimoto and K. Shudo: *Jpn. J. Cancer Res.* **82,** 665 (1991)].

Treatment of CHO cells for 2 hours with sodium chromate, a hexavalent chromium carcinogen, produced DNA single-strand breaks, DNA-protein cross-links, and chromium-DNA adducts. While the constitutive Grp 78 (BiP) level was not affected by the chromate, the inducibility of this Hsp was suppressed in a concentration- and time-dependent manner. The effects of chromate on *Grp 78* (BiP) induction correlated most closely with the presence of DNA-protein cross-links, but the suppression of total cytoplasmic RNA and mRNA synthesis correlated with the presence of chromium-DNA adducts. This indicates that chromate exerts a differential effect on the induction of the *Grp 78* gene and on general transcription [F. C. Manning and S. R. Patierno: *Mol.Carcinog.* **6,** 270 (1992).

Acute administration of the hepatocarcinogens, diethylnitrosamime, and 2-acetylaminofluorene was found to induce *Hsp* gene transcription in a dose- and time-dependent manner; the tumor promoter phenobarbital did not induce increased transcription. The greatest increase was found in the transcription of an Hsp 83 and a lesser increase in the transcription of Hsp 70. Increased levels of both Hsp's were observed during hepatic regeneration. These findings are similar to those with c-H-*ras* and c-*myc* expression in rat liver, suggesting a coordinated expression of these genes during early stages of hepatocarcinogenesis [B. I. Carr *et al.*: *Cancer Res.* **46,** 5106 (1986)].

CHAPTER 16

Extremely Low Frequency Electromagnetic Fields and Cancer

Bary W. Wilson and Jeffrey D. Saffer

1. INTRODUCTION

Because of the exceedingly small energies associated with power frequency (50 or 60 Hz) electric and magnetic fields (EMF), the possibility that these fields might be linked to increased cancer incidence was not seriously considered in the scientific community before the last decade. A series of epidemiologic studies (1–5), however, has led to considerable current debate as to whether exposure to extremely low frequency (ELF) electric and magnetic fields can be contributing factors to cancer risk in humans.

Before 1979, interest in biological interactions with ELF EMF centered on possible effects on several physiological processes, including nervous system function and behavior. First studied among these phenomena was the field-induced perception of light flashes known as phosphenes (6). These result from extremely low frequency sinusoidal or pulsed magnetic-field exposure (with field strengths of several hundred gauss) to the head. It is now known that physiological effects such as phosphenes and involuntary muscle contractions, which occur at still higher field strengths, are a result of the electric currents induced in the body by the time-varying magnetic fields (7, 8). As is discussed later, electrophysiological measurements have confirmed that weak fields can also affect neurological function (9).

Initial interest in cancer as a possible pathological effect of exposure, and in the magnetic-field component of EMF as a possible biologically active agent, was first prompted by an epidemiologic study by Wertheimer and Leeper (1). Their initial report was greeted with a great deal of skepticism from the scientific community, including many EMF researchers. The nonconventional statistical approach to analysis of the data and the fact that there did not appear to be plausible mechanisms by which magnetic-field exposure could increase cancer risk contributed to the skepticism. However, several subsequent epidemiologic studies considering surrogates for both occupational and residential EMF exposure also suggested an association between these indices and increased risk for certain cancers (2–4).

This chapter is a brief review of research that concerns the question of EMF and cancer. Epidemiologic data that have served to drive research in the area are considered, as are the theoretical objections raised by some as to the plausibility of biological or pathological effects from EMF exposure. Relevant laboratory studies conducted with both cellular and whole-animal models, and with human subjects, are discussed. Possible physical mechanisms by which the low-energy fields might be detected by, or otherwise interact with, biological organisms are considered, as are physiological processes by which the EMF fields may increase cancer risk.

In discussing possible adverse health effects from EMF exposure, it is important to note that beneficial applications of EMF in medical diagnostics and treatment have been actively sought and developed. Diagnostic procedures such as magnetic resonance imaging (MRI) involve short-term exposure to relatively strong magnetic and electromagnetic fields in the ELF and radiofrequency (RF) range. Therapeutic applications for low-strength EMF include devices that promote bone growth and are used to treat insomnia (10, 11).

Clinical experience with pulsed weak EMF, such as used in bone growth stimulators, has also been of benefit in helping to form hypotheses as to how EMF may affect cancer risk. There is now a substantial literature regarding specific characteristics of pulsed (broadband) magnetic fields that are most effective in stimulating growth of bone tissue into the gap between the opposing ends of a fracture. These data, along with knowledge gained in the study of magnetic-field–dependent navigation and homing in migrating birds and in certain reptiles, fish, and mammals, have been of value in the study of possible EMF effects on humans.

II. PHYSICAL PROPERTIES OF ELECTROMAGNETIC FIELDS

Time-varying EMF are characterized primarily in terms of their frequency and associated wavelength. Energy associated with these fields is proportional to frequency. In Figure 1, this energy is expressed in terms of electron volts. To appreciate the biological effects of EMF, it is important to distinguish between their associated photon energy and flux density. As is discussed later, characteristics of higher frequency radiative fields serve best to illustrate these important differences. Photon energy increases with frequency as the associated wavelength shortens. Field strength (of the electric-field component) or flux density (of the magnetic-field component), on the other hand, is a measure of the number of photons that pass through a given area in space in a given time without regard for their intrinsic energy.

At frequencies greater than approximately 10^{16} Hz (with wavelengths in the 10^{-10}-m range), electromagnetic radiation has sufficient energy to cause ionization by scattering electrons. At these energies, electromagnetic radiation (X-rays and gamma rays) can easily break chemical bonds in biological tissue, giving rise to highly reactive free radical species as well as causing direct damage to genetic material in cells. The term "radiation" is appropriately used at these frequencies. Effects of such fields are best described as resulting from the interaction of high-energy photons with matter.

Moving down the frequency spectrum, energy from ultraviolet (UV) light can cause chemical changes, but these fields are attenuated by biological tissue and do not penetrate very far below the surface. Nonetheless, overexposure to UV light is associated with skin cancer risk, especially in fair-skinned persons. At lower frequencies, the visible and infrared ranges, energy from electromagnetic radiation can be sensed as light and heat, each having profound effects on biological systems. Particle characteristics of EMF can be demonstrated at these lower energies by phenomena such as the photoelectric effect, wherein photons interact with electrons in certain metals on a discrete basis. Photon ejection of electrons from conductance bands in these metals is evidenced by resulting electric currents. However, electromagnetic radiation in the visible and ultraviolet light and lower frequency ranges is best conceptualized as being composed of waves. Wavelike

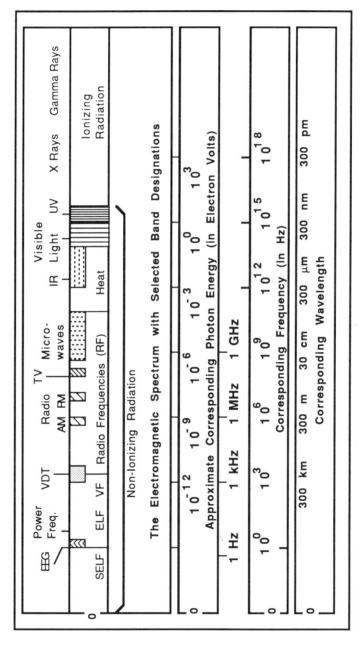

FIGURE 1. Electromagnetic spectrum showing selected band designations, as well as their corresponding frequencies, wavelengths, and approximate photon energies.

properties such as diffraction patterns are readily demonstrated for EMF in this frequency range.

In the microwave frequency regime (3×10^8 to 3×10^{11} Hz), irradiation of biological tissue with sufficient energy can cause heating, although the microwaves are not sensed directly as heat. At lower frequencies in the microwave band, tissue heating can still occur given sufficient energy, and the ability of RF fields to cause heating increases with frequency. In the ELF region of the electromagnetic spectrum (3–3000 Hz), wavelengths are long, of the order of several thousand kilometers. Fields are essentially nonradiative, and the electric- and magnetic-field components are largely decoupled.

For the purpose of this chapter, the term ELF is used to designate the range from 0 to 3000 Hz. Unless otherwise designated, the term EMF in this review refers to either the electric- or magnetic-field components, or to both. With regard to environmental EMF, and indeed, to certain of the pulsed fields used in laboratory and clinical studies, it should be noted that they often have frequency components that lie outside the ELF range. Such high-frequency components (extending into the megahertz range for certain household and industrial electrical devices) may be important in determining biological effects.

A. Properties of ELF Electromagnetic Fields

In a vacuum or in atmosphere, electric-field lines of force extend radially in all directions from an electric charge or charged object. A conducting object such as a human body, when placed in the electric field, causes substantial distortion of the field lines. Electric-field penetration of the body, however, is slight because impinging field lines cause charge within the conducting body to reorient so as to counter the external field. In time-varying electric fields, small internal body currents are created. Internal fields are small compared to the imposed external field, however, because of the attenuation of the field at the surface of the body.

Surface or internal body currents that do result from the presence of an external electric field flow primarily in the same direction as the overall field gradient (*e.g.*, from higher to lower potential). A well-documented effect of high-strength AC electric fields on the body is that of hair vibration (piloerection), which allows perception of the electric field at high field strengths (8).

Electric and magnetic fields are vector quantities having both magnitude and direction. Magnetic fields may be described in terms of their field strength (**H**) or their flux density (**B**). In vacuum (and for all practical purposes in atmosphere), the two quantities are related by the equation $\mathbf{B} = \mu_0\mathbf{H}$, where μ_0 is the permeability of free space and is equal to $4\pi \times 10^{-7}$.

Magnetic flux density is expressed in terms of tesla (T) or gauss (G), and can best be visualized as the density of magnetic flux lines passing through a given space. Although tesla is now the preferred unit in the scientific literature, gauss is the term more commonly used (1 tesla $= 10^4$ gauss); we use both terms here.

In contrast to electric fields, magnetic fields do not induce a surface charge. Magnetic fields penetrate the body with little or no attenuation because the permeability of biological tissue is essentially the same as that of air. Changing magnetic fields induce electric (E) fields in conducting bodies according to Faraday's law, which simply states that the electromotive force induced in a conductor by a magnetic field is proportional to the rate at which the magnetic field is changing. Thus, electromotive force is proportional to the time-rate of change of the magnetic field ($d\mathbf{B}/dt$) and is therefore, for a given frequency, also proportional to the amplitude of **B**.

Current induced in a conducting body by a magnetic field is proportional to the induced electric field, which in turn is proportional to the radius of the induced current path. Induced currents are inversely proportional to resistance along the current path, and circulate in the conductor in a plane at right angles (orthogonal) to the impinging field lines according to the right-hand rule. Thus, in determining induced currents from magnetic fields, the size of the test subject and frequency of the field are parameters that must be considered with flux density. A useful equation for calculating the approximate electric field induced in an object by an external magnetic field is

$$E = \omega \mathbf{B} \, (r/2)$$

where $\omega = 2\pi f$
  E is the induced electric field
  f is the frequency of the magnetic field in Hz
  $\mathbf{B}$ is magnetic-field flux density in T
  r is the effective radius of the conducting object at right angles to the magnetic-field direction.

Induced currents can be readily calculated if the conductivity (or resistance) of the object is known. For reviews of ELF EMF interactions with biological tissue, including many facets outside the scope of this present discussion, *see* Kaune and Anderson (12) and Tenforde (8). The geomagnetic field of the earth is of the order of 50 μT (0.5 G). It is primarily a non-time-varying (DC) field, with the angle of incidence to the surface of the earth increasing with latitude. Near the poles, the magnetic-field lines of force are almost perpendicular to the surface of the earth, while at the equator they are nearly parallel. Anthropogenic magnetic fields are primarily time varying at electric power–generating frequencies of 50 or 60 Hz and harmonics of those frequencies. Magnetic-field strength depends on proximity to current-carrying electrical conductors, such as powerlines and home appliances. Typical magnetic fields measured in residential settings range from 0.1 to 3 μT (1 to 30 mG) at 60 Hz (13).

Energy deposition into biological tissue from ELF electric or magnetic fields at typical human exposure levels is extremely low and is exceeded by the thermal energy already present at ambient temperature (see Figure 1). Based primarily on this fact, some scientists reject the possibility that these fields could have biological effects within certain constraints (14). Many of these objections are based on assumptions regarding cell shape, conductive properties, and intracellular organization, and thus are not informative with regard to complex biological organisms. Objections to meaningful EMF interactions with biological systems are often maintained despite the demonstrated ability of several species of animals to detect and use information from both the electric and magnetic components of these low-energy fields (7, 15).

III. EPIDEMIOLOGIC STUDIES

Research in the field of EMF interactions with biological systems during the last decade has been driven by results from epidemiologic studies, the first of which suggested an association between EMF exposure and leukemia and brain cancer in children. Subsequent studies have also suggested increased risk of brain cancer and leukemia in adults, as well as male breast cancer, prostate cancer, lymphomas, and melanoma in populations with putative increased occupational exposures to magnetic fields.

There are several important exceptions, but to date most epidemiologic studies, particularly those that have considered occupational exposure to EMF, have distinguished "exposed" or "higher exposure" groups from "nonexposed" or "lower exposure" groups by the use of surrogates rather than by direct measurements of the electric or magnetic fields. These surrogates reflect indirect estimates of the fields to which workers are exposed; the implicit assumption is that "dose", or something related directly to it, is reflected in the surrogate measure.

In residential studies, the surrogate most often used has been the configuration of electrical service wires outside the home. These external wiring configurations have been categorized by Wertheimer and Leeper (1), and this method of estimating long-term EMF exposure in homes has become known as the Wertheimer–Leeper wiring code. The wiring code is categorical with five levels of imputed exposure, from low to high, based on the numbers of transmission and distribution wires near the home, their gauge, distances to these wires, and whether or not they are buried. As is discussed later, in many instances this measure appears to be more closely associated with childhood leukemia incidence in residential epidemiologic studies than are magnetic fields themselves as determined by direct measurement.

In the study by Savitz *et al.* (2), residential magnetic-field measurements were obtained under low-power conditions (wherein power to the home was switched off to the extent possible at the distribution panel) and high-power conditions (wherein all home appliances and lights were turned on). Magnetic-field measurements were stratified into four categories: $<0.065\ \mu T$; 0.065 to $<0.1\ \mu T$; 0.1 to $0.25\mu T$; and $>0.25\ \mu T$. Correlation to observed cancer rates was elevated, but not statistically significant when data were analyzed using these categories. Nonsignificant increases in cancer were observed when comparing households in the lowest category to those in the three higher categories under low-power conditions (odds ratio: OR = 1.28–1.49). Trend tests for these comparisons were, however, significant. Although measurements have generally shown a weak association between magnetic-field strength and risk, there has been little association between measured electric fields and increased risk.

Among residential studies to date, perhaps the most informative was that by London *et al.* (4), who determined childhood leukemia risk related to wiring codes and measured magnetic fields in the homes of cases and controls in Los Angeles County, California. Although their data provided little support for an association between measured household magnetic fields and childhood leukemia, there was evidence for an association between wiring code and childhood leukemia, and also evidence for an association between use of certain electrical appliances by children and childhood leukemia.

When measured in residential epidemiologic studies, magnetic-field strengths in the home overall have generally shown weaker correlations with actual cancer incidence than do wiring code classifications. Some investigators have suggested that the surrogate measures, although crude, are more stable than short-term measurements and therefore may be more indicative of long-term exposures. It is also possible that the surrogate measures reflect some aspect of magnetic-field exposure that is more closely associated with increased risk than is the time-weighted average exposure to 60-Hz magnetic fields. (With few exceptions, measurements of field strength in studies to date are used to estimate a time-weighted average exposure at 60 Hz.) Other authors have suggested that the surrogates in the residential studies may reflect risk factors (as yet unknown) other than magnetic-field exposure and that therefore magnetic-field exposure does not constitute a risk.

A. Epidemiologic Studies on Electric Blanket Use

An interesting subset of the residential epidemiologic data are those that determined associations between adverse health outcomes and electric blanket use. Most electric blankets manufactured before 1989 generated magnetic fields near the blanket surface in the 3- to 30-μT range (16). Electric blankets commonly operate on a duty cycle, typically being switched on for approximately 50 to 100 sec then off for about the same time or longer, depending on the blanket controller setting and room temperature. These blankets thus represent relatively long, high–field strength exposures compared to ambient household magnetic fields. Considering their daily use, these blankets probably constituted the greatest single magnetic-field exposure source for most individuals who used them. Because individuals who use them may be readily distinguished from those who do not, their use has become a valuable indicator of exposure in residential epidemiologic studies.

Savitz *et al.* (17) reported that electric blanket use by the mother was associated with an increase in brain cancer in the offspring. In the more recent study on childhood leukemia by London *et al.* (4), cases were more likely to have used electric blankets than were controls. However, this odds ratio was unstable because of the small number of parents (7 cases and 1 control) reporting electric blanket use in children. Other studies considering electric blanket use as a source of EMF exposure include that by Verreault *et al.* (18), who reported on testicular cancer as associated with use of this appliance, and Vena *et al.* (19), who found no increase in breast cancer in postmenopausal women who used electric blankets. As is discussed later, Wilson *et al.* (20) found preliminary evidence for an effect of electric blanket use on melatonin rhythms in humans.

B. Occupational Epidemiologic Studies

In occupational studies, the surrogate most often used to estimate magnetic field exposure has been that of job title. Although limited in number, magnetic-field measurements to compare field exposures for different job titles in occupational settings have been reported. For example, Bowman *et al.* (21) measured magnetic fields in the work environments of people in occupations that have been shown by Savitz and Calle (22) to have increased leukemia risk. In the Bowman study, the geometric mean of 60-Hz magnetic fields in 67 occupational settings designated as used by "electrical workers" was 0.464 μT, with a range of 0 to 62.1 μT. Transmission station operators and overhead linemen had the highest exposures according to this study. Deadman *et al.* (23) also studied occupational EMF exposure, using a field meter that was worn by volunteers throughout their workday. These workers compared exposures in presumed exposed job categories to that in presumed nonexposed jobs. The geometric mean 60-Hz magnetic field among 20 subjects in "exposed" jobs was 1.66 μT; among 16 subjects in "nonexposed" jobs it was 0.16 μT.

C. Brain Cancer

In a number of case–control studies, elevated brain cancer incidence rates have been associated with occupations believed to have increased exposure to magnetic fields. As discussed earlier, where measurements have been made, persons in "electrical occupations" do tend to have increased exposure to these fields compared to those occupations classed as nonelectric. In at least one instance, when likely exposure was categorized, (24), there appeared to be a dose–response relationship between exposure and cancer risk.

Among the case–control studies of central nervous system (CNS) cancers are those of Speers and colleagues (25), who reported an odds ratio of greater than 13:1 for risk for gliomas among electrical utility employees; Pearce *et al.* (26), who reported that electrical engineers in New Zealand showed a 4.47-fold increased risk for brain tumors; and Mack *et al.* (27), who found excess astrocytomas in electrical occupations for those employed longer than 10 years. Compared to case–control studies of cancers of the CNS, cohort studies have suggested a generally lower risk and have been less likely to indicate statistically significant increases in risk. However, several of the more recent cohort studies, those done since 1990, have shown relative risks greater than 1.

D. Leukemia and Lymphoma

Increased leukemia incidence has been linked to electrical occupations in a number of studies, including those by Gilman *et al.* (28), Flodin *et al.* (29), Coggon *et al.* (30), Pearce *et al.* (26), and Garland *et al.* (31). In the latter study, age-adjusted leukemia incidence rates were determined for U.S. Navy personnel for more than 4 million person-years at risk between 1974 and 1984. The authors found a 2.4-fold increased risk (95% confidence interval: Cl = 1.0–5.0) for electrician's mates, with none of the other occupational specialties considered showing incidence greater than that expected. Among the studies cited, the highest reported odds ratio was 8.22 for chronic leukemia in EMF-exposed coal miners (28).

Several epidemiologic studies have also linked elevated mortality from lymphoma with electrical occupations. Most striking among these is a series of studies showing an apparent substantial increase in risk of non-Hodgkins lymphoma (NHL) in aluminum reduction plant pot-room workers. Originally reported from studies of workers in Washington State by Milham (32) and subsequently by Davis and Milham (33), increased NHL risk has also been reported by Spinelli *et al.* (34), who surveyed workers in a Canadian aluminum reduction plant.

Increased lymphoma in CFW mice chronically exposed to 60-Hz magnetic fields was reported recently by Mikhail and Fam (35). In light of the fact that pot-room workers are often exposed to ambient temperatures exceeding 100°F, it is interesting that one criticism of these latter studies has been the possibility that temperatures in the exposed animal cages were elevated from heat generated by the current in the magnetic-field coils.

Increase in risk for lymphomas as a consequence of EMF exposure appears consistent with the hypothesis that such exposure has a suppressive effect on immune function. Lymphoma incidence is known to be increased in immunocompromised populations (36). Immunosuppression in the case of EMF exposure may arise via reduction in melatonin synthesis or by direct action on T-cells, as was suggested by the *in vitro* studies of Lyle *et al.* (37).

E. Male Breast Cancer

When a rare cancer is linked with exposure to a specific agent, the association can lend credence to the hypothesis that the agent may be a carcinogen. Male breast cancer is a rare disease, and thus studies that suggest an association between magnetic-field exposure and this cancer are of particular interest. Stevens *et al.* (38, 39) suggested that increased breast cancer risk may result from EMF-induced changes in melatonin synthesis and release by the pineal gland. To date, three epidemiologic studies relevant to this hypothesis have been reported. A substantial body of data from laboratory studies is consistent with an effect of EMF exposure on male breast cancer, as suggested by the Stevens hypothesis (Figure 2).

In a study designed to specifically test the Stevens hypothesis, Demers *et al.* (3) compared exposures based on job category for 227 male breast cancer cases and 300

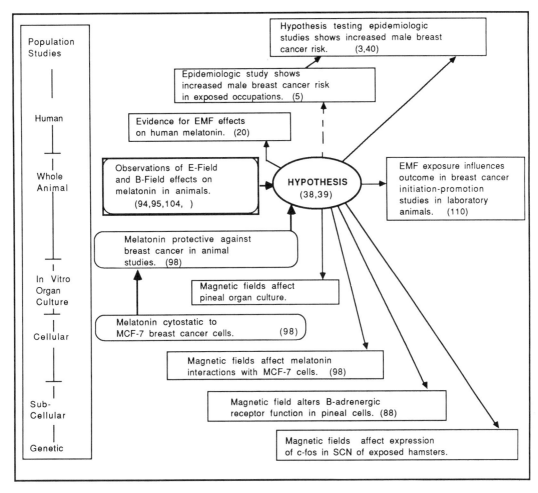

FIGURE 2. Overview of laboratory and epidemiologic studies consistent with the hypothesis that EMF exposure may increase breast cancer risk via effects on the neuroendocrine system. Numbers in parentheses refer to literature cited in the references.

controls. The highest risks (OR = 6.0; Cl = 1.7–21.5) were found for those in the electrical occupations described as electricians, telephone linemen, and electric power workers. A second related job category, radio and communications workers, with putatively increased exposure to higher frequency fields, also showed an increased risk (OR = 2.9; Cl = 0.8–10.2). The consolidated exposed group in these studies was also calculated to have an increased risk (OR = 1.8; Cl = 1.0–3.2) relative to assumed nonexposed job categories.

Tynes and Anderson (40) have reported breast cancer rates greater than expected in males working in designated electrical occupations in Norway. Overall, the risk ratio for male breast cancer in the combined electrical occupations grouping was 2.07. Electrical tram operators, for example, had an apparent 12-fold increase in their risk of breast cancer, the highest among the specific job classifications analyzed. Matanoski *et al.* (5, 41) published findings of breast cancer risk higher than expected in a large study of a telephone worker cohort. Highest risks for breast cancer was noted among office workers, who were in many cases exposed to rapidly changing ("spiky") fields generated by switching equipment.

F. Melanoma

Increased risk of malignant melanoma has been noted in several epidemiologic studies of electrically exposed workers. From a cohort study of telecommunication workers in Sweden, Vagero *et al.* (42) noted a statistically significant relative risk (SMR = 2.5) for malignant melanoma of the skin in telecommunications workers. Of all cancers considered, only melanoma and nodular lymphoma were increased in males. Melanoma was also increased in females (SMR = 2.8). Excess skin melanoma in electronics industry workers (42) and telecommunications workers (43) has been reported. A study of telecommunications workers in Canada by De Guire *et al.* (44) indicated an increased risk of melanoma for men (SIR = 2.7), but not for women. Swerdlow (45) found increased melanoma of the eye for electronics and electrical workers in the United Kingdom. Gallagher *et al.* (46), however, found no increased melanoma in electronics or electrical workers in western Canada. It has been pointed out that excess melanoma in electronics and telecommunications workers may be a consequence of their generally higher socioeconomic status (47).

The preceding discussion of epidemiologic findings is intended only as an introduction to underscore some of the following discussion. For more complete treatments of these data, see reviews by Walborg (48) and Theriault (49).

IV. OVERVIEW OF *IN VITRO STUDIES*

The extremely low energy of EMF in the ELF range precludes these fields from causing damage directly to the genome as does ionizing radiation. Because experimental results supported this hypothesis, investigations of the link between EMF and cancer have focused on proliferation-based models of carcinogenesis [reviewed by Cohen and Ellwein (50)]. In these models, increased cell proliferation can increase the likelihood of rare mutations arising from DNA synthesis and mitosis. Therefore, changes in cell proliferation and DNA synthesis have been of interest. More recently, much research has been directed at determining whether exposure to ELF magnetic fields can alter cellular function, as indicated by changes in gene expression, and whether the changes are caused by interference with intercellular or intracellular signaling processes.

In reviewing the research on the potential biological effects of ELF fields *in vitro,* it is important to note that the magnetic fields used in various studies differ in many aspects (*e.g.*, frequency, amplitude, pulse shape). Therefore, it is not always possible to compare related experiments directly. A similar situation exists for the biological systems; effects observed in one cell line are not necessarily expected to occur in another. Because most biological responses are common to all cells, however, some generalizations can be drawn.

A. ELF Magnetic Fields Are Not Directly Genotoxic

The link between ELF magnetic fields and cancer risk, if such a link exists, does not involve classic mutagenesis by these fields as a physical agent. The occurrence of single-strand DNA breaks in Chinese hamster ovary cells exposed to 60-Hz magnetic (0.1 or 2 mT) and electric (1 or 38 V/m) fields, alone or in combination, was not significantly different from that in unexposed control cells (51). Similarly, the frequency of chromosomal structural rearrangements in human peripheral lymphocytes exposed to a 60-Hz field (100–200 μT; 30 μA/cm^2) or a 50-Hz field (100–750 μT) did not differ relative to control cells (52, 53). The appearance of micronuclei, a sensitive indicator of chromosomal damage, was also unaffected in ELF field-exposed lymphocytes (54). Further, ELF fields do not alter the ability of cells to repair DNA damage from other agents (55, 56).

B. Altered Cell Proliferation

Even though ELF fields are not directly genotoxic, alterations in cell proliferation induced by the fields could affect the frequency of neoplastic events. The growth of embryonal carcinoma cells in the presence or absence of retinoic acid was promoted by a pulsed ELF field (57). An increased proliferation rate from ELF field exposure was suggested by the greater ability of two human colon cancer cell lines to form colonies in a clonogenicity assay following exposure as compared to unexposed cells (58). Changes in proliferation also occurred in human lymphocytes exposed to ELF fields; a pulsed ELF field increased phytohemagglutinin-induced proliferation (59); and a 50-Hz sinusoidal magnetic field enhanced cell cycle progression (53). Similarly, the rate of fibroblast proliferation in chicken tendon explants increased 32% with exposure to 1-Hz pulses at one field strength (7 mA/m^2), but no effect occurred at a lower field strength (1.8 mA/m^2), and proliferation decreased on exposure to higher strength fields (10 mA/m^2) (60).

Although increased proliferation at only the midlevel field strength could be interpreted as a "window" effect, the small changes involved must be viewed cautiously, particularly because negative results have been obtained by others. For example, no change in mitotic index (percent of cells undergoing mitosis) occurred in human peripheral lymphocytes exposed to a 60-Hz electromagnetic field (52); and proliferation of primary fibroblasts from rabbit marrow stroma was also unaffected by ELF fields (61). Nonetheless, altered cell proliferation remains a potential effect of ELF fields.

C. Altered DNA Synthesis

Consistent with increased cell proliferation, effects of ELF fields on DNA synthesis, as measured by the incorporation of radiolabeled thymidine, have also been reported (62, 63). DNA synthesis was slightly elevated in human fibroblasts exposed to a 76-Hz, 23-μT rms sine wave magnetic field (62). Exposure of the cells to other frequencies (15 Hz to 4 kHz) and field strengths (2.3–60 μT) produced similar small effects (62). For pulsed fields, specific field parameters were required to affect DNA synthesis. With a field of 20 μT at 100 Hz, only a 25-μsec pulse width elevated DNA synthesis 1.3-fold; other pulse widths from 6 to 125 μsec did not (63). Slight increases in DNA synthesis were noted at pulse frequencies of 10 or 100 Hz, but not at lower, intermediate, or higher frequencies. In contrast, varying the field strength of a 25-μsec pulse repeating at 100 Hz resulted in either an increase or an inhibition of DNA synthesis; at 20 μT, synthesis increased to a maximum of 1.3-fold, whereas at 200 μT synthesis was inhibited 20% (63).

In each of these experiments, the effect of ELF fields on DNA synthesis was minimal. Given the errors associated with these incorporation assays and the failure of the investigators to demonstrate consistent uptake of the labeled precursor in control and exposed cells, it is difficult to conclude a definitive effect on DNA synthesis.

V. EFFECTS OF EMF ON GENE EXPRESSION

A. General Changes in RNA

Evaluating the potential hazards (or benefits) of electromagnetic fields requires a full characterization of the affected cellular processes. In 1983, Goodman *et al.* (64) presented the first in a series of innovative studies examining changes in gene transcription caused by ELF fields. Recognizing that gene transcription would reflect cellular changes and perhaps represent initial effects, these researchers have produced a series of reports that have stimulated examination of the molecular events resulting from ELF field exposure. Reports from this group and others have characterized ELF field effects on RNA levels in general and on the amount of messenger RNA (mRNA) from specific genes. Understanding the basis for ELF field-induced changes in gene expression, particularly proto-oncogenes (*see* following), will be necessary to define the link, if any, between ELF fields and cancer.

In their original 1983 paper, Goodman *et al.* (64) reported that gene transcription in salivary gland cells from *Sciara coprophila* was increased by exposure to two different ELF magnetic fields, a 15-Hz pulse train (at a 19-mT peak) and a 72-Hz single-pulse waveform (3.5.mT peak). Autoradiography of the polytene chromosomes from cells grown in the presence of a radiolabeled RNA precursor demonstrated increased levels of RNA transcription following exposure to ELF fields (64). Because this method detects nascent RNA associated with the chromosome, the results indicate a change in RNA synthesis rate as opposed to decreased turnover of mature RNA. Analysis of the amount of radiolabel in different size classes showed that RNA in the 6S to 10S range was responsible for the observed increase (64). Although the authors suggested that this size class is consistent with mRNA, it would also include relatively abundant structural RNA such as 7S RNA.

The observation of increased RNA levels was expanded to test the effects of ELF fields of differing characteristics (65–67). Most of the fields tested resulted in increased RNA as measured by incorporation of labeled precursor, although with different efficacy. In each case, incorporation of label into 6S to 10S RNA increased most notably, with the incorporation into 20S to 5S RNA also showing a slight augmentation. In one experiment using a 1.5-Hz pulse train signal (1.5-mT peak), the authors examined RNA enriched for species containing poly(A) tails to demonstrate directly that mRNA levels were elevated in exposed cells (67). Despite the use of many different waveforms and frequencies, no conclusions could be drawn as to the relevant field parameters that induce the transcriptional changes. The difficulties in this regard include the lack of reproducibility, even though all work was done by the same group. In one instance (66), the 1.5-Hz pulse train signal (1.5-mT peak) was found to affect RNA synthesis less than a 72-Hz sine wave, but in another (67) the two fields gave equal responses. Furthermore, as pointed out by Phillips (68), the control cultures are treated inconsistently, making it difficult to evaluate the field conditions that result in changes in RNA levels.

Mammalian cells also respond to ELF fields by a general increase in RNA. Phillips and McChesney (69) exposed CCRF-CEM T-lymphoblastoid cells to the same 72-Hz pulse signal (3.5-mT peak field) used by Goodman *et al.* (64). Incorporation of labeled precursor into RNA was increased in exposed cells as compared to controls with a maximal increase of 3.2-fold occurring after a 2-hour exposure (69). The labeling of RNA in the exposed cells remained elevated 2.5-fold through 24 hours of exposure, except for a slight dip to 1.8-fold greater than control after a 16-hour exposure. In a population enriched for poly(A)-containing RNA, the amount of label was decreased in exposed cells relative to the controls after 30 min, but then increased by the same amount as the total by 2 hours (69). It is important to realize that assays of radiolabel incorporation measure the accumulation of RNA synthesized since the addition of the labeled precursor, not the total level of RNA in the cell.

Greene *et al.* (70) examined the effect of 60-Hz sine wave magnetic fields (1 mT) on the lymphocytic cell line HL-60. Exposed cells showed a transient 50 to 60% enhancement in radiolabel incorporation into total RNA relative to controls, with subsequent decline to baseline levels by the 18th hour. By comparing responses in different compartments of annular dishes, these investigators showed that the magnitude of the effect varied directly with the induced electric field. Therefore, it is imperative to consider the exposure geometry when evaluating the transcription studies.

B. Altered Expression of Specific RNA

The foregoing data indicate that accumulation of RNA can be affected by ELF fields. This effect may not be a general phenomenon, however. In their studies of dipteran chromosomes, Goodman and colleagues (64, 67, 71, 72) noted some specificity in the effect on transcription, with some regions showing enhanced synthesis while other loci appeared to be unaffected. Analysis of transcription on the X-chromosome indicated that ELF fields stimulated transcription at loci not detectably active in control cells as well as augmenting transcription at previously active loci (71). The specificity of the effect was dependent on the ELF signal used (71).

Specific transcriptional changes have also been evaluated in mammalian cells. Goodman *et al.* (73) exposed the human lymphocytic cell line HL-60 to several different ELF fields for 20 min. The fields were three asymmetric pulse signals (72-Hz single pulse, 3.5-mT peak; 15-Hz pulse train, 1.9-mT peak; 1.5-Hz pulse train, 0.38-mT peak) and two sine waves (60 Hz, 1.5-mT peak or 72 Hz, 1.1-mTt peak). The steady-state level of three transcripts (β-actin, histone H2B, and c-*myc*) were evaluated using dot blot analysis. Data demonstrating the specificity of each probe used were not presented. Expression of the genes was augmented in cells exposed to each field as compared to nonexposed cells. Curiously, all three genes showed essentially the same pattern of induction (73) (Figure 3). The magnitude of the induction was signal dependent; 60-Hz sine waves were more effective than 72-Hz sine waves, and the pulsed signals provided the smallest increase (73). Given the potential connection between ELF field exposure and cancer, observation of altered expression of c-*myc* has stimulated much interest in these effects.

To investigate further the frequency dependence of this phenomenon, the HL-60 cells were exposed to sine wave fields ranging from 15 to 150 Hz (74). As noted previously, the

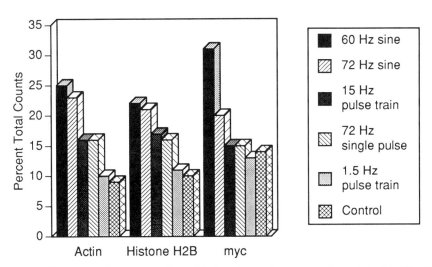

FIGURE 3. Effect of various magnetic-field signals on the expression of actin, histone H2B, and *myc* genes in HL-60 cells. [Adapted from R. Goodman, L.-X. Wei, J-C. Xu, and A. Henderson, *Biochim. Biophys. Acta* **1009**, 216 (1989).]

field-induced increases in expression of c-*myc* and histone H2B mRNA were identical. Exposure to a 45-Hz field produced the maximum effect, and the authors suggested a frequency "window". However, the change in frequency was accompanied by a change in field strength (from 0.2 mT at 15 Hz to 2.3 mT at 150 Hz), so that the difference in effect may not be solely the result of frequency dependence. Indeed, field strength- and time-dependent windows have also been reported in this system (72).

Because the c-*myc*, histone H2B, and β-actin are regulated by very different cellular stimuli, the identical stimulation of each gene by ELF fields suggests a general effect on basic cell properties rather than specific regulatory mechanisms. One, if not the only, case in which all three genes would show elevated expression is an increase in cell proliferation. Production of ribosomal RNA would also increase in this instance, but this was not observed in measurements of the incorporation of labeled precursors (65–67). It will be important to demonstrate in this system that ELF field-induced changes in expression of other transcribed genes are independent of c-*myc*, histone H2B, and β-actin. There are probably as many negative as there are positive regulatory systems in cells. Therefore, one should expect the expression of some genes to be decreased by the ELF fields and some to be unchanged. Goodman and Shirley-Henderson (72) did examine the expression of α-globin in the HL-60 cells, but because that gene is normally not expressed, the lack of expression in exposed cells was uninformative.

Work with the HL-60 cells by another group has yielded potentially contradictory results. The expression of c-*myc* in HL-60 cells exposed to ELF fields at 60 Hz (0.25–1 mT) for 15 to 60 min was unchanged (75). However, another lymphocytic cell line, Daudi, did exhibit an increase in the steady-state levels of c-*myc* following the same exposures. In general, the magnitude of the response varied directly with time and field strength. Czerska *et al.* (75) suggested the difference between the positive response in Daudi and the negative response in HL-60 was caused by translocation of the *myc* gene in the Daudi cells.

An ELF-field–induced increase in c-*myc* expression has also been observed in CEM-CM3 T-lymphoblastoid cells exposed to a 60-Hz, 100-μT magnetic field (76). The expression of two other proto-oncogenes, c-*fos* and c-*jun*, and the expression of protein kinase C (β-chain) were monitored in these cells as well. Both the steady-state levels of these RNA as measured by slot blots and their synthesis rates as measured by nuclear run-on assays were affected by the field. This combination of methods demonstrated that, in this case, the synthesis of these RNA, and not their stability, was being affected directly. Most importantly, the changes in expression of each gene were different; both the time course and the magnitude of the effect were gene specific. In contrast to the work just described, both positive and negative effects on transcription occurred in the CEM-CM3 cells. The responses of the genes to the field was also dependent on the cell density. This is particularly interesting because the cells had equal doubling times at both densities used, suggesting that the concentration of some growth factor in the medium may be important for the effect to occur. In this regard, the secretion of insulin-like growth factor II (IGF-II) and its accumulation in the medium of cells exposed to an electric field may help mediate the resulting proliferative response (77).

C. Summary of Transcription Effects

The studies reviewed above are potentially indicative of altered gene expression resulting from ELF magnetic-field exposure. Analysis of nascent RNA chains associated with the Sciara chromosomes (64, 67, 71, 72) and the nuclear run-on assays using

CEM-CM3 cells (76) suggest that the transcription process was directly affected in these cases. This change in RNA synthesis rate could be caused by direct stimulation of the transcription machinery by the applied ELF field or its induced currents; this is, however, unlikely. More reasonably, the ELF field alters the activity of specific transcription factors through signal transduction pathways. The observation of altered RNA synthesis rate for some genes does not rule out the possibility that changes in processing or stability can also play a role in the increased steady-state levels of RNA from these or other genes.

Even though the RNA assays indicate ELF field effects, there are clearly some issues that need clarification and resolution. In some cases, gene expression in exposed cells differs from controls by less than a factor of 2. Changes in RNA levels smaller than twofold cannot be reliably quantitated without painstaking efforts. In many of the published experiments, controls required for the assays performed were not reported.

On a more general level, the lack of a robust effect gives rise to other concerns. Cultured cells are sometimes exquisitely sensitive to their environment. The response of the cells to minor variations in culture conditions should be defined. For example, the use of separate incubators for control and ELF-exposed cells is often required. Even though extreme care can be taken to ensure the incubator temperatures (including recovery time after placing cells in the chamber) and CO_2 concentrations are equal, minor differences may remain. Questions remain about the ways in which cells respond to such subtle changes, and whether alterations in gene transcription are affected by small changes in these parameters. In light of the small magnitude of the effects reported, all possible confounding effects must be ruled out.

D. ELF Field Effects on Specific Proteins

As a logical extension to their analysis of RNA, Goodman and Henderson (78) demonstrated that exposure to ELF fields also results in changes in protein synthesis. Two-dimensional gels indicated that the pattern of proteins synthesized during a 45-min exposure were altered by the same fields used in the RNA studies. The changes were distinctive, depending on the field conditions. Although the observed changes in protein synthesis could result from initial effects on RNA levels, experiments reported to date do not distinguish between these and direct effects on translation.

In addition to the changes in protein expression observed by surveying protein patterns in two-dimensional gels, expression of specific proteins have also been investigated. Collagen production in bone fibroblasts was markedly increased by pulsed EMF in confluent cultures, even though their proliferation was not affected (61). In contrast, no ELF enhancement was observed in growing cells (61). Collagen expression in chicken tendon fibroblasts was stimulated by a 6-day exposure to pulsed EMF, whereas during a 1-day exposure collagen expression increased by only the same degree as the total proteins (79).

Ornithine decarboxylase (ODC) has been used as an enzyme marker for ELF field effects because its expression responds to many extracellular signals and is elevated in rapidly growing cells. ODC activity is increased in several cell lines exposed for 1 hour to a 60-Hz electric field relative to controls, the greatest stimulation (fivefold) occurring with a 10-mV/cm field (80). However, ODC activity was unchanged or even decreased in H35 rat hepatoma cells exposed for 2 or 3 hours, respectively (80).

ODC activity in murine L929 cells was increased following exposure of cells to either a 55- or 65-Hz magnetic field; maximal enhancement occurred with a 10-μT field applied for 4 hours (81). By switching between applied fields at each frequency, Litovitz *et al.* (81) showed the increased ODC activity required the field of a given frequency to be applied for a minimum of 10 sec (coherence time) for full effect; a partial effect occurred with a coherence time of 5 sec and no effect was observed for a 1-sec coherence time (81). This requirement that the field be applied for a minimum time is likely to reflect the fundamental mechanism of interaction between the applied field and the cell.

VI. MECHANISMS FOR EMF-INDUCED CELLULAR CHANGES

A. Modulation of Intracellular Calcium Concentration

Reports of ELF-induced alteration of calcium efflux from tissues (82–84) have led several investigators to hypothesize that changes in intracellular calcium during exposure to ELF fields may be responsible for many of the observed effects. To determine whether ELF fields do indeed alter intracellular calcium levels, Carson *et al.* (85) used a fluorescent indicator to monitor possible changes in intracellular calcium from exposure to ELF fields; a significant increase did in fact occur following exposure. Lymphocytes exposed to a 13.6-Hz, 20-μT peak sinusoidal magnetic field also exhibit enhanced calcium uptake relative to control cells; this effect occurred only when the field was applied during the incorporation of the labeled ions used to track uptake (37).

In rat lymphocytes exposed to a combination of a static magnetic field (23.4 μT) and a 16-Hz sine wave field (42.1 μT), the influx of calcium in response to mitogen stimulation was inhibited relative to control cells; exposure of the cells to either field alone resulted in no effect (86). With 60-Hz sinusoidal fields, a different picture emerged. Exposure of the rat lymphocytes to a 60-Hz, 22-mT field caused an enhancement of calcium uptake following mitogen stimulation (87). This augmentation of calcium uptake was specific for the plateau phase of calcium signaling and was directly proportional to the induced electric field (87). These results support the notion that alterations in intracellular calcium levels can occur as a result of exposure to ELF fields. The results may suggest that a calcium channel or another cell-surface receptor linked to a calcium channel is the ELF target.

B. Possible Direct Effects of ELF Fields on Cell-Surface Receptors

The concept that cell-surface receptors can be affected by ELF fields was first suggested by Luben *et al.* (88). In that work, the responses of the bone cell line MMB-1 to parathyroid hormone (PTH) *in vitro* were inhibited by a 72-Hz, single-pulse signal as well as a 15-Hz pulse train (same signals as used in the early transcription experiments). The fields reduced the cellular production of cAMP in response to PTH and blocked the inhibitory effects of the hormone on collagen synthesis (88). Notably, there was no effect of the field on inhibition of collagen synthesis by nuclear-acting 1,25-dihydroxyvitamin D_3, thus supporting a membrane-based effect for the action of the field on PTH responses. A similar inhibitory effect of pulsed ELF fields on PTH responses was observed in primary bone cell cultures (89). Figure 4 is a composite illustrating how changes to receptors or ion channels that span the cell membrane can have both short-term and longer effects on cell function. Longer term effects arise from second messenger–mediated phosphorylation of regulatory proteins in the nucleus, eventually resulting in affected protein synthesis.

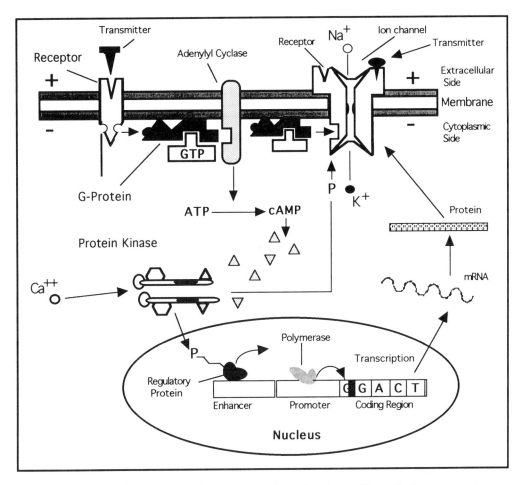

FIGURE 4. Composite diagram of various ways in which transmitters binding to receptors on the cell membrane can affect function of ion channels, including short-term effects such as direct binding to receptors on the ion channel, binding to other membrane receptors, which may result in regulation of the channel by G-protein, phosphorylation by protein kinase, and longer-term effects such as alteration in channel protein by control of regulatory elements in the nucleus.

VII. *IN VIVO* STUDIES

That EMF exposure can elicit responses in biological systems, including cultured cells, laboratory animals, and man, has been well demonstrated during the past decade in numerous studies using a variety of physiological, behavioral, and clinical endpoints. Whether or not such effects may be causally linked to cancer risk remains to be determined. However, several testable hypotheses for such a link have been proposed and are discussed next.

Nervous system responses to electric and magnetic fields, as determined by either direct electrophysiological measurements, behavioral changes, or endocrine endpoints in laboratory animals and man, have been demonstrated by a number of studies that were not specifically designed to provide information on possible cancer risk. Observation of these responses is of importance in development of the neuroendocrine hypothesis to account for possible increased cancer risk from EMF exposure. In humans, these studies include that of Bell *et al.* (90), who reported changes in human electroencephalogram (EEG) as a consequence of magnetic-field exposure, and of Graham *et al.* (91) on electric- and magnetic-field–induced changes in human cardiac interbeat interval. It is of interest that the latter, well-documented responses occur within a specific amplitude range and are most pronounced in response to intermittent field presentation.

In the preceding section, we reviewed cellular studies relevant to possible mechanisms by which EMF exposure may increase cancer risk. There are few animal studies bearing directly on this issue. Although there have been reports of increases in spontaneous tumor incidence from exposure to ELF magnetic fields, they have generally not been considered as significant because of questions regarding adequate control of exposure conditions. Several recently completed studies on the promotional and co-promotional effects of EMF, however, have given credence to the hypothesis that these fields may increase cancer risk via epigenetic mechanisms.

A. Cancer Co-Promotion Potential of EMF

McLean *et al.* (92) carried out a series of skin-painting studies to determine if exposure to magnetic fields could act as a co-promoter to increase skin cancer risk in chemically initiated animals. Mice were initiated with 7,12-dimethylbenz[*a*]anthracene and promoted thereafter with 12-*O*-tetradecanoylphorbol-13-acetate (TPA). In addition to TPA treatment, separate groups of animals were also exposed to 60-Hz magnetic fields of either 5 or 20 gauss (G). In the first of these experiments, reported in 1991, there was a slight decrease in the time to first tumor (latency) in the animals that were promoted with both magnetic-field exposure at 20 G and TPA as compared to animals promoted with TPA alone. In a replication of these studies, wherein the investigators used a decreased dose of both the initiator and TPA, there was an acceleration of papilloma growth early in the experiment, with the magnetic-field–exposed animals showing a shorter time to tumor. As in the first experiment, preliminary reports of this replicate study suggest that the overall tumor yield was not increased for the magnetic field–exposed animals as compared to controls (93).

B. Pineal Function and Cancer Risk

Among the endpoints investigated in EMF studies on animals and humans, those mediated by the nervous system have most consistently shown effects. An important manifestation of EMF interaction with the nervous system in these studies has been alteration in the circadian rhythm of melatonin synthesis and its release by the pineal gland. Because of the reported oncostatic properties of melatonin, its suppression by both electric-field exposure (94) and magnetic-field exposure (95) has been of interest relative to the question of EMF and cancer.

C. Melatonin As a Tumor-Suppressor

Melatonin is the principal hormone of the pineal gland. It is secreted on a circadian cycle with both blood and pineal concentrations increasing during the hours of darkness to peak between approximately 2 and 4 A.M., falling thereafter, and remaining low during the day. The timing and duration of the melatonin signal are believed to convey information about time of day and season to the internal organs of the body, and are important in synchronizing a number of other circadian and seasonal biological rhythms.

In mammals, melatonin rhythms appear to be determined by internal timing signals from the master clock of the suprachiasmatic nuclei in the hypothalamus and to be synchronized to the external day–night cycle by the onset of light and darkness. Melatonin can be found in nearly every tissue and in every body fluid. In many mammals, including rodents, melatonin is antigonadal. Overall, melatonin appears to suppress the activity of other endocrine organs.

An association between the pineal gland function and tumor growth was demonstrated some 70 years ago (96). The significance of this early work has been recognized during the last decade as evidence has mounted that the pineal hormone melatonin is protective against a number of neoplasms, including leukemia, breast and prostate cancers, and melanoma. In the case of chemically induced breast cancer models, there are now a number of studies that demonstrate, unequivocally, the protective effect of both endogenous and administered melatonin.

Several possible mechanisms have been proposed to account for the effect of melatonin on cancer growth. Hormone-dependent cancers, such as estrogen receptor–positive breast carcinoma and prostate adenocarcinomas, require adequate circulating concentrations of estrogen and testosterone, respectively, for growth and proliferation. One of the earliest recognized physiological roles for melatonin was that of antigonadal hormone. Thus, melatonin tends to reduce circulating levels of the gonadal steroids as well as prolactin.

Melatonin also is directly oncostatic against several cancer cell lines *in vitro*. Melatonin has been shown protective *in vivo*, whether produced endogenously or administered, against leukemia (97), breast cancer (98), melanoma (98), and prostate cancer (99).

A third general means by which melatonin may influence cancer risk is indirectly via modulation of the immune response (100). Results from a number of studies designed and carried out specifically to gather data on the interaction of melatonin with the immune system have suggested that this hormone may influence the activity of several components, including NK cell activity (101). In several of these studies, the timing of the melatonin administration was often critical in obtaining the immune system effects. It is of interest in this regard that McLean et *al.* (92) found an effect in natural killer (NK) cell activity in rats exposed to 60-Hz magnetic fields at 20 G.

D. EMF Effects on Melatonin Production

There are now more than two dozen published studies reporting effects of electric and magnetic fields on pineal gland function. Semm and coworkers (102) reported that specific cells in the pigeon pineal gland alter their firing rates in response to changes in the direction of the local static magnetic field. Subsequent work by Welker et *al.* (95) and by Olcese et *al.* (103) has shown that the rat can also respond to changes in the magnetic field by altering pineal gland function. Such alteration during the nighttime leads to a reduction in pineal melatonin concentrations. These studies, using DC magnetic fields, were aimed primarily at determining if rodents could detect magnetic field of the earth and use this information for navigation or homing.

Concurrent and independent work by Wilson et *al.* (104) showed that exposure to 60-Hz electric fields for 20 hours/day during a period of 3 weeks suppressed the nighttime rise in pineal melatonin in rats. This reduction appeared to be a threshold (all-or-none) response with onset at electric-field levels between 200 and 2000 V/m. Subsequent studies by this group showed that the effect was reversible with nighttime melatonin levels for exposed animals indistinguishable from those of controls within 3 days after cessation of exposure. Data shown in Figure 5 (105) are typical of the kinds of effects reported in

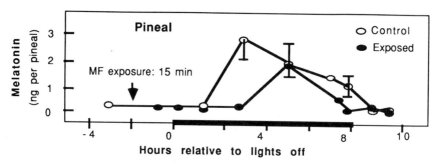

FIGURE 5. Melatonin concentrations as measured in the pineal glands of Djungarian hamsters during the dark period following 15 min of exposure to a 60-Hz magnetic field 2 h before onset of darkness. [Adapted from S. M. Yellon, *Annual Review of Research on Biological Effects of 50 and 60 Hz Electric and Magnetic Fields*, Milwankee, Wisconsin, 1991 (Abstr. A-25), p. A-25.]

studies of EMF effects on pineal gland function. In this experiment, exposure to a 60-Hz magnetic field for 15 min at 2 hour before onset of darkness resulted in a delay of the nightly peak in melatonin production as determined in both the pineal gland and blood.

In several studies, direct determination of *N*-acetyl transferase (NAT), the rate-limiting enzyme in the conversion of serotonin to melatonin, showed that its activity was suppressed by field exposure (94). This finding has been supported by the observation that serotonin, its metabolite 5-hydroxyindole acetic acid (106), and 5-methoxytryptophol (94) accumulate in the pineal gland on exposure to EMF. Both are produced via an enzymatic pathway that does not involve NAT and would be expected to accumulate in the face of decreased NAT activity.

E. Neuroendocrine Effects of EMF and the Melatonin Hypothesis

Given the various anticancer effects of melatonin, the finding that EMF exposure could reduce concentrations of this hormone in the pineal gland and blood has been of great interest in investigating whether or not EMF exposure may increase cancer risk. On the basis of observations that EMF exposure could reduce pineal melatonin concentrations in rats, Stevens (38) hypothesized that EMF may be a factor in increasing estrogen receptor–positive breast cancer risk by affecting melatonin concentrations in humans. This hypothesis was later extended to include prostate cancer in men and other hormone-dependent cancers in women (39, 107). Publication of these papers led to a number of epidemiologic and laboratory studies, as well as at least one neuroendocrine study in humans, that were designed to gather evidence to support or discount this hypothesis.

In the first such study, Leung and colleagues (108) chemically initiated female rats at 55 days of age with DMBA, followed by promotion with TPA in either in the presence or absence of 60-Hz electric fields. Results from the first of these studies were equivocal with a slight, but nonsignificant, increase in the number of mammary tumors per tumor-bearing animal in the electric-field–treated group. The initial study was followed by a second wherein the DMBA dose was reduced. Results from the second study were essentially the same as the first; there was a slight increase in the number of tumors per tumor-bearing animal. Analysis of the data from the two studies showed that they could be pooled; when this was done there was a statistically significant increase in the number of mammary tumors per tumor-bearing animal for the electric-field–exposed groups (109).

TABLE 1. Effect of Magnetic-Field Exposure on Tumor Latency and Burden in Rats Treated with N-nitroso-N-methylurea[a]

Group designation	Rats with tumors	Total tumors	Mean latency (days)
Control	27	31	74.4 ± 14.9
50-Hz MF (3 hours)	43	75	45.5 ± 11.7
Static MF (3 hours)	39	43	52.8 ± 17.1
50-Hz MF (30 min)	33	40	64.8 ± 10.5
Static MF (30 min)	32	36	65.4 ± 18.2

[a]Adapted from D. Beniashvili, V. G. Vilanishvili, and M. Z. Manabde, [*Cancer Lett.* **61**, 75 (1991)].

Experiments by Leung *et al.* were followed by those of Beniashvili (110), wherein N-nitroso-N-methylurea (NMU) was used instead of DMBA to initiate mammary tumors in groups of 50 rats each. This study design is particularly relevant because NMU-initiated mammary tumors are more sensitive to estrogen levels in the blood than are tumors induced with DMBA. Groups of animals were exposed to either 50-Hz or static magnetic fields for either 3 hours or 30 min per day. Table 1 shows data abstracted from the Beniashvili report. Tumor latency was decreased and tumor incidence increased in the magnetic-field–exposed animals. Groups of animals with 3 hours of exposure per day had higher incidence and shorter latency than groups with 30 min of exposure per day. Also, as would be anticipated by several models for mechanism of effect, static fields appeared to be less effective than sinusoidal (time-varying) fields in promotion of breast cancer in these studies. These authors did not measure melatonin in these studies, but noted that the outcome was consistent with the melatonin hypothesis for increased breast cancer risk.

VIII. EVIDENCE FOR EMF EFFECTS IN HUMANS

Experiments with animal models are valuable in determining possible consequences of weak EMF exposure on biological systems. The question as to whether these models are relevant to humans is best addressed by studies with human subjects. Few controlled laboratory experiments to determine EMF effects on humans have been conducted. As discussed earlier, clinical work on the use of EMF in bone healing and in treatment of insomnia and seizures constitutes strong evidence that humans can respond to these fields.

Human subject findings that have been reported from laboratory studies have focused on effects mediated by the nervous system: included are neurophysiological, neurobehavioral, and neuroendocrine investigations. Electric and magnetic fields (*e.g.,* 9 kV/m, 20 μT) have consistently shown an effect on heart rate by increasing the interbeat interval (91, 111). Electrophysiological measures have shown 60-Hz magnetic-field effects on event-related brain potentials. The amplitude of the major cognitive components (P300) was significantly increased by field exposure (111). Bell *et al.* (90) have reported that an 8-Hz magnetic field can affect EEG values in healthy individuals.

Wilson *et al.* (20) have reported changes in melatonin excretion in volunteers who used modified electric blankets. At onset of exposure, there was a short-term increase in excretion of the urinary metabolite 6-hydroxy melatonin sulfate. This was followed by a general decline in urinary excretion of this melatonin metabolite as exposure continued (for up to 10 weeks). At cessation of exposure, there was again a short-lived (5- to 8-day) increase in melatonin production. The magnitude of this increase was substantially higher than that of the first increase, and in some subjects was four to five times the amount measured for the evening before cessation of exposure.

In considering the area of possible EMF interactions with biological systems and the potential outcomes of these interactions in humans, whether beneficial or adverse, it is important to distinguish between biological (physiological) effects and health effects (pathology). A biological effect is defined here as a response by the organism that is within the normal physiological range of the parameter being measured. Increased circulating concentrations of epinephrine associated with a startle response, resulting in accelerated heart rate, dilation of the pupils, and heightened awareness, is an example of such a physiological effect. As they occur in normal life, such responses in and of themselves do not lead to disease. In an actual emergency, the body may well benefit from these "fight-or-flight" responses. Changes in physiological parameter observed in these human studies were all within normal physiological ranges, insofar as such ranges have been established.

Adverse health effects are defined as those that cause or contribute to eventual development of clinical disease or pathology in the organism. Continuing with the foregoing example, pathology would result from a situation wherein the animal was continuously exposed to stimuli that raised epinephrine levels, particularly if the animal found these stimuli adversive and could not, or perceived that it could not, escape. Depending on the animal or human model, specific pathologies that may result from such treatment over the longer term include heart disease and increased cancer risk, as well as various psychological symptoms.

IX. PHYSIOLOGICAL MECHANISMS OF EMF EFFECTS IN BIOLOGICAL SYSTEMS

Among the possible physiological mechanisms for biological effects of EMF exposure related to cancer is that of EMF effects on cell regulation. Adey and associates (*e.g.,* 88, 89) have been strong proponents of the view that magnetic-field signal transduction occurs at the cell membrane and that many of the subsequent biological effects observed in laboratory studies with cell cultures and whole animals may be plausibly or directly linked to perturbation of normal membrane events.

In early research bearing directly on the question of EMF interactions at the cell membrane, it was demonstrated that normal cell-to-cell passage of luciferin dye via gap junctions was impeded when cells were exposed to magnetic fields. Gap junctions are formed from protein as nearly tubular conduits that serve to pass small molecules from cell to cell. Because these connections pass through the nonconducting cell membranes, they also serve to electrically connect cells otherwise electrically isolated from one another. As discussed earlier, these connections must be considered in the simplifying assumptions made when attempting to construct theoretical models about what effects EMF exposure may have on extended aggregates of cells.

EMF-induced alterations in transmembrane signaling have been either postulated or directly demonstrated in connection with alterations in activity for a number of enzymes, including ODC and NAT.

At higher levels of tissue organization, there is a great deal of evidence that the nervous system can detect and respond to weak electromagnetic fields. Because of the linkages among the nervous, endocrine, and immune systems (112), nervous system effects may be expressed by changes in endocrine or immune function, both of which may affect cancer risk. Figure 6 illustrates how suppression or phase shifting of pineal melatonin production by EMF exposure may influence cancer risk (107).

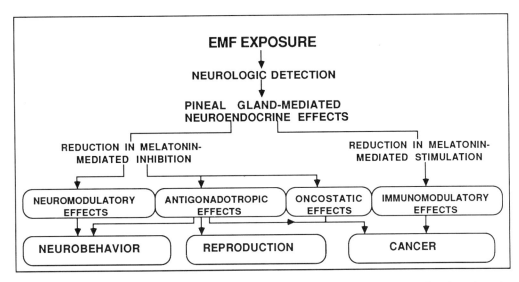

FIGURE 6. Schematic depicting various ways in which alterations in pineal melatonin synthesis may affect cancer risk, as suggested by the literature on melatonin effects. [Adapted from B. W. Wilson, R. G. Stevens, and L. E. Anderson, *Life Sci.* **45**, 319–1332 (1989).]

X. PHYSICAL MECHANISMS FOR EMF EFFECTS ON BIOLOGICAL SYSTEMS

A number of investigators have asserted that because of their exceedingly low energy, ELF EMF fields could have no effect on cell function. Such arguments are made primarily on thermodynamic grounds by noting that at the single-cell level energy associated with a 60-Hz magnetic field, for example, is many orders of magnitude less than the thermal energy already present at ambient temperatures. Therefore, these authors contend the thermal (kT) noise would make detection of any 60-Hz signal impossible.

Pilla (113), Adey (114), Weaver and Astumian (115), and others have presented cogent arguments that these objections do not apply to cellular arrays. Such arrays of cells organized in tissue are theoretically capable of detecting weak EMF signals. An important feature of such tissue is that the cells are generally in electrical contact via gap junctions, and such contact greatly increases the capability of arrays to detect weak signals. Additional arguments against the no-possible-effects position are based on the observation of magnetic materials in tissues that is of sufficient magnetic moment to transduce fields on the order of several hundred milligauss (116) and magnetic-field effects on free radical reactions (117). Detection of earth-strength magnetic fields is found in several species in the animal kingdom, and the means by which this detection occurs are, in some cases, fairly well understood (7, 8, 103). Thus, the generalization to whole animals of arguments based on assumptions about single cells appears invalid.

Determining the mode of interaction of weak magnetic fields with biological systems is of more than academic interest. This knowledge could be of value in deciding if eventual mitigation of magnetic fields is warranted as a protective measure. Most studied among the possible physical mechanisms are effects that fall into two broad categories. We will term these "electromagnetic", wherein effect arises from induced electric fields and their resulting currents, and purely "magnetic", wherein effect arises from magnetic-field interactions with biologically important ions or molecules. These are further defined and discussed next.

Pilla (113) proposed that induced electric fields and their associated currents flowing in the interstitial fluids between cells may affect normal cell function. Principal among the lines of evidence that the induced electric fields and currents are the determinant characteristics of EMF is the large body of data on the relative effectiveness of pulsed magnetic fields as compared to sinusoidal or static fields in stimulation of bone growth in humans (118) and laboratory animals. The relative effectiveness of pulsed fields as compared to sinusoidal fields of comparable amplitude in eliciting biological responses has been demonstrated in laboratory studies (87). Because electrical fields induced by pulsed fields are greater than those from sinusoidal fields of comparable amplitude, these findings are also evidence for induced currents as determinant. Pilla's model, for example, predicts that a signal-to-noise ratio of nearly 1:1 could be achieved when the applied magnetic field induced electrical fields in the body that were in the 10-mV/cm range. Such fields are induced by time rates of change in the 10^6 G/s range. That fields at this level can be detected by biological tissue is manifest by the clinical efficacy of bone growth stimulator devices that give rise to such electrical fields by magnetic induction.

Purely magnetic effects are defined here as those that may arise from the direct action of the magnetic field on the alignment, conformation, or motion of biologically important ions or molecules. Evidence that there may be purely magnetic effects on biological systems comes mainly from work on the detection of earth-strength fields by certain migrating birds (15) rats (103), and bees (119, 120). Because the magnetic field of the earth is essentially static, it cannot induce currents in slow-moving or stationary objects.

Direct detection of the magnetic field independent of its induced currents is consistent with the frequency and amplitude "windows" of sensitivity sometimes reported in EMF studies. Such windows are thought to result from the resonance conditions necessary for biologically important ions to experience motion as a result of the combined frequency of the imposed magnetic field and the strength of the static magnetic field. It should also be kept in mind, however, that apparent windows in response can be the result of signal processing by the nervous system. The human ability to detect visible light, which constitutes a narrow frequency window between the IR and UV wavelengths, is only one example of such processing. A special case of the purely magnetic effect that has recently received increased attention, that involving the magnetic material magnetite, is discussed in greater detail next.

A. Other Possible Physical Bases for EMF Detection

Magnetite is an inorganic iron compound, normally crystalline in form, that is either synthesized or sequestered by a number of animal species. Interaction of this magnetic material with the geomagnetic fields is known, or believed, to be important in adaptation strategies of several organisms, ranging from magnetotactic bacteria to certain migratory birds. Observation of magnetite crystals in the human brain by J. L. Kirschvink and coworkers has turned attention to the possibility that certain EMF-induced biological effects may be mediated by this compound. The hypothesis that magnetite is involved in detection of magnetic fields impinging on the organism is attractive because it circumvents many of the theoretical objections raised to interactions of magnetic fields with otherwise nonmagnetic (diamagnetic) biological tissue (121). Depending on the length and shape of the crystals, it is possible for them to experience a torque in weak magnetic fields in the same way that a compass needle aligns itself along the geomagnetic field lines of force. In higher animals, it is presumed that this motion may be detected within the cell or groups of cells and result in a signal, perhaps neurological, to which the animal may respond.

B. Free Radical Mechanisms

Several investigators have proposed that magnetic fields may interact with free radicals in tissue to slow their recombination rates (117). As an example of magnetic-field

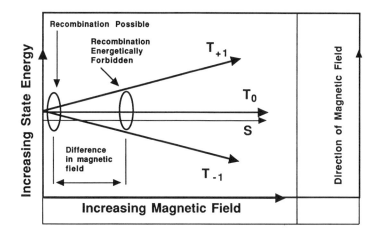

FIGURE 7. Diagram shows effect of magnetic field on the energy of triplet states. In the T_o state wherein spins are antiparallel, the field has no effect. For parallel spin triplet states, presence of the field reduces the number of potential free radical reaction partners by separating these states in energy. Matched spin pairs gain or lose energy compared to the T_o and singlet (S) states, depending on whether their projection in the direction of the incident magnetic field is additive or subtractive. [Adapted from K. McLauchlan, *Physics World (UK)*, Jan., 1 (1992).]

effects on free radical reactions, McLauchlan (117) cited the ability of a 60-Hz magnetic field to modulate free radical–dependent fluorescence from the reaction of pyrene with dicyanobenzene. Spins of unpaired electrons from the radicals interact with the magnetic field, yielding additional states (Figure 7). Splitting of the triplet states by the magnetic field reduces the concentration of potential recombination partners and thus slows the rate at which free radicals recombine to form neutral molecules.

In and of themselves, magnetic-field interactions with free radicals do not raise the theoretical objections based on thermodynamic considerations that have been cited against postulated effects on neutral molecules or alkali metal ions. Splitting of states is a low-energy process that simply interferes with recombination and prolongs the life of the free radical, a process normally measured in nanoseconds. Except as they may influence the concentrations of free radical precursors in solution, magnetic fields do not influence the formation of free radicals, and therefore their net effect may be to slightly increase concentrations of these species in biological tissue.

Stevens *et al.* (122) proposed that EMF exposure may affect cancer risk via free radical–dependent mechanisms. These authors noted that the presence of oxygen free radicals in cells increases oxidative stress and that EMF exposure may lead to increased free radical concentrations by interfering with calcium-dependent scavenging mechanisms. Free radical species are reactive and are known to be important as chemical cancer promoters (123). Compounds that scavenge oxygen free radicals, such as vitamins E and C, have been shown to be protective against cancers induced by DMBA. For a review of free radical and oxidative stress effects on cell growth and cancer in the context of EMF exposure, see Pascoe (124).

XI. CONCLUDING NOTE

A number of epidemiologic studies have shown an association between EMF exposure or exposure surrogates and increased risk for certain cancers. Whether this association represents a cause-and-effect linkage of EMF to cancer risk remains to be determined. Prospective epidemiologic studies, wherein field exposure is determined before occurrence of disease, are currently being planned or are under way. Because EMF exposures preceding diagnosis of the disease will be known in these studies instead of being inferred from later measurements, their outcome, whether positive or negative, will be important in eventually determining if a causal link exists between EMF exposure and cancer.

As determined by considering the time-weighted average exposure, the association between measured 60-Hz magnetic fields in residential studies and increased cancer risk is weak. Because of the absence of a strong correlation, and because occupational data have suggested that high-amplitude peak exposure, intermittent exposure, or exposure to fields with a high time rate of change or higher frequency components may better correlate with risk, interest in developing exposure metrics to take account of these latter characteristics for fields found in the environment has increased. Such exposure metrics reflect the assumption that induced currents are important in determining dose and are designed to quantify field attributes that relate most to change in the magnetic field flux density.

EMF exposure cannot cause direct chemical damage to the genome. However, studies both *in vitro* and *in vivo* have shown that weak electric and magnetic fields can interact with biological systems. Mechanisms for these effects likely involve cell membrane and second-messenger systems, and therefore could contribute to increased cancer risk via epigenetic processes. One epigenetic mechanism for which there is now support from both laboratory and epidemiologic data is the reduction of pineal melatonin secretion by exposure to EMF. On the basis of animal models and human studies, melatonin appears to be protective against many of the cancers associated with EMF exposure in epidemiologic studies.

Cell studies have provided evidence that EMF exposure may affect gene transcription and translation. Findings of alterations in NAT enzyme activity in animal studies are consistent with such effects. Recent reports indicate that EMF effects may extend to the expression of oncogenes or proto-oncogenes in certain cell types. Study of EMF effects on cellular regulatory mechanisms and gene expression promises to be a fruitful area for gaining knowledge of EMF interactions as well as gene function. Research in these areas must include repetition of critical findings to verify the existence of gene expression effects. These observations should then be extended to define the biological parameters necessary for the effects. To determine the link between these effects and cancer risk, cellular studies will likely require the development of new model systems; an ability to progress from cellular work to tissues and finally whole animals will be a key for this next generation of cellular tools.

Laboratory and clinical studies have demonstrated that EMF fields can interact with biological systems to affect cell growth and various neuroendocrine endpoints. There is not yet, however, much direct evidence for an effect on cancer risk. With few exceptions, the most relevant studies are those that tested fields as tumor promoters or co-promoters. EMF exposure has been reported to enhance onset of skin cancer (initiation with DMBA and promotion with TPA) and breast cancer (after initiation with DMBA or with NMU).

Induced current models for the interaction of EMF with biological systems are consistent with many of the data from clinical studies on bone healing, as well as with a variety of *in vitro* studies designed to directly determine if electrical currents were the active attribute of the fields. This model should be seriously considered where epidemiology has suggested an association between exposure and disease in environments in which strong or rapidly time-varying magnetic fields may be found.

It appears likely that more than one mechanism for the transduction of the EMF signals by biological systems will eventually emerge, as it is unlikely that a single mechanism could account for the various EMF effects in a variety of animals and over the wide range of field strengths and frequencies for which such effects have been observed.

Increased research in the area of EMF effects on biological systems is being driven by economic necessity as well as the possible health effects issue. Future research should concentrate on improved understanding of mechanisms, with the objective of determining what constitutes dose. Regardless of whether any increased cancer risk is eventually causally linked to EMF exposure, this research will provide valuable knowledge regarding biological responses to the changes made by man in his EMF environment.

ACKNOWLEDGMENT

This work was supported in part by the U.S. Department of Energy under contract DE-AC06-76RLO 1830.

REFERENCES

1. Wertheimer, N., and Leeper, E. L.: *Am. J. Epidemiol.* **109,** 273 (1979).
2. Savitz, D. A., Wachtel, H. A., Barnes, F., John, E. M., and Tvrdik, J. G.: *Am. J. Epidemiol.* **128,** 21 (1988).
3. Demers, P. A., Thomas,. D. B., Rosenblatt, K. A., Jimenez, L. M., McTiernan, A., Stalsberg, H., Stemhagen, A., Thompson, W. D., Curnen, M. G. M., Satariano, W., Audtin, D. F., Isacson, P., Greenberg, R. S., Key, C., Kolenel, L. N., and West, D. W.: *Am. J. Epidemiol.* **134,** 340 (1991).
4. London, S. J., Thomas, D. C., Bowman, J. D., Sobel, E., Cheng, T-C., and Peters, J. M.: *Am. J. Epidemiol.* **134,** 923 (1991).
5. Matanoski, G. M., Breysse, P. N., and Elliot, E. A.: *Lancet* **337,** 737 (1991).
6. d'Arsonval, A.: C. R. *Soc. Biol.* **3,** 451 (1896).
7. Tenforde, T. S.: Biological Responses to Static and Time-Varying Magnetic Fields. *In* "Electromagnetic Interaction with Biological Systems" (J. C. Lin, ed.). Plenum Press, New York, 1989, p. 83.
8. Tenforde, T. S.: *J. Electroanal. Chem.* **320,** 1 (1991).
9. Jaffe, R. A., Laszewski, B. L., Carr, D. B., and Phillips, R. D.: *Bioelectromagnetics* **1,** 131 (1979).
10. Bassett, C. A. L., Pilla, A. A., and Pawluk, R. J.: *Clin. Orthop.* **124,** 117 (1977).
11. Hajdukovic, R., Mitler, M. M., Pasch, B., and Erman, M.: *First World Congress for Electricity and Magnetism in Biology and Medicine, Lake Buena Vista, Florida, June 1992,* p. 92. (Abst.)
12. Kaune, W. T., and Anderson, L. E.: Physical Aspects of ELF Electric and Magnetic Fields: Measurement and Dosimetry. *In* "Extremely Low Frequency Electromagnetic Fields: The Question of Cancer" (B. W. Wilson, R. G. Stevens, and L. E. Anderson, eds.). Battelle Press, Columbus, Ohio, 1990, p. 17.
13. Kaune, W. T., Stevens, R. G., Callahan, N. J., Severson, R. K., and Thomas, D. B.: *Bioelectromagnetics* **8,** 315 (1987).
14. Adair, R. K.: *Phys. Rev.* A **43,** 1039 (1991).
15. Wiltschko, W., and Wiltschko, R.: Orientation by the Earth's Magnetic Field in Migrating Birds and Homing Pigeons. *In* "Progress in Biometeorology," Vol. 8, Effects of Atmospheric and Geophysical Variables in Biology and Medicine (H. Lieth, ed.). SPB Academic Publishing, The Hague, Netherlands, 1991, p. 31.
16. Florig, H. K., and Holberg, J. F.: *Health Phys.* **58,** 493 (1990).
17. Savitz, D. A., John, E. M., and Kleckner, R. C. *Am. J. Epidemiol.* **131,** 763 (1990).
18. Verreault, R., Weiss, N. S., and Hollenbach, K. A.: *Am. J. Epidemiol.* **131,** 759 (1990).
19. Vena, J. E., Graham, S., Hellmann, R., Swanson, M., and Brasure, J.: *Am. J. Epidemiol.* **132,** 791 (1990).
20. Wilson, B. W., Wright, C. W., Morris, J. E., Buschbom, R. L., Brown, D. P., Miller, D. L., Sommers-Flannigan, R., and Anderson, L. E.: *J. Pineal Res.* **9,** 259 (1990).
21. Bowman, J. D., Garabrant, D. H., Sobel, E., and Peters, J. M.: *Appl. Ind. Hyg.* **3,** 189 (1988).
22. Savitz, D. A., and Calle, E. E.: *J. Occup. Med.* **29,** 47 (1987).
23. Deadman, J. E., Camus, M., Armstrong, B. G., Héroux, P., Cyr, D., Plante, M., and Thériault, G.: *Am. Ind. Hyg. Assoc. J.* **49,** 409 (1988).
24. Lin, R., Dischinger, P. C., Conde, J., and Farrell, K. P.: *J. Occup. Med.* **217,** 413 (1985).
25. Speers, M. A., Dobbins, J. G., and Miller, V. S.: *Am. J. Ind. Med.* **13,** 629 (1988).
26. Pearce, N. E., Reif, J., and Frazer, J.: *Int. J. Epidemiol.* **18,** 55 (1989).

27. Mack, W., Preston-Martin, S., and Peters, J.: *Bioelectromagnetics* **12**, 57 (1991).
28. Gilman, P. A., Ames, R. G., and McCawley, A.: *J. Occup. Med.* **27**, 669 (1985).
29. Flodin, U., Fredrickson, M., Axelson, O., Persson, B., and Hardell, L.: *Arch. Environ. Health* **41**, 77 (1986).
30. Coggon, D., Pannet, B., Osmond, C., and Acheson, E. D.: *Br. J. Ind. Med.* **43**, 381 (1986).
31. Garland, F. C., Shaw, E., Gorham, E. D., Garland, C. F., White, M. R., and Sinsheimer, P. J.: *Am. J. Epidemiol.* **132**, 293 (1990).
32. Milham, S.: "Occupational Mortality in Washington State 1950–1971," Publication #76-175-A, B, C. National Institute for Occupational Safety and Health (NIOSH), Washington, D.C., 1976.
33. Davis, R. L., and Milham, S.: *Am. J. Ind. Hyg.* **18**, 79 (1990).
34. Spinelli, J., Band, P., Gallagher, R., Oleniuk, D., and Svirchev, L.: "Mortality and Cancer Incidence in Workers at the ALCAN Aluminum Plant in Kitimat, B.C. Final Report." Cancer Control Agency of British Columbia, Vancouver, 1989.
35. Mikhail, E. L., and Fam, W. Z.: *First World Congress for Electricity and Magnetism in Biology and Medicine, Lake Buena Vista, Florida, June 1992*, p. 28. (Abst.)
36. Gatti, R. A., and Good, R. A.: *Cancer (Philadelphia)* **28**, 89 (1971).
37. Lyle, D. B., Wang, X., Ayotte, R. D., Sheppard, A. R., and Adey, W. R.: *Bioelectromagnetics* **12**, 145 (1991).
38. Stevens, R. G.: *Am. J. Epidemiol.* **125**, 556 (1987).
39. Stevens, R. G., Davis, S., Thomas, D. B., Anderson, L. E., and Wilson, B. W.: *FASEB J.* **6**, 853 (1992).
40. Tynes, T., and Anderson, A.: *Lancet* **336**, 1596 (1990).
41. Matanoski, G. M.: *Environmental Update, September 1991*. Electric Power Research Institute, Palo Alto, California, 1991, p. 5. (Abst.)
42. Vagero, D., Ahlbom, A., Olin, R., and Sahlsten, S.: *Br. J. Ind. Med.* **42**, 191 (1985).
43. Vagero, D., Swerdlow, A. J., and Beral, V.: *Br. J. Indust. Med.* **47**, 317 (1990).
44. De Guire, L., Theriault, G., Iturra, H., Provenhers, S., Cyr, D., and Case, B. W.: *Br. J. Ind. Med.* **45**, 824 (1988).
45. Swerdlow, A. J.: *Am. J. Epidemiol.* **118**, 317 (1983).
46. Gallagher, R. P., Elwood, J. M., Rootman, J., Spinelli, J. J., Hill, G. B., Threlfall, W. J., and Birdsell, J. M.: *J. Natl. Cancer Inst.* **74**, 775 (1985).
47. Swerdlow, A. J.: *Ann. N.Y. Acad. Sci.* **609**, 235 (1990).
48. Walborg, E. F.: "Extremely Low Frequency Electromagnetic Fields and Cancer: Focus on Tumor Initiation, Promotion, and Progression". National Electrical Manufacturer's Association, Washington, D.C., 1991.
49. Theriault, G.: Health Effects of Electromagnetic Radiation on Workers: Epidemiologic Studies. *Proceedings of Scientific Workshop on Health Effects of Electromagnetic Radiation on Workers*. NIOSH, U.S. Department of Health and Human Services, Washington, D.C., 1991.
50. Cohen, S. M., and Ellwein, L. B.: *Cancer Res.* **51**, 6493 (1991).
51. Reese, J., Jostes, R., and Frazier, M. E.: *Bioelectromagnetics* **9**, 237 (1988).
52. Cohen, M. M., Kunska, A., Astemborski, J. A., McCulloch, D., and Paskewitz, D. A.: *Bioelectromagnetics* **7**, 415 (1986).
53. Rosenthal, M., and Obe, G.: *Mutat. Res.* **210**, 329 (1989).
54. Scarfi, M. R., Bersani, F., Cossarizza, A., Monti, D., Castellani, G., Cadosi, R., Franceschetti, G., and Franceschi, C.: *Biochem. Biophys. Res. Commun.* **176**, 194 (1991).
55. Cossarizza, A., Monti, D., Sola, P., Moschini, G., Cadossi, R., Bersani, F., and Franceschi, C.: *Radiat. Res.* **118**, 161 (1989).
56. Frazier, M. E., Reese, J. A., Morris, J. E., Jostes, R. F., and Miller, D. L.: *Bioelectromagnetics* **11**, 229 (1990).
57. Akamine, T., Muramatsu, H., Hamada, H., and Sakou T.: *J. Cell Physiol.* **124**, 247 (1985).
58. Phillips, J. L., Winters, W. D., and Rutledge, L.: *Int. J. Radiat. Biol.* **49**, 463 (1986).
59. Cossarizza, A., Monti, D., Besani, F., Cantini, M., Cadossi, R., and Sacchi, A.: *Biochem. Biophys. Res. Commun.* **160**, 692 (1989).
60. Cleary, S. F., Liu, L-M., Graham, R., and Diegelmann, R. F.: *Bioelectromagnetics* **9**, 183 (1988).
61. Farndale, R. W., and Murray, J. C.: *Calcif. Tissue Int.* **37**, 78 (1985).
62. Liboff, A. R., Williams, T., Strong, D. M., and Wistar, R.: *Science* **223**, 818 (1986).
63. Takahashi, K., Kaneko, I., Date, M., and Fukada, E.: *Experientia (Basel)* **42**, 185 (1986).
64. Goodman, R., Bassett, C. A. L., and Henderson, A.: *Science* **220**, 1283 (1983).
65. Goodman, R., and Henderson, A. S.: *Bioelectrochem. Bioenerg.* **15**, 39 (1986).
66. Goodman, R., and Henderson, A. S.: *Bioelectromagnetics* **7**, 23 (1986).
67. Goodman, R., and Henderson, A. S.: *J. Bioelectricity* **6**, 37 (1987).
68. Phillips, J. L.: Effects of Electromagnetic Field Exposure in Gene Transcription. *J. Cell. Biochem.* **51**, 381 (1993).

69. Phillips, J. L., and McChesney, L.: *Cancer Biochem. Biophys.* **12**, 1 (1991).
70. Greene, J. J., Skowronski, W. J., Mullins, J. M., and Nardone, R. M.: *Biochem. Biophys. Res. Commun.* **174**, 742 (1991).
71. Goodman, R., Abbott, J., and Henderson, A. S.: *Bioelectromagnetics* **8**, 1 (1987).
72. Goodman, R., and Shirley-Henderson, A.: *Bioelectrochem. Bioenerg.* **25**, 335 (1991).
73. Goodman, R., Wei, L-X., Xu, J-C., and Henderson, A.: *Biochim. Biophys. Acta* **1009**, 216 (1989).
74. Wei, L-W., Goodman, R., and Henderson, A.: *Bioelectromagnetics* **11**, 269 (1990).
75. Czerska, E., Casamento, J., Davis, C., Elson, E., Ning, J., and Swicord, M.: Effects of ELF on c-*myc* Oncogene Expression in Normal and Transformed Human Cells. *In* "Proceedings of the 1992 IEEE 18th Annu. Northeast Bioengineering Conference" (W. J. Ohley, ed.). IEEE, New York, 1993, p. 61.
76. Phillips, J. L., Haggren, W., Thomas, W. J., Ishida-Jones, T., and Adey, W. R.: *Biochim. Biophys. Acta* **1132**, 140 (1992).
77. Fitzsimmons, R., Strong, D., Mohan, S., and Baylink, D. J.: *J. Cell. Physiol.* **150**, 84 (1992).
78. Goodman, R., and Henderson, A. S.: *Proc. Natl. Acad. Sci. U.S.A.* **85**, 3928 (1988).
79. Murray, J. C., and Farndale, R. W. *Biochim. Biophys. Acta* **838**, 98 (1985).
80. Byus, C. V., Pieper, S. E., and Adey, W. R.: *Carcinogenesis* **8**, 1385 (1987).
81. Litovitz, T. A., Krause, D., and Mullins, J. M.: *Biochem. Biophys. Res. Commun.* **178**, 862 (1991).
82. Bawin, S. M., and Adey, W. R.: *Proc. Natl. Acad. Sci. U.S.A.* **73**, 1999 (1976).
83. Blackman, C. F., Benane, S. G., House, D. E., and Joines, W. T.: *Bioelectromagnetics* **6**, 1 (1985).
84. Blackman, C. F., Benane, S. G., Rabinowitz, J. R., House, D. E., and Joines, W. T.: *Bioelectromagnetics* **6**, 327 (1985).
85. Carson, J., Prato, F. S., Drost, D. J., Diesbourg, L. D., and Dixon, S. J.: *Am. J. Physiol.* **259**, C687 (1990).
86. Yost, M. G., and Liburdy, R. P.: *FEBS Lett.* **296**, 117 (1992).
87. Liburdy, R. P.: *FEBS Lett.* **301**, 53 (1992).
88. Luben, R. A., Cain, C. D., Chen, M. C-Y., Rosen, D. M., and Adey, W. R.: *Proc. Natl. Acad. Sci. U.S.A.* **79**, 4180 (1982).
89. Cain, C. D., Adey, W. R., and Luben, R. A.: *J. Bone Miner. Res.* **2**, 437 (1987).
90. Bell, G. B., Marino, A. A., Chesson, A. L, and Struve, F. A.: *Lancet* **338**, 251 (1991).
91. Graham, C., Cohen, H. D., Cook, M. R., Gerkovich, M. M., Riffle, D. R., and Hoffman, S. J.: *Proceedings of the Annual Meeting of the Bioelectromagnetic Society, June 23–27, 1991,*, p. 54. (Abst.)
92. McLean, J. R. N., Stuchly, M. A., Mitchel, R. E. J., Wilkinson, D., Yang, H., Goddard, D. W., Lecuyer, D. W., Schunk, M., Callary, E., and Morrison, D.: *Bioelectromagnetics* **12**, 272 (1991).
93. McLean, J. R. N., Thansandote, A., Stuchly, M. A., Goddard, D. W., Barnett, D., Lecuyer, D. W., and Mitchel, R. E. J.: *First World Congress for Electricity and Magnetism in Biology and Medicine, Lake Buena Vista, Florida, June 1992*, p. 107. (Abst.)
94. Wilson, B. W., Anderson, L. E., Hilton, D. I., and Phillips, R. D.: *Bioelectromagnetics* **2**, 371 (1981).
95. Welker, H. A., Semm, P., Willig, R. P., Commentz, J. C., Wiltschko, W., and Vollrath, L.: *Exp. Brain Res.* **50**, 426 (1983).
96. Georgiou, E.: *Z. Krebsforsch.* **38**, 562 (1929).
97. Buswell, R. S.: *Lancet* ii, 134 (1975).
98. Blask, D. E., Hill, S. M., and Pelletier, D. B.: Oncostatic Signaling by the Pineal Gland and Melatonin in the Control of Breast Cancer. *In* "The Pineal Gland and Cancer" (T. K. Das Gupta, A. Attanasio, and R. J. Reiter, eds.). Brain Research Promotion, London, 1988, p. 195.
99. Buzzell, G. R., Amerongon, H. M., and Toma, J. G.: Melatonin and the Growth of Duning R3327 Rat Prostatic Adenocarcinoma. *In* "The Pineal Gland and Cancer" (T. K. Das Gupta, A. Attanasio, and R. J. Reiter, eds.). Brain Research Promotion, London, 1988, p. 295.
100. Maestroni, G. J. M., and Conti, A.: *Immunology* **63**, 465 (1988).
101. Maestroni, G. J. M., Conti, A., and Pierpaoli, W.: *J. Neuroimmunol.* **13**, 19 (1986).
102. Semm, P., Schneider, T., and Vollrath, L.: *Nature (London)* **288**, 607 (1980).
103. Olcese, J., Reuss, S., and Semm, P.: *Life Sci.* **42**, 605 (1988).
104. Wilson, B. W., Anderson, L. E., Hilton, D. I., and Hewett, S.: *Bioelectromagnetics* **1**, 195 (1980).
105. Yellon, S. M.: An Acute 60-Hz Magnetic Field Exposure Suppresses the Nighttime Melatonin Rise in the Pineal and Circulation of the Adult Djungarian Hamster. *Annual Review of Research on Biological Effects of 50 and 60 Hz Electric and Magnetic Fields,* Milwaukee, Wisconsin, 1991, p. A-25. (Abstr. A-25)
106. Lerchl, A., Nonaka, K. O., and Reiter, R. J.: *J. Pineal Res.* **10**, 109 (1991).
107. Wilson, B. W., Stevens, R. G., and Anderson, L. E.: *Life Sci.* **45**, 319 (1989).
108. Leung, F. C., Rommereim, D. N., Stevens, R. G., Wilson, B. W., Buschbom, R. L., and Anderson, L. E.: *10th Annual Meeting of the Bioelectromagnetics Society,* June 1988, pp. 2-3 (Abstracts).
109. Wilson, B. W., Lueng, F., Buschbom, R., Stevens, R. G., Anderson, L. E., and Reiter, R. J.: Electric Fields, the Pineal Gland and Cancer. *In* "The Pineal Gland and Cancer" (T. K. Das Gupta, A. Attanasio, and R. J. Reiter, eds.). Brain Research Promotion, London, 1988, p. 245.

110. Beniashvili, D., Vilanishvili, V. G., and Manabde, M. Z.: *Cancer Lett.* **61,** 75 (1991).

111. Cook, M. R., Graham, C., Cohen, H. D., and Gerkovich, M. M.: *Bioelectromagnetics* **13,** 261 (1992).

112. Cotman, C. W., Brinton, R. E., Calaburda, A., McEwen, B., and Schneider, D. M.: "The Neuro-Immune-Endocrine Connection." Raven Press, New York, 1987.

113. Pilla, A. A.: *Ann. N.Y. Acad. Sci.* **238,** 149 (1974).

114. Adey, W. R.: *Neurochem. Res.* **13,** 671 (1988).

115. Weaver, J. C., and Astumian, R. D.: *Science* **247,** 459 (1990).

116. Kirschvink, J. L.: *Bioelectromagnetics* **10,** 239 (1989).

117. McLauchlan, K.: *Physics World* (*UK*) Jan. 1 (1992).

118. Fitton-Jackson, S., and Bassett, C. A. L.: The Response of Skeletal Tissue to Pulsed Magnetic Fields. *In* "Tissue Culture in Medical Research II" (R. J. Richard and K. T. Rajan, eds.). Pergamon Press, London, 1985, p. 21.

119. Walker, M. M., and Bitterman, M. E.: *J. Exp. Biol.* **145,** 489 (1989).

120. Kirschvink, J. L. and Kobayashi-Kirschvink, A.: *Am. Zool.* **31,** 169 (1991).

121. Kirschvink, J. L., and Kobayashi-Kirschvink, A.: *First World Congress for Electricity and Magnetism in Biology and Medicine, Lake Buena Vista, Florida, June 1992,* p. 13. (Abstr.)

122. Stevens, R. G., Wilson, B. W., and Anderson, L. E.: The Question of Cancer. *In* "Extremely Low Frequency Electromagnetic Fields: The Question of Cancer" (B. W. Wilson, R. G. Stevens, and L. E. Anderson, eds.). Battelle Press, Columbus, Ohio, 1990, p. 361.

123. Slaga, T. J., Klein-Szanto, A. J. P., Triplett, L. L., Yotti, L. P., and Trosko, J. E.: *Science* **213,** 1023 (1981).

124. Pascoe, G. A.: Calcium Homeostasis and Oxidative Stress *In* "Extremely Low Frequency Electromagnetic Fields: The Question of Cancer" (B. W. Wilson, R. G. Stevens, and L. E. Anderson, eds.). Battelle Press, Columbus, Ohio, 1990, p. 337.

Postscriptum: An Editor's Musings

The endeavor of bringing forth this volume received the visitation of an undue share of reverses and misfortunes, probably unknown in the *Annals of Editors' Odyssean Adventures*. The aim of this Postscriptum is to convey to the reader the unique "bittersweet flavor" of the editorial production of this book.

We, the Editors, were of course prepared to face and accept the "fact of life" that in our era *very few* authors (if any) deliver manuscripts on time. Because of the often conflicting obligations/commitments, complexities, and hurry in the lives of most scientists, timely delivery has become an almost inexistent, but cherished rarity—almost as rare as members of the now extinct species: the dodo. As we all know, self-imposed extensions of deadlines of several months, even up to a year (or more), are now common; this is a limiting factor which can become critical with a multiauthor book of this diversity and complexity. Also rare—by the way—are reference lists that are complete/spotlessly correct, as well as texts that are polished to a literary "high gloss". Yet the latter is of importance in the pursuit of Quality, where Form is inseparable from Essence.

To deal with these occurrences and to keep our task manageable we have developed a special literary style for effectively communicating with the laggards; we have termed this style, appropriate for such occasions, "impassioned plea". For those readers who wish to develop proficiency in this essential editorial style of letter-writing, we summarize here its main components: pathos, in the best tradition of the great Greek orators of antiquity; a sonorous call to the sense of civic duty as behooves a responsible member of the scientific community (devotion to Commitment, Deadline, and Peer Approval); an analysis of well-understood self-interest (of the authors', of course) heralding the benefits of their contributions to their careers and CVs—by brazenly promoting the value and merits of the book you are editing; and last, but not least, throwing yourself at their generosity and abjectly begging their understanding and mercy.

The necessity, indeed the requirement, that we do *in fact* obtain a chapter on *all* topics (as they now actually occur in the volume) devolved from the integrated, multidisciplinary character of the book. We felt that *all* factors/parameters must be represented without fail, and cross-referenced, in order to convey the vast and complete panorama of their (often interacting) influences on the chemical induction of cancer. Thus, unlike when gathering chapters for conference proceedings—where some invited contributions may be omitted/dropped from the Contents if manuscript delivery lags far behind a coordinated deadline—we felt we must ensure the presence of *all* chapters so as to avoid "mutilating" the essential nature/aim of this book. Considerable editorial and author effort was devoted to maintaining the up-to-dateness of all chapters during this lengthy struggle toward "seamless" continuity of acquisitioning and editing the chapters.

As the reader can see by now, we can be deemed to be reasonably well qualified for encounters with some hazards of editorial life—perhaps even greater than usual. But we could not foresee nor did we expect to be faced with the literary equivalents of the Four Horsemen of the Apocalypse: death, fire, breach of contract, and plagiarism. These and some Dragons related thereto are acid tests of an editor's mettle, but are also mileposts of forewarning to those who—perhaps not finding enough courage in their hearts—are not prepared to take up the sword to overcome and valiantly slay these creatures. This real-life imagery and the sketch below of a sampling of the factual events that occurred are presented to convey a sense of the obstacles that had to be actually faced and overcome during the production of this book.

First Horseman. At the beginning of this endeavor, sometime in early 1990, we had invited a prominent colleague—head of a well-known cancer institute abroad—to contribute a chapter in his scientific specialty. We were elated that he saw so much promise and importance in the design of the contents of the book that, on his own initiative, he proposed to commit several members of his institute to also cover additional chapters beyond the invited one. Alas, several months later we received the sad news of his sudden death from the senior member of the team of investigators in the institute (who had accepted the collective commitment). This senior member made a strong point to emphatically reassure us that—with the concurence of the newly-appointed acting head of the institute—the group's commitment for the writing of all those chapters did hold and that he would act as the liaison/coordinator between the group (his colleagues) and us, the Editors. Months then passed with periodic contacts between the group/the coordinator and us, and we were pleased with the assurances from them of the timely progress of the writings. One year passed. Since we still did not see any tangible evidence of actual chapters, we became—understandably—alarmed, and with this state of mind grew the frequency of our communications with them. We were then just a few months before the end of the second year and the thickness of the correspondence file (letters, FAXes, and phone conversation summaries) had grown to well over 1 inch. We felt we had no alternative but to impose a truly ultimate deadline—the end of the second year. The deadline came and the deadline passed: no manuscript(s), but neither any explanation. However, a totally unanticipated type of reply came to our pressing, strong letter: the reply (by FAX) contained a kind of apology, explaining that because of the vacation from which they were just returning, they were unable to deliver the manuscripts; we were being "assured", however, that at least two completed chapters were being edited by the acting head of the institute. Our utter dismay over their cavalier unreliability was expressed in no uncertain terms in our last letter to the group, in which letter we formally withdrew the invitation. Lo and behold, we were then entertained by them with what may be euphemistically seen as a display of *humeur noire*: they were *demanding* an apology from us (an unfulfilled dream, of course). We were, thus, back to ground zero with those chapters.

The heavy hand of the Angel of Death interfering in the fate of this endeavor was also seen in another chapter. This interference took the form of banishment of the most basic common sense, by bereavement. The writing of one chapter (on a biological parameter that modulates carcinogenesis) was being prepared by a colleague uniquely reputed in his area. This colleague also had a solid reputation for taking seriously his writing commitments, and we were pleased that he was truly enthusiastic about his forthcoming chapter. To assist his writing we supplemented his files with our extensive reprint collection in this area, beginning in about 1950. We knew that he was in remission from cancer; however, his remission appeared to hold since he had been able to undertake an extended visit to his country of origin in Europe. Because of his reputation of reliability we contacted him only twice, early during the year following our invitation to him. We received a shock in discovering late in the year a note in *Science* about his death, that occurred 2 months prior. We immediately contacted his spouse, only to learn the totally incredible fact that she had discarded all of his "old" reprints at home as well as the "papers" he had been working on, so as to make space for his "belongings" that she was pressed to remove from his institutional office he had occupied for close to 30 years.

Second Horseman. This undertaking also received two visitations from the Spirit of Fire. The more spectacular of these two was a forest fire in the West which threatened to engulf the home of one of our chapters' senior author. The prospect of the flames coming up the mountain necessitated the removal of all of the family's belongings from the home and their living on a houseboat for the weeks it took to bring the fire under control and to make the terrain passable again. Owing perhaps to the protective intercession of the Editors' Guardian Angel, the fire slowed down and was brought under control less than 50 feet from the house. The writing was delayed substantially, however, by this violence of the Spirit of Fire.

A Dragon, as per Introduction to the Third Horseman. There were two instances of "change of heart", where authors — committed in writing — later withdrew their commitments. The more interesting of the two involved one of the largest chapters and represents a textbook example of "Commitment by Relay", in the tradition of the Olympic runners carrying the torch. Our first author designate (Author A) withdrew the commitment after seven months, citing unforeseen family and professional obligations; fortunately, the collection of reprints and books supplied by us were returned expeditiously and were actually supplemented by more recent literature material from that colleague's files. Through consultation with several friends in the field we were able to identify a new presumptive author for the writing of the chapter. Upon contacting him (Author B), he readily and enthusiastically accepted the invitation and we then forwarded to him the enlarged literature files ("passing the torch") that had been returned to us by Author A. Lo and behold, the story does not end here, as we soon experienced an almost exact repetition of what happened with Author A. After about 10 months Author B withdrew his commitment, citing unforeseen professional obligations (dealing with research funding problems, in particular). Our tribulations at the hands of Author B did not end there, however, as we experienced difficulties having him return the literature files; in fact, we had to request the intercession of the colleagues who had recommended him to us. When the three packages containing the files were finally returned, we noticed that our original packing boxes had never been opened; Author B simply placed new address labels over the old labels for returning the packages. By repeating the search process again, we finally located our third — true — author designate (Author C) who abided by his commitment and brought the writing of the chapter to a good ending.

How little did we know that this series of withdrawals of commitment — painful as it was — was only a foretaste of the poisonous gift of the third horseman.

Third Horseman. By early spring of 1993 the entire book manuscript was ready for copyediting and typesetting. It was forwarded to what was at that time the Michigan-based division of a large Florida-headquartered scientific publisher (other than the original publisher of the previous volumes of the series) with which we had signed a Memorandum of Agreement. We were complimented on the care that went into the preparation of the manuscript, and also on its completeness and organization; the manuscript was essentially ready for production. After the usual preproduction checking and preliminary production-cost appraisal of newly acquisitioned book manuscripts, the entire manuscript file was transferred to headquarters where the corporation's editorial/ production facilities are located.

A production editor was assigned to the manuscript, and, as usual, extensive phone and correspondence contacts developed between the production editor and ourselves, establishing the general layout (2- *versus* 1-column page), typeface, headings, and other elements of book production style. Copyediting had begun; chapters of the copyedited manuscript were sent periodically to us with queries and for final approval. At about midcourse of this activity the final price of the book, to which our input was requested, was established. By the end of the copyediting stage we had arrived at a mutually agreed-upon production style. We were informed early fall that typesetting had begun.

In November of 1993, in mid-production, an unexpected shock descended upon us from a seemingly cloudless sky. We received a curt letter from the head of the Michigan-based corporate division, accompanied by a copy of an internal memo from headquarters to the division, informing us that the book is too long for them to realize any profit on the venture. The publisher gave us a choice: either shorten the manuscript by about 40% or find another publisher!

This flagrant breach of contract presented us with an impossible dilemma. To shorten the manuscript to that extent at this late date, was clearly a scientific and organizational impossibility. In addition, we felt we had a responsibility toward all the colleagues we had invited to author the chapters. Also, we were not prepared to lend our names to a book — stripped of any meaningful aim and coherence by the removal of integral parts of the text — just for the sake of producing another title. Thus, we felt we had no other choice but to seek a new publisher. However, the return of the manuscript, of the word processing disks thereof, most importantly of the original artwork of the illustrations, as well as the issuance by the publisher of the formal copyright release were not forthcoming. We had to seek and retain the services of a Florida-based forceful civil trial lawyer to recover/obtain these materials. We are grateful to our friend, Hank H. Gosch, for his help at this critical juncture of the endeavor in finding the right attorney for us and in establishing contact.

Peering into the misty infinity of probabilities, it may be a poetic fancy to believe that, with Birkhäuser (Springer International) as our new publisher, events have come full circle. This is how these events appear to the editor, JCA, to whom a particular Birkhäuser publication, in Switzerland, at the early stage of his scientific career [the reference (*Progr. Drug. Res.*, Vol. 4, E. Jucker, ed., Basel, 1962, pp. 407–581) at the end of the "theme quotation", in the front of the volume] bears a special significance. Harriet D. Shields acted as the indispensable catalyst for closing the circle by mediating our contact with Birkhäuser publishers. Actually, all volumes of this series, beginning with Volume I in 1968, bear the mark of her editorial coordination and oversight.

By late spring of 1994 the manuscript of this volume was typeset, and proofreading was started in early June.

Fourth Horseman. One late afternoon, at the end of summer in 1994, we were proofreading a large segment of the typeset text. This was a large chapter, and a scientifically complex one, so we had intentionally scheduled the proofreading of this chapter to the end. The Editors chose to proofread the entire typeset text of the book themselves, rather than returning each chapter to its author(s). While this was a somewhat grueling task, we felt that this was the only way that we could ensure uniformity of style and format throughout the book, note so far undetected spots where cross-referencing with other chapters might be needed, and perhaps even uncover unforeseen shortcomings.

As the story below demonstrates, this 3-month effort vastly justified itself. But, unknowing of what lay ahead, we were already savoring in our minds the end of our efforts – and the ensuing peace and relaxation – to complete the reading of the entire typeset proof for its return to the editorial coordinator.

This chapter was one of those which required substantial editing input. The author – a well-established name in the literature of this field and prominent in the scientific establishment in his country in Europe – overreached himself and submitted a manuscript that when typeset would have been almost twice as long as his allotted space in the book. The chapter was clearly in need of condensation. There were also some unusual turns in his use of the English language which needed editing. Because of the substantial editorial input to this chapter we were especially careful about the proofreading of the manuscript.

At some point during the proofreading of the pages, the need arose to verify a minor point in the terminology of that field. One of the Editors raised the point that our input into the revision/condensation of the manuscript could have introduced a terminological error at that particular spot. Two years earlier, at a FASEB meeting, we had purchased a highly-regarded fundamental textbook of that field, in anticipation of this chapter that we knew we would have to editorially evaluate and possibly process. As it will become evident below, it must have been the Editors' Guardian Angel who guided our decision to acquire *that particular* textbook. The verification of this minor terminological issue was the occasion of our first use of the textbook.

While verifying the terminology at that spot we immediately noticed the identity of wording in the texts of the typeset chapter and of the textbook. Our unbelieving eyes noted this exact identity not only in the text but also of the subtitles above and below that paragraph. Seized by a terrible premonition we then systematically compared the author's original manuscript to all topic-relevant chapters in the textbook. We discovered to our utter horror that the "author" of the chapter had plagiarized verbatim close to 90% of "his" manuscript from the textbook. It became clear then that the unusual turns in the use of the English language (mentioned above) introduced by the "author" represented intentional changes in the text, bumbling attempts to "cover his tracks" at plagiarism. Copies of the author's original manuscript and of relevant chapters in the textbook were subsequently submitted to 6 colleagues at different research institutes for confirmation of this unethical (and inept) misdeed. Their depositions, confirming the plagiarism, in the form of formal letters of testimony, are on file. It is a point of humor that our "author" abroad, when confronted with his misdeed, voiced in his defense that we did not provide him with an "Instructions to Authors"! He did inform us later (by FAX) that he would feel "uncomfortable" if "his" article would actually be published.

With the discarding of this typeset (but clearly unusable) chapter we were then – as a few times before – back to ground zero and in the "manuscript-acquisitioning mode" rather than in our real role as editors. But again, we were fortunate enough – in the midst of our pains and tribulations – that we were soon able to locate well-established presumptive authors for the writing of a new chapter. Since we were "burned" before, we made it a point to fully disclose the true, tragicomic history of this chapter to the new authors and ascertain that they would be able to give a very high priority to the writing of the new chapter. At the time of drafting this Postscriptum the completed new chapter is being typeset, and the long and complex history of the editing and production of this book appears now to approach a successful ending.

Beyond the forty-seven authors who parented the different chapters, this book had, at various stages of its writing and editing, many "midwives" who have helped to bring the product of this undertaking into the light of existence. The contributions of the latter individuals – some of which were indispensable for the success of this endeavor – are credited in the Acknowledgments.

The over five years spent on the acquisitioning of the chapters/sections, on their editorial preparation to integrate them into a multidisciplinary volume—as well as on the actual authoring/coauthoring of some of the chapters and "Notes"—required, from the Editors, a level of effort and total dedication for which they feel the qualifier "enormous" is possibly an understatement. This is because the sheer magnitude of the task—intellectual and "diplomatic"—was often mingled with frustration, stress, desperation, and, on occasion, humiliation. A sampling of such occurrences has been briefly sketched above. For the editor, JCA, these five years have been unforgettable years of a singular trial which truly tested his determination, physical stamina, and common sense. Indeed, a number of times the very feasibility of the whole endeavor appeared to hang on a thread. So JCA wishes to recognize those who contributed, during all these years, essential ingredients to hold body and mind together: Jessica Abreu, for the delicious and wholesome meals, cheerfully adjusted to his special health and nutritional requirements, that she has catered; the members of the Mill Run Dulcimer Band, for the Earth-grounded, hauntingly beautiful melodies which so often helped him to overcome the blues of desperation and also provided a counterpoint to the more austere, majestic beauty of the vast science panorama unfolding in many of the chapters—as well as for their friendship; Lisa Candelario, for her friendship, love, and encouragement, and for her supportive reassurances—call it faith—that, against all odds, this undertaking *will* be brought to completion.

Labor Omnia Vincit

Index

A

A (Agouti) locus, influence on tumor development, 465

2-AAF, *see* 2-Acetylaminofluorene

2-Acetylaminofluorene

antagonism in chemical carcinogenesis involving, 26, 28, 29

carcinogenesis in rat by

effect of body weight loss on mammary gland, 290, 291

effect of copper on, 344, 346

effect of dietary protein level on mammary gland, 290

effect of dietary tryptophan level on bladder and mammary gland, 308

effect of lead on, 350

effect of selenium on, 337–340

effect of strains, 456

hormonal enhancement of, 432, 434

hepatocarcinogenesis by, additivity in, 162

syncarcinogenesis with

chemical agents, 26, 28, 39, 45

ionizing radiations, 501

N-Acetyl-*l*-cysteine, 81, 82, 100, 101

Acridine orange, antagonism in chemical carcinogenesis involving, 27

ACTH (corticotropin)

endocrine feedback control, role in, 415–417

secretion by hypophysis, 409, 410

ACTH-releasing hormone (CRH)

endocrine feedback control, role in, 416

hypothalamic regulation by, 409

Actinomycin D

antagonism in chemical carcinogenesis involving, 34, 35

syncarcinogenesis involving, 34, 35

Additivity in carcinogenesis by chemical combinations, definition of, 186

Adenohypophysis, *see* Hypophysis, anatomical structure and function

S-Adenosylethionine, hepatic, increase by dietary ethionine plus copper, 346

S-Adenosylmethionine (Ado Met)

decarboxylation of, 295, 297

propylamino group donor, role as, 295, 305

transmethylation reactions, role in, 295, 305

S-Adenosylmethionine decarboxylase, 295, 297

Adenoviruses, 512, 574–577

transforming proteins of, 522, 575, 576

link to tumor-suppressor genes, 576, 577

Ado Met, *see* *S*-Adenosylmethionine

Adrenal glands

anatomical structure and functions, 410, 415–417

steroid hormones from, role in endocrine feedback control, 415–417; *see also* Glucocorticoids

AEV, *see* Avian erythroblastosis virus

AFB$_1$, *see* Aflatoxin/Aflatoxin-B$_1$

AFB$_2$, *see* Aflatoxin-B$_2$

Aflatoxin/Aflatoxin-B$_1$

antagonism in chemical carcinogenesis involving, 34, 35

effect of selenium on rat liver tumorigenesis by, 337–341

hepatitis B virus (HBV), potential syncarcinogenesis with, 172, 173; *see also* Synergism, aflatoxins and viral hepatitis, between

human liver cancer associated with, 299

role of dietary protein level in

binding to chromatin proteins by, 300

GGT liver foci induction by, 300, 301

liver tumorigenesis by, 299–301

syncarcinogenesis involving, 34, 35

Aflatoxin-B$_2$, syncarcinogenesis involving, 34, 35

Age, animal (chronological)

effect on tumorigenesis, 373–395

perinatal exposure, 388, 389

Aging/Aging process

benzo[*a*]pyrene-induced mouse skin tumorigenesis, effect on, 382